HANDBOOK OF PSYCHOLOGICAL AND EDUCATIONAL ASSESSMENT OF CHILDREN
Intelligence, Aptitude, and Achievement

HANDBOOK OF PSYCHOLOGICAL AND EDUCATIONAL ASSESSMENT OF CHILDREN

Intelligence, Aptitude, and Achievement

Second Edition

Edited by

Cecil R. Reynolds
Randy W. Kamphaus

THE GUILFORD PRESS

New York London

© 2003 The Guilford Press
A Division of Guilford Publications, Inc.
72 Spring Street, New York, NY 10012
www.guilford.com

Printed in the United States of America

This book is printed on acid-free paper.

Last digit is print number: 9 8 7 6 5 4 3 2 1

Library of Congress Cataloging-in-Publication Data

Handbook of psychological and educational assessment of children : intelligence, aptitude, and achievement / edited by Cecil R. Reynolds and Randy W. Kamphaus.— 2nd ed.
    p. cm.
  Includes bibliographical references and index.
  ISBN 1-57230-883-4 (alk. paper)
  1. Psychological tests for children. 2. Achievement tests. I. Reynolds, Cecil R., 1952–   II. Kamphaus, Randy W.
BF722.H33 2003
155.4'028'7—dc21

                          2003006119

This work is dedicated in recognition of the lifetime of work in the assessment, identification, and programming for gifted and talented children of Dr. E. Paul Torrance. An extraordinary scholar, pioneer, and mentor, his work has forever changed the landscape of gifted and talented education and how we think about children in general.

About the Editors

Cecil R. Reynolds, PhD, ABPN, ABPP, is Professor of Educational Psychology, Professor of Neuroscience, and a Distinguished Research Scholar at Texas A&M University. His primary research interests are in all aspects of psychological assessment, with particular emphasis on assessment of memory, emotional and affective states and traits, and issues of cultural bias in testing. Dr. Reynolds is the author of more than 300 scholarly publications and author or editor of 35 books, including *The Clinician's Guide to the Behavior Assessment System for Children* (2002, Guilford Press), *Clinical Applications of Continuous Performance Tests* (2001, Wiley), *Handbook of School Psychology* (1999, Wiley), the *Encyclopedia of Special Education* (2000, Wiley), and the *Handbook of Clinical Child Neuropsychology* (1997, Plenum Press). He is the author of several widely used tests of personality and behavior, including the *Behavior Assessment System for Children* and the *Revised Children's Manifest Anxiety Scale*. Dr. Reynolds is also senior author of the *Reynolds Intellectual Assessment Scales,* the *Test of Memory and Learning,* the *Clinical Assessment Scales for the Elderly,* and the forthcoming *Elderly Memory Schedule,* as well as coauthor of several computerized test interpretation systems. He has a clinical practice in Bastrop, Texas, where he treats trauma victims and individuals with traumatic brain injury.

Randy W. Kamphaus, PhD, is Professor and Head of the Department of Educational Psychology at the University of Georgia. A focus on issues related to clinical assessment has led him to pursue research in classification methods, differential diagnosis, test development, and learning disability and attention-deficit/hyperactivity disorder (ADHD) assessment. Dr. Kamphaus has served as principal investigator, coinvestigator, or consultant on federally funded research projects dealing with early intervention and prevention, child classification methods, prevalency of ADHD and conduct disorder in Latin America, and aggression reduction in schools. As a licensed psychologist and a Fellow of the American Psychological Association (APA), he has contributed extensively to his profession, and he is past president of the APA's Division of School Psychology. Dr. Kamphaus has also authored or coauthored five books, three psychological tests, more than 40 scientific journal articles, and more than 20 book chapters. He also participates in scholarship in the field through work as an editorial board member, associate editor, test reviewer, and newsletter editor.

Contributors

Wayne V. Adams, PhD, ABPP/CI, Department of Psychology, George Fox University, Portland, Oregon

Erin D. Bigler, PhD, Departments of Psychology and Neuroscience, Brigham Young University, Provo, Utah

Bruce A. Bracken, PhD, School of Education, The College of William and Mary, Williamsburg, Virginia

Brian R. Bryant, PhD, Department of Special Education, College of Education, University of Texas at Austin, Austin, Texas

Diane Pedrotty Bryant, PhD, Department of Special Education, College of Education, University of Texas at Austin, Austin, Texas

Christine W. Burns, PhD, Department of Psychiatry, University of Utah, Salt Lake City, Utah

Jeanne S. Chall, PhD (deceased), Harvard University, Cambridge, Massachusetts

Jack A. Cummings, PhD, Department of Counseling and Educational Psychology, School of Education, Indiana University, Bloomington, Indiana

Mary E. Curtis, PhD, Center for Special Education, Lesley University, Cambridge, Massachusetts

Rik C. D'Amato, PhD, Department of Educational Psychology, Teachers College, Ball State University, Muncie, Indiana

Joseph L. French, PhD, Department of Educational Psychology, Pennsylvania State University, University Park, Pennsylvania

Gilles E. Gignac, BA, Assessment Unit, Swinburne Centre for Neuropsychology, Swinburne University of Technology, Hawthorn, Victoria, Australia

Joseph J. Glutting, PhD, School of Education, University of Delaware, Newark, Delaware

Patricia A. Haensly, PhD, Department of Psychology, Western Washington University, Bellingham, Washington

Ronald K. Hambleton, PhD, School of Education, University of Massachusetts, Amherst, Massachusetts

Cheryl Nemeth Hendry, MEd, School Psychology Program, University of Georgia, Athens, Georgia

Jessica A. Hoida, MS, Department of Counseling and Educational Psychology, School of Education, Indiana University, Bloomington, Indiana

Mari Griffiths Irvin, EdD, Bernerd School of Education, University of the Pacific, San Francisco, California

Steven M. Kaiser, PhD, Utica Public Schools, Utica, New York

Randy W. Kamphaus, PhD, Department of Educational Psychology, University of Georgia, Athens, Georgia

Alan S. Kaufman, PhD, Child Study Center, Yale University School of Medicine, New Haven, Connecticut

James C. Kaufman, PhD, Learning Research Institute, California State University, San Bernardino, California

Timothy Z. Keith, PhD, Department of Educational Psychology, College of Education, University of Texas at Austin, Austin, Texas

Judith M. Kroese, PhD, Department of Special Education, Rehabilitation, and School Psychology, College of Education, University of Arizona, Tucson, Arizona

Elizabeth O. Lichtenberger, PhD, Department of Cognitive Science, Salk Institute for Biological Studies, San Diego, California

Gregory R. Machek, MS, Department of Counseling and Educational Psychology, School of Education, Indiana University, Bloomington, Indiana

C. Sue McCullough, PhD, College of Education and Human Services, Longwood University, Farmville, Virginia

Daniel C. Miller, PhD, Department of Psychology and Philosophy, Texas Women's University, Denton, Texas

Michael J. Miller, BS, Departments of Psychology and Neuroscience, Brigham Young University, Provo, Utah

Jack A. Naglieri, PhD, Department of Psychology, George Mason University, Fairfax, Virginia

Jason M. Nelson, MS, Department of Counseling and Educational Psychology, School of Education, Indiana University, Bloomington, Indiana

Salvador Hector Ochoa, PhD, Department of Educational Psychology, Texas A&M University, College Station, Texas

Blanca N. Palencia, MA, Division of Professional Psychology, University of Northern Colorado, Greeley, Colorado

Aurelio Prifitera, PhD, The Psychological Corporation, San Antonio, Texas

Cecil R. Reynolds, PhD, Department of Educational Psychology, College of Education, Texas A&M University, College Station, Texas

Cynthia A. Riccio, PhD, Department of Educational Psychology, College of Education, Texas A&M University, College Station, Texas

Gary J. Robertson, PhD, Wide Range, Inc., Tampa, Florida

Barbara A. Rothlisberg, PhD, Department of Educational Psychology, Teachers College, Ball State University, Muncie, Indiana

Joseph J. Ryan, PhD, Department of Psychology and Counselor Education, Central Missouri State University, Warrensburg, Missouri

Donald H. Saklofske, PhD, Department of Educational Psychology and Special Education, University of Saskatchewan, Saskatoon, Saskatchewan, Canada

Jonathan Sandoval, PhD, Division of Education, University of California at Davis, Davis, California

Kimberley Blaker Saye, MEd, Department of Educational Psychology, University of Georgia, Athens, Georgia

Jonathan W. Smith, PhD, Department of Psychology and Counselor Education, Central Missouri State University, Warrensburg, Missouri

Hoi K. Suen, PhD, Department of Educational Psychology, Pennsylvania State University, University Park, Pennsylvania

E. Paul Torrance, PhD, Georgia Studies of Creative Behavior, University of Georgia, Athens, Georgia

Philip A. Vernon, PhD, Department of Psychology, University of Western Ontario, London, Ontario, Canada

Marley W. Watkins, PhD, Departments of Education and School Psychology and of Special Education, Pennsylvania State University, University Park, Pennsylvania

Lawrence G. Weiss, PhD, The Psychological Corporation, San Antonio, Texas

Monica E. Wolfe, BA, Department of Educational Psychology, College of Education, Texas A&M University, College Station, Texas

Eric A. Youngstrom, PhD, Department of Psychology, Case Western Reserve University, Cleveland, Ohio

April Zenisky, MEd, School of Education, University of Massachusetts, Amherst, Massachusetts

Preface

The general area of psychological testing and assessment continues to be, as it has been for decades, the most prolific of research areas in psychology, as is evident by its representation in psychological journals. Although always controversial, psychological testing has nevertheless grown in its application to include evaluation and treatment of children's disorders of development, learning, and behavior. Tests continue to be published at an increasing rate. The scholarly literature on psychological testing of children has grown significantly over the past three decades and is rapidly becoming unmanageable. More than 40 different scholarly, refereed journals exist in North America alone that publish articles on psychological and educational assessment of children, making the task of the professor, the student, and the practitioner seem an impossible one. Hence, periodic comprehensive reviews of this massive literature seem necessary, albeit onerous. Such tasks require the work and the thoughts of many esteemed authors. In undertaking this task in the first edition, we endeavored to devise a work suitable for the professor as a reference, the student as a text, and the practitioner as a sourcebook and guide. In order to do this effectively, it seemed reasonable to separate the two major areas of assessment—intelligence and personality—into their own volumes. We have continued with this practice based upon the success in the first editions. This approach has allowed us the space for in-depth coverage, while retaining cohesion of topics in each book. The two volumes can thus be used in tandem or as separate units, depending on need.

Our hope for this two-volume handbook was to develop a broad-based resource for those individuals who are charged with the assessment of children and adolescents. We also wanted to develop a comprehensive resource for researchers who are studying various aspects of children's assessment and psychodiagnostics, and to provide breadth and depth of coverage of the major domains of children's assessment in a single source. These volumes include such diverse areas as academic achievement, intelligence, adaptive behavior, personality, and creativity assessment. Individual tests, such as the Wechsler Intelligence Scale for Children—Third Edition, the Kaufman Assessment Battery for Children, and the Rorschach, are given their own treatments, in addition to some general methods such as projective storytelling techniques. In each volume, the theoretical foundations and the measurement limitations of current approaches to the assessment of these latent constructs are addressed.

In order to ensure the volumes are authoritative, we sought out eminent scholars with a general command of assessment and a special expertise in research or practice in the area of their respective contributions. We have also sought new scholars, perhaps less well established, but whose thinking is clear, strong, and challenging on several fronts in formulating the second edition of each work. The chapters themselves purposely vary from an emphasis on specific applications in assessment to cutting-edge knowledge and critiques of research and statistical procedures. We hope that this scholarly emphasis will enhance the possibility of using the second edition of this two-volume handbook as a graduate-level text as it was so frequently adopted in its first edition. Because of its breadth, we think this text could be useful for courses in intellectual and personality assessment, practica and internship coursework, and courses on psychodiagnostics, psychopathology, and special education.

In the second edition, several chapters were added, a few deleted, and all but one revised to greater and lesser extents. Chapters on new instruments not in existence for the first edition, such as the Behavior Assessment System for Children and the Kaufman Adolescent and Adult Intelligence Test, are now treated in depth. We estimate the typical chapter contains one-third new material and some much more. With the various additions and deletions, more than half of the work is new. We intended to retain the best of the material from the first edition, and revise and update where new research and science so dictated.

We are deeply indebted to a number of individuals for assisting us with this at times overwhelming project. First of all, we wish to thank the authors of the various chapters for their extraordinary talent and patience with this arduous effort. We wish them continued success in all of their professional activities. We owe a great debt to Sharon Panulla, our original editor at The Guilford Press who signed the first edition of this work, and her successor, Chris Jennison, who followed the second edition through to its completion. We greatly appreciate their faith in giving us the opportunity to produce this work. We also thank Editor-in-Chief Seymour Weingarten for his concurrence, as well as his early thoughts on the organization and development of the first edition of this work. We are very appreciative of the efforts of our staff and students, especially Justine Hair, who assisted us in many ways through their organizational contributions and many trips to the library!

Finally, we wish to thank all of the researchers of the last century dating back to and including Sir Frances Galton and his modern-day counterpart, Arthur Jensen, as well as such clear thinkers in the field as John Carroll, John Horn, Anne Anastasi, and Raymond Cattell, for the great strides they have made in enhancing our ability to measure and consequently understand the nature of human behavior. To our common mentor, Alan S. Kaufman, we acknowledge a continuing debt for the superb model of scholarship that he continues to provide. However, it is to Julia and to Norma that we owe our greatest debts of gratitude. The strength they lend, the understanding they convey, and the support they give make our onerous schedules tolerable, and enable us to be so much more than we would be without them—thank you, again.

CECIL R. REYNOLDS
RANDY W. KAMPHAUS

Contents

III. ASSESSMENT OF ACADEMIC SKILLS

IV. SPECIAL TOPICS IN MENTAL TESTING

PART I

GENERAL ISSUES

1

A History of the Development of Psychological and Educational Testing

HOI K. SUEN
JOSEPH L. FRENCH

Assessment of human characteristics has been a part of life since the beginning of recorded history. In Eastern civilization, China has used an elaborate large-scale civil service examination system continuously for at least 3,000 years[1] (Bowman, 1989). Historically, somewhere between 200,000 and over 1 million examinees took part in these exams every 3 years (Ho, 1962). The system has had a profound influence on the cultural and political system, and social philosophy of China, as well as many other nations in the Far East (Miyazaki, 1981). Indirectly, it also influenced the development of the civil service examination system of the British East Indian Company, and subsequently the U.S. civil service exam system established in 1884.

In Western civilization, the earliest record of a large-scale systematic assessment of human abilities can be found in the book of Judges (Judges 12:4–6) in the Old Testament, in which the story was told of a battle between the Gileadites and the Ephraimites. The Gileadites had the Ephraimites surrounded against the River Jordan and were attempting to prevent the Ephraimites from escaping across the river. The problem was to identify who was an Ephramite. The two

peoples were the same in every respect, except that they pronounced the word "Shibboleth" differently: Whereas the Gileadites pronounced it with an "sh" sound, the Ephraimites pronounced it with an "s" sound. Thus, in order to identify escaping Ephraimites, suspected prisoners were asked if they were Ephraimites. If the answer was "nay," the prisoner was asked to say the word "shibboleth." Those who pronounced the word with the "s" sound were killed. The book of Judges reported that 42,000 individuals failed this "high-stakes" test and were thus killed.

From the Middle Ages until the end of the 19th century, there had been a few prominent cases of systematic assessment of individual characteristics in Western civilization, other than auditions for musicians and the occasional court jester. One such case was the testing method called "trial by ordeal." By the end of the first millennium, peasants in England were governed by the Anglo-Saxon laws of the time. The major purpose of these laws was to evaluate who among the accused was telling the truth. Under this approach, the accused was to perform a prescribed task called an "ordeal," and the result was used to determine whether the person was a liar. One such ordeal, for example, was to have the accused carry a red-hot iron for 3 yards. This was called the "fire test." Another ordeal was to have the accused plunge his or her hand into boiling water to take out a stone. If the wound healed in 3 days, the accused was judged to be telling the truth (Bishop, 1968). This was called the "hot water test." The belief underlying these test procedures was that if a person was telling the truth, God would protect him or her from harm, and the wound would thus heal quickly. These trial-by-ordeal methods and their accompanying rationale were later extended to the idea of "trial by combat" in duals of noblemen. One such example was the story of Tycho Brahe (1546–1601), the famous Danish astronomer, whose data were used by Johannes Kepler (1571–1630) to develop the laws governing planetary movements. When Tycho was a 20-year-old student at the University of Rostock, he had an argument with a fellow student during a dance as to who was the better mathematician. To determine this, they had a duel in which Tycho lost his nose, and he had to wear a gold and silver artificial nose for the remainder of his life (Boorstin, 1983, p. 306).

Perhaps the best-known case of systematic examination in the Middle Ages was the "testing" of witches. In 1484, two Dominican monks named Kraemer and Sprenger published a manuscript entitled *Malleus Malificarum* (*Hammer of Witches*). The book was intended to be a handbook on exorcism for monks in the Dominican order. However, the manuscript became very popular and was widely used throughout Europe. According to the manuscript, witches existed in every village and every farm, and witchcraft was "high treason against God's majesty." Accordingly, every witch and sorcerer should be identified and punished. In this manuscript, various testing procedures (including the trial-by-ordeal procedure) for the identification of witches were specifically prescribed. One of the most famous of these procedures was the "cold water test." In this test, the accused person was tied at the feet and hands and was lowered into cold water by a rope. This rope was tied around the accused's waist, and a knot was tied at a certain distance from the torso. If both knot and accused dipped beneath the

surface of the water, the accused was proven innocent. If the knot was dry, the accused was guilty. The theory behind this test was that if the accused were innocent, the spirit of the water, which represented the Biblical flood that washed away all sins, would consent to accept him or her. Another procedure was to search for an "evil mark" on the suspect's body. Based on the theory that witches would have "evil marks" on their bodies, juries of the suspects' sex would strip the bodies of the accused and examine them minutely for any "evil mark," which might include insensitive areas of skin, supernumerary nipples, and any unnatural excrescence. Other "assessment procedures" thus prescribed included various methods of torturing the woman until she "confessed." Kraemer and Sprenger recommended the use of tests over torturing because they believed that, with the assistance of the devil, witches might be insensitive to the pain of tortures. According to one source (Huxley, 1963, p. xix), several hundred thousand— perhaps as many as 1 million—persons (mostly women) in post-Reformation Europe were identified as witches (or sorcerers) through these testing methods and were exterminated.

In the United States, the cold water test was used in Connecticut shortly before the infamous 1692 witch trials at Salem Village in the Massachusetts Bay Colony. After reviewing traditional testing methods such as the cold water test, as well as the recommendations of such famous intellectuals of the time as Increase Mather (the first president of what was then Harvard College) and his son Cotton Mather (a prominent clergyman in Boston), the magistrates at the Salem Village trials determined that the cold water test was too crude and decided to use the "evil mark" method and the "touch test" (Starkey, 1963). The touch test was used when a victim was being tormented by the "spectral" form of the witch and was screaming, crying, and perhaps in convulsions. The suspected witch was directed to physically touch the victim. If the victim stopped the screaming and apparent convulsions when touched by the suspect, the suspect was judged to be a witch.

These testing procedures were largely related to the assessment of spiritual or moral characteristics, but not to the physical or mental abilities of a person. Although China has been testing individuals' mental abilities for over 3,000 years, the testing of mental abilities in Europe and the United States did not begin until the end of the 19th century. This lack of interest and development in the testing of mental abilities in Western civilization can be partly attributed to the belief—advocated by such influential philosophers as St. Augustine and St. Thomas Aquinas during the Middle Ages, and reinforced by the Roman Catholic Church—that only God could know such abilities and that humans should be concerned only about saving souls, not evaluating mental abilities. One such lack of recognition of individual differences in mental abilities can be found in the case of an 18th-century English astronomer. Freeman (1926) reported that in 1795, one of the observers working at the Greenwich Astronomical Observatory in England was found to differ from his colleagues in estimating the time it took a star to travel across a section of the sky. Individual differences were neither understood nor tolerated, and the observer was fired. It was not until 1822 that astronomers understood that different people have different reaction times, and began to take these individual differences into consideration when interpreting observational data.

In spite of this general lack of interest in the assessment of mental abilities, there were a few rare exceptions involving small numbers of people. These were mostly in the form of university and college examinations. Around 300 B.C., end-of-term examinations in the areas of grammar, geometry, rhetoric, and music were given to students at the Ephebic College in Athens. By 100 A.D., admissions tests were administered for entrance to the Ephebic College. By 1219, the University of Bologna in Italy implemented a systematic method of examining candidates for the Master of Law degree (Nitko, 1983). These were oral exams. Precise rules, and the exact time schedule for each step of the process, were carefully defined by 1275 (Pedersen, 1997, p. 263). Between 1750 and 1770, Cambridge University in England started a written examination system for its students; however, the system became a mere formality by 1780. By 1800, Oxford University initiated an alternative system of written exams, and soon both Cambridge and Oxford administered competence exams (Nitko, 1983).

Systematic large-scale testing of mental abilities in Europe and the United States emerged in the late 19th century. The first such testing programs were in the areas of intelligence, educational achievement, and personnel testing. The English geneticist Sir Francis Galton called for the testing of individual intelligence in 1890, and Alfred Binet and Theophile Simon developed the first intelligence test in 1904. In the area of academic achievement testing, Horace Mann, the secretary of the Massachusetts State Board of Education, called for oral and written teacher competency exams in 1837 (Nitko, 1983). Also significant was Joseph Rice's spelling test used to evaluate U.S. schools in 1893 (Rice, 1893). In the area of personnel testing, many authors of intelligence tests were also involved in the development of the Army Alpha and Beta Tests, the purpose of which was to determine the placement of army recruits in World War I. These tests were soon followed by a proliferation of a wide variety of instruments and assessment procedures. Today, hundreds of millions of standardized tests are administered in the United States alone every year.

THE EARLY DEVELOPMENT OF TESTING

The early mental testing activities were primarily interested in several areas: intelligence, academic achievement, physical attributes, personality, interests, and attitudes.

Individual Differences

Directors of early European psychological laboratories were primarily interested in discovering general laws to account for human behavior. In the 1870s, Galton proposed a new field of inquiry called "anthropometry," which was concerned with the measurement of human physical characteristics as they relate to human behaviors. In 1882, he opened his anthropometric laboratory at the South Kensington Museum in London; for a fee, anyone could have certain physical measurements made there, including tests of vision, hearing, and reaction time (Boorstin, 1974, p. 219). In the pursuit of these laws of human behaviors, it soon became apparent that individual differences in human ability necessarily had to be taken into account. The working partnerships that were established in these laboratories, as well as a fortuitous family relationship, substantially contributed to the investigative focus that eventually led to the development of the modem intelligence test. James McKeen Cattell, an American who was working as the first assistant to Wilhelm Wundt (the father of experimental psychology) in Germany, discovered the existence of individual differences in human sensation and perception. Because the problem of individual differences was assigned to the American Cattell, Wundt referred to the problem as "*ganzAmerikanisch*" (Boring, 1929). This focus on individual differences, which in Germany was initially concerned with measuring differences in individuals' reaction times, directed this line of research down a path that emphasized the measurement of human physical attributes.

At the same time in England, Charles Darwin, Alfred Wallace, Thomas Huxley, and Herbert Spencer were studying and formulating how physical characteristics were inherited. Galton, who was a grandson of Erasmus Darwin and half-cousin to Charles Darwin, became interested in extending his cousin's work on the inheritance of physical attributes to the inheritance of mental abilities (Freeman, 1926). To do this, Galton needed methods of measuring differences in mental abilities. He developed and presented some of these methods in his anthropometric laboratory. The measurement methodology developed by Galton focused primarily on the differences between people as manifested in physical and sensory tasks. Cattell, who had worked with Wundt, was briefly a lecturer at Cambridge University. It was at Cambridge in 1888 that he was associated with Galton. The two men were drawn together by their similar views and interests in investigating individual differences. Shortly thereafter, Cattell moved back to the United States, where he became a professor of psychology at the University of Pennsylvania. In 1891 Cattell moved to Columbia University, establishing a psychological laboratory there and remaining as its head for the next 26 years, until he was dismissed for his pacifistic views when the

United States entered World War I in 1917 (Boring, 1929). This association among Cattell, Wundt, and Galton not only provided a link between the German and English psychological laboratories, but also provided for the transportation across the Atlantic of European ideas mixed with the American interest in individual differences.

Cattell's initial interest at Columbia University in individual differences, melded with Gallon's interests in mental abilities, led to his publication of "Mental Tests and Measurements" (Cattell, 1890). This paper was the first to propose that mental abilities could be tested and objectively measured. The paper was essentially an initial list of tests that purported to measure mental functioning; the tests consisted primarily of tasks involving physical acuity and/or differences in individual physical reaction times. Cattell examined many college-age students at Columbia with his tests. Through his leadership, the American Psychological Association (APA) established a committee that in 1896 presented the membership with a list of recommended tests for measuring mental growth and ability in college students. These APA-recommended tests were simply extensions of the physical tests proposed by Cattell in 1890 (Freeman, 1926).

Intelligence

Most of the early American experimentation in mental functioning involved the measurement of these physical differences and attributes. Rarely was a test developed and given to people that did not primarily measure physical or sensory modalities. However, there were known problems with many of these tests, and a few divergent assessment techniques began to emerge. Bolton (1891) developed and used a memory test that required children to remember arithmetic digits. Ebbinghaus (1897) studied intellectual fatigue and memory loss. In Europe, Binet was experimenting with some new tasks. These required children to draw figures from memory that they had seen only for a brief period of time, to read and copy sentences, and to add numbers together. These were the first mental tasks that were not primarily measuring physical reactivity; as such, they were a break from the sensory tasks developed in the European laboratories.

Binet's efforts peaked in the development of the Binet–Simon Scale (Binet & Simon, 1905). The impetus for the construction of this test was given by the Minister of Public Instruction in Paris in 1904. The minister appointed a committee, of which Binet was a member, to find a way to separate children with mental retardation from normal children in the schools (Sattler, 1982). Originally, Binet's mental test results were to be used to determine how well children should achieve in school. Even with the emphasis on academics, the early Binet tasks were heavily influenced by physical measurement. Binet and Simon's 1905 scale consisted of 30 tests arranged in order of difficulty. The first of these required that a child follow with his or her eyes a lighted match. Henry H. Goddard, the director of research at the New Jersey Training School for Feeble-Minded Boys and Girls at Vineland, translated Binet's scale with the help of linguist Elizabeth Kite (Goddard, 1911). This translation was widely used in the United States (Freeman, 1926), until it was superseded by the more extensive revision made by Lewis Terman and his collaborators (Terman, 1916)—the Stanford Revision or the Stanford–Binet Scale.

Kuhlmann (1912) was one of the first to produce a useful American version of the Binet–Simon Scale. His later revision (Kuhlmann, 1922), published by the Educational Test Bureau, was frequently used for decades, especially for subjects with mental retardation below the educable level. Some attribute the eventually greater success of the Terman (1916) and Terman and Merrill (1937) versions of the Binet to the size and distribution of the publisher's sales force, and to Terman's longevity and productivity as an author of books and articles as well as tests. Even though the original Binet–Simon Scale had been through translation, extension, revision, and adaptation to the experience of American children, the influence of the European laboratories' concentration on physical attributes was still present in the protocol for the Stanford Revision. The following items were allotted space on the 1916 protocol where the information could be jotted down by the examiner: standing height, sitting height, weight, head circum-ference, right-hand grip strength, left-hand grip strength, and lung capacity. Among the items in the scale were comparing 3- and 15-gram weights, tying a bow knot, copying shapes, arranging given weights in order, and drawing shapes from memoery (Terman, 1916).

Other technical and psychometric advances were being made in both the United States and Europe that continued the development of mental testing beyond Binet's efforts. William Stem (1914) was the first person to use the term "mental quotient." His mental quotient was calculated by simply dividing a child's mental age by his or her chronological age. Thus a 12-year-old child whose mental age was 10 would have a mental quotient of .833. Terman thought that this method of measurement was substantially correct. Terman (1916) multiplied the mental quotient by 100, retaining only the whole number, and called the result the "intelligence quotient" (IQ).

The first point scale, instead of age scale, was developed by Yerkes, Bridges, and Hardwick (1915). When point scores for a child were compared to the average number of points of children the youngster's own age, the ratio was initially known as the "coefficient of intelligence." An average child would have a coefficient of 1.00, just as he or she would have an IQ of 100. The point scale was later developed into the Deviation IQ scores of today.

Academic Achievement

As early as 1865, the New York Board of Regents set examinations for elementary pupils. By 1878, examinations for secondary pupils were developed by the board. School exams were given in other states as well. An interesting early incident of social/political impact on academic achievement testing was the case of Samuel King, the superintendent of the Portland, Oregon, schools in the 1870s. In 1870, he decided to publish exam scores of pupils in newspapers. He was forced to resign by 1877, due to the outrage of parents and teachers over the publication of exam scores.

In 1877, Charles W. Eliot, the president of Harvard, advocated free public high school education to American children and suggested a need for a new system of examination. In 1890, Nicholas Butler proposed that since the federal government had no role in public education, a private central organization should be formed to administer examinations for college entrance (Boorstin, 1974). The College Entrance Examination Board was formed in 1899; in June 1901, it administered its first exam at 69 locations, including 2 in Europe. A total of 973 candidates from 237 schools took that exam, which consisted of traditional academic subjects, such as English and chemistry. The subjects tested were specified by about a dozen participating colleges. The exams were in essay format and were scored on a 100-point scale, with a 60 as the passing score. The aim of these exams was to provide the participating colleges with information on the performance on a standard set of academic subjects, because academic credits and grades in many of the newly formed high schools were often inflated by nonacademic courses (e.g., art, stenography, Red Cross, crafts, and hobbies). In 1924, the secretary of the College Entrance Examination Board summarized the board's plan to expand the exams in academic subjects to include tests of ethical behavior, physical health, powers of observation, mental alertness, ability to participate successfully in cooperative efforts or teamwork, skill in laboratory work, and facility in conversation in foreign language. In 1926, the board started experimenting with the new multiple-choice testing format in addition to essay questions. Carl Bingham was charged with developing the Scholastic Aptitude Test (SAT).[2]

In 1948, the Educational Testing Service (ETS) was founded. Its initial project was to develop and administer the SAT for the College Board. Within 2 months after its founding, it offered the Law School Aptitude Test (LSAT). A few months later, it was given a contract to develop the Medical College Aptitude Test (MCAT). The first president of ETS, Henry Chauncey, had envisioned a "Census of Abilities" to be implemented through ETS. The idea was to categorize, sort, and route the entire population of the nation by administering a series of multiple-choice mental tests to everyone, and then by suggesting, on the basis of the scores, what each person's role in society should be (Lemann, 1999, p. 5). Chauncey viewed such a process as "the moral equivalent of religion but based on reason and science rather than on sentiments and tradition" (Lemann, 1999, p. 69). In 1959, E. F. Linquist started the American College Testing (ACT) program to focus on the testing of academic achievements which was marketed primarily to nonselective public universities. The ACT program remains a competitor of ETS today.

Physical Attributes

In the area of employment, Edward Thomdike caught the attention of influential industrial leaders by saying that "Whatever exists at all exists in some amount," and that "to know it thoroughly involves knowing its quantity as well as its quality" (Thomdike, 1918, p. 16). Many people also agreed with Link, who believed that it would be "possible to select the right man for the right place" (Link, 1919, p. 293), and thereby to minimize industrial problems with manpower (and later womanpower). Early solutions primarily involved using graphology with completed application forms, and performing character analyses based on brief interviews.

Increasingly, through the first third of the 20th century, sales managers and marketing executives grasped at almost any straw to help them in hiring personnel and in helping those employees sell their products. Stereotypes played a major role in personnel selection. Norwegians, Greeks, and Russians were thought to be appropriate for most types of rough work, while the French and Irish were thought to be more capable of tasks requiring enthusiasm and artistry. Poles and Lithuanians were thought to be good mill workers, and Italians and Swedes good at railroad construction. Karen Blackford's plan, popularized in *The Job, the Man, and the Boss* (Blackford & Newcomb, 1919), advised managers about whom to hire by character analysis; books such as *Character Analysis: How to Read People at Sight* (Bush & Waugh, 1923) and *Plus + Selling* (Fosbroke, 1933) instructed salespersons about approaching customers according to their physical appearance. Fosbroke, for example, provided artists' conceptions of various kinds of buyers and attributed buying styles to physical characteristics such as the "sincere buyer," with a narrow-high forehead (case 28); the "tenacious buyer," with a wide medium-high forehead (case 29); the "slow-thinking yielding buyer," with a protruding forehead and light chin and jaw (case 33); and a "fast-thinking yielding buyer," with the same chin and jaw but a slanting forehead (case 35).

Scientists were making some headway, but development of better instruments for assessing personality and interests than these stereotypical judgments about ethnicity, body type, and hah" color took a long time. Personnel at the Carnegie Institute of Technology in Pittsburgh made major contributions to the advancement of assessment by starting a new Division of Applied Psychology that, among other tasks, was charged with developing tests for industry. Walter VanDyke Bingham came from Dartmouth in 1915 to head the organization, and soon had secured funding from nearly 30 firms to finance the work directed by Walter Dill Scott in the Bureau of Salesmanship Research (later known as the Bureau of Personnel Research) (Bingham, 1923a, 1923b).

Personality

During World War I, faced with an enormous number of interviews with military recruits to determine those who would be susceptible to wartime disorders, Robert Woodsworth formalized oral questions often posed by psychiatrists about worry, daydreaming, enuresis, and so on into 116 short questions (Woodworm, 1918), which could be administered to groups of people who could read and check "yes" or "no." Even though the scores turned out to be influenced by the situation (i.e., scores for many soldiers changed markedly after the Armistice), the work served as a basis for the Thurstone Personality Scale, the Allport Ascendance–Submission Test, and others.

One of Terman's students, Robert G. Bemreuter (1933), developed, as part of his 1931 doctoral dissertation, an instrument called simply the Personality Inventory. He pooled items from tests by Thurstone, Allport, and others to measure four traits: neurotic tendency, introversion, dominance, and self-sufficiency. "Personality inventory" became a generic term for such scales after Bemreuter's instrument became widely used in schools and industry through the 1930s

and 1940s. The availability of four scores from the Personality Inventory and the face validity of the 125 items probably contributed to its widespread use, although it contains some known psychometric problems. Another popular test of the time was the Humm–Wadsworth Temperament Scale (Humm & Wadsworth, 1935). It broke new ground with empirical keys based on the responses of groups of patients, criminals, and common persons thought to have one of seven psychiatric classifications. The first criterion-keyed personality test to withstand the tests of both time and peer critique was the Minnesota Multiphasic Personality Inventory (MMPI), which appeared in 1942. This self-report scale consisted of 495 items, which were to be answered "true," "false," or "cannot say." The MMPI was designed for use in diagnosing abnormal personality patterns, but was soon used with college students and in employee selection situations, where it did not prove to be as helpful. By the 1950s the Humm–Wadsworth Scale was dropping from use, but the MMPI was becoming very popular, and Bemreuter's Personality Inventory had sold over a million copies (Hathaway, 1964).

While personality inventories were being developed, a parallel development in the area of personality testing was that of projective tests. Projective testing arose in part from the desire for a test to yield insights into the structure of the whole personality. Frank (1939), who contributed one of the first major works in projectives, suggested that these tests are based both on Gestalt psychology (with its emphasis on the whole) and on psychoanalytic techniques of dream analysis. One of the first approaches to projective personality appraisal was through word association. In 1879, Galton developed a list of 86 stimulus words, all starting with the letter A (Forrest, 1974). Carl Jung (1910) provided stimulus words to represent "emotional complexes." Improving on earlier work, Jung analyzed reaction time, content, and physically observable tension as well as verbal responses. The list developed by Grace Kent and A. J. Rosanoff (1910), which avoided words likely to remind one of personal experiences, had objective scoring and norms and became popular in the United States. In 1921, Sidney Pressey produced a group-administered form of word association test, wherein subjects were asked to cross out one or more words in each series; the remaining words reflected things they worried about, liked, found unpleasant, or were nervous about (Pressey, 1921). Pressey's work led Payne (1928) to introduce a sentence completion technique, which became popular by the 1940s, when prominent psychologists advocated the technique.

Binet and other early test authors used meaningless inkblots to investigate imagination and fantasy (Tulchin, 1940). Hermann Rorschach, a Swiss psychiatrist, developed this method into a personality assessment tool (Rorschach, 1921). After trying many variations of blots with hospital patients, he settled on 10 blots. In the United States, Samuel J. Beck and Bruno Klopfer suggested more detailed scoring categories and helped the Rorschach technique gain in popularity by their speeches and writings in the late 1930s.

Morgan and Murray (1935) first presented the Thematic Apperception Test (TAT), which was not published by Harvard University Press until 8 years later (Murray, 1943). The TAT, stimulated by the work of Binet, Burt, and others who used pictures and stories about the pictures to study intellectual development, consists of 30 pictures. Subjects are asked to develop a story about each picture that describes the situation, events leading up to it, the outcome, and the thoughts and feelings of the people in the story. A number of other picture tests soon followed, such as Bellak and Bellak's (1952) pictures for children; Symonds's (1948) pictures for adolescents; and Shneidman's (1948) Make-A-Picture Story Test. Because of the many problems associated with projective tests—including the word association and sentence completion techniques, the inkblot technique, and the picture technique—they are not recommended today and are of historical interest only. Instead of regarding them as tests, we should view them as clinical tools that help clinicians generate hypotheses about an individual for further investigation (Anastasi, 1982).

Interests

Like many other aspects of vocational guidance, assessment of interests can be traced

back to the Boston Vocational Bureau and Frank Parsons. Parsons (1908) used interviews, questionnaires, and self-analysis in an eclectic approach to assess the aptitudes and interests of youths. E. L. Thorndike (1912) and T. L. Kelley (1914), however, were the first formal investigators of interests. Thorndike initiated studies about the relationship of interest to abilities; Kelley developed a questionnaire about things "liked and not liked." At Carnegie Tech, Bruce Moore (1921) distinguished different types of interests by separating social interests from mechanical interests of engineers. Meanwhile, C. S. Yoakum at Carnegie conducted a seminar in which graduate students identified about 1,000 items that eventually found their way into at least nine interest inventories (Campbell, 1971), among them the Strong Vocational Interest Blank (SVIB). Building on a 1924 thesis by Karl Cowdery, E. K. Strong produced the SVIB in 1927 and the manual a year later. The first scoring machines were used with the SVIB in 1930, but automated scoring was not available until 1946. Sales of the SVIB paralleled simplifications in scoring. Through the 1930s, about 40,000 booklets were printed each year. This jumped to about 300,000 in 1947.

The Kuder Interest Inventories (Kuder, 1934, 1948) have been used almost as long as the Strong series has. Strong approached the task of assessing interests by asking respondents to indicate whether they liked or disliked a wide variety of objects, activities, or types of persons commonly met in life, whereas Kuder asked respondents to indicate which of three items they would most and least like. In more recent times, inventories based on the techniques perfected by Strong have been developed, with items and keys for nonprofessional occupations.

THE CONFLUENCE OF DEVELOPMENTS IN MANY AREAS

With these early developments in mental testing, there was a rapid expansion of testing activities in the remainder of the 20th century. The National Industrial Conference Board (1948) found the use of all tests to be rising markedly during the 1940s. By the 1950s, 80 of the major companies used tests for employee selection (Scott, Clothier, & Spriegel, 1961). The tests used ranged from stenographic or clerical tests to intelligence tests, mechanical aptitude tests, personality or interest inventories, and trade, dexterity, or performance tests of various kinds.

From the early days to mental testing as we know it today, there have been many changes. These changes have been accelerated by the confluence of events and developments in many areas. Some of these events and developments include the occurrence of a number of significant sociopolitical events and currents; the development of statistical theories of test scores; the development of theories of validity; and the development of testing formats and technology.

Sociopolitical Changes

The 20th century witnessed many important social, political, and ideological events and changes. Many of these changes have had a profound impact on how mental testing has evolved and developed. Throughout most of human history, except for the Chinese civil service examination system, testing in general—including the witch tests and early mental tests—had always been conducted in a small-group setting, where a person or a small group of individuals to be assessed was asked to perform some task or provide some written or oral responses. A judge or a panel of judges would then evaluate the responses. The process was typically individualized, time-consuming, and inefficient. This was to change drastically in the 20th century in the United States, and subsequently elsewhere in the world.

One of the catalysts for the changes was the recruitment of mass armies. When the United States entered World War I in 1917, there was a need to classify and assign as quickly as possible millions of new army recruits—many of whom were non-English-speaking recent immigrants from Europe or from other continents. A massive sorting effort was needed. The inefficient individual or small-group testing approach was no longer adequate. To meet this need, a committee of the APA (the members of which included most of the early developers of intelligence tests) designed for the U.S. Army the Army Alpha Test for native English-speaking recruits and the Army Beta Test

for non-English-speaking recruits. These tests were designed for efficient large-group administrations. The objectives of these two tests were to identify so-called "mentally incompetent" individuals, and also to identify "officer material" from among the millions of recruits. Consequently, between 1917 and 1919, a total of 1,726,000 men took either the Army Alpha or Beta Test (Boorstin, 1983, p. 222; Fass, 1980). This was the first time in Western civilization that so many people needed to be and were administered a mental test within a very short time period. This mass-testing program inspired many other large-scale testing programs later, including the SAT program. The testing of large numbers of army recruits continued throughout the century and it has evolved into today's Armed Services Vocational Aptitude Battery (ASVAB) testing program.

Another major event that had an important impact on testing in the 20th century was the phenomenon of mass education. Throughout much of history, most people had little or no formal education. This was the case in the United States prior to the 20th century. In 1870, there were only 500 secondary schools and about 80,000 students. As of 1890, the total enrollment in U.S. public high schools was about 200,000. By 1910, there were 10,000 secondary schools and 900,000 students; by 1922, this had increased to over 2 million. Today, virtually all 14- to 17-year-olds attend high school. This increase can also be at least partly attributed to the dramatic immigration from Europe in the first decades of the century: Between 1901 and 1910 alone, nearly 9 million people migrated to the United States (Kownslar & Frizzle, 1967, pp. 600–601).

A similarly dramatic increase occurred in higher education. In 1890, a total of about 150,000 students enrolled in U.S. colleges and universities. This number had increased by 1922 to about 600,000. By 1935, there were a total of 1,500 colleges and universities, and the total enrollment was over 1 million students. The number of colleges and universities was to increase to about 2,000 by the 1960s and to about 2,500 by the 1970s; the total enrollment was to increase to over 3 million by the 1960s and to over 7 million by the 1970s. That is, the total college enrollment in the United States increased somewhere around 4,700% in the 70 years between 1890 and 1970 (Boorstin, 1974). The increases in public school and college enrollments were even more drastic in the second half of the 20th century, as the problem was further exacerbated by the GI Bill and the baby boom after World War II. Prior to the GI Bill, higher education was primarily accessible only to young men and women from well-to-do families. With the support for returning war veterans to attend college provided by the U.S. government through the GI Bill, enrollments in colleges increased drastically overnight. This was further compounded by the sudden increase in birth rate after World War II, leading to a large demographic cohort born in the 1950s and early 1960s. Enrollments in public schools and subsequently in colleges and universities continued to increase through the 1980s. As of 1999, the total student enrollment in kindergarten through college in the United States was about 67,870,000 (ETS, 1999). With mass public and higher education, there was a tremendous need for sorting, evaluating, classifying, program placement, admission, retention, scholarship awards, and so on. Consequently, millions upon millions of students in public schools, private schools, parochial schools, colleges, and universities need to be assessed in some form each year.

The increased need for mental ability testing in schools was not only prompted by the sheer increase in enrollment numbers. This increase was also exacerbated by various attempts at social and educational reforms, particularly toward the second half of the century. Federal laws intended to improve early childhood development have been passed; for example, Public Law (PL) 99-457 mandates that all children between the ages of 3 and 5 must be assessed to detect possible developmental problems. States have also mandated various tests for schools as part of school accountability concerns. Other social and educational reform programs, such as Head Start, Upward Bound, and Talent Search, have led to various mandatory achievement tests as part of program evaluation and accountability. Continual monitoring of school performances through comparisons across time, schools, districts, states, and countries have led to the need for numerous assessments and

tests. Many academic aptitude and achievement tests were subsequently developed to meet these needs.

The generally increased demands for intelligence, aptitude, and achievement tests were further encouraged and strongly influenced by several powerful, though not always mutually compatible, ideological concepts that have gained popularity in the 20th century. These include eugenics, equal opportunity, and meritocracy. During the first half of the century, the theory of eugenics gained popular support in Europe and the United States. Based on the belief in heredity, many believed that society could be ultimately improved by systematically sorting out those who were "superior" in some desired characteristics (e.g., intelligence) from those who were "inferior." The superior individuals would be encouraged to reproduce offspring, while the inferior ones would be discouraged from doing so. In the United States, mental tests would be the tool through which people's abilities could be sorted and a program of eugenics could be implemented. No such systematic social program was actually implemented in the United States (although this *was* done in Germany under Hitler, who used a criterion other than mental ability—namely, race/ethnicity). However, many of the early U.S. test developers, including some of the individuals in the early development of the SAT program, were motivated by this ideological vision in their efforts (Lemann, 1999). For instance, Benjamin Wood, one of the early pioneers of testing, advocated that individuals with inferior abilities (as indicated by low scores on intelligence tests) who had children had in effect committed crimes against humanity and should be punished by mandatory sterilization (Lemann, 1995a, 1995b). In the 1950s, in 25 of the 48 states, women with mental retardation had to be sterilized before they could be discharged from a school (institution). In later years, when such laws no longer existed, Christopher Shockley (the Nobel laureate who developed the transistor in the 1950s) persistently attempted to persuade Congress to set aside funds to pay individuals with below-100 IQ scores to undergo sterilization.

Another ideological force that has prompted the increase in testing activities was the concept of equal opportunity. The ideals of fairness and equal opportunity manifested themselves in two areas: civil service employment and education. During the 19th century, governmental jobs were dispensed primarily through patronage. With the election of Andrew Jackson in 1828, amid the loud cries of "Throw the rascals out," the spoils system had become firmly entrenched in American politics. During the mid-1800s, each president was besieged by numerous persons crying for a position on the government payroll. In 1872, President Ulysses S. Grant appointed the first Civil Service Commission to regulate and improve civil service through an examination system.[3] The U.S. system, however, was abandoned in 1875 because Congress, refusing to give up the patronage system, did not appropriate funds. In 1883, following the assassination of President James Garfield by a disappointed job seeker in 1881, Congress decided to pass and fund the Civil Service (Pendleton) Act to formally support the commission and the civil service examination system (U.S. Civil Service Commission, 1884).

The Pendleton Act had set the stage and tone for equal opportunity. This was to expand to the private sector. In the early 20th century, America was no longer going to tolerate the notion of robber barons building fortunes on the backs of children and immigrant labor. As industrial society and the U.S. economy flourished in the late 19th and early 20th centuries, many common men had opportunities for employment never known before. With geographic, economic, and social mobility came local autonomy, informal political and economic arrangements, increasingly radical labor unions, high rates of crime, corruption in government, and many other strains on society. Early in the 20th century, rapid growth and social unrest in the United States generated a "search for order" (Wiebe, 1967). In 1901, President Theodore Roosevelt began working toward two broad social aims. First, people were to be set free from the daily grind of toil and poverty. Second, immigrants were to be set free from the liabilities of their status as foreigners through new social legislation and the resources provided through public education. In 1916, Congress passed the Keating–Owen Child Labor Act; by 1918, all

states had enacted laws mandating child school attendance. Thus the concern for equality translated directly into increases in testing activities and in demands for public education, which in turn furthered the demands for testing.

Michael Young (1958) coined the term "meritocracy" in his mock sociology dissertation supposedly written in the year 2033. It describes a political system in which political power and wealth are distributed on the basis of intelligence, ability, and mental test scores. Although the United States has never had a hereditary aristocratic class in the sense of the European system, and in theory any American can achieve the Horatio Alger dream of moving from rags to riches, the primary roads toward success and political power prior to and during much of the early 20th century were in effect family connections, secondary education at private preparatory high schools, and college education in the private "Ivy League" colleges. Admissions into Ivy League colleges such as Harvard, Yale, and Princeton were primarily based on family legacy and attendance at private preparatory schools. Since the learning of academic skills was not emphasized, and the focus of college education was on character development for future leaders, it did not matter if students were not adequately prepared for college. Although the College Entrance Examination Board was formed in 1899 to establish and administer entrance exams for these colleges, the goal of these exams was efficiency of the admission process, not selection (since almost all young men with the right connections and preparatory school backgrounds were admitted). This was to change during the middle of the 20th century as the ideal of meritocracy started gaining ground in the United States. By the early 1960s, Ivy League universities started changing their admissions policy to accommodate both admissions through the traditional family connections and private prep school attendance approach, and admissions through outstanding SAT scores. Prestigious public universities, such as the University of California–Berkeley, did likewise. Test scores, particularly SAT scores, were to be the tool through which individuals were to be admitted into Ivy League institutions or prestigious public universities—the traditional ladders toward success, power, and wealth.[4]

The Development of Statistical Theories of Test Scores

Soon after the development of early mental tests at the beginning of the 20th century, the inherent limitation of the precision of scores was recognized. Test developers recognized that test scores contain errors, and that it is important to obtain accurate scores. The nature of score precision and measurement error was formalized by Charles Spearman (1904) when he explicated what has since become known as the true-score model. This model postulates that the observed score obtained from any administration of a test to an individual is composed of two parts: the true score of that individual, and a random error score. The smaller the random error score, the more accurate the observed score. When the test is administered to a number of individuals, there will be a variance of observed scores. This variance can also be decomposed into a variance of true scores and an error variance. The precision of test scores can then be described statistically by the proportion of the observed score variance that is true variance. This proportion is called the "reliability coefficient" or the "coefficient of precision" (Lord & Novick, 1968). Spearman's model was developed into classical test theory (CTT).

The focus of CTT is on the development of methods to estimate the reliability coefficient of test scores, from which other indicators of score precision (such as the standard error of measurement and confidence intervals) can be estimated. Statistically, the estimation of reliability coefficients was made possible by another earlier development. Galton discovered the concept of regression when he was investigating the effects of heredity. In 1896, Karl Pearson developed, based on Gallon's regression concept and the earlier work of the French mathematician A. Bravais in 1846, a statistical descriptor of the relationship between two variables (Boring, 1929)—known today as "Pearson's product–moment correlation coefficient" or simply "Pearson's r." The approach used in CTT is based on the use of two tests that meet a set of very re-strictive statistical assumptions known as parallel tests assumptions. If two such tests can be found and administered to the same group of individuals, the Pearson's r between the two sets of observed scores is mathematically equal to the reliability coefficient of the observed scores of either test. The problem then becomes one of trying to find two parallel tests. Two common methods of attempting to obtain classically parallel tests are the test–retest method and the equivalent-forms method. The correlations obtained from these methods are called "coefficient of stability" and "coefficient of equivalence," respectively. Both methods have serious conceptual and practical limitations (McDonald, 1999; Suen, 1991).

As CTT was being developed, it became apparent that the more items there are in a test, the less random error there is in the observed composite scores. Thus long tests tend to have higher reliability coefficients. In 1910, this relationship between test length and reliability coefficient was explicated mathematically by Spearman and by Brown independently (McDonald, 1999). The resulting formula has become known as the Spearman–Brown prophecy formula. With the development of this formula, the internal-consistency method—an alternative to the test–retest and equivalent-forms methods of obtaining parallel tests—became possible. One internal-consistency method is the split-half method, in which a single test is split into two halves, and each half-test is treated as if it is a parallel test. The Pearson's r between the scores of the two half-tests is then corrected through the Spearman–Brown formula. An alternative method is to treat each item in the test as a parallel single-item test and apply the Spearman–Brown formula to the average interitem correlation, the result from which has been referred to as the "standardized item alpha."

All these attempts to attain parallel tests suffer from a number of practical and theoretical problems, the most serious of which is the necessity of the very restrictive, unrealistic, and untestable parallel tests assumptions. A somewhat less restrictive set of assumptions, the essentially tau-equivalent assumptions, soon emerged; Kuder and Richardson (1937) then developed a set of reliability coefficients based on the internal-consistency strategy and these slightly less restrictive assumptions. The most commonly known of these coefficients is the Kuder–Richardson Formula 20 (KR_{20}), which can be used to estimate the reliability of the total scores from a test which consists of dichotomously scored (e.g., correct/incorrect) items. Luis Guttman (1945) developed the L_3 statistic, an extension of the KR_{20} to the general case beyond dichotomously scored items to include all types of items. Lee Cronbach (1951) popularized this statistic by introducing it in his 1951 paper under the name of "coefficient alpha." This has become known as "Cronbach's alpha reliability coefficient."

All these methods have a number of fundamental limitations. One limitation is the strong statistical assumptions necessary for these methods to work. Another is their inability to estimate beyond random errors. This renders these methods appropriate only for a relative interpretation of scores (i.e., norm-referenced interpretation). Another limitation is that these methods are applicable only to standardized paper-and-pencil tests; they cannot accommodate multifaceted testing conditions, such as the involvement of raters, direct observation of behavior, or complex testing designs. Yet another limitation is the implicit idea that reliability is an absolute property of a set of scores, regardless of interpretation and generalization. In the 1940s and 1950s, many researchers developed methods wherein one can estimate classical reliability coefficients under the less restrictive essentially tau-equivalent assumptions through the application of analysis-of-variance techniques (e.g., Hoyt's intraclass correlation). Based on these methods, Cronbach and his associates formalized the generalizability theory (GT) of measurement (Cronbach, Gleser, Nanda, & Rajaratnam, 1972). Based on analysis-of-variance methods, the GT allows for estimation of errors and reliability coefficients for any test/measurement conditions, regardless of design and conditions. For instance, it can accommodate performance assessment, athletic competitions, portfolio assessment, judgment-based assessment, and other complex test/assessment designs. It also explicitly recognizes that reliability is relative to score interpretation and intended degree of generalization. Thus there can be many different reliability coefficients for the same test, depending upon the intended use and interpretation. The statistical assumptions needed, randomly-parallel-tests assumptions, are substantially more realistic than those of CTT. Brennan (1983) described GT as a "liberalization" of classical theory. CTT in general, and Cronbach's alpha and KR_{20} in particular, proved to be special cases of GT.

Both CTT and GT focus on the precision of the observed score and its possible error. Neither attempts to estimate the true score directly. In 1904, along with the true-score model. Spearman developed the single-factor model of intelligence (later called g) through a method that later developed into factor analysis. This method attempts to identify the underlying theoretical latent trait (g) that presumably leads to the observed correlations among variables. Since the development of this method, many researchers have attempted to determine methods to estimate true scores or latent-trait scores directly from observed scores. One of the developments in the next several decades was the concept of an item characteristic curve (ICC). Specifically, the probability of a correct response to an item is related to the underlying true ability of the person in the form of a normal ogive function. Frederic Lord (1952) extended the ICC concept to develop a theoretical basis to estimate individuals' true scores directly, as well as the characteristics of the items simultaneously based on the observed responses to test items. Lord's theory was item response theory (IRT) or latent-trait theory. The statistical models developed by Lord were mathematically intractable (Warm, 1978) and were not practical until Alan Birnbaum suggested the use of a logistic approximation method in 1958 (see Lord & Novick, 1968). However, even with Birnbaum's simplified logistic approximation approach, IRT was still not practical because of its complex computational procedures until high-power computers became commonplace in the early 1980s. The complexity involved in estimating the parameters in IRT also depends on how items in a test are considered different from one another. We may consider items to differ in terms of difficulty, discrimination, and/or probability of a correct guess. Estimation is considerably simplified if we consider items to be different only in difficulties. The corresponding simplified statistical model is thus referred to as the one-parameter model. As we include additional parameters, whether we can find a unique solution in our estimation will depend on whether a number of assumptions are met. Therefore, the one-parameter model is most practical.

Independent of Lord's and Birnbaum's work, at the University of Copenhagen in Denmark between 1945 and 1948, Georg Rasch developed a statistical method to estimate individuals' latent abilities and items' difficulties simultaneously based on a logistic function between true ability score and the odds ratio of a correct response (see Rasch, 1980). Benjamin Wright brought this method to the United States in the 1970s and subsequently popularized it and became a strong advocate of this method, which is by now referred to as the Rasch model (Wright & Stone, 1979). It soon became clear that the Rasch model is mathematically equivalent to the one-parameter logistic IRT model. Because the IRT models and the Rasch model are based on the relationship between ability and responses to individual items (unlike CTT, which estimates reliability of the total score from a test containing fixed items), the application of IRT is not dependent on exactly which items are in a test. Thus IRT estimation methods are considered test-independent, making it possible to compare scores from different versions of a test consisting of different items and to implement computerized adaptive testing.

A limitation of these IRT and Rasch models is that they only apply to dichotomously and objectively scored items (i.e., items where no human rater is involved). Benjamin Wright and Geofferey Masters (1982) extended the Rasch model to accommodate polytomous rating scales such as Likert-type rating scales. The Wright and Masters method is appropriate for Likert-type scales but does not consider rating errors. Linacre (1989) built upon Wright and Masters's method and developed a many-faceted Rasch model. Linacre's method allows for the simultaneous estimation of individuals' abilities, items' difficulties (called "thresholds"), and raters' stringency or leniency.

The Development of Theories of Validity of Interpretation and Use

The use of mental tests is inherently an inferential activity. From a person's performance or responses to test items, we infer about a certain unobservable attitude, interest, ability, or other construct pertaining to that person. Furthermore, based on this inference, we make decisions or take actions about the individual. What makes such inferences and decisions meaningful and justified depends on the validity of our inferences from test scores to constructs. What constitutes validity has evolved and changed over the past century (Geisinger, 1992; Moss, 1992) as epistemology has changed.

During the 20th century, epistemology, the philosophy of science, has undergone several important changes. In the early part of the century, the most influential school of epistemology was that of logical positivism, which is attributed to a group of philosophers referred to as the Vienna circle. Logical positivism is also often (erroneously) attributed to Ludwig Wittgenstein (1922).[5] This philosophy holds that absolute truths and orders exist and can ultimately be discovered through logic, mathematics, and analysis of propositions through language. Empirical data are to be collected and analyzed logically through mathematical and statistical methods to reveal these truths. By the middle of the century, the thoughts of Karl Popper (1965) and Thomas Kuhn (1962) began to influence researchers and scholars. Popper suggested that truth is to be uncovered not through the search for direct proofs and empirical evidence, but through a process of falsification of theories. What is left standing becomes the best truth. Kuhn introduced the ideas of paradigms of beliefs and paradigm shifts: Knowledge is relative to a closed system called a "paradigm," and that knowledge is "gained" through the shifting of influence from one paradigm to another or from the merging of paradigms. Toward the last decades of the century, hermeneutics (e.g., Martin Heidegger) began to gain acceptance and influenced the way we seek knowledge in general. The observer and his or her subjective interpretation of events are inherently part of knowledge. Knowledge is to be gained through the generation, transmission, and acceptance of meaning. Knowledge is also manifested through language with different meanings for different observers. An interpretation can be "objective" and "valid," even if it is not verifiable (Dilthey, 1989). It is not concerned with verification, and it denies the possibility of objective knowledge. Instead, it argues that only a person who stands in history, subject to the prejudices of his or her age, can hope to understand it. As our understanding and our view of the nature of knowledge and our beliefs in what are the necessary conditions to demonstrate "truth" or knowledge changed throughout the 20th century, so did our concept of what constitutes a "valid" test and what needs to be done to validate a test correspondingly.

One of the earliest definitions of validity was provided by Hull (1928), who stated that a test is valid to the extent that it correlates with a test of free recall of the same material. A few years later, Bingham (1937) suggested what would later be called "concurrent validity" when he defined validity as the correlation of test scores with some other objective measure of that which the test is used to measure. Validity of a test was thus to be determined by a statistical correlation based on empirical data. This correlation coefficient was to be called the "validity coefficient" of the test and was considered a psychometric property of the test. This reflects the emphasis on mathematical models and empirical data at that time.

It soon became apparent that since the scores on a given test may have high statistical correlations with many other objective measures, a test could then have many validity coefficients. Guilford (1946) expressed this view when he stated that a test is valid for anything with which it correlates. Gulliksen (1950) expressed a similar view a few years later, when he suggested the concept of a criterion and proposed that the validity of a test is the correlation of the test with some criterion. This was empiricism at its extreme—in that we can in theory claim that a bathroom scale measures height among children, since the "scores" on the bathroom scale correlate well with height. The intention and content of the test are incidental and not considered at all.

The problems of this reliance on empirical validity coefficients without regard to content and intention became apparent to some in the 1930s and 1940s. One of the fundamental problems was the inherent tautology of the empirical concept of validity. If the validity of a test is determined by its correlation with some criterion measure, how do we determine the validity of the criterion measure? It became apparent that other means in addition to empirical validity coefficients are needed to determine validity. Garrett (1937) suggested the idea of intention as a component of validity when he defined validity as the extent to which the test measures what it purports to measure. This concept was later called "construct validity." Although Garrett's concept was appealing, there was no methodology available at that time to evaluate this idea of validity. While Garrett proposed the consideration of intention, Rulon (1946) proposed a role for subjective human judgment. Specifically, Rulon argued that when a test is reviewed by subject-matter experts who verify that its content represents a satisfactory sampling of the domain, the test is obviously valid. This concept was later to become "content validity."

In 1954, the APA formed a committee to establish technical standards for psychological tests. This committee summarized the various developments in the concept of validity and concluded that there were four types of validity: predictive, concurrent, construct, and content validities (APA, 1954). Predictive and concurrent validities were the empirical correlations of the early years. The difference between predictive and concurrent validity was in whether the criterion measure was given concurrently with the test or sometime in the future. Construct validity was essentially what was proposed by Garrett, and content validity corresponded to Rulon's concept.

During the 1950s, several important developments occurred that provided the methodology for construct validity. Cronbach and Meehl (1955) suggested the idea of a nomological net and the process of hypothesis testing as the means to establish construct validity. A few years later, Campbell and Fiske (1959) proposed the multitrait–multimethod matrix and the concepts of convergent and discriminant validity as other means of assessing construct validity. Meanwhile, after Spearman defined the single-factor model in 1904, much progress was made in factor-analytic techniques. This was to be used to examine the internal structure of a test as another approach to construct validity.

In 1966, the American Educational Research Association (AERA) and the National Council on Measurement in Education (NOME) joined the APA to form a joint committee to establish technical standards for testing (APA, 1966). In this new set of standards, the joint committee suggested that there are three types of validity: criterion-related, construct, and content validities. Essentially, they combined the previous predictive and concurrent validities into a single type called criterion-related validity. Meanwhile, since the method for determining construct validity was hypothesis testing, many new "types" of validity emerged in the literature, corresponding to the testing of different hypotheses. Also, during the 1960s, the civil rights movement and a number of litigations heightened the awareness of possible biases in testing. As tests were being used as the basis for important decisions about people's lives, questions were raised regarding fairness, bias, adverse impact, diagnostic utility, and social acceptability. The new joint committee for technical standards in 1974 recognized these concerns and advised test developers to consider adverse impact and test bias (APA, 1974).

In the 1980s, yet another new joint committee was formed to update technical standards (AERA, APA, & NCME, 1985). For the first time, validity was to be a joint responsibility of test developers and test users. The new standards suggested that test users should know the purposes of the test and the probable consequences of giving a test. More importantly, the new standards rejected the concept of three types of validity and suggested that there is only validity. Specifically, the new standards defined validity as

> the appropriateness, meaningfulness, and usefulness of the specific inferences from test scores. There are numerous validation processes to accumulate evidence. Some of these are provided by developers, others gathered by users. . . . Traditionally, the various means of accumulating validity evidence have been grouped into categories called *content-related, criterion-related, and construct-related evidence of validity*. These categories are convenient, . . . but the use of the category la-

bels does not imply that there are distinct types of validity or that a specific validation strategy is best for each specific inference or test use. (AERA et al., 1985, p. 9; italics in original)

Although validity was to be a unitary concept, researchers continued to propose new "types" of validity. When combined with concerns for test bias and adverse impact, and the emerging popularity of hermeneutics, the concepts of what is necessary for validity became murky and unwieldy. Samuel Messick (1989) proposed a faceted model of validity that combined all these concerns. He suggested that validity is to be established by examining four aspects of testing: (1) evidence to support interpretation; (2) consequences of the proposed interpretation; (3) evidence to support utility of the test; and (4) consequences in the proposed use of the test. This model gained wide acceptance in the next decade, although there were detractors. By 1999, a new joint committee completed another update of the technical standard. Messick's model was reflected in the new standards in the form of consequential validity. The new standards have also explicitly accepted the idea that a test may have many "validities." Specifically, the new joint committee has defined validity as

> the degree to which evidence and theory support the interpretations of test scores entailed by proposed uses of tests. . . . The process of validation involves accumulating evidence to provide a sound scientific basis for the proposed score interpretations. It is the interpretations of test scores required by proposed uses that are evaluated, not the test itself. When test scores are used or interpreted in more than one way, each intended interpretation must be validated. (AERA, APA, & NCME, 1999, p. 9)

Meanwhile, Lee Cronbach (1988) and Michael Kane (1992) proposed the idea that validity is a process of systematic arguments rather than types of validity or validation processes. This view is gaining acceptance today (e.g., Haertel, 1999). Interestingly, Cronbach, who had made many contributions to the concepts and methods of validity over half a century, observed that "validation was once a priestly mystery, a ritual performed behind the scenes, with the professional elite as witness and judge. Today, it is a public spectacle combining the attractions of chess and mud wrestling" (1988, p. 3).

The Development of Testing Formats and Technologies

Throughout most of human history, except for the Chinese civil service exams, testing was always conducted in a one-to-one or small-group setting. The person tested would be asked to perform some task or respond to some question. Additional tasks or questions would typically depend on some of the person's early responses. For example, in an oral examination at a university, a student would be asked a question by a single professor or a group of professors. Depending on the response, a follow-up question would be asked. In this manner, testing was mostly individual, customized, and based on performing some open-ended task. This was to change in the 20th century.

In terms of format, Ebbinghaus (1897) invented a new way of asking questions: the fill-in-the-blank format. This was a departure from the conventional open-ended oral or essay questions. Although fill-in-the-blank questions are still somewhat open-ended, the acceptable responses are more restricted. Sometime during World War I, the most restricted form of questions—the multiple-choice testing format—was invented. It is not clear exactly who invented this format. Some have attributed the invention to Henry Goddard; others have attributed it to Edward Thorndike. Other variants of multiple-choice, such as true-and-false, matching, and analogy formats, soon followed. Unlike open-ended questions, these new formats, often called "select-type items," can be administered efficiently to large numbers of people simultaneously because of the ease in administration and scoring.

In terms of the evolution of scoring methods, one of the first attempts at objective scoring was developed for the Chinese civil service exams. These exams were in essay format. In the last several centuries of these exams, copyists were employed to copy candidates' answers, and only the copies were given to the judges to evaluate. This system was intended to prevent the recognition of handwriting. In 1914, F. J. Kelly showed that the reliability of scores for free-response tests could be improved if scoring keys were employed (Nitko, 1983).

In spite of the efficiency of the new select-type formats, essay and oral exams and task performances remained the predominant methods of testing until 1937. However, in that year, the optical scanning machine was invented (DuBois, 1970). Combining the efficiency of the scanning technology with that of multiple-choice and other select-type items rendered these test formats quite practical for very large-scale testing. Since then, large-scale multiple-choice testing programs have proliferated (Angoff& Dyer, 1971). The development of high-power mainframe and personal computers in the following several decades has made the scoring and reporting of these types of tests even more efficient.

While select-type items provided an efficient testing approach, many observers in the last several decades of the century began to question the tradeoff. One concern was with the loss of the individually customized (or adaptive) assessments of the past. Although select-type items such as multiple-choice items are efficient (particularly when combined with scoring machines and computers), their efficiency is not optimal because every person must respond to all questions, regardless of the individual's ability and the difficulty of each question. The efficiency of the process would be further optimized if an individual only needed to respond to those questions the difficulties and informativeness of which matched the individual's level of ability—much in the same way professors base follow-up oral exam questions based on a student's ability, as manifested in the student's answers to previous questions. With the development of IRT and high-speed computers, this became possible in the last two decades, in the form of computerized adaptive testing. In this approach, computer algorithms based on IRT constantly "interact" with an examinee to evaluate the person's ability level based on the person's responses to previous questions, and select from a pool of items the next most appropriate question to match that person's ability level. This method can reduce testing time by about 80% for an individual examinee.

While the adaptive testing approach is an attempt to further optimize the efficiency of the testing process, others have questioned the validity of the large-scale testing approach based on select-type items. Concerns for such issues as authenticity, curricular validity, assessment of higher-order thinking skills, systemic validity, and so on have emerged in the last two decades. Many alternative approaches have been suggested and implemented, including such approaches as portfolio assessment, curriculum-based assessment, and performance-based assessment. With advances in computer technology, many of these alternative assessment approaches, which had previously been quite inefficient, have become possible. For performance assessment, for instance, various simulation computer programs have made it possible to assess performances in scientific experimentation, driving, and other skills. Scoring of alternative assessment has been made easier by such technologies as scoring algorithms and video technology. Portfolio assessment has been facilitated with the availability of the World Wide Web, where individuals can post electronic portfolios. Even the performance assessment of medical doctors has been facilitated by the development of computerized robotic mannequins and "standardized patients." There are more options in terms of approach, format, and technology at our disposal today for the assessment of human mental abilities than at any other time in history.

TESTING TODAY

From their relatively modest beginnings in European laboratories, mental testing activities have spread around the world and have become a major and constant facet of modern life. Also, it has become a major economic enterprise. Hundreds of millions of mental tests are being used every year in the United States alone for psychological treatments, a large variety of educational purposes, employment, licensure and certification of professionals, placement, and so on. The same phenomenon is repeated in virtually all developed and developing nations. In some countries (e.g., South Korea), the stakes involved in tests such as college entrance exams are so high that every year a number of young men and women commit suicide because of poor test scores. Government also regulates testing activities in many nations. For example, the Examination Yuan is one of five branches of government in Taiwan today.

As mental testing became more common-place and started to have an impact on individuals' lives and well-being, skepticism regarding its ability to guide decisions began to grow. Concerns for test quality and bias have led to a variety of responses. Over the past three decades, tests have become the object of many cases under litigation. Such cases have essentially rendered the judicial courts the final arbiters of quality, reliability, validity, and fairness in testing in many instances. These judgments, as well as the professional development and administration of many testing practices, are increasingly being guided by professional standards. These include the technical standards of the joint committees discussed earlier; the *Standards for Teacher Competence in Educational Assessment of Students* (American Federation of Teachers, NCME, & National Education Association, 1990); the *Code of Fair Testing Practices in Education* (AERA, APA, & NCME, 1988); and the *Code of Professional Responsibilities in Educational Measurement* (NCME, 1995). They also include laws such as the Americans with Disabilities Act (PL 99-457) and truth-in-testing laws, as well as government regulations such as the Equal Employment Opportunity Commission's (1978) regulation on employment testing. Many new concerns, such as opportunity-to-learn issues, have also been raised as a result of some of the court cases. Consumer advocates such as Ralph Nader, watchdog organizations such as Fair Test, and professional reviews such as the *Mental Measurement Yearbook* series (initiated by Oscar Bums in the 1930s) have constantly scrutinized the development and uses of tests. The widespread high-stakes testing activities have also spawned a new industry, in the form of test preparation and test coaching companies and publications. As the stakes in testing become higher in many areas, new methods of cheating continually emerge.

By all indications, the expansion of psychological and educational assessment activities will continue into the foreseeable future. As it expands, it is likely to continue to become more complex, involving sociopolitical and legal as well as scientific concerns. Its impact on our lives will continue to increase and to become even more pervasive. In fact, today we are so accustomed to the idea of mental testing in our daily lives that we have spawned yet another new industry:

mental testing as entertainment! Today, for our own amusement, we give our dogs canine IQ tests; we play with the nutrition IQ or word power tests in our magazines; we play board games such as Trivial Pursuit; and we watch TV quiz shows such as *Jeopardy* or *Who Wants to Be a Millionaire?*

ACKNOWLEDGMENTS

We wish to thank Jay T. Parkes, Steven C. Shatter, and Sang Ha Lee for their suggestions on an earlier draft of this chapter.

NOTES

1. DuBois (1970) suggested that the system had started over 4,000 years ago, in 2200 B.C. However, this conclusion was based on a single historic document that also contains some mythology. This conclusion has yet to be confirmed by other independent sources. Although the system was formally established in 1115 B.C., it did not become well-organized and was not offered on a regular basis until 605 A.D. under Emperor Yangdi of Sui, who also introduced the prestigious and coveted Jinshi (advanced scholar) degree (Burne, 1989).
2. What SAT stands for has undergone several iterations, depending upon the fashion of the time. Originally, SAT was the acronym for Scholastic Aptitude Test. After numerous studies and the success of such coaching programs as that of Stanley Kaplan, it was apparent that SAT scores could be increased through instruction. At some point, faced with this evidence that it does not measure "aptitude," SAT was said to stand for Scholastic Achievement Tests. Over the past decade, there has been a general movement among educators against objective multiple-choice "tests" such as the SAT in favor of authentic performance assessment, portfolio assessment, and other assessment techniques. Today SAT is considered to represent Scholastic Assessment Tests.
3. While mass testing was on the increase in the United States, interestingly, the historic Chinese civil service examination system was discontinued after 3,000 years in 1903 as part of an attempt toward political reform at the end of the Qing Dynasty. But the reform came too late, and the Qing Dynasty was overthrown in 1911. In the 1930s, the Nationalist government developed a different system of civil service exam, which continues today in Taiwan.
4. Until the 1950s, most public state universities had open admissions. The question of entrance exams for these universities was moot until later.
5. Although many have attributed logical positivism to Wittgenstein's book, Wittgenstein was technically not a logical positivist. A careful reading of Ch. 6 of his book *Tractatus Logico-Philosophicus* reveals that he rejected many of the premises of logical positivism.

REFERENCES

American Educational Research Association (AERA), American Psychological Association (APA), & National Council on Measurement in Education (NCME). (1985). *Standards for educational and psychological testing*. Washington, DC: Authors.

American Educational Research Association (AERA), American Psychological Association (APA), & National Council on Measurement in Education (NCME). (1988). *Code of fair testing practices in education*. Washington, DC: Authors.

American Educational Research Association (AERA), American Psychological Association (APA), & National Council on Measurement in Education (NCME). (1999). *Standards for educational and psychological testing*. Washington, DC: Authors.

American Federation of Teachers, National Council on Measurement in Education (NCME), & National Educational Association. (1990). *Standards for teacher competence in educational assessment of students*. Washington, DC: Authors.

American Psychological Association (APA). (1954). *Technical recommendations for psychological tests and diagnostic techniques*. Washington, DC: Author.

American Psychological Association (APA). (1966). *Standards for educational and psychological tests and manuals*. Washington, DC: Author.

American Psychological Association (APA). (1974). *Standards for educational and psychological tests and manuals*. Washington, DC: Author.

Anastasi, A. (1982). *Psychological testing* (5th ed.). New York: Macmillan.

Angoff, W. H., & Dyer, H. S. (1971). The admission testing program. In W. H. Angoff (Ed.), *The College Board Admission Testing Program: A technical report on research and development activities relating to the Scholastic Aptitude and Achievement Tests* (pp. 1–14). Princeton, NJ: Educational Testing Service.

Bellak, L., & Bellak, S. S. (1952). *Children's Apperception Test*. New York: CPS.

Bernreuter, R. G. (1933). The theory and construction of the Personality Inventory. *Journal of Social Psychology, 4*, 387–405.

Binet, A., & Simon, T. (1905). Methodes nouvelles pour le diagnostic du niveau intellectuel des anormaux. *L'Annee Psychologique, 11*, 191–244.

Bingham, W. V. (1923a). Cooperative business research. *Annals of the American Academy of Political Science, 110*, 179–189.

Bingham, W. V. (1923b). Psychology applied. *Scientific Monthly, 16*, 141–159.

Bingham, W. V. (1937). *Aptitude and aptitude testing*. New York: Harper.

Bishop, M. (1968). *The Middle Ages*. Boston: Houghton Mifflin.

Blackford, K. M. H., & Newcomb, A. (1919). *The job, the man, and the boss*. New York: Doubleday, Page.

Bolton, T. L. (1891). The growth of memory in school children. *American Journal of Psychology, 4,* 362–380.

Boorstin, D. J. (1974). *The Americans: The democratic experience*. New York: Vintage.

Boorstin, D. J. (1983). *The discoverers: A history of man's search to know his world and himself*. New York: Vintage.

Boring, E. G. (1929). *A history of experimental psychology*. New York: Appleton-Century.

Bowman, M. L. (1989). Testing individual differences in China. *American Psychologist, 44,* 576–57 S.

Brennan, R. L. (1983). *Elements of generalizability theory*. Iowa City, IA: American College Testing.

Burne, J. (Ed.). (1989). *Chronicle of the world*. New York: Prentice-Hall.

Bush, D. V., & Waugh, W. (1923). *Character analysis: How to read people at sight*. Chicago: Huron Press.

Campbell, D. P. (1971). *Handbook for the Strong Vocational Interest Blank*. Stanford, CA: Stanford University Press.

Campbell, D. T., & Fiske, D. W. (1959). Convergent and discriminant validity in the multitrait–multimethod matrix. *Psychological Bulletin, 56,* 81–105.

Cattell, J. M. (1890). Mental tests and measurements. *Minds, 15,* 373–380.

Cronbach, L. J. (1951). Coefficient alpha and the internal structure of tests. *Psychometrika, 16,* 297–334.

Cronbach, L. J. (1988). Five perspectives on the validity argument. In H. Wainer & H. I. Braun (Eds.), *Test validity* (pp. 3–17). Hillsdale, NJ: Eribaum.

Cronbach, L. J., Gleser, G. C., Nanda, H., & Rajaratnam, N. (1972). *The dependability of behavioral measurements: Theory of generalizability for scores and profiles*. New York: Wiley.

Cronbach, L. J., & Meehl, P. E. (1955). Construct validity in psychological tests. *Psychological Bulletin, 52,* 281–302.

Dilthey, W. (1989). *Introduction to the human sciences* (R. Makkreel, Trans.). Princeton, NJ: Princeton University Press.

DuBois, P. H. (1970). *A history of psychological testing*. Boston: Allyn & Bacon.

Ebbinghaus, H. (1897). Ueber eine neue Methode zur Pruning geistiger Fahigkeiten und ihre Anwendungbie Schulkindern. *Zeitschriftfur Psychologic, 13,* 401–459.

Educational Testing Service (ETS). (1999). *Breaking the mold: Assessment in a new century* (ETS 1999 Annual Report). Princeton, NJ: Author.

Equal Employment Opportunity Commission. (1978, August 25). Uniform guidelines on employee selection procedures. 43 Fed. Reg. 38290.

Fass, P. S. (1980). The IQ: A cultural and historical framework. *American Journal of Education, 88,* 431–458.

Forrest, D. W. (1974). *Francis Galton: The life and work of a Victorian genius*. New York: Taplinger.

Fosbroke, G. E. (1933). *Plus + selling*. Minneapolis, MN: Sales Engineering Institute.

Frank, L. K. (1939). Projective methods for the study of personality. *Journal of Psychology, 8,* 389–413.

Freeman, F. N. (1926). *Mental tests: Their history, principles and applications*. Boston: Houghton Mifflin.

Garrett, H. E. (1937). *Statistics in psychology and education*. New York: Longmans, Green.

Geisinger, K. F. (1992). The metamorphosis of test validation. *Educational Psychologist, 27*(2), 197–222.

Goddard, H. H. (1911). A revision of the Binet Scale. *Training School Bulletin, 8,* 56–62.

Guilford, J. P. (1946). New standards for test evaluation. *Educational and Psychological Measurement, 1,* 1–10.

Gulliksen. H. (1950). *Theory of mental tests*. New York: Wiley.

Guttman, L. (1945). A basis for analyzing test–retest reliability. *Psychometrika, 10,* 255–282.

Haertel, E. H. (1999). Validity arguments for high-stakes testing: In search of evidence. *Educational Measurement: Issues and Practice, 18*(4), 5–9.

Hathaway, S. R. (1964). MMPI: Professional use by professional people. *American Psychologist, 19,* 204–210.

Ho, P. T. (1962). *The ladder of success in imperial China: Aspects of social mobility, 1368–1911*. New York: Columbia University Press.

Hull. C. L. (1928). *Aptitude testing*. Yonkers, NY: World Book.

Humm, D. G., & Wadsworth, G. W. (1935). The Humm–Wadsworth Temperament Scale. *American Journal of Psychiatry, 92,* 163–200.

Huxley, A. (1963). Time Reading Program introduction. In M. L. Starkey, *The devil in Masssachusetts*. New York: Time.

Jung, C. G. (1910). The association method. *American Journal of Psychology, 21,* 219–269.

Kane, M. (1992). An argument-based approach to validity. *Psychological Bulletin, 112,* 527–535.

Kelley, T. L. (1914). *Educational guidance: An experimental study in the analysis and predcition of ability of high school pupils* (Contributions to Education No. 71). New York: Teachers College, Columbia University.

Kent, G. H., & Rosanoff, A. J. (1910). A study of association in insanity. *American Journal of Insanity, 67,* 317–390.

Kownslar, A. O., & Frizzle, D. B. (1967). *Discovering American history*. New York: Holt, Rinehart & Winston.

Kuder, G. F. (1934). *Kuder Preference Record—Vocational*. Chicago: Science Research Associates.

Kuder, G. F. (1948). *Kuder Preference Record—Personal*. Chicago: Science Research Associates.

Kuder, G. F., & Richardson, M. W. (1937). The theory of the estimation of test reliability. *Psychometrika, 2,* 151–160.

Kuhlmann, F. (1912). Binet–Simon's system for measuring the intelligence of children [Monograph supplement]. *Journal of Psycho-Asthenics, 1*(1), 76–92.

Kuhlmann, F. (1922). *Tests of mental development*. Minneapolis, MN: Educational Test Bureau.

Kuhn, T. S. (1962). *The structure of scientific revolutions*. Chicago: University of Chicago Press.

Lemann, N. (1995a, September). The great sorting. *The Atlantic Monthly,* pp. 84–100.

Lemann, N. (1995b, August). The structure of success in America. *The Atlantic Monthly*, pp. 41–60.

Lemann, N. (1999). *The big test: The secret history of the American meritocracy*. New York: Farrar, Straus & Giroux.

Linacre, J. M. (1989). *Many-faceted Rasch measurement*. Chicago: MESA Press.

Link, H. C. (1919). *Employment psychology: The application of scientific methods to the selection, training and grading of employees*. New York: Macmillan.

Lord, F. M. (1952). *A theory of test scores* (Psychometric Monograph No. 7).

Lord, F. M., & Novick, M. R. (1968). *Statistical theories of mental test scores, with contributions by Alan Birnbaum*. Reading, MA: Addison-Wesley.

McDonald, R. P. (1999). *Test theory: A unified treatment*. Mahwah, NJ: Eribaum.

Messick, S. (1989). Validity. In R. L. Linn (Ed.), *Educational measurement* (3rd ed., pp. 13–103). New York: Macmillan.

Miyazaki, I. (1981). *China's examination hell: The civil service examinations of imperial China* (C. Schirokauer, Trans.). New Haven, CT: Yale University Press.

Moore, B. V. (1921). Personnel selection of graduate engineers: The differentiation of apprentice engineers for training as salesmen, designers, and executives of production. *Psychological Monographs, 30*, 1–84.

Morgan, C., & Murray, H. A. (1935). A method for investigating phantasies: The Thematic Apperception Test. *Archives of Neurology and Psychiatry, 34*, 289–306.

Moss, P. A. (1992). Shifting conceptions of validity in educational measurement: Implications for performance assessment. *Review of Educational Research, 62*(3), 229–258.

Murray, H. A. (1943). *Thematic Apperception Test*. Cambridge, MA: Harvard University Press.

National Council on Measurement in Education (NCME). (1995). *Code of professional responsibilities in educational measurement*. Washington, DC: Author.

National Industrial Conference Board. (1948). *Experience with employment tests* (Studies in Personnel Policy No. 92). New York: Author.

Nitko, A. J. (1983). *Educational tests and measurement: An introduction*. New York: Harcourt Brace Jovanovich.

Parsons, F. (1908). *Choosing a vocation*. Boston: Houghton Mifflin.

Payne, A. F. (1928). *Sentence completions*. New York: New York Guidance Clinic.

Pedersen, O. (1997). *The first universities: Studium generate and the origins of university education in Europe*. New York: Cambridge University Press.

Popper, K. R. (1965). *The logic of scientific discovery*. New York: Harper & Row.

Pressey, S. L. (1921). A group scale for investigating the emotions. *Journal of Abnormal and Social Psychology, 16*, 55–64.

Rasch, G. (1980). *Probabilitic models for some intelligence and attainment tests*. Chicago: University of Chicago Press.

Rice, J. M. (1893). *The public school system of the United States*. New York: Century.

Rulon, P. J. (1946). On the validity of educational tests. *Harvard Educational Review, 16*, 290–296.

Rorschach, H. (1921). *Psychodiagnostik*. Bern: Bircher.

Sattler, J. M. (1982). *Assessment of children's intelligence and special abilities* (2nd ed.). Boston: Allyn & Bacon.

Scott, W. D., Clothier, R. C., & Spriegel, W. R. (1961). *Personnel management: Principles, practices, and a point of view* (6th ed.). New York: McGraw-Hill.

Shneidman, E. S. (1948). *The Make-a-Picture Story Test*. New York: Psychological Corporation.

Spearman, C. (1904). General intelligence objectively determined and measured. *American Journal of Psychology, 15*, 201–293.

Starkey, M. L. (1963). *The devil in Massachusetts*. New York: Time.

Stern, W. (1914). *The psychological methods of testing intelligence*. Baltimore: Warwick & York.

Suen, H. K. (1991). *Principles of test theories*. Mahwah, NJ: Eribaum.

Symonds, P. M. (1948). *Symonds Picture Story Test*. New York: Bureau of Publications, Teachers College, Columbia University.

Terman, L. M. (1916). *The measurement of intelligence*. Boston: Houghton Mifflin.

Terman, L. M., & Merrill, M. (1937). *Measuring intelligence*. Boston: Houghton Mifflin.

Thorndike, E. L. (1912). The permanence of interests and their relation to abilities. *Popular Science Monthly, 18*, 449–456.

Thorndike, E. L. (1918). The nature, purposes, and general methods of measurement of educational products. In G. M. Whiffle (Ed.), *Seventeenth yearbook, Part II* (pp. 16–24). Bloomington, IL: National Society for the Study of Education.

Tulchin, S. H. (1940). The preRorschach use of inkblot tests. *Rorschach Research Exchange, 4*, 1–7.

U.S. Civil Service Commission. (1884). *First annual report*. Washington, DC: U.S. Government Printing Office.

Warm, T. A. (1978). *A primer of item response theory*. Springfield, VA: National Technical Information Services.

Wiebe, R. (1967). *The search for order, 1877–1920*. New York: Hill & Wang.

Wittgenstein, L. (1922). *Tractatus logico-philosophicus* (German text with English transl. by C. K. Ogden and introduction by B. Russell). London: Routledge & Kegan Paul.

Woodworm, R. S. (1918). *Personal data sheet*. Chicago: Stoelting.

Wright, B. D., & Stone, M. H. (1979). *Best test design*. Chicago: MESA Press.

Wright, B. D., & Masters, G. N. (1984). *Rating scale analysis: Rasch measurement*. Chicago: MESA Press.

Yerkes, R. M., Bridges, J. W., & Hardwick, R. S. (1915). *A point scale for measuring mental ability*. Baltimore: Warwick & York.

Young, M. D. (1958). *The rise of the meritocracy, 1870–2033: An essay on education and equality*. London: Thames & Hudson.

2

A Practical Model for Test Development

GARY J. ROBERTSON

The development of educational and psychological tests occurs for a variety of purposes in a variety of settings. This chapter describes a practical model for developing tests that is applicable to many different types of tests in many different settings. Although the context used in this chapter is the development of standardized educational achievement and ability tests within commercial test-publishing firms, the core components of the model presented can be applied to virtually any test development enterprise—regardless of where the test is constructed or whether it is delivered to examinees printed in a booklet, presented orally to one individual at a time by a trained examiner, or displayed on a personal computer (PC) screen.

Test development requires knowledge of several academic disciplines honed by practical experience in an organization where tests are designed and produced. The most responsible positions in test development organizations are typically held by persons with advanced graduate training in educational psychology, measurement, psychometrics, statistics, and research methodology. For certain kinds of tests, other specialists are required. For example, educational achievement tests require experts in the curricular content areas assessed, whereas the development of psychological tests such as personality inventories requires a background in clinical psychology. Some test development operations are so small that only one or two specialists are needed, whereas very large test development organizations may employ many individuals with various types of specialized training. Skilled editorial, production, and clerical personnel are also required to undertake the many and varied tasks encountered in test development and test publishing.

In my chapter on test development written for the first edition of this handbook (Robertson, 1990), I made the statement that computers had lightened the test development workload during the preceding 25 years, but that test development was still largely a human-labor-intensive enterprise. Today I must say that although individuals are still required to develop tests, the technological advances in both PC hardware and software during the 1990s have resulted in significant changes in test development, as a direct result of the increased speed and efficiency with which information is received and processed.

Test development, along with many other areas of human endeavor, has benefited directly from the operation of Moore's law—which states that the number of transistors on a silicon computer chip doubles every 18 months, thereby cutting the cost per transistor by one-half (Moore, 1965). Translated into operational terms, this means that the PCs now at our individual desks or work stations can accommodate complex statistical algorithms and analyses once available only within centralized computer data-processing centers in universities or large test development organizations. Such advances, together with the changes occurring as a direct result of the Internet, have greatly increased the productivity of individuals engaged in test development. The changes we have witnessed during the past few years are undoubtedly only the beginning of even more dramatic changes to come in the years ahead.

QUALITY STANDARDS FOR TEST DEVELOPMENT

Although there are not and cannot be rigidly prescribed standards for test construction that are imposed uniformly upon all test publishers, both professional organizations and market forces encourage test developers to produce publications that meet accepted technical standards. For example, the American Educational Research Association (AERA), the American Psychological Association (APA), and the National Council on Measurement in Education (NCME) have produced various editions of joint technical standards for test use and development that date from 1954. A revised edition of these standards is issued about once every decade; at this writing, the latest version is the *Standards for Educational and Psychological Testing* (AERA, APA, & NCME, 1999). These standards have exerted a very positive influence on the development of commercially produced tests. The current standards represent a consensus among professionals in the three sponsoring organizations about the most desirable testing practices to follow in developing and using tests. However, because they are stated in rather broad, general terms, the standards still leave room for needed diversity in specific assessment applications.

Another professional organization having considerable direct influence on test development is the Buros Institute of Mental Measurements. The series of *Mental Measurements Yearbooks* published periodically since the 1930s by the Buros Institute has guided both test users and test developers in appropriate procedures for constructing and interpreting tests. Several professional journals also have periodic test reviews by recognized peer experts. Taken as a whole, test reviews have had a salutary effect on test publishing by calling attention both to exemplary practices and to errors of commission or omission.

Market forces have also operated, through a process akin to natural selection, to reward some tests with great longevity and to relegate others to relative obscurity at some point following their publication. Although neither test sales nor volume of test use is an automatic guarantee of technical quality, history has shown that tests with innovative content and technically sound underpinnings offering useful interpretive information have, with a few exceptions, enjoyed a high degree of market acceptance and longevity. Several tests in use today originated more than 50 or 75 years ago and, through successive revisions incorporating technical advances available at the time, have continued to evolve and find widespread market acceptance. Examples of such tests (by their current titles, but with their original publication dates) are the current editions of the Stanford–Binet Intelligence Scale (1916), the Stanford Achievement Test (1923), the College Board Scholastic Assessment Test (1926), and the Differential Aptitude Tests (1947), to mention but a few.

A PROCESS-BASED MODEL OF TEST DEVELOPMENT

The material presented in this chapter is organized around a model focused on the processes of test development outlined in Table 2.1. The steps in this model, which I have used throughout my career in test development, have functioned effectively with a wide assortment of test publications made available through commercial test publishers to school districts, psychologists, psychological clinics, business and industrial concerns, and government agencies.

TABLE 2.1. Steps in a Process-Based Model of Test Development

1. Gather preliminary ideas or proposals.
2. Evaluate the soundness of preliminary ideas or proposals (approve or reject).
3. Conclude formal publication arrangements.
4. Prepare test specifications.
5. Write items.
6. Conduct item tryout.
    a. Prepare tryout materials.
    b. Prepare tryout sample specifications.
    c. Recruit examiners and other participants.
    d. Administer the tryout items.
    e. Analyze tryout information and data.
7. Evaluate publication status following tryout.
8. Assemble final test form(s).
9. Conduct national standardization program.
    a. Prepare standardization sample specifications.
    b. Recruit participants.
    c. Prepare materials.
    d. Administer tests.
    e. Analyze data.
    f. Develop norms tables.
    g. Prepare supporting technical documentation (reliability, validity, differential-item-functioning [DIF] studies).
10. Prepare materials for final publication.
    a. Establish publication schedule.
    b. Write manual.
    c. Prepare test books and response forms.
    d. Manufacture materials for distribution.
11. Prepare marketing plan.
    a. Plan the marketing campaign.
    b. Initiate direct mail promotion.
    c. Initiate space advertising.
    d. Train sales staff.
    e. Attend professional meetings and conventions.
    f. Launch publication.

The remainder of this chapter is divided into sections that roughly parallel the steps outlined in Table 2.1. This process-based model follows a logical flow of activity, beginning with preliminary activities to define the nature and scope of a test publication, proceeding to item development and tryout, then to standardization and norms development, and finally to publication.

PRELIMINARY STEPS

All test publications begin with an idea or concept, which is refined until the essential characteristics are clear enough to permit the publisher to evaluate both its theoretical or pedagogical soundness and its anticipated financial return. Ideas for test publications often come from individuals outside the publisher's staff, who become authors if their publication ideas are accepted and published. Ideas for publications may also come from within a publisher's test development staff. The extent to which test publishers rely on outside authors as opposed to the internal professional staff varies considerably, depending upon the nature of a particular publisher's development and marketing staff resources. This section discusses the development and refinement of publication ideas, the evaluation of proposed publications, and the completion of formal arrangements for publication.

Development and Refinement of Publication Ideas

Ideas for test publications come from a variety of sources. Scholars such as university faculty members who are conducting various types of research constitute the main group of individuals outside a publisher's staff who submit publication proposals. Graduate students and teachers who may have designed a single measurement device for a specific area of inquiry or a specific assessment need constitute another significant group of individuals contacting publishers with new publication ideas. All of these proposals are intended to meet perceived areas of need where the available instrumentation is either of poor quality or entirely lacking. Publication ideas often evolve from within a publisher's staff, because both developmental and marketing staff members have the relevant product knowledge and market awareness to develop sound publication ideas. Publishers are now using more sophisticated market research methods to identify market needs and opportunities.

Test publication submissions range from one-paragraph descriptions supplied in short letters of inquiry to complete publication proposals with extensive documentation. An entire doctoral dissertation or report of a research study is frequently submitted to substantiate a proposal. Because there is wide variability in the nature and extent of material submitted with a publication proposal, publishers have developed guidelines for the type of information that should be submitted with a publication idea. An example of the type of information a publisher needs to evaluate a submission is shown in Table 2.2. Although all of the information listed in Table 2.2 may not be available, it represents an ideal that, if met, would provide most of the detailed information needed to evaluate thoroughly the soundness of a publication idea.

Frequently, the product that emerges as the final publication is rather different from the idea originally proposed. This occurs as a result of the refinement process that takes place once the publisher contributes additional ideas or market-related data that help to reshape or better define a publication. Most major test publications represent a blending of ideas and expertise from the original author(s) and the test publisher's professional development and marketing staffs. The nature of test publishing at present is such that the expertise, judgment, and experience of many different professional staff members are needed to launch a publication successfully. The decision to accept a publication is probably the most important decision a publisher makes, because the results of such decisions are what determine the professional reputation and financial success of a publishing firm. A key to the right publishing decisions lies in the procedures used to evaluate and screen publication submissions.

Evaluation of Proposed Publications

A first step in evaluating a proposed publication is to ascertain the extent to which it matches a particular publisher's general goals. Most test publishers specialize in certain types of publications. A publisher specializing in personality and clinical tests, for example, would probably not be interested in publishing a new type of group-administered diagnostic reading test. Such specialization among test publishers has occurred for both historical and economic reasons. What it means, however, is that different publishers fit into different niches of the market for testing materials, and hence have developed the specialization and expertise necessary to reach their particular market segment effectively.

TABLE 2.2. **Information Needed by Publishers to Evaluate Proposed Test Publications**

1. Description of the proposed test publication
   a. Statement of purpose, rationale, and need
   b. Age/grade range
   c. Structure/parts, subscales, or subtests
   d. Method of administration, with time required
   e. Method of scoring, with time required
   f. Qualifications needed for administering and scoring
2. Components
   a. Consumable print material—test books, answer sheets, and report forms
   b. Nonconsumable print material—test books, manuals, and interpretive aids
   c. Computer software for administering, scoring, and interpreting
   d. Manipulatives or other custom-designed manufactured items
3. Market information
   a. Targeted users/purchasers
   b. Targeted market segments
   c. Estimated market size
   d. Major competition
   e. Differential advantage of present product over competition
4. Accumulated research information
   a. Results of pilot studies
   b. Results of special research studies
   c. Research needed to complete product
5. Peer reviews/endorsements

Because resources are limited, test publishers must select publishing opportunities from among those available. This may be done either informally or in a more formal, structured way. Selection criteria typically include some evaluation of the proposed publication's theoretical soundness, as well as the extent to which it meets a market need. An attempt to gauge profitability may also be required before management reaches a final decision. A formal, systematic approach to evaluation increases the likelihood of selecting publications that will benefit the publisher both professionally and financially.

The nature of the system used to evaluate proposed publications will depend to some extent on the size of the publisher, with smaller publishers tending to favor less formal, less structured procedures, and larger publishers using more systematized, formal evaluation schemes. A system I have used successfully is based on an evaluation procedure centered around the four factors shown in Table 2.3. A rating system called the Proposed New Publication Rating Scale (PNPRS), designed to obtain ratings on these factors, is applied by one or more staff members to the proposed new product being evaluated. The PNPRS is structured to obtain information in four areas of major importance for evaluating new product proposals: Product Integrity, Marketability, Research and Development Capability, and Production Capability. Collectively, these four factors are known as Intangible Fac-

TABLE 2.3. Factors and Subfactors Constituting the Proposed New Publication Rating Scale (PNPRS)

Factor/subfactor	Weight
1. Product Integrity	20%
a. Theoretical soundness	
b. Ease of use	
c. Originality	
d. Author's credentials	
e. Proof of effectiveness	
f. Product longevity	
2. Marketability	40%
a. Size of market	
b. Relationship to market needs/wants	
c. Ease of market penetration	
d. Importance of consumables/services	
e. Price–value relationship	
f. Relationship to present customer–promotion mix	
g. Effect on sales of present products	
h. Order fulfillment demands	
3. Research and Development Capability	30%
a. Staff knowledge/skill	
b. Staff experience	
c. Managerial complexity	
d. Magnitude of project	
e. Time needed for development	
f. Availability of outside resource requirements	
g. Judged authorial compatibility	
4. Production Capability	10%
a. Staff knowledge/experience	
b. Inventory complexity	
c. Assembly requirements	
d. Current vendor capability	
e. Availability of outside resource requirements	

Note. The PNPRS was based on one proposed by O'Meara (1961) designed for consumer products.

tors; each of the factors and subfactors is rated on a numerical scale. A weighted composite score with a maximum value of 100 is derived, based on the weights shown in Table 2.3. Proposed publications at or above a specified "cut score" on the composite score have successfully met the first hurdle in the evaluation process. Proposals surviving this first stage are then evaluated extensively on several financial criteria. Various indices of projected product profitability and financial return are calculated. Those proposals whose profitability and financial return meet the level specified by the publisher are placed on an approved list. Developmental work begins as soon as the required financial and staff resources are available. Experience in using a particular evaluation system over time provides the data needed to set "cut score" and financial return rates that best serve a publisher's professional and financial interests. The evaluative factors shown in Table 2.3 are based on a system originally designed by O'Meara (1961), which he applied to the evaluation of consumer products.

Some publishers place the final publishing decisions in the hands of executive staff members who serve as a publications advisory board. Such groups typically consist of editorial and marketing executives who pass judgment on proposed publications. Various approaches are possible. One publisher may use only an executive advisory board; another may choose ratings or a combination of formal ratings and group evaluation. Publishers must first routinize the screening process, so that consistent methods are applied to all new publication submissions. Only a systematic approach to publication evaluation will result in generating dependable data that are useful to publishers in selecting successful publications.

Formal Arrangements for Publication

After a publisher has completed the evaluation of a proposed publication, a formal decision to accept or reject the proposal is made. If the proposal is rejected, then the prospective author(s) can, if desired, submit it to another publisher. If the proposal is accepted, then a contract is written to specify the exact terms of the relationship between the author(s) and the publisher. A contract is typically a work-for-hire agreement that contains the terms and conditions to which both parties are expected to adhere during the time period covered by the contract. Topics usually covered in a contract are such items as royalty rates, sharing of development costs, monetary advances to authors, and arrangements for revisions. In addition, some publishers include a time and task schedule for the entire development cycle. Due dates for critical items in the development schedule may also be added. Such a schedule seems to offer a number of obvious advantages, as well as to provide a time schedule to guide development of the publication. Contracts are frequently written to cover one edition of a test; however, multiple-edition contracts also exist. Authorized rights to revisions may be specified, but a new contract is usually needed to cover all aspects of a revision.

As soon as a contract has been signed by both author(s) and publisher, formal work on the publication commences. The master project budget developed during the financial analysis stage of the proposed product evaluation is used as a guide to financial planning and control. Once the preliminary steps of submission, evaluation, and contractual arrangements are concluded, content specifications and item development begin, unless these tasks have already been completed at the time of publication submission and require no further modification. The following section addresses these next steps.

CONTENT DEVELOPMENT

Once a decision to publish has been made and a formal agreement between the author(s) and publisher has been executed, content development begins. In some cases, content may have already been developed by the time a publication contract is signed. A first step in the development of content is the creation of a set of test specifications to guide the preparation of the test items. Such specifications, often termed a "blueprint," establish the basic content structure to guide item development. Once the scope of the content domain to be sampled by the test has been defined, test items can then be written. When an acceptable number of items have been prepared, critiqued, re-

vised, and edited, they are subsequently administered in a tryout edition for the purpose of obtaining statistical data that permit the determination of item quality. The final step in content development is the use of item analysis data to aid in the assembly of the final form(s) of the test. This section discusses a variety of issues pertaining to the various facets of content development.

Achievement and Ability Domains Defined

In keeping with the emphasis of this handbook, the specification of test content here is focused on two domains: educational achievement and cognitive ability. It is important to distinguish clearly between these two content domains. "Educational achievement" refers to skills and abilities developed as a result of direct instruction in a particular school subject or content area. "Cognitive ability," on the other hand, refers to content derived from psychological theory; such content is not directly taught, nor does it appear in specific curricula. Cognitive domains are defined from theoretical formulations of mental abilities and/or trait organization, not from skills and knowledge within specific curricula. Abilities in the cognitive domain are likely to cut across many different achievement domains (Millman & Greene, 1989).

Preparing Specifications for an Educational Achievement Test

Content domains for educational achievement tests can be broad, narrow, or somewhere in between, depending upon the purpose of the test. For teacher-made tests, a single textbook or curriculum guide will often suffice as the source for content specification. In the case of achievement tests developed for state or national use, the specification of test content is complicated by the diversity of curriculum content across school districts, states, and geographic regions. In any given curricular area, the multiplicity of textbooks and courses of study is truly staggering. Attempting to distill common elements from these diverse sources is the daunting task of the developer of a broad achievement test designed for state or national consumption.

A major factor affecting the structure of

test content domains is the interpretive information to be derived from a test. Two common types of information provided by tests are "norm-referenced" and "criterion-referenced" interpretations. Most tests are designed to provide either one type of information or the other; however, some tests have been designed to provide both types. Norm-referenced interpretations report an individual's rank within a specified norm group (e.g., "Ramon spelled as well as or better than 65% of third graders tested nationally"). Criterion-referenced interpretations report performance on a set of clearly defined learning tasks (e.g., "Ramon spelled 65% of the words on the third-grade word list correctly"). Thus the types of information provided by these two interpretive systems are quite different, and each type has different implications for test design.

In general, norm-referenced tests cover broad content domains with just a few items measuring each learning outcome, whereas criterion-referenced tests typically have rather narrow content domains with a relatively large number of items measuring each learning outcome or objective. The type of measurement desired has direct implications for the level of difficulty at which items are written: Norm-referenced tests deliberately require items of average difficulty for a particular reference group, and criterion-referenced tests allow the content domain to define item difficulty (Linn & Gronlund, 2000).

In addition to content, a second requirement for an effective test blueprint is the specification of appropriate so-called "process objectives." In cognitive learning, certain mental processes are frequently called upon as a student engages in various aspects of learning curricular content. Such mental processes as recalling, recognizing, defining, identifying, applying, analyzing, synthesizing, evaluating, generalizing, and predicting are examples of common process objectives (Thorndike & Hagen, 1977). These terms all attempt to describe overt, objectively verifiable behaviors that should occur if "learning" is really taking place in an instructional program. In a sense, these objectively verifiable behaviors become the means for assessing the degree to which learning is actually occurring in a specific curriculum.

An important influence on both education and test construction that deserves mention in connection with the specification of process objectives is Bloom's *Taxonomy of Educational Objectives,* particularly *Handbook I: Cognitive Domain* (Bloom, 1956). The six major categories of the cognitive domain, according to Bloom, are Knowledge, Comprehension, Application, Analysis, Synthesis, and Evaluation. The structure of knowledge that Bloom envisioned is hierarchical in nature, with the most basic requirement being the recall or recognition of certain facts (Knowledge). Knowledge was seen as a basic requirement necessary for the application of Comprehension, Application, Analysis, Synthesis, and Evaluation (see Bloom, Hastings, & Madaus, 1971, for more complete information pertaining to test development). Bloom's work made teachers and test developers aware of the desirability of including the so-called "higher order" cognitive processes both in education and in the assessment of educational outcomes. Not surprisingly, Bloom's work revealed that much of education dealt only with superficial recall and recognition of facts and information, with the result that the processes of Application, Analysis, Synthesis, and Evaluation generally received less emphasis than was ultimately thought desirable.

A necessary starting point in the development of an achievement test is a set of test specifications, or blueprint, showing the content and cognitive processes included along with the number of items desired. A convenient way to summarize this information is in a table of test specifications. An example of such specifications is shown in Table 2.4 for *KeyMath Revised NU: A Diagnostic Inventory of Essential Mathematics* (Connolly, 1997).

The KeyMath Revised NU is a norm-referenced, individually administered assessment of basic mathematical skills designed for kindergarten through eighth grade. The KeyMath Revised NU content structure is hierarchical in nature, starting at the highest level with three broad content groupings (Basic Concepts, Operations, and Applications), which in turn are divided into 13 strands, or subtests; these are further divided into 43 content domains, each of which has 6 items. Each of the items was prepared

TABLE 2.4. Partial Content Structure for KeyMath NU Revised: A Diagnostic Inventory of Essential Mathematics

Content Area	Content Strand (Subtest)	Domain	Illustrative Item Objective
			The student can . . .
1. Basic Concepts Subtests: 3 Domains: 11 Items: 66	1. Numeration Domains: 4 Items: 24	1. Numbers 0–9 Items: 6[a] 2. Numbers 0–99 3. Numbers 0–999 4. Multidigit Numbers	1-1. count objects (0–9 in a set). 2-1. order a set of two-digit numbers. 3-1. order a set of three-digit numbers. 4-1. rename a three-digit number.
	2. Rational Numbers Domains: 3 Items: 18	5. Fractions 6. Decimals 7. Percents	5-1. determine one-half of an even-numbered set of up to 10 objects. 6-1. express a fraction in its lowest terms. 7-1. order a set of decimal values from smallest to largest.
	3. Geometry Domains: 4 Items: 24	8. Spatial/attribute relations 9. Two-dimensional shapes 10. Coordinate geometry 11. Three-dimensional shapes	8-1. apply spatial relationship terms such as inside/outside and over/under to displays. 9-1. identify all triangles (or rectangles) in a set of figures. 10-1. identify the element in an array when given the row and column position. 11-1. name a shape when given a description of its faces.
2. Operations Subtests: 5 Domains: 15 Items: 90	4. Addition Domains: 3 Items: 18	12. Models and basic facts 13. Algorithm to add 14. Adding rational numbers	12-1. complete addition facts (0–9). 13-1. add two-digit numbers for a three-digit sum. 14-1. add fractions with like denominators.
	5. Subtraction Domains: 3 Items: 18	15. Models and basic facts 16. Algorithm to subtract 17. Subtracting rational numbers	15-1. compare sets of one to five objects. 16-1. subtract two-digit numbers when regrouping is required. 17-1. subtract fractions and mixed numbers.
	6. Multiplication Domains: 3 Items: 18	18. Models and basic facts 19. Algorithm to multiply 20. Multiplying rational numbers	18-1. complete multiplication facts (products 1–36). 19-1. multiply a two-digit number when regrouping is required. 20-1. multiply fractions.

(continued)

TABLE 2.4. *Continued*

Content Area	Content Strand (Subtest)	Domain	Illustrative Item Objective
2. Operations (*cont.*)	7. Division Domains: 3 Items: 18	21. Models and basic facts 22. Algorithm to divide 23. Dividing rational numbers	21-1. complete division facts (dividends 1–36). 22-1. divide a two-digit number when regrouping is required. 23-1. divide using decimal tenths as the divisor.
	8. Mental Computation Domains: 3 Items: 18	24. Computation chains 25. Whole numbers 26. Rational number	24-1. subtract 100 from a three-digit number. 25-1. mentally multiply with 100 as the factor. 26-1. mentally multiply a fraction and a whole number.
3. Applications Subtests: 5 Domains: 17 Items: 102	9. Measurement Domains: 4 Items: 24	27. Comparisons 28. Using nonstandard units 29. Using standard units—length 30. Using standard units—capacity	27-1. identify the longest and shortest objects in a set. 28-1. measure capacity using nonstandard units. 29-1. measure length using standard units (cm). 30-1. identify which standard unit is best to measure weight of given objects.
	10. Time and Money Domains: 4 Items: 24	31. Identifying passage of time 32. Using clocks 33. Monetary amounts to $1 34. Monetary amounts to $100	31-1. identify a season of the year. 32-1. tell time to the hour. 33-1. identify different coins by name. 34-1. combine coins and currency up to $5.
	11. Estimation Domains: 3 Items: 18	35. Whole and rational numbers 36. Measurement 37. Computation	35-1. estimate quantity (1–25). 36-1. estimate the height of a common object. 37-1. estimate the price per unit of given foodstuffs.
	12. Interpreting Data Domains: 3 Items: 18	38. Charts and tables 39. Graphs 40. Probability and statistics	38-1. interpret data presented as rows of one to nine objects. 39-1. interpret a simple bar graph to compare the frequency of different elements. 40-1. identify the range of a given distribution of scores.
	13. Problem Solving Domains: 3 Items: 18	41. Solving routine problems 42. Understanding nonroutine problems 43. Solving nonroutine problems	41-1. solve a simple subtraction word problem. 42-1. create an appropriate story for a given context and number sentence. 43-1. solve a routine two-step word problem that involves one-digit numbers.

Note. Adapted from Connolly (1988, 1997). Copyright 1988, 1997 by the American Guidance Service, Inc. Adapted with permission.
[a]Each domain contains six item objectives, only one of which is shown to illustrate each domain.

from an item behavioral objective similar to the examples shown in Table 2.4. Space limitations in Table 2.4 preclude showing all six item behavioral objectives for each content domain.

Figure 2.1 shows the complete content linkage for a single item in the KeyMath Revised NU. A similar content specification could be prepared for each of the 258 items in this test. The nature of the mathematics content is such that the exact specification of the hierarchical content levels (areas, stands, domains, and items) is precise and orderly. These specifications were prepared by the test's author after an extensive review of mathematics curricula and instructional materials, as well as consultation with nationally recognized mathematics curriculum experts (Connolly, 1997). Such a process is typically used to develop a nationally norm-referenced achievement test.

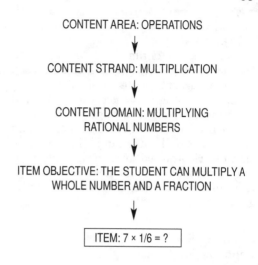

FIGURE 2.1. Levels of content specificity for a single item in the KeyMath Revised NU. Adapted from Connolly (1988, 1997). Copyright 1997 by American Guidance Service, Inc. Adapted by permission.

Writing Items for an Achievement Test

Once the set of test specifications, or blueprint, has been prepared, item development can begin. Before any test items are written, however, careful attention must be given to item format. If a test is to measure the desired learning outcomes effectively, the type(s) of items used must be chosen carefully. Objective-type item formats are favored by test publishers primarily for the advantages they offer in ease and consistency of scoring. Such items typically require the examinee either to *supply* a short answer, such as a number, a word, or a phrase, or to *select* an answer from a number of alternatives provided. True–false and multiple-choice items consisting of three, four, or five response alternatives are the two main types of selected response item formats. However, multiple-choice items are the most pervasive exemplars of selected response-type items present in published achievement tests, due to two major limitations of true–false items—namely, their susceptibility to guessing, and their limited usefulness for measuring a variety of learning outcomes. True–false items have, however, been used successfully in personality inventories.

Individually administered tests permit greater latitude in the types of items used than do group-administered tests, mainly

because an examiner is present to evaluate a student's response at the time it is given. For example, an individually administered achievement test may include mathematics items that require students to supply answers to problems, reading comprehension items that require students to select the main idea in a reading passage, and spelling items that require students to spell words dictated by the examiner. In a group-administered achievement test, on the other hand, the item format for these same tests would probably be restricted to multiple-choice, thereby permitting machine scoring of students' responses.

Regardless of the type of items selected, great care must be taken to write items that do in fact measure the intended learning outcomes in a clear, concise manner. Achievement test item writers must have adequate knowledge of the content domain being assessed and must understand the developmental characteristics of the examinees for whom the items are intended. In addition, item writers must possess good general writing skills, some creativity, and a basic knowledge of certain rules for writing effective test items. Several writers have provided excellent, extensive guidelines for writing good test items (e.g., Linn & Gronlund, 2000; Mehrens & Lehman, 1991;

Thorndike & Hagen, 1977; Wesman, 1971). An excellent, concise set of item-writing rules is outlined by Millman and Greene (1989). Item writing is a learned skill that depends upon writers' receiving adequate training in the necessary rules and procedures, along with supervision by an experienced item writer. Regardless of an item writer's skill, all test items must be subjected to rigorous editorial review and revision as needed before the items are administered in a tryout version to an appropriate group of examinees.

Preparing Specifications for a Cognitive Ability Test

As stated earlier, ability and aptitude tests are not based on knowledge or skills directly taught in a curriculum, but rely instead on theory for their specification. The developer of such a test applies either explicitly or implicitly a theoretical formulation, or rationale, to define the primary constituents of the trait or psychological construct for which the test is being designed. Past research frequently plays a significant role in informing the test developer of important elements that need to be included. In the area of human cognitive abilities, for example, studies of the organization of such abilities would probably be consulted by the developer of a test of general intellectual ability, in order to assist him or her in deciding which cognitive domains to sample for inclusion. Studies employing various factor-analytic methods have served to provide major insight into the structure and organization of such abilities. Two such investigations are cited here. There are other significant factor-analytic studies, most conducted on a smaller scale, that might be of special help to test developers; however, space limitations prevent their treatment here. Interested readers are referred to Carroll (1993) for information about such studies.

To date, the most ambitious efforts to define the scope and structure of human abilities have been the studies conducted by Guilford (1967, 1988) and his associates, and by Carroll (1993). Both of these investigations are of interest because they produced results that were quite different in attempting to define a theoretical structure of human abilities. Guilford's structure-of-in-tellect model (SIM) was developed principally during the 1950s and 1960s as an outgrowth of the Aptitudes Research Project at the University of Southern California Psychological Laboratory. The SIM, shown in Figure 2.2 on the next page, is a three-dimensional model defined by "contents," "operations," and "products." Each of the 180 cells is defined by a unique combination of the contents–operations–products dimensions of the model. The SIM has also been described by Guilford as an information-processing model of human cognition. The items commonly encountered on most ability tests can be isolated in one or more of the cells in the SIM. Guilford's research has resulted in a highly splintered view of human abilities. More recent reanalyses of Guilford's data have raised serious questions about the SIM and have suggested that its complexity may be an artifact of the particular type of factor-analytic methodology employed (Carroll, 1993).

An alternative formulation of the structure of human abilities has been proposed by Carroll (1993), who reanalyzed the results of 461 factor-analytic studies published between 1925 and 1987. Carroll's monumental effort resulted in a proposed model for the structure of human abilities, shown in Figure 2.3 on page 36. Essentially, Carroll's reanalysis of the data in these studies (including Guilford's) led him to formulate a hierarchical structure of abilities composed of three levels or strata. At the top of the model. Stratum III, is General Intelligence or g—the broadest of the ability factors identified, and correlated to varying degrees with the Broad Ability factors defined in Stratum II (fluid intelligence, crystallized intelligence, general memory and learning, broad visual perception, broad auditory perception, broad retrieval ability, and broad cognitive speediness). Narrower, more homogeneous factors, such as those identified in Stratum I, correspond to each of the Stratum II Broad Ability factors (examples of these are induction, language development, memory span, visualization, speech sound discrimination, originality/creativity, and numerical facility). The implication of this hierarchical model is that persons who score high on a narrow Stratum I factor (e.g., verbal language comprehension) will overlap substan-

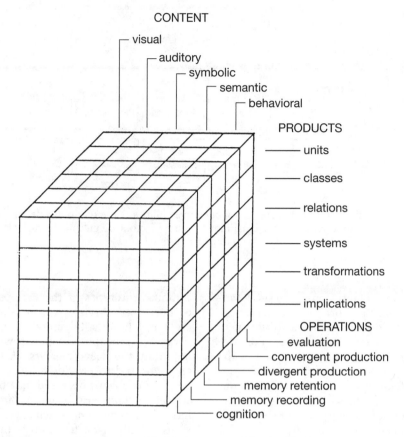

FIGURE 2.2. Structure-of-intellect model (SIM), as revised by Guilford (1988, p. 3). Copyright 1988 by *Educational and Psychological Measurement*. Reprinted by permission.

tially but not completely with those who score high on measures of the Broad Ability factor (Stratum II; e.g., crystallized intelligence), who will in turn overlap substantially but not completely with those who score high on Stratum III, General Intelligence or *g*.

For a test developer using Carroll's model of human abilities, it is possible to develop tests at three levels of generality–specificity by selecting one of the three strata, depending upon the tester's purpose. Thus a psychologist might elect to develop a test of General Intelligence at Level III, or a test of Crystallized Intelligence at Level II, or a test of Vocabulary at Level I. If the test developer is using Guilford's SIM, on the other hand, there is no hierarchical ordering of abilities to act as a guide. The SIM includes neither a broad *g* nor broad group factors. This implies that each of the 180 theoreti-

cally discrete abilities posited by the SIM is independent of all others, so the test developer would need to focus on the discrete cells of the SIM to generate different types of tests.

Writing Items for a Cognitive Ability Test

Both Guilford's taxonomic classification scheme in the SIM and Carroll's hierarchical model can aid the test developer in locating promising types of tests and items to consider for the ability domains to be tested. Another source for locating such material, based on work originally done by French, is the Kit of Factor-Referenced Cognitive Tests (Ekstrom, French, & Harman, 1976). The kit provides 72 tests measuring 25 factors identified in various factor-analytic studies of human abilities. Thorndike (1982) provided examples of the types of items fre-

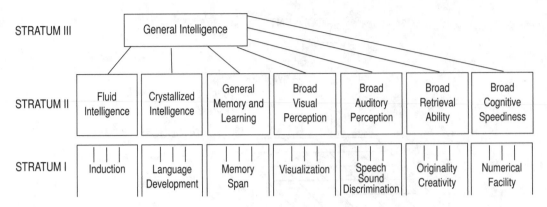

FIGURE 2.3. Carroll's hierarchical structure of cognitive abilities. Note that only one Stratum I factor is presented for illustrative purposes; the remaining Stratum I factors are given in Carroll (1993). Copyright 1993 by Cambridge University Press. Adapted by permission.

quently used in cognitive ability tests. Readers should consult Thorndike for actual examples of these items; the cognitive item types are summarized in Table 2.5. For convenience, the item types are classified by the type of content they employ—verbal, symbolic, and figural. These content dimensions should not be confused with ability factors identified by factor analysis; they are used as a classificatory aid for purposes of this discussion only.

Once the test specifications are complete, item development can begin. Before any items are written, it will be helpful to develop training materials specifying the exact procedures that are to be followed in developing the items. Such material should also contain prototypes of the various items to be developed. Many types of ability items are novel (especially figural or nonverbal) items. With inexperienced item writers, it is important to review their first efforts to create items and to provide feedback early, so that any problems observed may be corrected before item writing has progressed too far. Unlike achievement items, verbal ability items usually have few words in the item stem; the real challenge is generating attractive misleads or foils for these items. Generating three or four good foils often proves to be laborious and time-consuming. Editorial review by experienced item writers is essential in order to improve the quality of misleads. Frequently, trying out new items

TABLE 2.5. Types of Items Commonly Used in Ability Tests

	Content dimensions		
Item type	Verbal/semantic (words/sentences)	Symbolic (letters/numerals)	Figural/pictorial (geometric/abstract)
Analogies	×	×	×
Classification	×	×	×
Series completion	×	×	×
Matrices	×	×	×
Synonym/antonym	×		
Sentence completion	×		
Reasoning problems	×	×	
Disarranged stimuli	×	×	
Synthesis	×	×	×
Immediate/delayed recall	×	×	×
Spatial visualization: Two dimensions			×
Spatial visualization: Three dimensions			×

on a small sample of individuals prior to the formal item tryout yields dividends in improving item quality.

Additional Considerations in Item Development

Two additional considerations that must be taken into account in item development are addressed here: the number of items needed, and the final editorial review.

Number of Items Needed

In planning for item development, test developers always face the question of the number of items needed for tryout. Unfortunately, there is no exact formula or algorithm to assist test developers in answering this question. Factors that must be considered in arriving at an answer are as follows: (1) the age or grade range covered by the test; (2) the length of the test, including the number of forms if more than one form is being prepared; (3) experience and skill of the item writer(s); (4) novelty of the type(s) of items to be prepared; and (5) budgetary cost constraints. All of these factors must be weighed carefully in arriving at the total number of items needed. Cost considerations, including the availability of needed funds, definitely affect the scope of the test development enterprise and must be carefully considered at every step of the test development process. If artwork or illustrations are needed, one must proceed with caution, because costs for artwork (especially multicolor illustrations that require color separation) mount rapidly. It is important that the type of illustrative art selected be carefully investigated during the preliminary project-budgeting process, because changes made later are often at an increased cost and can soon exceed budgetary limitations. Other things being equal, a larger number of a new or novel type of item will be required than would be necessary for a more traditional item type. A new type of figural item, for example, would require more items for tryout than a familiar type of verbal item, such as multiple-choice vocabulary. An inexperienced item writer will generally need to produce more items than one who is experienced. In view of all the considerations mentioned, it is recommended as a general rule of thumb that a minimum of 25%–50% more items be prepared than are needed.

Final Editorial Review

The need for the test development process to include a thorough editorial review of all newly prepared items has been emphasized in the earlier sections addressing item development for achievement tests as well as for ability tests. Before the items are printed for item tryout, a final editorial review is essential. Ideally, this review should be performed by one or more seasoned item writers who were not involved in the initial item preparation and review process. In addition to a final content review, the items will also need copyediting to correct any problems with language mechanics or item structure. The keyed responses should also be verified one last time. For multiple-choice tests, the frequency with which the correct responses are distributed over the item alternative positions should be checked and, if necessary, switched, so that the correct alternatives are distributed randomly and evenly over all item response alternative positions. Besides the item content and editorial reviews, the item review for gender and ethnic bias must be completed at this stage, preferably before the final content and editorial reviews. The importance of these final item reviews cannot be overstressed. A flawed or poorly written item, if caught and corrected before item tryout, is one more potential item for the item pool used to construct the final test after the item tryout has been completed.

Item Tryout

Once the item development process has been completed, the items are ready for administration to the sample of individuals designated for tryout. The dimensions of the item tryout program will be determined by the following considerations: (1) the availability of funds for tryout; (2) the age or grade span for which data are needed; (3) the size of the tryout sample; and (4) the logistical details, such as time required, time of year, and various administrative arrangements. Each of these dimensions of the tryout program is discussed below.

Availability of Funds for Tryout

The availability of research and development funds from the publisher can certainly influence test development plans, including the scope of the item tryout program. To some extent, the characteristics of a particular test also determine the amount that will be spent on tryout. For example, when a publisher is norming an individually administered test, examiners must be paid for each examinee located and tested. For comprehensive test batteries, this fee can be as much as $50–$100 or more per examinee.

Table 2.6 shows the tryout budget for a hypothetical example, the individually administered ABC Achievement Test. For each expense category, the percentage it represents of the total tryout budget is also shown. This budget was based upon a plan to test 1,000 students, grades K–12, in 20 different schools.

Age or Grade Span

Serious consideration and careful planning must be given to the age or grade span for the tryout program. It is essential that items be tried out at the age or grade levels where they are intended to be used. Items should, as a rule, be tried out at enough age or grade levels to obtain sufficient data to permit decisions about the item to be made. Items for which some preliminary tryout data are already available can be targeted to the functional age or grade level more easily than can untried items. In the case of group tests, items may be repeated at adjacent test levels in order to obtain a broader spectrum of item performance data. For individually administered tests, the tailored testing format typically permits item data to be obtained across all functional age or grade levels.

Size of the Tryout Sample

The size of the group used for item analysis depends on both theoretical and practical considerations. Obviously, enough individuals must be tested to yield reasonably stable estimates of basic item statistics. Although no single number can be given, authorities agree that stable estimates of classical item difficulty and discrimination indices are possible with tryout sample sizes of about 200–500 individuals (Henrysson, 1971; Thorndike, 1982). As a general rule, the tryout sample should adequately represent the final target population of test takers. Thus the item tryout sample should match the final target population on relevant demographic variables, insofar as is possible. This ideal can frequently only be approximated in actual practice. For some group achievement and ability tests, it is necessary to include diverse types of schools from all major geographic regions even at the item tryout stage, in order to meet local school district requirements for representation in test research programs. Such requirements are often conditions imposed on the sale of materials after publication. Ethnic group item bias studies require careful advance planning, to insure that these populations are oversampled as needed to meet the min-

TABLE 2.6. Item Tryout Budget for the ABC Achievement Test

Type of expenditure	Explanation	Budgeted amount (in dollars)	Percentage of total budget
Incentive payments	Payments to participating schools	7,000	5.4
Clerical services	Payments to hourly clerical workers	19,000	14.6
Testing fees	Payments to examiners	50,000	38.5
Coordinator fees	Payments to coordinators	8,000	6.2
Content development	Item writing, expert consultation	16,000	12.3
Editing	Editing of items and other tryout materials	13,000	10.0
Printing	Preparation and printing	10,500	8.0
Shipping	Mailing materials to test sites	3,500	2.7
Miscellaneous	Unforeseen expenditures	3,000	2.3
Project total		130,000	100.0

Note. Dollar expenditures are stated as of year 2003 and may vary from the amounts shown, depending on a number of factors.

imum sample size requirements outlined above.

Practical Details

A number of practical details must be considered in planning and executing item analysis programs. Care must be taken to avoid overtaxing examinees by trying out too many items. If group tests are administered within a specified time limit, too many items per time unit will result in too many omissions of items at the end of the test, with the result that adequate item statistics will be unavailable. A good rule to follow is that of preparing multiple test forms whose length will permit about 90% of the examinees to finish all items within the allotted time period. Multiple forms of individual tests are also advisable when the testing period will last more than 1 to $1\frac{1}{2}$ hours, especially for younger students.

Another administrative detail that merits careful consideration is the time of year for which item analysis data are obtained. If the final test forms are intended for fall testing, then it is important that the item analysis program take place in the fall. This is particularly true for achievement tests, because differential growth rates in school subjects occur during the school year. Finally, it is important that directions, answer sheets or record forms, and other elements of the testing program be clearly prepared and well organized, so that testing will occur smoothly under relatively uniform conditions.

Statistical Analysis of Item Responses

As soon as the item tryout tests have been administered and scored, the statistical analysis of the test items can begin. Various statistical procedures have been developed to aid test developers in differentiating among items in terms of their utility or desirability for use in a particular test. "Classical" item analysis statistics have been in use in one form or another for the past 80 years. Item response theory (IRT) item analysis methodology has evolved over the past 40 years and includes various latent-trait models useful in item calibration. Test developers sometimes wonder which methodology to use—classical or IRT. I believe that both classical and IRT methodology provide useful information, for the reasons outlined below.

Classical Item Analysis

In classical item analysis, individuals who resemble as closely as possible those for whom the test is intended are identified and tested with the tryout items. For each item tried out, the following statistics are usually obtained:

1. Percentage choosing the item correctly.
2. Item–total test correlation (item discrimination).
3. Percentage choosing each distractor (for multiple-choice items only).

These statistics are obtained either for a single reference group of interest (e.g., first-year Spanish students, for tryout of items for a test designed to measure end-of-year achievement in first-year Spanish) or for multiple reference groups (e.g., successive age or grade groups for a test designed to span a broad age or grade range). The type of test determines whether a single set of item statistics or a set for each of several different groups of individuals is needed to evaluate the tryout items. It is important to remember that classical item analysis statistics do not generalize beyond the group on which they were based. Thus considerable care must be taken in recruiting the tryout sample, in order to make certain that the appropriate individuals are represented. Also, it is important that the range of ability in the tryout sample be similar to that in the target population for whom the test is intended. For example, item statistics based on a relatively homogeneous group of high-ability seventh-grade mathematics students will yield underestimates of item difficulty for a group of average seventh-grade mathematics students.

Multiple-reference-group item statistics have been especially useful for publishers of broad ability and achievement batteries, in which items are allocated to an appropriate level of a test based in part on their performance across several age or grade groups. In such applications, items must function satisfactorily in all age or grade groups where an item appears. In constructing a broad-gauge test of general cognitive ability, for example, items must show an increase in the percentage of individuals passing at successive ages in order to be retained for the final test. The percentage passing the item at each successive age can be plotted on cross-section graph paper, and a smoothed curve can be drawn by eye through the points. This is exactly the procedure used by Terman and Merrill (1937) in their revision of the Stanford–Binet Intelligence Scale. From percentage passing curves plotted for each item, the age where 50% of individuals answered the item correctly was determined. The "item age" determined in this way was subsequently used to assign items to age levels. This methodology was a crude precursor of the mathematically precise item–test regression analyses performed today in applications of IRT.

As an example, Table 2.7 shows a sample set of classical item statistics for a reading comprehension item administered to students in grades 4 and 5 in a tryout program. This item contains five multiple-choice options. As the data in Table 2.7 show, the item was answered by 1,600 students in grade 4 and 1,606 students in grade 5. The first line of statistical data ("No. answering") shows the number of students choosing each option. The second line ("Percent answering") shows the percent choosing each option, with about 45% choosing option 5, the correct answer. The third line shows the point–biserial r or item–total test correlation, which is negative for all options

except the correct answer, where it is .46. These results are quite good overall, and show that the four distractors are functioning as intended. Results are similar at grade 5—where the item is, as expected, easier than at grade 4, with 58% of the students answering correctly. Other things being equal, this item will probably be retained for inclusion in the final test.

IRT Item Analysis

The rapid increase in the availability and use of high-speed computers, especially the availability of software for PCs, has fueled advances in IRT methodology as well as the increased use of this technology. Known also as "item calibration," "latent-trait analysis," and "item characteristic curve theory," IRT is a type of item–test score regression that permits test items to be calibrated, or referenced, against the underlying latent trait measured by the test (Lord, 1980). Figure 2.4 shows an item characteristic curve for a reading comprehension test item. Essentially, the item characteristic curve shows the probability of passing the item as a function of reading comprehension ability, the underlying latent trait.

There are at least two distinct advantages of using IRT methods. First, items can be referenced to the ability scale for the underlying trait; thus it becomes possible to express item difficulty and person ability on the trait assessed by the item in common terms (i.e., similar scale units). This is a

TABLE 2.7. Classical Item Statistics for a Multiple-Choice Reading Comprehension Item Based on Tryout in Grades 4 and 5

	Answer options						Total
	1	2	3	4	5[a]	NR[b]	
Grade 4							
n (No. answering)	289	201	159	201	728	22	1,600
Percent answering	18.0	12.6	9.9	12.6	45.5	1.4	100.0
Point–biserial r	−.172	−.069	−.224	−.191	.464	−.035	—
Grade 5							
n (No. answering)	81	261	73	237	935	19	1,606
Percent answering	5.0	16.3	4.5	14.8	58.2	1.2	100.0
Point–biserial r	−.176	−.216	−.121	−.216	.461	−.030	—

[a]Correct response.
[b]No response given.

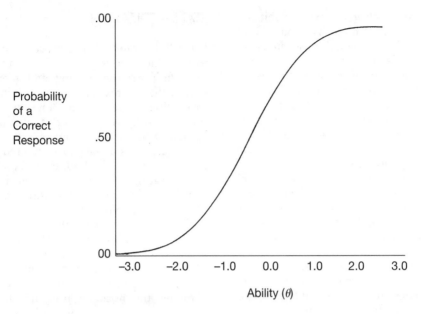

FIGURE 2.4. Item characteristic curve showing the relationship between item performance and ability (θ).

highly desirable feature from the standpoint of test development and is not easily accomplished with classical item analysis methods. Second, because IRT is essentially a type of regression procedure, item parameters remain invariant across groups of varying abilities (Lord, 1980). Unlike classical item analysis, in which item parameters change as the group upon which they are based changes, IRT frees estimates of item parameters from the ability level of the group upon which the estimates are based. Recall from the earlier discussion of classical item analysis the emphasis placed on carefully selecting item tryout samples to obtain participants whose characteristics match those of the final population of intended test takers. This sample matching has been stressed because classical item statistics are totally group-dependent. The benefits in test construction from both advantages of IRT mentioned above constitute persuasive arguments for the use of IRT methods in item analysis and selection.

The statistical algorithms used to calculate IRT item calibrations are so complex and labor-intensive that they must be performed by computer. Software now available permits such analyses to be done on desktop PCs. Examples of such software are WINSTEPS Version 3.02 (Linacre & Wright, 2000), which is useful in one-parameter item calibration; and BILOG 3.11 (Mislevy & Bock, 1990) and MULTILOG 6.3 (Thissen, 1995), both of which are useful for two- and three-parameter item calibration and estimation.

In summary, both classical and IRT methods provide valuable information about the functional utility of individual test items. The choice of methodology depends upon the sort of information needed and the nature of the underlying trait being assessed. Classical item analysis methods are especially helpful in the earlier stages of item development, when one is interested in obtaining a rough estimate of item difficulty and evaluating the functioning of distractors in multiple-choice items. IRT, on the other hand, offers advantages in the later stages of test development, when one is interested in using item calibration estimates to form final tests or scales.

Studies of Item Bias

The item tryout program is the ideal point in the test development process to investigate the extent to which items may exhibit bias toward members of minority groups. Both statistical and judgmental procedures are used to identify items that may be biased against minority group members. Statistical procedures are primarily concerned with investigating differences in the relative difficulty of items for persons from different ethnic, cultural, or experiential backgrounds. The statistical methodology used to investigate such differences is known technically by the term "differential item functioning" (DIF). Such methodology seeks to identify items where members of similar ability from different ethnic or cultural groups have different probabilities of success on the item in question (Anastasi & Urbina, 1997).

If DIF studies are undertaken, it is important to test an adequate number of minority group members to provide stable estimates of relevant statistical DIF indices. Depending upon the size and scope of the item tryout program, it may be necessary to oversample minority group members in order to have samples of sufficient size to produce stable statistical results. Planning for such studies must be undertaken early in the test development process, in order to make certain that adequate samples of minority group members are available at the time DIF studies are conducted.

As Camilli and Shepard (1994) point out, DIF analyses do not automatically "flag" biased items. Determination of bias goes beyond the statistics to investigate the reason for the observed difference; hence the identification of biased items relies on both statistical and judgmental criteria. IRT methodology, discussed earlier, has been used successfully to identify items meriting further review as possible sources of test bias. These methods and others are outlined in detail by Camilli and Shepard (1994); readers may wish to consult this material for much more detailed information than it is possible to provide here.

If panels of minority reviewers are needed to undertake subjective item reviews, then this activity must be completed prior to the time when such information is needed to select items for the final version of the test. The major test publishers commonly use both editorial review panels and statistical methods to locate and remove items judged to display bias toward minority group members.

STANDARDIZATION

"Standardization" is the process employed to introduce objectivity and uniformity into test administration, scoring, and interpretation. If the test results are to be meaningful, then different examiners must have the same carefully worked-out instructions for administering and scoring, in order to insure that the test data are gathered under uniform, standard conditions. Normative interpretation of performance on a test is possible only if these conditions are met (Anastasi & Urbina, 1997)

This section considers the various aspects of test standardization: assembly of the final test form(s), including directions for administering and scoring; selecting the standardization sample; obtaining informed consent; planning the norming program; norming samples for group and for individual tests; auxiliary studies; and norms development.

Assembly of Final Test Form(s)

Item analysis yields the information necessary to select the items for the final standardization edition of a test. Final test assembly begins by sorting the pool of tryout items into such classifications as "rejected," "salvageable with revision," and "acceptable." A work plan based on the test specifications is developed. Such a plan typically begins by allocating the "acceptable" items as required by the content specifications to one or more test forms being developed. If additional items are still needed to meet the test specifications, items are next drawn from the "salvageable with revision" category. If more items are required to meet the test blueprint than are available in the "acceptable" and "salvageable with revision" categories of the item tryout pool, additional items will have to be prepared and tried out before development of the final test form(s) can be completed. In order to avoid losing time and increasing development costs, it is recommended (as discussed earlier in "Additional Considerations in Item Development") that a sufficient surplus of items be tried out to allow for such attrition.

If multiple test forms are being developed and classical item analysis has been used, then items will need to be allocated from the tryout pool so that the alternate forms are as nearly identical as possible in content coverage, item difficulty, and item intercorrelations. Careful balancing of test forms using the item statistics mentioned will help insure that the final test forms meet the statistical requirements for parallel test forms—for example, that they have equal means, equal variances, and equal intercorrelations (Gulliksen, 1950).

If IRT item analysis is used and alternate forms are required, the need to match alternate forms on item parameter estimates is reduced. The reason is that once the items have been calibrated to the underlying ability scale, ability estimates produced by using subsets of these items, or "forms," are comparable and automatically adjust for any statistical differences inherent in the subset of items drawn from the total item pool (Hambleton, Swaminathan, & Rogers, 1991)

Calibration of the items using IRT permits items to be used for tailored testing (Lord, 1980)—more specifically termed "computerized adaptive testing," where the items can be stored in a computer item bank and selected for administration by computer as required to obtain an estimate of a person's ability. Theoretically, each examinee could be administered a different subset of items, or "form," from the pool, and the selection of each item could be based on the examinee's response to the previous item. IRT methods, as is true of classical item analysis, always rely heavily on providing an adequate sampling of content as outlined in the test specifications.

Once the item analysis has been completed, the final test form or forms for use in the standardization program are developed. A number of factors are considered in deciding how the standardization form(s) will be developed. Some of these factors include the number of topics to be sampled from the test specifications, the amount of time available for testing, the desired item difficulty level, the number and type of item formats used, and the number of items needed to meet minimum test reliability requirements.

Besides the assembly of the final test form(s), additional materials must be prepared for the standardization program. Included among such materials are the directions for administering the test, answer sheets (for group tests), record forms (for individually administered tests), and various other forms required for record-keeping purposes. In addition, for some individually administered tests, special manipulatives must be designed and manufactured.

It is essential that the directions for administering the test receive careful scrutiny before they are finalized. Thorough editing of all test directions is recommended before standardization, because the directions need to be in final form before normative data are gathered. The answer sheets developed for group-administered tests and the record forms designed for individually administered tests need not be in final form for publication, but it is essential that they be functional and easily used by both examinees and examiners. If test items use the completion or free-response format, as is frequently done in individual tests, then directions for recording and evaluating the examinees' responses must be developed. If responses are merely recorded, then it becomes possible to evaluate them later, after all responses obtained in the standardization program are analyzed.

Selecting the Standardization Sample

Selection of the test standardization sample begins with a carefully prepared plan for obtaining the individuals who will be tested. The elements necessary for a comprehensive standardization plan are discussed below, followed by separate sections devoted to standardization sampling plans for group-administered and individually administered tests.

Obtaining Informed Consent

Due to increased concern about the fairness of tests to various groups, including members of minority groups and individuals with physical and mental disabilities, several professional organizations have issued recommendations to insure that those who develop, administer, and interpret tests take precautions to use them wisely and treat all test takers fairly. For example, the "Ethical Principles of Psychologists and Code of Conduct" (APA, 2002), the *Code of Fair Testing Practices in Education* (Joint Committee on Testing Practices, 2003), and the *Standards for Educational and Psychological Testing* (AERA et al., 1999) all contain recommendations about informing test takers of the purpose of testing and the way in which the test results will be used, as well as the need to obtain the consent of the test takers (or their legal representatives) before tests are administered. For example, the *Standards for Educational and Psychological Testing* volume (AERA et al., 1999) contains this recommendation:

(Standard 8.4)
Informed consent should be obtained from test takers or their legal representatives before testing is done except (a) when testing without consent is mandated by law or governmental regulation, or (b) when testing is conducted as a regular part of the school activities, or (c) when consent is clearly implied.

In practice, Standard 8.4 has direct implications for test standardization programs. Parental consent is explicitly recommended for individually administered tests, where a relatively small number of students are selected for testing. For group tests, where all students in a class are tested, most school districts do not require signed parental permission for student participation; however, most districts inform students and parents about the nature of the testing and the purpose for which the results are being obtained. Students in many districts are excused from participating in group test standardization programs if such a request is made by a student or a parent.

The practical outcome of informed consent for test developers and publishers is that test standardization samples, for both group and individual test standardization programs, must consist of voluntary participants. For this reason, these samples cannot be considered random or true probability samples of examinees, in which each individual has an equal or known probability of being selected; as a result, the amount of error present in the norms cannot be specified. Therefore, it is imperative that test developers prepare special materials and make a special effort to communicate clearly with students and parents, in order to maximize standardization program participation rates.

Planning the Norming Program

A careful plan for obtaining the standardization sample is required, because for com-

mercially prepared tests, the test results obtained from the norm group are typically generalized to an entire national population referenced by age or grade. Thus it becomes essential that the norm group constitute a representative sample from the national population it represents. If such representation is to occur in the sample, then procedures must be spelled out from the start to insure that the norming sample is systematically and meticulously identified and tested. Control is sought over as many relevant factors as possible, in order to minimize the likelihood of introducing bias into the selection of the norming sample.

Every norming program is in fact a compromise between what is desirable from a strictly scientific perspective and what is realistically feasible—both within the practical constraints placed on the method of sampling examinees from a specified population, and within the limits of financial resources available for the norming program. The goal of all norming efforts should be to obtain the best standardization sample possible within the financial limitations of the project. A systematic, well-articulated sampling specification plan is the key to obtaining a standardization sample that is both scientifically defensible and practically obtainable.

Sampling specifications must carefully delineate the various population reference groups to be sampled. For educational and psychological tests, the two most common national reference groups are age and grade; however, in some instances local norm groups of various sorts may be the appropriate reference groups of interest. The specifications for obtaining national and local norm groups will, of necessity, differ considerably. The former usually require more complex, multistage sampling methods; the latter require simpler, less elaborate designs for obtaining norming samples. A well-prepared plan or design is essential in either case.

In addition to the reference group, the standardization sampling plan must specify the extent to which such demographic factors as socioeconomic status, gender, geographic region, urban versus rural residence, and race or ethnic group are to influence the selection of the sample. If the standardization sample is to represent a national population, then the success in representing that population will be judged by comparing the sample's demographic statistics with those of the national reference population of interest (typically defined by data from the most recent U.S. census). Obviously, it is essential to work out sampling procedures in advance, so that the demographic statistics for the standardization sample will compare as favorably as possible with those of the national reference population.

A careful plan must specify in detail the method to be used to obtain the sample. Although norm samples at one time were largely samples of convenience, their quality has improved dramatically over the past 35 years or so. The introduction of probability-sampling techniques by test publishers has substantially increased the precision of their test norms. Although probability-sampling methods are desirable because they permit estimation of the amount of error present in the norms (Angoff, 1971), as stated earlier, they present an ideal that can at best only be approximated in actual practice. This fact is illustrated by comparing the methods used to obtain norm samples for group-administered and individually administered tests. Although both types of tests usually share the goal of securing a norm sample representative of broad national age or grade reference groups, differences in test formats, together with their associated costs, necessitate the use of different sampling procedures for the two types of tests. Sampling procedures for each type of test are discussed separately in the next two sections.

Norming Samples for Group Tests

An important characteristic of group tests for norm sample ~election is their lower administrative cost per examinee when compared with individual tests. The very fact that individuals can be tested in naturally occurring units, such as grades or classes in schools, has an important bearing on the type of norming program that is practically and economically feasible. When schools or classes are used as the units to define the sample, then it becomes possible to use a type of probability sampling known technically as "multistage stratified random cluster sampling." This class of sampling methods has certain distinct advantages: (1) The process of selecting the elements of the sample is automatic and is not left up to idiosyncratic judgment or mere availability; (2) each element in the sample has a known probability of being selected; and (3) the known selection probabilities can be used to develop weights to correct for over- or underrepresentation within the sample when the norms are developed (Angoff, 1971).

Because schools and classes are naturally occurring units, or "clusters," an individual student is included in the norm sample because the student's class and school have been selected by the sampling procedure used. Although the goal may be, for example, to estimate the performance of all U.S. fourth-grade pupils on a reading test, it is not practically feasible to list all fourth-grade pupils in the United States and then draw a random sample from such a list. Instead, multistage sampling methods are used; these begin with a known, manageable listing, such as school districts. For efficiency, the school districts may be grouped in different ways (e.g., by size, socioeconomic status, geographic region, etc.). Once these subunits, or "strata," are formed, it then becomes possible to sample randomly from within the strata. Thus one proceeds via systematic sampling methods to schools, to classes, and finally to individual students within selected classes. These students then become participants in the norming program.

The use of a multistage cluster-sampling method, in conjunction with the decreased cost per student associated with group tests, results in much larger group test standardization samples than are employed for individually administered tests. Although size per se is not a guarantee of precision of the norms, well-designed group test standardization programs, in which 10,000–20,000 students per grade or age group are tested, permit more precise estimates of population performance than do individual test standardization efforts based on only a fraction of those numbers of individuals.

The use of sophisticated probability-sampling methods never permits an entirely precise estimate of the norms, however, because some schools and/or school districts refuse to participate. Thus, as stated earlier, despite attempts at randomized selection procedures, all norming programs consist of voluntary participants. It is important for test publishers to report the rate of acceptance of participation in the norming program, so that the extent to which the goals of the ideal probability-sampling model used can be ascertained for a particular norming enterprise.

Norming Samples for Individual Tests

The need to test each participant in the norming sample individually precludes the use of probability-sampling methods with individually administered tests. A procedure known as "quota sampling" is typically used in the selection of individual test standardization samples. For this procedure, a quota of examinees is assigned to each testing center participating in the norming program. It then becomes the responsibility of the test center supervisor to locate each person specified in the center's quota. The judgment of the supervisor is in effect the determining factor in deciding which individuals meet the criteria used to define the quota. Even if quasi-multistage sampling procedures similar to those used for group tests were feasible for individual tests, a quota sample is, in the final analysis, a voluntary sample. Examinees of school age can only be tested with parental consent, and securing examinees outside of school (e.g., adults) is totally dependent upon volunteers. Thus it is not possible to specify the precision of the norms for individual tests that use quota-sampling methods to designate norming samples (Angoff, 1971).

It is possible, however, to report the demographic composition of the norming sample, so that the representation of the sample can easily be compared with that of the entire U.S. population based on the latest U.S. census. Table 2.8 shows the target census goals stated as percentages of examinees tested for gender, race/ethnicity, socioeconomic status (parental educational attainment), and geographic region. These are frequently used criteria for evaluating the representation of both group-administered and individually administered elementary and secondary school-based test-norming programs.

One source of error present in individually administered norming programs is in the selection and matching of individuals for testing to the quota requirements for a particular standardization coordinator. A number of years ago, I developed a variation of the quota-sampling procedure in which individuals to be tested are selected randomly by computer from preassembled pools of available examinees. Although this method is not a true probability-sampling procedure, it minimizes the influence of subjective judgment, which is always present when a test center supervisor must locate examinees of a certain age, gender, ethnic group, urban or rural residence, and socioeconomic status. Experience has shown that substantial error is introduced in particular when local personnel must classify individuals in terms of socioeconomic status. Coding of demographic characteristics for the pool of possible examinees is accomplished by trained employees under the supervision of the pub-

TABLE 2.8. Examples of U.S. Census Targets Used to Structure and Evaluate the Demographic Characteristics of Test Standardization Programs, Ages 5–18 Years

I. Gender		II. Race/ethnic group	
Female	48.9%	African American	15.8%
Male	51.1%	Caucasian (European American)	65.7%
		Hispanic	13.5%
		Other	5.0%
III. Socioeconomic status (parental educational attainment)		IV. Geographic region	
Less than high school graduate	12.7%	Northeast	18.7%
High school graduate	32.5%	South	34.4%
Some college	30.1%	North Central	24.3%
College graduate (4-year)	24.7%	West	22.6%

Note. Target percentages are based on data from the U.S. Bureau of the Census (1997).

lisher. This procedure also saves considerable time, because each test center supervisor is told whom to test, instead of being asked to locate individuals who meet specified demographic characteristics. In addition, this procedure enables alternate examinees to be identified easily, should some of the primary test individuals be unavailable on the day the test is given. Although this procedure requires more lead time before testing, so that available examinees can be located and entered into a central computerized data bank, the increased accuracy and efficiency in conducting the actual testing program more than compensate for the extra time and cost needed to identify potential examinees. Use of a computerized database also facilitates record keeping during the time when standardization testing is occurring. Periodic updates of the demographic data for examinees tested can be used to check on demographic representation as desired. Filling gaps in the master sampling plan is thus greatly facilitated by the availability of a computerized database designed to summarize current demographic information at any point in time simply by accessing the online database.

As a general rule, individually administered tests employ a minimum of 100–200 examinees per grade or year of age. Compared with group tests, which typically test several thousand individuals per grade or year of age, individual tests are handicapped by their small standardization samples. To generalize from a sample of 100–200 children of age 10 to the entire population of U.S. 10-year-olds is, even with careful sample selection, difficult at best. Small samples are typically selected by proportionate allocation across test centers, according to census data such as those mentioned earlier and shown in Table 2.8. Once the sample has been selected, the quota for each test center can be recorded on a form such as that shown in Figure 2.5 and transmitted to the coordinator for each test center, who must make sure that each individual listed is located and tested. For example, the specification for one examinee shown in Figure 2.5 might be as follows:

Geographic region: North Central United States
Grade: 5

Ethnic group: African American
Parental education: High school graduate
Gender: Male

Such specific allocation procedures help insure that the census demographic characteristics are reflected as desired in the norming sample. Experience has shown such a procedure to work reasonably well in practice.

Finally, the standardization of any test, group or individual, is a complicated, expensive undertaking that depends upon qualified examiners as well as the cooperation of countless individuals—particularly the examinees and their parents, and of course the school administrators and teachers for school-based testing programs. Despite the most extensive, detailed plans, there will always be unforeseen circumstances to complicate what is already a complex procedure. One can only hope that the compromises inevitably required do not seriously impair the quality of the normative data, and that the sound judgment and good will of all persons participating in the norming program will bring the project to a successful completion.

Auxiliary Studies

Special studies must often be undertaken concurrently with the standardization program to provide data needed to support a test. For example, test–retest reliability studies with the same or an alternate test form are frequently needed. Other possible purposes for special studies include obtaining estimates of interrater reliability, equating old and new editions, equating forms or levels of a test, and correlating test results with external criteria (e.g., results of other standardized tests and/or course grades)

Examinees tested in these studies may either be selected from the regular standardization sample or obtained from supplementary sources. Criteria used to select these special study participants are usually less rigorous than those imposed on standardization sample participants. There is really no need to impose rigorous selection criteria on these studies unless there is a special reason to investigate certain properties of the test (e.g., validity with certain types of individuals). For most classical equating studies, it is desirable to test a wide range of ability,

ABC ACHIEVEMENT TEST   QUOTA/TESTING LOG SHEET   •   2004 STANDARDIZATION PROGRAM

CODES

PARENT EDUCATION LEVEL	ETHNIC GROUP
CG = COLLEGE GRADUATE (Bachelor's Degree or Higher)	AA = AFRICAN-AMERICAN
SC = SOME COLLEGE (Less than Bachelor's Degree)	HIS = HISPANIC
	CAU = CAUCASIAN (WHITE)
HSG = HIGH SCHOOL GRADUATE (No College)	OT = OTHER
<HSG = LESS THAN HS GRADUATE	GENDER
	M = MALE
	F = FEMALE

Phone: (999) 888-7777 Geographic Region: NE S (NC) W

Examiner/Coordinator K. L. Martin

Address 15 Easy St. Mytown IN 46404
         PO BOX/STREET   CITY   STATE   ZIP CODE

School District Mytown Community S.D.

City/State Mytown   IN 46404
            CITY   STATE

NUMBER OF STUDENTS TO BE TESTED

GRADE	GENDER		ETHNIC GROUP				PARENT EDUCATION			
	M	F	AA	HIS	CAU	OT	CG	SC	HSG	<HSG
2										
3										
4										
5	2	1	1	1	2			2		1
6	1	1	1				1	1		
7										
8										
9										
10										
11										
12										
TOTAL	3	2	2	1	2		1	3		1

STUDENT TESTING LOG SHEET

ID #	NAME OF STUDENT	DATE OF BIRTH			AGE		GRADE	GENDER*		ETHNIC GROUP*				PARENT EDUCATION*			
		MO	DAY	YEAR	YRS	MO		M	F	AA	HIS	CAU	OT	CG	SC	HSG	<HSG
00001	Rupert Johnson	2	26	--	11	1	5	✓		✓					✓		
00002	Caitlin Mathews	4	22	--	10	11	5		✓			✓				✓	
00003	Jeremy Price	11	15	--	10	5	5	✓				✓			✓		
00004	Rose Gonzales	7	18	--	11	9	6		✓		✓				✓		
00005	Foster Grant	1	15	--	12	2	6	✓		✓							✓

*Check the appropriate column.

FIGURE 2.5. Sample quota sheet used to transmit standardization sample demographic requirements and designate students to be tested.

in order to estimate equivalence at various points of the score scale with reasonable precision. For reliability studies, it is desirable to estimate reliability with individuals comparable in ability to those in the norming sample. Care should be taken to insure that the range of ability in the sample used to study reliability is not unduly restricted. The *Standards for Educational and Psychological Testing* (AERA et al., 1999) serves as a general guide to the types of additional data required at the time of test publication.

Development of Test Norms

As soon as the standardization testing has been completed, statistical analysis of the data gathered can begin. It is essential that the statistical analysis be carefully planned with respect to the types of norms required. Much time, effort, and expense can be spared by a comprehensive analysis of the data needed and the preparation of a well-articulated plan for norms development *before* any statistics are produced. The steps required to develop norms usually fall into the following general pattern: (1) data editing and checking, (2) data entry and scoring, (3) statistical analysis, (4) development of norms tables, and (5) analysis of data for supplementary studies. Each of these operations is discussed below.

Data Editing and Checking

Inspection, editing, and checking of the completed answer forms are especially important for individually administered tests that do not employ machine-scannable documents for recording examinee responses. Data recorded on the answer forms may need to be coded by hand before computer entry. For example, such demographic data as age/date of birth, grade, and other information may be given special numerical codes before data entry. The coding scheme must be carefully worked out to insure that all of the data needed for any part of the analysis are captured and coded at this time.

Response forms for individually administered tests should be checked to make certain that each individual tested meets the requirements originally established for the quota of examinees assigned to a particular test center. Also, response forms that are not

machine-scannable may need to be inspected to insure that basal and ceiling rules (if used) were properly followed, and that test administration generally seems to have been satisfactory. Occasionally, test item responses may need to be hand-scored or coded as correct–incorrect before computer entry can occur. In most cases, this first manual inspection by clerical personnel is done quickly and is designed to identify any gross anomalies that need attention before additional processing occurs.

For group tests and individually administered tests where responses have been recorded on machine-scannable test booklets or answer sheets, little manual inspection is required, because most checks can be performed by the computer if the data have been coded in preassigned grids on the booklets or answer sheets. In most cases, answer sheets for group tests have only to be batch-coded with a scannable document known as a "header sheet," and assembled for transport to the electronic equipment used to scan or "read" the marks coded on the sheets.

Data Entry and Scoring

If answer forms cannot be scanned by machine, the response recorded for each test item must be entered by hand into the computer before analysis can begin. Once the response record has been recorded on computer, raw scores can be produced by comparing each examinee's responses with the key programmed into the computer. As soon as raw scores are obtained and recorded, subsequent statistical analyses can be undertaken.

Machine-scannable answer sheets are designed to be scanned or "read" by high-speed electronic machines capable of processing several thousand sheets per hour of operation. These machines use either reflected or transmitted light to produce a computer record of answer sheet marks. Once these marks have been recorded, raw scores can be derived, and additional analyses can then be completed.

Statistical Analysis

As soon as raw scores are available, statistical analyses of various types may be conducted with the database. Such analyses often begin with basic information for each subtest, such as raw-score frequency distributions, cumulative percentages, means, and standard deviations. These data provide the basic descriptive statistical information essential to determine how the test has performed in the standardization program. Such data are usually obtained for subgroups of interest, such as each age or grade group tested. For multiscore tests, subtest intercorrelations may be important at this point and are usually generated as a part of the basic summary statistics. Demographic counts are often prepared along with the basic summary statistics.

Other types of analyses that are sometimes performed subsequent to the basic analyses include population subgroup analyses, item analyses, composite and total test score analyses, and factor analyses, to mention the more common types. When the norms tables become available, raw scores for the norms sample are usually converted to derived scores, so that several analyses may be performed with the normative scores instead of raw scores. The foregoing types of data analysis procedures are all essential prerequisites to the development of norms tables.

Changes in the way statistical analyses have been performed have continued to evolve since the first edition of this chapter appeared (Robertson, 1990). The operation of Moore's law, mentioned at the beginning of the present chapter as a significant stimulus for advances in computing technology, has resulted in vast increases in computer speed and memory capacity. Complex statistical analyses once available mainly to a limited number of individuals who had access to mainframe computers and customized programming, can now be performed on desktop PCs. Comprehensive statistical software packages such as SAS Systems, Version 8 (SAS Institute, 1999); SPSS for Windows, Rel. 10.0 (SPSS, 1999a); and SYSTAT 9 (SPSS, 1999b) can now execute almost any set of classical statistical analyses required by test developers. Anyone interested in developing a test can use these software packages (along with others that are narrower in scope) to accomplish what was once available only to the largest test publishers, thereby removing a significant barrier to entry into test development and test publication.

Development of Norms Tables

"Development of norms tables" refers to the process of preparing the tables of derived scores used to interpret performance on a test. Such tables form a major part of the test manual and must be offered at the time a norm-referenced test is released for general use.

Anastasi and Urbina (1997) offer a useful classification scheme for the most common types of derived scores. As summarized in Table 2.9, norms are of two basic types: "developmental" and "within-group." Developmental norms locate an individual along span or continuum of development. Age and grade equivalents are the most common examples of developmental norms. Both scales offer rather limited information, because they match an individual's performance to the typical or average performance of a particular age or grade group. For example, an age equivalent (mental age) of 5 years, 6 months on an intelligence test means that the individual's score corre-

TABLE 2.9. **Classification of Some Common Norm-Referenced Scores**

Type of comparison	Norm-referenced scores	Frame of reference
Developmental	Grade equivalents Age equivalents	Multiple grade groups Multiple age groups
Within-group	Percentile ranks, standard scores, stanines, T-scores	Single reference groups of any sort (age, grade, job applicants, admissions candidates, etc.)

Note. Based on Anastasi and Urbina (1997). Copyright 1997 by Prentice-Hall: Adapted by permission.

sponds to the typical or average score for children age 5 years, 6 months. A similar interpretation referenced to school grades can be offered for grade equivalents. Because developmental norms are tenuous from a psychometric perspective and cannot be manipulated easily from a statistical standpoint, within-group norms are generally preferred for test interpretation.

Within-group norms match an individual's performance to that of a single reference group of interest. Age and grade are two of the most common reference groups, but many others can be used. As shown in Table 2.9, there are several types of within-group normative scores to choose from, depending on the type of test and the interpretation to be made. Within-group norms can be applicable to any reference group of interest. Thus standard scores can be prepared for age groups, for grade groups, for job applicants, for licensure candidates, and so on.

Within-group norms yield more precise, psychometrically sound information than do developmental norms, because it becomes possible to place an individual more precisely within a reference group of particular interest. Percentile ranks, for example, show the rank of an individual in a typical group of 100 persons; standard scores convey information about the extent to which an individual's test performance deviates from the mean of a particular age or grade group, expressed in standard deviation units. Thus it becomes possible to describe a person's performance with more precision than is true of age and grade equivalents. It should be pointed out that Table 2.9 is merely suggestive of the more common types of within-group norms and is certainly not an exhaustive listing.

In the comparison of group and individual test standardization procedures made earlier, one major difference cited is that of sample size. This difference has a direct bearing on the ease of norms development. With their larger sample sizes, group test results are usually more stable across grade or age reference groups than are those for individual tests. Norms are much more stable and amenable to statistical treatment if they can be derived from a sample of 10,000–20,000 individuals per age or grade, for example, than for samples of 100–200 persons of a given age or grade. A procedure to compensate for small sample sizes has been proposed (Angoff & Robertson, 1987) and has been used successfully in several norming programs for individual tests.

The development of norms tables is both an art and a science. In the past, much of the work needed to develop norms tables was done by graphic methods, which required plotting data points and smoothing the curves by eye. Thus norms development was time-consuming and costly. Recently, computer programs that do the plotting, curve-fitting, and analytical smoothing have shown promise as tools to streamline norms development. The application of such sophisticated analytical procedures has increased substantially since the first edition of this chapter was published (Robertson, 1990).

Norms tables appearing in a test manual are the result of many complex, interrelated steps. These require that the norms developer have (1) a thorough knowledge of statistics and the ability to work with data; and (2) the skill to create norms that compensate and adjust as needed for anomalies present in the data, while at the same time preserving the fundamental integrity of the database.

If IRT-calibrated items are available—as mentioned in an earlier section (see "Assembly of Final Test Form(s)"), where computerized adaptive testing using item banks has been discussed—and if the underlying latent-trait scale has been normed on a suitable reference group, it then becomes possible to report norms on subsets of items drawn from the item bank. The only requirement is that all items present in the item bank be calibrated to the original IRT reference scale, so that the norms can be reported on any subset of items drawn from the item bank. Thus calibrated and normed item banks permit the generation of norms for a large number of different test forms constructed from an item bank (Hambleton et al., 1991). Development of computerized adaptive tests is feasible using specially prepared computer software such as Micro-CAT, distributed by Assessment Systems Corporation (1989).

Supplementary Studies

Reliability information and at least some validity data must be reported at the time the test is released. In some situations, certain research data must also be gathered to complete the norming process. These additional types of data and information needed are discussed below.

Reliability Information

Internal-consistency reliability estimates are routinely calculated at the time the norms are developed. Coefficient alpha reliabilities with their associated standard errors of measurement are determined for the various age, grade, or other relevant subgroups of the standardization sample for which norms are reported. Many individually administered tests also recommend and provide confidence intervals to aid users in score interpretation. Either the confidence bands must be developed, or the standard errors of measurement needed by users to form the bands must be calculated from the basic internal-consistency reliability indices. Alternate-form reliability coefficients and interrater reliability estimates both require specially designed studies to obtain data. Planning for these studies and recruiting participants must be done at the time the standardization sample is recruited.

Validity Information

Validity information about tests accumulates over time during the life of a test. Test developers must prioritize the various types of validity information to determine what is needed at the time of publication and what can be left either for postpublication research by the publisher or for other researchers to establish during the life of the test. Time and cost are significant factors contributing to the decision about the scope and extent of prepublication validity studies. For achievement tests, information about the selection, scope, and sequence of content is essential information that all users need at the time of publication. For individually administered achievement tests, correlations with other achievement tests and ability tests fall high on the priority list. For ability tests, in addition to correlation with other ability tests and achievement tests, results of various factor-analytic investigations (such as exploratory factor analysis and confirmatory factor analysis) may be

needed to help define the constructs measured by the tests. Other covariance structure analyses, known as "structural equation modeling" (SEM), may also be needed to aid in clarifying the causal relationships among the underlying factors (Byrne, 1994). The availability of various software packages for SEM analyses—such as EQS 5.7 (Multivariate Software, 1999) and LISREL 8.30 (Joreskog & Sorbom, 1996)—greatly facilitates the investigation of hypothesized relationships among test scores and other constructs, as Messick (1989) advocates in his discussion of nomological validity. Specially designed studies of convergent–discriminant validity may also be needed, although such comprehensive studies are most often required for personality tests (Anastasi & Urbina, 1997). All of these various studies need careful planning and execution to insure that the experimental designs used are appropriate for obtaining the data required.

Additional Research Studies

In order to complete the norming process, certain special studies may be needed. These mainly include various types of equating programs to equate multiple forms and multiple levels of a test. If IRT technology is used, then these types of classical test-equating programs will probably not be needed. Thus use of IRT can result in increased efficiency and cost reduction when compared with the operational requirements of classical test theory in these applications.

PUBLICATION

As soon as the standardization program's norms development and special studies are completed, final publication plans can be made. It is not always possible, especially for individually administered tests, to gauge the duration of the standardization program exactly; therefore, once that activity has been completed, more precise scheduling is possible. Additional activities leading toward final publication are as follows: establishing the publication schedule, producing publication components, developing the publication marketing plan, doing postpublication research, and evaluating the entire publication process. Each of these topics is discussed below, as is the scheduling of test revisions.

Establishing the Publication Schedule

The development of the final publication really occurs in two rather distinct phases. The first is the component development period, during which final manuscript copy for each component is created. The second is the production process, which begins with manuscript copy and terminates with printed and bound typeset materials ready for publication. Of these two phases of activity, the manuscript development phase usually cannot be scheduled as precisely as the final production phase.

Although the final publication schedule is typically set after standardization and norms development are completed, the schedule will need to be reviewed carefully; revised dates, as required, must be established after the final manuscript development phase is completed. Unforeseen delays in the preparation of final manuscript copy for publication components are not uncommon, despite the most careful planning.

An effective publication schedule must, first of all, be realistic. Establishing impossible due dates for the various activities of the final publication development process causes frustration and disillusionment in everyone, and can create serious staff morale problems. Furthermore, because marketing activities depend substantially on establishing a firm publication date, any delays can have an adverse impact on marketing activities planned to launch a new publication.

A second requisite for an effective publication schedule is that it be established jointly in a cooperative effort by those staff members who must adhere to it. Those persons who must actually do the day-to-day work are best informed and qualified to establish time requirements for various activities to be undertaken during final publication. A schedule imposed from above by management is almost always doomed to failure if it does not reflect the knowledge and experience of staff members, and if their endorsement and commitment are not secured before the schedule is set.

An example of a publication schedule is shown in Table 2.10 for hypothetical instrument, the ABC Achievement Test. Although this schedule was developed for illustrative purposes only, it is based on my own experience in developing similar schedules for actual test publications. Table 2.10 shows the completion dates for the various development tasks expressed in weeks prior to publication. For example, norms development is scheduled for completion 78 weeks prior to publication. Note that at this stage in the development process, each component must be scheduled separately; the publication date is really dependent upon the amount of time required to complete the test manual, the most complex component to be developed and published. Note also that all steps from typesetting through receipt of final print materials by the warehouse are production steps, whereas all prior steps are under the direction of the research and development staff. In this example, the various editing steps for the manual require 21 weeks to complete. This may seem excessive, but experience has proved otherwise, particularly for manuals similar in length to the one shown here. This schedule was developed with the assumption of a normal work flow in research and development, as well as in production. Completion of the publication within a shorter time span is feasible, but would result in increased expense and delay of other publications competing for staff time. It is assumed also in this example that the test plate book has been used in practically its final form during the standardization process and needs only minor changes for publication. Development of the examiner response form begins at about the same time as manuscript development for the manual, mainly because design details are needed to write certain sections of the manual describing the test and giving directions for administering and scoring.

Producing Publication Components

Producing test components is a highly complex, demanding task that requires specialized training in various technologies used in publishing. Production personnel typically begin with an edited manuscript and, through various processes, supervise the transformation of that manuscript into printed copy. The "manuscript" is now, cre-

TABLE 2.10. Final Publication Schedule for the ABC Achievement Test

Component	Activity	Completion time in weeks[a]
Manual (150 pages)	Norms development	P – 78
	Manuscript development, Chapters 1 and 2 (general background, administration, scoring)	P – 72
	Manuscript development, Chapters 3, 4, and 5 (technical and interpretive material)	P – 52
	Editing steps	P – 51 to P – 30
	Final copyediting, Chapters 1–5	P – 29
	Manuscript computer entry, Chapters 1–5	P – 25
	Proofreading, Chapters 1–5	P – 22
	Final printing proofs, Chapters 1–5	P – 11
	Printing	P–8
	Binding	P – 3
	Warehouse	P
Examiner response form	Basic layout, design	P – 72
	Computer entry	P – 26
	Final printing proof	P – 14
	Printing/packaging	P – 8
	Warehouse	P
Test plate book	Design cover/pages	P – 44
	Final edit of items and directions	P – 36
	Computer entry	P – 29
	Proof reading	P – 25
	Final printing proofs	P – 12
	Printing	P–8
	Binding	P–3
	Warehouse	P

[a]Completion time is in terms of weeks before publication; P – 78, for example, means 78 weeks prior to publication.

ated with word-processing software and may be downloaded onto a computer disk, and hence is usually not a true paper manuscript. Typesetting is now done by computer, sometimes by the publisher and sometimes by out-of-house vendors. Editors are now able to edit online and transfer the edited copy electronically to automated typesetting equipment, thus bypassing paper or "hard" copy. Computer interfaces now make it possible to develop norms on one computer and then transfer the norms tables to the computer used for typesetting. Thus computerization has streamlined the production process and eliminated many of the time-consuming steps once required when production relied primarily on "hard copy" proofs of text.

Manuals become more complex as the number of statistical tables and figures increases. Careful checking is required at the final proofing stage to make certain that ta-bles and figures are correctly placed. Special expertise is needed to design answer sheets and record forms. If machine-scannable forms are required, then care must be taken to design the forms according to the specifications of the scanner used. If manipulatives need to be designed and manufactured for individually administered tests, then considerable ingenuity and skill are required on the part of editorial and production personnel.

Developing the Publication Marketing Plan

As a publication approaches its final stages, a marketing plan is implemented. Two types of activities are commonly undertaken for test products: direct mail promotion and space advertising. If a publisher has a field sales force, these individuals will receive training in order to sell the new product to the appropriate clientele. Attending professional meetings is yet another way to advertise new products. These aspects of product marketing are discussed briefly below.

Direct Mail Promotion

Direct mail promotion relies on attractive, informative brochures sent to prospective test purchasers to convey product information. Mailing lists are available at a reasonable cost from commercial sources, so it becomes easy to reach potential purchasers as long as a mailing list is available. The publisher's catalog is also a major source of product information disseminated by direct mail.

Space Advertising

Space advertisements in journals, newsletters, convention programs, and professional magazines are also a commonly used source of new test product information. Care must be taken in preparing space ads to depict a publication honestly and correctly. This is especially difficult with small advertisements.

Field Sales Staff

The publisher's sales staff may engage in direct product sales to individuals by visiting school districts, state departments of education, or private practitioners, and by appearing at professional meetings and conventions (see below). The larger test publishers have carefully selected and trained sales personnel who present their products and conduct workshops in the uses of the new tests.

Professional Meetings and Conventions

Attendance at professional meetings and conventions provides a cost-effective means for publishers to reach significant numbers of individuals. Also, the fact that most meetings focus on a specific market segment means that publishers can target particular products for maximum exposure.

Doing Postpublication Research

For some publications, it is necessary to collect data following publication. Such data are usually needed to furnish evidence of validity. This is especially true for new tests that lack extensive validation. Postpublication research requires careful planning and attention if it is to meet the needs of a particular publication. Periodic updates to the manual, or even more extensive revisions to the manual, may be required. It is important that new data be disseminated as widely as possible.

Evaluating the Entire Publication Process

All publications seem to have their so-called "ups and downs." Some activities proceed smoothly according to plan; others may be more difficult than anticipated, thus requiring more time and incurring higher costs. All publications should be evaluated after their completion in an attempt to identify both successes and problems. Such an evaluation is not designed to assign blame or reprimand development personnel, but rather to develop an awareness of problems and ways to avoid them in the next publication. It is important that staff members understand the purpose of such analyses and approach them in a positive way.

Scheduling Test Revisions

Complete or partial revisions of tests are required periodically when there is good evidence that changes are needed. The two main reasons for revising a test are obsolescence of content and obsolescence of norms. In general, achievement tests are somewhat more sensitive to changes over time than are ability tests. Changes in curricular emphasis that affect user acceptance of an achievement test, as well as the usefulness of the norms, necessitate rather frequent revision; major test publishers now revise their comprehensive achievement batteries about every 5 years. Ability and aptitude tests are much less subject to problems stemming from dated content than are achievement tests, due primarily to the broader, more generalized nature of the cognitive abilities assessed. Norms for ability tests do, however, require regular updating to insure that they accurately describe the performance of the current population of users. Publishers usually review a number of different criteria in arriving at a decision to undertake the revision of a test.

CONCLUSION

The purpose of this chapter on test development has been to give readers a brief survey of the way in which commercial test publishers develop standardized tests—primarily achievement and ability tests, in keeping with the emphasis of this handbook. Although the actual procedures may vary to some extent, the material presented in this chapter represents the basic process adhered to by most commercial test publishers. Unfortunately, some topics, of necessity, have been either omitted or considered only briefly and superficially. Readers who desire additional information on any of the topics presented should consult the references, because most of these sources contain extensive information on various topics likely to be of interest to test developers and users.

REFERENCES

American Educational Research Association (AERA), American Psychological Association (APA), & National Council on Measurement in Education (NCME). (1999). *Standards for educational and psychological testing.* Washington, DC: Authors.

American Psychological Association (APA). (2002). Ethical principles of psychologists and code of conduct. *American Psychologist, 57,* 1060–1073.

Anastasi, A., & Urbina, 5. (1997). *Psychological testing* (7th ed.). Upper Saddle River, NJ: Prentice-Hall.

Angoff, W. H. (1971). Scales, norms, and equivalent scores. In R. L. Thorndike (Ed.), *Educational measurement* (2nd ed., pp. 508–600). Washington, DC: American Council on Education.

Angoff, W. H., & Robertson, G. J. (1987). A procedure for standardizing individually administered tests, normed by age or grade level. *Applied Psychological Measurement, 11*(1), 33–46.

Assessment Systems Corporation (1989). *MicroCAT* [Computer software]. St. Paul, MN: Author.

Bloom, B. M. (Ed.). (1956). *Taxonomy of educational objectives: Handbook I. Cognitive domain.* New York: McKay.

Bloom, B. M., Hastings, J. T., & Madaus, G. (1971). *Handbook on formative and summative evaluation of student learning.* New York: McGraw-Hill.

Byrne, B. M. (1994). *Structural equation modeling with EOS and EOS/windows.* Thousand Oaks, CA: Sage.

Carroll, J. B. (1993). *Human cognitive abilities: A survey of factor-analytic studies.* New York: Cambridge University Press.

Camilli, G. & Shepard, L. W. (1994). *Methods for identifying biased test items.* Newbury Park, CA: Sage.

Connolly, A. J. (1988, 1997). *KeyMath Revised NU: A diagnostic inventory of essential mathematics.* Circle Pines, MN: American Guidance Service.

Ekstrom, R. B., French, J. W., & Harman, H. H., with Dirmen, D. (1976). *Manual for kit of factor-referenced cognitive tests, 1976.* Princeton, NJ: Educational Testing Service.

Guilford, J. P. (1967). *The nature of human intelligence.* New York: McGraw-Hill.

Guilford, J. P. (1988). Some changes in the structure-of-intellect model. *Educational and psychological Measurement, 48,* 1–4.

Gulliksen, H. (1950). *Theory of mental tests.* New York: Wiley.

Hambleton, R. K., Swaminathan, H., & Rogers, H. J. (1991). *Fundamentals of item response theory.* Newbury Park, CA: Sage.

Henrysson, S. (1971). Gathering, analyzing, and using data on test items. In R. L. Thorndike (Ed.), *Educational measurement* (2nd ed., pp. 130–159). Washington, DC: American Council on Education.

Joint Committee on Testing Practices. (2003). *Code of Fair Testing Practices in Education.* Washington, DC: Author.

Joreskog, K. G., & Sorbom, D (1996). *LISREL 8.30,* [Computer software]. Lincolnwood, IL: Scientific Software International.

Linacre, J. M., & Wright, B. D. (2000). *WINSTEPS Version 3.02* [Computer software]. Chicago: MESA Press.

Linn, R. L., & Gronlund, N. (2000). *Measurement and assessment in teaching* (8th ed.). Upper Saddle River, NJ: Merrill/Prentice-Hall.

Lord, F. M. (1980). *Applications of item response theory to practical testing problems.* Hillsdale, NJ: Erlbaum.

Mehrens, W. & Lehman, I. (1991). *Measurement and evaluation in education and psychology* (4th ed.). New York: Holt, Rinehart & Winston.

Messick, S. (1989). Validity. In R. L. Linn (Ed.), *Educational measurement* (3rd ed., pp. 13–103). New York: Macmillan.

Millman, J., & Greene, J. (1989). The specification and development of tests of achievement and ability. In R. L. Linn (Ed.), *Educational measurement* (3rd ed., pp. 335–366). New York: Macmillan.

Mislevy, R. J., & Bock, D. R. (1998). *BILOG 3.11* [Computer software]. Lincolnwood, IL: Scientific Software International.

Moore, G. (1965). Cramming more components onto integrated circuits. *Electronics, 38*(8), 114–116.

Multivariate Software. (1999). *EQS 5.7* [Computer software]. Encino, CA: Author.

O'Meara, J. T., Jr. (1961, January–February). Selecting profitable products. *Harvard Business Review,* pp. 83–89.

Robertson, G. J. (1990). A practical model for test development. In C. R. Reynolds & R. W. Kamphaus (Eds.), *Handbook of psychological and educational assessment of children: Intelligence and achievement* (pp. 62–85). New York: Guilford Press.

SAS Institute. (1999). *SAS Systems, Version 8* [Computer software]. Cary, NC: Author.

SPSS. (1999a). *SPSS for Windows, Rel. 10.0* [Computer software]. Chicago: Author.

SPSS. (1999). *SYSTAT 9* [Computer software]. Chicago: SPSS, Inc.

Terman, L. M., & Merrill, M. M. (1937). *Measuring intelligence.* Boston: Houghton Mifflin.

Thissen, D. M. (1995). *MULTILOG 6.3.* [Computer software]. Lincolnwood, IL: Scientific Software International.

Thorndike, R. L. (1982). *Applied psychometrics.* New York: Wiley.

Thorndike, R. L., & Hagen, E. P. (1977). *Measurement and evaluation in psychology and education* (4th ed.). New York: Wiley.

U.S. Bureau of the Census. (1997, March). *Current population survey* [Machine-readable data file]. Washington, DC: Author.

Wesman, A. G. (1971). Writing the test item. In R. L. Thorndike (Ed.), *Educational measurement* (2nd ed., pp. 81–129). Washington, DC: American Council on Education.

3

Legal and Ethical Issues in the Assessment of Children

JONATHAN SANDOVAL
MARI GRIFFITHS IRVIN

Before I built a wall I'd ask to know
What I was walling in or walling out,
And to whom I was like to give offense.
—Frost (1939, p. 47)

There is nothing illegal about a test. The right to construct and publish a test is guaranteed under the First Amendment of the U.S. Constitution, which protects freedom of speech. However, using a test may bring about situations that jeopardize three important rights held by individuals: the right to equal protection, the right to due process, and the right to privacy. Most of the legal issues in testing are results of legislation, regulation, or litigation directed at securing these rights when tests are used to make decisions about individuals. To the extent that tests become walls or barriers keeping people in or out of programs, they may give offense and stimulate legal challenges.

The first two individual rights—that is, to equal protection and due process—are set forth by the Fourteenth Amendment of the U.S. Constitution. This amendment reads in part, "No state shall . . . deprive any person of life, liberty, or property without due process of law, nor deny any person within its jurisdiction, the equal protection of the laws." The equal protection clause of the amendment has been interpreted to mean that with respect to governmental actions

(which includes actions by school personnel), an individual should enjoy the same rights and receive the same benefits or burdens as all other citizens, unless it may be shown that there is a valid reason to withhold those rights or to single out an individual or a class of individuals for differential treatment.[1] When a test is used (even in part, along with other information) to assign a different treatment, such as a special education or to promote or assign an individual to a different job classification, then the use of the test must be strongly justified, and the test must be shown to be valid for the purposes for which it is used. Thus test use that results in minority group members' disproportionately receiving benefits or not receiving them creates a situation where it is possible that the equal protection principle is being violated, unless it can be shown that the differential representation is a valid and reasonable outcome.

Due process rights, which are protected by the Fifth Amendment, may be divided into two categories: procedural due process and substantive due process (Reutter, 1985). "Procedural due process" means that an individual has the right to protest and be heard prior to any action taken with respect to him or her. As a result, individuals must be informed before any procedure may be instituted that potentially deprives them of protected interests in liberty or property, and have a right to examine and comment on any evidence used to justify the deprivation. In addition, individuals may have a right to a fair and impartial hearing prior to the action. In the case of psychological or educational assessment, the Individuals with Disabilities Education Act (IDEA)[2] requires that individuals (or their parents) must give permission prior to testing and be informed of the results of any test that may be used to make a change in educational or other placement, and must have access to an unbiased hearing.

"Substantive due process" means that individuals may not have rights and privileges arbitrarily or unreasonably removed from them, and that the government cannot act capriciously or unfairly in dealing with individuals. Once, again, if a test is used to make a decision that denies rights and privileges, it must be valid and fair. Substantive due process rights and equal protection rights are related, because they both protect citizens from arbitrary and discriminatory treatment.

There is no mention of the right or privacy in the U.S. Constitution. The right to privacy is, however, inherent in several provisions of the Bill of Rights, and the U.S. Supreme Court has consistently ruled in favor of protecting the privacy of individuals. There are limits, though (see *Bowers v. Hardwick*, 1986). The court, announcing the decision in *Griswold v. Connecticut* (1965), suggested that there exist within the Bill of Rights guarantees creating zones of privacy: the First Amendment, protecting the rights of association (friends); the Third Amendment, prohibiting the intrusion of the government in quartering soldiers without the consent of the property's owner (home); the Fourth Amendment, protecting against unreasonable search and seizure (home and possessions); and the Fifth Amendment, protecting an individual against self-incrimination (attitudes, opinions, and beliefs). Privacy is also considered to be one aspect of liberty protected by the due process clause of the Fourteenth Amendment, according to Justice Brennan (*Carey v. Population Services International*, 1977). Other scholars (e.g., Kemer-

er & Deutsch, 1979) point to privacy as an unmentioned individual right that the government cannot remove, according to the Ninth Amendment. Substantive due process is also linked to the protection of privacy. With the passing of time, the courts have begun to protect the right to privacy, and legislative action has created privacy rights in various spheres. (The advent of computer data bases and the Internet has stimulated numerous new problems.) Increasingly, an individual has the right to choose whether, when, and how behaviors, attitudes, beliefs, and opinions are to be shared with others. The control of revealing test results, as one example of private data, rests with the individual under the right to privacy.

SPECIFIC ISSUES RELATED TO EQUAL PROTECTION

Whether or not a test is valid and reliable for members of particular groups becomes an issue of equal protection when the use of that test results in the denial of rights and benefits to individuals belonging to that group. The key sign of a violation of these rights is that a disproportionate number of group members are either receiving or being denied access to a program or benefit.

The Civil Rights Act of 1964 was a major landmark in the securing of constitutional rights by various minority groups. Its titles, particularly Title IV, spelled out that individuals cannot be discriminated against or deprived of the equal protection of the law on the basis of race or color in educational institutions. It specified that racially discriminatory impact—that is, events resulting in smaller percentages of minority group members' receiving benefits than would be expected by their numbers in the population—may signal an illegal practice. Although originally directed at the practice of racial segregation at the school site level, a number of complaints related to other educational practices have been brought to court, charging a violation of this statute.

Tracking and Testing Members of Language Minority Groups

Legal challenges and related legislative provisions have resulted in the generally accepted principle that children whose primary language is other than English should be tested in their first or predominant language. The first major court case questioning educational practice relevant to language minority children was *Lau v. Nichols* (1974), wherein the U.S. Supreme Court held that English instruction for Chinese-speaking children amounted to depriving these children of the benefits of education. Complaints were then filed that generalized this principle to the testing of non-English-speaking children. Landmark cases were *Diana v. State Board of Education* (1970), *Covarrubias v. San Diego Unified School District* (1971), and *Guadalupe Organization Inc. v. Tempe Elementary School District No. 3* (1972). These cases were brought on behalf of Hispanic children who had been placed in special education classrooms for students classified as "educable mentally retarded (EMR)," in districts where the results of tests administered in English were used in making the decision. Hispanic children were overrepresented in such classrooms. All of these cases were settled out of court with an agreement that children be tested only in their primary language. It was further agreed that a fair and proper assessment of a non-English-speaking child for special education would begin with a determination of the child's primary language, prior to using that language for assessment. A proper assessment would include the evaluation of adaptive behavior and the use of nonverbal tests and materials. The defendants further agreed to reevaluate the children previously classified as "EMR," to reintegrate into regular classrooms all misclassified children, and to monitor the proportion of the minorities placed in special classes. It was agreed that any disproportionate numbers of Hispanic children in special education would be explained and justified in keeping with equal protection principles. It was reaffirmed in the settlements that intelligence tests should not be the primary or only basis for making this diagnosis. In addition, procedural due process rights to prior notice, informed consent, and open, impartial hearings in the parent's language were reasserted (Prasse, 1984). The provisions of these settlements soon found their way into law within the IDEA, which requires testing in the child's "native language or other mode of communication, unless it is clearly not feasible to do so" (IDEA, 1997, § 300.532).

Tracking and Testing Members of Ethnic Minority Groups

The landmark event signaling a change in the civil rights of minorities was the famous case of *Brown v. Board of Education* (1954), in which the U.S. Supreme Court ruled that segregated schools and unequal educational opportunities for black children were not constitutionally permissible. In the decade following that decision, schools resisted the mandate, and some districts used intelligence and achievement tests to maintain a segregated school system. An early case addressing this practice was *Stell v. Savannah–Chatham County Board of Education* (1965). The Fifth Circuit held that individual students could be assigned to different schools on the basis of intelligence or achievement if the program was uniformly administered and race was not a factor in making the assignment (see Bersoff, 1979). Since race was established to be a factor in the procedure under adjudication, the court ruled for the plaintiffs.

By far the most influential case securing equal opportunity for black students was *Hobson v. Hanson* (1967). In this case, the District of Columbia was challenged for using standardized group tests to place children into academic tracks. The case was begun by the discovery of a disproportionate number of black children in the lower tracks. One of the tracks, labeled the "special academic" track, was equivalent to the "EMR" classification in other parts of the country. Although the criteria for being placed in one of the tracks included teacher and counselor evaluations, estimates of grades, school history, and physical condition, testing was determined to be one of the most important factors in an assignment. When disproportional impact is discovered, as it was in this case, it is important for the court to determine whether or not the classification has a rational, valid basis. The court ruled against the school district, and found that the tracking system was indefensible because students were placed in the tracks on the basis of traits that were not relevant. The court decided that the standardized group aptitude tests were inappropriate (i.e., not valid), because the tests were standardized on white middle-class children and could not be appropriately generalized to black children. This notion of standardization became the first legal definition of test bias or lack of validity. In the decision, the court particularly disapproved of the inflexibility of the tracking system and its stigmatizing effect on black children. Because placement in a lower track was perceived to be harmful, the issue of equal educational opportunity was identified. In addition, the judge criticized the practice of using ability tests as the sole basis (or a major factor) for deciding on placement.

Prasse (1984) points out two ironies in the court's decision. First, it ruled that because the tests did not access "innate ability," they could not form the basis of a tracking system; a system based on measures of innate ability presumably might be legal. Few psychologists believe that measures of innate ability exist. Second, because individual tests had been used to identify misplacement, many psychologists believed that the decision actually supported test use. In later cases, this fact would not prove to be important. (In the *Larry P.* case, discussed in the next section, the plaintiffs also used individual test results to indicate that the children were misplaced.)

Another important case brought under Title VII of the Civil Rights Act of 1964, but under the section forbidding discriminatory practices in employment, was *Griggs v. Duke Power Co.* (1971). Although this litigation did not have to do with children, it established a precedent regarding a number of principles related to achievement testing. In this suit, a group of black employees challenged the use of intelligence tests as one device to determine job categories (e.g., coal shoveler) and promotion in a power plant. In ruling in favor of the plaintiffs, the U.S. Supreme Court noted that even though there was no explicit intent to discriminate, the number of black workerss holding low-paying jobs and the disproportionate infrequency of promotions to supervisor earned by black employers indicated unfairness; moreover, any requirement for promotion must show a clear and manifest relationship to job success. The burden of proof—here, of demonstrating test validity by correlating test results to job performance—was placed on the employers (or users of tests). If a test could not be shown to have demonstrated concurrent validity with respect to relevant performance, its use was illegal. In this instance, of course, IQ tests could not be shown to correlate very highly with physical performance, and the defendants lost. This case was particularly important because tests were directly implicated in illegal practice for the first time. A similar case brought 4 years later, *Albemarle Paper Co. v. Moody* (1975), resulted in the same judgment. In this opinion, however, the U.S. Supreme Court explicitly noted the American Psychological Association's (APA's) test standards as appropriate to follow in planning studies to determine the job-related validity of employment tests.

Another case a year later, *Washington v. Davis* (1976), upheld the use of ability tests for screening applicants for police training in Washington, D.C. Although black applicants failed the test in disproportionately high numbers, the test was determined by the court to have content validity and to predict grades in the police academy. As an equal protection case it was important, because the U.S. Supreme Court rejected the notion that disproportional impact alone was enough to signal an illegal practice, but ruled that the plaintiffs must prove intent to discriminate instead of intent to predict accurately. A second case concerning selection in a police department, *Guardians Association of New York City v. Civil Service Commission* (1981), resulted in the U.S. Supreme Court's concluding that content-oriented validation methods were appropriate for establishing the validity of certain kinds of tests. However, the court acknowledged that construct validity is perhaps more appropriate than content validity for abstract abilities (e.g., intelligence) (see Bersoff, 1981).

Issues of Ethnic Bias in Individual Intelligence Tests

The major cases in which the use of intelligence tests with children has received judicial attention are *Larry P. v. Riles* (1979) and *PASE v. Hannon* (1980). Both have been the subjects of numerous articles (e.g., Bersoff, 1979, 1981, 1982; Condras, 1980;

Lambert, 1981; Sattler, 1981, 1982) and an excellent comprehensive book (Elliott, 1987). Both of these cases were decided in federal district courts and were not appealed to the U.S. Supreme Court, although *Larry P.* went to the Federal Circuit Court of Appeals. In both cases, attorneys for the plaintiffs, who were black children assigned to "EMR" classes, sought to lay the blame for disproportionate black assignment to such classes on the intelligence tests used by school psychologists in the process in determining eligibility. The two cases were decided differently, however, with the California Ninth Circuit federal court ruling in *Larry P.* that IQ tests should not be used with black children, and the Illinois federal court ruling in favor of the defense in *PASE* and vindicating the use of standardized IQ tests. Elliott (1987) outlines a number of differences in context and in lines of argument and evidence between the two cases, which led in all likelihood to the conflicting decisions. Of most relevance for assessment, the *Larry P.* trial focused on several issues in test bias: the historical background of test development (i.e., the "racist" attitudes of the early pioneers of the American testing movement); the inclusion of black children in the standardization sample (important because of *Hobson*); the selection of items for the tests (items were selected to minimize sex differences, but no such parallel effort was directed at race differences); the failure to tap the "black experience pool" in developing items; and, most importantly, the internal and external validity of tests (Elliott, 1987). The attorneys for the plaintiffs convinced the court that the tests had not been validated for the specific purpose of selecting children from each minority group who are unable to profit from instruction in regular classes with remedial instruction. The court accepted as relevant only studies correlating black children's test scores with classroom grades. It also accepted the plaintiffs' arguments on other validity issues, rather than evidence from the defendants' witnesses, particularly evidence on internal validity (similarity of item performance between races) (Bersoff, 1979).

The *PASE* case differed, in that the court did not accept that a difference in performance on IQ measures automatically indicated test bias (Elliott, 1987). For the first time, a judge requested information on item performance by the two races. When little was forthcoming, he proceeded to perform an "armchair" analysis of the items and used this rational approach as the main justification for his decision. Test validity for the different groups, in this instance, was defined as internal validity and differential item response. This type of evidence, item performance on achievement and ability tests, will continue to be important in the future.

California has had to continue reporting on the representation of black children in special education. Because of continued overrepresentation, the Ninth Circuit Court issued a new ruling in the fall of 1986—extending the ban against using intelligence tests to the testing of black children for any special education purpose within the public schools (except placement in programs for gifted children), and indicating that no records on intelligence test results could be kept by the schools. Black parents could not even be asked to permit intelligence testing (Landers, 1986). The court later ruled in 1992 (a ruling that was upheld by the Ninth Circuit Court of Appeals) that plaintiffs in another case (*Crawford v. Honig,* 1994) representing black children with learning disabilities (LDs) were not bound by the 1986 order, and that parents could give permission for testing. The order was viewed as applying to the use of intelligence tests in assigning children to "dead-end EMR classes" only. Neither side has chosen to appeal these cases further.

Two principles seem to have emerged from these cases and have been explicitly codified in IDEA and in Section 504 of the Rehabilitation Act of 1973: Namely, tests must be validated for the specific purpose for which they are used, and should not be discriminatory. The process of determining whether a test is biased is a long and controversial one (Flaughter, 1978; Reynolds & Kaiser, 1990; see also Reynolds & Kaiser, Chapter 22, this volume). Neither the law nor the courts have indicated what level of validity must obtain before a test may be used and considered nondiscriminatory.

The validity of a test can seldom be established with a single correlation, however, and correlations can be misleading when a criterion is inappropriate. Validity would seem to be best thought of as a judgment about a test made on the basis of the preponderance of empirical evidence (Messick, 1995). Furthermore, this judgment probably should be made by professionals, not by the courts. In other domains, the court has left educational decisions to professionals.

The concept of fairness in testing has been given a prominent place in the most recent revision of the *Standards for Educational and Psychological Testing* (American Educational Research Association [AERA], APA, & National Council on Measurement in Education [NCME], 1999). Four views of fairness are discussed: fairness as lack of bias; fairness as equitable treatment in the testing process; fairness in equality of outcomes of testing; and fairness as opportunity to learn. The standards acknowledge that it is unlikely that consensus will be reached about the correctness of the various views. The standards do call for a careful examination of validity evidence for subgroups of examinees if there is reason to believe that a test does not have the same meaning across subgroups.

Issues related to grouping and placement practices were also raised in *Marshall v. Georgia* (1984). In this case, the plaintiffs representing black school children alleged that the students were improperly assigned to achievement groups in regular education, overrepresented in "EMR" classrooms, and underrepresented in special education classrooms for children with LDs. The case has parallels to *Hobson* and to *Larry P.* that have been thoroughly explored by Reschly, Kicklighter, and McKee (1988a, 1988b, 1988c). In this case—as well as in a similar Florida case, *S-1 v. Turlington* (1979)—IQ tests were not the central issue (Reschly et al., 1988c). The emphasis in these trials was on illustrating that children's placements were legitimately related to educational needs. The court ruled in *Marshall* that overrepresentation was not discriminatory; in *S-1*, the case was dismissed. Both decisions upheld the notion of multidisciplinary assessment, and granted that professionals should have reasonable latitude in selecting and using individual tests.

Testing Individuals with Disabilities

When IDEA was reauthorized in 1997 (PL 105-17), Congress added a number of new provisions (Jacob-Timm & Hartshorne, 1998; Telzrow, 1999). Part B of IDEA requires that tests for a child with sensory, motor, or speech impairments be selected so as to insure that the results accurately reflect the child's aptitude, achievement level, or whatever it purports to measure, rather than reflecting primarily the impaired skills.

Of particular relevance to assessment was the IDEA mandate that students with disabilities participate in state and local assessment programs with appropriate accommodations or through alternative assessments as determined by individual education program teams. Pratt and Moreland (1998) have reviewed the differing accommodations appropriate for various disabling conditions, such as relaxing limits or appointing a nondisabled individual to assist with the administration and recording of responses. Unfortunately, the influence of most accommodations on test scores is not well documented (Geisinger, 1994; Pratt & Moreland, 1998). One response to giving accommodations on a test is to "flag" the results, indicating that the test was administered under nonstandard conditions. This practice is contentious, however. Individuals with disabling conditions argue that flagging calls attention to modifications intended to eliminate bias from testing, and thus results in unfair and discriminatory practices. On the other hand, Section 4.5 of the Code of Professional Responsibilities in Education Measurement calls on test administrators to notify those who use the results if any nonstandard or delimiting conditions occur during testing (Joint Committee on Testing Practices, 1996). These disputes are finding their way into court.

Another aspect of the 1997 reauthorization of IDEA was to reduce the requirements for reevaluation, once a child has been placed in special education. Existing data, including test results, can be used to justify continued eligibility. This change can reduce the amount of testing done in special education, but not everyone agrees that this is necessarily a good idea (Telzrow, 1999). The law reflects a change in point of view that focuses on using tests to improve the educational outcomes for children with disabilities, and opens the door to more academic testing, curriculum-based measurement, and functional behavioral assessment.

Other Testing Cases

Achievement tests, either locally produced or nationally standardized, have been used with increasing frequency to verify students' competency—typically for high school graduation, but also for promotion at lower grade levels (Lerner, 1981). Although this practice has been viewed with some skepticism by psychologists (e.g., Glass & Ellwein, 1986), indications are that it will continue for some time.

In practice, use of these competency tests has had a disproportionate impact on members of minority groups, and complaints have resulted (DeMers & Bersoff, 1985). It is noteworthy that similar competency tests have been developed for teachers, and these tests have also been challenged in the courts (e.g., *United States v. Chesterfield County School District*, 1973).

The most prominent case involving competency tests for graduation has been *Debra P. v. Turlington* (1983). In this case, the Florida State Department of Education had to demonstrate that its functional literacy examination, used to establish eligibility for a high school diploma, was a fair test of what was actually taught in the schools. The plaintiffs, noting a disparate impact on black students, challenged this requirement; they lost, because the defendants presented a convincing validation study. The court also accepted testimony that the test, as an objective standard, could help remedy the vestiges of past segregation. A parallel Texas case was dismissed recently by a federal judge (Schmidt, 2000). Tests of achievement and other curriculum-based measures seem to be much easier to defend against legal challenge than do aptitude or ability tests (Galagan, 1985). It remains to be seen how defensible school readiness tests and minimum-competency tests used for school promotion may be, inasmuch as there have been no notable challenges to these procedures (Smith & Jenkins, 1980).

An infamous validity case, involving a suit brought by Golden Rule Insurance Company against Educational Testing Service (ETS) and the Illinois Department of Insurance over the use of the Multistate Insurance Licensing Examination, was resolved by specifying one criterion of test bias and suggesting how much of a difference in item performance between groups would be permissible (see Anrig, 1987; Rooney, 1987). This case, like *PASE*, went beyond the examination of group differences in the test scores to define bias and turned to item performance. The *Golden Rule* settlement, in addition to calling for the disclosure of results after tests have been administered, also required that item statistics be calculated separately for test takers from minority groups, and that these item statistics be used to construct new tests. The new tests would be developed so that there would be no more than a 15% disparity in the pass rate of test takers from majority and minority groups, and so that the pass rate would be greater than 40%. This procedure of using test items on which black and white performance was most similar became the focus for draft legislation in New York and elsewhere, inasmuch as it was advocated as a means to correct for racial bias by the National Center for Fair and Open Testing. The president of ETS (Anrig, 1987) later repudiated the settlement, arguing that "The procedure ignores the possibility that differences in performance may validly reflect real differences in knowledge or skill. . . . The National Council on Measurement in Education has written that such general use [of the procedure] would undermine the construct validity of tests and might even worsen group differences" (p. 3). Anrig reported that ETS was beginning to use other statistical procedures (the Mantel–Haenszel method) to match individuals in terms of relevant knowledge and skill before comparing their item performance. APA's Committee on Psychological Tests and Assessment also criticized the *Golden Rule* procedure (Denton, 1987).

In spite of the phrase's appearance in a number of court decisions and its occurrence in a number of laws, exactly what it means for a test to be "valid for the purpose for which it is used" has not yet been specified. Since standards change, however, perhaps the most reasonable approach would be to require that a test meet the standards set forth by professional organizations. In fact, legislation in New York in the late 1970s proposed just this, and the courts subsequently began to reference the then-current version of the AERA/APA/NCME *Standards for Educational and Psychologi-*

cal Testing as a reasonable authoritative basis for judging evidence and making decisions on validity issues (Lerner, 1978).

Cases Mandating Assessment

In a somewhat ironic turn of events, some cases have been settled that seemingly mandate the use of tests by psychologists. In an early case, *Frederick L. v. Thomas* (1976), the plaintiffs, children with LDs in Philadelphia, charged that they were being denied equal protection rights to education because they had not been screened and identified as disabled and thus eligible for special classes (see Tillery & Carfioli, 1986). The court ruled that the school district should develop an identification process presumably based on screening and individual testing, since the court pointed out that parent and teacher referral was not adequate. The court left the details of the plan to the district and its professionals, however, and did not require tests per se.

Another related New York case, *Lora v. Board of Education of City of New York* (1978), involved black and Hispanic children classified as "emotionally disturbed." Their attorneys claimed that the overuse of culturally biased tests led to disproportionate placement in special day schools (Wood, Johnson, & Jenkins, 1986). The court chose to focus on the failure to follow acceptable practice in the use of tests (such as the assessment of minority group members by majority group members and the failure to perform annual reviews), rather than on the adequacy of the tests themselves. As a result, the ruling required a more comprehensive evaluation procedure to be put in place that involved more use of psychologists and tests. A related case, *Luke S. v. Nix* (1981), led to similar reforms in Louisiana (Taylor, Tucker, & Galagan, 1986).

ISSUES RELATED TO PROCEDURAL DUE PROCESS

In order for an individual to protest and be heard about any test-based decision that has been made about him or her, the individual must be informed about the test. To make an effective protest, the individual should have access to the information that has been

generated by the test and the validity of that information. Procedural safeguards for parents have been set up by law (IDEA) and the courts (Buss, 1975); these include the right (1) to be notified of procedures in advance, (2) to submit evidence, (3) to cross-examine witnesses, (4) to be represented by a lawyer, (5) to have a case decided by an independent and impartial hearing officer, (6) to examine all school records, (7) to receive a state-provided independent psychological examination, and (8) to appeal. How far a tested administrator must go in providing test information has been the subject of several legislative mandates and court cases. In the achievement domain, test critics have worked for full disclosure of test items and correct answers under the banner of "truth in testing." A landmark law passed in New York in 1979 (a similar but less stringent law was passed in California in the same year) requires testing companies to release general statistics about the test to the public; to identify the test items used in assessment; and (for an individual examinee, upon request) to provide the individual's answers and the keyed correct answers. The rationale is that the examinee may then challenge any of the answers and should have the right to protest effectively any test score. This legislation at present only applies to tests used for admissions purposes, but the practice has been established and may be expanded to other kinds of tests.

The *Golden Rule* case, described above, has been one of several that have explored whether or not a test taker or his or her guardians may examine test protocols and individual test responses. The courts generally have held that the individual's right to protest holds priority over the copyrights of test publishers and/or the privacy rights of the examiner.

The most important guarantor of the right to inspect and correct educational records is the Family Educational Rights and Privacy Act of 1974 (PL 93-380), commonly known as the "Buckley Amendment." This law gives parents (or individuals over the age of 18) the right to inspect, review, and amend all educational records pertaining to their children (or themselves). Similar provisions have been incorporated into IDEA. For the purposes of this discussion, the most important issue springing from these two pieces of legislation is whether or not test protocols and/or individual item responses must be revealed to parents. In the past, if a psychologist were to grant access to protocols, he or she might violate professional ethics related to safeguarding psychological tests (to be discussed later). Recently, however, ethical standards are being modified to permit disclosure. The Buckley Amendment does not require a psychologist's private notes (i.e., notes that are not shown to anyone and are in the sole possession of the psychologist) to be revealed. But records that are used in the provision of treatment to the student (such as special education) may be reviewed by an appropriate professional of the student's choice. Since psychologists' reports and often the protocols are shown to others in the schools (e.g., the multidisciplinary team), and constitute the basis of treatment decisions, presumably they must be revealed. The question of whether they may be directly revealed to parents still remains. In *Detroit Edison v. NLRB* (1979), the U.S. Supreme Court did indicate in a case related to testing that the federal statutory obligation to reveal information takes precedence over the ethical standards of a private group (in this case, the APA). The court in *Lora* indicated that the failure to provide unspecified clinical records to parents would be a violation of due process rights. Spitzzeri (1987) reported an Illinois case, somewhat clouded by the fact that the plaintiff's mother held a doctorate in counseling psychology, in which the parents won the right to inspect the specific Rorschach responses elicited from their daughter (*John K. and Mary K. v. Board of Education for School District #65, 1987*). The principal rationale for the decision was that the test protocol was created to evaluate the child, and that it must be available for review to protect due process rights. New issues may be raised in the future with the use of computerized testing (Burke & Normand, 1987). If a computerized output is used, must it be revealed? Probably so (Walker & Myrick, 1985).

APA's Division of School Psychology has adopted the position that parents should be given the right to inspect protocols under appropriate professional supervision, but should not be given photocopies of complete protocols or permitted to copy extended portions of protocols word for word (Martin, 1986). In situations in which secure testing material is subpoenaed for a legal proceeding, an editorial in the *American Psychologist* (Fowler, 1999) suggests that psychologists ask the court to deliver these materials only to psychologists or other professionals who are bound by a duty to protect them. If this request is refused and they are to be delivered to nonqualified legal counsel, the psychologist should request "that a protective order be issued prohibiting parties from making copies of the materials, requiring that the materials be returned to the psychologists at the close of litigation, and ordering that the record be sealed if test questions or answers are admitted as part of the public record" (Fowler, 1999, p. 1078).

ISSUES RELATED TO PRIVACY

Both the test giver and the test taker have right of privacy, although, as we have seen above, the test giver's rights may be secondary. The most sweeping laws that have addressed this issue are IDEA, the Buckley Amendment, and the "Hatch Amendment" (i.e., Sections 439(a) and (b) of the General Education Provisions Act, PL 90-247), all of which require parental permission to be secured before any kind of testing takes place or before any release of information is given to a third party. The Hatch Amendment requires permission for psychological testing if the primary purpose is to reveal information concerning "mental and psychological problems potentially embarrassing to the student or his [*sic*] family" (Section 439(b)(2)), among other sorts of information. This requirement is broad in impact for psychologists.

Test responses may be considered to be privileged information given to a psychologist by a client, and to that extent they may be protected from the disclosure to other parties, given that a psychologist has such privileges of confidentiality. It is clear that parents must give permission before any testing can take place; once the testing has occurred, however, the extent to which the information developed during the process of testing must be reported back is not as clear.

Although the information is privileged in most states, psychologists are bound to report indications of child abuse or indications that children constitute a danger to themselves or others (i.e., are suicidal or homicidal). To the degree that the test may reveal such tendencies or situations, a psychologist may be bound to break this confidence (e.g., *Phillis P. v. Clairmont Unified School District*, 1986, involving a school psychologist).

DeMers and Bersoff (1985) have pointed out that informed consent has three elements: knowledge, voluntariness, and competence. To give consent, an individual must understand what will be done, why it will be done, and how it will be done. Furthermore, the consent must not be obtained under any duress, and the individual must be legally competent. Obviously, informed consent means that psychologists must work hard to explain their procedures in language that parents can understand (Pryzwansky & Bersoff, 1978).

An issue that has not been adequately determined—either legally, religiously, psychologically, or otherwise—is the age at which a child is capable of giving consent for testing or any psychological procedure (Grisso & Vierling, 1978; Melton, Koocher, & Saks, 1983). The age of 18 is most often cited in legislation (e.g., the Buckley Amendment), but if one were to keep within the spirit of the law, one might give children the option to consent whenever they individually seem able to rationally understand the request.

ISSUES RELATED TO MALPRACTICE

What constitutes malpractice with respect to psychological testing? A tort occurs when a professional acts negligently in the provision of services and harm has resulted to the client. Negligence may be an act of omission, such as failure to include an appropriate test in a battery, or an act of commission, such as using an inappropriate test. Not performing up to standards could occur in any of a number of areas, such as explaining the testing procedure to the client or representatives inadequately, selecting testing materials that are not appropriate, administering the test incorrectly, selecting a faulty computer scoring/interpreting system, or interpreting test data incorrectly (Walker & Myrick, 1985).

Besides negligence, another tortious act is defamation (i.e., libel or slander). In one case, a psychologist was sued, unsuccessfully, for reporting that a child was a "high-grade moron" (McDermott, 1972). However, reporting test results that may be perceived as defamatory (or injurious to the reputation of an individual) is not illegal if the results are transmitted to a professional or another person with a legitimate interest in the child (McDermott, 1972).

Torts actions in the courts are generally decided on the basis of whether or not other competent professionals would have made the same decisions or would have reached the same conclusions as the person under question. (Other defenses against negligence and defamation are used first, of course—e.g., establishing that an injury did not occur.) Once again, professional standards become important in determining whether or not a professional has been acting correctly and whether or not the harm done to the client would have been avoided by most other professionals. A consideration of legal issues soon turns into a consideration of ethics.

RELATIONSHIP OF LAW AND ETHICS

There is often overlap in conceptual understanding when "law" and "ethics" are discussed. Both are related to values identifying that which is "the good." "Values" generally are reflections of strong feeling that can be supported by rational justification. More critically, they imply preferences that specify a course of action (Kieffer, 1979). "Ethics" are judgments of value or of obligation. The focus of ethics is on what ought to be, in contrast to what is (Steininger, Newell, & Garcia, 1984). Ethical reasoning, then, is the process by which the individual resolves conflicts in values and makes decisions for what ought to be done.

"Laws" may be defined as values or ethical judgments that have societal sanction. When a value or ethical judgment is elevated to the status of law, a given individual's rejection of that value or judgment does not excuse the person from societal responsibility under the law. By contrast, a professional "code of ethics" reflects values and ethical judgments that individuals voluntarily assume when they join the particular professional group. In some states, however, the professional standard of practice embodied in such ethical principles is accepted as the minimal legal standard of practice. When this is the case, violation of a professional ethical standard affects the individual's ability to function professionally, whether or not the person is a member of the professional organization (APA, 2002).

PROFESSIONAL ETHICAL STANDARDS

The ethical task in regard to assessment is to identify that which is valued without sanction of law, and, if necessary, to resolve conflicts in values so that professional behavior may be enacted in the effort to attain the ideal of what ought to be done. It will be recognized that "what is" is often not "what should be." Ethical behavior represents an individual's self-conscious attempt to reach the ideal behaviorally.

The APA and the National Association of School Psychologists (NASP), the two largest national associations with members who assess children, have each developed standards for professional conduct that are binding on their members (APA, 2002; NASP, 2000). Each of these documents contains sections relative to assessment goals and activities. In addition, as mentioned earlier in this chapter, standards for educational and psychological testing have been developed jointly by three national professional organizations: the AERA, the APA, and the NCME (AERA et al., 1999). Each of these documents has undergone revision in recent years, and future revisions are anticipated as knowledge and professional practice values change.

"Ethical Principles of Psychologists and Code of Conduct" (APA, 2002) is the most recent version of the professional standards affecting members of APA. The preamble and general principles of the document identify the values of importance to professional psychologists, and serve an aspirational function to guide psychologists to attain the highest ideals of psychology. These ideals include the increase of scientific and professional knowledge of behavior; the application of that knowledge to improve the conditions of individuals, organizations, and society; the respect for civil and human rights, as well as for freedom of professional inquiry and expression; and the attempt to help the public in making informed judgments and choices concerning human behavior. Five general principles govern the actions of psychologists: beneficence and nonmaleficence; fidelity and responsibility; integrity; justice; and respect for people's rights and dignity. The APA ethical standards have been operationalized into an enforceable code of conduct, which in some states may be legally applied to psychologists whether or not they are APA members.

Members of NASP are subject to ethical principles, the most recent statement approved for implementation in 2001. Two underlying assumptions serve as the foundation for this code of conduct, that "school psychologists will act as advocates for their students/clients" and "at the very least, school psychologists will do no harm" (NASP, 2000, p. 13, p. 654). An earlier version of the NASP statement of professional ethics spoke specifically of "the uncertainties associated with delivery of psychological services in a situation where rights of the student, the parent, the school and society may conflict" (NASP, 1985, p. 2). The 2000 document refers to the obligation of school psychologists to "'speak up' for the needs and rights of their students/clients even at times when it may be difficult to do so. . . . Given one's employment situation and the array of recommendations, events may develop in which the ethical course of action is unclear" (NASP, 2000, p. 14). In contrast to the APA (2002) document, the NASP (2000) document, though not as explicit as its predecessor, is sensitive to the fact that school psychologists are most frequently employees who must function within an organizational setting where the primary mission is not that of providing psychological services.

"Specialty Guidelines for the Delivery of Services by School Psychologists" (APA, 1981) and "Standards for the Provision of School Psychological Services" (part of NASP, 2000) are documents acknowledging that state statutes, not professional psychological associations, govern the services provided by school psychologists. It is recognized that these guidelines are "advisory" to the governing organizations; nonetheless, specific guidelines are set forth for the provision of school psychological services, including assessment activities. It is expected that members of the individual psychological associations will work to implement their particular guidelines in the school districts of their employment. Although there are some differences in the specificity contained within the guidelines, there is much commonality in the values stressed as critical for the delivery of adequate school psychological services.

Another set of guidelines with specific direction for persons involved in the psychological assessment of children was published by the APA Office of Ethnic Minority Affairs. This document, "Guidelines for Providers of Psychological Services to Ethnic, Linguistic, and Culturally Diverse Populations" (APA, 1993), goes beyond the expectation for sensitivity to the needs of many client groups. More critically, they stress the need for competency in skills in working with many persons who represent increasing constituencies among the receivers of psychological services. Historically, persons who are not representative of the dominant culture in any of several ways have been poorly served by psychologists, even by those who have claimed an advocacy role on their behalf, because of knowledge and skill deficits on the providers' part.

The jointly prepared *Standards for Educational and Psychological Testing* volume (AERA et al., 1999) provides the greatest degree of specificity regarding the comprehensive nature of the assessment effort. The focus is exclusively on "tests" (which are defined broadly enough to encompass a variety of assessment techniques and methodologies). *Guidelines for Computer Based Tests and Interpretations* (APA, 1987) was also developed to give specific direction in response to the increasing usage of technology in various aspects of the assessment process. The language in these two documents tends to be much more operational than that in the APA and NASP statements of ethical principles.

SPECIFIC ETHICAL ISSUES IN REGARD TO ASSESSMENT OF CHILDREN

A review of the statements of values contained in these professional standards of conduct and guidelines to professional practice leads to the identification of some specific ethical issues in regard to assessment in general and the assessment of children in particular.

Test Construction

Psychologists are expected to use scientific procedures and to observe organizational standards in the development of assessment techniques (APA, 2002). The *Standards for Educational and Psychological Testing* volume (AERA et al., 1999) is the most comprehensive statement of ethical practice regarding all aspects of test construction. In addition, commentary is provided that facilitates the reader's understanding of the standards' intent.

Test Publication

Technical manuals and users' guides should be provided to prospective test users at the time a test is published or released. These manuals should contain all relevant information needed by the test giver, whose responsibility is to determine whether the test is reliable and valid for the purpose intended in any given situation. Promotional material about a given test should be accurate, not intended to mislead, and supported by the research base of the instrument. If test misuse can be anticipated, the test manual should provide specific cautions about such possible misuse (AERA et al., 1999).

Test Usage

Ysseldyke and Algozzine (1982) point out that tests deficient in validity or reliability or with poorly developed norms are commonly administered to children for special education purposes. They claim that evidence is often not provided by the publishers of many of these instruments to support their claims for validity, reliability, or standardization. Current professional ethics codes specify that assessment procedures and test selection should be made with attention to validity and reliability for the purpose intended (APA, 1981, 2002; NASP, 2000) and should be research-based (NASP, 2000). Obsolete measures are not to be used (APA, 1981).

Furthermore, the selection of assessment techniques and rationale for interpretation for any given evaluation should reflect appropriate understanding of differences in age, gender, socioeconomic status, sexual orientation, and cultural and ethnic backgrounds (APA, 2002; NASP, 2000), as well as differences in religion, disability, and language (APA, 2002). The new APA ethics code focuses on psychologists' use of assessment methods in a manner "appropriate to an individual's language preference and competence" (Standard 9.02c), and acknowledges that appropriate tests for some diverse populations may not be developed. In such instances, psychologists "document the efforts they made and the result of those efforts, clarify the probable impact of their limited information on the reliability and validity of their opinions, and appropriately limit the nature and extent of their conclusions or recommendations" (Standard 9.01b). School psychologists are expected to use test results with observations and background information for appropriate interpretation, and interventions are to be appropriate, given the problem presented and the data gathered (NASP, 1997).

Validity for Testing Purpose

Cole (1981) raised another issue in the choice of assessment tools. She distinguished between questions of technical validity of a given test and the question of whether a test should be used, even if it is valid. She quoted Messick (1975, p. 962) in her discussion of this distinction:

> First, is the test any good as a measure of the characteristic it is interpreted to assess? Second, should the test be used for the proposed purpose? The first question is a technical and scientific one and may be answered by appraising evidence bearing on the test's psychometric properties, especially construct validity. The second question is an ethical one, and its answer requires an evaluation of the potential consequences of testing in terms of social values.

Cole continued her argument about the limits of validity by citing an example that goes beyond the argument in the *Larry P.* case in the presentation of testing as an activity with social policy implications:

> As members of a scientific community, testing scholars clearly value scientific evidence on whether a test is accurate for some intended inference. For example, an intelligence test might accurately (validly) identify mentally retarded children. However, if a test is accurate (valid), validity theory does not say whether the use of the test, or the whole system in which the test use is embedded, will produce a social good or a social evil. Thus, the use of a valid intelligence test to identify mentally retarded children for assignments to a special educational intervention does not ensure that the special intervention will provide the education the children need. (Cole, 1981, p. 1068)

In this regard, the standards for the provision of school psychological services published by NASP (2000) state that assessment techniques should be used that increase the probability of effective interventions and follow-up.

Nonbiased Assessment

The "Guidelines for Providers of Psychological Services to Ethnic, Linguistic, and Culturally Diverse Populations" document states general principles that are intended to be aspirational and to provide suggestions for psychologists working with such populations (APA, 1993). The documents setting forth ethical principles for both APA (2002) and NASP (2000) mention the responsibility of psychologists to insure that appropriate instruments and methodologies are used in the assessment of clients; the APA (2002) ethics code stresses the need to extend this responsibility to forensic assessment services.

However, the *Standards for Educational and Psychological Testing* volume (AERA et al., 1999) is the most explicit in regard to nonbiased assessment. These standards include not only those related to the assessment of persons from racial/ethnic minority groups and of lower socioeconomic status; specific attention is also called to the particular needs of persons in linguistic minority groups and persons who have disabling conditions. Clients are to be tested in their dominant language or an alternative communication system, as required; modifications of the conditions under which the test is administered should be considered for persons with disabilities.

Yet there remain many unanswered, even unresearched questions about the effect of such nonstandardized accommodations upon the ability to use such test data. Does the test still measure that which was intended by the test developer (i.e., has the validity of the instrument been altered)? Because the ethical standards do not provide case-specific answers to many of the questions that will confront an ethically sensitive psychologist regarding the use of a given instrument in a specific situation, caution is advised when tests are administered to persons whose particular linguistic or disabling condition is not represented in the standardized sample.

Although the various standards provide cautions to the practicing psychologist about the need to use assessment instruments that are culture-fair, Ysseldyke and Algozzine (1982) reviewed the literature available at that time and concluded that there is little agreement among the experts as to the definition of a "fair test." They went on to cite Petersen and Novick's (1976) belief that some of the models are in themselves internally contradictory. It is probably safe to say that these issues raised over 20 years ago have still not been adequately addressed.

Decision Making

In most instances, testing is done to gather data that are needed to make a decision about a child. Thus the choice of assessment instruments should be based at least in part on the type of decision that needs to be made (Ysseldyke & Algozzine, 1982). When the assessment data are obtained through means other than empirically standardized tests—methods that include interview and behavioral observation techniques—special cautions are warranted. Such techniques should yield multiple hypotheses regarding the child's behavior, with each hypothesis modifiable on the basis of further information, and decision making should include consideration of the decision's context.

There are also multiple postassessment decision-making variables. Some of these variables reside in the decision makers themselves. For example, who are the decision makers? Aside from the persons legally required for decision making, ethical decisions may need to be made about who the decision makers should be. How do the decision makers see their responsibility? What personal meanings do they assign to the decision-making process? What decision-making process will be used? Do all concerned parties understand the assessment results? The professional ethical codes (APA, 2002; NASP, 2000) tend to address the last question most directly, specifying that psychologists have the responsibility to ensure that assessment results and recommended interventions be presented in a manner conducive to the understanding of both the clients and the decision makers.

Informed Consent

DeMers (1986) has defined "informed consent" as "the receipt of specific permission to do something following a complete explanation of the nature, purpose, and potential risks involved" (p. 45). Law regulating assessment tends to be explicit about the age or competency conditions that affect who must give informed consent for assessment to occur. But the ethical guidelines regarding informed consent contain some ambiguity. The NASP ethical principles state that when a party other than the child/student initiates services, it is the responsibility of the school psychologist to make "every effort to secure voluntary participation of the child" (NASP, 2000, p. 20). DeMers, Fiorello, and Langer (1992) addressed this issue even in the assessment of preschoolers, and it becomes especially pertinent for older children and adolescents. What action is a psychologist to take when a parent gives consent for the assessment and a "mature" child does not wish the assessment to take place? Although it appears to be assumed in professional practice that parents/guardians "always" act with the best interest of their children at heart, it is realistic to assume that such is not always the case. Scholten, Pettifor, Norrie, and Cole (1993) explored some of the dilemmas faced by school practitioners in dealing with informed consent.

Invasion of Privacy

As with informed consent, the implicit assumption in law and ethical codes is that parents are to serve as their children's agents in the actualization of the children's right to privacy. Psychologists might well consider the possibility that the parents' right to determine when and under what circumstances consent is provided, and their legal right to obtain information about their children, may in reality violate the children's right to privacy. In a similar manner, obtaining information from a child even when parental consent is given may violate the privacy rights of a parent or guardian.

Exposure of Self to Others

The assessment process may be considered a "probe" that results in the exposure of self to others and hence represents a threat to the invasion of privacy. When assessment is warranted by the need for information to be used in decision making, just how much assessment information is needed may be a matter of professional judgment. A good rule of thumb may be that only the information actually needed for good decision making should be obtained in response to the referral concern or the presenting problem. This guideline, if practiced conscientiously, may result in considerably less "testing" per se. A corollary outcome might be the freeing up of some psychological service time—a scarce resource in most professional settings.

Self-Confrontation

The assessment process may result in a type of self-confrontation experience for a client—an experience that may be of positive or negative value to the client. Because it is difficult to predict how clients will experience themselves in such circumstances, it may be necessary for the psychologist to consider either possibility in any given situation. The degree of feedback to a child about the testing results should be considered in this light. To what degree should the "right to know" be tempered by the psychologist's judgment of a minor client's ability to profit from the assessment experience? Of ethical importance is that the client may have provided "informed consent" without a full understanding of the impact of the process upon the self; hence an unknown "risk" may result, even when every attempt has been made to inform the client's parent/guardian fully before obtaining consent for assessment.

Confidentiality

Parents/guardians have the legal right to obtain information about the assessment results of their minor children. Except under specific circumstances, such as suspected child abuse or the voluntary waiver of parental right, they similarly have the right to determine to whom and under what conditions these results are disseminated to others. However, in relation to the confidentiality issue as well as to other matters regarding a multiple-client system, the psychologist needs to be sensitive to the possibility of ethical violation of children's rights when the parents' legal rights are upheld. The increase in the number of separated, blended, or shared-custody families requires psychologists who work with children as their clients to be particularly attentive to the rights of the children in the process of assessment and the use of data collected. This may be particularly true in work with children whose behaviors or disorders are found more frequently in families where the biological parents have separated, are divorced, or exhibit high degrees of marital stress (Barkley, 1997). The NASP "Principles for Professional Ethics" document specially assigns school psychologists the responsibility for attempting "to resolve situations in which there are divided or conflicting interests in a manner that is mutually beneficial and protects the rights of all parties involved" (NASP, 2000, p. 17).

Even when parent–child conflict of interest is not an issue, it is good practice for the psychologist to advise the minor child of the rights of certain other persons to the results of assessment efforts. A case can be made for doing this at an early stage in the development of the assessment relationship between child and psychologist, as a corollary to the informed consent process.

The psychologist is also responsible for seeing that assessment records, including technological data management material, are maintained in a manner that will insure confidentiality (APA, 1981, 2002; NASP, 2000). The provision of confidentiality in assessment records may extend to the systematic review and possible destruction of information that is not longer appropriate, as these ethical standards also attend to this issue. Again, even when a psychologist is an employee with limited input into the policy development of the organization, the psychologist has the responsibility to seek resolution of matters that invoke professional ethical conflict (NASP, 2000).

Reporting of Results

Much of the material previously presented and discussed relates to the reporting of assessment results. Obviously, results should be reported in a manner that respects clients' right to full explanations of the nature and purpose of the techniques in language the clients can understand, unless an explicit exception to this right has been agreed upon in advance. When explanations are to be provided by others, psychologists establish procedures for insuring the adequacy of these explanations. All the major ethical standards documents state that in reporting assessment results, psychologists need to indicate any reservations that exist regarding validity or reliability because of the circumstances of the assessment or the inappropriateness of the norms for the person tested. Furthermore, technological assistance obtained in the scoring, analysis, report writing, or interpretation of test data is to be obtained only if a psychologist assumes full responsibility for the use of such aid.

Competence of Examiner

IDEA requires that a multidisciplinary team is to be used in the assessment process when educational decisions are to be made for children entitled to public educational services, but only professionally trained persons are to use assessment techniques (APA, 1981, 2002; NASP, 2000). If the assessment need is outside the scope of a psychologist's training, the psychologist is to refer the client to another professional who is competent to provide the needed service. The various ethical standards also require psycholo-

gists to keep current in the use of professional skills, including those involved in assessment.

Allocation of Limited Resources

As in bioethical cases involving medically related decision making (Kieffer, 1979), psychological assessment services most frequently involve the allocation of limited organizational resources. Agencies such as schools generally do not have an abundance of psychological services personnel; thus a psychologist's time represents financial expenditure. Within this framework, a school psychologist often has to face a decision regarding the amount of time needed to be spent conducting the psychological assessment of a child. The issue of how best to respond appropriately to a referral concern within the context of gathering sufficient valid and reliable data for decision making represents an almost daily tension for the psychologist who works in an environment where he or she does not have autonomy over the expenditure of professional time. How much information is sufficient? What is the ethical cost–benefit ratio of the expenditure of time for one client in relation to the need to serve many clients?

Possible Conflict between Law and Ethics

Psychologists in public and private practice have the responsibility of adhering to federal, state and local laws and ordinances governing their practice. If such laws are in conflict with existing ethical guidelines, both the APA (2002) and NASP (2000) ethical codes direct psychologists to proceed toward resolution of such conflict through positive, respected, and legal channels.

BEYOND CODES OF ETHICS

Although the professional guidelines for assessment appear explicit, full and careful reading of the documents reveals that more than factual determinations must be made in many instances if a psychologist is to function ethically. In the various codes and standards, the psychologist is directed to respect certain values in relation to professional practice, but no process is prescribed to aid the psychologist in the operational-ization of this value system. In order to re-solve some conflicts in values that affect professional practice, the psychologist must sometimes (perhaps often) make judgments that go beyond the explicit guidance provid-ed by codes of ethics.

Furthermore, the attentive reader of such codes will discover that certain statements in such documents appear to rely on utilitarian ethical theory: The "right" course of action in a given situation is that which results when the most "good" can be anticipated to result from the action. Other statements in the same codes of ethics appear to be deon-tological or principle-directed; that is, the rightness of a given action is independent of the consequence that results from the action. In a given real-life moral dilemma, the psy-chologist committed to acting ethically may choose different courses of action, depend-ing upon whether principle alone or antici-pated consequences from the action deter-mine the "ought" in the situation. Thus the choice of different behaviors may result in different consequences; yet each choice may be the "right" choice, given the ethical theo-ry underlying the behavior selected.

Ethical codes are limited to consensus statements that have been professionally validated by the majority of psychologists regarding certain values (Eberlein, 1987). However, the limitations involved in relying on codes of ethics alone to provide ethical direction should not result in cynicism on the part of a psychologist who is committed to acting ethically. Rather, it should be rec-ognized that a primary function of such codes is to sensitize the individual to the ethical dimensions of providing psychologi-cal services.

Self-conscious (i.e., reflective, deliberate) processing and identification of personal and professional values are prerequisites to the development of ethical reasoning skills. This process needs to begin with an ac-knowledgment that some decisions with ethical dimensions are made unknowingly. Because of a psychologist's own internaliza-tion of values developed through the early socialization and educational processes, as well as those acquired through professional education, the psychologist may often be unaware that such "decisions" have been made or how they are made.

The ethical reasoning process in the pro-fessional workplace has received increasing attention in recent years. The teaching of applied ethics in universities and profession-al schools has had a cross-disciplinary em-phasis (Hastings Center Institute, 1980), but formal training in ethical decision mak-ing has not, until fairly recently, had wide-spread emphasis in clinical and school psy-chology graduate training programs (Nagle, 1987; Tymchuk et al., 1982). The need for ethics education for psychologists became a topic of professional concern in the 1980s (Handelsman, 1986; Nagle, 1987; Stein-inger et al., 1984; Tannebaum, Greene, & Glickman 1989; Woody, 1989). Problem-solving methodologies were developed that allowed for systematic and case-specific consideration of alternative courses of ac-tion in the working through of ethical dilemmas (Keith-Spiegel & Koocher, 1985; Kitchener, 1984; Tymchuk, 1986). The de-velopment of problem-solving and decision-making skills enables psychologists to func-tion more in the present tense as they encounter ethical questions in practice.

Increasingly, it is recognized that practic-ing psychologists have the responsibility to go beyond ethical codes and more static de-cision-making models in resolving the com-plex ethical dilemmas that appear to be in-creasingly common in their professional experience (O'Neill, 1998). The legal man-dates and multiple-client systems involved in providing services to families (Curtis & Batsche, 1991; Hansen, Green, & Kutner, 1989) and in delivering various types of ed-ucationally related services (Howe & Mira-montes, 1992; Paul, Berger, Osnes, Mar-tinez, & Morse, 1997) as members of multidisciplinary teams present most school psychologists with everyday dilemmas. The professional literature of the 1990s docu-mented practitioners' need for a dynamic approach to ethical problem solving (Fiedler & Prasse, 1996; Gutkin & Rey-nolds, 1998; Jacob-Timm, 1999; Prillel-tensky, 1991; Tabachnick, Keith-Spiegel, & Pope, 1991a, 1991b), and also provided some educational resources specifically de-signed for the preservice and in-service eth-ical development of psychologists (Bersoff, 1995; Canter, Bennet, Jones, & Nagy, 1994; Jacob-Timm & Hartshorne, 1998; Plante, 1998).

The "how" of teaching ethical practice to psychologists in training, in addition to the specificity of content, is also relevant. Keith-Spiegel, Tabachnick, and Allen (1999) surveyed undergraduates in psychology to obtain their views of their professors as "ethical beings," and found them to be sensitive and negatively evaluative of many of the behaviors not discussed in the professional literature as problematic by academic psychologists. Kitchener (1992) contended that professors' ethical or unethical interactions with their own graduate students in professional psychology influence the students' ethical behavior. This includes how faculty members deal with students when students engage in unethical or unprofessional conduct. Kitchener argued that the behaviors and attitudes of faculty members serve as a type of ethical "content" for students in training. "Virtue ethics" (Jordan & Meara, 1990)—an approach to the "doing" of ethics that focuses on the characteristics of the person rather than on actions alone—may be particularly relevant when there is recognition of the effect of modeling behavior on the teaching of ethics to future professional psychologists

Booth (1996) has developed an approach to the ethical decision-making process that provides practical guidelines for situations when ethical principles are in conflict. Johnson and Corser (1998) suggested that a series of "hearings" convened by students before a mock ethics panel would provide a realistic arena for the discussion of salient ethical issues likely to be encountered by the students in their future professional practice. Case vignettes organized in response to current specific ethical standards, such as those developed by Nagy (2000), continue to represent a popular approach to the teaching of professional psychology's ethical content.

The attention to the development of ethical sensitivity and decision making for psychologists is international in scope (Booth, 1996; Oakland, Goldman & Bischoff, 1997; O'Neill, 1998). Clearly, for those psychologists who find themselves enmeshed in the natural environments of school and family as they attempt to work through the issues involving the assessment of children, the ethical challenge is continually present. Fortunately, the resources available for meeting this challenge are expanding.

NOTES

1. In *San Antonio Independent School District v. Rodriguez* (1973), the U.S. Supreme Court ruled that education is not a fundamental right for purposes of equal protection analysis. This ruling weakened the constitutional basis for challenging testing procedures. Bersoff (1979) has pointed out that federal statutes extending equal protection guarantees to the educational domain have become the more usual basis for litigation. Another U.S. Supreme Court case, *Plyler v. Doe* (1982), suggests that the right to education is protected by the equal protection clause. Under state constitutions (e.g., California's), however, education is a fundamental right, and any procedure affecting access to education is subject to strict scrutiny. Any classification that affects access to education should receive heightened attention.

2. The IDEA was formerly known as the Education for All Handicapped Children Act of 1975 (Public Law [PL] 94-142). The name of the act was changed effective October 1, 1990, by the Education for the Handicapped Act Amendments of 1990 (PL 101-476).

REFERENCES

Albemarle Paper Co. v. Moody, 422 U.S. 405 (1975).

American Educational Research Association (AERA), American Psychological Association (APA), & National Council on Measurement in Education (NCME). (1999). *Standards for educational and psychological testing.* Washington, DC: Authors.

American Psychological Association (APA). (1981). Specialty guidelines for the delivery of services by school psychologists. *American Psychologist, 36,* 670–681.

American Psychological Association (APA). (1987). *Guidelines for computer based tests and interpretations.* Washington, DC: Author.

American Psychological Association (APA). (1993). Guidelines for providers of psychological services to ethnic, linguistic, and culturally diverse populations. *American Psychologist, 48,* 45–48.

American Psychological Association (APA). (2002). Ethical principles of psychologists and code of conduct. *American Psychologist, 57,* 1060–1073.

Anrig, G. R. (1987, January). *Golden Rule:* Second thoughts. *APA Monitor,* pp. 1–3.

Barkley, R. A. (1997). Attention-deficit/hyperactivity disorder. In E. J. Mash & L. G. Terdal (Eds.), *Assessment of childhood disorders* (3rd ed., pp. 7–129). New York: Guilford Press.

Bersoff, D. N. (1979). Regarding psychologists testily: Legal regulation of psychological assessment in the public schools. *Maryland Law Review, 39,* 27–120.

Bersoff, D. N. (1981). Testing and the law. *American Psychologist, 36*, 1047–1056.

Bersoff, D. N. (1982). The legal regulation of school psychology. In C. R. Reynolds & T. B. Gutkin (Eds.), *The handbook of school psychology* (pp. 1043–1074). New York: Wiley.

Bersoff, D. N. (Ed.). (1995). *Ethical conflicts in psychology.* Washington, DC: American Psychological Association.

Booth, R. (1996). Hands up all those in favour of ethics. *Irish Journal of Psychology, 17*(2), 110–125.

Bowers v. Hardwick, 106 S.Ct. 2841 (1986).

Brown v. Board of Education, 347 U.S. 483 (1954).

Burke, M. J., & Normand, J. (1987). Computerized psychological testing: Overview and critique. *Professional Psychology: Research and Practice, 18*, 42–51.

Buss, W. (1975). What procedural due process means to a school psychologist: A dialogue. *Journal of School Psychology, 13*, 298–310.

Canter, M. G., Bennett, B. E., Jones, S. E., & Nagy, T. F. (1994). *Ethics for psychologists: A commentary on the APA ethics code.* Washington, DC: American Psychological Association.

Carey v. Population Services International Inc., 431 U.S. 678 (1977).

Civil Rights Act of 1964, § 701 et seq., 701(b) as amended, 42 U.S.C.A. § 2000 et seq., 2000e(b); U.S.C.A. Const. Amend. 14.

Cole, N. (1981). Bias in testing. *American Psychologist, 35*, 1067–1077.

Condras, J. (1980). Personal reflections on the *Larry P.* trial and its aftermath. *School Psychology Review, 9*, 154 158.

Covarrubias v. San Diego Unified School District, Civ. No. 70-394-S (S.D. Cal. filed Feb. 1971) (settled by consent decree, July 31, 1972).

Crawford v. Honig, 37 F.3d 485 (9th Cir. 1994).

Curtis, M. J., & Batsche, G. M. (1991). Meeting the needs of children and families: Opportunities and challenges for school psychology training programs. *School Psychology Review, 20*, 565–577.

Debra P. v. Turlington, 564 F. Supp. 177 (1983), aff'd, 703 F.2d 1405 (1984).

DeMers, S. T. (1986). Legal and ethical issues in child and adolescent personality assessment. In H. Knoff (Ed.), *The assessment of child and adolescent personality* (pp. 35–55). New York: Guilford Press.

DeMers, S. T., & Bersoff, D. (1985). Legal issues in school psychological practice. In J. R. Bergan (Ed.), *School psychology in contemporary society: An introduction* (pp. 319–339). Columbus, OH: Merrill.

DeMers, S. T., Fiorello, C., & Langer, K. L. (1992). Legal and ethical issues in preschool assessment. In E. V. Nuttall, I. Romero, & J. Kalesnik (Eds.) *Assessing and screening preschoolers: Psychological and educational dimensions* (pp. 43–54). Needham Heights, MA: Allyn & Bacon.

Denton, L. (1987, September). Testing panel weighs science, social factors. *APA Monitor*, p. 39.

Detroit Edison v. NLRB, 440 U.S. 301 (1979).

Diana v. State Board of Education, C.A. No. C-70-37 (N.D. Cal. July 1970) (settled by consent decree).

Eberlein, L. (1987). Introducing ethics to beginning psychologists: A problem-solving approach. *Professional Psychology: Research and Practice, 18*, 353–359.

Education for All Handicapped Children Act of 1975, PL 94-142, 20 U.S.C. § 1401 (1975).

Education for the Handicapped Act Amendments of 1990, PL 101-476, 901(a), 104 Stat. 1103, 1141–1142 (1990).

Elliott, R. (1987). *Litigating intelligence.* Dover, MA: Auburn House.

Family Educational Rights and Privacy Act of 1974, PL 93-380, 20 U.S.C. § 1232g (1974).

Fiedler, C. R., & Prasse, D. P. (1996). Legal and ethical issues in the educational assessment and programming for youth with emotional or behavioral disorders. In M. J. Breen & C. R. Fiedler (Eds.), *Behavioral approach to assessment of youth with emotional /behavioral disorders: A handbook for school-based practitioners* (pp. 23–79). Austin, TX: Pro-Ed.

Flaughter, R. L. (1978). The many definitions of test bias. *American Psychologist, 33*, 671–679.

Fowler, R. D. (1999). Test security: Protecting the integrity of tests [Editorial]. *American Psychologist, 54*, 1078.

Frederick L. v. Thomas, 419 F. Supp. 960 (E.D. Pa. 1976), aff'd on appeal, 557 F.2d 373 (1977).

Frost, R. (1939). Mending wall. In *Collected poems of Robert Frost* (pp. 47–48). New York: Halcyon House.

Galagan, J. E. (1985). Psychoeducational testing: Turn out the lights, the party's over. *Exceptional Children, 52*, 288–299.

Geisinger, K. F. (1994). Psychometric issues in testing students with disabilities. *Applied Measurement in Education, 7*, 121–140.

General Education Provisions Act, PL 90-247, 20 U.S.C. § 1232h (as amended, 1975).

Glass, G. U., & Ellwein, M. C. (1986, December). *Reform by raising test standards: Evaluation comment.* Los Angeles, CA: UCLA Center for the Study of Evaluation.

Golden Rule Ins. Co. et al. v. Washburn et al., No. 419-76 (Ill. 7th Jud. Cir. Ct. Sagamon County, settled on October 10, 1984).

Griggs v. Duke Power Co., 401 U.S. 424 (1971).

Grisso, T., & Vierling, L. (1978). Minors' consent to treatment: A developmental perspective. *Professional Psychology, 9*, 412–427.

Griswold v. Connecticut, 381 U.S. 479 (1965).

Guadalupe Organization Inc. v. Tempe Elementary School District No. 3, 587 F.2d 1022 (9th Cir. 1972).

Guardians Association of New York City v. Civil Service Commission, 630 F.2d 79 (2d Cir. 1980), cert. denied, 49 U.S.L.W. 3932 (June 15, 1981).

Gutkin, T. B., & Reynolds, C. R. (Eds.). (1998). *The handbook of school psychology* (3rd ed.). New York: Wiley.

Handelsman, M. M. (1986). Problems with ethics training by "osmosis." *Professional Psychology: Research and Practice, 17,* 371–372.

Hansen, J. C., Green, S., & Kutner, K. B. (1989). Ethical isues facing school psychologists working with families. *Professional School Psychology, 4,* 245–255.

Hastings Center Institute of Society, Ethics, and the

Life Sciences. (1980). *The teaching of ethics in higher education.* Hastings-on-Hudson, NY: Author.

Hobson v. Hanson, 269 F. Supp. 401 (D.C. 1967).

Howe, K. R., & Miramontes, O. B. (1992). *The ethics of special education.* New York: Teachers College Press.

Individuals with Disabilities Education Act (IDEA), PL 105-17, § 614, 11 Stat. 81 (1997).

Jacob-Timm, S. (1999). Ethically challenging situations encountered by school psychologists. *Psychology in the Schools, 36,* 205–217.

Jacob-Timm, S., & Hartshorne, T. S. (1998). *Ethics and law for school psychologists* (3rd ed.). New York: Wiley.

John K. and Mary K. v. Board of Education for School District #65, Cook County, 504 N.E. 2d 797 (Ill. App. 1 Dist. 1987).

Johnson, W. B., & Corser, R. (1998). Learning ethics the hard way: Facing the ethics committee. *Teaching of Psychology, 25,* 26–28.

Jordan, A. E., & Meara, N. M. (1990). Ethics and the professional practice of psychologists: The role of virtues and principles. *Professional Psychology: Research and Practice, 21,* 107–114.

Joint Committee on Testing Practices. (1996). *The rights and responsibilities of test takers.* Washington, DC: American Psychological Association.

Keith-Spiegel, P., & Koocher, G. P. (1985). *Ethics in psychology: Professional standards and cases.* New York: Random House.

Keith-Spiegel, P. C., Tabachnick, B. G., & Allen, M. (1999). Ethics in academia: Students' views of professors' actions. In D. N. Bersoff (Ed.), *Ethical conflicts in psychology* (pp. 465–471). Washington, DC: American Psychological Association.

Kemerer, F. R., & Deutsch, K. L. (1979). *Constitutional rights and student life.* St. Paul, MN: West.

Kieffer, G. H. (1979). *Bioethics: A textbook of issues.* Reading, MA: Addison-Wesley.

Kitchener, K. S. (1984). Intuition, critical evaluation, and ethical principles: The foundation for ethical decisions in counseling psychology. *The Counseling Psychologist, 12,* 43–55.

Kitchener, K. S. (1992). Psychology as teacher and mentor: Affirming ethical values throughout the curriculum. *Professional Psychology: Research and Practice, 23,* 190–195.

Lambert, N. (1981). Psychological evidence in *Larry P. v. Wilson Riles:* An evaluation by a witness for the defense. *American Psychologist, 36,* 937–952.

Landers, S. (1986, December). Judge reiterates I.Q. test ban. *APA Monitor,* p. 12.

Larry P. v. Riles, 343 F. Supp. 1306 (N.D. Cal. 1972) (order granting preliminary injunction), aff'd, 502 F.2d 963 (9th Cir. 1974), 495 F. Supp. 926 (N. D. Cal. 1979) (decision on merits), aff'd, No. 80-427 (9th Cir. Jan. 23, 1984), No. C-71-2270 RFP (Sept. 25, 1986) (order modifying judgment), 793 f.2d 969 (9th Cir 1994).

Lau v. Nichols, 414 U.S. 563 (1974).

Lerner, B. (1978). The Supreme Court and the APA, AERA, NCME test standards: Past references and future possibilities. *American Psychologist, 33,* 915–919.

Lerner, B. (1981). The minimum competency testing movement: Social, scientific and legal implications. *American Psychologist, 36,* 1057–1066.

Lora v. Board of Education of City of New York, 456 F. Supp. 1211, 1227 (E.D. N.Y. 1978).

Luke S. v. Nix, Civil Action No. 81-1331 (E.D. La. 1981).

Marshall v. Georgia, No. CV 482-233 (S.D. Ga. 1984).

Martin, R. P. (1986, February). Ethics column. *The School Psychologist,* pp. 1, 7.

McDermott, P. (1972). Law, liability, and the school psychologist: Malpractice and liability. *Journal of School Psychology, 10,* 397–407.

Melton, G. B., Koocher, G. P., & Saks, M. J. (Eds.). (1983). *Children's competence to consent.* New York: Plenum Press.

Messick, S. (1975). The standard problem: Meaning and values in measurement and evaluation. *American Psychologist, 30,* 955–966.

Messick, S. (1995). Validity of psychological assessment. *American Psychologist, 50,* 741–749.

Nagle, R. J. (1987). Ethics training in school psychology. *Professional School Psychology, 2,* 163–171.

Nagy, T. F. (2000). *Ethics in plain English: An illustrative casebook for psychologists.* Washington, DC: American Psychological Association.

National Association of School Psychologists (NASP). (1985). *Professional conduct manual.* Washington, DC: Author.

National Association of School Psychologists (NASP). (2000). *Professional conduct manual.* Bethesda, MD: Author.

Oakland, T., Goldman, S., & Bischoff, H. (1997). Code of ethics of the International School Psychology Association. *School Psychology International, 18,* 291–298.

O'Neill, P. (1998). Teaching ethics: The utility of the CPA code. *Canadian Psychology, 39,* 194–201.

Paul, J. L., Berger, N. H., Osnes, P. G., Martinez, Y. G., & Morse, W. C. (Eds.). (1997). *Ethics and decision making in local schools: Inclusion, policy, and reform.* Baltimore: Brookes.

PASE v. Hannon, 506 F. Supp. 831 (N.D. Ill. 1980).

Petersen, N. S., & Novick, M. R. (1976). An evaluation of some models for culture-fair selection. *Journal of Educational Measurement, 13,* 3–29.

Phillis P. v. Clairmont Unified School District, 183 Cal. App. 3d 1193 (1986).

Plante, T. G. (1998). Teaching a course on psychology ethics to undergraduates: An experiential model. *Teaching of Psychology, 25,* 286–287.

Plyler v. Doe, 457 U.S. 202, 102 S. Ct. 2382 (1982).

Prasse, D. P. (1984). School psychology and the law. In J. E. Ysseldyke (Ed.), *School psychology: The state of the art* (pp. 245–278). Minneapolis: National School Psychology Inservice Training Network, University of Minnesota.

Pratt, S. I., & Moreland, K. L. (1998). Individuals with other characteristics. In J. Sandoval, C. L. Frisby, K. F. Geisinger, J. D. Scheuneman, & J. R. Grenier (Eds.), *Test interpretation and diversity* (pp. 349–271). Washington, DC: American Psychological Association.

Prilleltensky, I. (1991). The social ethics of school psychology: A priority for the 1990's. *School Psychology Quarterly, 6,* 200–222.

Pryzwansky, W., & Bersoff, D. (1978). Parental consent for psychological evaluations: Legal, ethical and practical considerations. *Journal of School Psychology, 16*, 274–281.

Rehabilitation Act of 1973, Section 504, 29 U.S.C. § 794 (1973).

Reschly, D. J., Kicklighter, R., & McKee, P. (1988a). Recent placement litigation, Part I: Regular education grouping comparison of *Marshall* (1984, 1985) and *Hobson* (1967, 1969). *School Psychology Review, 17*, 9–21.

Reschly, D. J., Kicklighter, R., & McKee, P. (1988b). Recent placement litigation, Part II: Minority EMR overrepresentation: Comparison of *Larry P.* (1979, 1984, 1986) with *Marshall* (1984, 1985) and *S-1* (1986). *School Psychology Review, 17*, 22–38.

Reschly, D. J., Kicklighter, R., & McKee, P. (1988c). Recent placement litigation, Part III: Analysis of differences in *Larry P., Marshall,* and *S-1* and implications for future practices. *School Psychology Review, 17*, 39–50.

Reutter, E. E. (1985). *The law of public education* (3rd ed.). Mineola, NY: Foundation Press.

Reynolds, C. R., & Kaiser, S. M. (1990). Bias in assessment of aptitude. In C. R. Reynolds & R. W. Kamphaus (Eds.), *Handbook of psychological and educational assessment of children: Intelligence and achievement* (pp. 611–653). New York: Guilford Press.

Rooney, J. P. (1987). Golden Rule on "Golden Rule." *Educational Measurement: Issues and Practice, 6*(2), 9–12.

S-1 v. Turlington, No. 79-8020-Civ-CA QPB (S.D. Fla. June 15, 1979) (order granting preliminary injunction), aff'd, 635 F.2d 342 (5th Cir. 1981).

San Antonio Independent School District v. Rodriguez, 411 U.S. 1, 28 (1973).

Sattler, J. R. (1981). Intelligence tests on trial: An interview with judges Robert F. Peckham and John F. Brady. *Journal of School Psychology, 19*, 359–369.

Sattler, J. R. (1982). The psychologist in court: Personal reflections of one expert witness in the case of *Larry P. et al. v. Wilson Riles et al. School Psychology Review, 11*, 306–318.

Schmidt, P. (2000, January 10). Texas test required for high-school graduation does not discriminate, judge rules. *The Chronicle of Higher Education,* p. 2.

Scholten, T., Pettifor, J., Norrie, B., & Cole, E. (1993). Ethical issues in school psychological consultation: Can every expert consult? *Canadian Journal of School Psychology, 9*, 100–109.

Smith, J. D., & Jenkins, D. S. (1980). Minimum competency testing and handicapped students. *Exceptional Children, 46*, 440–443.

Spitzzeri, A. A. (1987, January). Court upholds releasing raw test data. *NASP Communique,* p. 5.

Steininger, M., Newell, J. D., & Garcia, L. T. (1984). *Ethical issues in psychology.* Homewood, IL: Dorsey Press.

Stell v. Savannah–Chatham County Board of Education, 255 F. Supp. 83 (S.D. Ga. 1965).

Tabachnick, B. G., Keith-Spiegel, P., & Pope, K. S. (1991a). Ethics of teaching: Beliefs and behaviors of psychologists as educators. *American Psychologist, 46*, 506–515.

Tabachnick, B. G., Keith-Spiegel, P., & Pope, K. S. (1991b). Ethics of teaching: Beliefs and behaviors of psychologists as educators. *American Psychologist, 46*, 802–809.

Tannenbaum, S. I., Greene, V. J., & Glickman, A. S. (1989). The ethical reasoning process in an organizational consulting situation. *Professional Psychology: Research and Practice, 20*, 229–235.

Taylor, J. M., Tucker, J. A., & Galagan, J. E. (1986). The *Luke S.* class action suit: A lesson in system change. *Exceptional Children, 52*, 376–382.

Telzrow, C. F. (1999). IDEA amendments of 1997: Promise or pitfall for special education reform? *Journal of School Psychology, 37*, 7–28.

Tillery, W. L., & Carfioli, J. C. (1986). *Frederick L.*: A review of the litigation in context. *Exceptional Children, 52*, 367–375.

Tymchuk, A. J. (1986). Guidelines for ethical decision making. *Canadian Psychology, 27*, 36–43.

Tymchuk, A. J., Drapkin, R., Major-Kingsley, S., Ackerman, A. B., Coffinan, E. W., & Baum, M. S. (1982). Ethical decision making and psychologists' attitudes toward training in ethics. *Professional Psychology, 13*, 412–421.

United States v. Chesterfield County School District, 484 F.2d 70 (4th Cir. 1973).

Walker, N. W., & Myrick, C. C. (1985). Ethical considerations in the use of computers in psychological testing and assessment. *Journal of School Psychology, 23*, 51–57.

Washington v. Davis, 426 U.S. 229 (1976).

Wood, F. H., Johnson, J. L., & Jenkins, J. R. (1986). The *Lora* case: Nonbiased referral, assessment, and placement procedures. *Exceptional Children, 52*, 323–331.

Woody, R. H. (1989). Public policy, ethics, government, and law. *Professional School Psychology, 4*, 75–83.

Ysseldyke, J. E., & Algozzine, B. (1982). *Critical issues in special and remedial education.* Boston: Houghton Mifflin.

4

Measurement and Design Issues in Child Assessment Research

TIMOTHY Z. KEITH
CECIL R. REYNOLDS

Both the content and the quality of published child assessment research are diverse. Investigators in this field conduct research on instruments as diverse as projective personality measures, intelligence tests, and rating scales. And this research ranges from the simple correlation of one measure with another to sophisticated investigations of the relation between evoked cortical potentials and measured intelligence. Given the diversity in assessment research, it may seem fruitless to attempt to survey the body of research and come up with recommendations. Nevertheless, there do seem to be a number of problems common to much assessment research; several of these are discussed briefly below.

This chapter first focuses on needs in the design of child assessment research, such as the need for consistency between research design and available theory. We then briefly skim over the normal basics of measurement research—reliability and validity—so that we can concentrate on several other topics in more depth. In particular, we discuss several complex research methods that are becoming increasingly common in assessment research (e.g., exploratory and confirmatory factor analysis, multiple regression analysis,

and structural equation modeling), and we discuss one productive avenue of assessment research (test bias methods).

PROBLEMS AND NEEDS IN CHILD ASSESSMENT RESEARCH

Consistency with Theory

All too frequently, child assessment research seems to pay little attention to relevant theory. Consider the following hypothetical, but realistic, examples.

1. Researchers administer several measures each of achievement and intelligence, and then use multiple regression analysis to predict each measure from the others.
2. Researchers discover mean score ethnic group differences on a new test of intelligence (or achievement); they conclude that the test may be biased.

The common difficulty with these two studies is the unclear role of theory in the development of the research problem and interpretation of the results. In the first example, the researchers have essentially predicted everything from everything, a confusing process that quickly will become unmanageable. It is as if the researchers cannot decide which variable—achievement or intelligence—is the "cause" and which is the "effect." Yet a cursory glance at available theories of learning (e.g., Carroll, 1963; Walberg, 1981) suggests that intelligence should only be used to predict achievement, not the reverse.

This example also illustrates some of the frustrations and problems in assessment research. Much of this research is nonexperimental in nature. There is no active manipulation of an independent variable, after which change in the dependent variable can be measured. Rather, each variable—achievement and intelligence—is measured, with the researchers deciding which is the independent (cause) and which is the dependent variable (effect). As noted elsewhere (e.g., Keith, 1999), theory is especially important for the valid analysis of nonexperimental research. Even so, when researchers are seeking *causal* explanations of observed relations, caution is necessary even in the face of a theory with strong intuitive appeal. Reynolds (1999) has discussed this issue and provided examples of false leads in both recent and remote literature.

The second example (test bias research) is almost atheoretical. Theories of intelligence and achievement consistently acknowledge the importance of home environment for the development of skills. It is also well known that there are unfortunate differences in the environments of U.S. ethnic groups. If home environment affects these skills, and if there are differences in the home environments of different groups, then group intelligence or achievement differences should not be surprising. Indeed, this is one reason why the mean-score definition of test bias is almost universally rejected (cf. Kamphaus, 2001, p. 153).

Assessment research should also be consistent with—or at least consider—basic measurement theory (and statistical reality). Consider the following two examples.

1. A new intelligence test is administered to a group of students who were classified as gifted, in part because of their scores on another commonly used intelligence scale. The new scale produces lower scores, on average, than did the previous measure.

2. An achievement test is administered to the same group; its correlation with the intelligence test, although statistically significant, is of only moderate magnitude, and is considerably less than with normal samples.

Given these results (and they are to be expected), many readers and too many researchers would conclude that caution is warranted in using and interpreting the new intelligence scale, but this conclusion might well be completely erroneous. (A quick perusal of validity research with almost any new test following its introduction would show that neither of these examples is unusual.) Such a conclusion is not warranted because similar results would be expected on purely statistical grounds. In the first example, we would expect the group to score lower on the second test as a result of regression to the mean. Any group that is discrepant from the mean will probably score closer to the mean upon the administration of a second test. It matters little whether the same test is administered twice or whether two different tests are administered (although we would expect to see less change if one test were administered twice). Regression to the mean occurs; it is a statistical fact, and one that *must* be recognized in research of this type. The degree of change from one administration to the next depends primarily on the correlation between the two measures (which in turn depends on the reliability of measurement, the stability of the trait being measured, and the time lapse between measures; cf. Linn, 1980, and Roberts, 1980) and the degree of discrepancy from the mean.

In the second example, we would also expect a lower correlation between the two tests, simply because of the reduction in variance resulting from using a selected group (in this case, gifted students). There is less variation (i.e., lower variance and standard deviation) in the selected group, and since the correlation between the two measures depends in part on the degree of variation, it too is lowered. Indeed, Linn (1983) has shown how a substantial positive correlation between two tests can become a large negative correlation simply as a result of a preselected sample and restricted range!

Researchers who conduct research with such discrepant groups must be aware when statistical phenomena such as regression to the mean and restriction of range are operating, and must take those phenomena into account when interpreting results.

Consistency with Practice

Assessment research should be more consistent with normal assessment practice. It is not unusual to see research in which a criterion such as achievement is predicted from a variety of other measures. For example, stepwise multiple regression analysis might be used to predict teacher ratings of achievement from the subtest scores of an intelligence test and an achievement test. In such an analysis, the first variable to enter the equation would probably be one of the achievement subtests, followed by whichever measure correlated well with the criterion but was least redundant with the first-loading subtest; a nonverbal intelligence subtest would be a likely candidate. The end result would be a hodge-podge of achievement and intelligence subtests predicting teacher ratings. Such research is often conducted to provide information about the validity of one of the instruments being used, but it is debatable whether the research as outlined provides that information.

The question addressed by such research is this: Which subset of the two tests used can best predict teacher ratings of achievement? Unfortunately, this research bears little resemblance to normal practice, and therefore tells us little beyond the efficiency of group prediction (we discuss additional objections later). Few psychologists use bits and pieces of instruments in their assessment. School psychologists, for example, commonly administer standardized tests of intelligence and achievement to children who are referred for school problems; they then combine that information with observations, background information, and interview information before making a prediction about a child's future performance. If the goal in the present example is to learn something about the validity of the achievement test in this process, a better approach might be to use hierarchical multiple regres-

sion analysis (discussed later) to determine whether the achievement measure improves the prediction of ratings above that accomplished by the intelligence measure alone. This approach is slightly more consistent with practice than is the initial stepwise approach. Even so, there are inconsistencies of which readers and researchers alike should be aware: The regression approach seeks to *reduce* redundancy among measures, whereas redundancy is often *desired* in actual assessment practice (Keith, 1987, p. 284). Nevertheless, other things being equal, when assessment research is consistent with normal practice, it will inform such practice more than when it is not. Phillips's (1999) research-in-action approach has much to offer academics and practitioners alike in this arena.

Hypothesis Testing

Another area of need in much assessment research is the use of a hypothesis-testing approach. As an example, researchers might administer a new intelligence test to a sample of 50 children, along with commonly used measures of intelligence and achievement, in an effort to investigate the validity of the new scale. In a normal population, all of the correlations among these instruments would probably be significant, and all too often the researchers would conclude with some vague statements about the research's supporting the validity of the new scale.

A central problem with this type of research is that no real hypothesis is being tested. Simply reporting the significance of correlations does little to inform decisions about validity. Yet a very salient hypothesis could be tested: whether this new scale measures intelligence rather than simply academic achievement. Since correlations can be computed between the new scale and both an existing intelligence test and an existing achievement test, the researchers could easily compare the two correlations. If the intelligence–intelligence correlation were significantly higher than the intelligence–achievement correlation, the researchers would have better evidence of the validity of the new intelligence scale. Such research might be particularly salient when there is debate concerning what the new scale in fact measures (for more information concerning hypothesis testing in corre-lational analysis, see Lindeman, Meranda, & Gold, 1980, pp. 49–54).

The problem of no testable hypothesis is not necessarily a function of the type of analysis being performed. Sophisticated factor analyses can suffer from the same faults. A joint factor analysis of the Wechsler Intelligence Scale for Children—Third Edition (WISC-III), the Kaufman Adolescent and Adult Intelligence Test (KAIT), and the Wechsler Individual Achievement Test—Second Edition (WIAT-II) would tell us little if interpreted in the usual fashion (i.e., performing the analysis and naming factors), because without a specific purpose it makes little sense to factor-analyze intelligence and achievement tests in combination. On the other hand, if we were testing whether the WISC-III Verbal tests were better measures of achievement or intelligence, such an analysis might be very useful (cf. Keith, 1997).

It is easier to draw meaningful conclusions from research results when that research has tested *specific hypotheses* or research questions. And this seemingly obvious statement applies to assessment research just as it does other types of research. For this reason, Landy (1986) argued that the traditional validity "trinity"—content, concurrent, and construct validity—be replaced with a general hypothesis-testing approach. We also argue for that approach, or, alternatively, for a research question approach (e.g., "What are we assessing? Why are we assessing it?"). In line with current psychometric thought that all validity is a subset of construct validity, using a carefully constructed research question approach may well lead to more and empirically validated applications of tests as well.

RESEARCH METHODOLOGIES

The Basics of Assessment Research

Reliability

"Reliability" of measurement refers to the accuracy, reproducibility, or constancy of a test score derived from some specified device. If one gave the same test over and over (with no effects from the repeated testing), would the results be the same each time? To what degree would the results of the assessments differ? Although various methods are used to estimate reliability, all attempt to address this essential question. The topic of reliability is well covered in most introductory assessment texts, and only a few salient points are made here.

If reliability can be considered constancy of measurement from a conceptual level, at a theoretical level it is defined as the square of the correlation of obtained scores with true scores (Kenny, 1979, Ch. 5; Kerlinger & Lee, 2000, Ch. 27). Of course we never know the true scores, so the best we can do is to *estimate* the reliability of a test. We do so through a variety of methods—correlating alternate forms of a test, or correlating odd with even items—but in each case we are attempting to estimate the same basic construct: the extent to which obtained scores correspond with true scores.

Each method of estimating reliability does so slightly differently, and as a result is also confounded with other information. Test–retest reliability estimation is a function both of the reliability of the test *and* of the stability of the construct being measured, for example, and these confounding factors should be considered when one is evaluating the adequacy of a reliability coefficient.

The need for reliable assessment devices is universal across types of measurement. It is just as important to establish the reliability of observational, curriculum-based, performance, and personality assessments as it is to establish the reliability of normative achievement tests. Furthermore, although the methods of calculating reliability may differ for different types of assessment, most still fit within the traditional triad (internal-consistency, test–retest, and alternate-forms).

Finally, it is worth reiterating that all we can do is to *estimate* the reliability of scores of a test with a particular sample, at a particular time. Despite common usage to the contrary, it is not the test that is reliable, but a particular set of scores that may or may not be reliable (Thompson & Vacha-Haase, 2000).

Validity

All readers are no doubt familiar with the traditional categorizations of validity: content, criterion-related (including concurrent and predictive), and construct validity. More recent views note the unitary nature of validity, and the focus on validity as support for inferences about test scores: "an integrated evaluative judgment of the degree to which empirical evidence and theoretical rationales support the *adequacy* and *appropriateness* of *inferences* and *actions* based on test scores or other modes of assessment (Messick, 1989, p. 13; emphasis in original).

Only recently have test manuals begun to discuss the validity of test score interpretations in line with these newer views of validity as a more fluid psychometric construct (e.g., Reynolds, 2002; Woodcock, McGrew, & Mather, 2001). Like reliability, these topics are well covered in most basic tests, and only a few points are made here. For a detailed review of history and current thinking about validity, see Kane (2001).

Variance Definitions of Reliability and Validity

Classical test theory's variance definition of reliability and validity is useful for understanding these two constructs and the relation between them. Briefly, a person's score on a test is a product of two things: that person's true (but unknown) score, and error. Similarly, the variance in a set of scores is a function of true-score variance (V_t) and error variance (V_e):

$$V = V_t + V_e$$

This relation is displayed pictorially in Figure 4.1. According to this definition, reliability is simply the proportion of true-score variance (V_t) to total variance (V). If a test is error-laden, it is unreliable. Conversely, if scores on a test are primarily the result of the test takers' *true* scores, those scores are relatively reliable.

The true-score variance, a reflection of the reliability of the test, may also be subdivided. Suppose we administer several measures of reading comprehension. One measure requires a child to read a passage and point to a picture that describes the passage read; one requires the child to fill in a blank with a missing word; and the third requires the child to act out a sentence or passage (e.g., "Stick out your tongue"). Each method mea-

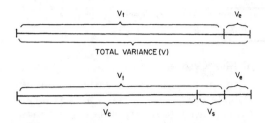

FIGURE 4.1. Variance definitions of reliability and validity. Variance in test scores may be due to true-score variation (V_t) or error variance (V_e). True-score variation may be further divided into common variance (V_c) and specific or unique variance (V_s), as in the bottom half of the figure. Reliability is a function of V_t; validity is a function of V_c.

sures reading comprehension, and may do so very reliably. But each method also measures something else in addition to reading comprehension. In the first case, the child has to comprehend the passage, but also has to be able to recognize and interpret a picture depicting that passage; in the third measure, we are also requiring the child to be able to translate the passage into action. In other words, each method measures reading comprehension, but each also measures something *specific* or unique to that measure, although both components may be measured reliably. Of course, the degree to which each test measures reading comprehension is the "validity" of that test. In Figure 4.1, we can further divide the V_t (reliability) into the variance each measure shares with the other (V_c, or common variance—in this example, representing reading comprehension), and the variance that is specific to the test (V_s, representing pictorial understanding, etc.). As is the case with reliability, the validity of the test may be thought of as the proportion of common variance to total variance (V_c/V). The relation of validity to reliability is clear with this definition; we may consider validity as simply a subset of reliability. This, then, is the reason for the rule learned (and often confused) by students of measurement: A test cannot be valid unless it is reliable (or "all valid tests are reliable; unreliable tests are not valid; and reliable tests may or may not be valid"—Salvia & Ysseldyke, 2001, p. 155). For a more complete discussion of these issues, refer to Guilford (1954), Keith (in preparation), or Kerlinger and Lee (2000, Chs. 27, 28).

Factor Analysis

Factor analysis is an increasingly common tool in assessment research. Thirty years ago it was unusual to see reports of factor analyses in the research literature, but now they are almost commonplace. The introduction of new intelligence tests and other theory-derived measures are generally greeted by a flurry of factor analyses to determine whether the tests measure what they are designed to measure. The use of factor analysis to create composite variables (e.g., from several survey items) is also becoming more commonplace (cf. Keith & Cool, 1992).

Factor analysis is useful because it can help answer the central question of validity—what it is that we are measuring. There are two primary types of factor analysis. Exploratory factor analysis is more common, but confirmatory factor analysis, a newer and much more theory-bound approach, has also become an important tool in assessment research.

Exploratory Factor Analysis

Mathematically, exploratory factor analysis is nothing more than a reduction technique; it reduces many measures into few. It does so by grouping together those measures or scales that correlate highly with each other, and by grouping them separately from tests with which they do not correlate. Essentially, factor analysis is an efficient method of establishing convergent and discriminant validity.

Psychologically, we believe that factor analysis helps establish what it is that those various scales measure, or the underlying "traits" or skills that result in the scores we get when we administer the tests. The primary reason why two scales correlate highly is that they measure the same thing (or they measure two variables that are influenced by some common third variable). And if those two scales do not correlate well with two other tests, a primary reason is that they measure something fundamentally different, especially if all four scales are measured using similar methods. Tests that measure something in common form a factor in a factor analysis; tests that measure something different form a separate factor.

An Informal Analysis

Table 4.1 shows a hypothetical correlation matrix for six tests, including three reading and three mathematics tests. The correlations are made up, and are for illustration only; correlation matrices are never this neat. An inspection of the matrix shows that the three reading tests correlate highly with each other (in the .553–.631 range), and that the three arithmetic tests correlate highly with each other (.548–.620), but that the reading tests do not correlate well with the arithmetic tests (.000–.176). We have in essence two clusters of tests, reading and arithmetic, and this "eyeball factor analysis" can serve as the conceptual basis for understanding factor analysis. Factor analysis does something like this eyeball analysis, but efficiently and mathematically.

A Primer on How to Conduct a Factor Analysis

In practice, factor analysis is conducted using computers, and there are many pro-

TABLE 4.1. Hypothetical Correlations among Six Reading and Mathematics Tests

Test	1	2	3	4	5	6
1. Mathematics Reasoning	1.000					
2. Arithmetic Computation 1	**.620**	1.000				
3. Arithmetic Computation 2	**.588**	**.548**	1.000			
4. Reading Comprehension 1	.158	.098	.057	1.000		
5. Reading Comprehension 2	.176	.113	.070	*.631*	1.000	
6. Reading Recognition	.087	.035	.000	*.553*	*.574*	1.000

Note. The Arithmetic "factor" is in **boldface**, whereas the Reading "factor" is in *bold italics*.

grams available to do a variety of types of factor analyses. The correlation matrix shown in Table 4.1 was used as the input for a factor analysis conducted with the Statistical Package for the Social Sciences (SPSS) subprogram Factor. A number of choices are required in using this or other such programs. The first choice is the type of analysis to be conducted. Here we have used principal-factors analysis (PFA, also known as principal-axis factoring), probably the most common technique. The essential features of PFA may be illustrated by contrasting it with another common procedure, principal-components analysis (PCA). Although these two procedures often produce similar results, they are conceptually very different. PCA analyzes all the variance in the set of scores (or V from Figure 4.1), whereas PFA endeavors to analyze only the variance that is common among the measures (V_c in Figure 4.1). To accomplish these ends, PCA performs the analysis on the correlation matrix. PFA also begins with the correlation matrix, but substitutes an initial estimate of the common variance, squared multiple correlations (the square of the multiple correlation obtained when each measure in the factor analysis is predicted from all other measures) in the diagonal of the correlation matrix, rather than the 1.00's normally there. In other words, each measure in the PFA is predicted from all other measures, and the square of the multiple-correlation coefficient is used as the initial estimate of the common variance, or communality. The square of the multiple-correlation coefficient predicting math reasoning from arithmetic computation 1 and 2, reading comprehension 1 and 2, and reading recognition ($R^2 = .485$) would be inserted in place of 1.00 in the top left (row 1, column 1) of Table 4.1. These values are used as initial estimates, and the program then gradually improves these estimates through a series of iterations. Thus articles discussing PFA will often note parenthetically "communalities estimated by squared multiple correlation" or "R^2 in the diagonal," and those using PCA will note "1.00's in the diagonal."

How many factors? Once a factor method has been chosen, the next choice required is the number of factors to be retained in the factor analysis. Remember that the mathematical purpose of factor analysis is to reduce many things into a few, so some reduction is necessary. But how much reduction? There are no hard-and-fast rules, and therefore the process is a mixture of habit, subjectivity, and judgment. Probably the most common method is to retain factors with eigenvalues greater than 1.00. An eigenvalue may be thought of as an indication of the size of (variance accounted for by) a factor, and these are computed as an initial step in the factor analysis. Factors with eigenvalues of less than 1.00 are generally considered trivial, and, in this approach, are not analyzed. For the data presented in Table 4.1, the first three eigenvalues were 2.45, 1.91, and 0.46; if we were using the eigenvalue criterion, we would retain only two factors in the factor analysis.

Another common technique for determining the number of factors to retain is the scree test (Cattell, 1966), in which the eigenvalues are plotted and the decision about how many factors to retain is based on changes in the slope of the line drawn through the eigenvalues; this graph is then referred to as a "scree plot" (for more information, see Cattell, 1966; Kim & Mueller, 1978). It is also common for researchers to decide in advance, based on theory, how many factors to retain. In the present example, it would be perfectly reasonable to decide to retain only two factors, believing that one should represent reading and the other mathematics. Finally, it is common to combine these and other methods of deciding how many factors to retain, or to compare several approaches and use the one whose results make the most "psychological sense."

Factor rotation. The factor analyst also needs to choose a technique for rotating the factors, because the initial results of the factor analysis, without rotation, are often uninterruptible. Table 4.2 shows the initial results of a factor analysis of the six reading and arithmetic tests from the correlation matrix in Table 4.1. We have used PFA (communalities estimated by squared multiple correlations) and retained two factors. The "factor loadings" are shown in Table 4.2, and they represent the correlations of each test with the two hypothetical factors.

TABLE 4.2. Unrotated Factor Loadings of Six Reading and Mathematics Tests

Test	Factor 1	Factor 2
1. Mathematics Reasoning	.658	.489
2. Arithmetic Computation 1	.569	.502
3. Arithmetic Computation 2	.511	.514
4. Reading Comprehension 1	.605	−.491
5. Reading Comprehension 2	.638	−.498
6. Reading Recognition	.506	−.504

An examination of the factor loadings helps us name the factors, because it helps us understand the trait, skill, or characteristic measured by each factor. But the results shown in Table 4.2 do not provide much illumination; all of the tests load highly on the first factor, and there is a mixture of high positive and high negative loadings on factor 2.

Suppose, however, we plot the factor loadings shown in Table 4.2, using the two values for each test as points on x and y axes, with the axes representing the two factors. This has been done in Figure 4.2. The x axis represents factor 1, and the y axis factor 2. The point shown for test 1 (Math Reasoning), then, represents a value of .658 on factor 1 (x) and .489 on factor 2 (y). With this graphic representation of factors, two clusters of tests again become evident. And since the placement of the axes is arbitrary, we are free, now that we have the points plotted, to *rotate* the axes to make the factors more interpretable. In the bottom of Figure 4.2, we have simply rotated the x and y axes a few degrees clockwise— the old axes are shown as a dotted line, the new axes as solid lines. With this rotation, we see that factor 1 is primarily related to tests 4, 5, and 6, and factor 2 to tests 1, 2, and 3. And with the rotated axes, the factor loadings also become more interpretable. With rotation, the reading tests (4–6) load highly on factor 1, and the arithmetic tests (1–3) load highly on factor 2 (the rotated factor loadings are shown in Table 4.3).

There are, of course, different methods available for rotation. The graphic method used in this example is one method, but it is difficult when the factors are not so clear-cut and when there are more than two factors. It is also too disconcertingly subjective

for many researchers (although it is less subjective than presented here; cf. Carroll, 1985, 1993; Harman, 1976; Thurstone, 1947). Analytic methods are therefore more common. Orthogonal rotation techniques (e.g., varimax) are quite common; they simply specify that the factors are uncorrelated, or, graphically, that the factors are perpendicular (90° apart, as in Figure 4.2). Oblique rotations, allowing the factors to be correlated, are more common among British researchers (e.g., Eysenck, 1979).

Oblique rotations are probably more theoretically defensible when we are analyzing things like intelligence tests, because we know that the different components of intel-

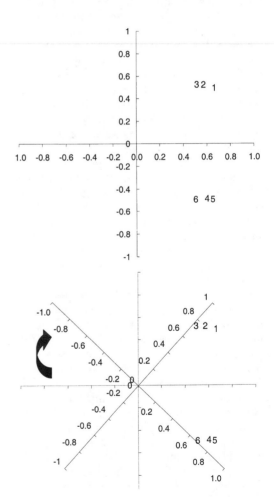

FIGURE 4.2. The unrotated factor solution of six hypothetical reading and arithmetic tests (top). In the bottom half of the figure, the reference axes were rotated 42° clockwise to allow easier interpretation of the factors.

TABLE 4.3. Rotated Factor Loadings for the Six Reading and Mathematics Tests

Test	Factor 1	Factor 2
1. Mathematics Reasoning	.123	.810
2. Arithmetic Computation 1	.051	.757
3. Arithmetic Computation 2	.001	.725
4. Reading Comprehension 1	.775	.078
5. Reading Comprehension 2	.804	.095
6. Reading Recognition	.714	−.001

ligence (e.g., verbal and nonverbal intelligence) are correlated (because they both also measure general intelligence), but orthogonal rotations are generally easier to interpret. They are also often more useful clinically, since they maximize the distinctions that can be made among theoretically related constructs. Nevertheless, in our experience, the two types of rotations often yield similar results. Of course, if a *hierarchical* factor analysis is desired (a factor analysis of factors), then the rotation should be oblique because it is the correlations among factors that are used as the input for the second-order factor analysis. Indeed, it is generally recognized that g, or general intelligence, is best conceived as a higher-order factor resulting from oblique rotation of first- or higher-order factors (Carroll, 1993).

Interpretation. Choosing a factoring method, the number of factors, and the rotation method will produce a unique solution for a given set of data. And then comes the hard, but subjective and enjoyable, part: interpreting and naming the factors. Factors are named according to the tests that load highly on them; based on what we know about the tests themselves (what they measure), we can infer something about the factors. If three tests that measure crystallized intelligence load on the same factor, then that factor may well be a crystallized-intelligence factor. With our reading–arithmetic example, this is an easy process. We have three reading tests on one factor, and three math tests on another; Reading Achievement and Math Achievement are obvious names for the factors.

In practice, of course, things are never this easy. Tests generally measure a number

of different skills. And the factors are never as clean as shown in this example; rather, some loadings on a factor may be large, others moderate, and still others small. The job of the factor analyst is to try to consider all the possible skills or abilities that those tests constituting a factor have in common, and contrast those to the skills shared by tests that do not load on the factor and tests that form different factors. Obviously, the process is subjective and inexact, and this is both a problem and an allure of factor analysis: It is not automatic; instead, it requires skill and judgment. But as a result, different analysts from different orientations may come up with different names, and therefore interpretations, of different factors. For example, the mysterious third (or fourth) factor of the original WISC and its revisions has been variously interpreted as reflecting freedom from distractibility, short-term or working memory, the ability to manipulate numbers mentally, or quantitative reasoning (Kaufman, 1994; Keith & Witta, 1997; Kranzler, 1997).

Table 4.4 shows the results of an exploratory factor analysis of the WISC-III standardization data. The overall covariance matrix from the research reported in Keith and Witta (1997) using the WISC-III standardization data was used as input for the factor analysis, which was PFA followed by varimax rotation. We decided in advance to interpret the four-factor solution, based on other research supporting such a solution (Keith & Witta, 1997; Wechsler, 1991).

The rotated first factor included significant loadings (defined here as ≥.35) by all of the Verbal tests except Digit Span, and high loadings by all of those except Arithmetic. Although the factor included a small significant loading by Picture Completion, the factor is obviously a verbal factor and is traditionally labeled Verbal Comprehension. Factor 2 included significant loadings by all of the Performance tests except Coding and Symbol Search and was labeled Perceptual Organization to reflect its nonverbal content. The third factor included high loadings by Coding and Symbol Search, the two tests that form the WISC-III Processing Speed Index.

The fourth factor nicely illustrates the difficulties in interpreting factor-analytic results. It included strong loadings by Arith-

TABLE 4.4. Rotated Factor Loadings for the WISC-III

Subtest	Factor 1	Factor 2	Factor 3	Factor 4
Information	**.710**	.287	.096	.250
Similarities	**.718**	.285	.088	.232
Arithmetic	**.425**	.274	.164	**.660**
Vocabulary	**.798**	.223	.165	.185
Comprehension	**.645**	.199	.188	.169
Digit Span	.252	.178	.178	**.372**
Picture Completion	**.381**	**.540**	.079	.096
Coding	.110	.130	**.757**	.096
Picture Arrangement	.331	**.383**	.255	.061
Block Design	.287	**.690**	.170	.261
Object Assembly	.250	**.672**	.144	.126
Symbol Search	.195	.348	**.589**	.198
Mazes	.064	**.371**	.127	.098

Note. Significant loadings (≥.35) are in **boldface**.

metic, and a smaller but significant loading by Digit Span. This factor has traditionally been labeled Freedom from Distractibility, because it is assumed that in order to perform well on the tests that load on it consistently (Digit Span and Arithmetic), a child must be able to tune out distractions and concentrate. But the two tests also require short-term memory skills and the ability to manipulate numbers, so naming this factor Memory or Quantitative would also be reasonable. This difficulty with interpreting the fourth factor illustrates the subjectivity of the technique. Different researchers from different orientations can interpret essentially the same factor structure as meaning different things. It is also a truism of factor analysis that "you only get out of the analysis what you put into it." A nonverbal subtest will behave differently in a factor analysis if analyzed with nothing but verbal subtests than if it is analyzed with an assortment of verbal and nonverbal scales. The subtests that make up this fourth factor would undoubtedly behave differently if they were factor-analyzed with a larger assortment of quantitative and memory tests.

Factor analysis is a major method of establishing construct validity for new tests or scales. In particular, the factor analysis of new instruments in common with better-understood measures can lead to a better understanding of what these new scales measure (e.g., Woodcock, 1990). Finally, the use of factor analysis as a preliminary step in research is likely to increase, and should lead

to better measurement of constructs of interest. For example, initial factor analysis of survey items can help a researcher decide which items may be best combined to create a composite variable (cf. Keith & Cool, 1992). For more information about exploratory factor analysis, see Comrey and Lee (1992) or some of the other sources cited in this section. See also Kerlinger (1986) and Kerlinger and Lee (2000) for an excellent introduction to the method; indeed, much of our beginning discussion on the topic was informed by Kerlinger (1986).

Confirmatory Factor Analysis

Exploratory factor analysis is common in assessment research with children, and a newer form of factor analysis, confirmatory factor analysis, is becoming increasingly commonplace as well. For those who are disturbed by the subjectivity and looseness of exploratory factor analysis, the confirmatory form can be more reassuring. Unfortunately, it is also more difficult to perform, and can be abused just as exploratory analysis can be, especially if one is too rigid in applying or interpreting the results—typically just the opposite problem of the abuses of exploratory analysis.

In exploratory factor analysis, the researcher decides the technique, the criteria for choosing the number of factors, and the method of rotation. The results of the analysis are then subjectively compared to the expected results, often the actual or theoretical structure of the test being analyzed. In confirmatory factor analysis, the researcher specifies in advance the number of factors, which tests load on those factors, and the relations among the factors (i.e., correlated or uncorrelated factors). Tests that are not expected to load on a factor are specified in advance as having loadings of 0 on that factor. The results of the analyses include statistics to describe the extent to which the factor structure specified in advance (called the "theoretical model") fits the data analyzed, and how the model might be modified to fit the data better. These fit indices can be thought of as measures of the "correctness" of the model, and are derived by comparing the original correlation (or, more accurately, covariance) matrix with the matrix that would result if the model proposed were correct.

Confirmatory factor analysis also allows the testing of hierarchical factor models with any number of levels of factors (for examples, see Keith, 1997). Furthermore, it tests all levels of the hierarchical analysis in combination. In contrast, for hierarchical exploratory analyses, one level of factors is commonly derived along with the correlations among those factors. The factor correlations are then factor-analyzed in a second step.

An Example: Confirmatory Analysis of the WISC-III

A simplified example will help illustrate confirmatory factor analysis. Figure 4.3 is a pictorial representation of the theoretical structure of the WISC-III. The ovals in the figure represent the "latent" or "unmeasured" variables, or the factors. The variables enclosed in rectangles represent the measured variables—the subtests for which scores are generated when the test is given. According to this model, the test first measures g, or general intelligence. At the second level, there are four factors: a Verbal factor, a Nonverbal factor, a third factor of unknown origin, and a Perceptual Speed factor. These factors correspond to the Verbal Comprehension, Perceptual Organization, Freedom from Distractibility, and Processing Speed index scores obtained on the WISC-III, respectively. At the third level are the 13 WISC-III subtests. The arrows in the

model point from the factors to the tests, which may seem unusual at first glance. But this direction nicely illustrates an implicit assumption of factor analysis: The factors represent the constructs that underlie our measurement; they are what we are most interested in because they lead to or cause the scores we get on tests. The factors are reflections of properties of the individuals we are assessing—collections of skills and abilities, traits, or characteristics. Those underlying abilities, often termed "latent traits," are what we are most interested in assessing.

The averaged covariance matrix (from Keith & Witta, 1997) was used as input into the Amos computer program (Arbuckle & Wothke, 1999) to test the model shown in Figure 4.3. Amos, which stands for *Analysis of moment structures*, is one of numerous programs for analyzing structural equation models or covariance structures—a technique that subsumes confirmatory factor analysis. A chief advantage of Amos is that one specifies the model to be tested via drawings such as the one in Figure 4.3.

Fit of the model. Figure 4.4 shows some of the results of the analysis. The "goodness-of-fit" data are listed underneath the factor model, and they suggest that this strict factor model provides a relatively good fit to the standardization data. One measure of fit compares chi squared (χ^2) to the degrees of freedom; if the χ^2 is large in comparison to the degrees of freedom, the null hypothesis that the model fits the data is rejected. The probability listed next also involves a comparison of these two values, and may be thought of in some sense as the probability that the model is correct. Thus, unlike many other types of analyses, what is desired is a *low* χ^2 and a *high* ($\geq .05$) probability. However, both the probability and the χ^2 are dependent on sample size; even good models may be rejected with large samples such as that used here. To illustrate, if we had specified an *n* of 200 for these analyses (the sample size for each of the 11 age levels), rather than the total *n* (2,200), the χ^2 would be 35.95 and *p* > .05. For this reason, χ^2 is generally not an appropriate test of significance when large samples are used—although it, along with the degrees of freedom, is often very useful for comparing two competing, nested models (i.e., when one

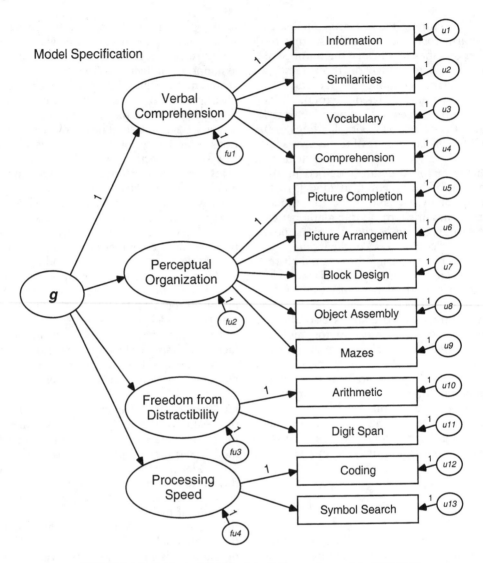

FIGURE 4.3. A hierarchical model of the structure of the WISC-III.

model is a subset of another; Bentler & Bonett, 1980).

Two other fit indices are shown in the model, although there are dozens to choose from. The comparative fit index (CFI) is one of several fit indices that compare the existing model with a "null" or "independence" model—one in which all variables are assumed to be uncorrelated (although other baseline models can be used for comparison). The CFI is designed to provide a population estimate of the improvement in fit over the null model. Although the CFI is not independent of sample size (Tanaka, 1993), is much less affected by it than is χ^2. Values

of the CFI approaching 1.00 suggest a better fit; common rules of thumb suggest that values over .95 represent a good fit of the model to the data, and values over .90 represent an adequate fit (cf. Hayduk, 1996, p. 219). Another problem with χ^2 and its associated probability is that p is the probability that a model fits perfectly in the population, even though most researchers would argue that a model is only designed to *approximate* reality. The root mean square error of approximation (RMSEA), shown next in Figure 4.4, is designed to assess the approximate fit of a model, and may thus provide a more reasonable standard for evaluating

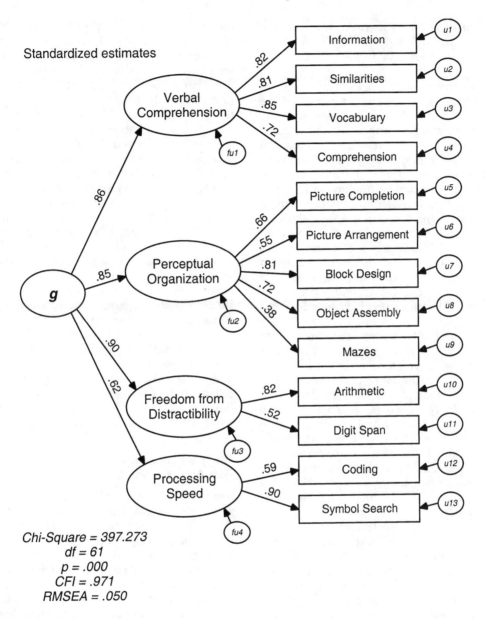

FIGURE 4.4. Standardized estimates for a hierarchical, four-factor confirmatory factor analysis of the WISC-III.

models. RMSEAs below .05 suggest a "close fit of the model in relation to the degrees of freedom" (Browne & Cudeck, 1993, p. 144)—in other words, a good approximation—and RMSEAs below .08 suggest a reasonable fit, with those above .10 representing a poor fit (Browne & Cudeck, 1993). Research with the RMSEA supports these rules of thumb (i.e., values below .05 suggesting a good fit; Hu & Bentler, 1999), as well as its use as an overall measure of model fit (Fan, Thompson, & Wang, 1999). Other advantages of the RMSEA include the ability to calculate confidence intervals around it; the ability to use it "to test a null hypothesis of poor fit," (Loehlin, 1998, p. 77); and the ability to conduct power calculations using RMSEA (MacCallum, Browne, & Sugawara, 1996). Again, there are dozens of possible fit indices, and this is an area of constant flux. At any rate, the CFI and RMSEA suggest that the WISC-III model provides a good fit to the data.

Interpretation and respecification. Given this adequate fit, we can next turn to the factor loadings. All of those loadings are significant ($t > 2.0$), and all are substantial. Vocabulary has the strongest loading on Verbal, and Block Design has the strongest loading on Nonverbal. Interestingly, Arithmetic has the strongest loading on the third factor, with a considerably smaller loading by Digit Span. Processing Speed shows a large loading by Symbol Search and a smaller loading by Coding. None of these results are surprising, and are generally consistent with the earlier exploratory analyses. Of more interest are the second-order factor loadings. All four factors have high loadings on the *g* factor. Interestingly, however, the third factor has the strongest loading on this factor (.90)—a finding suggesting that, at least in the "pure" form analyzed here, this factor is probably more cognitive and less behavioral than the name "Freedom from Distractibility" suggests. Given the high *g* loading of this factor and the difference in loadings of the two subtests (Arithmetic considerably higher than Digit Span) on the factor, the name Quantitative may be more appropriate (see Keith & Witta, 1997, for more detail and additional possible interpretations).

Other results reported by Amos (e.g., modification indices and residuals) may provide hints about how the model proposed could be modified to fit the data better. For example, the standardized residual covariances (a comparison of the predicted to the original covariance matrices, standardized) from this analysis suggest that the model shown here does not adequately account for the correlations between Picture Arrangement and the two Processing Speed tests. Again, this information can be useful in the modification of a model; however, all such modifications should also be theoretically defensible (MacCallum, 1986).

Uses of Confirmatory Factor Analysis

With its ability to test the adequacy of specific models, confirmatory factor analysis can provide a considerably stronger test of

the underlying structure of scale than exploratory factor analysis, and can be especially useful for tests (such as most modern intelligence tests) that are based on a well-articulated underlying theory. More importantly, it can be used to compare, and thus test the viability of, alternative competing models. Confirmatory analysis is an extremely powerful and flexible methodology, and one that can be used to test alternative theoretical models, the convergence versus divergence of factors across tests, the equivalence of factors across groups, and the viability of the theories underlying tests (for examples, see Keith, 1997). Joint confirmatory analyses of multiple tests should go far toward answering nagging questions—such as those touched on here—about exactly what skills tests are measuring, and they should do so much more completely than confirmatory analyses of tests in isolation (e.g., Keith, Kranzler, & Flanagan, 2001).

Obviously, this short discussion has only touched on confirmatory factor analysis and its uses. Fortunately, there are many excellent sources for more detail and illustrations of the method (e.g., Keith, 1997; Kline, 1998; Loehlin, 1998).

Multiple Regression Analysis, Path Analysis, and SEM

Multiple regression analysis has also become a common technique in child assessment research. Like ordinary correlation and regression, multiple regression allows us to estimate the extent to which a test is related to other measures of the same or related constructs. The difference between the two techniques is that in simple regression we are limited to two variables, whereas in multiple regression we can have multiple predictors of an outcome. In the traditional validity trinity, multiple regression can help establish criterion-related validity more powerfully in many cases than simple regression can. It is also a very general and flexible technique; it is a near-direct implementation of the general linear model, which subsumes most statistics of interest in assessment. Unfortunately, this generality may make the technique confusing for the novice; multiple regression can be conducted in a variety of fashions, and when completed, there are a variety of statistics that can be interpreted.

Multiple Regression: An Introductory Example

A researcher is interested in determining whether and to what extent children's eighth-grade achievement can be predicted from their second-grade intellectual ability and achievement scores. Table 4.5 shows a fictitious correlation matrix among second-grade intelligence (Ability), second-grade achievement (Ach-2), and eighth-grade achievement (Ach-8) for 200 children.

Using simple regression, our best method of predicting Ach-8 would be from Ach-2. But it also appears that we could predict almost as successfully by using Ability; perhaps we could predict even more accurately using both. This is exactly what multiple regression does; it predicts a criterion from the best linear combination of predictor variables. When multiple regression is used to predict Ach-8 from Ach-2 and Ability, the multiple correlation increases significantly, from .65 (simple r between Ach-8 and Ach-2) to .69 (multiple r, or R); the two variables together account for close to 50% of the variance in Ach-8 ($R^2 = .48$). Interestingly, if the two predictor variables, Ability and Ach-2, were *less* highly correlated with each other, the two would have a higher multiple correlation with Ach-8 (assuming that their correlations with Ach-8 remained constant).

A common question in this type of analysis is the following: Which variable is most important in the prediction of Ach-8? Unfortunately, the answer depends on how the regression analysis is conducted and what is interpreted. If we were to use stepwise regression (a common approach), we would find that Ach-2 explained 42% of the variance in Ach-8, and that Ability Explained only approximately 5% more variance (these do not sum to 48% because of errors from rounding); Ach-2 is clearly more im-

portant in this approach. On the other hand, we could reason that Ability is theoretically prior to achievement, and that it should therefore enter the regression equation first. Using this approach, we would find that Ability explained 38% of the variance in Ach-8 and that Ach-2 explained 9% more; Ability seems more important in this approach. To confuse matters further, we could also interpret the beta (β) weights from this analysis rather than the R^2 (β's are standardized partial-regression coefficients; they—or their unstandardized counterparts, b weights—could be used in actual prediction equations to predict an *individual's* Ach-8 from that person's ability and Ach-2). Using this approach, we would find β's of .32 for ability and .42 for Ach-2, suggesting that both are important in predicting Ach-8, with Ach-2 slightly more important.

Prediction versus Explanation

Stepwise Regression

Stepwise regression is, unfortunately, a common multiple-regression approach in assessment research, but methodologists generally discourage its use for all but a small portion of such research (e.g., Cohen & Cohen, 1983, Ch. 3; Keith, in preparation; Pedhazur, 1997, Ch. 8; Thompson, 1998). The reason for this condemnation, and also possibly for the popularity of the approach, is that stepwise regression is an atheoretical approach.

In stepwise regression, the data, rather than the researcher, decide the order in which variables are entered into the regression equation (and we have already seen how order of entry can affect our conclusions). The variable with the highest correlation with the criterion is the first to enter the regression equation. The multiple-regression program then calculates the semipartial correlations between each of the remaining variables and the criterion (the semipartial correlation is the correlation of each variable with the criterion, *with the effects of the variable already in the equation removed* from each variable). The variable that can explain the most additional variance is entered next. The joint effects of these two variables are then removed from all of the other correlations, and the vari-

TABLE 4.5. Fictitious Correlations among Second-Grade Intellectual Ability, Second-Grade Achievement (Ach-2), and Eighth-Grade Achievement (Ach-8)

Variable	Ability	Ach-2	Ach-8
Ability	1.00	—	—
Ach-2	.70	1.00	—
Ach-8	.62	.65	1.00

able that can account for the next highest amount of variance is added. The process continues until some criterion for stopping is reached. Common criteria are that only a certain number of variables are allowed to enter the equation, or some value is set by which R^2 must increase before a variable is entered.

This may seem a perfectly reasonable approach: "Let the data decide!" And it may be reasonable, if our interest is in prediction only. In the present example, if our only interest were the best prediction of eighth-grade achievement, then second-grade achievement would seem to offer the single best predictor of the two variables we have used in the equation (but remember that these data are fictitious).

In many cases, however, our intent is not simply prediction, but rather understanding. We may be interested in knowing which variables influence eighth-grade achievement, and how that influence works; or we may be interested in the extent to which second-grade achievement affects eighth-grade achievement, after controlling for the important background variable of ability. In either of these cases, we are concerned with more than prediction; we are interested in understanding or explaining Ach-8, and stepwise regression does not generally help in this regard.

There are a number of reasons why stepwise regression is not appropriate when we are interested in going beyond prediction, but the most important is that the technique does not generally encompass available theory or previous research. We do not have room to enumerate the reasons here, but multiple regression can produce very misleading results if not guided by theory, or at least by logic. Anything can be regressed against anything, but unless there is some logic for regressing one thing against another, the results are meaningless. Regression results are also very much dependent on the variables used in the analysis. Because the technique looks for *nonredundant* predictors, a variable can look like a good or a poor predictor, depending on the choice of the other predictor variables. If we want to interpret regression results as showing the effect or influence of one variable on another (an explanatory approach), then theory must guide both the selection on variables

and their order of entry into the regression equation. For a more complete discussion of the need for theory, see Cohen and Cohen (1983), Keith (in preparation), or Pedhazur (1997). For an even more damning critique of stepwise methods, see Thompson (1998).

Hierarchical Regression

One approach that can incorporate theory, and that therefore is useful when explanation is desired, is hierarchical (or sequential) regression. This technique involves entering the variables, either one at a time or in groups, in a predetermined order; changes in R^2 are interpreted as reflections of the importance of each predictor variable. The technique thus has some similarities to stepwise regression, but it is the researcher, not the data, who decides the order in which variables are entered into the equation.

The order of variables' entry in multiple regression makes a great deal of difference in the variance they explain. The overlapping circles shown in Figure 4.5 illustrate why. In the figure, each circle represents the variance of a variable, and the overlap among the circles represents the variance they share (their covariance, or correlation). For the sake of consistency, we label these variables Ability, Ach-2, and Ach-8 (the overlap is not intended to be drawn to scale). Some of the variance in Ability is shared with Ach-8, as depicted by the horizontally hatched overlap between the two variables. Some of the variance in Ach-2 is shared with Ach-8, as depicted by the vertically hatched area. Finally, some of the variance is shared among all three variables, as depicted by the double-hatched area of overlap; it is this area of overlap that makes the difference in R^2, depending on the order of variables' entry. Using this increase-in-R^2 approach, the first variable to enter the equation (Ability or Ach-2) would be attributed this variance and the second variable would not be attributed any of the variance shared by all three variables. This treatment of shared variance is why the order of variables' entry into the regression equation can have such important effects on the conclusions we draw from the analyses.

We should note that although changes in R^2 (ΔR^2) are often used in hierarchical regression as indicators of the "importance"

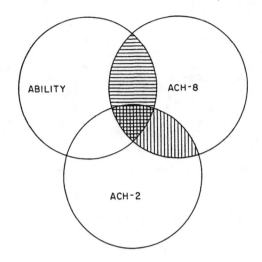

FIGURE 4.5. Unique and shared variance among second-grade intellectual ability (Ability), second-grade achievement (Ach-2), and eighth-grade achievement (Ach-8). The areas of overlap (common variance) are not drawn to scale.

of variables, there are serious problems with this approach. Many writers have commented on the importance of variables with small ΔR^2's (e.g., Gage, 1978; Rosenthal & Rubin, 1979), and Darlington (1990) demonstrated why ΔR^2 provides an underestimate of "importance" (see also Keith, in preparation). In fact, $\sqrt{\Delta R^2}$ is probably a better measure of the importance of variables entered in a hierarchical regression.

Forced-Entry Regression

Another theory-based approach to regression is the third method alluded to above, forced-entry (or simultaneous) multiple regression. With forced-entry regression, all variables are forced into the regression equation in a single step. The regression coefficients (β, b, and the statistical significance of b) are used to judge the importance of variables. With β, the standardized regression coefficient, all variables are on the same standardized scale, and thus it is relatively easy to compare coefficients for their "importance;" order of entry is not an issue because all variables enter the equation at the same time. In fact, standardized regression coefficients (β) work fairly well as a measure of relative importance, unless the predictor variables are highly intercorrelat-

ed. Semipartial correlations or the t values associated with the unstandardized coefficients (b; $t = [b/SE_b]$) may also be used (Darlington, 1990; Keith, in preparation).

Path Analysis

Another theory-based approach to regression is a technique known alternately as "path analysis," "causal modeling," or "structural equation modeling." In general, path analysis may be considered the simplest form of structural equation modeling. The simplest form of path analysis, in turn, uses multiple regression and is a good method for illustrating and understanding multiple regression.

An Example of Path Analysis

Path analysis begins with a theory displayed figurally as a path model. Essentially, a path model explicitly defines the researchers' theory of which variables affect which (or "cause" and "effect"), with decisions of causal ordering made on the basis of formal and informal theory, time precedence, previous research, and logic. Figure 4.6 shows a path model to explain Ach-8 as a function of Ability and Ach-2. An arrow or path is drawn from Ability to Ach-2, based on presumed time precedence and theory. Ability appears to be fairly stable from at least a preschool level (cf. Jensen, 1980, Ch. 7), and it therefore makes sense to place it before the achievement variables, which are primarily products of schooling. In addition, theories of school learning generally recognize ability or aptitude as an influence on learning or achievement (cf. Carroll, 1963; Walberg, 1981). Paths are drawn from Ability and Ach-2 to Ach-8 for similar reasons, and because second-grade achievement obviously occurs before eighth-grade achievement.

Given the viability of a number of assumptions (e.g., one-way causal flow), the standardized paths may be estimated by the β weights from forced-entry regression; these are also inserted in Figure 4.6 (the unstandardized paths may be estimated using the b's). The paths to Ach-8 have been estimated by regressing it on Ability and Ach-2, and the path from Ability to Ach-2 has been estimated by regressing Ach-2 on Ability.

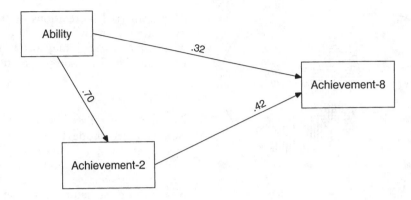

FIGURE 4.6. Path analysis of the effects of Ability and Ach-2 on Ach-8.

The standardized paths are interpreted as the portion of a standard deviation (SD) unit increase (or decrease, in the case of negative paths) in the effect for each SD change in the cause. In other words, each SD increase in Ach-2 will increase Ach-8 by 0.42 SD.

Advantages and More Complex Procedures

One advantage of path analysis over other regression approaches is that it allows one to focus on indirect effects. In Figure 4.6, for example, Ability has a direct effect on Ach-8 (β = .32), but Ability also affects Ach-2, which in turn affects Ach-8; this indirect effect of Ability on Ach-8 may be calculated by multiplying the two paths (.70 × .42 = .30).

Path analysis has other advantages as well. It requires an explicit, graphic statement of a researcher's theory of cause and effect, and its interpretation is straightforward; for this reason, path analysis avoids many of the ambiguities that can result from multiple regression. Because of these and other advantages, Keith (1988) recommended it as the technique of choice when conducting explanatory analysis using nonexperimental data, and Cohen and Cohen (1983) went even further: ". . . it seems clear to us that nonexperimental inference that is not consistent with its [path or causal analysis's] fundamental principles is simply invalid" (p. 14). The biggest danger in path analysis is when an important common cause (a variable that affects both the primary cause and effect of interest) is not in-

cluded in the model. But in a way, this too is an advantage of path analysis; this danger threatens all nonexperimental analyses in which the results are interpreted as one variable's affecting or influencing another (see Keith, 1999). Because path analysis requires a graphic presentation of what affects what, it is often easier to spot a missing variable than with ordinary multiple regression. As shown throughout this chapter, path models—whether analyzed or not—are also useful heuristic devices.

When the assumptions that underlie multiple regression (e.g., reliably measured variables, uncorrelated errors of measurement) are not met, other techniques can be used to estimate the paths. In its most powerful form, structural equation modeling uses programs like Amos to perform joint confirmatory factor analysis (the measurement model) and path analysis (the structural model). The measurement model cleanses the variables of their error to get closer to the construct level; the structural model estimates the effects of the *constructs* on each other. If multiple measures of the three variables shown in Figure 4.6 were available, latent-variable structural equation modeling would come closer to telling us the effect of "true" second-grade ability on "true" eighth-grade achievement.[1]

An Example Comparing Various Regression Approaches

Table 4.6 shows the correlations among the variables Ability, Academic Motivation, Amount of Academic Coursework, and

TABLE 4.6. Correlations among Intellectual Ability, Motivation, Academic Coursework, and Academic Achievement for 200 High School Students

Variable	1	2	3	4
1. Ability	1.00	—	—	—
2. Motivation	.21	1.00	—	—
3. Coursework	.50	.38	1.00	—
4. Achievement	.74	.26	.62	1.00

Note. Data from Keith and Cool (1992).

Academic Achievement for a sample of high school students (the correlations are taken from a larger matrix reported in Keith & Cool, 1992; the sample size was really more than 20,000, but for the purposes of illustration we have used a sample size of 200). Ability, Motivation, and Coursework are commonly recognized influences on learning (or Achievement), and appear frequently in theories of school learning (e.g., Walberg, 1981); they are also commonly used as predictors of achievement. In our first analysis, we used stepwise multiple regression to predict Achievement from these three variables. Ability was the first variable to enter the equation ($R^2 = .54$), followed by Coursework ($\Delta R^2 = .08$, $p < .01$); Motivation did not lead to a statistically significant increase in the variance explained, and therefore did not enter the equation. Our best conclusion from these results would be that of the predictor variables used, Ability and Coursework are the best predictors of achievement.

We could easily argue that the order of entry for the stepwise regression is wrong; available theory, research, and logic suggest that Ability affects Motivation, which in turn affects Coursework and Achievement. The three variables were entered in that order in the second step of these analyses (hierarchical regression). Ability entered the equation first, with the same results, of course, as in the stepwise analysis. When Motivation entered the equation second, it did explain a small but statistically significant amount of additional variance (change in $R^2 = .01$, $p < .05$); Coursework was entered last, and also statistically significantly increased the variance explained (R^2 change $= .07$, $p < .01$). Our conclusion from this analysis would be that all three variables appear to affect Achievement.

As the third step in this set of analyses, the variables were analyzed via forced-entry regression. For this analysis, the standardized regression (β) coefficients to Achievement were .57 (from Ability), .02 (Motivation), and .32 (Coursework). The Ability and Coursework regression (b) coefficients were statistically significant, whereas the Motivation coefficient was not. The forced-entry regression's results were therefore inconsistent with the hierarchical regression's results, despite our insistence that these methods are more appropriate than the stepwise approach. Which results are "correct"?

As the fourth step in this set of analyses, the variables were put into the path model shown in Figure 4.7. To solve for the path model, Ability, Motivation, and Coursework were regressed against Achievement via forced-entry regression, and the β weights were used as estimates of the paths to achievement. Ability and Motivation were regressed on Coursework to estimate the paths to Coursework, and Ability was regressed on Motivation to estimate the path to Motivation from Ability. The results of the path analysis are also shown in Figure 4.7, and they may lead to a richer understanding of how the three variables of interest affect Achievement. All of the paths in the model are significant, with the exception of the path from Motivation to Achievement. From a path-analytic orientation, we would conclude that Motivation has no significant *direct* effect on Achievement.

Motivation does appear, however, to have *indirect* effects on Achievement: Motivation affects Coursework ($\beta = .28$), which in turn affects Achievement ($\beta = .32$). Table 4.7 shows the direct (path), indirect, and total (direct + indirect) effect for each of the three variables on achievement; all of the *total* effects are statistically significant. The path results, then, if fully interpreted, would lead to conclusions similar to those of both other theoretical approaches, even though those two approaches (hierarchical and forced-entry regression) appeared inconsistent with each other. Furthermore, the path results also suggest how those effects may operate. It appears that Motivation affects Achievement primarily indirectly: Highly motivated students take more academic courses, and that Coursework increases their Achieve-

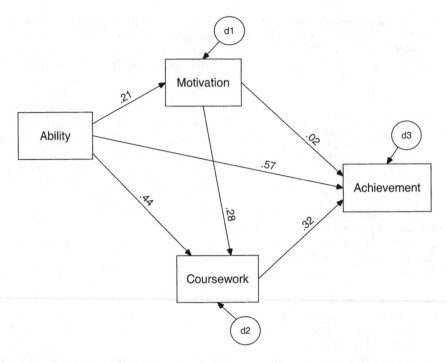

FIGURE 4.7. Effects of Ability, Motivation, and Coursework on Achievement in high school. Data from Keith and Cool (1992).

ment (for additional detail, see Keith, 1999, in preparation; Kline, 1998; Loehlin, 1998).

This example may seem far removed from assessment and assessment research. Assessment, however, provides the basis for intervention. Successful interventions need to be based on a solid research understanding of just what influences the characteristic we are trying to change (such as achievement). It makes little difference if a variable is a good predictor of that characteristic; if it is not a meaningful *influence* on that characteristic, manipulating it will not produce the desired outcome. Theory and research are crucial to the design of interventions.

TABLE 4.7. Direct, Indirect, and Total Effects of Ability, Motivation, and Academic Coursework on Achievement

Variable	Direct effects	Indirect effects	Total effects
Ability	.57*	.17*	.74*
Motivation	.02	.09*	.11*
Coursework	.32*	—	.32*

*$p < .05$.

Use of Regression in Clinical Diagnosis and Classification Studies

One common use of multiple regression in assessment research is in classification or diagnostic studies. Researchers might use a regression-based technique to see which subset of a larger set of tests could best predict which children are classified as having mental retardation and which as having learning disabilities. Many such studies use related techniques, such as discriminant analysis or logistic regression, in which the criterion of interest is a nominal-level variable (e.g., the two diagnostic categories just mentioned) rather than a continuous variable. The similarities across the techniques are more important at this point than the differences, and all these methods are commonly used in diagnostic studies.

Psychologists have long studied the ability of various tests and other diagnostic methods to differentiate one class of psychopathological disorders from another and to classify individuals correctly into one diagnostic group or another. To their credit, researchers have recently brought to bear sophisticated multivariate techniques directly to the problem of diagnosis and classification of mental disorders; most such investigations involve regression analysis or related methods. In the quest to provide accurate diagnosis and a breadth of research findings, a large array of behaviors is evaluated in the typical study. For example, Rourke (1975), in discussing more than 20 years of research in differential diagnosis, reported that children seen in his laboratory and clinic were administered, on a routine basis, "the WISC, the Peabody Picture Vocabulary Test, the Halstead Neuropsychological Test Battery for Children, an examination for sensory-perceptual disturbances, the Klove–Mathews Motor Steadiness Battery, and a number of other tests for receptive and expressive language abilities" (p. 912). Multiple regression would seem an ideal technique for analyzing such data. But this and related methods are very powerful analytical tools that take advantage not only of fluctuations in performance, but also any *chance* relations (i.e., correlated error variance) to maximize discriminability and thus determine group membership. Unfortunately, if a large set of variables is used along with a small group of subjects, those subjects can easily be grouped and classified purely on the basis of random or chance variation! The need for large numbers of subjects in such research is crucial.

In the study of clinical disorders, however, one is frequently limited to relatively small samples of convenience rather than larger random samples of design. Although most researchers acknowledge this difficulty, many apparently do not realize the devastating effects that low subject-to-variable ratios (i.e., the number of variables approaching the number of subjects) have on the generalizability of studies of differential diagnosis. This is not to say that some excellent studies have not been completed. Studies of discriminability by Satz and his colleagues (e.g., Satz & Friel, 1974) use large numbers of variables but have considerable subject populations. Large-n studies of clinical populations are the exception rather than the rule, however. Some of the problems encountered in such studies are discussed below (see also Darlington, 1990; Thompson, 1998; Willson & Reynolds, 1982).

Shrinkage and Other Problems

Several considerations are important when one is predicting group membership (e.g., making a diagnosis) from a predictor set of variables (e.g., the clinical assessment). First, procedures that use samples from a target population always involve sampling error in the estimation of the relations being examined. This means that results are expected to fluctuate from sample to sample, due to the random differences inherent in the samples. The usual measure of a prediction's accuracy in multiple regression is the squared multiple correlation (R^2). In applying results of a particular sample to a second sample, R^2 is expected to decrease, since multiple regression is a maximizing operation—R^2 was made as big as possible for the first sample, because multiple regression capitalizes on chance variation in addition to true relations among variables. It is highly unlikely that the same fit of the data will occur in a second sample.

A second consideration occurs when the prediction uses a strategy for selecting a smaller number of variables from the larger predictor set, such as stepwise regression or discriminant analysis. When numerous predictors are available, stepwise procedures maximize the probability of selecting predictors that do not predict well in the population but, by chance, correlate highly with the outcome in the particular sample being used. We are only interested in the correlation of *true*-score variance among any set of variables, but due to chance fluctuation in data, error variances occasionally correlate. Multivariate methods, particularly stepwise techniques, take maximum advantage of these correlated error variances—correlations that cannot generalize beyond the sample.

The degree of decease in R^2 from sample to population can be estimated. The most common estimate, due to Wherry (1931; see also Lord & Novick, 1968, p. 286) is

$$\hat{R}^2 = 1 - (1 - R^2)\frac{(n-1)}{(n-K-1)}$$

In this equation, n is the number of observations; K is the number of predictors; R^2 is the observed squared multiple correlation between outcome and predictors; and $\hat{R}^2$ is the estimate of the *population* squared multiple correlation (called the "shrunken R^2"). This formula may be applied to multiple regression or discriminant analysis. The essence of this formula is that as sample size (n) becomes small in relation to the number of predictors (K), the shrunken R^2 becomes considerably smaller than the original R^2.

Cattin (1980) suggested that with a small n and a large K, another approximation should be used:

$$\hat{R}^2 = \frac{(n - K - 3)\rho^4 + \rho^4}{(n - 2K - 2)\rho^2 + K}$$

where

$$\rho^2 = 1 - \frac{(n - 3)}{n - K - 1}(1 - R^2)$$

$$\left[1 + \frac{2(1 - R^2)}{n - K - 1} + \frac{8(1 - R^2)^2}{(n - K + 1)(n - K + 3)}\right]$$

Although $\hat{R}^2$ is a biased estimate, the amount of bias is on the order of .01–.02 for $n = 60$ and $K = 50$.

Of special interest is the case where there are more predictors than people; for the equation above, the shrunken R^2 may become negative or greater than 1.00. Mathematically, with more predictors than observations of the outcome, there is no unique solution to a best prediction. In discriminant analysis, having more predictors than subjects will result in perfect classification *entirely at random*! This perfect prediction is a result of having more parameters to estimate than data points to use in the estimation, not because of some true relation between the predictors and groups. Since it is mathematically impossible to estimate all regression coefficients, there will be $K/n = K!/[n!(n - K!)]$ different solutions that would provide perfect classification in this case, but would not be expected to generalize to any other samples. Even when there are fewer predictors (e.g., test scores) than people, the shrunken R^2 estimate will rapidly approach 0 as the number of predictors becomes a significant proportion of the number of subjects.

Multiple regression, logistic regression, and discriminant analysis have been discussed interchangeably to this point, but there are differences among the three techniques. For those familiar with multiple regression, logistic regression may be easier to understand than discriminant analysis. When there are only two groups, either logistic regression or discriminant analysis may be used; at this time, discriminant analysis may be more useful with more than two groups (although the method of logistic regression with more than two groups is developing rapidly). Furthermore, if the groups used form a continuous variable (e.g., children with severe, moderate, and mild mental retardation), ordinary multiple regression may be used. For logistic regression, there are various methods for estimating an analogue to R^2 (Menard, 1995). In discriminant analysis, R^2 can be calculated from the canonical correlation (R_c; see Cooley & Lohnes, 1971, p. 170), but their squared sum (R^2_c) is the maximum possible R^2. R^2_c may be useful as a liberal estimate of R^2, because if it can be shown that R^2_c is near 0, there is no need to estimate the study's R^2, which will produce an even smaller estimate of R^2. Whichever method is used, the important point is that shrinkage will occur in prediction research, and its effects will be dramatic if n is small in relation to K.

Effects of Shrinkage in Diagnostic Research

Willson and Reynolds (1982) assessed the effects of sample size and the application of these regression-based procedures on the outcome of nine studies of diagnostic classification in various clinical journals. Of the 17 R^2's obtainable from the nine studies, 12 were initially significant. After correcting for shrinkage, however, Willson and Reynolds reported that only between 4 and 8 of these 12 R^2's were significant (depending on whether R^2 was corrected for the original full set of predictors or only the number used in the final prediction equation). Thus half the results reported in these studies may be attributed to chance correlations! Under the most optimistic of circumstances, the upper limit of the shrunken R^2 estimate showed a mean $\hat{R}^2$ of .37 versus a mean obtained R^2 of .48 for all studies considered. The lower-bound estimate of the shrunken R^2 estimate yielded even more pessimistic results, demonstrating a mean value of only .25. Thus, when one is using powerful multivariate techniques, the chance variation that can *appear* to be reliable discrimination is rather considerable. The importance of large subject-to-variable ratios and proper cross-validation becomes immediately obvious in considering the results summarized here (for more detail, see Willson & Reynolds, 1982).

It must be reiterated that the shrinkage occurs in research in which correlation maximizing procedures have been used: stepwise multiple regression, stepwise discriminant analysis, and canonical correlation. The R^2 does not shrink in a fixed-variable study in which all variables are included and in which order is unimportant (a balanced analysis-of-variance design) or in which order is predetermined (path analysis or other theory-bound regression approach). Diagnosis seeks to find the best empirical discriminators, but it is most prey to chance.

It should also be stressed that shrinkage and related problems with stepwise approaches not only are problems with diagnostic research, but apply to all uses of stepwise-regression-based techniques. Shrinkage would also occur in a stepwise analysis predicting achievement test scores from several other measures. Still, these problems are particularly salient for the diagnostic literature, with its common reliance on small samples. Furthermore, diagnostic research seems so applicable to everyday psychological practice; it is therefore particularly dangerous to neglect this very real and common danger in such research.

The Need for Cross-Validation

The estimation of a population or shrunken R^2 and the expected misclassification rate are methods of correcting for the tendency of stepwise regression to capitalize on chance variation. But the procedures only provide estimates of shrinkage, and are far from perfect. A better method of estimating shrinkage is through cross-validation, in which the regression weights and variance estimates from one sample are then tested on another sample.

Cross-validation requires two independent samples. Ideally, both samples are drawn independently from the same population, but often a single sample is split in half. In either case, the regression equation and statistics are computed for one sample (the screening sample), and then the equation is applied to the second sample (the cross-validation sample) to predict scores on the outcome (or group membership, as appropriate). Those predicted scores are then correlated with the actual outcome scores, with the resulting correlation producing an excellent estimate of the shrunken R (for more information, see Pedhazur, 1997, Ch. 8). Indeed, the shrunken R^2 discussed above is really just a one-sample estimate of this correlation between predicted and actual scores. Unfortunately, in clinical samples the n is typically so small that splitting it is not a good idea. Two-sample cross-validation, in which two separate samples are drawn from the same population, is then the preferred approach.

Researchers should cross-validate prediction studies prior to publication. The Selz and Reitan (1979) research is an example where this procedure was followed, with quite credible results. We recognize that it is difficult to obtain subjects with rare disorders, but holding results until a second population is sampled would result in no real loss to our discipline. On the contrary, there would be a net gain, since only the cross-validated results would be published. The external validity of prediction studies would also be stronger.

Cross-validation is especially important for practicing clinicians. When actuarial rules for the diagnosis of psychological disorders appear in refereed professional journals, those in applied settings, especially those keeping closest to current developments in the field, may feel confident in applying such rules in the diagnosis and treatment of their clients. But in the absence of proper cross-validation, diagnoses or classifications may be made on the basis of random relations—an unacceptable situation for all involved, but especially for the individuals under study. Caution is needed on the part of researchers and clinicians alike.

Researchers need to be extremely cautious when subject-to-variable ratios are less than 10:1. When cross-validation is not possible and the results are important enough to be published without cross-validation, estimates of shrinkage in R^2 and the subsequent decrease in classification accuracy should be conveyed, and clear, appropriate cautions should be provided to clinicians.

TEST BIAS RESEARCH

As noted earlier in this chapter, many observers mistakenly take research showing mean differences across ethnic or related groups in levels of performance on a psychological test as being proof that the test is "biased" against one or more of these groups. Such simple comparisons err in assuming that demographically derived groups of individuals *cannot* differ on any psychological attribute, and hence that any differences revealed by a test mean the test is faulty. In fact, groups may or may not differ; there is a cadre of research methods available to determine whether, when group differences are located, the differences are real ones (requiring additional explanation) or artifacts due to a biased test. Tests can be examined for bias at the level of either the total test or any of its subscales. As a concept for study, "bias" must first be defined, however.

The term "bias" carries many different connotations for the lay public and for professionals in any number of disciplines. To the legal mind, it denotes illegal discriminatory practices, whereas to the lay mind it may conjure up notions of prejudicial attitudes. Much of the rancor in psychology and education regarding proper definitions of test bias is due to the divergent uses of this term in general, but especially by professionals in the same and related academic fields. Contrary to more common or lay usages of the term, the term "bias" should be used in discussions of educational and psychological tests in its widely recognized, distinct *statistical* sense. "Bias" denotes constant or systematic error, as opposed to chance or random error, in the estimation of some value; in test bias research, this constant or systematic error is usually due to group membership or some other nominal variable, and occurs in the estimation of a score on a psychological or educational test.

Other uses of this term in research on the differential or cross-group validity of tests are unacceptable from a scientific perspec-

tive, for two primary reasons: (1) The imprecise nature of other uses of the term makes empirical investigation and rational inquiry exceedingly difficult; and (2) other uses invoke moral and value systems that are the subject of intense, polemic, emotional debate without a mechanism for rational resolution. Here we note briefly the more common and promising methods for research on bias in assessment research. Methods for evaluating *item* bias are specifically not reviewed, and the interested reader is referred to Berk (1982) for an excellent review of item bias methodology. Reynolds (1982, 2000) has provided chapters on methods for detecting bias in a variety of cognitive and personality measures. A review of the outcomes of bias research is provided by Reynolds and Kaiser in Chapter 22 of the current volume.

Research Methods for Detecting Bias

Internal Indices of Bias

Item bias studies evaluate the bias internal to the test at the level of the individual item, but deal principally with bias in test content (content validity). Construct validity across groups, on the other hand, is assessed primarily through internal analyses of tests taken as a whole. Bias exists in regard to construct validity of a test whenever that test can be shown to measure different hypothetical traits or constructs for one group than it does for another group, or to assess the same construct but with differing degrees of accuracy (Reynolds, 2000; Reynolds, Lowe, & Saenz, 1999).

Factor-Analytic Methods

One of the more popular and necessary empirical approaches to investigating construct validity, and therefore construct bias, is factor analysis. As noted earlier, factor analysis identifies clusters of test items or subtests that correlate highly with one another and less so with other subtests or items. Consistent factor-analytic results across populations provide strong evidence that whatever is being measured by an instrument is being measured in the same manner, and is in fact the same construct, within each group. If factor-analytic results are constant across groups, then one may have greater confidence that the individuals in each group perceive and interpret the test materials in a similar manner. The information derived from comparative factor analyses across populations is directly relevant to the use of educational and psychological tests in diagnosis and decision making.

Exploratory methods. Both general methods of factor analysis can be used in test bias research. When exploratory factor analysis is used, the focus is generally on the *similarity* (or lack of similarity) of factor structures across groups. There are, in turn, a number of methods for determining factorial similarity across groups. These methods differ primarily along two lines: whether they allow estimates of shared variance between factors, and what the various assumptions underlying their use are. With large samples, various indices of factorial similarity typically produce consistent findings (Reynolds & Harding, 1983). In small-sample studies, multiple methods of evaluation are necessary to guard against the overinterpretation of what may simply be sampling error.

The Pearson correlation can be used to examine directly the comparability of factor loadings on a single factor for two groups. The correlation coefficient between pairs of factor loadings for corresponding factors has been used in some previous work; however, in the comparison of factor loadings, assumptions of normality or linearity are likely to be violated. Transformation of the factor loadings using Fisher z transformation prior to computing r helps to correct some of these flaws, but is not completely satisfactory. Other, more appropriate indices of factorial similarity exist and are no more difficult to determine than the Pearson r in most cases.

One popular index of factorial similarity is the coefficient of congruence (r_c). It is similar to the Pearson r, and is based on the relation between pairs of factor loadings for corresponding factors. When one is determining the degree of similarity of two factors, an r_c value of .90 or higher is typically (although arbitrarily) taken to indicate equivalence of the factors in question or factorial invariance across groups (Cattell, 1978; Harman, 1976). The coefficient of congruence is calculated by the following equation:

$$r_c = \frac{\sum ab}{\sqrt{\sum a^2 \sum b^2}}$$

where a represents the factor loading of a variable for one sample, and b represents the factor loading of the same variable for the second sample on the same factor.

Cattell (1978) described a useful nonparametric index for factor comparison, known as the salient-variable-similarity index (s). The calculation of s is straightforward, with one exception. In the determination of s, one first proceeds by classifying each variable by its factor loading as being salient or nonsalient and as being positive or negative, depending on the sign of the variable's loading. After reviewing several other options, Cattell recommended a cutoff value of .10 to indicate a variable with a salient loading. Although .10 is probably the best choice for item factor analyses (or with subscales, in the case of personality scales), it is probably too liberal when examining subscales of cognitive batteries with high subtest reliabilities and a large general factor, especially given the sensitive nature of questions of potential bias. In the latter case, investigators should consider adopting more conservative values: from .15 to .25 for positive salience and −.15 to −.25 for negative salience.

Many other methods of determining the similarity of factors exist, and a complete review of these techniques cannot be undertaken here. Configurative matching methods or the use of Cattell's coefficient of pattern similarity (r) are but two prominent examples. These and others are reviewed by Cattell (1978). The methods noted above, however, will be adequate for the vast majority of cases (especially if analyses are based on covariance matrices), and are certainly the most common procedures in the test bias literature. When one is using these indices of factorial similarity to evaluate overall results of an analysis, not only should individual factors be compared; the comparison of communalities and of unique–specific variances may also be appropriate, especially in the case of diagnostic psychological tests. See Fan, Willson, and Reynolds (1995) for an illustration of many of these methods.

Confirmatory methods. Confirmatory factor-analytic methods can also be used to test for construct bias. Briefly, simultaneous (or multisample) factor analyses are performed in the separate groups. With confirmatory analysis, the focus is on *differences* in factor structures across groups. Parameters, such as factor loadings, are constrained to be equal across groups, and the fit of such models compared to models without these equality constraints; $\Delta\chi^2$ is often used to determine the statistical significance of the constraints. If constraining factor loadings across groups results in a statistically significant increase in $\Delta\chi2$, the results suggest that the test is not measuring the same construct across groups, and thus may be biased. Various degrees of consistency may be specified and tested, including first- and second-order factor loadings, factor variances, factor correlations, and unique and error variances. Keith and colleagues (1995) provide an illustration of confirmatory factor analysis to test for bias.

Comparing Internal-Consistency Estimates

The previously offered definition of bias in construct validity requires equivalence in the "accuracy" of measurement across groups for nonbiased assessment. Essentially, this means that any error due to domain sampling in the choice of items for the test must be constant across groups. The proper test of this condition is the comparison of internal-consistency reliability estimates (r_{xx}) or alternate-form correlations (r_{ab}) across groups; the two require different statistical procedures.

Internal consistency. Internal-consistency reliability estimates are such coefficients as Cronbach's alpha, Kuder–Richardson 20 (KR_{20}), KR_{21}, odd–even correlations with length corrections, or estimates derived through analysis of variance. Typically, the preferred estimate of r_{xx} is Cronbach's coefficient alpha or KR_{20}, a special case of alpha. Alpha has a variety of advantages; for example, it is the mean of all possible split-half correlations for a test, and is also representative of the predicted correlation be-

tween true alternate forms of a test. Feldt (1969) provided a technique that can be used to determine the significance of the difference between alpha or KR_{20} reliabilities on a single test for two groups. Although this technique was originally devised as a test of the hypothesis that alpha or KR_{20} is the same for two tests, the assumptions underlying Feldt's test are even more closely met by those of a single psychological or educational test and two independent samples (L. S. Feldt, personal communication, 1980). The test statistic is given by the ratio of 1 – alpha for the first group over 1 – alpha for the second group:

$$F = \frac{1 - alpha_1}{1 - alpha_2}$$

In this formula, $alpha_1$ is the reliability coefficient of the test being studied for group 1, and $alpha_2$ is the same reliability coefficient as calculated for the second group. KR_{20} reliabilities may be used in the equation as well. The test statistic will be distributed as F with $n_1 - 1$ degrees of freedom in the numerator and $n_2 - 1$ degrees of freedom in the denominator. The expression 1 – alpha represents an error variance term, and the largest variance is always placed over the smallest variance.

Alternate forms. Comparison of correlations between alternate forms of a test across groups may be needed in cases where alpha or KR_{20} is inappropriate or for some reason not available. With two samples, alternate-form correlations are calculated separately for each group, producing two independent correlations. The standard statistical test for the differences between independent correlations is then calculated (e.g., Bruning & Kintz, 1997).

When a significant difference between alternate-form reliability estimates for two groups occurs, several other possibilities must be considered prior to concluding that bias exists. The tests under consideration must be shown to be actual alternate forms for at least one of the two groups. Before two tests can be considered alternate forms, they must in fact be sampling items from the same domain. Other methodological problems that apply generally to the investigation of alternate-form reliability also will apply. Comparison of test–retest correlations across groups may also be of interest and can be conducted in the same matter. Whether a test–retest correlation is an appropriate measure of a test's reliability, however, should be evaluated carefully. Unless the trait the test is measuring is assumed to be stable, test–retest correlations speak more directly to the stability of the trait under consideration than to the accuracy of the measuring device.

Correlation of Age with Raw Scores

A potentially valuable technique for investigating the construct validity of aptitude or intelligence tests is the evaluation of the relation between raw scores and age. Virtually all theories of early cognitive development suggest that scores on tests of mental ability during childhood should increase with age. If a test is a valid measure of mental ability, then performance on the test—as measured by raw scores—should show a substantial correlation with age when data are compared across age levels. If a test is measuring some construct of mental ability in a uniform manner *across groups,* then the correlation of raw scores with chronological age should be constant across groups.

Kinship Correlations and Differences

Jensen (1980) proposed that "the construct validity of a test in any two population groups is reinforced if the test scores show the same kinship correlations (or absolute differences) in both groups" (p. 427). The use of kinship correlation to test for bias is relatively complex and involves calculation of heritability estimated across groups. Structural equation modeling and confirmatory factor analysis are increasingly used in heritability research (e.g., Thompson, Detterman, & Plomin, 1991); they should also prove useful in test bias research comparing heritabilities and kinship correlations across groups.

Multitrait–Multimethod Validation

One of the most convincing techniques for establishing the construct validity of psychological tests is through the use of a multitrait–multimethod validity matrix. This technique evaluates both the convergent and divergent validity of a test with multiple methods of assessment. That is, predictions regarding what will correlate with the test score are evaluated, along with predictions regarding what the test *will not* correlate with (an equally important facet of validity); multiple methods of assessment are used, so that the observed relations are not artifacts of a common assessment method. Multiple methods are used to assess what we think are multiple traits. So, for example, we could use both test scores and teacher ratings (methods) to assess both reading and mathematics achievements (traits). The resulting correlation matrix would be a multitrait–multimethod matrix.

Both exploratory and confirmatory methods can be used to factor-analyze multitrait–multimethod matrices (e.g., Wothke, 1996). The methods are complex and still under development. The procedures, however, have great potential for the ultimate resolution of the question of bias.

External Indices of Bias

The defining of bias with regard to the relation between a test score and some later level of performance on a criterion measure has produced considerable debate among scholars in the fields of measurement and assessment (see, e.g., Reynolds, 1982; Reynolds et al., 1999). Although this debate has generated a number of selection models from which to examine bias, selection models focus on the decision-making system and not on the test itself. In fact, these selection models are all completely external to the issue of test bias, because each of the models deals solely with value systems and the statistical manipulations necessary to make the test score conform to those values. In contrast, none of the various selection models of "bias" deals with constant error in the estimation of some criterion score (by an aptitude or other predictor test) as a function of group membership. But test bias deals directly with constant or systematic error in the estimation of some true value as a function of group membership. Within the context of *predictive* validity, bias is concerned with systematic error in the estimation of performance on some criterion measure (i.e., constant over- or underprediction).

Since the present section is concerned with statistical bias, and not the social or political justifications of any one particular selection model, a test is considered biased with respect to predictive validity if the inference drawn from the test score is not made with the smallest feasible *random* error, or if there is *constant* error in an inference or prediction as a function of membership in a particular group (Reynolds et al., 1999).

Evaluating Bias in Prediction

The evaluation of bias in prediction under this definition (the regression definition) is quite straightforward. With simple regressions, predictions take the form of $Y_i = a + bX_i$, where a is the intercept, or constant, and b is the regression coefficient. When this equation is graphed (forming a regression line), b represents the slope of the regression line and a the Y intercept. Since our definition of bias in predictive validity requires errors in prediction to be independent of group membership, the regression line formed for any pair of variables must be the same for *each group* for which prediction is to be made. Whenever the slope or the intercept differs significantly across groups, there is bias in prediction if one attempts to use a regression equation based on the combined groups. When the regression equations for two (or more) groups are equivalent, prediction is the same for all groups. This condition is referred to as "homogeneity of regression across groups" (see Reynolds & Kaiser, Chapter 22, this volume, and Reynolds, 2000, for illustrations of these methods).

In the evaluation of slope and intercept values, several techniques have been employed in the research literature. Keith (in preparation) and Pedhazur (1997, Ch. 14) have described the regression method for testing the equivalence of regression equations across groups (for an example, see Kranzler, Miller, & Jordan, 1999). Another method, described by Potthoff (1966; also detailed in Reynolds, 1982) allows the simultaneous test of the equivalence of regression coefficients and intercepts across K independent groups with a single F ratio. If a significant F results, researchers may then test the slopes and intercepts separately if

they desire information concerning which value differs. When homogeneity of regression does not occur, three basic conditions can result: (1) Intercept constants differ, (2) regression coefficients (slopes) differ, or (3) slopes and intercepts both differ. A final method uses multisample path analysis. Briefly (and similar to a multisample confirmatory factor analysis), a path model is estimated across groups, with the paths and intercepts constrained to be equal across groups. All methods may be generalized to more than one independent variable. With multiple *dependent* variables, multisample structural equation modeling may be especially useful.

Testing for Equivalence of Validity Coefficients

The correlation between a test score and a criterion variable, whether measured concurrently or at a future time, is typically referred to as a "validity coefficient" (r_{xy}) and is a direct measure of the magnitude of the relation between two variables. Thus another method for detecting bias in predictive (or concurrent) validity is the comparison of validity coefficients across groups. The procedure described in an earlier section of this chapter for comparing alternate-form reliabilities may also be used to test the hypothesis that r_{xy} is the same for two groups.

Some researchers, in evaluating validity coefficients across groups, have compared each correlation to 0; if one correlation deviates significantly from 0 and the other does not, they have concluded that bias exists. As Humphreys (1973) has explained so eloquently (and as we have suggested in the section "Problems and Needs in Child Assessment Research"), the testing of each correlation for significance is incorrect. To determine whether two correlations are different, they must be compared directly with one another and not separately against hypothetical population values of zero. The many defects in the latter approach have been amply explained by Humphreys and are not reiterated here. Other questions must be considered in comparing the correlations directly with one another, however, such as whether to make corrections for unreliability, restriction of range, and other study-specific elements prior to making the actual comparisons. The particular questions involved, and whether the analyses are directed at questions of theory or those of practice, will influence the outcome of these deliberations.

Path Models of Bias

The concept of bias, and especially predictive bias, may be explained using the concepts of path analysis and latent variables discussed earlier. One such model has been briefly discussed and is illustrated in Figure 4.8. In this model, bias exists when the path from the test (in this case, an intelligence test) to some criterion it should predict (e.g., Achievement) differs across groups, or when the intercepts differ across groups.

Another model of bias is illustrated in Figure 4.9. This figure shows two models in which an intelligence test (Ability) is the predictor of interest and Achievement is the criterion (the models used here are based on ones in Birnbaum, 1981, and Linn, 1984). Group Membership is the dichotomous bias variable, coded 0 for all those who are members of one group (e.g., the minority group) and 1 for all those who are members of another group (e.g., the majority group). The Ability variable enclosed in a rectangle represents measured Ability (the scores on

an intelligence test), whereas the circled Ability variable represents *true* Ability (the latent variable or factor). The top half of the figure shows a no-bias model. Group Membership may affect true Ability (path a), but it only affects measured Ability (and measured Achievement) through true Ability. The bottom half of the figure shows a model in which there is bias in the intelligence test. Group Membership affects true Ability (a), but it also affects measured Ability *independent* of true Ability (path d). To the extent that d deviates from 0, the intelligence test is biased; the errors of measurement are related to Group Membership.

Given a model such as that displayed at the top of Figure 4.9 (the no-bias model), Birnbaum (1979, 1981) and Linn (1984) have illustrated a paradox that results from analyses of predictive bias. Assume that path b is less than 1.00 (i.e., the test is less than perfectly reliable), that path a is not equal to 0 (i.e, there is a correlation between Group Membership and true Ability), and that path c is not equal to 0 (true Ability affects Achievement)—all reasonable assumptions. Given these conditions, it can be shown that if group 1 scores lower on the intelligence test than group 2, then

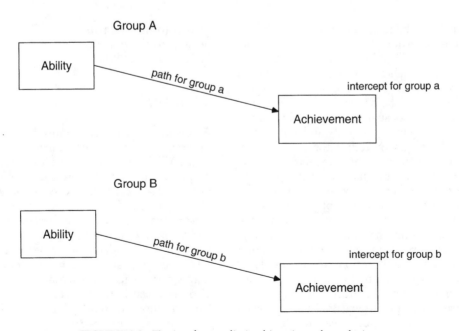

FIGURE 4.8. Testing for predictive bias via path analysis.

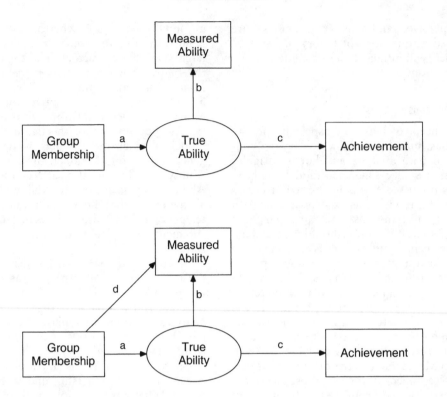

FIGURE 4.9. Another path model of bias. The top model shows a condition of no bias; Group Membership may affect true Ability, but does not affect measured Ability except through true Ability. The bottom model depicts a condition in which the intelligence test is biased; Group Membership affects measured Ability directly. The models used here are based on ones in Birnbaum (1981) and Linn (1984).

group 1 will be lower in measured Achievement than group 2 members *of the same measured Ability,* but that group 2 members will be higher in measured Ability than group 1 members *of the same measured Achievement.* The first part of this paradox would seem to suggest bias in the intelligence test against group 1, and the second half against group 2, but the paradox occurs in the absence of any bias. Furthermore, the second half of this paradox (group 2 members higher in measured Ability than group 1 members of the same measured Achievement) is equivalent to the common finding that intelligence tests overpredict the performance of minority group members on the criterion (see Reynolds & Kaiser, Chapter 22, this volume). That common finding may therefore not suggest any reverse bias, but rather simply be a consequence of imperfect measurement. The models shown in Figure 4.9 can also be ex-

tended to include paths from Group Membership to the outcome variables (see Keith & Reynolds, 1990).

SUMMARY

Assessments of children must be grounded in research if those assessments are to be valid. We have focused here on a diversity of issues in assessment research. We have presented several complex research methodologies (multiple-regression analysis and factor analysis) that are becoming more widely used. Our emphasis has been on providing a basic understanding of those methods, focusing more often on conceptual than on statistical understanding. We have also discussed both the promises and problems of those methods. We have also focused on a research area—test bias—that has generated intense controversy, but has also been extremely productive. This avenue of research illustrates well how multiple methods and procedures can be used to focus on the same research question. Finally, we have briefly covered several basic points about reliability and validity that we believe are often overlooked and that are important for understanding these all-important topics. Our assumption, in all of these presentations, has been that these are topics with which consumers of research (and those who conduct research) will need to be increasingly familiar.

We reemphasize the problems and needs that seem to be too common in child assessment research: Such research needs more consistency with theory and practice, and it should more often involve the testing of hypotheses. Still, much excellent child assessment research is being conducted, and this can form an excellent basis for practice. In order to use this research as a guide for assessment, however, practitioners will need to evaluate it—to separate the wheat from the chaff. We hope that the topics presented here will help in that evaluation.

NOTE

1. Indeed, latent-variable structural equation modeling would be a good choice for estimating this model, because it can allow for correlations among the error and unique variances (the invalidity in Figure 4.1) of variables. If the same or similar achievement measures were administered in second and eighth grades, some of the correlation between the two tests would be due to the correlation between true second-grade achievement and true eighth-grade achievement. But some of the correlation would be the result of correlations between errors of measurement at the two times and between the specific variances of the test at the two times.

REFERENCES

Arbuckle, J. L., & Wothke, W. (1999). *Amos 4.0 user's guide.* Chicago: Smallwaters.

Bentler, P. M., & Bonett, D. G. (1980). Significance tests and goodness of fit in the analysis of covariance structures. *Psychological Bulletin, 88,* 588–606.

Berk, R. A. (1982). *Handbook of methods for detecting test bias.* Baltimore: Johns Hopkins University Press.

Birnbaum, M. H. (1979). Procedures for the detection and correction of salary inequities. In T. H. Pezzullo & B. E. Brittingham (Eds.), *Salary equity* (pp. 121–144). Lexington, MA: Lexington Books.

Birnbaum, M. H. (1981). Reply to McLaughlin: Proper path models for theoretical partialling. *American Psychologist, 36,* 1193–1195.

Browne, M. W., & Cudeck, R. (1993). Alternative ways of assessing model fit. In K. A. Bollen & J. S. Long (Eds.), *Testing structural equation models* (pp. 136–162). Newbury Park, CA: Sage.

Bruning, J. L., & Kintz, B. L. (1997). *Computational handbook of statistics* (4th ed.). New York: Longman.

Carroll, J. B. (1963). A model for school learning. *Teachers College Record, 723–733.*

Carroll, J. B. (1985). Exploratory factor analysis: A tutorial. In D. K. Detterman (Ed.), *Current topics in human intelligence: Vol. 1. Research methodology* (pp. 25–58). Norwood, NJ: Ablex.

Carroll, J. B. (1993). *Human cognitive abilities: A survey of factor-analytic studies.* New York: Cambridge University Press.

Cattell, R. B. (1966). The scree test for the number of factors. *Multivariate Behavioral Research, 1,* 245–276.

Cattell, R. B. (1978). *The scientific use of factor analysis in behavioral and life sciences.* New York: Plenum Press.

Cattin, P. (1980). Note on the estimation of the squared cross-validated multiple correlation of a regression model. *Psychological Bulletin, 87,* 63–65.

Cohen, J., & Cohen, P. (1983). *Applied multiple regression/correlation analysis for the behavioral sciences* (2nd ed.). Hillsdale, NJ: Erlbaum.

Comrey, A. L., & Lee, H. B. (1992). *A first course in factor analysis* (2nd ed.). Mahwah, NJ: Erlbaum.

Cooley, W. W., & Lohnes, P. R. (1971). *Multivariate data analysis.* New York: Wiley.

Darlington, R. B. (1990). *Regression and linear models.* New York: McGraw-Hill.

Eysenck, H. J. (1979). *The structure and measurement of intelligence.* New York: Springer-Verlag.

Fan, X., Thompson, B., & Wang, L. (1999). Effects of sample size, estimation methods, and model specification on structural equation modeling fit indexes. *Structural Equation Modeling, 6,* 56–83.

Fan, X., Willson, V. L., & Reynolds, C. R. (1995). Assessing the similarity of the factor structure of the K-ABC for African-American and white children. *Journal of Psychoeducational Assessment, 13,* 120–131.

Feldt, L. S. (1969). A test of the hypothesis that Cronbach's alpha or Kuder–Richardson coefficient twenty is the same for two tests. *Psychometrika, 34,* 363–373.

Gage, N. L. (1978). *The scientific basis of the art of teaching.* New York: Teachers College Press.

Guilford, J. P. (1954). *Psychometric methods* (2nd ed.). New York: McGraw-Hill.

Harman, H. (1976). *Modern factor analysis* (2nd ed.) Chicago: University of Chicago Press.

Hayduk, L. A. (1996). *LISREL issues, debates, and strategies.* Baltimore: Johns Hopkins University Press.

Hu, L. & Bentler, P. M. (1999). Cutoff criteria for fit

indexes in covariance structure analysis: Conventional criteria versus new alternatives. *Structural Equation Modeling, 6,* 1–55.

Humphreys, L. G. (1973). Statistical definitions of test validity for minority groups. *Journal of Applied Psychology, 58,* 1–4.

Jensen, A. R. (1980). *Bias in mental testing.* New York: Free Press.

Kamphaus, R. W. (2001). *Clinical assessment of child and adolescent intelligence* (2nd ed.). Boston: Allyn & Bacon.

Kane, M. T. (2001). Current concerns in validity theory. *Journal of Educational Measurement, 38,* 319–342.

Kaufman, A. S. (1994). *Intelligent testing with the WISC-III.* New York: Wiley.

Keith, T. Z. (1987). Assessment research: An assessment and recommended interventions. *School Psychology Review, 16,* 276–289.

Keith, T. Z. (1988). Path analysis: An introduction for school psychologists. *School Psychology Review, 17,* 343–362.

Keith, T. Z. (1997). Using confirmatory factor analysis to aid in understanding the constructs measured by intelligence tests. In D. P. Flanagan, J. L. Genshaft, & P. L. Harrison (Eds.), *Contemporary intellectual assessment: Theories, tests, and issues* (pp. 373–402). New York: Guilford Press.

Keith, T. Z. (1999). Structural equation modeling in school psychology. In C. R. Reynolds & T. B. Gutkin (Eds.), *The handbook of school psychology* (3rd ed., pp. 78–107). New York: Wiley.

Keith, T. Z. (in preparation). *Multiple regression and beyond: A conceptual introduction to multiple regression, confirmatory factor analysis, and structural equation modeling.* Boston: Allyn & Bacon.

Keith, T. Z., & Cool, V. A. (1992). Testing models of school learning: Effects of quality of instruction, motivation, academic coursework, and homework on academic achievement. *School Psychology Quarterly, 7,* 207–226.

Keith, T. Z., Fugate, M. H., DeGraff, M., Diamond, C. M., Shadrach, E. A., & Stevens, M. L. (1995). Using multi-sample confirmatory factor analysis to test for construct bias: An example using the K-ABC. *Journal of Psychoeducational Assessment, 13,* 347–364.

Keith, T. Z., Kranzler, J. H., & Flanagan, D. P. (2001). What does the Cognitive Assessment System (CAS) measure? Joint confirmatory factor analysis of the CAS and the Woodcock–Johnson Tests of Cognitive Ability (3rd edition). *School Psychology Review, 30,* 89–119.

Keith, T. Z., & Reynolds, C. R. (1990). Measurement and design issues in child assessment research. In C. R. Reynolds & R. W. Kamphaus (Eds.), *Handbook of psychological and educational assessment of children: Intelligence and achievement.* New York: Guilford Press.

Keith, T. Z., & Witta, L. (1997). Hierarchical and cross-age confirmatory factor analysis of the WISC-III: What does it measure? *School Psychology Quarterly, 12,* 89–107.

Kenny, D. A. (1979). *Correlation and causality.* New York: Wiley.

Kerlinger, F. N. (1986). *Foundations of behavioral research* (3rd ed.). New York: Holt, Rinehart & Winston.

Kerlinger, F. N. & Lee, H. B. (2000). *Foundations of behavioral research* (4th ed.). New York: Harcourt College.

Kim, J. O., & Mueller, C. W. (1978). *Factor analysis: Statistical methods and practical issues.* Beverly Hills, CA: Sage.

Kline, R. B. (1998). *Principles and practice of structural equation modeling.* New York: Guilford Press.

Kranzler, J. H. (1997). What does the WISC-III measure? Comments on the relationship between intelligence, working memory capacity, and information processing speed and efficiency. *School Psychology Quarterly, 12,* 110–116.

Kranzler, J. H., Miller, M. D., & Jordan, L. (1999). An examination of racial/ethnic and gender bias on curriculum-based measurement of reading. *School Psychology Quarterly, 14,* 327–342.

Landy, F. J. (1986). Stamp collecting versus science: Validation as hypothesis testing. *American Psychologist, 41,* 1183–1192.

Lindeman, R. H., Merenda, P. F. & Gold, R. Z. (1980). *Introduction to bivariate and multivariate analysis.* Glenview, IL: Scott, Foresman.

Linn, R. L. (1980). Discussion: Regression toward the mean and the interval between test administrations. In G. Echternacht (Ed.), *New directions for testing and measurement: No. 8. Measurement aspects of Title I evaluations* (pp. 83–89). San Francisco: Jossey-Bass.

Linn, R. L. (1983). Pearson selection formulas: Implications for studies of predictive bias and estimates of educational effects in selected samples. *Journal of Educational Measurement, 20,* 1–14.

Linn, R. L. (1984). Selection bias: Multiple meanings. *Journal of Educational Measurement, 21,* 33–47.

Loehlin, J. C. (1998). *Latent variable models: An introduction to factor, path, and structural analysis* (3rd ed.). Hillsdale, NJ: Erlbaum.

Lord, F. M., & Novick, M. R. (1968). *Statistical theories of mental tests.* Reading, MA: Addison-Wesley.

MacCallum, R. C. (1986). Specification searches in covariance structure modeling. *Psychological Bulletin, 100,* 107–120.

MacCallum, R. C., Browne, M. W., & Sugawara, H. M. (1996). Power analysis and determination of sample size for covariance structure modeling. *Psychological Science, 1,* 130–149.

Menard, S. (1995). *Applied logistic regression analysis.* Thousand Oaks, CA: Sage.

Messick, S. (1989). Validity. In R. L. Linn (Ed.), *Educational measurement* (3rd ed., pp. 13–103). New York: Macmillan.

Pedhazur, E. J. (1997). *Multiple regression in behavioral research: Prediction and explanation* (3rd ed.). New York: Holt, Rinehart & Winston.

Phillips, B. N. (1999). Strengthening the links between science and practice: Reading, evaluating, and applying research in school psychology. In C. R. Reynolds & T. B. Gutkin (Eds.), *The handbook of school psychology* (pp. 56–77). New York: Wiley.

Potthoff, R. F. (1966). *Statistical aspects of the prob-*

lem of bias in psychological tests (Institute of Statistics Mimeo Series No. 479). Chapel Hill: Department of Statistics, University of North Carolina.

Reynolds, C. R. (1982). Methods for detecting construct and predictive bias. In R. A. Berk (Ed.), *Handbook of methods for detecting test bias* (pp. 192–227). Baltimore: John Hopkins University Press.

Reynolds, C. R. (1999). Inferring causality from relational data and designs: Historical and contemporary lessons for research and clinical practice. *The Clinical Neuropsychologist, 13,* 386–395.

Reynolds, C. R. (2000). Methods for detecting and evaluating bias in neuropsychological tests. In E. Fletcher-Janzen, T. Strickland, & C. R. Reynolds (Eds.), *The handbook of cross-cultural neuropsychology* (pp. 249–286). New York: Kluwer Academic/Plenum Press.

Reynolds, C. R. (2002). *Comprehensive Trail-Making Test.* Austin, TX: Pro-Ed.

Reynolds, C. R., & Harding, R. D. (1983). Outcome in two large sample studies of factorial similarity under six methods of comparison. *Educational and Psychological Measurement, 43,* 723–278.

Reynolds, C. R., Lowe, P. A., & Saenz, A. L (1999). The problem of bias in psychological assessment. In C. R. Reynolds & T. B. Gutkin (Eds.), *The handbook of school psychology* (3rd ed., pp. 549–595). New York: Wiley.

Roberts, A. O. H. (1980). Regression toward the mean and the regression-effect bias. In G. Echternacht (Ed.), *New directions for testing and measurement: Vol. 8. Measurement aspects of Title I evaluations* (pp. 59–82). San Francisco: Jossey-Bass.

Rosenthal, R., & Rubin, D. B. (1979). A note on percent variance explained as a measure of the importance of effects. *Journal of Applied Social Psychology, 9,* 395–396.

Rourke, B. P. (1975). Brain–behavior relationships in children with learning disabilities: A research program. *American Psychologist, 30,* 911–920.

Salvia, J., & Ysseldyke, J. E. (2001). *Assessment in special and remedial education* (8th ed.). Boston: Houghton Mifflin.

Satz, P., & Friel, J. (1974). Some predictive antecedents of specific disability: A preliminary two year follow-up. *Journal of Learning Disabilities, 7,* 437–444.

Selz, M., & Reitan, R. M. (1979). Rules for neuropsy-

chological diagnosis: Classification of brain functions in older children. *Journal of Consulting and Clinical Psychology, 47,* 358–364.

Tanaka, J. S. (1993). Multifaceted conceptions of fit in structural equation models. In K. S. Bollen & J. S. Long (Eds.), *Testing structural equation models* (pp. 10–39). Newbury Park, CA: Sage.

Thompson, B. (1998, April). *Five methodology errors in educational research: The pantheon of statistical significance and other faux pas.* Invited address presented at the annual meeting of the American Educational Research Association, San Diego, CA. (ERIC Document Reproduction Service No. ED 419 023)

Thompson, B., & Vacha-Haase, T. (2000). Psychometrics IS datametrics: The test is not reliable. *Educational and Psychological Measurement, 60,* 174–195.

Thompson, L. A., Detterman, D. K., & Plomin, R. (1991). Associations between cognitive abilities and scholastic achievement: Genetic overlap but environmental differences. *Psychological Science, 2,* 158–165.

Thurstone, L. L. (1947). *Multiple factor analysis.* Chicago: University of Chicago Press.

Walberg, H. J. (1981). A psychological theory of education productivity. In F. H. Farley & N. Gordon (Eds.), *Psychology and education.* Berkeley: McCutchan.

Wechsler, D. (1991). *Manual for the Wechsler Intelligence Scale for Children—Third Edition.* New York: Psychological Corporation.

Wherry, R. J., Sr. (1931). A new formula for predicting the shrinkage of the coefficient for multiple correlation. *Annals of Mathematical Statistics, 2,* 440–457.

Willson, V. L., & Reynolds, C. R. (1982). Methodological and statistical problems in determining membership in clinical populations. *Clinical Neuropsychology, 4,* 134–138.

Woodcock, R. W. (1990). Theoretical foundations of the WJ-R measures of cognitive ability. *Journal of Psychoeducational Assessment, 8,* 231–258.

Woodcock, R. W., McGrew, K. S., & Mather, N. (2001). *Woodcock–Johnson III Tests of Cognitive Abilities.* Itasca, IL: Riverside.

Wothke, W. (1996). Models for multitrait-multimethod matrix analysis. In G. A. Marcoulides & R. E. Schumacker (Eds.), *Advanced structural equation modeling* (pp. 7–56). Mahwah, NJ: Erlbaum.

PART II

ASSESSMENT OF INTELLIGENCE AND LEARNING STYLES/STRATEGIES

5

Clinical Interpretation of the Wechsler Intelligence Scale for Children—Third Edition (WISC-III) Index Scores

LAWRENCE G. WEISS
DONALD H. SAKLOFSKE
AURELIO PRIFITERA

The Wechsler Intelligence Scale for Children—Third Edition (WISC-III; Wechsler, 1991) is probably already well known to the readers of this chapter. In fact, the Wechsler scales for assessing intelligence in both children and adults remain among the most often used tests of their kind. For decades, university graduate programs in psychology, including school and clinical psychology, have trained students in the administration, scoring, and interpretation of the WISC-III and its predecessors. Note, for example, that Sattler's (2001) most recent text on cognitive assessment includes three chapters on the WISC-III (and two on the Wechsler Adult Intelligence Scale—Third Edition [WAIS-III]), in contrast to one (or less than one) chapter for any of the other current intelligence tests. Although the legacy of the Wechsler scales essentially began in 1939 with the publication of the Wechsler–Bellevue and continues to the present, each revision has added to that legacy with significant improvements based in clinical research and psychometric advancements. The inclusion of four composite scores based on factor analyses; the added focus on working memory and speed of information processing; and new subtests such as Symbol Search in the WISC-III, and Matrix Reasoning and Letter–Number Sequencing in the WAIS-III, are examples of these changes from the original test. There are exciting prospects for future revisions of these tests, including, in the near future, the Wechsler Preschool and Primary Scale of Intelligence—Third Edition and WISC-IV. Clinical research being conducted as we write will determine whether the advances made in the WAIS-III in terms of new working memory subtests (Letter–Number Sequencing) and new fluid reasoning subtests (Matrix Reasoning) can be applied to children with the WISC-IV.

THE WECHSLER INTELLIGENCE SCALES IN THE CONTEXT OF PSYCHOLOGICAL MEASUREMENT AND ASSESSMENT: CRITICAL VIEWS

Meyer and colleagues (2001) concluded that "formal assessment is a vital element in psychology's professional heritage and a central part of professional practice today" (p. 155). A comprehensive psychological assessment of a child includes the collection of information from different sources (e.g., parents, teachers, the child) and through the use of different methods (e.g., tests, observations, interviews) that reflect characteristics of the child (e.g., intelligence, personality, motivation) and the child's context (e.g., home, school). There is certainly general agreement that the assessment of children's intelligence provides valuable information of relevance to most diagnostic decision needs, as well as for formulating prevention and intervention strategies. Intelligence is one of the most important variables in accounting for individual differences, and although much still needs to be learned about intelligence, we also know and can use a great deal in our descriptions and understanding of children (Deary, 2001; Neisser et al, 1996; Saklofske, 1996).

Wechsler's Definition of Intelligence

As stated above, the WISC-III and its predecessors, the original WISC (Wechsler, 1949) and the WISC-R (Wechsler, 1974), are the most frequently employed individually administered, standardized intelligence tests in use today. Yet—or perhaps because of the widespread use of the WISC-III by school and clinical psychologists—the question posed by some is whether the Wechsler tests have now outlived their usefulness for assessing children's intelligence in both research and applied settings. One criticism is directed at the very definition in which the WISC-III is grounded. In turn, this has led to challenges in the way the Wechsler scales represent and summarize a child's cognitive and intellectual abilities (i.e., via IQ scores). David Wechsler (1944) defined intelligence as "an aggregrate and global entity": "the capacity of the individual to act purposefully, to think rationally, and to deal effectively with his or her environment" (p. 3). This definition is still applied to the current WISC-III, as it was to earlier versions. Wechsler operationalized this definition through the calculation of the Full Scale IQ (FSIQ). However, he further argued for the need to reflect two broad factors in the assessment of intelligence. The ability to use words and symbols is summarized by the Verbal IQ (VIQ), while the ability to manipulate objects and perceive visual patterns comprises the Performance IQ (PIQ).

But the debates heard in the latter part of the 20th century, and extending into the 21st, have in part focused on whether intelligence can be meaningfully or even best represented by a single summary score (such as the FSIQ) versus a number of separate scores. Current research in cognitive psychology and neuropsychology has resulted in new models for describing intelligence. Some of the most recently published intelligence tests that have been presented to clinical and school psychologists reflect these alternative perspectives, such as the Woodcock–Johnson Psycho-Educational Battery—III (WJ-III; Woodcock, McGrew, & Mather, 2001) based on the Cattell–Horn–Carroll model, and the Cognitive Assessment System (Naglieri & Das, 1997) grounded in Luria's PASS model (i.e., planning, attention, simultaneous and sequential processing). Of interest is that all these tests also allow for the calculation of a summary or composite measure of ability. It would seem that the debate begun by Spearman, Thorndike, and Thurstone early in the 20th century has been partially resolved. There is good evidence that more cognitively complex measures tend to correlate and yield a general factor (see Carroll, 1993). Demonstrating that there is a general factor in many of these tests is no longer so much the critical question. However, the four-factor structure of the WISC-III, and the recommended use of the General Ability Index (GAI; see below) when a composite score is required, do raise questions about the current relevance of and need for the VIQ and PIQ scores. These issues are discussed further later in this chapter.

Clinical Relevance and Efficacy

From another perspective, psychologists are required to demonstrate the clinical utility of their assessments as they contribute to diagnosis and appropriate programming. A critical question now asked by practicing psychologists is whether the tests available for their use have "meaningful" diagnostic and prescriptive validity, as well as sound psychometric properties. Many significant changes in psychological science, as well as in applied and professional assessment practice requirements, have occurred since the publication of the WISC in 1949 and the WISC-R in 1974. In fact, each revision of the Wechsler intelligence scales has been subjected to close scrutiny within both professional and public circles. The practicing psychologist must always remain aware of all these evaluations, whether positive or negative, if they are professionally and competently to serve the best interests of the children they are requested to assess. Thus it is not sufficient to state that "I only use the WISC-III because that is what I was trained to do," "I feel comfortable with it," "It tells me all I need to know about a child's intelligence," or "I haven't the time to learn new tests." Alternatively, it would be unwise to state that "I don't use the WISC-III because it doesn't really measure children's intelligence," "The WISC-III is a poor test to use with [a particular ethnic, linguistic, or special needs group]," "I don't believe in a test that gives IQ scores," or "The ideas in the WISC-III are old." Rather, the WISC-III, like any intelligence test, must be evaluated in terms of what it does well and what other tests may do more or less well. Of course, it should also be remembered that intelligence tests do not exist in isolation from the world of children or their home and school environments (Sattler, 2001). Thus all intelligence tests and test results must also be examined and interpreted both in context and in relation to the results of empirically validated research findings.

Intelligence tests have their critics, and the Wechsler family of tests have not been exempted in this regard. In spite of the criticisms, after over 10 years and with a lineage of some 60 years, the WISC-III has demonstrated that it is a psychometrically sound and clinically useful measure of children's intelligence. The very evolution of psychological assessment (and of some of the expectations described above) has made it necessary for the Wechsler scales to continue to evolve. Hundreds of studies have appeared in the research literature supporting the reliability, validity, and clinical value of the WISC-III; many other publications have presented findings that sharpen our use of the test. Several books have been published that provide sound guides to the clinical uses and interpretations of WISC-III test data (e.g., Kaufman, 1994; Prifitera &

Saklofske, 1998). All this has led Sattler and Saklofske (2001b) to conclude:

> The WISC-III has been well-received by those who use tests to evaluate children's and adolescents' intellectual ability. It has excellent standardization, reliability and concurrent and construct validity and useful administrative and scoring guidelines are provided. The manual is outstanding, and much thought and preparation have gone into the revision. The WISC-III will serve as a valuable instrument in the assessment of children's intelligence for many years to come. (p. 262)

Another significant advance in the last decade has been the linking of the Wechsler ability tests to other measures that appear important for diagnosis. The Wechsler intelligence tests have been integrated into a kind of assessment battery that will provide a much more powerful assessment capability for the practitioner. For example, the WISC-III has been linked with the WISC-III as a Process Instrument (WISC-III-PI; Kaplan, Fein, Kramer, Delis, & Morris, 1999), the Wechsler Individual Achievement Test (WIAT; Psychological Corporation, 1992), and the Children's Memory Scale (CMS; Cohen, 1997). The WIAT-II (Psychological Corporation, 2001) in turn is linked with the Process Assessment of the Learner (PAL; Berninger, 2001) and several PAL-based teaching programs for reading, writing, and arithmetic (Berninger, 1998; see also Berninger, Stage, Smith, & Hildebrand, 2001; Busse, Berninger, Smith, & Hildebrand, 2001)). The WAIS-III has been linked with the Wechsler Memory Scale—Third Edition (WMS-III; Wechsler, 1997b) and the WIAT.

STRUCTURE OF THE WISC-III

The changes made to the WISC-III, in relation to the WISC-R, are familiar to psychologists. The most significant changes to the WISC-III, besides the updating of norms (see Flynn, 1984, 1998, for discussions of IQ changes) and the addition of the Symbol Search subtest, have been the ways in which a child's cognitive abilities can now be represented. The FSIQ, VIQ, and PIQ were retained because they are still widely used. For example, school psychologists rely very much on these scores for diagnostic and placement decisions. Overall ability measures provide the guideposts in the assessment of the "two tails" of the ability spectrum (Robinson, Zigler, & Gallagher, 2001). The VIQ and PIQ are still considered useful in the assessment of children who present with various disabilities ranging from hearing impairments to language disorders (see Prifitera & Saklofske, 1998).

However, the emergence of a four-factor structure now also permits the reporting of Index scores, including the Verbal Comprehension Index (VCI), the Perceptual Organization Index (POI), the Freedom from Distractibility Index (FDI) or Working Memory Index (WMI), and the Processing Speed Index (PSI). As we later discuss in greater detail, the Index scores appear to offer an improved means of describing a child's cognitive abilities. Both the VCI and POI are argued to provide purer measures of what was previously measured by the VIQ and PIQ. This is because the emphases on speed and memory have been separated into other factors. Such information is especially useful for both a priori and a posteriori hypothesis testing. Subtest analysis, as well as other "pattern analyses" based on various combinations of subtests, may also be used either for hypothesis generation or as another

> bit of data converging on a particular hypothesis. Of course, psychologists must be careful about jumping to unsubstantiated 'stock' conclusions (e.g., 'everybody knows that Picture Arrangement measures social judgement') regarding the meaning of subtest score differences (Kamphaus, 1998); interpretation is the crux of the assessment endeavor . . . (Kamphaus, 2001, p. ix)

The usual tables reporting statistically significant score discrepancies have been supplemented in the WISC-III technical manual (Wechsler, 1991) with tables showing the frequency of IQ and Index score differences. The addition of these base rate tables permits the psychologist to determine not only whether score differences are statistically significant, but also how frequently they appear. Thus the inclusion of the factorially derived Index scores, with this supporting information, gives the psychologist more specific information on which to base clinical interpretations of a child's cognitive functioning.

The inclusion of both IQ and Index scores on the WISC-III offers the clinician greater options for scoring and interpretation. This is represented in Figure 5.1. However, as we discuss later, we strongly encourage psychologists to consider the Index scores as primary for interpretative purposes.

CHAPTER OBJECTIVES

So what can we say about the WISC-III that has not already been discussed in recent journal articles and books (e.g., Hildebrand & Ledbetter, 2001; Kaufman, 1994; Prifitera & Saklofske, 1998; Sattler & Saklofske, 2001a, 2001b, 2001c). Rather than reviewing this work again, we have chosen to focus the remainder of this chapter on several key features of the WISC-III and to provide some new information for practicing psychologists that we trust will assist in the complex tasks of diagnosis and assessment. In particular, we do the following:

- Review general interpretative strategies for the WISC-III.
- Discuss the relevance of the factor-derived Index scores in contrast to VIQ and PIQ.
- Present the GAI and contrast it to the FSIQ.
- Suggest when the GAI and FSIQ are or are not appropriate summary measures.
- Provide new tables for using the GAI to "predict" WIAT-II scores.
- Discuss the interpretation of the FDI and PSI.
- Discuss the role of working memory and processing speed in higher-order cognitive processing.
- Compare clinical versus factorial models of assessment.

GENERAL INTERPRETATIVE STRATEGIES

It has been common practice that reports of children's intellectual functioning should begin with a discussion of the most global score and proceed in successive levels to less global, more specific scores (e.g., Kaufman, 1994). But is it best to begin one's prereport investigation of a child's WISC-III profile at

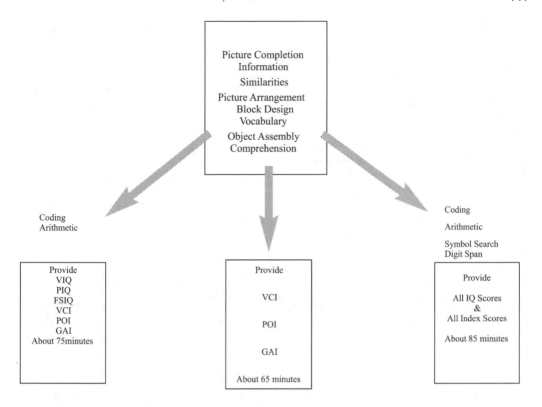

FIGURE 5.1. WISC-III Administration and score options.

the Full Scale level and proceed with an analysis of the scores in the same top-down manner? Whereas the clinical utility and meaningfulness of WISC-III test scores for an individual child may be gleaned at the subtest, Index, and IQ levels, it is also necessary to insure that the psychometric premises on which the WISC-III is founded are met. In order to determine whether the global scores are valid, or which global scores to focus interpretation upon (e.g., VIQ, PIQ, or the Index scores), it is necessary to begin the investigation at a more detailed level and build up to the global interpretations. For example, a VIQ–PIQ discrepancy of 37 points may render the FSIQ less meaningful as an overall summary of intellectual ability (e.g., VIQ = 79, PIQ = 116, FSIQ = 90). In this case, the FSIQ does not capture the child's general cognitive functioning, nor does it reflect the child's abilities based on either the Verbal or Performance scales. This is further indicated by the fact that such a difference is both statistically significant ($p < .05$ for an 11-point difference at all ages) and extremely rare

(occurring in less than 1% of the standardization sample). However, this does not necessarily negate the importance and clinical value of a discrepant finding. For example, in cases of recent lateralized brain trauma, the presence of a large discrepancy may be very meaningful. Rather, the presence of a large Verbal–Performance discrepancy makes interpretation of the child's overall intellectual abilities more complex.

In the same manner, widely divergent subtest scores may also complicate the interpretation of the VIQ, the PIQ, or both as summary measures. Combining scores on the Verbal subtests (or the Performance subtests) that range from 6 to 16 (Information = 16, Arithmetic = 6, Vocabulary = 10, Similarities = 7, Comprehension = 14) would provide an average composite score that would not adequately represent the child's general verbal reasoning abilities.

Similarly, any factor-based score such as the PSI essentially "disintegrates" when, for example, a scaled score of 15 is obtained for Symbol Search versus 7 for Coding. Again this does not negate the potential clinical usefulness of the subtest findings and the hypotheses that may be generated, as long as the test was properly administered and scored, the testing conditions were adequate, and the examinee was motivated and seemed to understand the task demands. It might be that graphomotor difficulties underlie such discrepant scores, or that the child is meticulous when copying figures (at the expense of speed). Thus it may be less than meaningful to combine subtest scores to yield either Index or IQ scores if there are wide differences between them. Once the investigation is accomplished in this detailed, bottom-up manner, an integrated report may then be written in the traditional top-down manner, focusing on the most appropriate global scores when and where appropriate.

Investigation of WISC-III scores should also be conducted within an ecological context. Interpretations of score patterns may vary, depending on the sociocultural background, family educational values, pattern of academic strengths and weaknesses, test session compliance, motivation, and psychiatric and medical history (e.g., Oakland & Glutting, 1998; Puente & Salazar, 1998; Sattler, 2001). A common mistake is to offer stock interpretations of score patterns that do not vary as a function of such mediating influences on the expression of intelligent behavior. Probably all psychologists have had numerous opportunities to comment on children who perform contrary to expectations on the WISC-III (e.g., "He missed two of the more simple Arithmetic items but was successful on all of the others," or "She completed the Block Design and Object Assembly tasks quickly and efficiently, in contrast to teacher reports describing her disorganization and confusion with new tasks and her inability to form and use effective problem-solving strategies"). Not only will interpretations differ in relation to the examinee's personal context and history, but the examiner's expectations of the likeliness of finding certain patterns will be influenced by the referral information and ecological context (e.g., "Given his serious hearing impairment since an early age, I would hypothesize that his Verbal test scores are likely to be lower than his Performance scores"). As Kamphaus (2001) points out, an anticipated or hypothesized pattern of

strengths and weaknesses that is based on such factors and that is subsequently observed in the test data leads to a more meaningful and valid interpretation than the same pattern identified through a "buckshot" approach of comparing all possible test scores.

The following section discusses interpretative strategies for the broader IQ and Index scores that take these issues into account. In particular, we contend that the Index scores are likely to provide more clinically relevant information and should be the preferred "units" for describing broad abilities.

INTERPRETING IQ VERSUS INDEX SCORES

The introduction of Index scores with normative tables occurred with the WISC-III, following the results of both exploratory and confirmatory factor analyses. Earlier versions of the WISC were grounded in the three IQ scores, and sometimes on some nonstandardized subtest patterns described in the research literature. Now, when one is using the WISC-III, it is first necessary to determine whether the IQ or Index scores will be the main focus of interpretation. Probably the major reasons why many psychologists continue to use the IQ scores are that (1) they are familiar, and (2) they are still accepted and expected in the reports written for some institutions such as schools. In addition, the VIQ and PIQ may continue to receive some preference because they form the basis for generating the FSIQ, which again is often used by school and clinical psychologists for describing children's intelligence. The FSIQ, and sometimes the VIQ or PIQ, are usually compared with scores on standardized achievement tests (e.g., the WIAT-II) to assess ability–achievement discrepancies, which in turn may alert a psychologist to a possible learning difficulty.

Increasing numbers of psychologists, however, are employing the WISC-III to focus on the Index scores from the start. Thus they begin the assessment of children with the purpose of measuring verbal ability as reflected in the VCI, nonverbal reasoning as tapped by the POI, and (when relevant to the referral question) the FDI and PSI factors. Thus it is less a question of investigating scoring options after the test has been administered than of deciding in advance what information will be or needs to be gleaned from the test in order to describe a child's current intellectual functioning.

VIQ or VCI?

An initial goal is to determine whether the VIQ is a valid and appropriate indicator of verbal reasoning ability, or whether interpretation should focus upon the VCI . Typically, the VIQ score has been considered the best indicator of verbal reasoning ability. However, in some cases the VCI may be a better estimate of a child's verbal ability. This can occur if the Arithmetic subtest score is significantly different from the other Verbal subtest scores.

The VIQ and VCI differ only because the Arithmetic subtest scaled score enters the calculation of the VIQ score but not the VCI score. Therefore, if the Arithmetic subtest score reflects a significant weakness among a child's scores on the five Verbal subtests, then his or her VIQ score will be less than the VCI score. This tends to occur more often with students in special education programs than with those in regular education programs. For example, Prifitera and Dersh (1993) reported that children diagnosed with learning disablilities earned their lowest scores on the Arithmetic subtest. This is in part due to the finding that the Arithmetic subtest taps problems with attention, concentration, and working memory, as well as reasoning and thinking with numbers. In turn, this has the potential to lower the VIQ and also the FSIQ. As psychometric studies have demonstrated, the four-factor model that best describes the pattern of WISC-III subtests shows that Arithmetic and Digit Span load on the factor termed Freedom from Distractibility. Thus the Arithmetic subtest is not as highly correlated with verbal reasoning as are the other Verbal subtests; in fact, it loads on another factor that is summarized by a separate Index score (the FDI). The VCI excludes Arithmetic and is, in essence, a *purer* measure of verbal reasoning than VIQ is. In such a case, the VCI may be a "fairer" way to represent the child's overall verbal reasoning ability, since it is less affected by the specific measures of attention, concentration, and working memory (Prifitera, Weiss, & Saklofske, 1998).

Therefore, if the Arithmetic subtest scaled score is significantly different from the child's mean of the five Verbal subtest scores, then the VCI score can be considered a better estimate of verbal reasoning than the VIQ score. Table B.3 in the WISC-III manual (Wechsler, 1991) provides the needed data for making this comparison. This applies regardless of whether the Arithmetic subtest score is significantly lower or higher than the mean of the five Verbal subtests. Thus children who happen to possess an isolated strength with numbers or have exceptionally well-developed working memory, for example, in the context of generally average or even lower-than-average overall ability, will have their VIQ (and FSIQ) scores pushed upward by this one task, perhaps resulting in the setting of less accurate expectations.

Other strategies for interpreting WISC-III profiles recommend that the VCI score be utilized when there is a large amount of *scatter* among the five subtests entering the VIQ (Kaufman, 1994) . Verbal scatter is determined by subtracting the highest from the lowest Verbal subtest scaled scores. If the scatter is large among the five subtests entering the VIQ, then the VCI might be emphasized in favor of the VIQ. However, if the scatter is the result of, say, a very high score on the Comprehension subtest and a very low score on the Information subtest, then the VCI will not provide a better estimate of verbal reasoning than the VIQ. This is because the highest and lowest subtests (Comprehension and Information, in this example) are both included in the VCI as well as in the VIQ. In fact, this would be true if the large scatter were caused by any subtest other than Arithmetic. The decision to use the VCI may then hinge on the discovery of a significant difference between Arithmetic and the mean of the five regular Verbal subtests. Alternatively, large Verbal scatter (8 points or more) that *is* caused by a much higher or lower Arithmetic score would also be an appropriate basis for selecting the VCI over the VIQ. However, we recommend that the VCI be used routinely to describe verbal reasoning ability.

PIQ or POI?

On the Performance side, the PIQ and POI scores differ only because the Coding subtest scaled score enters the calculation of the PIQ score but not the POI score. If the Coding subtest scaled score reflects a significant weakness among a child's scores on the five Performance subtests, then his or her PIQ score will be less than the POI score. Again, this may more often be the case among some students with special needs, such as children with attention-deficit/hyperactivity disorder (ADHD) (Prifitera & Dersh, 1993; Schwean & Saklofske, 1998). The Coding subtest taps speed of information processing, and can lower PIQ and FSIQ scores if the student has a relative weakness in this domain; the reverse is true if this is an area of relative strength, as may be found in some children with developmental disabilities. Also, the Coding subtest is not as highly correlated with nonverbal intelligence as are the other Performance subtests, but rather loads most highly on the factor that yields the PSI.

In profiles where there is a discrepancy between Coding and the other subtests constituting the PIQ, the POI may then be a "fairer" or at least more accurate way to represent a summary estimate of the child's overall nonverbal reasoning ability. It has been suggested that the POI is a *purer* measure of nonverbal reasoning than the PIQ (Prifitera et al., 1998). So if the Coding subtest score is significantly different from the other Performance subtest scores, then the POI may be a better indicator of overall nonverbal reasoning ability, and interpretation should focus upon the POI. Again, this strategy applies regardless of whether the Coding subtest scaled score is significantly lower or higher than the mean of the five Performance subtests. Table B.3 of the WISC-III manual (Wechsler, 1991) also gives the necessary data to determine whether Coding produces a significant difference in the child's Performance profile. Thus we recommend that POI be routinely used to summarize nonverbal, perceptual organization ability.

As an additional note, Kaufman (1994) has recommended that the Symbol Search subtest be routinely substituted for Coding when the purpose is to calculate the PIQ. This is based on data from the U.S. standardization study, which showed that Symbol Search correlated higher with PIQ and loaded more highly on the Performance factor than did Coding. These results were also observed in the Canadian standardization of the WISC-III. Tables have subsequently been published to permit the substitution of Symbol Search when one is calculating PIQ and FSIQ in both the United States (Reynolds, Sanchez, & Wilson, 1996) and Canada (Saklofske, Hildebrand, Reynolds, & Wilson, 1998). Although this may be a preferred practice when it is necessary to report the PIQ, the more important point is that both these subtests define a more or less unique processing speed factor. Thus, again, using the POI and allowing both Coding and Symbol Search to define the PSI will potentially provide more meaningful information to the psychologist.

DETERMINING THE BEST WAY TO SUMMARIZE GENERAL INTELLECTUAL ABILITY: THE GAI

Historically, the FSIQ score has been the only method available within the Wechsler scales for summarizing overall or general cognitive ability. This is due both to the model of intelligence proposed by David Wechsler ("an aggregate and global entity") and the fact that correlations among the 13 subtests are high, as are the correlation between each of the subtests and the FSIQ (ranging from .31 to .74). Thus, for any given profile, if VIQ and PIQ are each unitary constructs and are not substantially different from each other, then the best estimate of overall ability is indeed the FSIQ. This is because the FSIQ incorporates not only verbal and nonverbal reasoning, but elements of working memory (Arithmetic) and processing speed (Coding), which are also considered important to overall intelligence (see discussion below).

However, we have previously suggested that the FSIQ is not necessarily the best way to summarize overall ability when the VCI and POI are better estimates of verbal and nonverbal reasoning than the VIQ and PIQ scores, respectively (Prifitera et al., 1998). In fact, when a child's verbal reasoning ability is not fully represented by the VIQ, it may not make a good deal of sense to summarize his or her intelligence with a composite score that includes the same subtests constituting the VIQ! It may be equally difficult to defend using the FSIQ when nonverbal reasoning is less well represented by the PIQ. Furthermore, if the intent of the assessment is to make full use of the Index scores for interpretation, then having particular tests such as Arithmetic and Coding serve more than one purpose may confuse or confound this purpose.

In these situations, it would be more appropriate to utilize an alternative composite score derived from the four subtests that enter the VCI and the four subtests that enter the POI. As noted earlier, this composite is referred to as the GAI, in order to distinguish it from the traditional 10-subtest FSIQ. The GAI score is an eight-subtest composite that *excludes* Arithmetic and Coding, which load on the FDI and PSI, respectively. Those subtests that load on the VCI and POI also account for the most variance when one is estimating FSIQ. The Arithmetic and Digit Span subtests better define the FDI, and the Symbol Search and Coding subtests load on the PSI. Thus this process allows the examiner to estimate a general level of ability, as well as to use the four Index scores to examine individual differences in cognitive ability more closely, given that there is now no subtest overlap. Of relevance is that the GAI and FSIQ were found to correlate .98 in the Canadian standardization sample (Weiss, Saklofske, Prifitera, Chen, & Hildebrand, 1999); this suggests that both measures provide excellent estimates of general mental ability as reflected by the content of the WISC-III. This same procedure has recently been recommended for use with the WAIS-III, where the VCI and POI consist of only three subtests each (Tulsky, Saklofske, Wilkins, & Weiss, 2001).

GAI Norms Tables

We have previously provided national GAI norms for WISC-III practitioners in the United States (Prifitera, Weiss, & Saklofske, 1998), and these are repeated here in Table 5.1 for the convenience of the reader.[1] We

have also recently published national GAI norms for Canadian children, and interested readers are referred to our article published in the *Canadian Journal of School Psychology* (Weiss et al., 1999)

To use Table 5.1, first calculate the General Ability Sum of Scaled Scores (GASSS) by adding the scaled scores for the following eight subtests: Picture Completion, Information, Similarities, Picture Arrangement, Block Design, Vocabulary, Object Assembly, and Comprehension. Find the resulting GASSS in one of the columns labeled "Sum of scaled scores" in Table 5.1, and read across the row to determine the GAI score, associated percentile rank, and confidence interval. Estimates of overall intelligence calculated in this way should *always* be clearly identified as GAI (not FSIQ) scores in psychological and educational reports.

When to Select the GAI to Represent General Intellectual Ability on the WISC-III

We recommend that the GAI be reported under any of the following conditions:

1. When interpretation of verbal abilities focuses on the VCI rather than the VIQ—in other words, when Arithmetic is significantly different from the mean of a student's five Verbal subtest scaled scores.
2. When POI is interpreted rather than the PIQ—that is, when Coding is significantly different from the mean of a student's five Performance subtests.
3. When both VIQ and PIQ are abandoned in favor of interpreting VCI and POI.

When a decision is made to report the GAI in lieu of the FSIQ, it is better to avoid viewing it only as a novelty item (some type of supplemental or alternative score), with "real-life" decisions still being based on the FSIQ. When the GAI is selected on the basis of the decision steps listed above, it is because a psychologist has determined that it represents the best summary of a student's overall intelligence and, when clinically appropriate, should be given primary consideration in most relevant psychological, educational, and vocational decisions. We

TABLE 5.1. GAI Equivalents of Sums of Scaled Scores

Sum of scaled scores	GAI	Percentile rank	Confidence interval 90%	Confidence interval 95%	Sum of scaled scores	GAI	Percentile rank	Confidence interval 90%	Confidence interval 95%
8	50	0.0	47–58	46–59	51	78	7	74–84	73–85
9	50	0.0	47–58	46–59	52	79	8	75–85	74–86
10	50	0.0	47–58	46–59	53	79	8	75–85	74–86
11	50	0.0	47–58	46–59	54	80	9	76–86	75–87
12	50	0.0	47–58	46–59	55	81	10	77–87	76–88
13	50	0.0	47–58	46–59	56	81	10	77–87	76–88
14	50	0.0	47–58	46–59	57	82	12	78–88	77–89
15	50	0.0	47–58	46–59	58	83	13	79–89	78–90
16	50	0.0	47–58	46–59	59	84	14	80–90	79–91
17	51	0.1	48–59	47–60	60	84	14	80–90	79–91
18	52	0.1	49–60	48–61	61	85	16	80–91	80–92
19	53	0.1	50–61	49–62	62	86	18	81–92	80–93
20	54	0.1	51–62	50–63	63	87	19	82–93	81–94
21	55	0.1	52–63	51–63	64	88	21	83–94	82–95
22	56	0.2	53–63	52–64	65	88	21	83–94	82–95
23	57	0.2	54–64	53–65	66	89	23	84–95	83–96
24	58	0.3	55–65	54–66	67	90	25	85–96	84–97
25	58	0.3	55–65	54–66	68	91	27	86–97	85–98
26	59	0.3	56–66	55–67	69	91	27	86–97	85–98
27	60	0.4	57–67	56–68	70	92	30	87–98	86–99
28	61	0.5	58–68	57–69	71	93	32	88–99	87–100
29	62	1	59–69	58–70	72	94	34	89–100	88–101
30	63	1	60–70	59–71	73	94	34	89–100	88–101
31	63	1	60–70	59–71	74	95	37	90–101	89–101
32	64	1	61–71	60–72	75	96	39	91–101	90–102
33	64	1	61–71	60–72	76	97	42	92–102	91–103
34	65	1	61–72	61–73	77	98	45	93–103	92–104
35	66	1	62–73	61–74	78	98	45	93–103	92–104
36	67	1	63–74	62–75	79	99	47	94–104	93–105
37	67	1	63–74	62–75	80	100	50	95–105	94–106
38	68	2	64–75	63–76	81	101	53	96–106	95–107
39	69	2	65–76	64–77	82	102	55	97–107	96–108
40	70	2	66–77	65–78	83	103	58	98–108	97–109
41	70	2	66–77	65–78	84	103	58	98–108	97–109
42	71	3	67–78	66–79	85	104	61	99–109	98–110
43	72	3	68–79	67–80	86	105	63	99–110	99–111
44	73	4	69–80	68–81	87	106	66	100–111	99–112
45	74	4	70–81	69–82	88	107	68	101–112	100–113
46	75	5	71–82	70–82	89	107	68	101–112	100–113
47	75	5	71–82	70–82	90	108	70	102–113	101–114
48	76	5	72–82	71–83	91	109	73	103–114	102–115
49	77	6	73–83	72–84	92	109	73	103–114	102–115
50	77	6	73–83	72–84	93	110	75	104–115	103–116
94	111	77	105–116	104–117	124	138	99	131–141	130–142
95	112	79	106–117	105–118	125	139	99.5	132–142	131–143
96	112	79	106–117	105–118	126	140	99.6	133–143	132–144
97	113	81	107–118	106–119	127	141	99.7	134–144	133–145
98	114	82	108–119	107–120	128	142	99.7	135–145	134–146
99	115	84	109–120	108–120	129	143	99.8	136–146	135–147
100	116	86	110–120	109–121	130	143	99.8	136–146	135–147
101	117	87	111–121	110–122	131	144	99.8	137–147	136–148
102	118	88	112–122	111–123	132	145	99.9	137–148	137–149
103	119	90	113–123	112–124	133	146	99.9	138–149	137–150
104	119	90	113–123	112–124	134	147	99.9	139–150	138–151
105	120	91	114–124	113–125	135	148	99.9	140–151	139–152

TABLE 5.1. *Continued*

Sum of scaled scores	GAI	Percentile rank	Confidence interval 90%	Confidence interval 95%	Sum of scaled scores	GAI	Percentile rank	Confidence interval 90%	Confidence interval 95%
106	121	92	115–125	114–126	136	149	99.9	141–152	140–153
107	122	93	116–126	115–127	137	150	100	142–153	141–154
108	122	93	116–126	115–127	138	150	100	142–153	141–154
109	123	94	117–127	116–128	139	150	100	142–153	141–154
110	124	95	118–128	117–129	140	150	100	142–153	141–154
111	125	95	118–129	118–130	141	150	100	142–153	141–154
112	126	96	119–130	118–131	142	150	100	142–153	141–154
113	127	96	120–131	119–132	143	150	100	142–153	141–154
114	128	97	121–132	120–133	144	150	100	142–153	141–154
115	129	97	122–133	121–134	145	150	100	142–153	141–154
116	130	98	123–134	122–135	146	150	100	142–153	141–154
117	131	98	124–135	123–136	147	150	100	142–153	141–154
118	132	98	125–136	124–137	148	150	100	142–153	141–154
119	133	99	126–137	125–138	149	150	100	142–153	141–154
120	134	99	127–138	126–139	150	150	100	142–153	141–154
121	135	99	128–139	127–139	151	150	100	142–153	141–154
122	136	99	129–139	128–140	152	150	100	142–153	141–154
123	137	99	130–140	129–141					

recommend that, when appropriate, the GAI be used to determine eligibility for services and placement decisions in the same manner as the FSIQ is used when that score is appropriate (e.g., when Arithmetic and Coding are not significantly divergent from the respective composites).

What are the likely consequences of using the GAI in educational decisions? In some special education cases, the GAI will result in a slightly higher estimate of overall intellectual ability than the FSIQ. This will occur when Arithmetic, Coding, or both are significantly below their respective scale means and thus lower the FSIQ score. In determining eligibility to receive services for learning disabilities, this is likely to increase the discrepancy between achievement and ability as estimated by the GAI, thus increasing some students' chances of receiving special assistance. In placement decisions concerning entrance into programs for gifted and talented students, high-functioning students with learning disabilities may also have a better chance of being determined eligible based on the GAI score rather than the FSIQ score. Several studies have reported that children with ADHD tend to earn lower scores on both the FDI and PSI, suggest-

ing that they may also tend to have slightly higher GAI than FSIQ scores (Schwean & Saklofske, 1998). This is even more apparent when both VIQ and PIQ scores are found to be lower than VCI and POI scores (Prifitera & Dersh, 1993; Schwean, Saklofske, Yackulic, & Quinn, 1993). Since there is also some evidence that children identified as gifted tend to score lower on Coding (and Symbol Search) (Wechsler, 1991, p. 210), the GAI score may also boost some children over their school district's preset cutoff score for entrance into programs for gifted and talented students. Of course, the situation can be different for any given student, especially those whose Arithmetic and/or Coding subtest scaled scores are significantly higher than their respective composite means. However, the decision of which summary score to use should be based on the decision steps listed above and not on the desired outcome.

On the low end of the distribution, the situation is less clear. Although the GAI score may tend to be higher than the FSIQ among certain populations receiving special education, there is also some evidence that very low-functioning children tend to score higher on Coding (and Symbol Search) than on other subtests (Wechsler, 1991, p. 210). This may be because these tasks are similar to the matching and copying drills used in many classrooms for students with mental retardation, and are highly practiced skills. As well, it should be remembered that both of these subtests are cognitively very simple, as the aim is to measure processing speed. Thus, for some children in the intellectually deficient range (FSIQ < 70), the GAI score may tend to be lower than the FSIQ score. On the other hand, neither the GAI nor the FSIQ may provide a reasonable summary score if either of the Verbal or Performance scores falls outside the range of mental retardation, and/or if there is a significant and rarely observed discrepancy between them. In this instance, the best description of the child's cognitive abilities may be provided by the Index or VIQ and PIQ scores (Kamphaus, 2001; Spruill, 1998). But an intelligence test score alone should never be the sole basis for "designating" a child or determining his or her educational or vocational placement. Placement decisions for children with mental retardation should also be based on measures of adaptive functioning, such as the Vineland Adaptive Behavior Scales (Sparrow, Balla, & Cicchetti, 1984) or the Adaptive Behavior Assessment System (Harrison & Oakland, 2000).

More to the point, there is not much evidence that IQ or Index scores varying by only a few points have much impact on diagnostic accuracy. So there really is no clinically significant or meaningfully useful distinction between an FSIQ of 55 and a GAI of 53, or an FSIQ of 106 and a GAI of 109. Even though cutoff scores are used for selection or placement purposes, there is really no statistical or clinically discernible difference between an IQ of 130 (which might be the minimum score needed for entry into a gifted education program) and 129! Remember, there are many combinations of subtest scores that can yield either an FSIQ or GAI of 70, 100, 120, and so on. Only at the extreme ends of the FSIQ or GAI range would one also expect all of the subtest scores to be either uniformly very high or very low. And, again, remember that 100 people all earning a FSIQ or GAI score of 100 (mean score or 50th percentile) may also vary in as many ways as there are individual differences variables. Every teacher

can recall four (or many) children with average IQ scores: one who failed and dropped out of school; one who completed high school and works as a salesperson; another who went to a university, earned a teaching degree, and is now a teacher; and yet another who didn't complete high school, but now is an internationally successful artist! This may be a good point to stress that tests themselves do not make decisions (e.g., diagnostic, placement). Decision making is our responsibility as psychologists, and thus we must use tests such as the WISC-III and the information (e.g., VCI, GAI, Vocabulary, qualitative observations) gleaned from them to serve the best interests of children.

One final comment about the GAI is in order. We have described this eight-subtest composite as a purer measure of general cognitive ability than the traditional FSIQ. However, this is in no way meant to imply that we think GAI is a measure of true, innate ability! Like the FSIQ, the GAI is a summary measure of *expressed* (phenotypic) abilities reflected on the WISC-III, which are known to be affected by education, environment, and various personality factors that can moderate the expression of intelligent behavior. Our discussion of GAI as a purer measure of intelligence is meant only to imply a *psychometric* pureness relative to the FSIQ—which can be unduly influenced by certain subtests reflecting working memory and speed of information processing.

DETERMINING WHEN AND WHEN NOT TO SUMMARIZE OVERALL INTELLECTUAL ABILITY

Before one rushes to interpret overall intellectual ability in terms of either the FSIQ or GAI, there is another important question to consider: Do these summary measures represent an "aggregate and global" measure of cognitive ability for the child at hand? Although we have alluded to this issue in the previous pages, it is worth revisiting this critical point and drawing some firm conclusions. For each profile, are the Verbal and Performance scale scores sufficiently similar so that the Full Scale score is clinically meaningful? If the student scores very differently on the Verbal and Performance subtests, then the Full Scale score is simply the average of two widely divergent sets of abilities and therefore not very meaningful as a summary of overall intelligence. For example, if a child's VIQ score is 83 and PIQ score is 120, then the Full Scale score of 100, although a numerically accurate summary, is very misleading from any clinical or practical perspective. Of course, the problem is the same whether one is interpreting the FSIQ or the GAI.

When the Verbal–Performance discrepancy is large, the Full Scale score either should not be reported or should only be reported with appropriate cautions. In these situations it is best to state in the report that, for example, "Johnny's nonverbal reasoning abilities are much better developed than his verbal reasoning abilities, and this unique set of thinking and reasoning skills makes his overall intellectual functioning difficult to summarize by a single score." Then the evaluator should go on to describe his performance on the appropriate Verbal (VIQ or VCI) and Performance (PIQ or POI) composites separately.

How Large a Discrepancy Is Meaningful?

What size Verbal–Performance discrepancy invalidates the Full Scale score? Although a 12-point discrepancy is statistically significant at the $p < .05$ level for both VIQ–PIQ and VCI–POI discrepancies, differences of this size are not uncommon. In fact, more than one-third of the children in the WISC-III standardization sample obtained Verbal–Performance splits of 12 points or greater (Wechsler, 1991, p. 262). (Remember, of course, that this is a 12-point difference in either direction. As a general rule, dividing by 2 will give an approximate estimate of a one-tailed or directional difference.) This occurs because the formula for statistical significance takes into account the size of the sample, and a Verbal–Performance discrepancy of the same size will be more statistically significant in larger samples. With the 2,200 children in the WISC-III standardization sample, a Verbal–Performance difference of only 12 points was significant. Interestingly, in the military, where tens of thousands of recruits are tested annually, a difference of only 2 or 3 points between IQ scores may be statistical-

ly significant—but it is probably not clinically meaningful. This is why many researchers are moving away from a rigid reliance only on traditional criteria of statistical significance when evaluating data. With large samples, we can determine the clinical relevance of a difference by the frequency with which differences of that size occur in the sample. Often we say that if the difference occurs in 10% of cases or fewer, then it is considered less common (or rare) and therefore potentially to be clinically meaningful, or at least to warrant further examination. But even this 10% criterion is rather arbitrary.

As a general rule of thumb, we think that a 20-point Verbal–Performance discrepancy should raise "red flags" in the examiner's mind. A 20-point or greater VIQ–PIQ discrepancy was obtained by approximately 12% of the WISC-III standardization sample. A 20-point or greater VCI–POI discrepancy was obtained by about 14% of the sample. Less than 10% of the sample obtained 22-point or greater discrepancies on either of these measures (Wechsler, 1991, p. 262). It should also be recalled that these percentages do not take the direction of the difference into account, and therefore should be halved (approximately) to determine the percentage of children in the total standardization sample who presented with differences in either direction (e.g., VIQ > PIQ, PIQ > VIQ).

General Mental Ability Estimates and Demographic Factors

The situation becomes more complicated, however, when we take into account sociocultural factors such as the racial/ethnic group of the student, the educational level of the student's parents, and the direction of the difference (Verbal < Performance or vice versa) (Weiss, Prifitera, & Dersh, 1995). Table 5.2 presents cumulative percentages of VIQ–PIQ and VCI–POI discrepancies by direction for all Hispanic children in the WISC-III standardization sample ($n = 242$). Table 5.3 presents the same information for all African American children in the standardization sample ($n = 338$). Note that these data are especially compelling, because these samples were very closely representative of the U.S. population percentages

TABLE 5.2. Cumulative Percentages of WISC-III VIQ–PIQ and VCI–POI Discrepancies in Hispanic Children ($n = 242$)

Amount of discrepancy	IQ discrepancies[a]		Index discrepancies[b]	
	VIQ > PIQ	PIQ > VIQ	VCI > POI	POI > VCI
36	0.0	0.0	0.0	0.8
35	0.0	0.0	0.0	1.2
34	0.0	0.4	0.0	1.2
33	0.0	0.4	0.0	1.2
32	0.4	0.4	0.0	1.7
31	0.4	1.2	0.4	2.5
30	0.4	1.7	0.4	2.9
29	0.4	2.1	0.4	3.3
28	0.4	2.1	1.2	3.3
27	0.4	2.1	1.2	3.7
26	1.7	3.3	1.2	3.7
25	1.7	4.1	1.2	4.5
24	1.7	6.2	1.7	5.0
23	1.7	8.3	1.7	5.8
22	2.5	9.9	1.7	7.0
21	2.5	11.6	2.5	9.9
20	2.5	13.6	2.9	12.0
19	2.9	14.9	3.3	12.8
18	3.3	15.7	4.1	14.5
17	3.3	17.4	4.1	16.1
16	3.3	18.6	4.5	18.6
15	4.1	20.2	4.5	21.1
14	4.5	22.3	5.0	22.3
13	5.8	25.6	5.8	22.7
12	5.8	28.9	7.0	26.9
11	7.0	33.1	8.3	30.6
10	7.9	34.7	9.1	35.1
9	8.3	37.2	9.9	38.0
8	9.9	39.7	12.0	39.3
7	11.6	41.7	14.5	42.6
6	14.0	46.7	16.5	45.9
5	15.3	52.5	18.6	50.4
4	18.2	56.2	20.7	56.6
3	20.7	61.2	22.3	60.7
2	24.0	64.5	23.1	65.7
1	26.4	69.0	26.4	70.2

Note. Data and table copyright 1994 by The Psychological Corporation. All rights reserved. Reprinted by permission.
[a]VIQ = PIQ for 4.6% of the sample.
[b]VCI = POI for 3.4% of the sample.

of Hispanics and African Americans in terms of region of the country and parental education level, and contained equal numbers of subjects at each year of age between 6 and 16. These data are reproduced here in order to encourage culturally sensitive assessment decisions.

Most experienced examiners are aware that Hispanic children tend to score higher on the Performance than on the Verbal sub-

tests. As shown in Table 5.2, 69% of the Hispanic sample obtained higher PIQ than VIQ scores. On average, Hispanic children scored approximately 5 points higher on PIQ than on VIQ, and 5½ points higher on POI than on VCI. A 20-point PIQ > VIQ difference was obtained by 13.6% of the Hispanic sample, and a 20-point POI > VCI difference was obtained by 12% of this sample. Less than 10% of the Hispanic

TABLE 5.3. Cumulative Percentages of WISC-III VIQ–PIQ and VCI–POI Discrepancies in African American Children (n = 338)

Amount of discrepancy	IQ discrepancies[a]		Index discrepancies[b]	
	VIQ > PIQ	PIQ > VIQ	VCI > POI	POI > VCI
31	0.0	0.3	0.0	0.0
30	0.0	0.3	0.3	0.0
29	0.3	0.3	1.2	0.0
28	0.3	0.6	1.5	0.0
27	1.5	0.6	2.1	0.0
26	1.8	0.6	2.7	0.3
25	3.0	0.9	4.4	0.6
24	3.8	1.5	4.7	0.6
23	5.0	2.1	5.9	0.6
22	5.6	2.7	6.8	2.7
21	6.5	3.3	8.0	3.6
20	7.7	4.4	8.9	4.1
19	9.8	4.4	10.4	4.4
18	10.9	5.6	10.7	4.7
17	12.1	6.8	12.4	5.6
16	13.3	7.4	15.1	6.5
15	14.5	8.6	16.3	8.3
14	16.6	10.7	19.2	9.5
13	18.3	11.2	21.9	11.8
12	19.5	13.0	23.7	13.3
11	22.8	13.9	28.4	13.6
10	25.4	14.8	30.5	16.0
9	27.8	16.3	35.2	16.6
8	32.8	18.6	37.6	18.0
7	36.1	21.9	39.1	20.1
6	39.9	24.3	42.6	22.5
5	42.6	28.4	45.0	23.1
4	47.0	30.2	49.4	26.6
3	50.9	32.0	53.8	29.3
2	53.6	36.7	58.3	32.0
1	57.1	40.5	61.8	34.9

Note. Data and table copyright 1994 by The Psychological Corporation. All rights reserved. Reprinted by permission.
[a]VIQ = PIQ for 2.4% of the sample.
[b]VCI = POI for 3.3% of the sample.

sample obtained PIQ > VIQ discrepancies of 22 points or more, and POI > VCI discrepancies of 21 points or more.

Table 5.4 shows the mean discrepancy scores by parental education level for the Hispanic and African American samples. A clear trend is evident for the Hispanic sample: The lower the level of parental education, the larger the mean Performance > Verbal discrepancy. Thus examiners should expect larger Performance > Verbal discrepancies to occur more frequently among Hispanic children whose parents have less education. On the other hand, even moderate discrepancies of this type may be viewed

with suspicion in Hispanic children whose parents have graduated from college.

Even very large Performance > Verbal discrepancies, however, may be given psychoeducational meaning only within the context of the full clinical picture. Hispanic children who have been speaking English as a second language for 3–5 years, for example, may appear bilingual in normal conversation but continue to experience difficulty with tasks that require abstract verbal reasoning in English (e.g., the Similarities and Comprehension subtests). Practitioners must use appropriate clinical sensitivity when interpreting individual Verbal–Perfor-

TABLE 5.4. Means and Standard Deviations for WISC-III VIQ–PIQ and VCI–POI Discrepancies in Hispanic and African American Samples by Parental Education Level and Overall

Parental education level (years)	Hispanic		African American	
	VIQ–PIQ	VCI–POI	VIQ–PIQ	VCI–POI
<9	−8.6 (10.9) $n = 73$	−8.7 (11.4) $n = 73$	4.7 (11.6) $n = 23$	5.5 (11.9) $n = 23$
9–11	−5.7 (9.4) $n = 57$	−5.3 (9.8) $n = 57$	1.4 10.8) $n = 78$	2.5 (11.4) $n = 78$
12	−4.7 (13.7) $n = 65$	−4.3 (13.7) $n = 65$	2.6 (11.9) $n = 142$	3.4 (11.7) $n = 142$
13–15	−2.6 (8.9) $n = 35$	−1.5 (8.8) $n = 35$	1.8 (12.7) $n = 65$	3.5 (12.5) $n = 65$
>15	0.2 (11.8) $n = 12$	0.2 (13.4) $n = 12$	1.8 (11.1) $n = 30$	2.6 (12.9) $n = 30$
Overall	−5.6 (11.4) $n = 242$	−5.2 (11.7) $n = 242$	2.2 (11.7) $n = 338$	3.3 (11.8) $n = 338$

Note. Negative signs indicate Verbal < Performance. Data and table copyright 1994 by The Psychological Corporation. All rights reserved. Reprinted by permission.

mance discrepancies, taking into account the level of acculturation (as suggested by the age at which English was first taught, value placed on English-language development in the home, parental education level, etc.), in order to help differentiate among language loss, delayed language development, and other possible interpretations.

Only 26% of the Hispanic sample obtained a Verbal score higher than the Performance score. Less than 10% of the Hispanic sample obtained VIQ > PIQ discrepancies of 8 points or more, and VCI > POI discrepancies of 9 points or more. For a Hispanic child, therefore, a VIQ of 100 and PIQ of 92 are rare and may indicate a clinically meaningful discrepancy between the child's verbal and nonverbal reasoning abilities. This is true even though an 8- or 9-point difference is not statistically significant. Relying purely on the criterion of statistical significance, or general base rate tables, would cause examiners to miss these cases.

As shown in Table 5.3, there was a general tendency for African American children to score higher on Verbal than on Performance subtests. Fifty-seven percent of the

African American children obtained higher VIQ than PIQ scores, and approximately 62% obtained higher VCI than POI scores. On average, African American children scored approximately 2 points higher on VIQ than on PIQ, and 3 points higher on VCI than on POI. Less than 10% of the African American sample obtained VIQ > PIQ splits of 19 points or greater, and VCI > POI splits of 20 points or more. Thus, when an examiner identifies discrepancies of this magnitude in an African American child, he or she may consider any Full Scale score to be an inappropriate summary of overall intelligence, and proceed with exploring the possible meaning of this discrepancy for the child's psychoeducational functioning.

Performance > Verbal discrepancies occur less often among African American children. PIQ > VIQ differences of 15 points or greater, and POI > VCI splits of 14 points or more, were obtained by less than 10% of the African American sample. Again, practitioners should be careful not to ignore moderate Performance > Verbal discrepancies in African American children, as they occur infrequently.

Finally, as suggested earlier, these critical values should not be applied in a rigid fashion. There is nothing "magical," "exact," or "definite" about a 22-point discrepancy, for example, that makes a child noticeably different from a child with a 19- or 20-point discrepancy. Rather, differences that are either or both statistically different and infrequent should alert the psychologist to the potential relevance of this observation for describing and understanding children's cognitive abilities in relation to their academic, social, and personal needs. As always, test results must be interpreted in the context of a full sensitivity toward a child's culture, combined with an understanding of his or her medical and educational history, parental and environmental factors, and premorbid level of functioning.

ABILITY–ACHIEVEMENT DISCREPANCIES: THE GAI AND WIAT-II

Most state departments of education require evidence of a significant discrepancy between a student's ability and achievement in one or more content areas defined under the Individuals with Disabilities Education Act (IDEA; Public Law 101-476, 1990) and its amendments in order to qualify the student for special educational services. To accomplish this comparison, some states use the simple-difference method, while others use the predicted-difference method (see Gridley & Roid, 1998).

Simple-Difference Method

The simple-difference method involves subtracting the student's ability score (such as the WISC-III FSIQ) from the child's score on a nationally standardized achievement test (such as the WIAT-II or WJ-III). Usually, students with a 15-point difference or greater are deemed to qualify for services, depending on the state. The following description and tables focus on the WISC-III and the recently published WIAT-II, since the two tests were examined together in a linking study during the standardization of the WIAT-II. The WIAT-II is an improved achievement measure with extended diagnostic capabilities. This will increase the likelihood that psychologists will use both

tests when assessing intelligence and achievement.

In order for practitioners to utilize the simple-difference method most effectively, it is also important to know the magnitude of the difference between ability and achievement required for statistical significance, and the frequency with which a difference of that magnitude occurs in the population. This information has not previously been available for the GAI score. Table 5.5 shows the differences between WISC-III GAI scores and obtained WIAT-II subtest and composite standard scores required for statistical significance for children in two age bands. For a 9-year-old child, a GAI score of 95 and a WIAT-II Word Reading standard score of 85 (a 10-point difference) would be considered a significant difference at the $p < .05$ level. Table 5.6 shows the differences between WISC-III GAI scores and WIAT-II subtest and composite standard scores obtained by various percentages of children. As shown in this table, a 10-point difference between GAI and Word Reading was obtained by 17% of the children in the linking study of the WISC-III and WIAT-II.

Predicted-Difference Method

In the predicted-difference method, the ability score is used to predict the student's expected score on the achievement test (based on statistical regression equations or their equivalents). This predicted achievement score is then compared to the student's actual achievement score, and the difference is evaluated for significance. This method is preferred on statistical grounds, but it requires the use of ability and achievement tests that have been conormed on the same national sample, which was done with the WIAT-II and WISC-III. To date, the necessary information to use the GAI in ability–achievement discrepancy analyses has not been available.

In this chapter, we extend our previous work with the GAI by providing tables for predicting WIAT-II achievement scores based on the WISC-III GAI score, and analyzing the difference. Table 5.7 shows WIAT-II subtest and composite standard scores predicted from WISC-III GAI scores for children ages 6 through 16. The examiner looks up the student's obtained GAI score

TABLE 5.5. Differences between WISC-III GAI and WIAT–II Subtest and Composite Standard Scores Required for Statistical Significance (Simple-Difference Method)

Subtests/composites	Ages 6:0–11:11[a]		Ages 12:0–16:11[a]	
	p	GAI	p	GAI
Subtests				
Word Reading	.05	8.32	.05	8.56
	.01	10.95	.01	11.27
Numerical Operations	.05	12.34	.05	9.71
	.01	16.25	.01	12.79
Reading Comprehension	.05	9.00	.05	8.87
	.01	11.84	.01	11.68
Spelling	.05	9.56	.05	9.86
	.01	12.59	.01	12.98
Pseudoword Decoding	.05	8.32	.05	7.94
	.01	10.95	.01	10.45
Math Reasoning	.05	10.24	.05	9.90
	.01	13.48	.01	13.03
Written Expression	.05	13.07	.05	12.49
	0.01	17.21	.01	16.44
Listening Comprehension	.05	14.42	.05	14.05
	.01	18.98	.01	18.50
Oral Expression	.05	12.38	.05	12.94
	0.01	16.30	.01	17.04
Composites				
Reading	.05	7.78	.05	7.78
	.01	10.24	.01	10.24
Mathematics	.05	9.84	.05	8.25
	.01	12.95	.01	10.86
Written Language	.05	9.89	.05	9.64
	.01	13.02	.01	12.70
Oral Language	.05	11.46	.05	11.66
	.01	15.08	.01	15.35
Total	.05	7.78	.05	7.04
	0.01	10.24	.01	9.27

Note. Data and table copyright 2001 by The Psychological Corporation. All rights reserved. Reprinted by permission.
[a]Ages are given in years:months.

in this table, and then reads across the row to the predicted achievement score. For example, according to this table, a child with a GAI score of 90 is predicted to have a Reading Comprehension standard score of 94. This is due to a statistical phenomenon known as "regression to the mean." Let's say this child obtained a Reading Comprehension score of 79. The simple difference between his or her GAI (90) and Reading Comprehension (79) scores would be 11 points, but the difference between the pre-

dicted (94) and obtained (79) Reading Comprehension scores would be 15 points. Note, however, that for children with ability scores above 100, the regression-to-the-mean phenomenon works in reverse, so that the difference between predicted and obtained achievement scores would be smaller than the simple difference.

Tables 5.8 and 5.9 parallel Tables 5.5 and 5.6, except that these tables are for use with the predicted-difference method. Table 5.8 shows the differences between predicted

TABLE 5.6. Differences between WISC-III GAI and WIAT–II Subtest and Composite Standard Scores Obtained by Various Percentages of Children in the Linking Sample (Simple-Difference Method)

Subtests/composites	Percentage[a]								
	25	20	15	10	5	4	3	2	1
Subtests									
Word Reading	9	11	14	17	22	24	26	28	32
Numerical Operations	10	12	15	18	24	25	27	30	34
Reading Comprehension	9	11	13	16	21	22	24	26	30
Spelling	10	13	16	19	25	26	28	31	35
Pseudoword Decoding	10	12	16	19	25	26	28	31	35
Math Reasoning	8	10	12	15	19	20	21	23	27
Written Expression	10	12	15	19	25	26	28	31	35
Listening Comprehension	8	10	12	15	19	21	22	24	27
Oral Expression	10	13	16	20	25	27	29	32	36
Composites									
Reading	9	11	13	16	21	22	24	26	30
Mathematics	8	10	13	16	20	22	23	25	29
Written Language	10	12	15	18	24	25	27	30	34
Oral Language	8	10	12	15	20	21	23	25	28
Total	7	9	11	14	18	19	21	23	26

Note. Data and table copyright 2001 by The Psychological Corporation. All rights reserved. Reprinted by permission.
[a]Percentage of children whose obtained achievement score was below their GAI score by the specified amounts.

and actual WIAT-II subtest and composite standard scores required for statistical significance in two age bands. Table 5.9 shows the differences between predicted and actual WIAT-II subtest and composite standard scores obtained by various percentages of children

These tables have been created by the same statistical methods, and are based on the same nationally representative WISC-III–WIAT-II linking sample (*n* = 775), as described in the WIAT-II technical manual (Psychological Corporation, 2001) for the prediction of WIAT-II achievement scores from the WISC-III FSIQ. Of particular note about the methodology is the fact that this sample was also used to revalidate the WISC-III norms so that they would be current with the WIAT-II norms developed 10 years later. A recalibration of approximately 2–3 points is built into Table 5.7, which shows WIAT-II achievement scores predicted from *obtained* WISC-III GAI scores. Thus WISC-III–WIAT-II discrepancy scores derived from the predicted-difference method are based on ability and achievement scores that were conormed at the same point in time.

Although the methods described here to determine ability–achievement discrepancies are statistically sound and represent best current practice, some cautionary notes about this approach to special education assessment are in order. Practitioners must clearly understand that ability–achievement discrepancies are used only to determine eligibility to receive special education services, and that determining eligibility based on this criterion may not always equate to a diagnosis of learning disability. Although assessments of intellectual potential and academic achievement are essential components of an overall evaluation of the total student, the presence of an ability–achievement discrepancy is not sufficient to diagnose a learning disability. A diagnosis of learning disability requires evidence of impairment in the core cognitive processes that underlie the academic skill in question. For example, we know that specific language impairments in preschoolers are often precursors to learning disorders in school, and that deficits in rapid automatized naming and pseudoword decoding are strong predictors of latter reading disorders in early elementary school. The next frontier in school psy-

TABLE 5.7. WIAT-II Subtest and Composite Standard Scores Predicted from the WISC-III GAI Scores for Children Ages 6 Years, 0 Months to 16 Years, 11 Months

	Subtest total raw scores									Composite standard scores					
GAI score	Word Read.	Num. Ops.	Read. Comp.	Spell.	Pseudowd. Decod.	Math Reason.	Written Expr.	Listen. Comp.	Oral Expr.	Read.	Math	Written Lang.	Oral Lang.	Total	GAI score
40	63	67	60	69	69	55	69	56	71	60	58	67	57	54	40
41	64	67	60	70	70	56	69	57	71	61	59	67	58	55	41
42	65	68	61	70	70	57	70	58	72	62	60	68	59	56	42
43	65	69	62	71	71	57	70	59	72	62	60	68	60	56	43
44	66	69	62	71	71	58	71	59	73	63	61	69	60	57	44
45	66	70	63	72	72	59	71	60	73	64	62	69	61	58	45
46	67	70	64	72	72	60	72	61	74	64	62	70	62	59	46
47	67	71	64	73	73	60	72	61	74	65	63	70	62	59	47
48	68	71	65	73	73	61	73	62	75	65	64	71	63	60	48
49	69	72	66	74	74	62	73	63	75	66	64	71	64	61	49
50	69	72	66	74	74	62	74	63	75	67	65	72	64	61	50
51	70	73	67	75	75	63	74	64	76	67	66	72	65	62	51
52	70	73	67	75	75	64	75	65	76	68	66	73	66	63	52
53	71	74	68	76	76	65	75	65	77	69	67	74	66	64	53
54	72	74	69	76	76	65	76	66	77	69	68	74	67	64	54
55	72	75	69	77	77	66	76	67	78	70	68	75	68	65	55
56	73	75	70	77	77	67	77	68	78	70	69	75	68	66	56
57	73	76	71	78	78	67	77	68	79	71	70	76	69	67	57
58	74	76	71	78	78	68	78	69	79	72	70	76	70	67	58
59	74	77	72	79	78	69	78	70	80	72	71	77	70	68	59
60	75	77	73	79	79	70	79	70	80	73	72	77	71	69	60
61	76	78	73	80	79	70	79	71	81	74	72	78	72	69	61
62	76	78	74	80	80	71	80	72	81	74	73	78	72	70	62
63	77	79	74	81	80	72	80	72	81	75	74	79	73	71	63
64	77	80	75	81	81	72	81	73	82	75	74	79	74	72	64
65	78	80	76	82	81	73	81	74	82	76	75	80	74	72	65
66	79	81	76	82	82	74	82	74	83	77	76	80	75	73	66
67	79	81	77	83	82	74	82	75	83	77	76	81	76	74	67
68	80	82	78	83	83	75	83	76	84	78	77	81	76	75	68
69	80	82	78	84	83	76	83	77	84	79	78	82	77	75	69
70	81	83	79	84	84	77	84	77	85	79	78	83	78	76	70
71	81	83	80	84	84	77	84	78	85	80	79	83	78	77	71
72	82	84	80	85	85	78	85	79	86	81	80	84	79	77	72
73	83	84	81	85	85	79	85	79	86	81	80	84	80	78	73
74	83	85	81	86	86	79	86	80	87	82	81	85	80	79	74
75	84	85	82	86	86	80	86	81	87	82	82	85	81	80	75
76	84	86	83	87	87	81	87	81	87	83	82	86	82	80	76
77	85	86	83	87	87	82	87	82	88	84	83	86	82	81	77
78	85	87	84	88	88	82	88	83	88	84	84	87	83	82	78
79	86	87	85	88	88	83	88	83	89	85	84	87	84	83	79
80	87	88	85	89	89	84	89	84	89	86	85	88	84	83	80
81	87	88	86	89	89	84	89	85	90	86	86	88	85	84	81
82	88	89	87	90	90	85	90	85	90	87	86	89	86	85	82
83	88	90	87	90	90	86	90	86	91	87	87	89	87	85	83
84	89	90	88	91	91	87	91	87	91	88	87	90	87	86	84
85	90	91	89	91	91	87	91	88	92	89	88	90	88	87	85
86	90	91	89	92	92	88	92	88	92	89	89	91	89	88	86
87	91	92	90	92	92	89	92	89	93	90	89	92	89	88	87
88	91	92	90	93	93	89	93	90	93	91	90	92	90	89	88
89	92	93	91	93	93	90	93	90	94	91	91	93	91	90	89
90	92	93	92	94	94	91	94	91	94	92	91	93	91	91	90
91	93	94	92	94	94	91	94	92	94	92	92	94	92	91	91
92	94	94	93	95	95	92	95	92	95	93	93	94	93	92	92
93	94	95	94	95	95	93	95	93	95	94	93	95	93	93	93
94	95	95	94	96	96	94	96	94	96	94	94	95	94	93	94
95	95	96	95	96	96	94	96	94	96	95	95	96	95	94	95
96	96	96	96	97	97	95	97	95	97	96	95	96	95	95	96
97	97	97	96	97	97	96	97	96	97	96	96	97	96	96	97
98	97	97	97	98	98	96	98	97	98	97	97	97	97	96	98
99	98	98	97	98	98	97	98	97	98	97	97	98	97	97	99
100	98	98	98	99	99	98	99	98	99	98	98	98	98	98	100
101	99	99	99	99	99	99	99	99	99	99	99	99	99	99	101
102	99	99	99	100	100	99	100	99	100	99	99	99	99	99	102

TABLE 5.7. *Continued*

	Subtest total raw scores									Composite standard scores					
GAI score	Word Read.	Num. Ops.	Read. Comp.	Spell.	Pseudowd. Decod.	Math Reason.	Written Expr.	Listen. Comp.	Oral Expr.	Read.	Math	Written Lang.	Oral Lang.	Total	GAI score
103	100	100	100	100	100	100	100	100	100	100	100	100	100	100	103
104	101	101	101	100	100	101	100	101	100	101	101	101	101	101	104
105	101	101	101	101	101	101	101	101	101	101	101	101	101	101	105
106	102	102	102	101	101	102	101	102	101	102	102	102	102	102	106
107	102	102	103	102	102	103	102	103	102	103	103	102	103	103	107
108	103	103	103	102	102	104	102	103	102	103	103	103	103	104	108
109	103	103	104	103	103	104	103	104	103	104	104	103	104	104	109
110	104	104	104	103	103	105	103	105	103	104	105	104·	105	105	110
111	105	104	105	104	104	106	104	106	104	105	105	104	105	106	111
112	105	105	106	104	104	106	104	106	104	106	106	105	106	107	112
113	106	105	106	105	105	107	105	107	105	106	107	105	107	107	113
114	106	106	107	105	105	108	105	108	105	107	107	106	107	108	114
115	107	106	108	106	106	109	106	108	106	108	108	106	108	109	115
116	108	107	108	106	106	109	106	109	106	108	109	107	109	109	116
117	108	107	109	107	107	110	107	110	106	109	109	107	109	110	117
118	109	108	110	107	107	111	107	110	107	109	110	108	110	111	118
119	109	108	110	108	108	111	108	111	107	110	111	108	111	112	119
120	110	109	111	108	108	112	108	112	108	111	111	109	111	112	120
121	110	109	111	109	109	113	109	112	108	111	112	110	112	113	121
122	111	110	112	109	109	113	109	113	109	112	113	110	113	114	122
123	112	111	113	110	110	114	110	114	109	113	113	111	114	115	123
124	112	111	113	110	110	115	110	115	110	113	114	111	114	115	124
125	113	112	114	111	111	116	111	115	110	114	114	112	115	116	125
126	113	112	115	111	111	116	111	116	111	114	115	112	116	117	126
127	114	113	115	112	112	117	112	117	111	115	116	113	116	117	127
128	115	113	116	112	112	118	112	117	112	116	116	113	117	118	128
129	115	114	117	113	113	118	113	118	112	116	117	114	118	119	129
130	116	114	117	113	113	119	113	119	113	117	118	114	118	120	130
131	116	115	118	114	114	120	114	119	113	118	118	115	119	120	131
132	117	115	119	114	114	121	114	120	113	118	119	115	120	121	132
133	117	116	119	115	115	121	115	121	114	119	120	116	120	122	133
134	118	116	120	115	115	122	115	121	114	119	120	116	121	123	134
135	119	117	120	116	116	123	116	122	115	120	121	117	122	123	135
136	119	117	121	116	116	123	116	123	115	121	122	117	122	124	136
137	120	118	122	116	117	124	117	123	116	121	122	118	123	125	137
138	120	118	122	117	117	125	117	124	116	122	123	119	124	125	138
139	121	119	123	117	118	126	118	125	117	123	124	119	124	126	139
140	121	119	124	118	118	126	118	126	117	123	124	120	125	127	140
141	122	120	124	118	119	127	119	126	118	124	125	120	126	128	141
142	123	120	125	119	119	128	119	127	118	125	126	121	126	128	142
143	123	121	126	119	120	128	120	128	119	125	126	121	127	129	143
144	124	122	126	120	120	129	120	128	119	126	127	122	128	130	144
145	124	122	127	120	121	130	121	129	119	126	128	122	128	131	145
146	125	123	127	121	121	130	121	130	120	127	128	123	129	131	146
147	126	123	128	121	122	131	122	130	120	128	129	123	130	132	147
148	126	124	129	122	122	132	122	131	121	128	130	124	130	133	148
149	127	124	129	122	122	133	123	132	121	129	130	124	131	133	149
150	127	125	130	123	123	133	123	132	122	130	131	125	132	134	150
151	128	125	131	123	123	134	124	133	122	130	132	125	132	135	151
152	128	126	131	124	124	135	124	134	123	131	132	126	133	136	152
153	129	126	132	124	124	135	125	135	123	131	133	127	134	136	153
154	130	127	133	125	125	136	125	135	124	132	134	127	134	137	154
155	130	127	133	125	125	137	126	136	124	133	134	128	135	138	155
156	131	128	134	126	126	138	126	137	125	133	135	128	136	139	156
157	131	128	134	126	126	138	127	137	125	134	136	129	136	139	157
158	132	129	135	127	127	139	127	138	125	135	136	129	137	140	158
159	133	129	136	127	127	140	128	139	126	135	137	130	138	141	159
160	133	130	136	128	128	140	128	139	126	136	138	130	138	141	160

Note. Based on the correlations between WIAT–II standard scores and WISC–III GAI scores in the linking sample (*n* = 775). Presented in the order shown in the table, the correlations for the nine WIAT–II subtests were .581, .525, .638, .485, .489, .709, .492, .691, and .463, and the correlations for the five WIAT–II composites were .629, .659, .530, .675, and .727. Predicted scores include an adjustment for the difference between norming dates (refer to WIAT-II manual [Psychological Corporation, 2001, p. 153] for details). Data and table copyright 2001 by The Psychological Corporation. All rights reserved. Reprinted by permission.

TABLE 5.8. Differences between Predicted and Actual WIAT–II Subtest and Composite Standard Scores Required for Statistical Significance Using WISC-III GAI Score (Predicted-Difference Method)

Subtests/composites	Ages 6:0–11:11[a]		Ages 12:0–16:11[a]	
	p	GAI	p	GAI
Subtests				
Word Reading	.05	6.43	.05	7.00
	.01	8.46	.01	9.22
Numerical Operations	.05	10.95	.05	8.38
	.01	14.41	.01	11.03
Reading Comprehension	.05	7.38	.05	7.63
	.01	9.72	.01	10.05
Spelling	.05	7.78	.05	8.22
	.01	10.24	.01	10.82
Pseudoword Decoding	.05	6.04	.05	6.02
	.01	7.95	.01	7.92
Math Reasoning	.05	9.19	.05	8.95
	.01	12.10	.01	11.78
Written Expression	.05	11.77	.05	11.37
	.01	15.49	.01	14.96
Listening Comprehension	.05	13.58	.05	13.44
	.01	17.88	.01	17.69
Oral Expression	.05	11.10	.05	11.70
	.01	14.61	.01	15.40
Composites				
Reading	.05	5.80	.05	6.33
	.01	7.63	.01	8.33
Mathematics	.05	8.51	.05	6.96
	.01	11.21	.01	9.17
Written Language	.05	8.26	.05	8.12
	.01	10.87	.01	10.69
Oral Language	.05	10.45	.05	10.75
	.01	13.76	.01	14.16
Total	.05	6.30	.05	5.84
	.01	8.29	.01	7.69

Note. Data and table copyright 2001 by The Psychological Corporation. All rights reserved. Reprinted by permission.
[a]Ages are given in years:months.

chology may be the early identification of students with learning disabilities *before* the cumulative effects of the disabilities result in discrepancies between their ability and achievement.

For some children with learning disabilities or attentional disorders, the GAI partly removes the impact of their disabilities on the estimate of intelligence. Thus the GAI is useful in evaluating the impact of such disabilities on intelligence, and the procedures described here are appropriate when one is

determining eligibility for special education services. As described below, however, working memory and processing speed are essential to a more complete and integrated view of intelligence.

STRATEGIES FOR INTERPRETING THE FDI

The most crucial element in the proper interpretation of the FDI score is the examiner's knowledge that this index does not in

TABLE 5.9. Differences between Predicted and Actual WIAT-II Subtest and Composite Standard Scores Obtained by Various Percentages of Children in the Linking Sample Based on WISC-III GAI Scores (Predicted-Difference Method)

Subtests/composites	Percentage[a]								
	25	20	15	10	5	4	3	2	1
Subtests									
Word Reading	8	10	13	16	20	21	23	25	28
Numerical Operations	9	11	13	16	21	22	24	26	30
Reading Comprehension	8	10	12	15	19	20	22	24	27
Spelling	9	11	13	17	21	23	25	27	30
Pseudoword Decoding	9	11	13	17	21	23	24	27	30
Math Reasoning	7	9	11	14	17	18	20	22	25
Written Expression	9	11	13	17	21	23	24	27	30
Listening Comprehension	7	9	11	14	18	19	20	22	25
Oral Expression	9	11	14	17	22	23	25	27	31
Composites									
Reading	8	10	12	15	19	20	22	24	27
Mathematics	8	9	12	14	19	20	21	23	26
Written Language	9	11	13	16	21	22	24	26	30
Oral Language	7	9	11	14	18	19	21	23	26
Total	7	9	11	13	17	18	19	21	24

Note. Data and table copyright 2001 by The Psychological Corporation. All rights reserved. Reprinted by permission.
[a]Percentage of children whose obtained achievement standard score was below their GAI score by the specified amounts.

fact measure distractibility. This composite was originally named "Freedom from Distractibility" in the interest of simplicity (Cohen, 1959), and the name was retained in the WISC-III for reasons of historical continuity. But "Freedom from Distractibility" is a misleading name for this construct, because it may tend to encourage naive interpretations on the part of lay readers of WISC-III reports (e.g., teachers, parents, principals, and even pediatricians), as well as some inexperienced or poorly trained examiners!

This composite of Arithmetic and Digit Span is better conceptualized as a measure of working memory (i.e., WMI), as has been demonstrated on the WAIS-III (Wechsler, 1997a). "Working memory" is the ability to hold information in mind temporarily while performing some operation or manipulation with that information, or engaging in an interfering task, and then accurately reproducing the information or correctly acting on it. Working memory can be thought of as mental control involving reasonably higher-order tasks (rather than rote tasks), and it presumes attention and concentration. Thus

this index measures the ability to sustain attention, concentrate, and exert mental control. In the WAIS-III (Wechsler, 1997a), a composite of the Arithmetic, Digit Span, and Letter–Number Sequencing subtests has been renamed the WMI. One might expect the WISC-IV to do the same.

Digit Span backward is an excellent example of a task designed to tap working memory, because the student must hold in his or her short-term memory store a string of numbers while reversing the sequence, and then must correctly reproduce the numbers in the new order. The Arithmetic subtest is a more ecologically valid working memory task than Digit Span backward. We are frequently called upon to mentally calculate arithmetic problems in real-life situations. Some examples include checking change at the grocery store, estimating driving time at a certain rate of speed, halving the ingredients for a cake recipe, remembering a telephone number to call while entering the security code on the front door, or even figuring out what combination of touchdowns and field goals a losing football team needs to score in order to win the game. For students who have not learned grade-level skills related to arithmetic calculation and mathematical operations, or for students with a primary mathematical disability, the Arithmetic subtest may not be an accurate indication of working memory. An alternate hypothesis, however, is that such a student may have had difficulty in acquiring the requisite mathematical concepts because of the deficit in working memory. The point is that the Arithmetic subtest assesses a complex set of cognitive skills and abilities, and a low score may have several appropriate interpretations, depending on the clinical context.

It should also be remembered that both the Arithmetic and Digit Span subtests tap only verbal working memory, and not spatial or visual working memory. Working memory does not involve only numbers. Other examples include writing the main points of a teacher's lecture in a notebook while continuing to attend to the lecture, or keeping a three-part homework assignment in mind while recording the first two parts in an assignment pad, or keeping in mind the next points one wants to make while explaining one's first point. Clearly, a serious deficit in working memory can have major implications in a student's academic life, and can create difficulties in daily life functioning as well as in many vocational settings.

Children with learning or attentional disorders may be more likely to experience problems with working memory, as suggested by significantly lower scores on the WISC-III FDI (Wechsler, 1991). However, this must be demonstrated to be the case with each individual, rather than being assumed to apply to all children with a particular diagnosis or being used as a diagnostic "marker" (see Kaufman, 1994). Children with serious deficits in working memory are academically challenged, but not necessarily because of lower intelligence. A weakness in working memory may make the processing of complex information more time-consuming and drain the student's mental energies more quickly as compared to other children of the same age, perhaps contributing to more frequent errors on a variety of learning tasks. Executive function system deficits in planning, organization, and the ability to shift cognitive sets should also be evaluated with these children.

At home, these children can appear oppositional when they fail to "remember" that they were supposed to clean their room after watching a TV show, or "forget" a second instruction while performing the first task or chore assigned. Some of these children are dismayed by the way ideas seem to fly out of their minds, while others willingly accept the role of the class clown (or worse) cast upon them by others. When the FDI is low, practitioners should question teachers and parents about these behaviors and help them reframe the problem. Viewing these children as simply distractible oversimplifies the problem and leads to treatment strategies designed to reduce extraneous stimulation, which will largely be ineffective. Even worse, viewing these children as oppositional leads to inappropriate treatment recommendations designed to shape behavioral compliance. Even when these behavioral strategies are based on principles of positive reinforcement (not always likely in the home), the children's self-esteem can suffer whey they continue to "forget" despite putting forth their best effort.

To evaluate the FDI as a possible strength or weakness in the profile, the FDI score can be compared to the VCI and POI scores. If the FDI score is significantly higher or lower than either the VCI or POI score, then FDI is considered a relative strength or weakness respectively. Table B.1 in the WISC-III manual (Wechsler, 1991, p. 261) shows the differences between factor-based Index scores required for statistical significance, and Table B.2 (Wechsler, 1991, p. 262) shows the base rate of occurrence of differences of various magnitudes. If a good portable rule of thumb is needed for hypothesis generation, a difference of 15 points (or one standard deviation) makes a good deal of sense. A difference of this magnitude or greater between FDI and VCI is significant and was obtained by 27% of the standardization sample, and a 15-point or more difference between FDI and POI was obtained by approximately 32% of the sample. As also shown in Table B.1, however, the critical differences for significance at the $p < .05$ level showed considerable variation by age. For example, a difference between the FDI and VCI of 15 points was needed at age 7, whereas a difference of only 11 points was significant at age 15.

Thus the astute examiner will refer to the appropriate tables.

Of course, interpretation of the FDI presumes that this Index is valid. If the Arithmetic and Digit Span subtest scaled scores are very different from each other, then the FDI score can only represent the average of two widely divergent sets of abilities and will therefore have little intrinsic meaning. These two subtests load on the same factor in factor analyses of the WISC-III, yet correlate only moderately ($r = .43$ across ages). So divergent scores are certainly possible.

How large a difference is required before the FDI should be abandoned as an interpretable score? Table 5.10 shows percentages of the WISC-III standardization sample obtaining various Arithmetic–Digit Span discrepancies. As shown in the table, approximately 17.5% of the sample obtained a 5-point difference or greater. Furthermore, it would appear clinically inappropriate to us to report that a child has obtained an average score on the FDI when the Arithmetic and Digit Span subtest scaled scores are 7 and 12, respectively—a difference of 5 points. (Other examiners may consult this table and choose different guidelines, depending on the context within which the profile is being interpreted.) When the Arithmetic and Digit Span subtest scaled scores are 5 points or more apart, then these subtests should be interpreted independently. Both these subtests measure attention, concentration, and mental control, but the Arithmetic subtest also measures specific skills in numerical operations and mathematics reasoning. Table B.3 of the WISC-III manual (Wechsler, 1991) can be consulted to determine whether either subtest constitutes a significant strength or weakness in a child's profile.

Let's consider the case when Digit Span is a weakness and Arithmetic is not. The Digit Span subtest is a direct assessment of short-term auditory memory; performance on this subtest requires attention, concentration, and mental control, and can be influenced by the ability to sequence information correctly. If performance on Digit Span backward is also impaired, then the working memory interpretation is further supported. However, the interpretation varies, depending on the absolute elevation of these subtests. If Arithmetic is in the average range

TABLE 5.10. Cumulative Percentages of the WISC-III Standardization Sample Obtaining Various Coding–Symbol Search (CD-SS) Discrepancies and Various Arithmetic–Digit Span (AR-DS) Discrepancies

Difference[a]	CD-SS	AR-DS
11	0.5	0.2
10	1.2	0.8
9	2.6	1.7
8	4.0	3.6
7	6.9	6.2
6	11.0	10.1
5	17.5	17.5
4	27.8	29.4
3	43.2	43.7
2	63.7	66.4
1	88.2	89.3
0	100.0	100.0

Note. Data and table copyright 1997 by The Psychological Corporation. All rights reserved. Reprinted by permission.
[a]Absolute value of the difference.

and Digit Span is below average, then the working memory interpretation is primary. If, however, Arithmetic is in the above-average range and Digit Span is significantly lower but still within the average range, this may suggest better-developed skills in numerical calculation or mathematics reasoning, rather than a deficit in working memory.

As noted above, Digit Span backward is an excellent example of a working memory task. The requirement to manipulate (e.g., reverse) the digits in Digit Span backward makes this a more difficult working memory task than Digit Span forward, in which numbers are simply repeated in sequence. Digit Span backward is a purer measure of mental control than Digit Span forward. Both tasks tap short-term auditory memory, numerical sequencing ability, attention, and concentration, but Digit Span backward demands more working memory to complete successfully. For this reason, it is often helpful to examine a student's performance on Digit Span backward and Digit Span forward separately. Even when FDI is not a specific deficiency in the profile, a Digit Span backward scaled score that is much lower than the Digit Span forward scaled score raises the question of a relative weakness in working memory. Tables B.6 and B.7

in the WISC-III manual (Wechsler, 1991) provide the needed information to assess discrepancies between Digit Span forward and backward.

On the other hand, if Arithmetic is a weakness and Digit Span is not, then there is less evidence of a deficit in working memory. This is especially true if performance on Digit Span backward is not impaired. In this case, an examiner may suspect poorly developed skills in numerical calculation or mathematics reasoning, and perhaps even a specific learning disability in math. This warrants further study, perhaps with an achievement test that has broader coverage of the domain of arithmetic.

STRATEGIES FOR INTERPRETING THE PSI

On the surface, the Coding and Symbol Search subtests are simple visual scanning and tracking tasks. A direct test of speed and accuracy, the Coding subtest assesses ability in quickly and correctly scanning and sequencing simple visual information. Performance on this subtest may also be influenced by short-term visual memory, attention, or visual–motor coordination. The Symbol Search subtest requires the student to inspect several sets of symbols and indicate whether special target symbols appear in each set. Also a direct test of speed and accuracy, this subtest assesses scanning speed and sequential tracking of simple visual information. Performance on this subtest may be influenced by visual discrimination and visual–motor coordination.

Yet it could be a mistake to think of the PSI as a measure of simple clerical functions that are not especially related to intelligence. There is consistent evidence that both simple and choice reaction time correlate about .20 or slightly higher with scores from intelligence tests, whereas inspection time (hypothesized by some to be a measure of the rate that information is processed) correlates about .40 with intelligence test scores (see Deary, 2001; Deary & Stough, 1996). Performance on the PSI is an indication of the rapidity with which a student can process simple or routine information without making errors. Because learning often involves a combination of routine information processing (such as reading) and complex information processing (such as reasoning), a weakness in the speed of processing routine information may make the task of comprehending novel information more time-consuming and difficult. A weakness in simple visual scanning and tracking may leave a child less time and mental energy for the complex task of understanding new material. This is the way in which these lower-order processing abilities are related to higher-order cognitive functioning.

A pattern in which processing speed abilities are lower than reasoning abilities is more common among students who are experiencing academic difficulties in the classroom than among those who are not (Wechsler, 1991, p. 213). Research studies have also indicated that children with ADHD earn their lowest WISC-III scores on the PSI (Prifitera & Dersh, 1993; Schwean et al., 1993). Although little research exists on this topic, it is possible to hypothesize that children with processing speed deficits may learn less material in the same amount of time, or may take longer to learn the same amount of material, than those without processing speed deficits may. We think that children with these deficits may also mentally tire more easily because of the additional cognitive effort required to perform routine tasks, and that this could lead to more frequent errors, less time spent studying, and possible expressions of frustration. Conversely, a strength in processing speed may facilitate the acquisition of new information. However, a caution is given here: There is also evidence that reaction time is similarly correlated with IQ scores from both speeded and nonspeeded tests.

The PSI score can be compared to the VCI and POI scores in order to evaluate it as a possible strength or weakness in the profile. If the PSI score is significantly higher or lower than either the VCI or POI score, then PSI is considered a relative strength or weakness, respectively. Tables B.1 and B.2 of the WISC-III manual (Wechsler, 1991) provide the necessary data for evaluating comparisons between these index scores. As a rule of thumb, a 15-point or more difference may be sufficient to generate a hypothesis of a relative weakness in processing speed functions. Differences of this magnitude or greater are statistically significant at the $p < .05$ level and were obtained by slightly more than one-third of the standardization sample. Larger differences, of course, generate more serious concerns about a deficit in this area. In the standardization sample, PSI–POI or PSI–VCI discrepancies of 20 points or more occured in approximately 21% and 24% of cases, respectively, while discrepancies of 25 points were observed in about 12% and 13% of cases, respectively.

We raise a caution here similar to the one we have raised regarding the differences between the two subtests (Arithmetic and Digit Span) defining the FDI: If the Coding and Symbol Search subtest scaled scores are very different from each other, then the PSI will have little intrinsic meaning and should not be interpreted as a unitary construct. Table 5.10 shows percentages of the WISC-III standardization sample obtaining various Coding–Symbol Search discrepancies. We recommend that a difference of 5 or more points between Coding and Symbol Search should raise strong concerns about interpreting the PSI as a unitary construct. Actually, a difference between these two subtests of only 4 points is significant at the $p < .05$ level (see Table B.4 of the WISC-III manual), but a difference of this size or greater was obtained by more than one out of every four children (27.7%) in the standardization sample. Only 17% of the sample obtained a 5-point difference or greater. If the difference between Coding and Symbol Search is 5 points or greater, then the PSI may not be considered valid, and these two subtests are best interpreted separately.

An examiner who is considering possible reasons for a disparity in performance on these two subtests should note that both of them measure skills in quickly scanning and correctly sequencing simple visual information, and that each can be influenced by attention, psychomotor speed, and visual–motor coordination. They differ, however, in the content of the stimulus material. The Coding subtest includes symbolic content, while the content of the Symbol Search subtest is purely figural. The symbolic content of the Coding B subtest, for example, allows the child to form paired associations between the numbers and shapes. To the extent that a student adopts this approach to the Coding subtest, it is sensitive to the student's ability to learn these associations, and performance can be influenced by a weakness in short-term visual memory of the learned associations. The Symbol Search subtest is not affected by associative learning and may be a purer measure of psychomotor speed than the Coding subtest. The Symbol Search subtest also does not require fine motor skills (e.g., drawing), as does Coding. Because the Symbol Search symbols are complex and similar in appearance, however, the Symbol Search subtest may be more readily influenced by the student's visual discrimination skills than the Coding subtest.

Only careful observation of the student's approach to these tasks can shed further light on these alternative hypotheses for explaining the differential performance observed on these two subtests. For example, did the child form the relevant associations in the Coding task? Did he or she remember them? Did the child refer to the key throughout the Coding task? Did he or she have difficulty manipulating the pencil? Were discrimination errors made in the Symbol Search subtest? Did the child not make errors on Symbol Search, but work too slowly and fail to complete a sufficient number of items? Answers to these questions, based not on the test scores but on astute observations of the child's behavior during testing, are clues to unearth the explanation for large observed differences between the Coding and Symbol Search subtests. This strategy is referred to as the "process approach" (Kaplan, Fein, Morris, & Delis, 1991), in that it emphasizes the process by which the student approaches the solution to the task, rather than the score he or she obtained.

THE DYNAMIC INTERPLAY OF WORKING MEMORY AND PROCESSING SPEED

Contrary to popular opinion, the FDI and PSI scores should not be considered minor players in the assessment of intelligence. There are large and obvious age-related trends in processing speed, which are accompanied by age-related changes in the number of transient connections to the central nervous system and increases in myelinization. Several investigators have found that measures of infant processing speed predict later IQ scores (e.g., Dougherty & Haith, 1997), and WISC-III PSI scores have been shown to be potentially sensitive to neurological disorders such as epilepsy (Wechsler, 1991). PSI scores also have been shown to be higher for children with mental retardation and lower for gifted children than their other Index scores (Wechsler, 1991). In samples with learning disabilities and ADHD, both PSI and FDI scores were found to be lower than their VCI and POI scores, as well as lower than those of the normal population (Prifitera & Dersh, 1993; Schwean et al. 1993). Perhaps most interestingly for school psychologists and specialists, several researchers have found that the FDI contributes the second largest amount of variance, after the VCI, to the prediction of reading, writing, and mathematics scores on the WIAT and other measures of achievement (Hale, Fiorello, Kavanagh, Hoeppner, & Gaither, 2001; Konold, 1999).

Thus it is not surprising that speed of information processing and short-term memory are included as components of most psychometric models of intelligence, such as the Gf-Gc theory (Carroll, 1993). However, working memory should not be confused with many of the short-term memory measures included in the Gf-Gc model. Working memory is much more complex than the temporary storage and retrieval of auditory or visual information. Working memory involves the manipulation of information in temporary storage, and as such is very closely related to reasoning.

Furthermore, the interpretation by some of factor-analytically derived models of intelligence is that each factor is a unique source of variance, contributing independently to general intelligence. However, this would not seem to be the case from two perspectives. First, a g factor tends to emerge whenever a number of cognitively complex variables are factor-analyzed (Carroll, 1993). The basis for the FSIQ and GAI on the WISC-III is the fact that the VIQ and PIQ, and the four Index scores, while tapping variance that is unique or exclusive to each, are all positively correlated. Moreover, the subtests are all more or less positively correlated (while also demonstrating subtest specificity), with those subtests defining a particular factor correlating even more highly.

Second, clinical research in developmental cognitive neuropsychology suggests a more dynamic picture—one that practicing psychologists attempt to construct in their everyday clinical assessment practice. Fry and Hale (1996) administered measures of processing speed, working memory, and fluid intelligence to children and adolescents between 7 and 19 years of age. Structural equation modeling provided evidence that age-related increases in speed of processing were associated with increases in working memory capacity, which in turn were associated with higher scores on measures of fluid reasoning. This study shows that as children develop normally, more rapid processing of information results in more effective use of working memory, which enhances performance on many reasoning tasks. This study led Kail (2000) to conclude: "Processing speed is not simply one of many different independent factors that contribute to intelligence; instead processing speed is thought to be linked causally to other elements of intelligence" (p. 58). This dynamic model of cognitive information processing suggests that language and reading impairments, which interfere with the rapid processing of information, may burden the working memory structures and reduce a student's capacity for comprehension and new learning. This is an area that is ripe for research.

FACTOR-ANALYTIC VERSUS CLINICAL MODELS OF ASSESSMENT

Most factor-analytic studies of the WISC-III have supported the four-factor structure (Blaha & Wallbrown, 1996; Konold, Kush, & Canivez, 1997; Kush et al., 2001; Roid, Prifitera, & Weiss, 1993; Roid & Worrall, 1996; Sattler & Saklofske, 2001b; Wechsler, 1991), although others have supported a three-factor structure (Logerquist-Hansen & Barona, 1994; Reynolds & Ford, 1994; Sattler, 1992). In spite of this strong empirical support for the factor structure of the WISC-III, we have previously argued that factor analysis should not be the sole criterion for determining how to summarize test performance, but that this decision should be informed by clinically meaningful patterns in the performance of diagnostic groups as well (Prifitera et al., 1998).

Perhaps one dramatic example of this point involves the WMS-III. In this test, the immediate and delayed conditions of each memory task correlate highly with each other, because the subject's score in the delayed condition is dependent on the extent of learning that occurred in the immediate condition. Thus separate immediate and delayed memory factors cannot be identified in factor analyses of the WMS-III (Millis, Melina, Bowers, & Ricker, 1999; Price, Tulsky, Millis, & Weiss, in press). In spite of this, there is general agreement that it is important to measure immediate and delayed memory separately, because they represent different neuropsychological functions and show different patterns of impairment across various types of dementia (see Tulsky et al., in press).

Based on numerous factor analyses of many different intelligence tests, a taxonomy of intelligence known as Gf-Gc theory has been proposed (Horn & Noll, 1997). This structure has undergone several modifications over the decades, and is now known as the Cattell–Horn–Carroll model (Carroll, 1993). The model includes many narrowly defined subfactors of intelligence, perhaps the most important of which are fluid reasoning, crystalized intelligence, broad visualization, short-term memory, and processing speed. As we have argued above, short-term memory (either immediate or delayed) is not the same construct as working memory, and the latter has important clinical correlates with many psychoeducational and neuropsychological disorders.

More importantly, we would strongly argue that the goal of a clinical assessment is not simply to measure all of the factors and subfactors in the Cattell–Horn–Carroll model, as some seem to suggest (Flanagan, 2000). Rather, the goal of any meaningful evaluation is to target assessment to the specific cognitive processes underlying the clinical issue for which the child was referred. The practitioner's decision about which tests and subtests to administer to a given child must not be governed by statistical models (e.g., factor analysis) used to summarize patterns of correlations among subtests in nonclinical individuals. Such decisions are best made with clinical knowledge

of how meaningful patterns in performance vary among diagnostically relevant groups. The present chapter has elaborated on the relevance of the WISC-III Index scores to important clinical issues.

CONCLUSION

Certainly no intelligence test should be used as a stand-alone assessment, and in this regard all evaluations essentially involve a cross-battery approach. In fact, this was Wechsler's original intention when he gathered together a dozen tasks designed to tap different underlying cognitive functions into one battery, and began to examine profiles for clinically meaningful variations. Wechsler continued his search for clinically meaningful facets of intelligent behavior by incorporating memory into his battery of tests with the WMS, and later expanded his thinking to include the nonintellective or noncognitive factors that would further describe individual differences and have relevance in clinical diagnosis. Efforts to link intelligence to other human factors, such as personality (Collis & Messick, 2001; Saklofske & Zeidner, 1995; Sternberg, 1995), are now becoming commonplace.

Future research might examine the factor structure of the WISC-III when it is administered together with its intended complements (e.g., the WIAT-II, the WISC-III PI, NEPSY, and the CMS), and might evaluate profile differences across clinical groups. This approach has already shown considerable promise with the WAIS-III and WMS-III (Tulsky et al., in press). There continues to be strong research and clinical support for using the WISC-III as an individually administered, standardized intelligence test. In the hands of the skilled clinician, the WISC-III will continue to provide significant information about children's intellectual abilities. The WISC-IV promises even further advances in that regard, and so the legacy continues.

NOTE

1. GAI reliability coefficients for ages 6–16 are as follows: .95, .94, .96, .95, .95, .95, .96, .95, .95, .97, and .96. These were calculated

from the subtest reliabilities reported in the WISC-III manual (Wechsler, 1991), using the formula for the reliability of a composite (Nunnally, 1978). The average GAI reliability was computed using Fisher's z transformations for ages 6–11 as $r = .95$, and for ages 12–16 as $r = .96$. These average reliabilities by two age bands were used in the calculations for Table 5.5.

REFERENCES

Berninger, V. W. (1998). *Process Assessment of the Learner (PAL): Guides for reading and writing intervention.* San Antonio, TX: Psychological Corporation.

Berninger, V. W. (2001). *Process Assessment of the Learner Test Battery for Reading and Writing (PAL-RW).* San Antonio, TX: Psychological Corporation.

Berninger, V. W., Stage, S. A., Smith, D. R., & Hildebrand, D. (2001). Assessment of reading and writing intervention: A three-tier model for prevention and remediation. In J. W. Andrews, D. H. Saklofske, & H. L. Janzen (Eds.), *Handbook of psychoeducational assessment: Ability, achievement, and behavior in children* (pp. 195–223). San Diego, CA: Academic Press.

Busse, J., Berninger, V. W., Smith, D. R., & Hildebrand, D. (2001). Assessment of math talent and disability: A developmental model. In J. W. Andrews, D. H. Saklofske, & H. L. Janzen (Eds.), *Handbook of psychoeducational assessment: Ability, achievement, and behavior in children* (pp. 225–253). San Diego, CA: Academic Press.

Blaha, J., & Wallbrown, F. H. (1996). Hierarchical factor structure of the Wechsler Intelligence Scale for Children—III. *Psychological Assessment, 8,* 214–218.

Carroll, J. B. (1993). *Human cognitive abilities: A survey of factor-analytic studies.* New York: Cambridge University Press.

Cohen, J. (1959). The factorial structure of the WISC at ages 7-6, 10-6, and 13-16. *Journal of Consulting Psychology, 23,* 285–299.

Cohen, M. (1997). *Manual for the Children's Memory Scale.* San Antonio, TX: Psychological Corporation.

Collis, J. M., & Messick, S. J. (Eds.). (2001). *Intelligence and personality.* Mahwah, NJ: Erlbaum.

Deary, I. J. (2001). *Intelligence: A very short introduction.* Oxford: Oxford University Press.

Deary, I. J., & Stough, C. (1996). Intelligence and inspection time: Achievements, prospects, and problems. *American Psychologist, 51,* 599–608.

Dougherty, T. M., & Haith, M. M. (1997). Infant expectations and reaction times as predictors of childhood speed of processing and IQ. *Developmental Psychology, 33*(1), 146–155.

Flanagan, D. P., McGrew, K. S., & Ortiz, S. O. (2000). *The Wechsler intelligence scales and Gf-Gc theory: A contemporary approach to interpretation.* Boston: Allyn & Bacon.

Flynn, J. R. (1984). The mean IQ of Americans: Massive gains 1932 to 1978. *Psychological Bulletin, 95,* 29–51.

Flynn, J. R. (1998). IQ gains over time: Toward finding the causes. In U. Neisser (Ed.), *The rising curve: Long-term gains in IQ and related measures* (pp. 25–66). Washington, DC: American Psychological Association.

Fry, A. F., & Hale, S. (1996). Processing speed, working memory, and fluid intelligence: Evidence for a developmental cascade. *Psychological Science, 7*(4), 237–241.

Gridley, B. E., & Roid, G. H. (1998). The use of the WISC-III with achievement tests. In A. Prifitera & D. H. Saklofske (Eds.), *WISC-III clinical use and interpretation: Scientist–practitioner perspectives* (pp. 249–288). San Diego, CA: Academic Press

Hale, J. B., Fiorello, C. A., Kavanagh, J. A., Hoeppner, J. B., & Gaither, R. A. (2001). WISC-III predictors of academic achievement for children with learning disabilities: Are global and factor scores comparable? *School Psychology Quarterly, 16*(1), 31–55.

Harrison, P. L., & Oakland, T. (2000). *Adaptive Behavior Assessment System manual.* San Antonio, TX: Psychological Corporation.

Hildebrand, D. K., & Ledbetter, M. F. (2001). Assessing children's intelligence and memory: The Wechsler Intelligence Scale for Children—Third Edition and the Children's Memory Scale. In J. W. Andrews, D. H. Saklofske, & H. L. Janzen (Eds.), *Handbook of psychoeducational assessment: Ability, achievement, and behavior in children* (pp. 13–32). San Diego, CA: Academic Press.

Horn, J. L., & Noll, J. (1997). Human cognitive capabilities: Gf-Gc theory. In D. P. Flanagan, J. L Genshaft, & P. L. Harrison (Eds.), *Contemporary intellectual assessment: Theories, tests, and issues* (pp. 53–91). New York: Guilford Press.

Individuals with Disabilities Education Act Amendments of 1991, PL No. 102-150, 105 Stat. 587 (1992).

Individuals with Disabilities Education Act Amendments of 1997, 20 U. S. C. 1400 et seq. (Fed. Reg. 64, 1999).

Kail, R. (2000). Speed of information processing: Developmental change and links to intelligence. *Journal of Psychology, 38*(1), 51–61.

Kamphaus, R. W. (1998). Intelligence test interpretation: Acting in the absence of evidence. In A. Prifitera & D. H. Saklofske (Eds.), *WISC-III clinical use and interpretation: Scientist–practitioner perspectives* (pp. 39–57). San Diego, CA: Academic Press.

Kamphaus, R. W. (2001). *Clinical assessment of child and adolescent intelligence* (2nd ed). Needham Heights, MA: Allyn & Bacon.

Kaplan, E., Fein, D., Kramer, J., Delis, D., & Morris, R. (1999). *Manual for the WISC-III-PI.* San Antonio, TX: Psychological Corporation.

Kaplan, E., Fein, D., Morris, R., & Delis, D. (1991). *Manual for the WAIS-R as a neuropsychological instrument.* San Antonio, TX: Psychological Corporation.

Kaufman, A. S. (1994). *Intelligent testing with the WISC-III.* New York: Wiley.

Konold, T. R. (1999). Evaluating discrepancy analysis

with the WISC-III and WIAT. *Journal of Psychoeducational Assessment, 17*, 24–35.

Konold, T. R., Kush, J. C., & Canivez, G. L. (1997). Factor replication of the WISC-III in three independent samples of children receiving special education. *Journal of Psychoeducational Assessment, 15*, 123–137.

Kush, J. C., Watkins, M. W., Ward, T. J., Ward, S. B., Canivez, G. L., & Worrell, F. C. (2001). Construct validity of the WISC-III for white and black students from the WISC-III standardization sample and for black students referred for psychological evaluation. *School Psychology Review, 30*(1), 70–88.

Logerquist-Hansen, S., & Barona, A. (1994, August). *Factor structure of the Wechsler Intelligence Scale for Children—III for Hispanic and non-Hispanic white children with learning diabilities.* Paper presented at the annual meeting of the American Psychological Association, Los Angeles.

Meyer, G. J., Finn, S. E., Eyde, L. D., Kay, G. G., Moreland, K. L., Dies, R. R., Eisman, E. J., Kubiszyn, T. W., & Reed, G. M. (2001). Psychological testing and psychological assessment: A review of evidence and issues. *American Psychologist, 56*, 128–165.

Millis, S., Melina, A., Bowers, D., & Ricker, J. (1999). Confirmatory factor analysis of the Wechsler Memory Scale—III. *Journal of Clinical and Experimental Neuropsychology, 21*(1), 87–93.

Naglieri, J. A., & Das, J. P. (1997). *Cognitive Assessment System.* Itasca, IL: Riverside.

Neisser, U., Boodoo, G., Bouchard, T. J., Jr., Boykin, A. W., Brody, N., Ceci, S. J., Halpern, D. F., Loehlin, J. C., Perloff, R., Sternberg, R. J., & Urbina, S. (1996). Intelligence: Knowns and unknowns. *American Psychologist, 51*, 77–101.

Nunnally, J. (1978). *Psychometric theory* (2nd ed.). New York: McGraw-Hill.

Oakland, T., & Glutting, J. (1998). Assessment of test behaviors with the WISC-III. In A. Prifeitera & D. H. Saklofske (Eds.), *WISC-III clinical use and interpretation: Scientist–practitioner perspectives* (pp. 289–310). San Diego, CA: Academic Press.

Price, L., Tulsky, D., Millis, S., & Weiss, L (in press). Redefining the factor structure of the Wechsler Memory Scale—III: Confirmatory factor analysis with cross validation. *Journal of Clinical and Experimental Neuropsychology.*

Prifitera, A., & Dersh, J. (1992). Base rates of WISC-III diagnostic subtest patterns among normal, learning disabled, and ADHD samples. *Journal of Psychoeducational Assessment Monograph Series*, pp. 43–55.

Prifitera, A., & Saklofske, D. H. (Eds.). (1998). *WISC-III clinical use and interpretation: Scientist–practitioner perspectives.* San Diego, CA: Academic Press.

Prifitera, A., Weiss, L. G., & Saklofske, D. H. (1998). The WISC-III in context. In A. Prifitera & D. H. Saklofske (Eds.), *WISC-III clinical use and interpretation: Scientist–practitioner perspectives* (pp. 1–38). San Diego, CA: Academic Press.

Psychological Corporation. (1992). *Manual for the Wechsler Individual Achievement Test.* San Antonio, TX: Author.

Psychological Corporation. (2001). *Manual for the Wechsler Individual Achievement Test—Second Edition.* San Antonio, TX: Author.

Puente, A. E., & Salazar, G. D. (1998). Assessment of minority and culturally diverse children. In A. Prifitera & D. H. Saklofske (Eds.), *WISC-III clinical use and interpretation: Scientist–practitioner perspectives* (pp. 227–248). San Diego, CA: Academic Press.

Reynolds, C. R., & Ford, L. (1994). Comparative three-factor solutions of the WISC-III and WISC-R at 11 age levels between $6\frac{1}{2}$ and $16\frac{1}{2}$ years. *Archives of Clinical Neuropsychology, 9*, 553–570.

Reynolds, C. R., Sanchez, S., & Wilson, V. L. (1996). Normative tables for calculating the WISC-III Performance and Full Scale IQ's when Symbol Search is substituted for Coding. *Psychological Assessment, 8*, 378–382.

Robinson, N. M., Zigler, E., & Gallagher, J. J. (2001). Two tails of the normal curve: Similarities and differences in the study of mental retardation and giftedness. *American Psychologist, 55*, 1413–1424.

Roid, G. H., Prifitera, A., & Weiss, L. G. (1993). Replication of the WISC-III factor structure in an independent sample. *Journal of Psychoeducational Assessment Monograph Series*, pp. 6–21.

Roid, G. H., & Worrall, W. (1996, August). *Equivalence of factor structure in the U. S. and Canada editions of the WISC-III.* Paper presented at the annual meeting of the American Psychological Association, Toronto.

Saklofske, D. H. (1996). Using WISC-III Canadian study results in academic research. In D. Wechsler (Ed.), *WISC-III manual Canadian supplement* (pp. 5–13). Toronto: Psychological Corporation.

Saklofske, D. H., Hildebrand, D. K., Reynolds, C. R., & Wilson, V. (1998). Substituting symbol search for coding on the WISC-III; Canadian normative tables for Performance and Full Scale IQ scores. *Canadian Journal of Behavioural Science, 30*, 57–68.

Saklofske, D. H., & Zeider, M. (Eds.). (1995). *International handbook of personality and intelligence.* New York: Plenum Press.

Sattler, J. M. (1992). *Assessment of children* (3rd ed.). San Diego, CA: Author.

Sattler, J. M. (2001). *Assessment of children: Cognitive applications* (4th ed.). San Diego, CA: Author.

Sattler, J. M., & Saklofske, D. H. (2001a). Interpreting the WISC-III. In J. M. Sattler, *Assessment of children: Cognitive applications* (4th ed., pp. 298–334). San Diego, CA: Author.

Sattler, J. M., & Saklofske, D. H. (2001b). Wechsler Intelligence Scale for Children—III (WISC-III): Description. In J. M. Sattler, *Assessment of children: Cognitive applications* (4th ed., pp. 220–297) San Diego, CA: Author.

Sattler, J. M., & Saklofske, D. H. (2001c). WISC-III subtests. In J. M. Sattler, *Assessment of children: Cognitive applications* (4th ed., pp. 266–297). San Diego, CA: Author.

Schwean, V. L., & Saklofske, D. H. (1998). WISC-III assessment of children with attention deficit/hyperactivity disorder. In A. Prifitera & D. H. Saklofske (Eds.), *WISC-III clinical use and interpretation: Sci-*

entist–practitioner perspectives (pp. 91–118). San Diego, CA: Academic Press.

Schwean, V. L., Saklofske, D. H., Yackulic, R. A., & Quinn, D. (1993). WISC-III performance of ADHD boys: Cognitive, intellectual, and behavioral comparisons. *Journal of Psychoeducational Assessment Monograph,* pp. 6–21.

Sparrow, S. S., Balla, D. A., & Cicchetti, D. A. (1984). *Vineland Adaptive Behavior Scales.* Circle Pines, MN: American Guidance Service.

Spruill, J. (1998). Assessment of mental retardation with the WISC-III. In A. Prifitera & D. H. Saklofske (Eds.), *WISC-III clinical use and interpretation: Scientist–practitioner perspectives* (pp. 73–90). San Diego, CA: Academic Press.

Sternberg, R. J. (1995). *In search of the human mind.* Fort Worth, TX: Harcourt Brace College.

Tulsky, D. S., Saklofske, D. H., Heaton, R. K., Chelune, G. J., Ivnik, R. J., Prifitera, A., Bornstein, R., & Ledbetter, M. F. (Eds.). (2003). *Clinical interpretation of the WAIS-III and WMS-III.* San Diego, CA: Academic Press.

Tulsky, D. S., Saklofske, D. H., Wilkins, C., & Weiss, L. G. (2001). Development of a General Ability Index for the WAIS-III. *Psychological Assessment, 13,* 566–571.

Wechsler, D. (1944). *The measurement of adult intelligence.* Baltimore: Williams & Wilkins.

Wechsler, D. (1949). *Manual for the Wechsler Intelligence Scale for Children.* New York: Psychological Corporation.

Wechsler, D. (1974). *Manual for the Wechsler Intelligence Scale for Children—Revised.* New York: Psychological Corporation.

Wechsler, D. (1991). *Manual for the Wechsler Intelligence Scale for Children—Third Edition.* San Antonio, TX: Psychological Corporation.

Wechsler, D. (1997a). *Manual for the Wechsler Adult Intelligence Scale—Third Edition.* San Antonio, TX: Psychological Corporation.

Wechsler, D. (1997b). *Manual for the Wechsler Memory Scale—Third Edition.* San Antonio, TX: Psychological Corporation.

Weiss, L. G., Prifitera, A., & Dersh, J. (1995). *Base rates of WISC-III Verbal–Performance discrepancies in Hispanic and African American children.* Unpublished manuscript.

Weiss, L. G., Saklofske, D. H., Prifitera, A., Chen, H., & Hildebrand, D. K. (1999). The calculation of the WISC-III General Ability Index using Canadian norms. *Canadian Journal of School Psychology, 14*(2), 1–9.

Woodcock, R. W., McGrew, K. S., & Mather, N. (2001). *The Woodcock–Johnson Psycho-Educational Battery—III.* Itasca, IL: Riverside.

6

Assessing the Intelligence of Adolescents with the Wechsler Adult Intelligence Scale—Third Edition (WAIS-III)

JOSEPH J. RYAN
JONATHAN W. SMITH

HISTORY

During his career, David Wechsler provided psychological services in the U.S. Army, as well as in the Bureau of Child Guidance, the Brooklyn Jewish Social Service Agency, and Bellevue Hospital in New York City. In many instances, he was asked to evaluate the intellectual functioning of adolescent and adult clients, in order to assist with appropriate disposition. The assessment process was often demanding and complex, since many of these individuals' problems included psychosis, mental retardation, brain damage, and/or illiteracy. Moreover, the intelligence tests available in the 1920s and 1930s had limited norms, were designed for children, overemphasized verbal ability or speed of performance, yielded scores of questionable validity (e.g., the "mental age" construct was inappropriate for teenagers and adults), and/or were viewed by some examinees as childish or foolish. From his experiences as a practitioner, Wechsler concluded that a new test designed specifically for adolescent and adult examinees should be developed. The new test needed to possess face validity, to place less emphasis on time limits, and to provide a reasonably diverse coverage of the ability spectrum (including measurement of both verbal and nonverbal functions).

According to Wechsler (1944), "Intelligence is the aggregate or global capacity of the individual to act purposefully, to think rationally and to deal effectively with his environment" (p. 3). This definition includes cognitive, emotional, and motivational factors, and argues that intelligence is multifaceted, multidetermined, and part of personality as a whole. To measure intelligence so defined, Wechsler appropriated tasks from published scales such as the Stanford–Binet Intelligence Scale, the Army Alpha and Beta Tests, the Kohs Block Designs, and the Army Individual Performance Scale (AIPS). Because he wanted to assess intellectual ability in a reasonably comprehensive manner, he used items from the Stanford–Binet and the Army Alpha Test to construct a Verbal scale, whereas components from the Kohs Block Designs, the Army Beta Test, and the AIPS were used to create a Performance scale. The Verbal and Performance Scales were thought to contribute equally to overall intellectual ability and were combined to provide an index of general intelligence.

Wechsler's approach to test construction emphasized practicality and clinical utility, but he did not ignore the major theories of intelligence promulgated by contemporary scholars such as Charles E. Spearman and E. L. Thorndike. Basically, Spearman (1927) believed that intelligence was most accurately described by a pervasive general factor (i.e., *g*), which was the brain's overall capacity to perform intellectual work. According to Spearman, this factor accounted for the observation that an examinee's score on one ability test will tend to correlate highly with scores on other ability tests (e.g., IQ is highly correlated with scores on aptitude, achievement, and memory tests). Conversely, Thorndike felt that intelligence was most accurately characterized by examination of a series of distinct abilities, including the facility for abstract thinking and the capacity to use symbols, manipulate objects, and deal effectively with people (see Wechsler, 1944).

In 1939, Wechsler introduced his new test and designated it the Wechsler–Bellevue Intelligence Scale, Form I (WB-I; Wechsler, 1939). This instrument, which was named after its author and the Bellevue Hospital (where he was then employed as chief psychologist), was considered a unique clinical tool because it possessed good face validity, grouped items into 11 subtests, and yielded deviation IQs instead of mental age values. The influence of Spearman was evident in the global or *g* score produced by the WB-I, the Full Scale IQ. The impact of Thorndike was seen in the individual subtests and separate IQs for the Verbal and Performance scales. Although the WB-I enjoyed wide popularity among psychologists in the United States, it had numerous shortcomings that needed to be rectified. For example, the norms were not representative of the U.S. population, since they were based on only 1,081 European Americans from the greater New York City area. In 1955, the Wechsler Adult Intelligence Scale (WAIS; Wechsler, 1955) was published as a replacement for the WB-I. The WAIS used a nationally stratified normative sample and measured a wider range of cognitive functions than its predecessor. In 1981, the WAIS was superseded by an updated and restandardized version

known as the Wechsler Adult Intelligence Scale—Revised (WAIS-R; Wechsler, 1981). Although Wechsler died in 1981, the Psychological Corporation continued his work and in 1997 produced the latest and most sophisticated version of the scale, which is known as the Wechsler Adult Intelligence Scale—Third Edition (WAIS-III; Wechsler, 1997a). The WAIS-III is now the gold standard for the intellectual assessment of adolescents and adults, with few exceptions (e.g., persons with severe mental retardation).

STRUCTURE OF THE WAIS-III

The WAIS-III is an individually administered examination for persons 16–89 years of age. It consists of 11 standard subtests, 2 supplementary subtests, and 1 optional subtest. The Verbal IQ is based on Vocabulary, Similarities, Arithmetic, Digit Span, Information, and Comprehension, while the Performance IQ is calculated using Picture Completion, Digit Symbol–Coding, Block Design, Matrix Reasoning, and Picture Arrangement. A global Full Scale IQ is obtained by combining scores on the 11 standard subtests. The three IQs have a mean of 100 and a standard deviation of 15; the 14 subtests yield scaled scores with a mean of 10 and a standard deviation of 3. The supplementary subtests are Letter–Number Sequencing and Symbol Search. The former subtest may be used to calculate the Verbal IQ only when it replaces Digit Span. Replacement is justified when the Digit Span subtest has been invalidated because of an interruption in test procedure or some other violation of standardized administration. The Symbol Search subtest may be used to obtain the Performance IQ only for a spoiled Digit Symbol–Coding administration. The optional subtest, Object Assembly, may replace any spoiled Performance scale subtest for examinees in the age range 16–74 years.

In addition to IQ values, the WAIS-III provides four other subtest composites, which have been designated as Index scores. They are based on the results of a series of factor analyses performed on participants from the standardization sample (Psychological Corporation, 1997) and allow for the assessment of more refined domains of cognitive functioning than the traditional IQs. The Verbal Comprehension Index (VCI) includes Vocabulary, Similarities, and Information, and the Perceptual Organization Index (POI) consists of Picture Completion, Block Design, and Matrix Reasoning. The Working Memory Index (WMI) and the Processing Speed Index (PSI) involve, respectively, Arithmetic, Digit Span, and Letter–Number Sequencing, and Digit Symbol–Coding and Symbol Search. Each Index has a mean of 100 and a standard deviation of 15. In some situations, an examiner may wish to obtain the Indexes as well as the traditional IQs. In order to accomplish this goal, it is necessary to administer 13 of the 14 WAIS-III subtests. The Object Assembly subtest remains optional and does not need to be administered in order to obtain either the IQs or Indexes.

Finally, two optional procedures that are not used in IQ or Index computation may be used to clarify results of the Digit Symbol–Coding subtest. The Digit Symbol–Incidental Learning procedure evaluates an examinee's immediate recall of the standard stimuli (i.e., nine number–symbol pairs) used in the Digit Symbol–Coding subtest. The Digit Symbol–Copy procedure requires the examinee to copy symbols as quickly as possible without the need to form number–symbol associations. It is sometime possible to ascertain the reason for poor performance (e.g., poor incidental memory or motor slowing) on the Digit Symbol–Coding subtest by comparing the results of these optional procedures. Table 6.1 presents a brief description of the WAIS-III subtests, the optional procedures for Digit Symbol–Coding, the IQs, and the Indexes.

STANDARDIZATION

The WAIS-III was standardized on a representative sample of 2,450 individuals who were stratified on sex, age (13 groups), race/ethnicity (European Americans, African Americans, Hispanics, and other), education (five groups), and geographic region of residence (four regions), according to 1995 data provided by the U.S. Bureau of the Census. Persons with positive histories of medical and/or psychiatric conditions that could potentially affect intellectual functioning were excluded from the sample. Table 6.2 presents the demographic characteristics of the WAIS-III standardization group. Note that parental education was used for the 400 participants in the age range 16–19 and that the race/ethnicity breakdown of the adolescent participants was 68.3% European American, 16% African American, 11.8% Hispanic, and 4% other.

REASONS FOR ADMINISTERING THE WAIS-III

There are many reasons for administering the WAIS-III to an adolescent or young adult. In vocational or educational guidance, a measure of adaptive capacity is important, because general intelligence sets broad limits on the kind of occupation or training that an individual may be expected to pursue with reasonable success. In young persons with suspected or confirmed brain injury, attention-deficit/hyperactivity disorder (ADHD), and/or learning disabilities, the WAIS-III often provides useful information concerning the examinees' approach to problem situations, language proficiency, and cognitive strengths and weaknesses. In skilled hands, the WAIS-III can assist with the formulation of educational and/or vocational interventions.

For many referrals, interpretations based at least in part on WAIS-III scores may be used to assist with disability determination and/or placement, whether educational or vocational (Kaufman, 1990). The fact that the WAIS-III was conormed with the Wechsler Memory Scale—Third Edition (WMS-III; Wechsler, 1997b) and linked with the Wechsler Individual Achievement Test (WIAT; Psychological Corporation, 1992) for persons 16–19 years of age should not be overlooked. These established associations with other tests indicate that the WAIS-III is probably the most appropriate intelligence measure when referrals involve memory impairment or deficiencies in academic achievement. Because of the high correlation between IQ and memory and between IQ and academic performance, the inclusion of the WAIS-III in a test battery allows a clinician to determine whether an examinee's memory skills and/or achievement scores are commensurate with his or her level of intelligence.

TABLE 6.1. Subtests, Optional Procedures, Indexes, and IQs for the WAIS-III

WAIS-III component	Description
Picture Completion	Twenty-five drawings of people, animals, and common objects, each with a missing part that must be identified within 20 seconds. It contributes to the POI, Performance IQ, and Full Scale IQ. It appears to measure attention/concentration, visual memory, and the ability to visually distinguish essential from nonessential details.
Vocabulary	Thirty-three words arranged in order of increasing difficulty to be defined orally by the examinee. It contributes to the VCI, Verbal IQ, and Full Scale IQ. It appears to measure word knowledge, verbal conceptualization, and (to a lesser extent) verbal reasoning. It is also considered a measure of crystallized intelligence.
Digit Symbol–Coding	Referring to a key with number–symbol pairs, the examinee copies the symbols corresponding to their numbers as rapidly as possible. The task has a 120-second time limit. It contributes to the PSI, Performance IQ, and Full Scale IQ. It measures clerical/handwriting speed, visual scanning, attention/concentration, visual memory, sequencing, the ability to remain free from distraction, and (to some extent) facility with numbers.
Similarities	The examinee is presented 19 or fewer word pairs and asked to identify the similarities between each pair. It contributes to the VCI, Verbal IQ, and Full Scale IQ. It appears to measure primarily verbal conceptualization and verbal reasoning. Performance on this subtest requires both crystallized and fluid abilities.
Block Design	This task requires the reproduction of 24 or fewer design patterns using colored blocks within specified time limits. It contributes to the POI, Performance IQ, and Full Scale IQ. It appears to measure visual–spatial problem solving, constructional ability, spatial visualization, and nonverbal concept formation. It is a complex task that requires, at least in part, the application of fluid intellectual abilities.
Arithmetic	Contains 23 arithmetic problems that require counting, addition, subtraction, multiplication, or basic probability. Each item is timed, and the computational levels do not exceed the eighth grade. It contributes to the WMI, Verbal IQ, and Full Scale IQ. It appears to measure computational skills and facility with numbers, as well as attention/concentration, short-term memory, sequencing, and the ability to work under time pressure. In addition to computation skills, it requires the application of fluid intellectual abilities.
Matrix Reasoning	Consists of 26 multiple-choice items that require pattern completion, serial reasoning, and/or classification. The examinee responds by pointing to or saying the correct response to each item. It contributes to the POI, Performance IQ, and Full Scale IQ. It appears to measure nonverbal reasoning, fluid intelligence, and spatial visualization.
Digit Span	Consists of separate digits-forward and digits-backward components, each requiring the examinee to repeat strings of digits in a prescribed sequence. It contributes to the WMI, Verbal IQ, and Full Scale IQ. It appears to measure attention/concentration, short-term memory, mental tracking and sequencing, facility with numbers, and internal visual scanning.
Information	Consists of 28 orally presented questions about well-known historical figures and common objects, events, and places. It contributes to the VCI, Verbal IQ, and Full Scale IQ. It appears to measure long-term memory and fund of general information. It is accurately described as a measure of crystallized ability.

TABLE 6.1. *Continued*

WAIS-III component	Description
Picture Arrangement	Eleven individual sets of pictures are presented in mixed-up order, and the examinee rearranges each set into a logical sequence within a specified time frame. It contributes to the Performance IQ and Full Scale IQ. It appears to measure visual sequencing and nonverbal reasoning applied to social situations. It taps both crystallized and fluid abilities.
Comprehension	Contains 16 questions dealing with everyday problem situations and two items that require interpretation of proverbs. It contributes to the Verbal IQ and Full Scale IQ. It appears to measure common sense, knowledge of social conventionalities, abstract thinking, verbal reasoning, and verbal conceptualization. It has been designated as a measure of crystallized intelligence.
Symbol Search	Each of the 60 items is composed of two symbols on the left side of a page and five on the right. The examinee decides whether either symbol on the left also appears on the right. The time limit is 120 seconds. It is a supplementary subtest that can replace Digit Symbol–Coding, if the latter is spoiled. It contributes to the PSI and, when substituted for Digit Symbol–Coding, the Performance IQ and Full Scale IQ. It appears to measure perceptual discrimination, clerical speed, visual scanning, attention/concentration, and the ability to remain free from distraction.
Letter–Number Sequencing	Each of the seven items requires the examinee to listen to a series of letters and numbers and than repeat the material with numbers in ascending order and letters in alphabetical order. It is a supplementary subtest that can replace Digit Span, if the latter is spoiled. It contributes to the WMI and, when substituted for Digit Span, the Verbal IQ and Full Scale IQ. It appears to measure auditory tracking, mental flexibility, facility with numbers attention/concentration, and sequencing. Visual–spatial ability and speed of mental processing may also be measured by this subtest.
Object Assembly	Contains five jigsaw puzzles that must be constructed within specific time limits. As an optional subtest, it may be administered for clinical reasons and, for examinees in the 16–74 age range, as a substitute for any spoiled Performance scale subtest. If used as a substitute, it contributes to the Performance IQ and Full Scale IQ. It appears to measure constructional ability, fluid ability, visual organization, and appreciation of part–whole relationships.
Digit Symbol–Incidental Learning	This is an optional procedure that may be administered immediately after Digit Symbol–Coding. It requires the examinee to remember individual symbols and number–symbol pairs from the Digit Symbol–Coding subtest. It appears to measure incidental learning of rehearsed material.
Digit Symbol–Copy	This is an optional procedure that may be administered at the end of the WAIS-III. It presents the same symbols that are used in the Digit Symbol–Coding subtest, but this time the examinee simply copies as many as possible in 90 seconds. It appears to measure perceptual and graphomotor speed.
Verbal IQ	A summary score traditionally based on Information, Comprehension, Arithmetic, Similarities, Digit Span, and Vocabulary. It measures general intelligence, with an emphasis on previously learned and stored verbal information and ideas. To a lesser extent, it reflects working memory and basic mental arithmetic skills.
Performance IQ	A summary score based on Picture Completion, Digit Symbol–Coding, Block Design, Matrix Reasoning, and Picture Arrangement. It measures perceptual organization, fluid reasoning, and attention to details. To a lesser extent, it reflects clerical processing speed.

(continues)

TABLE 6.1. *Continued*

WAIS-III component	Description
Full Scale IQ	Consists of the six Verbal scale and five Performance scale subtests described above. It provides a global estimate of psychometric intelligence.
Verbal Comprehension Index (VCI)	Consists of the Vocabulary, Similarities, and Information subtests, and appears to provide a relatively pure measure of verbal knowledge and the ability to apply this material across situations. This composite is a good measure of crystallized intelligence.
Perceptual Organization Index (POI)	Consists of the Picture Completion, Block Design, and Matrix Reasoning subtests. Although fluid intelligence is measured by this composite, it also provides a reasonably detailed assessment of an examinee's ability to interpret and organize visually presented material.
Working Memory Index (WMI)	Consists of the Arithmetic, Digit Span, and Letter–Number Sequencing subtests, and appears to measure attention, numerical proficiency, quantitative reasoning, auditory short-term memory, sequencing, and information processing.
Processing Speed Index (PSI)	Consists of the Digit Symbol–Coding and Symbol Search subtests, and appears to measure visual scanning, clerical speed, and the ability to process visual information rapidly.

Note. From Wechsler (1997a). Copyright 1997 by The Psychological Corporation. Adapted by permission.

RELIABILITY

WAIS-III internal consistency was assessed for the IQs, Indexes, and subtests with the split-half reliability coefficient (Psychological Corporation, 1997). This type of reliability measures consistency with regard to item content and is obtained from a single administration of the WAIS-III. The Full Scale reliability coefficients are ≥.97 across the entire age range in the standardization sample. On the Verbal scale, the coefficients across the age range are ≥.96; on the Performance scale, they are ≥.93. For the VCI, POI, WMI, and PSI, the reliability coefficients across the age range are ≥.94, ≥.90, ≥.91, and ≥.86, respectively. Among the subtests, those in the Verbal scale are generally more reliable than those in the Performance scale. For persons in the age range 16–17 years, the most reliable subtests are Vocabulary (.90) and Digit Span (.90), whereas the least reliable is Picture Arrangement (.70). In the age range 18–19 years, the most reliable subtest is Vocabulary (.93), and the least reliable is Object Assembly (.70).

Standard Error of Measurement

The standard error of measurement (SEM) reflects the reliability of the individual score and is simply the standard deviation of the distribution of error scores. It is expressed in terms of confidence limits that are placed around the obtained score. The larger the SEM, the larger the confidence limits, and the less precise the score. The average SEM for the Full Scale IQ across all age groups in the standardization sample is 2.30. The average SEM is smaller for the Verbal scale (2.55) than for the Performance scale (3.67). For the Indexes, the average SEMs are slightly larger, indicating that these composites are less precise than the IQs. The average SEM is 3.01 for the VCI, 3.95 for the POI, 3.84 for the WMI, and 5.13 for the PSI. Among the individual subtests, Vocabulary has the smallest average SEM (0.79), whereas Object Assembly has the largest (1.66). For persons in the age range 16–17, the SEMs are slightly larger for the IQs, the Indexes, and 10 of the 14 subtests. For persons 18–19 years of age, the Verbal IQ and WMI have slightly smaller SEMs than the

TABLE 6.2. Characteristics of the WAIS-III Normative Sample

Demographic variable	Description
Age	The 13 age ranges were: 16–17, 18–19, 20–24, 25–29, 30–34, 35–44, 45–54, 65–69, 70–74, 75–79, 80–89.
Sex	The numbers of males and females in each age range were as follows: 16–64 years = 100 males and 100 females; 65–69 years = 90 males and 110 females; 70–74 years = 88 males and 112 females; 75–79 years = 83 males and 117 females; 80–84 years = 54 males and 96 females; 85–89 years = 32 males and 68 females.
Race/ethnicity	European Americans = 1,925; African Americans = 279; Hispanics = 181; and other racial/ethnic groups = 65.
Education	Individuals in the age range 16–19 were classified according to years of parental education. The five categories used in standardization were as follows: ≤8 years = 284; 9–11 years = 289; 12 years = 853; 13–15 years = 579; and ≥16 years = 445.
Geographic region	Standardization participants were recruited from the following regions: 9 Northeastern states, 12 North Central states, 17 Southern states, and 12 Western states.

Note. From The Psychological Corporation (1997). Copyright 1997 by The Psychological Corporation. Adapted by permission.

average of the standardization sample. Six of the 14 subtests also have slightly smaller SEMs than the overall average.

Test–Retest Stability

To evaluate the stability of scores over time, the WAIS-III was administered to 394 individuals on two occasions with an average retest interval of 34.6 days (Psychological Corporation, 1997). For purposes of statistical analysis, the sample was divided into four age groups: 16–29 years, 30–54 years, 55–74 years, and 75–89 years. Corrected stability coefficients ranged from .94 to .97 for the Verbal IQ, from .88 to .92 for the Performance IQ, and from .95 to .97 for the Full Scale IQ. Stability coefficients were also high for the Indexes, with ranges from .92 to .96 for the VCI, from .83 to .92 for the POI, from .87 to .93 for the WMI, and from .84 to .90 for the PSI. Among the Verbal scale subtests, Vocabulary (ranging from .89 to .94) and Information (ranging from .93 to .94) were the most stable across the four age groups. Digit Symbol–Coding was the most stable (ranging from .81 to .91) of the Performance scale subtests.

For those who work with adolescents, information concerning test–retest changes for persons 16–29 years of age is of most interest. Among these individuals, the average increases on the Verbal, Performance, and Full Scale IQs were 3.2 points, 8.2 points, and 5.7 points, respectively. These retest changes, which were greater on the Performance scale than on the Verbal scale, probably reflect practice effects. On the VCI, the average point gain from test to retest was 2.5, while average increases were 7.3 for the POI, 2.9 for the WMI, and 6.0 for the PSI. Of the seven Verbal scale subtests, Vocabulary (0.2) and Letter–Number Sequencing (0.1) demonstrated the smallest average retest gains, whereas Information, Arithmetic, and Similarities had the largest mean retest gains (0.6). Within the Performance scale, the smallest average gain was on Matrix Reasoning (0.1), and the largest retest gains (2.3) were on Picture Completion and Object Assembly.

In work with individual examinees, it is often necessary to interpret observed changes in WAIS-III scores from serial evaluations. Thus it is important to ascertain whether score changes reflect chance variation/practice effects or a meaningful improvement or decline in intellectual functioning. The information in Table 6.3 reports base rate data for the magnitude of test–retest change that occurred in ≤15% and ≤5% of the 394 participants in the stability study reported above (Barrett, Chelune, Naugle, Tulsky, & Ledbetter,

2000; Psychological Corporation, 1997). For example, if an examinee's Full Scale IQ declines by 7 points on retest, Table 6.3 tells us that a loss of this magnitude is highly unusual, having occurred in fewer than 5% of the currently available test–retest cases. On the other hand, if an examinee improves his or her Full Scale IQ by 15 points, Table 6.3 indicates that a gain of this magnitude is highly unusual and very likely not to be the result of chance variation or practice effects. When unusual test–retest gains or losses occur, they must be carefully evaluated in order to determine their cause. The proper way to approach this task is to interpret gains and losses in conjunction with information from medical, social, and educational sources, as well as behavioral observations during testing and the examinee's verbal report. Whenever appropriate, specialized assessment procedures may provide useful information concerning the cause of unusual test–retest change. Finally, it is noted that the cutoffs provided in Table 6.3 are based on an average retest interval of approximately 5 weeks and may not generalize to longer intervals (e.g., months or years). Previous research with the Wechsler scales suggest that (1) once retest intervals exceed 12 months, practice effects are far less pronounced; and (2) the cutoffs provided in Table 6.3 are probably not accurate for retest intervals that exceed 6 months (Kaufman, 1990).

TABLE 6.3. Magnitude of Test–Retest Change Necessary to Exceed 15% and 5% Base Rate Expectations in Either Direction

Score	15% $\leq$	15% $\geq$	5% $\leq$	5% $\geq$
IQs				
Verbal	–3	9	–6	12
Performance	1	16	–4	21
Full Scale	1	11	–3	14
Indexes				
VCI	–4	9	–8	13
POI	–2	17	–7	22
WMI	–6	11	–11	16
PSI	–3	15	–8	20

Note. From Barrett, Chelune, Naugle, Tulsky, and Ledbetter (2000). Adapted by permission of the authors.

VALIDITY

The "validity" of a test refers to the extent to which it measures what it claims to measure and the appropriateness with which inferences can be made on the basis of the results. Support for the validity of the WAIS-III as a psychometric and clinical measure of intelligence is impressive, as discussed below.

Content Validity

The Psychological Corporation conducted extensive literature reviews to identify any problems with items from previous editions of the Wechsler scales of adult intelligence. Experts were then asked to review potential WAIS-III items, to design new items, and to assist in updating old items. The results of item tryout studies and pilot studies were also subjected to careful review. From these efforts, the Psychological Corporation concluded that the WAIS-III has an appropriate level of content validity.

Concurrent Validity

When the WAIS-III and other tests of intelligence are administered at approximately the same time, high positive correlations consistently emerge. For example, the WAIS-III Full Scale IQ correlated .88, .93, and .88, respectively, with composite scores from the Wechsler Intelligence Scale for Children—Third Edition (WISC-III), the WAIS-R, and the Stanford–Binet, Fourth Edition (Psychological Corporation, 1997). WAIS-III scores also demonstrated meaningful associations with tests of school-related performance. For a group of examinees 16–19 years of age, correlation coefficients between the WIAT composites for Reading, Mathematics, Language, and Writing and the WAIS-III Full Scale IQ ranged from .68 to .81 (Psychological Corporation, 1997). Thus it is possible to formulate reasonably accurate predictions about an examinee's achievement test performance, based on knowledge of his or her WAIS-III results. It is also worth noting that for individuals $\geq$25 years of age, the Verbal, Performance, and Full Scale IQs correlated with level of education .55, .46, and .55, respectively (Tulsky & Ledbetter, 2000). The relationship between scores from the WMS-III (Wechsler, 1997b) and the WAIS-III provide additional evidence of concurrent validity. Correlation coefficients between the eight memory scores and the Full Scale IQ were moderately high and ranged from .36 to .68 (Psychological Corporation, 1997). These findings indicate that the WAIS-III and WMS-III are meaningfully associated, although they appear to be measuring different constructs.

Construct Validity

The 14 WAIS-III subtests are significantly intercorrelated. The Verbal scale subtests are more highly associated with each other than they are with the Performance scale subtests. Likewise, the Performance scale subtests tend to be more highly associated with each other than they are with the Verbal scale subtests. These observations support the premise that a pervasive, general intelligence factor underlies the WAIS-III, and that the pattern of associations among the subtests is consistent with expectations based on practical knowledge and psychological theory. The pattern of intercorrelations constitutes evidence of convergent and discriminant validity

Factor analysis provides additional evidence of construct validity. An exploratory factor analysis of the WAIS-III standardization sample using 13 subtests (Object Assembly was omitted) was reported in the *WAIS-III–WMS-III Technical Manual* (Psychological Corporation, 1997), while a similar analysis on the same sample using all 14 subtests was provided by Sattler and Ryan (1999). For the total standardization sample, these analyses identified four robust factors. The Verbal Comprehension factor was composed of Information, Vocabulary, Similarities, and Comprehension, while the Perceptual Organization factor consisted of Picture Completion, Block Design, Matrix Reasoning, and Picture Arrangement. The third and fourth factors, Working Memory and Processing Speed, included Arithmetic, Digit Span, and Letter–Number Sequencing and Digit Symbol–Coding and Symbol Search, respectively. This four-factor model was also supported by a subsequent confirmatory factor analysis using the standardization participants (Psychological Corporation, 1997).

The Verbal Comprehension and Perceptual Organization factors bear a close resemblance to the Verbal and Performance scales, providing construct validity support for interpretation of the Verbal and Performance IQs. In addition, the magnitude of the subtest loadings on the first unrotated factor, which included all 14 subtests, supports the validity of the Full Scale IQ and indicates that 50% of the variance in WAIS-III performance may be attributed to the construct of general intelligence or *g* (Sattler & Ryan, 1999). In addition to the exploratory factor analyses, the results of a confirmatory factor analysis supported the validity of regrouping the WAIS-III subtests into four clusters (Verbal Comprehension, Perceptual Organization, Working Memory, and Processing Speed) when test results are interpreted for individual examinees (Psychological Corporation, 1997; Ward, Ryan, & Axelrod, 2000).

The validity of WAIS-III subtests, Indexes, and IQs may be evaluated within a theoretical framework, such as the Horn–Cattell theory of fluid (Gf) and crystallized (Gc) intelligence (Horn & Noll, 1997). This theory holds that human ability can be divided into the primary components of Gf and Gc, although the model recognizes the importance of several other kinds of intelligence. Gf involves the ability to learn, solve novel problems, and think abstractly. It tends to decline with advancing age and is disrupted by damage to the brain. Gc involves primarily the use of previously learned and stored verbal information, shows little or no deterioration with advancing age, and demonstrates less of a decline following brain injury than does Gf.

Most of the WAIS-III subtests cannot be assigned unequivocally to either the Gf or Gc category (Horn & Noll, 1997). Nevertheless, a liberal application of Gf-Gc theory suggests that the Verbal scale subtests, with the exception of Letter–Number Sequencing, may be considered as measures of Gc, whereas the Performance scale subtests may be designated as measures of Gf. For example, there were no meaningful age effects in the standardization sample on the Verbal scale subtests of Information and Vocabulary, since it took about the same number of raw-score points to earn scaled scores at the 50th percentile, regardless of an examinee's age. The situation was markedly different for older and younger standardization participants on the Performance scale subtests. For persons in the age range 16–17 years, it took 17 raw-score points on Matrix Reasoning and 40 raw-score points on Block Design to achieve at the 50th percentile. Conversely, in the age range 85–89 years it took only 7 and 23 raw-score points, respectively, on Matrix Reasoning and Block Design to reach the 50th percentile. These observations suggest that the relationship of age to Gf is distinctively different from the corresponding relationship of age to Gc (Ryan, Sattler, & Lopez, 2000).

ADMINISTRATION AND SCORING

For a valid administration of the WAIS-III, an examinee should be fluent in English and possess adequate vision, hearing, and motor functions. When giving the scale to English-speaking persons from countries other than the United States, the examiner must be alert to the possibility that failure on certain test items (e.g., Information subtest items 10 and 11) may reflect cultural loading, not an intellectual limitation. When administering the WAIS-III to Asian Americans and Native Americans, the examiner should keep in mind that these groups were not well represented in the standardization sample. Therefore, some of the responses given by these examinees may need to be interpreted within an appropriate cultural context.

Persons who plan on administering the WAIS-III must be thoroughly familiar with the instructions and procedures contained in the *WAIS-III Administration and Scoring Manual* (Wechsler, 1997a), including the proper sequence of subtest administration; subtest starting points and discontinuance rules; the precise time limits required for administration of individual items; and situations in which to utilize the supplementary and optional subtests. The examiner will need two No. 2 pencils without erasers and a stopwatch to insure accurate timing on five subtests and one optional procedure. In addition to obtaining a comfortable, quiet, and properly furnished (i.e., an appropriate table and chairs) room, the practitioner must schedule sufficient time to complete the examination. Based on data collected

during standardization of the WAIS-III, administration of the 13 subtests that yield both the IQs and Indexes requires anywhere from 65 to 95 minutes (Wechsler, 1997a). However, when one is assessing persons with psychiatric, medical, and/or neurological disorders, administration time may be increased. In a sample of 62 patients with a variety of diagnoses, administration of the 13 subtests required from 61 to 144 minutes (Ryan, Lopez, & Werth, 1998).

The WAIS-III is a complex instrument. The examiner must collect detailed behavioral observations and record the examinee's responses during testing. Moreover, he or she must simultaneously manipulate the test materials, the administration manual, and a stopwatch. Before administering the WAIS-III, examiners should have passed a formal graduate course in intelligence assessment and/or have successfully completed numerous supervised practice administrations. The Sattler and Ryan (1999) "Administration Checklist for the WAIS-III" provides a useful guide for assessing the adequacy of an examiner's administration skills. Finally, examiners from the field of applied psychology should read and adhere to the "Ethical Principles of Psychologists and Code of Conduct" (American Psychological Association, 2002), with particular attention to Ethical Standard 9, "Assessment." Professional counselors should follow the guidelines provided in the American Counseling Association's "Code of Ethics and Standards of Practice" (Herlihy & Corey, 1996), especially Section E, "Evaluation, Assessment, and Interpretation."

For proper WAIS-III administration, it is important that a good working relationship be established. To develop rapport, a conversational, nonthreatening, and interactive approach is helpful. A warm, supportive, yet firm manner can facilitate the assessment process. Examinees often say and do things that are humorous, and the examiner should not be afraid to laugh or reply in kind. The skilled examiner will encourage the examinee to work efficiently, will respond to questions (without giving away test answers), and will be attentive to the examinee's needs (e.g., redirection or a bathroom break). Verbal and nonverbal reinforcement should be given freely throughout the session to promote a high degree of effort from the examinee. However, reinforcement should not be contingent on whether the examinee's response is correct or incorrect.

The detailed instructions provided in the *WAIS-III Administration and Scoring Manual* (Wechsler, 1997a) should be read verbatim when the examiner is giving each subtest. To insure standardized procedures, it is important that the rules concerning order of subtest administration, as well as those for starting, reversing, and discontinuing each subtest, are followed precisely. Repetition of instructions and test items is allowed for all subtests except Digit Span and Letter–Number Sequencing. However, it should be kept in mind that on the Arithmetic subtest, timing always begins at the end of the first reading of the problem.

It is sometimes necessary to use probing questions or queries to help clarify incomplete or vague responses. The *WAIS-III Administration and Scoring Manual* (Wechsler, 1997a) provides examples and guidelines concerning when to initiate the process and what to say. For instance, in the scoring sections when the notation "(Q)" follows a sample response, this indicates a need to query. In these cases, it is permissible to make statements such as "Explain what you mean," or "Tell me more about it." The Vocabulary, Comprehension, and Similarities subtests require the most frequent queries.

Scoring the WAIS-III is a demanding task that requires attention to detail and thorough familiarity with both the *WAIS-III Administration and Scoring Manual* (Wechsler, 1997a) and the *WAIS-III–WMS-III Technical Manual* (Psychological Corporation, 1997). To score a complete administration, the examiner will perform over 45 calculations and more than 200 numerical entries. He or she will also plot about 20 individual scores and consult as many as 16 tables. During this process, it is possible to convert scores incorrectly, give inappropriate credit to individual items, fail to credit correct responses, and make mistakes when adding raw points and scaled scores. Obviously, it is essential that examiners allow themselves sufficient time to carry out their duties in a conscientious manner. The Psychological Corporation has produced one or more computer programs to assist in scoring the WAIS-III. However, even with the use of computerized scoring programs

that eliminate the need to perform calculations, make numerical entries, and consult numerous conversion tables, it remains the examiner's responsibility to score individual responses accurately and to input raw scores correctly into the program.

CHOOSING BETWEEN THE WAIS-III AND WISC-III

Both the WISC-III (Wechsler, 1991) and the WAIS-III can be administered to 16-year-old examinees. At times one must decide which of these tests is most appropriate for a given individual. Based on purely psychometric considerations (e.g., Full Scale floor and ceiling effects), the WISC-III is probably better for adolescents who are below average in intellectual ability, whereas the WAIS-III appears to be more appropriate for adolescents with above-average ability (Sattler & Ryan, 1999). In the first instance, the WISC-III provides a lower floor than the WAIS-III and therefore allows for a more thorough sampling of an examinee's performance at the lower end of the ability spectrum. In the second instance, the WAIS-III provides a higher ceiling than the WISC-III, thereby reducing the possibility that a bright adolescent will "top out" on one or more subtests. One can select either the WAIS-III or the WISC-III when an examinee is likely to possess average intelligence. The latter conclusion is based on research with 16-year-olds that administered the two tests to a sample of 184 examinees over a retest interval of 2–12 weeks (Psychological Corporation, 1997). Results indicated that the two scales yielded comparable IQs (e.g., for the Full Scale IQ, WISC-III $M = 103.9$, $SD = 15.2$; WAIS-III $M = 104.6$, $SD = 15.1$).

APPLICATION OF THE WAIS-III

Analysis of WAIS-III results may be accomplished by a hypothesis-driven interpretative approach that considers both the quantitative and qualitative aspects of performance. The first step is to evaluate the variability between and among subtests. This is done to determine whether the IQ and Indexes "hang together" and provide adequate estimates of the abilities they purport to measure. For instance, if the individual subtest scores comprising an IQ or Index cluster around their respective scaled score means, unusual intersubtest scatter is absent, and each composite score may be interpreted in the standard fashion. Conversely, if marked intersubtest scatter is present, the examiner cannot be sure that the composite is mea-

suring a unitary entity, and interpretation of the IQ or Index may be problematic.

Table 6.4 provides an illustrative, hypothetical example of a protocol in which six of the WAIS-III composites reflect extreme intersubtest scatter. Our position is to question whether a composite score based on a group of subtests provides a meaningful di-

TABLE 6.4. Illustrative WAIS-III Results

Subtests, scales, and Indexes	Scaled scores	Mean	Differences
Verbal scale			
Vocabulary	4	10	−6.0
Similarities	16	10	6.0
Arithmetic	10	10	0.0
Digit Span	12	10	0.2
Information	9	10	−1.0
Comprehension	10	10	0.0
Letter–Number Sequencing	9	10	−1.0
Range of the six standard subtests = 12			
Performance scale			
Picture Completion	14	9.7	4.3
Digit Symbol–Coding	3	9.7	−6.7
Block Design	10	9.7	0.3
Matrix Reasoning	4	9.7	−5.7
Picture Arrangement	15	9.7	5.3
Symbol Search	12	9.7	2.3
Range of the five standard subtests = 12			
VCI			
Information	9	9.7	−0.7
Vocabulary	4	9.7	−5.7
Similarities	16	9.7	6.3
Range of the three standard subtests = 12			
POI			
Picture Completion	14	9.3	4.7
Block Design	10	9.3	0.7
Matrix Reasoning	4	9.3	−5.7
Range of the three standard subtests = 10			
WMI			
Arithmetic	10	10.3	−0.3
Digit Span	12	10.3	1.7
Letter–Number Sequencing	9	10.3	−1.3
Range of the three standard subtests = 3			
PSI			
Digit Symbol–Coding	3	7.5	−4.5
Symbol Search	12	7.5	4.5
Range of the two standard subtests = 9			

Note. Verbal IQ = 100; Performance IQ = 94.

mension of ability whenever the degree of scatter within the composite equals or exceeds that for 95% of the standardization sample participants. The use of the 95% base rate figure as a definition of "extreme intersubtest scatter" is rather conservative and reflects the our personal preference. However, the decision as to what constitutes "extreme" rests with the individual examiner. It may be argued that when the goal of assessment is to formulate a conclusive diagnosis, a strict criterion (i.e., ≤5%) is appropriate. Conversely, when the WAIS-III is administered for screening or some other less crucial purpose, a more liberal criterion will suffice (Kaufman, 1990).

To return to the example in Table 6.4, it can be seen that on the Verbal scale there are two 6-point deviations from the mean of the seven subtests, one positive (indicating a profile strength) and one negative (indicating a profile weakness). Table B.3 in the *WAIS-III Administration and Scoring Manual* (Wechsler, 1997a) indicates that when seven Verbal subtests are administered, unusually large deviations (those that occurred in 5% or fewer of the standardization participants) range from 3.00 points on Vocabulary to 4.43 points on Digit Span. In the current profile, the –6.0 point deviation for Vocabulary and the +6-point deviation for Similarities are both highly unusual, having occurred in fewer than 1% of the standardization sample. The presence of marked intersubtest scatter indicates that the Verbal IQ of 100 is probably not measuring a unitary construct and should not be taken as conclusive evidence that this examinee has average verbal abilities. On the Performance scale, large deviations from the mean are found on Digit Symbol–Coding (–6.7), Matrix Reasoning (–5.7), Picture Arrangement (5.3), and Picture Completion (4.3). Table 6.5 shows that when Symbol Search is administered alone with the five standard Performance subtests, deviations that equal or exceed those for 95% of persons in the standardization sample range from 3.57 points on Symbol Search to 4.14 points on Digit Symbol–Coding. Table 6.5 also indicates that each of the four subtest deviations listed above is unusually large and was obtained by fewer than 5% of the WAIS-III normative group. Thus the Performance IQ of 94 is probably not reflecting a unitary en-

TABLE 6.5. Differences between Individual Subtest Scaled Scores and Mean Scaled Score for Five Standard Performance Scale Subtests Plus Symbol Search That Occurred in ≤5% of the Standardization Sample

Subtest	Deviation from the mean
Picture Completion	3.93
Digit Symbol–Coding	4.14
Block Design	3.65
Matrix Reasoning	3.79
Picture Arrangement	4.03
Symbol Search	3.57

Note. From LoBello, Thompson, and Evani (1998). Copyright 1998 by The Psychoeducational Corporation. Adapted by permission.

tity, and this composite should not be taken as conclusive evidence that the examinee has average nonverbal abilities.

In the example above, separate means for the seven Verbal and six Performance subtests were utilized. We could have taken an alternative approach and used the mean of all 13 subtests for the deviation score analysis. This would have produced essentially the same pattern and magnitude of deviation scores that were obtained with separate Verbal and Performance means. The only time that it is essential to use separate means is when the Verbal and Performance IQs are markedly discrepant; that is, Verbal IQ minus Performance IQ ≥ ±19 points (see Sattler & Ryan, 1999, p. 1253). The analysis above also utilized means based on seven Verbal scale subtests and six Performance scale subtests. This approach may be followed as long as the supplementary subtests of Letter–Number Sequencing and Symbol Search do not show unusually large deviations from their respective scale means (i.e., a difference from the mean that occurred in 5% or fewer of persons in the standardization sample).

Further inspection of Table 6.4 suggests that extreme intersubtest scatter characterizes the VCI, POI, and PSI. For example, Vocabulary and Similarities deviate by approximately 6 points from the mean of the three VCI subtests. Examination of Table 6.6 indicates that deviations of this magnitude were obtained by 5% or fewer of participants in the standardization sample, and that the VCI probably does not represent a unitary construct. Specifically, deviations from the mean greater than or equal to 2.56, 2.51, and 2.22 points are considered unusual for the Vocabulary, Information, and Similarities subtests, respectively. The appropriate critical values presented in Table 6.6 indicate that extreme intersubtest scatter is also present among the components of both the POI and the PSI. However, the WMI contains relatively little scatter and appears to represent a unitary entity, since none of the subtests in this composite deviate meaningfully from their overall mean. A traditional interpretation of the WMI thus appears justified.

A less time-consuming—and, in most cases, similarly effective—method for determining whether or not subtest composites represent unitary constructs was recommended by Kaufman and Lichtenberger (1999). To evaluate the utility of the Verbal IQ, the scaled score range on the six subtests used to compute the composite is examined (note that Letter–Number Sequencing is not included). The range is found by

subtracting the lowest of the six subtests from the highest of these subtest scores. If the range is ≥8 scaled score points, the Verbal IQ is probably not interpretable. The Performance scale range is obtained by subtracting the highest of the five subtest scores used to obtain the IQ from the lowest of these scores (note that Symbol Search is not included). A range of ≥8 scaled score points suggests that the Performance IQ is not a unitary construct. To check on the validity of the Indexes, the examiner should calculate the ranges for each composite and determine whether each equals or exceeds the following cutoff: VCI, ≥5 scaled score points; PCI, ≥6 scaled score points; WMI, ≥6 scaled score points; and PSI, ≥4 scaled score points. Application of these cutoffs to the data in Table 6.4 leads to the same conclusion as the deviation analysis provided in the previous paragraphs: There is an unusual amount of scatter in five of the six composite scores. Only the WMI reflects a unitary entity that can be easily interpreted. We recommend that the Kaufman and Lichtenberger method of evaluating scatter by inspection of range statistics be used in conjunction with subtest deviation analysis. In some situations, deviation analysis will be too conservative and make profile analysis unnecessarily difficult. Therefore, if deviation analysis suggests that a composite (i.e., an IQ or Index) should be disregarded because it does not appear to represent a unitary construct, but inspection of the range statistic indicates the opposite conclusion, the examiner has the option of accepting either interpretation.

Table 6.4 presents a protocol with extreme intersubtest scatter—evidence of an unusual WAIS-III performance. In most cases, however, the standard composites usually "hang together" according to the guidelines provided above. Consider the set of illustrative WAIS-III results given in Table 6.7. Within the Verbal scale, only Comprehension shows an unusually large deviation from the mean of the seven subtests (i.e., 4.86). Table B.3 in the *WAIS-III Administration and Scoring Manual* shows that a deviation score this large occurred in <2% of the standardization sample participants. This noteworthy strength would be highlighted if a written report of the WAIS-III results were prepared. However, we feel that

TABLE 6.6. Differences between Individual Subtest Scaled Scores and Mean Scaled Score for Each WAIS-III Factor-Based Composite That Occurred in ≤5% of the Standardization Sample

Index subtest	Deviation from the mean
VCI	
Vocabulary	2.56
Information	2.51
Similarities	2.22
POI	
Picture Completion	3.50
Block Design	3.09
Matrix Reasoning	3.23
WMI	
Arithmetic	3.32
Digit Span	3.14
Letter–Number Sequencing	3.24
PSI	
Digit Symbol–Coding	2.46
Symbol Search	2.46

Note. From Sattler (2001). Copyright 2001 by the author. Adapted by permission.

TABLE 6.7. Illustrative WAIS-III Results

Subtests, scales, and Indexes	Scaled scores	Mean	Differences
Verbal scale			
Vocabulary	14	12.14	1.86
Similarities	10	12.14	–2.14
Arithmetic	13	12.14	0.86
Digit Span	11	12.14	–1.14
Information	10	12.14	–2.14
Comprehension	17	12.14	4.86
Letter–Number Sequencing	10	12.14	–2.14
Range of the six standard subtests = 7			
Performance scale			
Picture Completion	9	10.67	–1.67
Digit Symbol–Coding	9	10.67	–1.67
Block Design	13	10.67	2.33
Matrix Reasoning	11	10.67	0.33
Picture Arrangement	13	10.67	2.33
Symbol Search	9	10.67	–1.67
Range of the five standard subtests = 4			
VCI			
Information	10	11.33	–1.33
Vocabulary	14	11.33	2.67
Similarities	10	11.33	–1.33
Range of the three standard subtests = 4			
POI			
Picture Completion	9	11.00	–2.00
Block Design	13	11.00	2.00
Matrix Reasoning	11	11.00	0.00
Range of the three standard subtests = 4			
WMI			
Arithmetic	13	11.33	1.67
Digit Span	11	11.33	-0.33
Letter–Number Sequencing	10	11.33	–1.33
Range of the three standard subtests = 3			
PSI			
Digit Symbol–Coding	9	9.00	0.00
Symbol Search	9	9.00	0.00
Range of the two standard subtests = 0			

Note. Verbal IQ = 115; Performance IQ = 106; VCI = 107; POI = 105; WMI = 108; PSI = 93.

the single atypical score on Comprehension does not preclude interpretation of the Verbal IQ as a unitary entity. Thus the Verbal IQ may be interpreted as a measure of general intelligence, with an emphasis on previously learned and stored verbal information and ideas. This decision was based on the fact that (1) the range of scaled scores (i.e., 7 points) on the six subtests constituting the Verbal IQ is below the cutoff of ≥8 points (Kaufman & Lichtenberger, 1999); and (2) the Indexes (i.e., VCI = 107 and WMI = 105) that constitute the Verbal scale are not significantly different from one another (see Table B.1 in the *WAIS-III Administration and Scoring Manual*).

Inspection of the Performance subtests reveals minimal scatter, with a scaled score range of 4; no unusual deviations from the mean of the seven subtests; and a nonsignificant (i.e., $p < .05$; see Table B.1 in the *WAIS-III Administration and Scoring Manual*) discrepancy between the Indexes (POI = 105; PSI = 93) that constitute the Performance scale. Therefore, the Performance IQ may be interpreted as a unitary construct that reflects perceptual organization, fluid reasoning, and attention to details.

The next step in WAIS-III analysis deals with the Indexes. Inspection of the VCI subtests indicates that the Vocabulary score deviates (i.e., 2.67) from the appropriate mean by an unusually large degree, exceeding that of 95% of the standardization sample participants (see Table 6.6). However, since the range of scores across the three subtests is below the recommended cutoff of ≥ 5 points, the examiner may elect to accept the VCI as a unitary entity. Further inspection of Table 6.7 indicates that none of the POI, WMI, or PSI subtests produced unusually large deviations from their respective means. Moreover, the range statistic for each subtest combination falls within acceptable limits as defined by Kaufman and Lichtenberger (1999).

In the present example, it has been determined that each WAIS-III IQ and Index appears to represent a reasonable estimate of the construct it purports to measure. The next step in the interpretative process is to examine the relationship between the Verbal and Performance IQs and between and among the four Index scores. Table 6.7 shows that the Verbal and Performance IQs differ by 9 points. Table B.1 in the *WAIS-III Administration and Scoring Manual* indicates that a difference of this magnitude is reliable at the 95% level. Therefore, this discrepancy did not result from measurement error and probably reflects a true difference in how the examine demonstrates his or her intelligence. Nevertheless, Table D.4 in the *WAIS-III–WMS-III Technical Manual* indicates that an IQ difference of 9 points, regardless of the direction (i.e., Verbal > Performance or Performance < Verbal), occurred in 48.4% of individuals in the standardization sample with a Full Scale IQ in the high average range (i.e., 110–119). This base rate figure indicates that the 9-point difference is not unusual (we consider a difference to be unusual if it occurred in $\leq 5\%$ of the standardization sample), and that the Full Scale IQ provides a reasonable estimate of the examinee's overall cognitive functioning. This interpretative step continues with the determination of any potentially important relationships between and among the four Indexes. When Table B.1 in the *WAIS-III Administration and Scoring Manual* is consulted, it can be seen that the VCI and the WMI are both significantly greater than the PSI.

Once the decision has been made to interpret the individual IQs and Indexes, it is necessary to convert each value to an ability level, according to Table 2.3 in the *WAIS-III Administration and Scoring Manual*. Next, each IQ and Index is assigned a percentile rank and banded by the 95% confidence limits. The percentile conversions are found in Table 2.2, and the confidence intervals are provided in Tables A.3 through A.9, of the *WAIS-III Administration and Scoring Manual*. It is noted that the confidence limits provided by the test publisher are based on the standard error of estimation (SEE), not the SEM discussed previously and presented in Table 3.4 of the *WAIS-III–WMS-III Technical Manual*. This should not concern the reader, since the SEE and the SEM are interpreted in exactly the same manner and yield highly similar confidence intervals, especially for IQs and Indexes within the middle portion of the ability distribution. For those who prefer using the SEM, confidence intervals based on this statistic for all age groups in the standardization sample are provided in Table 0–1 of Sattler and Ryan (1999).

The preceding discussion has focused on quantitative aspects of WAIS-III interpretation. However, purely numerical scores are frequently insufficient for understanding an individual's problems during a cognitive examination. This is especially true of examinees with neurological and psychiatric conditions. Thus qualitative information gleaned from behavioral observations and responses to individual test items may provide insight into an examinee's cultural background, cognitive deficits, sensory-perceptual limitations, thought processes, and/or mental status. It is also important to document the nature and effectiveness of the strategies that an individual uses to either pass or fail a test item. Table 6.8 provides examples of qualitative errors that might be observed during a WAIS-III administration.

INTERPRETATION OF THE WAIS-III

To interpret the WAIS-III properly, it is necessary to utilize an approach that integrates historical information, behavioral observations, and the quantitative aspects of test performance. If possible, the qualitative features of the examinee's performance should also be incorporated. This requires the gathering of pertinent behavioral observations during test administration, as well as scrutiny of data from the examinee's medical, educational, and social histories. This information is then used to formulate hypotheses or expectations about the examinee's test performance using a sequential process. Before the WAIS-III is scored, a priori hypotheses are developed to explain the Full Scale IQ, Verbal and Performance IQs, Indexes, scores on combinations of subtests, scores on single subtests, and the specific characteristics of individual item responses. Next, the WAIS-III scores are calculated, and the a priori hypotheses are tested against the obtained results. If the a priori expectations and hypotheses do not account for the data, the examiner formulates a posteriori explanations for the findings. These hypotheses may also be offered at the composite, subtest combination, and single-subtest levels. At this stage in the process, it may be necessary to collect additional data (e.g., administration of language or achievement tests) to test or support the a priori and a posteriori explanations. Finally, the examiner draws conclusions and writes his or her report. It is best to place emphasis on explanations that are supported by at least two pieces of evidence (e.g., history, behavioral observations, supplementary test data). Let's apply this approach to a WAIS-III protocol obtained from an actual examinee.

TABLE 6.8. **Examples of Qualitative Errors Associated with Selected WAIS-III Subtests**

Subtest	Error and hypothesized interpretation
Similarities	*Stimulus-bound response:* An examinee provides common associations to word pairs, not similarities. For example, in response to item 10, the examinee states, "Chair you sit on, and table you eat on." Sometimes given by people with concrete thinking, persons with low general intelligence, and/or patients with brain damage.
Digit Span	*Incorrect sequencing:* An examinee recalls all the elements in a digit series, but fails to maintain the order of presentation. When this happens frequently during test administration, it may be associated with a learning disability or possibly an anxiety state.
Letter–Number Sequencing	*Auditory discrimination problems:* An examinee with intact auditory attention/concentration may repeat incorrect letters. For example, on the second trial of item 2, the examinee may hear "d" as "t."
Block Design	*Broken gestalts:* An examinee fails to maintain the 2 × 2 or 3 × 3 configuration of one or more designs. Seen occasionally in the records of persons with marked visual–spatial impairment. May suggest the presence of brain damage.
Matrix Reasoning	*Positional preferences:* An examinee shows a consistent tendency to prefer answers on one side of the page. May reflect visual scanning problems.
Digit Symbol–Coding	*Associating the wrong symbol with a number:* Suggests failure to comprehend instructions, inattention, or visual scanning problems.

CASE EXAMPLE

This section describes the WAIS-III results of D. W., a 17-year-old male who was in the ninth grade at a public school in the Midwest. During his grammar school years, he was diagnosed with ADHD and prescribed Ritalin. There were no apparent problems until he stopped taking the medication approximately 3 months prior to this referral. According to his parents and teachers, the youngster's everyday behavior and performance in school deteriorated significantly once the medication was terminated. The examinee's mother described him as distractible, forgetful, intrusive, impulsive, and unable to follow either oral or written directions. She noted that his listening skills were poor and that he frequently needed to have oral questions and directions repeated. He was always "on the go" and didn't sit still or follow through with chores, assignments, or homework.

The examinee was enrolled in remedial reading and remedial mathematics classes. The teacher reported that D. W. exhibited numerous problems in the classroom, including poor concentration, inadequate listening skills, failure to remember two- or three-step directions, impulsivity, and a tendency to rush through assignments with little regard for accuracy or quality of work. However, he was able to attend and deal more successfully with class assignments when seated close to the teacher. Specific problems were noted in reading and mathematics. When reading, he often lost his place and frequently omitted, substituted, or inserted words or sounds. When performing basic arithmetic problems, he sometimes omitted necessary steps or carried out the operations in the wrong order.

During the WAIS-III examination, D. W. was alert, cooperative, and friendly. He appeared motivated to perform the majority of tasks, but also displayed restlessness and often experienced some difficulty remembering instructions. On the Arithmetic subtest, he showed a short attention span and a tendency either to guess impulsively at items or to give up without trying. He was unsuccessful at solving problems that involved basic subtraction, multiplication, and/or division. These failures seemed to reflect a mixture of impulsive responding, careless-ness, and possibly an inadequate mastery of rudimentary mathematical skills (e.g., basic division combinations). During completion of the Digit Symbol–Coding subtest, he twice associated the wrong symbol with a number, and on one occasion he added an extra line to the symbol he was copying. During the Digit Span subtest, he was able to focus attention and perform normally on items that were relatively simple and involved only rote memorization (i.e., he successfully repeated 7 digits forward). Conversely, when the task required internal visualization and mental manipulation, his performance suffered (i.e., he successfully repeated only 3 digits in reverse order). There was also one instance during backward Digit Span when he appeared to lose set and momentarily lapsed into giving them forward.

With this background information and these behavioral observations, we can formulate a series of reasonable a priori hypotheses to explain D. W.'s WAIS-III performance. To arrive at such hypotheses, an examiner needs a working knowledge of the pertinent assessment literature (e.g., Kaufman & Lichtenberger, 1999; Psychological Corporation, 1997; Sattler & Ryan, 1999) and a full appreciation of the particular condition or disorder under study (e.g., American Psychiatric Association, 2000; Fisher, 1998). Listed below are some expectations and hypotheses presented in a sequential manner, starting with the most global score:

1. D. W. should achieve a Full Scale IQ that falls within the average range. This hypothesis is based on the literature indicating that individuals with ADHD usually exhibit normal psychometric intelligence.

2. Comparable achievement is expected on the Verbal and Performance IQs. The literature sometimes indicates a tendency for groups of individuals with ADHD to exhibit a Performance IQ > Verbal IQ pattern, but the magnitude of this difference is typically not significant from a statistical standpoint.

3. The WMI and the PSI are expected to be significantly lower than the VCI and the POI. The literature indicates that individuals with ADHD tend to perform relatively poorly on subtests that are sensitive to

problems with attention/concentration and response inhibition.

4. D. W.'s performance on subtests that are highly sensitive to deficits in attention/concentration and the ability to remain free from distraction (Arithmetic, Digit Span, Letter–Number Sequencing, Picture Completion, Digit Symbol–Coding, and Symbol Search) will be impaired, relative to the appropriate average subtest score. Likewise, subtests that reflect a facility with numbers and sequential reasoning (Arithmetic, Digit Span, Letter–Number Sequencing, Picture Arrangement, and Digit Symbol–Coding) will be performed poorly, relative to the appropriate average subtest score. Finally, performance on subtests that require memory (Information, Arithmetic, Digit Span, Picture Completion, Digit Symbol–Coding, and Letter–Number Sequencing) will suggest impairment, relative to the appropriate average subtest score. The use of these subtest combinations is based on the ADHD literature, D. W.'s educational and medical histories, and behavioral observations collected during the examination. The specific subtest combinations are taken, with slight modification, from Table 4.16 (Abilities Shared by Two or More WAIS-III Verbal and Performance Subtests) in Kaufman and Lichtenberger (1998).

5. D. W.'s Digit Span performance should be atypical in two ways. First, there should be a large discrepancy between the forward and backward spans; second, there should be sequencing errors in his digit recollections. These predictions are based on a review of the pertinent literature, the examinee's history, and behavioral observations during the examination.

Once the WAIS-III scores have been calculated, some of these hypotheses will be supported and others will not. However, by formulating these predictions, we have attempted to integrate external information with the test results and focus our attention on the complete array of information provided by the WAIS-III.

The second step in the interpretative process is to determine whether D. W.'s summary scores represent valid estimates of the constructs they purport to measure. Table 6.9 summarizes the quantitative and qualitative features of D. W.'s WAIS-III performance. Analysis begins with calculation of the Verbal scale range, a value derived by subtracting the lowest score (Arithmetic = 6) from the highest score (Comprehension = 16). The range of 10 suggests the presence of marked variability within the profile. Analysis continues with inspection of the values provided in the "Differences" column of Table 6.9. These scores indicate the amount that each subtest deviates from the mean of the seven Verbal scale subtests and constitutes an additional way to assess intersubtest scatter in the profile. For the Verbal scale subtests, these numbers are compared to the values in Table B.3 of the *WAIS-III Administration and Scoring Manual*. As can be seen, the scores on the Similarities (3.71 points), Arithmetic (–4.29 points), and Comprehension (5.71 points) subtests deviate meaningfully from the Verbal scale mean of 10.29 points. These are judged to be meaningful deviations because 5% or fewer of the standardization sample participants had deviation scores that equaled or exceeded 3.29 points on Similarities, 3.57 points on Arithmetic, and 3.57 points on Comprehension. These findings indicate that the Verbal IQ does not measure a unitary ability.

Intersubtest scatter on the Performance scale may be evaluated by inspection of the range statistic (Block Design minus Picture Completion = 8) and by comparing the deviation scores in the "Differences" column of Table 6.9 with the values provided in Table 6.5. The range indicates that a considerable degree of variability characterizes the profile, but deviation score analysis reveals that only Block Design (4.17) is markedly discrepant with the Performance Scale mean. If a conservative approach is taken (and it is always up to the examiner whether a liberal, moderate, or conservative interpretation is utilized), these findings suggest that the Performance IQ may not represent a unitary construct and probably should not be interpreted.

The third step focuses on the four Indexes, three of which do not appear to represent unitary constructs. Examination of the VCI subtests (see Table 6.9) reveals a range of 5 (Similarities minus Information), which equals the suggested cutoff for extreme scatter presented above. Comparing the deviation scores in the "Differences" column of

TABLE 6.9. WAIS-III Results for D. W.

Subtests, scales, and Indexes	Scaled scores	Mean	Differences
Verbal scale			
Vocabulary	12	10.29	1.71
Similarities	14	10.29	3.71
Arithmetic	6	10.29	−4.29
Digit Span	8	10.29	−2.29
Information	9	10.29	−1.29
Comprehension	16	10.29	5.71
Letter–Number Sequencing	7	10.29	−3.29
Range of the six standard subtests = 10			
Performance scale			
Picture Completion	7	10.83	−3.83
Digit Symbol–Coding	7	10.83	−3.83
Block Design	15	10.83	4.17
Matrix Reasoning	13	10.83	2.17
Picture Arrangement	10	10.83	-0.83
Symbol Search	13	10.83	2.17
Range of the five standard subtests = 8			
VCI			
Information	9	11.67	2.67
Vocabulary	12	11.67	0.33
Similarities	14	11.67	2.33
Range of the three standard subtests = 5			
POI			
Picture Completion	7	11.67	−4.67
Block Design	15	11.67	3.33
Matrix Reasoning	13	11.67	1.33
Range of the three standard subtests = 8			
WMI			
Arithmetic	6	7.00	−1.00
Digit Span	8	7.00	1.00
Letter–Number Sequencing	7	7.00	0.00
Range of the three standard subtests = 2			
PSI			
Digit Symbol–Coding	7	10.00	−3.00
Symbol Search	13	10.00	3.00
Range of the two standard subtests = 6			

Note. Verbal IQ = 104; Performance IQ = 102; Full Scale IQ = 103; VCI = 109; POI = 109; WMI = 82; PSI = 99.

Some qualitative features of D. W.'s responses were as follows:

Arithmetic: responded rapidly to some items without apparent reflection; made careless errors, such as 30 ÷ 6 = "6."
Digit Symbol–Coding: Two symbol substitution errors and one design elaboration.
Digit Span (forward correct maximum = 7):

4-1-7-9-3-8-6	Repeated as "4-9-7-1-3-8-6"
5-8-1-9-2-6-4-7	Repeated as "5-8-9-1-6-2-4-7"
3-8-2-9-5-1-7-4	Repeated as "3-8-2-5-9-1-7-4"

Digit Span (backward correct maximum = 3):

3-2-7-9	Repeated as "9-2-7-3"
4-9-6-8	Repeated as "4-6-8-9"

Table 6.9 with the values provided in Table 6.6 indicates that both Similarities (2.33) and Information (2.67) differ meaningfully from the mean of the VCI subtests. These are considered meaningful departures, because 5% or fewer of the standardization participants had deviation scores that equaled or exceeded 2.22 points on Similarities and 2.51 points on Information. The POI is also characterized by an unusually high degree of intersubtest scatter, as evidenced by a range (Block Design minus Picture Completion) of 8 points. Moreover, ipsative analysis indicates that the Picture Completion (−4.67) and Block Design (3.33) scores differ meaningfully from the mean of the POI subtests. Table 6.6 indicates that 5% or fewer of the standardization sample had deviation scores that equaled or exceeded 3.50 on Picture Completion and 3.09 on Block Design. Like the VCI and POI, the PSI represents an average of diverse abilities. The range (Symbol Search minus Digit Symbol–Coding) of 6 points exceeds the cutoff recommended in the preceding section, and both components of the PSI differ meaningfully from the average subtest score. Table 6.6 indicates that 5% or fewer of the standardization participants had deviation scores on Symbol Search and Digit Symbol–Coding equal to or greater than 2.46 points.

As indicated above, the VCI, POI, and PSI do not represent unitary constructs. On the other hand, the WMI emerges as a cohesive ability dimension. The scaled score range (Digit Span minus Arithmetic) within this subtest cluster is only 2, and none of the three components differs meaningfully from the overall mean.

The fourth step in WAIS-III interpretation involves testing a priori expectations and hypotheses against the actual scores obtained by the examinee. As shown in Table 6.9, the Full Scale IQ falls within the average range, and the difference between the Verbal and Performance IQs is negligible. Hypotheses 1 and 2 are confirmed. Thus, in terms of the major summary scores gleaned from the WAIS-III, D. W.'s achievement levels are consistent with those in the literature describing groups of children and adolescents with a diagnosis of ADHD.

To address hypothesis 3, it is necessary to consult Table B.1 in the *WAIS-III Administration and Scoring Manual*. By reading down the appropriate columns in the table, one can determine that the WMI is significantly lower than the other three composites. Following the same procedure makes it apparent that the PSI differs only from the WMI, with the former representing a significantly higher level of achievement. Therefore, the VCI, POI, and PSI all reflect comparable performance, whereas WMI performance emerges as a distinct weakness. These findings confirm our expectations for the WMI, but not for the PSI. The lack of confirmation of the PSI hypothesis should come as no surprise, since profile analysis has indicated that for D. W. this composite does not provide a cohesive estimate of the construct of interest and should not be interpreted in the standard fashion.

To address each part of hypothesis 4, it is necessary to consult Table 6.10 and then to apply a simple rule of thumb recommended by Kaufman and Lichtenberger (1999). First, to use Table 6.10, we must read down

TABLE 6.10. Differences Required for Significance at $p = .05$ When Each Verbal and Performance Subtest Score is Compared to the Appropriate Scale Mean

Subtest	Difference from the mean	Subtest	Difference from the mean
Vocabulary	2.09	Picture Completion	3.02
Similarities	2.76	Digit Symbol–Coding	2.91
Arithmetic	2.66	Block Design	2.81
Digit Span	2.39	Matrix Reasoning	2.50
Information	2.33	Picture Arrangement	3.57
Comprehension	2.95	Symbol Search	3.37
Letter–Number Sequencing	3.15		

Note. From Sattler (2001). Copyright 2001 by the author. Adapted by permission.

the two left columns to determine whether the score on a Verbal scale subtest differs significantly from the mean of the seven Verbal scale subtests. Next, we must read down the two right columns to determine whether a Performance scale subtest differs significantly from the mean of six Performance scale subtests. Each instance where a subtest differs significantly (i.e., $p = .05$) from the appropriate scale mean is recorded. The second step involves applying the following rule of thumb to each subtest combination:

a. At least one subtest is significantly below the appropriate scale mean.
b. At least four subtests must be below the appropriate scale mean.
c. Only one subtest may equal or exceed the appropriate scale mean.

The first part of hypothesis 4 focuses on a subtest combination that is thought to measure attention/concentration and the ability to remain free from distraction (Arithmetic, Digit Span, Letter–Number Sequencing, Picture Completion, Digit Symbol–Coding, and Symbol Search). Table 6.10 indicates that the scores of four subtests (Arithmetic, Letter–Number Sequencing, Picture Completion, and Digit Symbol–Coding) are significantly different from their respective scale means. For example, the deviation score of –4.29 for Arithmetic exceeds the tabled value of 2.66, indicating that the Arithmetic score is significantly below the Verbal scale mean. Likewise, the deviation score for Picture Completion of –3.83 exceeds the tabled value of –3.02, indicating that the Picture Completion score is significantly below the Performance scale mean. Once requirement a has been met, we determine how many of the subtests are below their respective scale means. In this case, five of the six subtest scores are below the appropriate mean and therefore requirement b has been met. Finally, requirement c has been met, since only the score on Symbol Search exceeds the appropriate scale mean. These findings support the first part of hypothesis 4; they indicate that D. W.'s performance on subtests that are highly sensitive to deficits in attention/concentration and the ability to remain free from distraction represents a weakness in the overall profile.

When the same procedures are applied to the subtest grouping that measures facility with numbers and sequential reasoning (Arithmetic, Digit Span, Letter–Number Sequencing, Picture Arrangement, and Digit Symbol–Coding), three subtests are found to be significantly below the appropriate scale mean, and all five are below their appropriate scale mean. The second part of hypothesis 4 is confirmed, since D. W.'s facility with numbers and his sequencing abilities represent a weak area within his profile. The third part of hypothesis D predicts that D. W. should perform poorly on subtests placing a premium on memory and recall ability (Information, Arithmetic, Digit Span, Letter–Number Sequencing, Picture Completion, and Digit Symbol–Coding). When the three steps presented above are applied to the profile, four of the six subtest scores are found to be significantly different from the appropriate mean value, and all six are below the appropriate scale mean. The hypothesis is supported, in that D. W. shows a definite weakness on memory sensitive subtests.

With respect to hypothesis 5, results of the Digit Span subtest provide strong support for the predicted superiority of digits forward (i.e., longest correct span = 7) over digits backward (i.e., longest correct span = 3), as well as the presence of sequencing errors (see Table 6.9).

D. W.'s WAIS-III profile contains three noteworthy strengths that have not been predicted on an a priori basis. Inspection of the Verbal scale subtests reveals that the Comprehension and Similarities subtests are at the 91st and 98th percentiles, while on the Performance scale the Block Design subtest is at the 95th percentile. To explain these meaningful strengths, it is necessary to formulate at least two a posteriori hypotheses. Listed below are the a posteriori hypotheses, both focusing on subtest combinations:

1. D. W.'s good scores on Similarities, Comprehension, and Block Design may be explained by a well-developed capacity to engage in verbal and nonverbal concept formation and reasoning.
2. D. W.'s good score on the Block Design subtest reflects, in addition to a strength in nonverbal concept formation, a well-developed capacity to deal with prob-

lems and situations that require spatial visualization skills.

To test a posteriori hypothesis 2, we need to examine performance on the four subtests (Similarities, Vocabulary, Comprehension, and Block Design) that appear to measure the construct of interest (see Table 6.1). First, we must consult Table 6.10 and read down the two left columns to determine whether each Verbal subtest score differs significantly from the mean of the seven Verbal scale subtests. Next, we must read down the two right columns in the table to see whether Block Design differs significantly from the mean of six Performance scale subtests. The second step involves applying a simple rule of thumb to the subtest combination. Note that this rule is different from the one set forth earlier, because we are now looking for a "strength" in the profile and because the present subtest combination has only four components. The following rule of thumb comes from Kaufman and Lichtenberger (1999):

a. At least one subtest is significantly above the appropriate scale mean.
b. At least three subtests must be above the appropriate scale mean.
c. Only one subtest may be equivalent to the appropriate scale mean.

When these steps are applied to the present subtest combination, three of the components are found to be significantly above the appropriate scale mean, and all four are above their respective scale means. Hypothesis 1 is confirmed, and it may be concluded that D. W. has demonstrated a well-developed capacity and overall strength to engage in verbal and nonverbal concept formation and reasoning.

To test a posteriori hypothesis 2, we need to examine performance on the three subtests (Block Design, Matrix Reasoning, and Symbol Search) that appear to measure the construct of spatial visualization (see Table 6.1). First, we must consult Table 6.10 and read down the two right columns to determine whether each subtest score differs significantly from the mean of six Performance scale subtests. The second step involves applying a simple rule of thumb to the subtest combination. Note that this rule

is different from the preceding one, because the present subtest combination has only three components. The following rule of thumb comes from Kaufman and Lichtenberger (1999):

a. At least one subtest is significantly above the appropriate scale mean.
b. At least three subtests must be above the appropriate scale mean.
c. Only one subtest may be equivalent to the appropriate scale mean.

When these steps are applied to the present subtest combination, one of the components is found to be significantly above the scale mean, while the remaining two are above the scale mean. A posteriori hypothesis 2 is confirmed, and it may be concluded that D. W. has demonstrated a well-developed capacity for dealing with tasks that require spatial visualization skills.

In most assessment situations, the next step in test interpretation involves the collection of additional data to corroborate the a priori and a posteriori hypotheses. This is usually an easy task, since the WAIS-III is almost always administered as part of a test battery. When one is evaluating an individual with suspected or diagnosed ADHD, a test battery may include measures of attention/concentration, academic proficiency, language, memory, visual–spatial ability, executive functions, and personality. Observations of school behavior and parent and teacher ratings are also obtained.

THE WAIS-III REPORT

The WAIS-III was administered to D. W. in order to gain insights into his cognitive and adaptive abilities. However, test scores by themselves have little meaning and must be translated so that the referral source can utilize the information they provide. This requires formulating conclusions and the preparation of a professional report. The following paragraphs attempt to demonstrate this process with respect to the WAIS-III. The sample report excerpted below is incomplete and omits important information (e.g., background information, reason for referral, behavioral observations, mental status, etc.) that must be included in a professional report. The reader is referred to Sattler (1992), Kaufman (1994), and Kamphaus (1993) for detailed examples of how to present assessment findings.

Reporting IQs

Excerpt from D. W.'s Report

On the WAIS-III, D. W. achieved a Verbal IQ of 104, a Performance IQ of 102, and a Full Scale IQ of 103. The chances that the range of scores from 99 to 107 includes his true IQ are about 95 out of 100. His overall achievement is classified in the average range and ranked at the 58th percentile. Although he was mildly restless and occasionally forgot instructions, he was never markedly distracted, and he attempted the majority of tasks with a good deal of effort. Therefore, these results appear to be a valid and reliable reflection of his current level of cognitive functioning in a medication-free state.

Comment

It is important to provide the sophisticated reader with traditional IQs. D. W. was referred for evaluation by his school district, and there was a clear expectation that such information would be forthcoming. Also, it is recognized that the Verbal and Performance IQs probably do not represent unitary constructs. However, for practical reasons this potential problem is dealt with in another section of the report. The goal of this paragraph is to communicate information concerning D. W.'s general intellectual level. Finally, the results are considered valid and reliable because D. W. was alert, cooperative, and friendly. Moreover, his test-taking motivation was usually adequate; he was able to work for over 90 minutes in order to complete the entire scale; and the three IQs were in line with expectations (i.e., a priori hypotheses 1 and 2) concerning the level and pattern of performance.

Intersubtest Scatter

Excerpt from D. W.'s Report

The distribution of subtest scores was characterized by a high degree of intersubtest scatter,

with scores that ranged from 16 (98th percentile) to 6 (9th percentile). A scatter range of this magnitude (i.e., 16 − 6 = 10) or larger occurred in fewer than 11% of the standardization sample. This finding is somewhat unusual and suggests that the composite IQs, three of the four Indexes, and the relationship between the various scales and Indexes (e.g., Verbal IQ–Performance IQ discrepancy) may not provide accurate descriptions of D. W.'s intellectual strengths and weaknesses. In order to explain the scaled score fluctuations, the 13 WAIS-III subtests have been reorganized into specific categories according to theoretical and practical considerations.

Comment

This paragraph informs the reader that there was considerable scatter across the 13 subtests, and that the Full Scale IQ, traditional Verbal–Performance IQ dichotomy, and Index score discrepancies, if accepted at face value, may lead to erroneous conclusions about the examinee. The base rate data describing the magnitude of scatter were obtained from Table B.5 in the *WAIS-III Administration and Scoring Manual*. This kind of information should help the reader put statements such as "high degree" into a meaningful context and improve communication. Finally, the reader is told that the WAIS-III results will be carefully evaluated, using clinical judgment, common sense, and a working knowledge of psychological theory and research in order to reveal the dynamics of D.W.'s scaled score profile.

Profile Analysis

Excerpt from D. W.'s Report

D. W. demonstrated several meaningful strengths and weaknesses across the 13 WAIS-III subtests. His capacity for concept formation and reasoning appeared well developed, regardless of whether the tasks were exclusively verbal in nature (i.e., oral questions) or involved primarily the manipulation of nonverbal stimuli. He performed within the superior range on a task that reflects knowledge and appreciation of social conventionalities and the ability to supply solutions to hypothetical everyday problems (98th percentile). Above-average achievement emerged on a measure of verbal abstraction (91st percentile), and also on a subtest that requires the reproduction of abstract patterns using colored blocks (95th percentile). A solidly average performance was noted on a task of vocabulary knowledge that required D. W. to orally define a series of words (75th percentile). Another area of strength within the profile was evidenced on tasks that require spatial visualization. His abilities to appreciate complex visual–spatial relationships (95th percentile), to engage in rapid visual scanning and symbol recognition (84th percentile), and to perform nonverbal, visual problem solving (84th percentile) were all above average.

Solidly average achievement (50th percentile) was obtained on a task that requires temporal sequencing and the ability to plan and anticipate within a social context. Thus, when presented with sets of pictures and instructed to put each group in order so it depicts the most sensible story, he quickly and efficiently rearranged the stimuli into logical sequences. He also demonstrated an average fund (37th percentile) of general information about people, places, and events. For example, he knew that Lincoln was president of the United States during the Civil War, that Rome is the capital of Italy, and that the first Olympic games were held in Greece.

D. W. experienced difficulty with subtests that are sensitive to deficits in attention/concentration, short-term auditory memory, auditory sequencing, and/or facility with numbers. When asked to solve a series of mental arithmetic problems, his overall achievement was well below average (9th percentile) and characterized by reduced attentiveness, guessing, carelessness, and a poor mastery of mathematical operations. The low score is consistent with his academic history, while his test-taking behavior suggested that he had a negative "mindset" when it came to mathematics. The very idea of solving arithmetic problems caused his attention to wander and his achievement motivation to drop. His total score on a task of digit repetition was in the low average range (25th percentile). However, this score is misleading, because he repeated in proper order 7 digits forward but only 3 digits backward. This is an unusual finding, because the former score is normal, whereas the latter is deficient. A backward span of 3 or less was obtained by only 3% of 16- to 17-year-old participants in the WAIS-III standardization sample. Also noted were sequencing errors in his forward and backward digit spans. This is a common error for someone with a history of school learning problems. When order of recall was ignored, he actually repeated 8 digits forward and 4 backward. These observations suggest that D. W.'s auditory attention is basically normal when the task requires passive recall (i.e., digits forward) without information processing (i.e., digits backward), but is impaired when the task involves rote memorization plus information processing. Performance on the Letter–Number Sequencing subtest, a measure of auditory attention/concentration, short-term memory, and information processing, was below average (16th percentile) and consistent with the preceding interpretation. The latter task required D. W. to listen to series of random numbers and letters, and then to repeat the numbers in ascending order and the letters in alphabetical order.

On nonverbal subtests that, among other things, measure attention/concentration, memory, and/or facility with numbers, his achievement levels represented a weakness in the overall profile. When asked to identify omitted parts in pictures of common objects and settings, his performance suggested difficulties with visual attention and/or visual memory (16th percentile). Likewise, when asked to rapidly reproduce symbols that were paired with corresponding numbers in a key, his performance was below average (16th percentile). Behavioral observations during this task raised the possibility of poor short-term memory for the associated number–symbol pairs. On two occasions, he associated the same incorrect symbol with the number "four," although he immediately noticed each error and made the necessary correction. He also embellished one symbol by adding an extra line. Because these errors required time to commit, notice, and correct, they reduced the overall time available to complete the subtest.

Comment

This section describes D. W.'s achievement levels and highlights his strong reasoning, concept formation, and spatial visualization abilities. It also documents his deficits on tasks of attention/concentration, facility with numbers, auditory sequencing, and memory. Where appropriate, attempts were made to integrate history, behavioral observations, and the examiner's subjective impressions. Base rate information taken from Table B.6 in the *WAIS-III Administration and Scoring Manual* was utilized to clarify the term "unusual" in describing the relationship between scores on digits forward and digits backward. Although it is usually preferable to stress traditional composite scores when one is interpreting WAIS-III results, this was not possible with D. W., because the IQs and three of the Indexes represented averages of diverse abilities rather than unitary constructs. Also, separate interpretations were provided for the Information and Picture Arrangement subtests, because they were performed in an adequate manner and represented neither an asset nor a deficit.

Overall Conclusions

Excerpt from D. W.'s Report

D. W. performed within the average range of intelligence, as evidenced by a Verbal IQ of 104 (61st percentile), a Performance IQ of 102 (55th percentile), and a Full Scale IQ of 103 (58th percentile). The distribution of subtest scores was characterized by an unusual degree of scatter, suggesting that these summary values do not provide an accurate description of his intellectual strengths and weaknesses. However, regrouping of the 13 subtests according to theoretical and practical considerations yields a clinically meaningful picture of D. W's WAIS-III performance.

D. W. displayed noteworthy strengths on verbal and nonverbal tasks requiring reasoning, concept formation, and spatial visualization. Within this area, his most noteworthy strength was on a task that reflects knowledge and appreciation of social conventionalities. When compared to that of participants ages 16–17 in the WAIS-III standardization sample, his level of achievement was at the 98th percentile. On other measures that assess reasoning ability applied to social situations and fund of general information, his scores were age-appropriate and within the average range.

Important weaknesses emerged on verbal and nonverbal measures that require attention/concentration, short-term memory, auditory sequencing, and/or a facility with numbers. For example, his poorest performance was on a task of mental arithmetic calcula-

tion, since he demonstrated a very limited mastery of the necessary problem-solving concepts (9th percentile) and simultaneously displayed a negative mental set toward the subject of mathematics. Although he earned poor scores on tests of attention/concentration and auditory short-term memory, examination of individual item responses yielded a potentially important observation. Specifically, auditory attention was normal when the task required passive recall, but impaired when the task involved multiple operations (such as rote memorization, sequencing, and information processing).

Comment

These paragraphs summarize the most important results and interpretations gleaned from the WAIS-III. However, in most clinical situations, an examiner would not be forced to base his or her opinions on a single instrument. Instead, the WAIS-III is typically a component of an extensive test battery that taps such important functions as memory, learning, academic achievement, and the examinee's self-perceptions. The WAIS-III supplementary procedures of Digit Symbol–Learning and Digit Symbol–Copy, along with parent and teacher behavior rating scales, would be administered as part of a properly constructed battery. Data from these measures can be integrated with the client's background information and behavioral observations to support, clarify, or refute the hypotheses generated from the WAIS-III. Finally, it should be noted that diagnostic assertions were not contained in the present report. This is because empirical evidence is insufficient, at this moment in time, to justify use of the WAIS-III as a diagnostic indicator of ADHD or to use the instrument to discriminate between various subtypes of the disorder. The WAIS-III should be viewed as an excellent tool for describing an individual's intellectual strengths and weaknesses, not for diagnosing psychiatric or neurological disorders.

REFERENCES

American Psychiatric Association. (1994). *Diagnostic and statistical manual of mental disorders* (4th ed.). Washington, DC: Author.

American Psychological Association. (2002). Ethical principles of psychologists and code of conduct. *American Psychologist, 57,* 1060–1073.

Barrett, G., Chelune, G., Naugle, R., Tulsky, D., & Ledbetter, M. (2000, February). *Test–retest characteristics and measures of meaningful change for the Wechsler Adult Intelligence Scale—III.* Poster presented at the 28th annual conference of the International Neuropsychological Society, Denver, CO.

Fisher, B. C. (1998). *Attention deficit disorder misdiagnosis: Approaching ADD from a brain–behavior/neuropsychological perspective for assessment and treatment.* Boca Raton, FL: CRC Press.

Herlihy, B., & Corey, G. (1996). *ACA ethical standards casebook* (5th ed.). Alexandria, VA: American Counseling Association.

Horn, J. L., & Noll, J. (1997). Human cognitive capabilities: Gf-Gc theory. In D. P. Flanagan, J. L. Genshaft, & P. L. Harrison (Eds.). *Contemporary intellectual assessment: Theory, tests, and issues.* New York: Guilford Press.

Kamphaus, R. W. (1993). *Clinical assessment of children's intelligence.* Boston: Allyn & Bacon.

Kaufman, A. S. (1990). *Assessing adolescent and adult intelligence.* Boston: Allyn & Bacon.

Kaufman, A. S. (1994). *Intelligent testing with the WISC-III.* New York: Wiley.

Kaufman, A. S., & Lichtenberger, E. O. (1999). Intellectual assessment. In A. S. Bellack & M. Hersen (Eds.-in-Chief) & C. R. Reynolds (Ed.), *Comprehensive clinical psychology: Vol. 4. Assessment.* New York: Pergamon Press.

LoBello, S., Thompson, A. P., & Evani, V. (1998). Supplementary WAIS-III tables for determining subtest strengths and weaknesses. *Journal of Psychoeducational Assessment, 16,* 196–200.

Psychological Corporation. (1992). *Wechsler Individual Achievement Test.* San AntonPio, TX: Author.

Psychological Corporation. (1997). *WAIS-III–WMS-III Technical Manual.* San Antonio, TX: Author.

Ryan, J. J., Lopez, S. J., & Werth, T. R. (1998). Administration time estimates for WAIS-III subtests, scales, and short forms in a clinical sample. *Journal of Psychoeducational Assessment, 16,* 315–323.

Ryan, J. J., Sattler, J. M., & Lopez, S. J. (2000). Age effects on Wechsler Adult Intelligence Scale—III subtests. *Archives of Clinical Neuropsychology, 15,* 311–317.

Sattler, J. M. (1992). *Assessment of children: Revised and updated third edition.* San Diego, CA: Author.

Sattler, J. M. (2001). *Assessment of children: Cognitive applications* (4th ed.). San Diego, CA: Author.

Sattler, J. M., & Ryan, J. J. (1999). *Assessment of children: Revised and updated third edition, WAIS-III supplement.* San Diego, CA: Authors.

Spearman, C. E. (1927). *The abilities of man.* New York: Macmillan.

Tulsky, D. S., & Ledbetter, M. F. (2000). Updating to the WAIS-III and WMS-III: Consideration for research and clinical practice. *Psychological Assessment, 12,* 253–262.

Ward, L. C., Ryan, J. J., & Axelrod, B. N. (2000). Confirmatory factor analyses of the WAIS-III standardization data. *Psychological Assessment, 12,* 341–345.

Wechsler, D. (1939). *Wechsler–Bellevue Intelligence Scale.* New York: The Psychological Corporation.

Wechsler, D. (1944). *Measurement of adult intelligence.* Baltimore: Williams & Wilkins.

Wechsler, D. (1955). *WAIS manual.* New York: Psychological Corporation.

Wechsler, D. (1981). *WAIS-R manual.* New York: Psychological Corporation

Wechsler, D. (1991). *WISC-III manual.* San Antonio, TX: Psychological Corporation.

Wechsler, D. (1997a). *WAIS-III administration and scoring manual.* San Antonio, TX: Psychological Corporation.

Wechsler, D. (1997b). *WMS-III administration and scoring manual.* San Antonio, TX: Psychological Corporation.

7

Assessing the Intelligence of Adolescents with the Kaufman Adolescent and Adult Intelligence Test (KAIT)

JAMES C. KAUFMAN
ELIZABETH O. LICHTENBERGER
ALAN S. KAUFMAN

The Kaufman Adolescent and Adult Intelligence Test (KAIT; Kaufman & Kaufman, 1993) was developed with several purposes in mind. The Kaufmans wanted to construct a test battery that was based on intellectual theory and would account for developmental changes in intelligence. In addition, they wanted this test to provide important clinical and neuropsychological information (Lichtenberger, 2001).

THEORETICAL FRAMEWORK

The KAIT is based on an integration of three cognitive and neuropsychological theories: (1) Horn and Cattell's (1966, 1967) theory of fluid (Gf) and crystallized (Gc) intelligence; (2) Luria's (1966, 1980) definition of planning ability; and (3) the formal-operational stage of development according to Piaget's (1972) theory. Each of these theories is explored in greater detail.

The Horn–Cattell theory is the foundation for organizing and interpreting the KAIT subtests. The theory used in the KAIT is the original formulation of the fluid–crystallized distinction, referred to as the Gf-Gc theory (Horn & Cattell, 1966). Fluid ability measures adaptability and flexibility when one is solving novel problems, using both verbal and nonverbal stimuli to do so; crystallized ability measures acquired concepts, knowledge, and problem-solving ability when one is using stimuli that are dependent on schooling, acculturation, and verbal-conceptual development for success. Horn's expanded model (Horn & Hofer, 1992; Horn & Noll, 1997), although still referred to as Gf-Gc theory, divided cognitive abilities into nine separate abilities instead of two. The KAIT scales were designed to measure the broader, more general versions of Gf and Gc as originally conceptualized by Cattell and Horn.

The Kaufmans made the decision to focus on the original model instead of the expanded model, because of the belief that assessing these two broader abilities would enhance the value of the KAIT as a clinical measure of adolescent and adult problem-solving ability. Measuring each of nine abilities, they argued, would decrease the practical utility of the test by making the tasks less relevant to problems encountered in real life (Kaufman & Kaufman, 1997). In addition, they adhered to David Wechsler's deep-seated belief that the best way to develop a clinically rich instrument is to offer complex measurement of a few broad constructs rather than many narrow constructs (Kaufman, 2000).

Although not as central in defining KAIT as the Horn–Cattell theory, both Luria's (1980) definition of planning ability and Piaget's (1972) stage of formal operations also helped to guide the development of the test. Luria (1973) described the basic building blocks of intelligence as being cognitive processes that enable people to perform certain distinctive tasks. Planning ability is one of these central blocks. Planning is associated with certain developmental changes in the brain that emerge at the age of 11 or 12. Similarly, Piaget's formal-operational stage begins to emerge at about the same age. Both Luria's conception of planning ability and Piaget's concept of formal operations are centered around similar ideas, such as decision making and evaluating hypotheses. Therefore, to reflect the very important changes that are crucial to adult development and take place in the brain at this age, Kaufman and Kaufman (1993) decided that their adolescent and adult test should assess intelligence in individuals beginning at age 11, since this is a theoretically meaningful age distinction. Because the Kaufmans used the Piaget and Luria theories as "entry-level" requirements for a task's inclusion in the KAIT, this further insured that the KAIT would meet its goal of measuring broad, complex constructs. Even the Crystallized subtests deliberately measure some reasoning ability, in order to be advanced enough to measure formal operations and planning ability (Kaufman, 2000).

ORGANIZATION OF THE KAIT

The KAIT is a standardized measure of old (Crystallized) and new (Fluid) learning for individuals ages 11–85+. The combination of these two types of abilities (Composite) may be considered general intelligence. It provides three global IQ scores: Fluid, Crystallized, and Composite. Each of these is a standard score with a mean of 100 and a standard deviation of 15.

As shown in Table 7.1, the KAIT is organized into a Core Battery and an Extended

TABLE 7.1. Outline of KAIT Subtests

Core Battery

Crystallized subtests: Definitions, Auditory Comprehension, Double Meanings
Fluid subtests: Rebus Learning, Logical Steps, Mystery Codes

Expanded Battery

Crystallized subtests: As above, plus Auditory Delayed Recall, Famous Faces
Fluid subtests: As above, plus Rebus Delayed Recall, Memory for Block Design

Supplemental Subtest

Mental Status

Battery. The Core Battery comprises two scales, Crystallized and Fluid, which contain three subtests each. The three Crystallized subtests are Definitions, Auditory Comprehension, and Double Meanings. In Definitions, examinees identify a word by studying the word shown with some of its letters missing, and hearing or reading a clue about its meaning. In Auditory Comprehension, examinees listen to a recording of a news story and then answer literal and inferential questions about the story. In Double Meanings, examinees study two sets of word clues and then must think of a word with two meanings that relates closely to both sets of clues.

The three Fluid subtests in the Core Battery are Rebus Learning, Logical Steps, and Mystery Codes. In Rebus Learning, examinees learn words or concepts associated with a particular rebus (drawing), and then "read" phrases and sentences composed of these rebuses. In Logical Steps, examinees are presented with logical premises both visually and aurally, and then respond to questions by making use of these logical premises. In Mystery Codes, examinees study clues associated with a set of pictorial stimuli, and then decipher the code for a novel pictorial stimulus.

The Extended Battery comprises 10 subtests. It includes the six Fluid and Crystallized scales mentioned above, plus two additional Crystallized subtests (Auditory Delayed Recall and Famous Faces) and two Fluid subtests (Rebus Delayed Recall and Memory for Block Design). In Auditory Delayed Recall, examinees answer literal and inferential questions about the news stories that were heard approximately 25 minutes earlier during the Auditory Comprehension subtest. In Famous Faces, examinees name people of current or historical fame, based on their photographs and a verbal clue about them. In Rebus Delayed Recall, examinees "read" phrases and sentences composed of the rebuses they learned about 45 minutes earlier during the Rebus Learning subtest. In Memory for Block Design, examinees study a printed abstract design that is exposed briefly; they then reconstruct the design from memory, using six yellow and black wooden blocks and a tray. The delayed-recall subtests allow for a comparison of performance on immediate- and delayed-recall tasks. Furthermore, the inclusion of the delayed-recall tasks—which are administered without prior warning about 25 and 45 minutes after the administration of the original subtests—expands the Horn (1989) abilities measured by the KAIT whenever the Expanded Battery is given.

In addition to the broad Gf and Gc abilities measured by the IQ scales, the delayed-recall subtests offer reasonably pure measurement of an ability that Horn (1985, 1989) calls "long-term storage and retrieval." This long-term memory ability, labeled *Glr* in the Woodcock–Johnson—Revised (WJ-R) and Woodcock–Johnson—Third Edition (WJ-III), taps into the ability to store information and then retrieve it as needed (Woodcock, 1990, p. 234). The KAIT also includes a supplemental Mental Status exam, in which examinees answer simple questions which assess attention and orientation to the world. This Mental Status subtest is a standardized, normed test that is utilized for people with neurological impairment. Although it is not included in the composite scores with the other KAIT subtests, it may provide important neuropsychological information.

PSYCHOMETRIC PROPERTIES

Standardization

The KAIT's standardization sample was composed of 2,000 adolescents and adults, selected according to 1988 U.S. Census data. The sample was stratified on the variables of gender, race/ethnic group, geographic region, and socioeconomic status (educational attainment). This large sample was divided into 14 age groups between 11 and 85+, with 100–250 participants in each age group. The matches for geographic region were close for the North Central and South regions, but the sample was underrepresented in the Northeast and overrepresented in the West (Kaufman & Kaufman, 1993).

Types of Scores

The KAIT yields several types of scores, including raw scores, scaled scores, and IQs. Raw scores are not norm-referenced, and are therefore not interpretable. Thus it is necessary to transform the raw scores into some kind of standard scores (in this case, either scaled scores or IQs). Scaled scores are the standard scores for each subtest; they have a mean of 10 and a standard deviation of 3. IQs are obtained by adding the scaled scores and transforming them into a standard score for each IQ scale (Fluid, Crystallized, Composite). The IQs have a mean of 100 and a standard deviation of 15 (Lichtenberger, Broadbooks, & Kaufman, 2000).

Reliability

The KAIT has strong reliability. The standardization data showed that mean split-half reliability coefficients for the Crystallized, Fluid, and Composite IQs were .95, .95, and .97, respectively. For the 10 individual subtests, the mean split-half reliability coefficients ranged from .71 on Auditory Delayed Recall to .93 on Rebus Learning (median = .90). Mean test–retest reliability coefficients, based on 153 individuals identified as "normal" in three age groups (11–19, 20–54, and 55–85+) who were retested after a 1-month interval, were .94 for Crystallized IQ, .87 for Fluid IQ, and .94 for Composite IQ. Mean test–retest reliability values for each of the 10 individual subtests ranged from .63 on Auditory Delayed Recall to .95 on Definitions (median = .78). An additional study of 120 European Americans found slightly lower test–retest reliabilities (in the .80s), but concluded that the KAIT was a reliable measure (Pinion, 1995).

Construct Validity

The construct validity of the Crystallized and Fluid scales was supported by exploratory and confirmatory factor analysis. Two-factor solutions were identified for the total standardization sample, as well as for separate groups of European Americans, African Americans, and Hispanics, and males and females (Gonzalez, Adir, Kaufman, & McLean, 1995; A. S. Kaufman, McLean, & Kaufman, 1995). In addition, Caruso and Jacob-Timm (2001) conducted confirmatory factor analysis using a normative sample of 375 adolescents ages 11–14 years and a cross-validation sample of 60 sixth and eighth graders. They tested three factor models: a single-factor model of general intelligence (g), an orthogonal Gf-Gc model, and an oblique Gf-Gc model. The orthogonal model fit both samples poorly, while the g model only fit the cross-validation sample. The oblique model, however, fit both samples (and fit significantly better than the g model in both samples).

The KAIT manual (Kaufman & Kaufman, 1993) provides strong evidence for the construct validity of the scale, using the entire standardization sample. However, because people from different ethnic groups often perform differently on tests of intelligence, it is important to extend the construct validity of the KAIT to examine the differential construct validity for separate ethnic groups. Here we discuss the KAIT's construct validity in samples of European Americans, African Americans, and Hispanics (A. S. Kaufman, Kaufman, & McLean, 1995).

The construct validity of the overall KAIT standardization sample is evident from the results of factor analysis, which identified clear-cut crystallized (Gc) and fluid (Gf) factors across the entire KAIT age range. The individual KAIT Crystallized and Fluid subtests load most strongly on the Crystallized and Fluid factors, respectively. A. S. Kaufman, Kaufman, and McLean (1995) analyzed a sample of 1,535 European Americans, 226 African Americans, and 140 Hispanics to determine whether the validity of the Gc and Gf constructs would hold for the groups separately. Consistent results were found across analyses when different types of factor-analytic rotational procedures were used. For each of the three ethnic group samples, all KAIT Crystallized subtests loaded primarily on the Gc factor, and all KAIT Fluid subtests loaded primarily on the Gf factor. With both the varimax and promax rotations, there were secondary loadings for some subtests in the different ethnic groups. Specifically, in the varimax rotation, the Double Meanings subtest was weighted .60 on Gc and .53 on Gf for African Americans. For Hispanics, Rebus Learning had about equal loadings on both factors (.53 on Gf and .42 on Gc). However, the promax rotation gave more decisive splits for the subtests on each of the factors. Considerable congruence between the pairs of factors indicated that the empirically defined dimensions were quite similar for all three subject groups. Thus the results of this study support the construct validity of the KAIT for separate groups of European Americans, African Americans, and Hispanics.

The construct validity of the KAIT was further demonstrated through concurrent validity—its correlations with other measures of adolescent and adult intelligence (Kaufman & Kaufman, 1993). In four samples of participants (ages 16–19, 20–34, 35–49, and 50–83), the Composite IQ of the KAIT correlated from .83 to .88 with the Full Scale IQ of the Wechsler Adult Intelligence Scale—Revised (WAIS-R; Wechsler, 1981). In a sample of 79 adolescents and adults, the KAIT Composite IQ was found to correlate .87 with the Stanford–Binet Intelligence Scale: Fourth Edition (Thorndike, Hagen, & Sattler, 1986). In a sample of 124 normal 11- to 12-year-olds, the KAIT composite was found to correlate .66 with the Kaufman Assessment Battery for Children (K-ABC) Mental Processing Composite, but showed a stronger correlation ($r = .82$) with the K-ABC Achievement scale (Kaufman & Kaufman, 1993). In a sample of 30 sixth graders and 30 eighth graders (Vo, Weisenberger, Becker, & Jacob-Timm, 1999), the KAIT Composite IQ and Crystallized IQ correlated strongly with the Full Scale IQ and Verbal IQ, respectively, on the Wechsler Intelligence Scale for Children—Third Edition (WISC-III; Wechsler,

1991). In this same sample, the KAIT Fluid IQ had a moderately strong correlation with the Performance IQ on the WISC-III. In a sample of 50 preadolescents and adolescents, 33 with scholastic concerns and 17 with central nervous system disorders, the KAIT showed acceptable concurrent validity with the WISC-III (Woodrich & Kush, 1998).

DEVELOPMENTAL TRENDS ON THE KAIT

Crystallized abilities have been noted to be fairly well maintained throughout the lifespan, but fluid abilities are not as stable, peaking in adolescence or early adulthood before dropping steadily through the lifespan (Horn, 1989; Kaufman & Lichtenberger, 1999, 2002). To analyze age trends in the KAIT standardization data, a separate set of "all-adult" norms was developed to provide the means with which to compare performance on the KAIT subtests and IQ scales (Kaufman & Kaufman, 1993). Data from 1,500 individuals between ages 17 and 85+ were merged to create the all-adult norms. The IQs from this new all-adult normative group were also adjusted for years of education, so that this would not be a confounding variable in analyses.

Analyses of the Crystallized and Fluid scales across ages 17 to 85+ produced results that generally conformed to those reported in previous investigations. Crystallized abilities generally increase through age 50, but do not drop noticeably until age 75 and older. The fluid abilities, on the other hand, do appear to peak in the early 20s, then plateau from the mid–20s through the mid–50s, and finally begin to drop steadily after age 55. These findings were consistent for males and females (Kaufman & Horn, 1996). Kaufman and Kaufman (1997) hypothesize that the fluid aspects of some of the KAIT Crystallized subtests may have contributed to the accelerated age-related decline in scores on these subtests.

GENDER AND ETHNICITY DIFFERENCES

Gender Differences

Gender differences on Crystallized and Fluid IQ for ages 17–94 on the KAIT were examined for 716 males and 784 females. When the data were adjusted for educational attainment, less than 1 IQ point separated males and females for both IQ scores. Males averaged 100.4 on Fluid IQ and 99.8 on Crystallized IQ, while females averaged 99.6 on Fluid IQ and 100.1 on Crystallized IQ (J. C. Kaufman, Chen, & Kaufman, 1995; Kaufman & Horn, 1996; Kaufman & Lichtenberger, 2002, Table 4.1). However, several KAIT subtests did produce gender differences that were large enough to be meaningful: Memory for Block Design, Famous Faces, and Logical Steps. On each of these subtests, males scored higher than females by about 0.2 to 0.4 standard deviation (SD). These results of specific subtests do not contradict the lack of differences on the global Fluid and Crystallized IQs; two of the three subtests that favored males are on the Extended Battery, but not the Core Battery, and do not contribute to the KAIT IQs.

The results of gender differences on the KAIT (as on the Wechsler scales) are of limited generalizability regarding a theoretical understanding of male versus female intellectual functions. The results are contaminated because test developers have avoided or minimized gender bias whenever possible when selecting tasks and items. Thus the lack of meaningful gender differences in global IQs is undoubtedly an artifact of the specific subtests included in the KAIT and Wechsler scales; to some extent, differences in subtest scores (such as the KAIT Famous Faces subtest and the similar Information subtest on the WISC-III and WAIS-III) may be an artifact of the specific items chosen for each subtest. However, it is possible to reach some hypotheses about "true" male–female differences on some of the subtests (Kaufman, McLean, & Reynolds, 1988). It is hard to imagine how any items on the KAIT Memory for Block Design subtest (or the related Wechsler Block Design subtest, which also consistently produces differences favoring males over females) could have been eliminated due to gender bias (or any other kind of bias) because of the abstract, nonmeaningful nature of the stimuli.

Consequently, it seems reasonable to conclude that adolescent and adult males are superior to adolescent and adult females in the skills assessed by the Wechsler Block Design subtest and the KAIT Memory for Block Design subtest. In contrast, females outstrip males on clerical and psychomotor tasks, such as the Wechsler Coding and Digit Symbol subtests; these results with individually administered, clinical instruments are quite consistent with the bulk of the cognitive literature on gender differences (Kaufman & Lichtenberger, 2002, Ch. 4). However, even the Wechsler and KAIT subtests that yielded the largest gender differences produced differences of about 0.40 to 0.50 *SD*, which reflect small (or at best moderate) effect sizes (McLean, 1995)—discrepancies that are too small to be of very much clinical value.

Ethnicity Differences

Differences between European Americans and African Americans on the KAIT were examined in a sample of 1,547 European Americans (575 ages 11–24 years and 972 ages 25–94 years) and 241 African Americans (117 ages 11–24 years and 124 ages 25–94 years). Without educational adjustment, European Americans scored approximately 11–12 IQ points higher than African Americans in the 11–24 age group. At ages 25–94 years, European Americans scored approximately 13–14 IQ points higher than African Americans (J. C. Kaufman et al., 1995). Once adjustments for educational attainment were made, these differences were reduced to approximately 8–9 points for ages 11–24 and approximately 10 points for ages 25–94 (A. S. Kaufman, McLean, & Kaufman, 1995). A multivariate analysis with educational attainment covaried found that the only significant difference between these two groups with increasing age was a reduced difference in the Famous Faces (Crystallized) subtest (J. C. Kaufman, McLean, Kaufman, & Kaufman, 1994). In comparison, European Americans outscored African Americans on the four WAIS-III Indexes by between 12 and 15 points (Manly, Heaton, & Taylor, 2000).

Without educational adjustment, European Americans scored approximately 12–13 points higher on Crystallized IQ than Hispanics ages 11–24 years, and approximately 9 points higher on Fluid IQ. At ages 25–94 years, European Americans scored approximately 17 points higher than Hispanics on Crystallized IQ, and approximately 10 points higher on Fluid IQ (J. C. Kaufman et al., 1995). When adjustments were made for educational attainment, these differences were reduced to approximately 6 points for ages 11–24 and approximately 9 points for ages 25–94 (J. C. Kaufman et al., 1995).

It is worth noting that Hispanics scored about 4 points higher on Fluid IQ than Crystallized IQ at ages 11–24 and almost 6 points higher at ages 25–94, without an adjustment for education (A. S. Kaufman, Kaufman, & McLean, 1995). These differences resemble the magnitude of Performance > Verbal differences on the WISC-III and WAIS-III, although Fluid IQ is not the same as Performance IQ; they load on separate factors (A. S. Kaufman, Ishikuma, & Kaufman, 1994), and the Fluid subtests require verbal ability for success (Kaufman & Lichtenberger, 2002).

ASSESSING INDIVIDUALS WITH SPECIAL NEEDS

Individuals who are referred for evaluation may have special needs that must be addressed during the testing. For example, examinees may be bilingual, or they may have language or hearing impairment, learning disabilities, or dementia. Many KAIT subtests are sensitive to these needs. For instance, much verbal expression is required on only one Core Battery subtest (Rebus Learning), allowing for smoother assessment of individuals with expressive language problems. To help bilingual individuals, responses may be given in a foreign language or sign language (except on the Definitions subtest), and on teaching items, the examiner may use a foreign language or sign language to help teach the task if necessary.

Although the KAIT inherently facilitates its own use when working with individuals with special needs, sometimes it will be necessary to modify standardized procedures to accommodate an individual. Some ways in which one may change standardized procedures include the following: omitting or substituting certain subtests (e.g., omitting Definitions for someone with a spelling disability; omitting Auditory Comprehension or Logical Steps for someone with moderate to severe impairment in hearing or receptive language); extending the test session over more than one session; and removing time limits for individuals with moderate to severe motor impairments. However, when any standardized procedures are changed, it is always important to note the modifications made. Also, once standardized procedures have not been followed, the norms for the test may not be appropriate. Clinical judgment should be exercised in determining whether norms are appropriate to use if modifications are made in the standardized procedures.

There has been some research on learning disabilities and the KAIT. Kaufman and Kaufman (1993) reported that in a small sample of 14 adolescents with reading disabilities, there were no differences between this sample and matched controls. However, they did report that one trend was evident: The Fluid scale scores were significantly higher than those on the Crystallized scale. Another study examined 21 remedial undergraduate students, 35 average students, and 10 honors students, and found that the KAIT discriminated between the honors students and the other two groups (Shaughnessy & Moore, 1994).

In a study examining the performance of 30 college students with learning disabilities to 30 students without learning disabilities on the KAIT and WAIS-R, interesting nonsignificant differences were found (Morgan, Sullivan, Darden, & Gregg, 1997). The participants with learning disabilities had been previously diagnosed. Morgan and colleagues found that there were no differences between the two groups on the following: WAIS-R Full Scale IQ, Verbal IQ, and Performance IQ, and KAIT Composite, Crystallized, and Fluid scales. However, when the scales of the KAIT were compared to the scales of the WAIS-R, one significant difference was found: In both the groups (those with and those without learning disabilities), the WAIS-R Performance IQ was significantly higher than the KAIT Fluid IQ. Possible explanations for the differences between these two scales include the following: (1) The KAIT has newer norms, and (2) the Fluid subtests are more novel than the Performance subtests (Morgan et al., 1997).

Because these results demonstrate that the KAIT offers results comparable to those obtained with the WAIS-R, the new format of the KAIT, which has less emphasis on expressive language, appears to be a valuable addition to the assessment battery for learning disabilities.

STRENGTHS AND A WEAKNESS OF THE KAIT

The KAIT has currently been in use for a decade, and there have been several published reviews since the test became available for use in 1993. In addition, we have used the KAIT in clinical evaluations, research, and teaching, and have supervised graduate students in administration, scoring, and interpretation of the instrument. Thus the following overview of the advantages and one disadvantage of the KAIT is based both on these published reviews (Brown, 1994; Dumont & Hagberg, 1994; Flanagan, Alfonso, & Flanagan, 1994) and on our own experience with the test. The strengths and the one weakness are grouped into the following categories: test development; administration and scoring; standardization; validity and reliability; and interpretation.

The KAIT has some significant strengths that we have noted, although there are no weaknesses that we consider major. The strengths we want to emphasize include the following: the test's development from current cognitive and neuropsychological theory; the ease of administration and scoring for examiners; the excellent psychometric properties and standardization sample; the test's outstanding use with gifted and college-educated examinees, and the neuropsychological data that can be gained from the Expanded Battery. Although we did not find any significant weaknesses in the KAIT, it is always important to keep in mind that no test, the KAIT included, measures all cognitive abilities. Thus supplemental data (e.g., behavioral observations, additional test scores) should always be used in conjunction with scores from intelligence tests to confirm hypotheses about an individual's abilities. One weakness specific to the KAIT is that, due to inadequate floors for certain age levels and the difficulty of the test for persons who have not reached the formal-operational stage of development, the KAIT is probably not the best instrument to be used for individuals with very low functioning.

ILLUSTRATIVE CASE REPORT

Here is an illustrative case report for a young woman with reading difficulties who was considering applying to medical school.

Name: Aviva Katz
Date of evaluation: 08/08/01
Chronological age: 22 years, 1 month
Date of birth: 07/08/79

REFERRAL AND BACKGROUND INFORMATION

Ms. Katz was referred for evaluation by the Counseling Center at XYZ University. Ms. Katz graduated from the university 4 months ago and is currently thinking of applying to medical school. She stated that she has had some difficulty with her schoolwork in the past, and she would like to know what her intellectual and achievement abilities are before she applies to medical school. More specifically, Ms. Katz reported that reading has always been a problem for her and that she has difficulty comprehending what she reads. She also stated that she has difficulty concentrating, is easily distracted, and takes a long time on tests. These reported difficulties are troubling to Ms. Katz, and she would like to know what her strengths and weaknesses are and whether she has a learning disability.

Ms. Katz was originally from the Midwest and moved to the West Coast when she was 18 to attend the university. Her immediate family still lives in the Midwest, and she does not have any relatives on the West Coast. However, Ms. Katz reported that she has a lot of friends from school and that she enjoys living here. She currently lives alone and works full-time as a research associate in a biology lab. She has worked there for $2\frac{1}{2}$ years; she stated that she really likes her job, and that her boss says she works hard and does a good job. Ms. Katz would like to continue working in research until she attends medical school.

Ms. Katz's parents were divorced when she was quite young. Her father received custody of her and her sister, and they both lived with him and his second wife until they went away to college. Ms. Katz reported that although her mother did not raise her, she has maintained contact with her; she continues to see her on occasion, and speaks to her on the phone fairly regularly. Ms. Katz is the younger of two children. Her sister, Allison, is 28 years old and currently teaches high school Spanish. Ms. Katz said that she and her sister are not very close, and their stepmother confirmed this when interviewed.

Both Ms. Katz and her stepmother reported that Allison had been tested for a learning disability when she was a freshman in college, and that "some type of learning problem was found." Neither of them recalled what the exact problem was, but they both said that as a result of the testing, Allison was allotted more time on certain types of exams.

Ms. Katz reported that her mother had an uneventful pregnancy and delivery with her. Overall, Ms. Katz's developmental and medical history are unremarkable. She reached all of the developmental milestones within a normal time frame and has not had any major illnesses. Ms. Katz did report that as a young child, she had her tonsils out and tubes placed in her ears. She also stated that she had her hearing tested in junior high, and that the results suggested she had a minor hearing impairment. This was not followed up with at the time; however, Ms. Katz was referred for a hearing evaluation as part of the present assessment.

Both Ms. Katz and her stepmother reported that Ms. Katz did well in elementary school and junior high school, but that she had some difficulty in high school. She has always done well in math, science, and activities involving memory, but she never enjoyed reading and writing. Ms. Katz received good grades until her sophomore year in high school, when her grades began to fall. Her father and stepmother reported that she was too focused on her social life and was not putting enough into her schoolwork. As a result, they moved her in the middle of the year to a private school that was more structured and emphasized academics. Although initially angry, upset, and fairly oppositional, Ms. Katz eventually adjusted to her new school and was able to improve her grades in just a few months.

Ms. Katz reported having some of the same

academic difficulties in college. She said that she had difficulty with reading, and that she did well in her science lab courses but not as well in the lecture portion of the class. An interview with one of Ms. Katz's professors, Dr. Cooper, supported this information. Dr. Cooper taught Advanced Chemistry, which he described as a "very difficult course that few students earn A's in." He recalled that most of the students received a C in the course, as did Ms. Katz. Dr. Cooper also reported that Ms. Katz received a B in the lab section that went with the course. Dr. Cooper described the lab course as "difficult and complicated." In the lab, students were responsible for performing technically difficult experiments; Dr. Cooper noted that "Ms. Katz did a good job, worked well with her lab partner, and got things done." On the written exams in class, Ms. Katz's performance was mixed. She did poorly on the first exam, but obtained average grades on the next two exams. The exams primarily required essay and short-answer responses, and Dr. Cooper felt that Ms. Katz did not express her knowledge well on the exams. When he talked to her, it was clear that she understood what she was doing and why, but she did not reveal this on the exams. Dr. Cooper contrasted Ms. Katz's clear understanding and comprehension with those of other students in the class. He said that many of the students did not "grasp" what they were doing in lab and lecture, and that they did not understand the theory behind the tasks, but that Ms. Katz did.

APPEARANCE AND BEHAVIORAL CHARACTERISTICS

Ms. Katz is an attractive young woman with a fair complexion and long black hair. She was neatly groomed and dressed casually. Ms. Katz appeared to be eager to participate in the testing and put forth much effort. Initially she was rather shy, but she was both friendly and cooperative. Ms. Katz made a moderate amount of eye contact and generally spoke in a very quiet voice. She stated that she was nervous about being tested, and that she did not really like categorizing her intelligence abilities into a "number," but that she understood the importance of the testing and knew that it would help answer her questions.

Ms. Katz approached all of the tasks on the subtests in a serious manner. She did not give up easily and persevered even when tasks were difficult for her. In fact, Ms. Katz sometimes had to be told it was "OK" to give up on a task when it was clear to the examiner that she could not do the problem. Ms. Katz's problem-solving style was cautious and extremely slow, especially on tasks that required her to calculate problems on paper rather than in her head. On average, she took more time to solve problems than most people do. Even though she was slow, she did not seem to be frustrated with herself or the task; in fact, she was quite patient.

As the testing progressed, Ms. Katz appeared to feel more comfortable with the examiner. She became more verbal, friendly, and relaxed; however, her approach to the subtests did not change. Ms. Katz continued to work hard, and she seemed to feel a little more confident. In the beginning of testing, she had difficulty saying that she did not know an answer or that she wanted to move on, but as time passed she appeared to feel more comfortable communicating her needs. Overall, Ms. Katz pushed herself and was embarrassed and/or hard on herself when she did not know an answer. Feedback from the examiner and verbal encouragement seemed to put her at ease. In general, Ms. Katz's motivation and drive were notable throughout the testing.

TESTS ADMINISTERED

Kaufman Adolescent and Adult Intelligence Test (KAIT)
Woodcock–Johnson—Revised (WJ-R) Tests of Achievement
Woodcock–Johnson—Revised (WJ-R) Tests of Cognitive Abilities, selected subtests
Kaufman Brief Intelligence Test (K-BIT), Matrices subtest

TEST RESULTS AND INTERPRETATION

Ms. Katz was administered the KAIT, which measures two types of problem solving: the ability to be adaptable and flexible when faced with novel problems (fluid intelligence), and the ability to call upon school learning and acculturation experiences to answer school-related problems (crystallized intelligence). Ms. Katz's KAIT Composite IQ of 105 ± 5 (a combination of fluid and crystallized abilities) classifies her intelligence as average and, over- all, ranks her at the 63rd percentile compared to other young adults. Ms. Katz earned a sig- nificantly higher KAIT Fluid IQ (111 ± 6; 77th percentile, high average) than Crystallized 1Q (99 ± 6; 47th percentile, average), indicating that she performs better when solving novel problems than when answering questions that are dependent on schooling and acculturation. The difference of 12 points in favor of her flu- id abilities, though statistically significant, is not unusually large; that is, many people Ms. Katz's age display discrepancies of that magni- tude. However, the gap between her fluid and crystallized intelligence is probably larger than the scores would indicate. She performed well (84th percentile) on a supplementary test of fluid ability (copying abstract block designs from memory), and poorly (25th percentile) on a supplementary test of crystallized ability (identifying pictures of famous people). Nei- ther of these scores is included in the IQ com- putations.

Also, Ms. Katz had a significant weakness relative to her high average level of fluid intel- ligence (50th percentile) on a KAIT Fluid sub- test that measures logical thinking and de- pends heavily on verbal comprehension. Her relatively low score may have resulted primar- ily from an auditory processing deficit. This possibility, which was suspected from interac- tions with Ms. Katz, was investigated by ad- ministering the two-subtest Auditory Process- ing scale of the WJ-R Tests of Cognitive Ability. She scored in the average range on both subtests, earning an overall standard score of 102 ±10 (55th percentile). Those test results reveal intact auditory processing abili- ty, although other possible explanations for her relatively low score on the fluid subtest, such as subtle hearing loss, need to be further investigated. (The evaluation from University Medical Clinic, conducted during the course of this assessment, is not interpretable without a written report.)

Because of the uncertainty about Ms. Katz's true level of fluid intelligence, additional, var- ied measures of novel problem-solving ability were administered to her. She scored at the 79th percentile on the K-BIT Matrices task, a measure of reasoning with abstract stimuli, and she performed phenomenally well on two subtests from the WJ-R Tests of Cognitive Ability: a test requiring her to learn words

paired with abstract symbols (99.9th per- centile), and a measure of her conceptual de- velopment (99th percentile).

Overall, Ms. Katz's performance on fluid tasks converged at a high average to superior level of functioning. She performed at a com- parable level on KAIT subtests that assess de- layed recall of information learned about 30–45 minutes previously. She surpassed 91% of young adults on two tasks: one that re- quired her to recall the verbal concepts associ- ated with abstract symbols, and another that assessed her ability to retrieve from long-term storage information from mock news stories that were presented by cassette. Her outstand- ing long-term memory for material taught re- cently indicates a good ability to understand and remember information that is taught in a classroom. Her strong fluid ability reveals ex- treme capability for excelling in solving new problems, and especially for being adaptable and flexible when exposed to new material. Both of these assets predict success in medical school.

These areas of strength are in contrast to her low average ability to respond quickly within the visual–motor modality (WJ-R Pro- cessing Speed standard score of 89 ± 6) and to her average crystallized abilities. Furthermore, she has a weak fund of information (31st per- centile, on the average), as demonstrated on two KAIT subtests: the Famous Faces task (a test of general factual knowledge) and a differ- ent task assessing word knowledge. This area of weakness is fairly pervasive, as evidenced by her performance on the WJ-R Tests of Achievement Knowledge cluster (standard score of 98 ± 6, surpassing 46% of young adults). Consistent with her college major in chemistry, her current success at her job as a research associate at a chemistry laboratory, and her interest in pursuing a career in medi- cine is the fact that she performed better on science items (60th percentile) than on items pertaining to social studies (47th percentile) or humanities (34th percentile).

Ms. Katz's achievement in the area of ex- pressing her ideas in writing is outstanding (99.6th percentile), although she has difficulty when she is required to write down her ideas as rapidly as possible (23rd percentile). The latter problem is consistent with the relative weakness she demonstrated on the WJ-R visu- al–motor processing tasks, indicating that her cognitive deficit translates directly into the academic arena. Notably, Ms. Katz performed well on a highly speeded test of fluid ability on the KAIT (84th percentile in figuring out codes), indicating that her deficit pertains to speed of *motor* processing, not speed of *mental* processing. She is aware of her general deficit in response speed, and commented several times about how long it takes her to complete tasks and express her ideas. Her concern about not being able to express her ideas appropriately seems unfounded, however. Her level of performance on the test of written comprehension (which is untimed and does not penalize spelling or other mechanical errors) was truly exceptional. Ms. Katz's difficulty seems to be expressing her ideas under extreme time pressure, particularly in writing.

Like her writing abilities, Ms. Katz's reading skills varied considerably, ranging from the 43rd percentile on a test of passage comprehension to the 99th percentile on a test of word decoding. The latter test requires a person to use knowledge of phonetics to sound out nonsense words (a novel task that relates to her excellent fluid ability); she evidently has the ability to apply her strengths to classroom tasks. Overall, she demonstrated better basic reading decoding skills (95th percentile) than reading comprehension abilities (48th percentile). These findings are consistent with her stepmother's description of Ms. Katz as having reading problems as a child and young adolescent—specifically, reading slowly, in word-by-word fashion. Ms. Katz's math abilities revealed the same pattern she showed in reading: better performance on basic computational and quantitative skills (91st percentile) than on the application of those concepts to the solving of applied math problems (58th percentile). Note that even her areas of relative academic weaknesses are comfortably within the average range when compared to the school-related skills of other young adults about Ms. Katz's age.

DIAGNOSTIC IMPRESSIONS

Because Ms. Katz does not have discrepancies between her ability and achievement, she cannot be considered to have a "learning disability" in the conventional sense. She does have a clear-cut deficit in visual–motor processing speed—a deficiency that translates directly to

classroom performance when she must express her ideas rapidly in written format. Her limited visual–motor processing capacities are likely to impair her ability to express her knowledge base under certain circumstances, making it more difficult for her to perform well in graduate school courses that assess knowledge by highly speeded exams. On the other hand, Ms. Katz demonstrates excellent skills in delayed recall of information and fluid thinking, and is outstanding at communicating her ideas in writing, all of which portend well for her success in medical school.

Ms. Katz is a dedicated student who takes her schoolwork seriously. She gave full effort during the extensive testing sessions at our clinic; she also indicated clearly that she wants to understand her assets and deficits, and learn how to take an active role in overcoming her limitations. Any accommodations that a medical school can make to enhance her performance in classwork and allow her to demonstrate her knowledge by a wider variety of measurement techniques that do not stress speeded responses will be efforts well spent and much appreciated by Ms. Katz. It is the conclusion of the staff of this clinic that Ms. Katz is a good medical school risk, aided to a great deal by her motivation and willingness to work hard and take responsibility for her own successes or failures.

RECOMMENDATIONS

The following recommendations and accommodations should facilitate Ms. Katz's comprehension and further enhance her learning.

1. Ms. Katz is average in her ability to understand what she has reads. Her reflective and slow cognitive style and difficulties with reading (e.g., not enjoying it) have affected her acquisition of general factual information, including vocabulary. When compared to other medical students in this respect, Ms. Katz will be below average. Therefore, Ms. Katz should plan to allot a considerable amount of extra time for both reading and writing assignments.

2. Ms. Katz would benefit from developing an individualized learning/studying approach in order to enhance her ability to learn. For example, she should take notes on all material that she studies, organizing the facts in a mean-

ingful and understandable manner. Ms. Katz should review these notes while studying and before taking an exam.

3. Also, rather than just reading and rereading pages in a text or pages of notes, Ms. Katz should make up tests for herself and then write out the answers to these test.

4. An appointment for a thorough hearing evaluation by an audiologist should be made. The hearing test that was conducted at the time of this assessment does not provide enough information for us to definitively rule out a hearing impairment. There appears to be more than enough information in Ms. Katz's history to warrant pursuing such an evaluation. As a young child, Ms. Katz had a number of earaches and eventually had to have tubes placed in her ears. Ms. Katz also reported that in junior high school she had a hearing screening that suggested the presence of a hearing deficit. Ms. Katz's stepmother stated that she feels Ms. Katz has trouble distinguishing background noise from what is being said to her. Furthermore, it was noted during this assessment that Ms. Katz spoke in an extremely soft voice. Much of her communication was nonverbal and gestural. In fact, Ms. Katz would not give a verbal response if a gesture would suffice.

5. Ms. Katz's specific learning problems require modification of procedures for assessing her ability. She should be allowed to demonstrated her knowledge under conditions that permit her to write her responses, whether short answers or long essays, under untimed conditions.

6. Ms. Katz should take a graduate course in biology before applying to medical school, to see whether she is able to do the work, and possibly to improve her grade point average. If she does well, her grade may be submitted to a medical school as an indicator of what she is capable of doing at this level.

7. Ms. Katz should consider going to medical school on a part-time basis. Attending school part-time would allow her to take only a couple of classes at a time, giving her more time to study and the opportunity to learn under less pressure.

ACKNOWLEDGMENTS

We would like to thank Kristee A. Beres, Nadeen L. Kaufman, Shauna Cooper, and Allison Kaufman.

REFERENCES:

Brown, D. T. (1994). Review of the Kaufman Adolescent and Adult Intelligence Test (KAIT). *Journal of School Psychology, 32,* 85–99.

Caruso, J. C., & Jacob-Timm, S. (2001). Confirmatory factor analysis of the Kaufman Adolescent and Adult Intelligence Test with young adolescents. *Assessment, 8,* 11–17.

Dumont, R., & Hagberg, C. (1994). Test reviews: Kaufman Adolescent and Adult Intelligence Test. *Journal of Psychoeducational Assessment, 12,* 190–196.

Flanagan, D. P., Alfonso, V. C., & Flanagan, R. (1994). A review of the Kaufman Adolescent and Adult Intelligence Test: An advance in cognitive assessment? *School Psychology Review, 23,* 512–525.

Gonzalez, J., Adir, Y., Kaufman, A. S., & McLean, J. E. (1995, February). *Race and gender differences in cognitive factors: A neuropsychological interpretation.* Paper presented at the annual meeting of the International Neuropsychological Society, Seattle, WA.

Horn, J. L. (1985). Remodeling old models of intelligence. In B. B. Wolman (Ed.), *Handbook of intelligence* (pp. 267–300). New York: Wiley.

Horn, J. L. (1989). Cognitive diversity: A framework of learning. In P. L. Ackerman, R. J. Sternberg, & R. Glaser (Eds.), *Learning and individual differences* (pp. 61–116). New York: Freeman.

Horn, J. L., & Cattell, R. B. (1966). Refinement and test of the theory of fluid and crystallized intelligence. *Journal of Educational Psychology, 57,* 253–270.

Horn, J. L., & Cattell, R. B. (1967). Age differences in fluid and crystallized intelligence. *Acta Psychologica, 26,* 107–129.

Horn, J. L., & Hofer, S. M. (1992). Major abilities and development in the adult period. In R. J. Sternberg & C. A. Berg (Eds.), *Intellectual development* (pp. 44–99). New York: Cambridge University Press.

Horn, J. L., & Noll, J. (1997). Human cognitive capabilities: Gf-Gc In theory. D. P. Flanagan, J. L. Genshaft, & P. L. Harrison (Eds.), *Contemporary intellectual assessment: Theories, tests and issues* (pp. 53–91). New York: Guilford Press.

Kaufman, A. S. (2000). Tests of intelligence. In R. J. Sternberg (Ed.), *Handbook of intelligence* (pp. 445–476). New York: Cambridge University Press.

Kaufman, A. S., & Horn, J. L. (1996). Age changes on test of fluid and crystallized ability for females and males on the Kaufman Adolescent and Adult Intelligence Test (KAIT) at ages 17 to 94 years. *Archives of Clinical Neuropsychology, 11,* 97–121.

Kaufman, A. S., Ishikuma, T., & Kaufman, N. L. (1994). A Horn analysis of the factors measured by the WAIS-R, KAIT, and two brief tests for normal adolescents and adults. *Assessment, 1,* 353–366.

Kaufman, A. S., Kaufman, J. C., & McLean, J. E. (1995). Factor structure of the Kaufman Adolescent and Adult Intelligence Test (KAIT) for whites, African Americans, and Hispanics. *Educational and Psychological Measurement, 55,* 365–376.

Kaufman, A. S., & Kaufman, N. L. (1993). *Manual for Kaufman Adolescent and Adult Intelligence Test (KAIT)*. Circle Pines, MN: American Guidance Service.

Kaufman, A. S., & Kaufman, N. L. (1997). The Kaufman Adolescent and Adult Intelligence Test (KAIT). In D. P. Flanagan, J. L. Genshaft, & P. L Harrison (Eds.), *Contemporary intellectual assessment: Theories, tests, and issues* (pp. 209–229). New York: Guilford Press.

Kaufman, A. S., & Lichtenberger, E. O. (1999). *Essentials of WAIS-III assessment*. New York: Wiley.

Kaufman, A. S., & Lichtenberger, E. O. (2002). *Assessing adolescent and adult intelligence* (2nd ed.). Boston: Allyn & Bacon.

Kaufman, A. S., McLean, J. E., & Kaufman, J. C. (1995). The fluid and crystallized abilities of white, black, and Hispanic adolescents and adults, both with and without an education covariate. *Journal of Clinical Psychology, 51*, 637–647.

Kaufman, A. S., McLean, J. E., & Reynolds, C. R. (1988). Sex, race, residence, region, and educational differences on the WAIS-R subtests. *Journal of Clinical Psychology, 44*, 231–248.

Kaufman, J. C., Chen, T. H., & Kaufman, A. S. (1995). Ethnic group, education, and gender differences on six Horn abilities for adolescents and adults. *Journal of Psychoeducational Assessment, 13*, 49–65.

Kaufman, J. C., McLean, J. E., Kaufman, A. S., & Kaufman, N. L. (1994). White–black and white–Hispanic differences on fluid and crystallized abilities by age across the 11- to 94-year range. *Psychological Reports, 75*, 1279–1288.

Lichtenberger, E. O. (2001). The Kaufman tests—K-ABC and KAIT. In A. S. Kaufman & N. L. Kaufman (Eds.), *Specific learning disabilities and difficulties in children and adolescents: Psychological assessment and evaluation* (pp. 97–140). New York: Cambridge University Press.

Lichtenberger, E. O., Broadbooks, D. A., & Kaufman, A. S. (2000). *Essentials of cognitive assessment with the KAIT and other Kaufman tests*. New York: Wiley.

Luria, A. R. (1966). *Human brain and psychological processes*. New York: Harper & Row.

Luria, A. R. (1973). *The working brain: An introduction to neuropsychology*. New York: Basic Books.

Luria, A. R. (1980). *Higher cortical functions in man* (2nd ed.). New York: Basic Books.

Manly, J. J., Heaton, R. K., & Taylor, M. J. (2000, August). The effects of demographic variables and the development of demographically adjusted norms for the WAIS-III and WMS-III. In D. S. Tulsky & D. Saklofske (Chairs), *The clinical interpretation of the WAIS-III and WMS-III: New research findings*. Symposium presented at the annual meeting of the American Psychological Association, Washington, DC.

McLean, J. E. (1995). *Improving education through action research*. Thousand Oaks, CA: Corwin.

Morgan, A. W., Sullivan, S. A., Darden, C., & Gregg, N. (1997). Measuring the intelligence of college students with learning disabilities: A comparison of results obtained on the WAIS-R and the KAIT. *Journal of Learning Disabilities, 30*, 560–565.

Piaget, J. (1972). Intellectual evolution from adolescence to adulthood. *Human Development, 15*, 1–12.

Pinion, G. A. (1995). *Test–retest reliability of the Kaufman Adolescent and Adult Intelligence Test*. Unpublished doctoral dissertation, Oklahoma State University.

Shaughnessy, M. F., & Moore, J. N. (1994). The KAIT with developmental students, honor students, and freshmen. *Psychology in the Schools, 31*, 286–287.

Thorndike, R. L., Hagen, E. P., & Sattler, J. M. (1986). *Stanford–Binet Intelligence Scale: Fourth Edition*. Chicago: Riverside.

Vo, D. H., Weisenberger, J. L., Becker, R., & Jacob-Timm, S. (1999). Concurrent validity of the KAIT for students in grade six and eight. *Journal of Psychoeducational Assessment, 17*, 152–162.

Wechsler, D. (1981). *Manual for the Wechsler Adult Intelligence Scale—Revised (WAIS-R)*. San Antonio, TX: Psychological Corporation.

Wechsler, D. (1991). *Manual for the Wechsler Intelligence Scale for Children—Third Edition (WISC-III)*. San Antonio, TX: Psychological Corporation.

Woodcock, R. W. (1990). Theoretical foundations of the WJ-R measures of cognitive ability. *Journal of Psychoeducational Assessment, 8*, 231–258.

Woodrich, D. L., & Kush, J. C. (1998). Kaufman Adolescent and Adult Intelligence Test (KAIT): Concurrent validity of fluid ability for preadolescents and adolescents with central nervous system disorders and scholastic concerns. *Journal of Psychoeducational Assessment, 16*, 215–225.

8

Preschool Intellectual Assessment

KIMBERLEY BLAKER SAYE

Early intervention programs are increasingly interesting and important in the realm of education (Culbertson & Willis, 1993). Research supports the notion of intervening as early as possible in a child's life, in order to minimize lasting effects of the child's difficulties (Kenny & Culbertson, 1993). Much legislation has now been passed recognizing the need for early diagnosis of developmental delays and providing funds for screening preschool children. Today states are required under the Individuals with Disabilities Education Act (IDEA), Part B, to provide intervention services for children ages 3–5 with disabilities. They are offered services under the same categories as older children. Public Law (PL) 102-119 has created an additional category for children ages 3–5 who have developmental delays. This category includes children who are experiencing delays in physical, cognitive, communicative, social, emotional, or adaptive development (Nagle, 2000). Under PL 99-457, states are offered funds in order to create and implement intervention services to children from birth (McLinden & Prasse, 1991). The current popular focus on early intervention has resulted in the need for school psychologists and other qualified

personnel to become familiar with tests suitable for infants and preschoolers.

Preschool assessment can take place for many reasons. Assessments in educational settings are often used for screening, diagnosis, and placement decisions; remediation of problem areas; and curriculum planning and evaluation (Nagle, 2000). The National Association of School Psychologists (NASP) has issued an early childhood assessment position statement that endorses multidisciplinary team assessments including multiple procedures and sources of information across multiple settings. A comprehensive picture of a child's abilities should be sought, and this assessment should be linked to intervention strategies (Bracken, Bagnato, & Barnett, 1991).

Infant and preschool assessment methods can look very different from "typical" school-age assessments. Infant and preschool assessments must typically be more dynamic in nature, because infants and preschoolers often do not yet understand why they must sit at a table and answer questions, doing their best throughout the assessment. In addition, such issues as reliabilities, test floors, and item gradients often present psychometric problems in the testing of very young children. Because of these inherent difficulties, "alternative" methods are often employed alongside, or in place of, "traditional" methods when infants and preschoolers are assessed. Examples of such "alternative" methods include play-based assessment, parent interviews, child observations, rating scales, and curriculum-based assessment (Nagle, 2000). Nagle's (2000) review indicates that these "alternative" measures should be used in addition to the more traditional tests, as they can also provide valuable information regarding a child's functioning. In order to provide early intervention services, most states require standardized assessment data to show eligibility. The more traditional tests are used for this purpose, though the "gold standard" assessment would include additional measures (parent interviews, rating scales, observations, etc.).

Although it is recognized that screening, remediation of problem areas, and curriculum planning and evaluation are important parts of the early intervention process, this chapter's focus is on the diagnostic assessment of preschool cognitive ability. Moreover, the chapter focuses on more traditional intelligence tests, rather than "developmental" or curriculum-based measures. The reader is strongly encouraged to use a broad range of assessment measures— including parent and teacher reports, observations, and "alternative" measures—to get a complete picture of a child's functioning. No assumption is made that the intelligence tests discussed are the only true measure of a child's development. They are simply additional tools (though often mandated by state eligibility requirements) that help a multidisciplinary team reach decisions for early intervention purposes.

SPECIAL CONSIDERATIONS IN PRESCHOOL TEST ADMINISTRATION

Developmental Influences

Normal developmental transitions affect the motivation, interest, and cooperation of young children (Culbertson & Willis, 1993). Often they will not have typical school-age testing behavior. Especially if children have never been in a school setting

before, the idea of sitting down at a table and doing activities an examiner requests can be foreign to them. They may not want to make the transition from certain subtests, yet may refuse to try other subtests. When children are learning to say "no," they may exert themselves forcefully and appear oppositional. They can also be egocentric and only understand their own needs, not those of others (Kamphaus, Dresden, & Kaufman, 1993). In addition, children often have normal fears (e.g., fear of separation from their parents), especially in strange situations. Because children may experience a great deal of change in a very short amount of time, their development can be rapid and uneven. Moreover, at different ages, different areas of development may be assessed (Hynd & Semrud-Clikeman, 1993).

Further developmental issues may include varying degrees of sociability, depending on how much interaction children have had with other children and with adults. Children with little interpersonal experience may react with fear or hostility to the demands an examiner is making of them. Depending on their experiences, children may be unfamiliar with the materials used in the test kits and may not understand how to manipulate the items. In addition, young children have physiological issues that change with age. For example, a child may be taking naps, may be undergoing toilet training, or may need several snacks throughout the morning. Attention span can be short and activity level can be high; both of these factors also change with age. Finally, young children can be susceptible to influences of extraneous variables, such as noise outside the testing room, the decorations on the wall, and so forth (Kamphaus et al., 1993). An examiner should be aware of all these developmental influences and be flexible enough to adapt the testing to each child's particular characteristics. For further reading on examinee characteristics, see Bracken (2000).

Examiner Characteristics

The development of rapport is especially important with young children. According to Kamphaus and colleagues (1993), examiners should approach the assessment in a "friendly, cheerful, relaxed, warm, natural, reassuring, encouraging, and patient" (p. 57) way. Kamphaus and colleagues further indicate that better rapport will be established if the examiner is sincerely interested in the child and is responsive to his or her needs and temperament. Something an examiner often overlooks when first performing assessments with young children is his or her clothing. With children of this age, the examiner may be playing on the floor with them or squatting down to greet them. Restrictive or overly elaborate clothing is not appropriate in these instances. Clothing should be professional, but comfortable enough to allow the examiner to play on the floor. Simple clothes and jewelry that will not distract a child are best. Another thing to consider in building rapport with young children is to become aware of things that young children enjoy; knowledge of a child's favorite cartoon character or book may go a long way toward building rapport. Furthermore, the tests should be introduced to the child in an honest but non-threatening way (Bracken, 2000). Squatting to the child's level and speaking naturally should help maintain rapport. The examiner should introduce the tests in such a way that the child is interested and motivated to perform well.

To facilitate the testing process, the examiner should do several things. First, of course, he or she should be familiar with the tests to be administered. Great familiarity with the tests allows the examiner to focus more on the child's behavior. Also, a 3-year-old child is not going to sit patiently while the examiner fumbles for the next item booklet needed; therefore, having needed items accessible is important to a successful administration. Second, well-developed behavior management skills can be important to maintain rapport when the child becomes frustrated, bored, or oppositional. Third, the examiner should be familiar with the typical developmental characteristics of young children (Bracken, 2000). With adequate working knowledge of these characteristics, the examiner can then say whether a child's behavior appears typical or atypical. Fourth, the examiner should be approachable, yet should clearly be in charge. Bracken (2000) says examiners should avoid making requests implying that the child has a right to refuse, such as "Would you like to try the next one?" Instead, examiners should use the approach of making simple directives, such as "Try the next one," and offering the child a choice only if he or she truly has one. Fifth, Bracken and Walker (1997) note that using humor can create an enjoyable atmosphere. Finally, and perhaps most obviously, the examiner should enjoy working with the preschool population. These children can be a true delight to work with, but they also present their own unique challenges that can frustrate examiners.

Environmental Characteristics

Kamphaus and colleagues (1993) provide a good list of characteristics that the "gold standard" testing room should have. Some of these include having the room be free from interruption, well lit, pleasantly but minimally decorated, and equipped with child-sized furniture. Things that can be done to minimize distraction while maintaining comfort are usually good options. Testing materials should be child-appropriate (e.g., large crayons and pencils), and materials should be placed so they are readily accessible to the examiner but out of the child's reach. Finally, the timing of the assessment should be planned around the child's sleeping and eating schedules.

CONDITIONS FOR TEST ADMINISTRATION

To get the best performance out of a preschool child, it is often necessary to break the testing session down into a few briefer sessions over the span of a day or a few days. If a child starts to become uncooperative, sometimes a brief break or a change in scenery, such as going for a walk or playing a game on the floor, can be helpful. Breaks should be used judiciously, however. The primary purpose of a break is to maximize the child's ability to perform well (Kamphaus et al., 1993). The examiner should watch for signs that the child needs a break, and offer one accordingly (at a good stopping point, when possible). Social rewards, such as smiles and saying encouraging things, can be helpful in maintaining rapport and motivation; tangible rewards, such as stickers, are also useful. The examiner should be sure to reward the child for effort, not correct responses. Another thing to consider in administering the tests is to control the pacing of the test. If the examiner senses that the child is feeling overwhelmed, slowing the pace a bit may help. However, if the child is beginning to fidget and appears to have trouble paying attention, increasing the pace may be beneficial. If a child is shy or reticent, it may help to warm the child up by beginning with a test that requires little or no verbal communication. Such tests include the Bracken Basic Concepts Scale—Revised (BBCS-R; see discussion later in this chapter), the Peabody Picture Vocabulary Test—Third Edition (PPVT-III), and the Beery–Buktenica Developmental Test of Visual–Motor Integration. Because these tests require only pointing or drawing, they can serve as good "ice breakers" for the testing process.

TEST CHARACTERISTICS AND PSYCHOMETRICS

With many different tests available with which to assess preschool populations, how does one choose the best? Bracken (1987) has proposed standards for minimal levels of technical adequacy. These standards are presented below, along with a description of the psychometric properties evaluated.

Test Floors

A "test floor" indicates how well a test provides meaningful scores at low levels of functioning (Bracken, 2000). That is, are there enough easy items to differentiate between abilities at the low end of the average range and those that are below average? The floor is found by determining the lowest IQ score that would be obtained ($M = 100$, $SD = 15$) if an examinee were to pass only one item on each subtest. Adequately sensitive tests will yield a standard score 2 standard deviations (SDs) or more below the mean (a standard score of 70 or below). If the test does not generate a standard score of 2 SDs or more below the mean, it does not have a sensitive floor, and cannot accurately identify very delayed functioning. This is important, because scores may be inflated due to poor psychometric properties

of the test and thus may not adequately identify those children in need of intensive services. Bracken (2000) states that this problem is especially apparent for children below age 4, and that tests must be examined carefully for children younger than age 4, especially if they are thought to have low functioning.

Test Ceilings

The concept of a "test ceiling" is similar to that of a test floor, though this problem occurs at the upper end of the normal distribution. Tests intended to identify giftedness, which is usually defined as 2 SDs above the mean (standard score of 130 or above), should provide accurate scores at and above this level (Bracken, 2000). Ceilings are not as widespread a problem in preschool testing, but examiners should check on this anyway. Some tests, such as the Differential Ability Scales (DAS; see later discussion), have subtests that are discontinued for older preschool children for this reason.

Item Gradients

As shown in Bracken (1987), an "item gradient" measures how quickly standard scores change as a result of one item. For example, does answering one additional item correctly raise one's score from a 94 to a 104, or does answering one additional item correctly simply raise one's score from a 94 to a 96? This is an extremely important consideration when one is choosing a test for a preschool assessment. The larger the change is in a resulting standard score from one test to another, the less sensitive the test is to subtle differences in a child's abilities. Examiners should look at norm tables in the manuals to determine which tests have item gradients that are too steep. Bracken (1987) recommends that an increase or decrease of a single raw score should not alter the corresponding standard score by more than 0.33 SD.

Reliability

"Reliability" refers to the stability of the test score over time. With multiple testings, one would expect a child's scores to hover around a given value, the child's true score.

The closer the test scores are upon retest, the higher the reliability. Similarly, one would expect scores on similar tasks to obtain similar results, which is a measure of internal consistency. If test scores are to be valuable in documenting progress or making predictions about future performance, the scores need to be reasonably stable over time (Hynd & Semrud-Clikeman, 1993). Hynd and Semrud-Clikeman (1993) also mention that attentional difficulties can decrease test–retest reliability, because tests are often made up of fewer items in order to keep a child's attention. They note further that test–retest reliability often increases over the course of development. Bracken (1987) has set .90 as his standard for internal consistency and stability. According to him, subtest and composite reliabilities should approximate .80.

Validity

"Validity" indicates to us how well a test measures what it purports to measure (Kamphaus, 2001). Validity documentation is one of the most important sections included in test manuals. Few numerical guidelines can be found for the interpretation of validity coefficients, but the examiner should examine the studies cited in the manuals and determine whether there is adequate evidence of validity. Most preschool tests of intellectual functioning include measures of construct validity, concurrent validity, and predictive validity. Predictive validity is weak for preschoolers, according to Flanagan and Alfonso (1995). First, prediction assumes that what is measured is stable; this is not as certain with preschool children (because their development occurs so rapidly) as it is with older children or adults. Second, the quality of the tests may vary across age and ability levels, due both to reliability and to the possibility that test items may not measure the same constructs at different ages. Hynd and Semrud-Clikeman (1993) note that in order to get the best possible sample of a child's abilities (especially if the child may have intellectual deficiencies), the examiner may have to take a more proactive role in the assessment. However, the more the examiner "interferes," the more the assessment is not standardized, and validity may be affected. The examiner should be aware of this possibility when trying to obtain a good sample of a child's abilities.

Norms Tables

Bracken (2000) states that some tables of norms for preschool tests are too broad to be sensitive to the rapid growth and development that occur early in life. He suggests that norms tables not exceed 3-month intervals, and that these intervals be even briefer (e.g., 1–2 months) for younger ages. It is important to examine the norms tables to be sure that no extreme jumps occur when a child moves to a higher age table.

Test Directions and Procedures

Finally, Bracken (2000) recommends finding tests with simple directions, including demonstration and sample items that allow the examiner to be sure that the child understands what he or she is supposed to do before performing the task for credit. That is, the examiner must make sure that the basic test concepts presented to the child can be understood by the child. If not, then the test does not measure what it is intending to measure.

REVIEW OF COMMON PRESCHOOL INTELLIGENCE TESTS

Now that the basic psychometric properties have been covered, a review is presented of traditional intelligence tests that can be used with preschool-age children.

Differential Ability Scales

The DAS (Elliott, 1990) is an individually administered test of intellectual ability and achievement that can be used with chidren ages 2 years, 6 months through 17 years, 11 months. It is a revision of the British Ability Scales (Elliott, Murray, & Pearson, 1979). The DAS is theoretically based on the Cattell–Horn–Carroll g factor of general intelligence. The DAS can be used to make diagnostic decisions, to evaluate strengths and weaknesses, and (along with other data) to classify children. The Cognitive Battery has 17 subtests divided into two levels: the

Preschool Level, which is subsequently divided into the Lower and Upper Preschool Levels, and the School-Age Level, for children ages 6 years to 17 years, 11 months. This discussion is limited to the Preschool Level.

Children ages 2 years, 6 months through 3 years, 5 months are administered four subtests that yield the General Conceptual Ability (GCA) composite. Two diagnostic subtests are also available. Children ages 3 years, 6 months through 5 years, 11 months (Upper Preschool Level) are administered six subtests and can be given five diagnostic subtests. Tests at the Upper Preschool Level take 25–65 minutes to administer. At this level, two cluster scores are obtained in addition to the GCA; these are Verbal Ability and Nonverbal Ability.

The DAS kit includes a manual, an introductory and technical handbook, three stimulus booklets, picture similarities cards, picture stimulus cards, a box of small toys, foam blocks, plastic blocks, counting chips, wood blocks, sorting chips, and a tray with wooden pieces. Lower Preschool Level tasks include building designs with wood blocks, answering questions to determine receptive vocabulary knowledge, placing similar pictures together, and naming objects. Upper Preschool Level activities include performing tasks as instructed, placing similar pictures together, naming objects, making designs out of blocks, performing simple quantitative problems, and copying geometric designs. A stopwatch is also needed. The most difficult aspect of DAS administration is switching between the different booklets and different test materials. However, the test is stimulating and appears fun for children. With practice, the administration becomes easier.

Test Administration and Scoring

The tests are given in a specified order, with starting points delineated by age. Instead of hard-and-fast stopping points, the DAS includes decision points based upon age. At each decision point, if the child has fewer than three questions wrong, testing is continued to the next decision point. If the child has fewer than three questions correct, then testing drops back to the previous starting point. These are clearly marked, and "discontinue" criteria are stated directly on the record form. Items are generally scored dichotomously, and ability scores are calculated based on raw scores and the item set administered. Ability scores are then transformed into T-scores. T-scores for each cluster are then added together, and then standard scores are found from the sums of T-scores.

Test Standardization

The DAS was standardized with a sample of 3,475 children ages 2 years, 6 months through 17 years, 11 months. There were equal numbers of boys and girls in the sample. There were 175 cases for each 6-month age group from ages 2 years, 6 months through 4 years, 11 months, and there were 200 cases per year from ages 5 years through 17 years, 11 months. The sample was stratified on race/ethnicity, parental education, geographic region, and educational preschool enrollment, and was based on 1988 U.S. census information.

Reliability

The DAS technical manual describes the reliabilities of the DAS. For the preschool age group, internal consistency estimates of subtests range from a low of .68 for Block Building at ages 2 years, 6 months to a high of .90 for Pattern Construction at age 5 years. Generally, internal consistency estimates are in the low .80s. The GCA score shows higher ratings, at about .90. As expected, test–retest reliability coefficients increase with age. At ages $3\frac{1}{2}$ to $4\frac{1}{2}$ years, correlations range from .56 for Picture Similarities to .81 for Verbal Comprehension. The GCA test–retest correlation over a period of 2–6 weeks was good at .90. At ages 5 to $6\frac{1}{2}$ years, test–retest correlations increase. In general, the DAS shows high reliability.

Validity

The DAS was given in a counterbalanced order with the Wechsler Preschool and Primary Scale of Intelligence—Revised (WPPSI-R; see later discussion) to a sample of 62 children. For 4- and 5-year-olds, the GCA of the DAS correlated .89 with the

Full Scale IQ of the WPPSI-R, indicating that the DAS and the WPPSI-R measure many of the same constructs. The DAS GCA correlated adequately (.77) with the Stanford–Binet Intelligence Scale: Fourth Edition (SB4; see later discussion) Composite score. With 3- to 5-year-olds, correlations between the WPPSI-R and the DAS are not quite as high but are still adequate, with the correlation between the total scores being .81. These scores indicate that the DAS is a valid measure for assessing cognitive functioning at the preschool level.

Summary

The DAS is a valid, reliable measure used to assess cognitive functioning in preschool children (Kamphaus, 2001). It yields one or two standard scores, depending on whether the Cognitive Battery is administered at the Upper or Lower Preschool Level. The DAS has a great number of pieces that the examiner must keep track of, but the pieces are colorful and are very reminiscent of toys, which helps a child stay interested. The drawings and photos are colorful for the most part, and children seem to enjoy the Verbal Comprehension subtest especially well. Almost every subtest has something for a child to manipulate, which makes the process more enjoyable. Administration can be difficult and takes some practice. The starting, stopping, and decision points are different from those of many other tests and require some study. Also, the answers to some of the block designs are given from the child's point of view, and it would have been helpful to have them from the examiner's point of view. However, the test seems fun for children and moves at a relatively fast pace. The DAS Lower Preschool Level should take about 40 minutes to administer. The Upper Preschool Level can usually be finished within 90 minutes.

Wechsler Preschool and Primary Scale of Intelligence—Third Edition

The WPPSI-III (Wechsler, 2002a, 2002b, 2002c) is the revised version of the WPPSI-R (Wechsler, 1989). It is an individually administered test of cognitive ability that can be used with children ages 2 years, 6 months through 7 years, 3 months. The WPPSI-III is an extension of the WPPSI-R and adds new subtests and child-friendly materials. Those persons familiar with the WISC-III or the WAIS-III would immediately recognize the majority of the tasks and would have little trouble adapting to the WPPSI-III. The WPPSI-III has two core batteries to be used based on the child's age; one battery (four core subtests) is used for children 2 years, 6 months to 3 years, 11 months and the other battery (seven core subtests) is used with children 4 years, 0 months to 7 years, 3 months. The WPPSI-III includes more appealing and colorful artwork than the WPPSI-R, simpler language in instructions, elimination of bonus points for speeded items, more practice or teaching items, and extended floors and ceilings.

Like other Wechsler scales, the WPPSI-III yields three standard scores: the Full Scale IQ, the Performance IQ, and the Verbal IQ. Additionally, the upper level yields a Processing Speed Quotient and the lower level yields a General Language Composite. Subtest tasks include putting puzzles together, making patterns out of blocks, completing patterns, and forming groups of objects with common characteristics. Verbal tasks include measures of receptive vocabulary, giving answers to general information questions, and identifying concepts described in a series of clues. The Processing Speed Quotient includes Symbol Search and Coding Items, like those found on the WISC-III. There are additional supplemental subtests (to create 14 subtests in all) to provide additional information about the child's cognitive abilities. These supplemental tests provide a broader sampling of abilities and may also be substituted for core subtests. The WPPSI-III is organized much like the other Wechsler tests, with alternating Performance and Verbal subtests.

The WPPSI-III is intended to be used to measure intellectual ability. It can be used for diagnosis of giftedness, developmental delays, and mental retardation; for program placement; for assessment of change; and for research.

The test kit for the WPPSI-III consists of an administration and scoring manual (which has a "cracked" cover that allows it to stand), a technical and interpretive manual, two stimulus books, 14 puzzles in a plastic case, blocks for Block Design, two child-appropriate pencils without erasers, and scoring templates. In addition, record forms and response booklets are used in the administration. A stopwatch is also needed, as responses to all of the Performance subtests are timed. This is a lot of equipment to keep up with, but the WPPSI-III is an interesting test.

Test Administration and Scoring

The core subtests of the lower level of the WPPSI-III generally take between 30 and 45 minutes to administer. The core battery of the upper level generally takes between 45 minutes to 1 hour to administer. The WPPSI-III subtests are administered in alternating Performance-Verbal fashion, as noted above. Regarding the lower level, there are five subtests in all (Picture Naming is optional). The first subtest administered is Receptive Vocabulary, which requires the child to point to the correct picture on a sheet. This does not require a verbal response, and so may be helpful for shy children. The artwork has been updated and looks more like artwork in storybooks. Starting and stopping points are given both in the manual and on the record form. Correct responses are in red on the record form. Additionally, most items at this level are printed in the record form to make administration more examiner-friendly. Block design items are shown from the examiner's perspective on the record form to further aid the examiner. Administration of Object Assembly is quite different from previous versions of Object Assembly. The puzzles are laid out in a line by a number found on the back. They must be laid out and turned over in a specific fashion that requires some practice. There is no layout shield and no schematic drawing to lay out each puzzle. Having only four core subtests and requiring minimal verbal responses is helpful.

Regarding the upper level, there are 14 subtests in all (Symbol Search, Comprehension, Picture Completion, Similarities, and Object Assembly are supplementary, and Receptive Vocabulary and Picture Naming are optional). The first subtest administered is Block Design, which is like a game, involves manipulatives, and does not require verbal responses from the child. Most children seem to find it enjoyable. Starting and stopping points are given in the manual and are nicely located on the record form for ease of use.

Most of the subtests have a type of practice item—an item where the correct answer can be "taught" to the child if he or she misses the item. This is especially important with preschoolers, as it allows them to practice the task and come to an understanding of the requirements. A child can be asked to elaborate on an answer by saying "Tell me more about it," and a "Q" should be marked on the record form.

After the raw scores are obtained by adding up the individual scores, they are converted to scaled scores. The Performance score is found by adding all of the scaled scores for core Performance tasks; the Verbal score is likewise found by adding all of the scaled scores for the core Verbal tasks. At the upper level, the Processing Speed Quotient is found by adding Symbol Search and Coding scores. The Full Scale score is the sum of the Verbal and Performance scores as well as the Coding score. IQ scores are obtained from the Full Scale, Performance, and Verbal sums of scaled scores via a table in the manual.

Test Standardization

The WPPSI-III was standardized with a sample of 1,700 children ages 2 years, 6 months through 7 years, 3 months. There were equal numbers of boys and girls in the sample. The sample was representative of the U.S. population of children at these ages. The sample was stratified on demographic variables (such as age, sex, parent education level, and geographic region), based on 2000 U.S. Census information. Children who were non-English speaking, had physical impairments (e.g., upper extremity impairment or uncorrected vision or hearing loss), or had psychiatric or neurological issues were excluded from the standardization sample.

Reliability

Greater confidence that an observed score is representative of a child's true ability can be obtained with higher reliabilities. Split-half reliabilities of individual tests for the age groups $2\frac{1}{2}$ years to 7 years, 3 months range from a low of .84 to a high of .96. The IQ scores show high split-half reliabilities, with an average of .93 for Performance IQ, .95 for Verbal IQ, and .96 for Full Scale IQ. The Processing Speed Quotient shows average split-half reliability of .89, and the General Language Quotient has split-half reliability of .93. These are high reliabilities for the composite scores, and thus the IQ scores should serve as better estimates of a child's true scores than the individual subtest scores do. Test–retest stability coefficients for the Performance IQ, Verbal IQ, and Full Scale IQ are high, at .86, .91, and .92, respectively. The WPPSI-III shows very high reliability overall.

Validity

In order to determine whether the WPPSI-III measures the same constructs as the WPPSI-R, a study was conducted with a sample of 176 children chosen to be representative of the U.S. population according to 2000 census data. These children were administered the WPPSI-III and the WPPSI-R 1–8 weeks apart. The correlations found between the WPPSI-III and WPPSI-R Performance IQ, Verbal IQ, and Full Scale IQ were .70, .86, and .85, respectively. These correlations indicate that the same constructs are most likely being measured by both tests. Correlations between the WPPSI-III and WISC-III scores were also high at .89. The WPPSI-III FSIQ and DAS GCA correlate at .87. These correlations and other good studies mentioned in the WPPSI-III technical manual indicate that the WPPSI-III is a valid measure for assessing cognitive functioning. The technical manual gives many studies of the use of the WPPSI-III with special populations.

Summary

The WPPSI-III is a reliable and valid measure that can be used with preschool children to assess cognitive functioning. It yields three standard scores in Performance and Verbal areas and in a Full Scale composite, as well as a Processing Speed Quotient. The WPPSI-III has many pieces to work with, but this helps make it interesting to a young child. The pieces and drawings have been revised to be colorful and engaging. The addition of picture items and minimal verbal responses, especially for younger

children, is a good adaptation. Splitting the test into a lower level and an upper level appears to be a very helpful revision. Administration can be a bit burdensome for a new examiner, but is mastered with some repetition. For those familiar with the other Wechsler tests, the WPPSI-III should pose few problems in administration, as it is similar to the WISC-III and WAIS-III in style. The WPPSI-III has one drawback: It can take more than an hour to administer the core and supplemental tests, and young children may not be able to sit and work for that long. Two sessions may be required to finish the entire battery.

Woodcock–Johnson III Tests of Cognitive Abilities

The Woodcock–Johnson III Tests of Cognitive Abilities (WJ-III COG; Woodcock, McGrew, & Mather, 2001) is a revision of the WJ-R COG (Woodcock & Johnson, 1989). The WJ-III COG is an individual assessment battery based on Cattell–Horn–Carroll theory. It is useful for ages 2 through 90. Standard scores are obtained for general intelligence, Verbal Ability, Thinking Ability, and Cognitive Efficiency. It also gives cluster standard scores (including measures of verbal comprehension, knowlege, long-term memory retrieval, visual–spatial thinking, auditory processing, fluid reasoning, processing speed, and short-term memory), as well as clinical clusters (such as a measure of phonemic awareness). There are two batteries for the WJ-III COG. The Standard Battery includes tests 1 through 10, and the Extended Battery includes tests 11 through 20. The examiner's manual (Mather & Woodcock, 2001) gives lists of the abilities measured by the battery and of which tests measure each ability, to allow the examiner to select specific tests to administer.

The WJ-III COG, according to the examiner's manual, can be used to determine strengths and weaknesses, to gather information to help in placement or diagnostic decisions, and to gain information regarding an individual's impairment. It can also be used to describe ability–achievement discrepancies, to plan educational programming, and to aid in research, among other things.

Little material is needed in order to give the battery: a comprehensive test record, a subject response booklet, two easel-backed ring binders that hold test questions, an audiocassette that is used for some tests, and a stopwatch. In addition, the test kit includes a technical manual, an examiner's manual, a computerized scoring program, scoring guides made of sturdy plastic, and an examiner's training workbook.

It should take roughly 1 hour to administer all of the Standard Battery, and roughly 2 hours to adminster the Extended Battery. Young children, of course, may need additional time due to some of their characteristics, such as being hesitant to respond, giving multiple answers, and requiring more queries for their responses.

Test Administration and Scoring

Each page in the two easel-backed ring binders provides instructions to the examiner. The first page in each binder gives general test instructions, as well as suggested starting points for testing, depending on an examinee's estimated ability level. For some tests, basals and ceilings must be reached. These criteria can be found in each test in the test book and also in the test record. The examiner's manual gives much detail about what to do when there are no apparent basals or ceilings, or when there are two apparent basals or ceilings. Some tests have time limits, designated by a drawing of a stopwatch. Some tests require the use of the audiocassette recording provided with the test kit. A checklist is also provided on the front of the test record on which to describe the examinee's qualitative behavior, such as diligence in responding and distractibility. An important feature for young children is that sample items are included with which to familiarize the children with the task at hand.

The Standard Battery includes 10 tests, all coming from the easel-backed binders or audiotape. Each test has a suggested starting point for preschool children, and some tests (on the first page after the tabbed page) have general instructions for accommodating preschool children. It is important to read this information and be familiar with it before testing begins, in order to proceed through the battery fluently.

Because of the wide range of tests on the WJ-III COG, scoring processes are not discussed in detail in this chapter. Scoring is simple, however, and instructions are clear on the test record. The Compuscore program (Schrank & Woodcock, 2001) is a vital part of the WJ-III COG. No hand-scoring option is available. For some, this may be a drawback; however, the Compuscore program is relatively easy to use and produces score reports quickly. It usually asks the examiner to input numbers that are in shaded boxes on the test record, or to input numbers from a special "Software Score Entry" box on the test record. The examiner's manual gives a great deal of information on interpreting the scores obtained from the test and is very helpful. When one is interpreting scores, this is the best source at which to look. A worksheet is given in the appendix to aid in diagnosis.

Test Standardization

According to the technical manual for the WJ-III COG, the norms were based on a large sample of 8,818 subjects. This sample was stratified on 10 factors and was representative of the United States. The preschool sample had 1,143 children ages 2–5 years who were not enrolled in kindergarten. The age 2 category had the smallest number of subjects, with 259. There were 310 children at age 3, 394 at age 4, and 373 at age 5.

Reliability

Reliability statistics for age 2 years are not available for tests 2, 6, 7, 9, 10, 14, 15, 16, 19, or 20. At age 3 years, reliability information is not available for tests 9, 10, 15, 19, or 20. At age 4, only test 20 has no reliability information. At ages 2 and 3, there is no reliability information for the General Intellectual Ability score (Extended Battery); at age 2, there is no such information for the General Intellectual Ability score (Standard Battery). When one looks past this, however, the median split-half test reliabilities fall mostly above .80. The cluster scores, which are recommended for interpretation, are mostly .90 and higher.

Validity

The items in the WJ-III COG were selected for inclusion if they were considered representative of factors of the Cattell–Horn–

Carroll theory. For external validation, special validity samples of preschool children were administered the WJ-III COG, the WJ-III Tests of Achievement (ACH), the WPPSI-R, and the DAS. The Extended Battery WJ-III COG General Intellectual Ability scores correlated .73 with the DAS GCA score, and .74 with the WPPSI-R Full Scale IQ. The Standard Battery WJ-III COG General Intellectual Ability scores correlated .67 with the DAS GCA score and .73 with the WPPSI-R Full Scale IQ. The tests thus seem to be adequately measuring similar constructs at the preschool level.

Summary

The WJ-III COG is an individually administered test of cognitive functioning that can be used with children as young as 2 years of age. This test is advantageous in that it is easy to administer; there are few pieces of which to keep track. The WJ-III COG also yields several clusters of scores that can be useful diagnostically. It is also strongly theory-driven. Finally, the computerized scoring program is easy and relatively quick to use.

The WJ-III COG does have some weaknesses when the test is used with preschoolers. It seems that some of the tests do not have adequate floors to be sensitive to variations in children's abilities. Also, some of the directions and tasks required seem too sophisticated for very young children to understand. For example, the Verbal Comprehension test requires four parts to be administered in order to get a score for that test. The parts require a child to recognize pictures, to give synonyms and antonyms of words, and to finish analogies. However, some of the tests, such as the General Information test, do seem more appropriate for use with very young children. It is best to use professional judgment and to consider the tests with reliability information when deciding which ones to give. Another drawback is that the instructions can be long, which makes them difficult for preschoolers to understand and attend to. Also, many tests require spoken responses from the child, which can pose a problem if the child is reticent. Finally, although the easel-backed binders are easy to use, they are not very exciting to a child who has not yet learned to sit still, look at pages of books, and respond to questions from an adult; the absence of ma-nipulatives can make the tests less interesting and captivating to such a child.

Stanford–Binet Intelligence Scale: Fourth Edition

The SB4 (Thorndike, Hagen, & Sattler, 1986) is an individually administered test of intellectual ability. It can be used with persons ages 2 to adult. There are 15 subtests, which measure four cognitive areas: Verbal Reasoning, Abstract/Visual Reasoning, Quantitative Reasoning, and Short-Term Memory. A Composite score is also obtained.

The SB4 is a revision of the Stanford–Binet Intelligence Scale: Form L-M (SB-LM; Thorndike, 1973). According to its developers (Thorndike et al., 1986), the SB4 is broader in coverage, is more flexible to administer, and gives a more detailed diagnostic assessment than the previous forms. The SB4 can be used to help identify children in need of special services. It can also differentiate between students with mental retardation and those with learning disabilities.

The SB4 consists of an administration and scoring guide, a technical manual, the record booklet, four item books, a set of beads and a stick, a set of dice, a set of green blocks, a formboard with pieces, a picture, and a set of cubes with a different design on each side. For some children, scissors and paper will be needed. A stopwatch and pencil are also necessary. Like some of the tests discussed earlier, the SB4 has a lot of items with which to keep up, but young children generally enjoy having things to manipulate.

Test Administration and Scoring

Test items are arranged by levels, which are indicated by letters. A basal of two complete levels correct, and a ceiling of three out of four items (or all four items) incorrect in two consecutive levels, must be obtained for each test. After the first test, Vocabulary, is administered, the ceiling of that test is combined with the person's chronological age to reach a starting-level guideline for the remaining subtests. The table for determining the starting level is given on the record form. If the starting level does not seem appropriate after a few subtest administrations, the level can be adjusted by the examiner. The starting level was designed to present items that are neither too hard nor too easy for an examinee; this saves time and prevents boredom, discouragement, or frustration.

According to the administration guide, some problems exist when the SB4 is used with children at age 2. Zero scores occur frequently, especially on novel tasks. This frequency of zero scores makes it impossible for the SB4 to discriminate adequately among the lowest-scoring 10%–15% of 2-year-olds. Zero scores also occur at age 3, though they are less frequent. The SB4 cannot discriminate among the lowest-scoring 2% of 3-year-olds. This information should be taken into consideration when one is selecting a test for a 2- or 3-year-old, especially if the child is believed to have very low functioning.

The administration and scoring guide gives good detail regarding administration and expanded scoring guidelines for some of the tests. There is also a section on testing preschoolers that offers good advice to the examiner.

Subtest raw scores may be converted to Standard Age Scores using tables in the back of the administration and scoring guide. A computer software scoring program (Four Score; Riverside, 2000) is available and is a quicker, easier way to score the test.

Test Standardization

The eight SB4 subtests for ages 2–5 (Vocabulary, Comprehension, Absurdities, Pattern Analysis, Copying, Quantitative, Bead Memory, and Memory for Sentences) were normed on a sample of 226 children at age 2, 278 at age 3, 397 at age 4, and 460 at age 5. The sample was representative of the U.S. population, according to the 1980 U.S. Census, and was stratified on geographic region, community size, ethnic group, age, and gender.

Reliability

The reliability information provided in the technical manual for the SB4 was noted to be somewhat inflated due to statistical procedures used. The values listed in the tables of this manual are therefore considered to be high estimates of the SB4's reliability. Most of the internal-consistency indices for individual subtests at ages 2–5 are in the mid-.80s, with a low of .74 at age 2 on the Copying subtest, and a high of .91 at age 3 on the Absurdities subtest. The area scores are slightly better, with average indices in the high .80s to low .90s. The Composite score shows greater reliability, with a low of .95 at age 2 and a high of .97 at ages 4 and 5. In addition, test–retest reliability was found to be adequate, though the sample for this study was small. Reliabilities ranged from a low of .71 for the Quantitative Reasoning area (which is not surprising, as this area consists of only one subtest at the preschool level) and a high of .91 for the Composite score.

Validity

A sample of 139 children was given both the SB4 and the SB-LM. The correlation between the Composite scores of these tests was adequate, with an r of .81; the subtests did not show correlations as high, however. Another sample of 205 children was given the SB4 and the WISC-R. The Full Scale IQ of the WISC-R correlated .83 with the Composite score of the SB4. A third sample of 75 children was given the SB4 and the WPPSI. The Full Scale IQ of the WPPSI correlated .80 with the Composite score of the SB4. The correlations between the SB4 Composite score and the corresponding scores of the other tests are adequate and indicate that the tests are generally measuring the same constructs.

Summary

The SB4 is a test of cognitive ability that can be used with preschool-age children. However, it is unable to discriminate adequately among the lowest-scoring 10%–15% of 2-year-olds and among the lowest-scoring 2% of 3-year-olds; it is therefore suggested that another test be used, or that the SB4 information be supplemented, when a preschool child who is thought to have low functioning needs to be tested. The SB4 has a strength in that it tailors the items, by way of the starting point, to a child's ability level rather than the child's chronological age. One weakness is that the SB4 can seem less like a game to preschool children, which can cause their interest to wane (Kamphaus, 2001). Another weakness is that it may be difficult to obtain basals on some of the tests. Also, the item books can be cumbersome, and it can be difficult to find the starting points. The samples are usually found at the beginning of the subtest, and then the examiner must flip to the pages with the examinee's starting level. This takes time and can be frustrating for a new examiner. Moreover, if it is necessary to drop back a level to establish a basal, one must sometimes change tasks, which can be confusing to the child. If the starting level seems high, the examiner should drop back a level or two on subsequent subtests. Practice with the SB4 is highly recommended. The test is discussed more extensively by Youngstrom, Glutting, and Watkins (Chapter 10, this volume).

At the time of this writing, the SB5 is being developed. The standardization version shows great promise of being very preschooler-friendly, with multicolored drawings, toys, and lots of manipulatives.

Bracken Basic Concept Scale—Revised

Though it is not a traditional intelligence test, the BBCS-R (Bracken, 1998) is an individually administered test used to assess the development of basic concepts (such as colors, size, numbers, and time) in young children. It can be a useful cognitive screening tool, and is often a great test with which to begin an assessment. It yields a standard score similar to an IQ score to give an estimate of cognitive ability. The BBCS-R is used with children ages 2 years, 6 months through 7 years, 11 months. The BBCS-R measures basic concepts in 11 areas; these basic concepts are related to intelligence, academic achievement, and language development. The first six subtests make up the School Readiness Composite (SRC), which allows the examiner to assess the child's knowledge of concepts helpful to his or her entering school. Bracken (1998) asserts in the BBCS-R manual that a preschool child's knowledge of basic concepts is very important to assess. In addition to concept acquisition, the BBCS-R measures receptive language abilities. The SRC is reported as a standard score; a standard score is also reported for the total test.

The BBCS-R serves five basic assessment purposes, according to the examiner's manual. First, it can be used as part of a compre-hensive speech–language assessment, assessing in part the child's receptive language ability. The BBCS-R is also useful in screening for possible cognitive-developmental delays or exceptionalities, such as learning disabilities or giftedness. In addition, the BBCS-R is useful in curriculum-based assessment, school readiness screening, and clinical and educational research.

The BBCS-R is a revision of the earlier BBCS (Bracken, 1984). The revision was undertaken to improve the scale with updated norms and materials. It also has new features, such as a larger examiner's manual, a stimulus manual with full-color art, 50 more items to enhance the assessment of abilities, and a Spanish adaptation of the items as well as a Spanish record form.

The test kit consists of three things. First is the examiner's manual, which has detailed information regarding administration, scoring, and interpretation procedures. Technical information, such as test development, standardization, and norms, can also be found here. The Spanish edition is also discussed in the manual. Second, the stimulus manual is an easy-to-use easel-backed manual, with full-color pictures for all items. Each subtest has a numbered tab for ease of reference. The pictures are bright and simple. Third is the record form, which comes in both English and Spanish versions. The form has administration, recording, and scoring directions for the test in general and for each specific subtest. The first page includes an area in which to record all scores, as well as a profile chart and a place for ipsative subtest score analysis.

The BBCS-R should take roughly 30 minutes to administer, though the time will vary depending on the age and ability of the child, as well as the examiner's skill. Administration of the SRC should take about 15 minutes. As noted throughout this chapter, preschool-age children are often more difficult to manage, and typically have not been socialized to sit still and perform tasks asked of them; this can lengthen the administration time. However, the BBCS-R is a good test with which to start a battery, because the pictures are colorful and child-friendly, and a child does not have to say much. He or she merely points to one of four pictures in the easel that fits the description read by the examiner. This allows the hesitant or slow-to-warm-up child additional time to become comfortable with the examiner and the testing process.

Test Administration and Scoring

Trial items are used to acquaint the child with the testing procedure. Once the child understands that he or she is to point in response to the examiner's questions, the testing begins. Repetition of items is allowed. Directions are the same at the beginning of each subtest in order to reorient the child to the task, but may be shortened during each subtest once the examiner is sure that the child understands the task. A dichotomous scoring criterion is used. The correct answer is printed in blue on the record form to aid the examiner.

Subtests 1–6, which are Colors, Letters, Numbers/Counting, Sizes, Comparisons, and Shapes, constitute the SRC. Each child is administered these subtests beginning with item 1. Items are administered until the child misses three items in a row, which is the ceiling, or completes the subtest. Starting points for subtests 7–11, which are Direction/Position, Self-/Social Awareness, Texture/Material, Quantity, and Time/Sequence, are determined by adding up the raw scores for subtests 1–6 and using the Start Point Table on page 4 of the record form to determine the letter or number of the starting item for the remaining subtests. A basal of three items in a row passed, and a ceiling of three items in a row failed, must be established for these subtests. All items below the basal are considered to be correct. The examiner's manual gives several examples of working with basals and ceilings. Scaled score tables and standard score tables based on chronological age are found in the back of the examiner's manual.

Test Standardization

The BBCS-R research included nationwide tryout and standardization phases (Bracken, 1998). The standardization, validity, and reliability research occurred in the fall of 1997. Participants were more than 1,100 children between the ages of 2 years, 6 months and 8 years, 0 months. The sample was representative of the general U.S. population, according to the 1995 U.S. Census

update. Children were not excluded if they were receiving special education services (such children accounted for 4% of the sample) or if they were receiving services for the gifted and talented (such children accounted for 1.7% of the sample).

Reliability

The BBCS-R examiner's manual includes measures of internal consistency (split-half) and test–retest reliability. The range of split-half reliability coefficients reported is good, at .78 to .98 for the subtests and .96 to .99 for the total test. The test–retest reliabilities range from a low of .78 on Quantity and Time/Sequence to a high of .88 for the SRC. Test–retest reliability for the total test is good at .94.

Validity

The BBCS-R manual includes several measures of validity, including concurrent, predictive, and construct validity. Concurrent validity was evaluated by comparing scores on the BBCS-R with scores on the BBCS, the WPPSI-R, and the DAS. All comparisons showed no significant differences between the means of the BBCS-R and the other tests at the .05 level. Predictive validity was also supported. As for construct validity, the BBCS-R was compared to other instruments used to measure receptive language and basic concepts. The correlations between the BBCS-R and the other tests seem to indicate that the BBCS-R is indeed a measure of basic concepts and receptive language.

Summary

The BBCS-R is a test that shows good measures of reliability and validity and is useful for assessing the development of preschoolers. The BBCS-R is advantageous in many ways. First, it is easy to administer and it is colorful, which makes it more stimulating and interesting to a preschool child's eye. It also does not require a verbal response, and so can be a valuable instrument to "warm up" a child or to assess children with social phobia or autism. It can be a good cognitive screener as well. It includes a Spanish form and culturally diverse pictures, as well as trial items. In addition, the record form is clear and easy to use. One limitation is that children with limited visual or auditory acuity may be at a disadvantage, as questions are read aloud and a choice must be made between pictures. Also, children who understand little English may be at a disadvantage when assessed with the English version, because it emphasizes English language and concept development. From an examiner's standpoint, the directions become tedious, as they are the same for each test; however, they can be shortened once a child fully understands what is required of him or her.

The Battelle Developmental Inventory

The Battelle Developmental Inventory (BDI; Newborg, Stock, Wnek, Guidubaldi, & Svinicki, 1984) is an individually administered battery of tests that assesses primary developmental skills in children from birth to age 8. Although it is not a traditional intelligence test, the BDI yields a cognitive measure in addition to its measures of adaptive and developmental abilities. Each domain of the BDI is contained in a separate spiral-bound book for ease of administration.

The authors of the BDI discuss several features that make the BDI user-friendly. First, the assessment procedures are such that many sources are used to gather information about a child. There is a structured test format for individual work with the child, along with directions to observe the child and interview the child's caregivers. Second, the authors mention a 3-point scoring system that allows more sensitive reporting of the child's abilities. Also, there are modifications listed that will aid the examiner in adapting each part of the test for children with a wide range of disabling conditions. Finally, the BDI is compatible with the content and organization of early childhood education programs, and can aid in planning a child's curriculum.

There are many applications for the BDI in a wide range of settings. For example, it can be used to identify strengths and weaknesses in very young children, including those with disabilities. It can be used for general screening, such as that taking place before kindergarten placement. It can also be helpful for instructional planning and development and for measuring student progress (e.g., examining the effects of a new educational program).

There are five domains in the full BDI: Personal–Social, Adaptive, Motor, Communication, and Cognitive, with specific skill areas below each domain. This review is limited to the Cognitive domain. The Cognitive domain consists of 56 items that measure conceptual skills and abilities. This domain is further broken down into four specific skill areas: (1) Perceptual Discrimination, (2) Memory, (3) Reasoning and Academic Skills, and (4) Conceptual Development. Examples of items from these skill areas include matching geometric forms; repeating digits and recalling objects to obtain measures of auditory and visual memory; answering questions about basic concepts, such as "What flies?" and "Why . . . ?" questions; and showing an understanding of such concepts as "big" and "little," "longer" and "shorter," "more" and "less," and early number concepts.

Test Administration and Scoring

The BDI requires a lot of material to administer. The kit is large and bulky, and not all items are included; the examiner must provide certain items, such as ones that demonstrate different textures. In other words, this test cannot be picked up and administered with little forethought. Administration time varies, with a usual maximum of 30–45 minutes for the Cognitive domain.

Items are scored 0, 1, or 2 for failure, partial success, or successful completion, respectively. Criteria for these categories are listed in the manual and are not on the test protocol. Two successful completions in a row at a particular age level are required to get a basal, and two consecutive wrong responses at a particular age level are required to obtain a ceiling. Results for the domain and the subtests are given in standard scores, which are referred to as Developmental Quotients (DQs). Age equivalents are given for the entire domain, but not for each subscale.

Test Standardization

The BDI is a relatively old test, having undergone standardization in 1982 and 1983. A total of 800 children were included in the sample, and they were stratified and composed in order to approximate 1980 U.S.

Census data. They were not stratified on the basis of socioeconomic status, however. About 50 boys and 50 girls were included at each age level.

Reliability

The BDI shows very good reliability, with extremely high coefficients, such as .99 for the BDI total score. Interrater reliability is also high. The standard errors of measurement (SEMs) reported in the manual, however, are perhaps erroneously small. McLinden (1989, cited in Kamphaus, 2001) suggested that the SEMs given are actually the standard errors of the mean, and he gave larger and more realistic SEMs in his article.

Validity

Most validity studies cited by Kamphaus (2001) showed that the BDI has adequate concurrent validity. For example, the BDI Cognitive domain DQ was shown to be correlated .38 with the PPVT-R and .31 with the Stanford–Binet Third Edition Vocabulary subtest. The BDI Cognitive domain DQ and the Bayley Scales of Infant Development Mental score correlated highly, at .93. However, Oehler-Stinnett (1989) suggested that the BDI only has evidence for modest criterion-related validity. She found that the BDI Cognitive domain DQ did not correlate as highly as expected with the Stanford–Binet and WISC-R. She concluded that this means the BDI Cognitive domain is not tapping the same cognitive skills as these other two tests tap.

Summary

The BDI is an individually administered measure of early academic and cognitive skills. The Cognitive domain is usually administered in roughly 30 minutes. Children generally find the test interesting, because it involves many different materials. However, the BDI requires some practice before administration can be fluid. In particular, studying the criteria for failure and success on each item is important. Also, the test does include many parts, and the examiner has to "juggle" these parts quickly and smoothly, especially with an active child. An examiner may find it helpful to have an as-

sistant in the room to help keep the child occupied while the examiner is setting up for the next section.

One drawback for the test is that the standard scores (the DQs) reach a minimum at 65. In order to get lower scores, a complicated formula is given, and these transformed scores are not recommended for use other than by the examiner. Sometimes the DQ scores can be misinterpreted as intelligence quotient (IQ) scores, which is not accurate. Another drawback is that some of the items can be quite verbally loaded. If a child has difficulty expressing him- or herself, or if a speech problem exists that makes understanding the child difficult, the child typically does not do well.

However, an advantage of the BDI is that it can be used with children who are not yet capable of doing tasks that are required by other tests, such as the WPPSI-R. It also has a fairly short administration time, and children's interest is usually maintained by the tasks at hand.

CONCLUSION

More and more emphasis is being placed on early intervention and early identification of developmental delays. As more and more people become aware of, and as research continues to show the benefits of, early intervention, the need for school psychologists and other qualified personnel to administer cognitive tests to the preschool population will only increase. Though there are many caveats to the assessment of preschool children, this kind of assessment can ultimately be beneficial to such children and their families. As long as intelligence tests such as the ones described are not given any more power than they are due (i.e., they are used in conjunction with other tests, observations, and rating scales), and as long as an examiner bases the choice of such tests on a child's presenting problems, they definitely have a solid place in the assessment process. Examiners need to remember to use these tests intelligently. Considering the points discussed in this chapter should help examiners make informed decisions regarding test selection, and should help them be better prepared to encounter the challenges and delights of preschool children.

REFERENCES

Bracken, B. A. (1984). *Bracken Basic Concept Scale.* San Antonio, TX: Psychological Corporation.

Bracken, B. A. (1987). Limitations of preschool instruments and standards for minimal levels of technical adequacy. *Journal of Psychoeducational Assessment, 4,* 313–326.

Bracken, B. A. (1998). *Bracken Basic Concept Scale—Revised.* San Antonio, TX: Psychological Corporation.

Bracken, B. A. (2000). Maximizing construct relevant assessment: The optimal preschool testing situation. In B. A. Bracken (Ed.), *The psychoeducational assessment of preschool children* (pp. 33–44). Boston: Allyn & Bacon.

Bracken, B. A., Bagnato, S. J., & Barnett, D. W. (1991, March 24). *Early childhood assessment.* Position statement adopted by the National Association of School Psychologists Delegate Assembly.

Bracken, B. A., & Walker, K. C. (1997). The utility of intelligence tests for preschool children. In D. P. Flanagan, J. L. Genshaft, & P. L. Harrison (Eds.), *Contemporary intellectual assessment: Theories, tests, and issues* (pp. 484–502). New York: Guilford Press.

Culbertson, J. L., & Willis, D. J. (1993). Introduction to testing young children. In J. L. Culbertson & D. J. Willis (Eds.), *Testing young children: A reference guide for developmental, psychoeducational, and psychosocial assessments* (pp. 1–10). Austin, TX: Pro-Ed.

Elliott, C. D. (1990). *Differential Ability Scales.* San Antonio, TX: Psychological Corporation.

Elliott, C. D., Murray, D. J., & Pearson, L. S. (1979). *British Ability Scales: Directions for administering and scoring (Manual 3).* Windsor, England: National Foundation for Educational Research.

Flanagan, D. P., & Alfonso, V. C. (1995). A critical review of the technical characteristics of new and recently revised intelligence tests for preschool children. *Journal of Psychoeducational Assessment, 13,* 66–90.

Hynd, G. W., & Semrud-Clikeman, M. (1993). Developmental considerations in cognitive assessment of young children. In J. L. Culbertson & D. J. Willis (Eds.), *Testing young children: A reference guide for developmental, psychoeducational, and psychosocial assessments* (pp. 11–28). Austin, TX: Pro-Ed.

Kamphaus, R. K. (2001). *Clinical assessment of child and adolescent intelligence* (2nd ed.). Boston: Allyn & Bacon.

Kamphaus, R. K., Dresden, J., & Kaufman, A. S. (1993). Clinical and psychometric considerations in the cognitive assessment of preschool children. In J. L. Culbertson & D. J. Willis (Eds.), *Testing young children: A reference guide for developmental, psychoeducational, and psychosocial assessments* (pp. 55–72). Austin, TX: Pro-Ed.

Kenny, T. K., & Culbertson, J. L. (1993). Developmental screening for preschoolers. In J. L. Culbertson &

D. J. Willis (Eds.), *Testing young children: A reference guide for developmental, psychoeducational, and psychosocial assessments* (pp. 73–100). Austin, TX: Pro-Ed.

Mather, N., & Woodcock, R. W. (2001). *Examiner's manual: Woodcock–Johnson III Tests of Cognitive Abilities.* Itasca, IL: Riverside.

McLinden, S. E. (1989). An evaluation of the Battelle Developmental Inventory for determining special education eligibility. *Journal of Psychoeducational Assessment, 7,* 66–73.

McLinden, S. E., & Prasse, D. P. (1991). Providing services to infants and toddlers under PL 99-457: Training needs of school psychologists. *School Psychology Review, 20*(1), 37–48.

Nagle, R. J. (2000). Issues in preschool assessment. In B. A. Bracken (Ed.), *The psychoeducational assessment of preschool children* (pp. 19–32). Boston: Allyn & Bacon.

Newborg, J., Stock, J. R., Wnek, L., Guidubaldi, J., & Svinicki, J. (1984). *Battelle Developmental Inventory examiner's manual.* Allen, TX: DLM Teaching Resources.

Oehler-Stinnett, J. (1989). Review of the Battelle Developmental Inventory. In J. C. Conoley & J. J. Kramer (Eds.), *The tenth mental measurement yearbook* (pp. 66–70). Lincoln: University of Nebraska Press.

Riverside Publishing Company. (2000). *Four Score (Version 1. 0)* [Computer software]. Chicago: Author.

Schrank, F. A., & Woodcock, R. W. (2001). *Woodcock– Johnson III: WJ-III Compuscore and Profiles Program* [Computer software]. Itasca, IL: Riverside.

Thorndike, R. L. (1973). *Stanford–Binet Intelligence Scale: Form L-M, 1972 norms tables.* Boston: Houghton Mifflin.

Thorndike, R. L., Hagen, E. P., & Sattler, J. M. (1986). *Stanford–Binet Intelligence Scale: Fourth Edition.* Chicago: Riverside.

Wechsler, D. (1989). *Wechsler Preschool and Primary Scale of Intelligence—Revised.* San Antonio, TX: Psychological Corporation.

Wechsler, D. (1991). *Wechsler Intelligence Scale for Children—Third Edition.* San Antonio, TX: Psychological Corporation.

Wechsler, D. (2002a). *Wechsler Preschool and Primary Scale of Intelligence—Third Edition.* San Antonio, TX: Psychological Corporation.

Wechsler, D. (2000b). *WPPSI-III administration and scoring manual.* San Antonio, TX: Psychological Corporation.

Wechsler, D. (2000c). *WPPSI-III technical and interpretive manual.* San Antonio, TX: Psychological Corporation.

Woodcock, R. W., & Johnson, M. B. (1989). *Woodcock–Johnson Tests of Cognitive Ability—Revised.* Itasca, IL: Riverside.

Woodcock, R. W., McGrew, K. S., & Mather, N. (2001). *Woodcock–Johnson III Tests of Cognitive Abilities.* Itasca, IL: Riverside.

9

Clinical Assessment Practice with the Kaufman Assessment Battery for Children (K-ABC)

RANDY W. KAMPHAUS

The Kaufman Assessment Battery for Children (K-ABC; Kaufman & Kaufman, 1983) has been the subject of scores of research investigations, and is still being used in schools and clinics. In particular, Flanagan (1995) identified the K-ABC as the test of choice for the assessment of intelligence in preschool bilingual children. That the K-ABC has many features to recommend it for clinical assessment is clear from its theoretical foundation, psychometric qualities, administration procedures, and task selection. The intelligence or Mental Processing scales are derived from an aggregate of theories of neuropsychological processing, depending heavily on the cerebral specialization work of Sperry and the neurological research of Luria. The separate processing scales focus on the *process* used to solve a problem (linear/analytic/*sequential,* akin to left-hemisphere thinking, vs. Gestalt/holistic/*simultaneous,* or right-hemisphere processing).

The K-ABC Mental Processing scales are primarily nonverbal. This reflects a deliberate decision by the test authors to enhance fair assessment of minority group members, bilingual children, individuals with speech or language difficulties, and youngsters with learning disabilities, all of whom may fail verbal, fact-oriented items because of their low *achievement,* not low intelligence. The verbal and factual items are included on the K-ABC, but on separate Achievement scales, to facilitate assessment of learning disabilities as well as a fairer estimate of intellectual functioning in minority group members.

Psychometrically, the K-ABC has been praised by Anastasi (1988) as "an innovative, cognitive assessment battery whose development meets high standards of technical quality" (pp. 269–270). A strong empirical foundation is necessary for any test to realize its clinical potential. The K-ABC has other features that make it useful clinically—for example, the inclusion of "teaching items" to help insure that each child understands task demands; a varying set of tasks based on the child's developmental level; several novel subtests and others with a strong research basis; and the use of photographs for several tasks to provide realistic stimuli for evoking clinical responses.

Negative aspects of the K-ABC include a limited "floor" on several subtests for very young children; insufficient "ceiling" to challenge gifted youngsters above the age of 10; the question of whether "ability" and

204

"achievement" can be neatly divided into separate components; and the question of whether the Mental Processing scales truly measure the intended processes, or some other set of skills such as semantic memory and nonverbal reasoning (Keith & Dunbar, 1984). In this chapter, I attempt to integrate the diverse features of the K-ABC as I discuss the test's applicability for clinical assessment of children with special needs. I also consider the use of K-ABC short forms for screening of exceptional children.

CHILDREN WITH MENTAL RETARDATION

If nothing else, an intelligence test must be able to differentiate mental retardation from intellectual normality; it was the need for the accurate diagnosis of mental retardation that led to the development of intelli-

gence tests such as the Binet scales (Binet & Simon, 1905). The K-ABC should yield scores at or near the second percentile rank (standard score ≅ 70) for groups of children who are referred for suspected mental retardation or have already been identified as having mental retardation. Unfortunately, data on referred populations are not available, and data for previously identified children with mental retardation are available, but tainted by confounding variables.

K-ABC data for samples of previously identified children with mental retardation are shown in Table 9.1. Note that the mean Mental Processing Composites (MPCs) range from the middle 60s to about 70. Although these means are acceptable and indicate the K-ABC's utility for these children, they are likely to be abnormally high because of confounding variables such as regression effects and selection bias. For

TABLE 9.1. K-ABC Global Scale and Subtest Standard Score Means for Samples of Children with Mental Retardation

	Sample			
Scale of subtest	Naglieri, 1985a (n = 33)	Nelson, Obrzut, & Cummings, 1984 (n = 30)	Naglieri, 1985a (n = 37)	Obrzut, Nelson, & Obrzut, 1990 (n = 29)
Global scales				
Sequential Processing	77.9	72.4	67.2	72.4
Simultaneous Processing	81.9	72.8	67.7	72.8
Mental Processing Composite	77.8	69.7	65.1	69.7
Achievement	69.7	58.3	64.0	58.3
Mental Processing subtests				
3. Hand Movements	6.9	—	—	7.2
4. Gestalt Closure	8.2	—	—	6.6
5. Number Recall	6.0	—	—	4.0
6. Triangles	7.1	—	—	5.2
7. Word Order	6.1	—	—	4.9
8. Matrix Analogies	6.4	—	—	7.0
9. Spatial Memory	7.0	—	—	5.2
10. Photo Series	7.4	—	—	4.5
Achievement subtests				
12. Faces and Places	78.9	—	—	65.9
13. Arithmetic	75.2	—	—	66.0
14. Riddles	78.5	—	—	70.7
15. Reading/Decoding	70.8	—	—	64.6
16. Reading/Understanding	68.0	—	—	62.6

Note. From Kamphaus and Reynolds (1987, p. 71). Copyright 1987 by American Guidance Service. Reprinted by permission.

example, every experienced psychologist knows that when children with mental retardation are reevaluated, some are declassified; that is, they obtain IQ scores considerably higher than 70. (Adaptive behavior must also be taken into account in classification of mental retardation, of course.) This result is expected, since scores from repeated testings regress toward the mean due to lack of perfect reliability. Since the Wechsler tests do not correlate perfectly with themselves in reevaluations, reevaluation scores will usually be higher than initial evaluation scores, or they will move toward the mean.

The K-ABC was standardized with a sample that overlapped the standardization sample of the Vineland Adaptive Behavior Scales (Sparrow, Balla, & Cicchetti, 1984). The overlap was large enough and the characteristics of the standardization samples of both instruments were similar enough for their normative base to be considered comparable. Thus direct comparisons can be made between the K-ABC and the Vineland—a useful comparison for the classification of mental retardation. The Vineland manuals supply tables indicating differences between K-ABC and Vineland scores that are required for statistical significance.

On the other hand, the K-ABC has some practical limitations that examiners must consider in using the test to diagnose mental retardation. First is the issue of subtest floor. Kamphaus and Reynolds (1987) note that the K-ABC lacks easy items for some children with low functioning. In other words, a 5-year-old child with mental retardation may obtain too many raw scores of 0. This lack of floor is less likely to occur for an 8-year-old child. Second, the K-ABC composite score norms usually do not go below a standard score of 55, making the K-ABC less useful for the diagnosis of moderate or severe levels of retardation. Tests such as the Stanford–Binet Intelligence Scale: Fourth Edition may be better suited for the purpose, since its Composite score norms often go down as low as a standard score of 36. However, a test should never be selected primarily because scores have been extrapolated to very low or high levels. The Stanford–Binet, for example, has questionable norms (Reynolds, 1987); its scale structure

has dubious construct validity support (Reynolds, Kamphaus, & Rosenthal, 1988); and its stability has been challenged for preschool children (Bauer & Smith, 1988). In comparison to the K-ABC's stability for preschool children, the Stanford–Binet did poorly over a 1-year interval for 28 children ages about 4–6 years: The K-ABC MPC produced a test–retest coefficient of .93, whereas the Stanford–Binet Test Composite yielded a value of .20 (Bauer & Smith, 1988).

Although the K-ABC appears appropriate for the diagnosis of mild retardation, there are some cautions for examiners to keep in mind. The K-ABC may not yield scores low enough to diagnose moderate levels of mental retardation. In addition, the K-ABC may yield too many raw scores of 0 for younger children with mental retardation. The examiner who keeps these cautions in clear focus will find the K-ABC appropriate and useful for the diagnosis of mild retardation with many referral cases.

CHILDREN WITH LEARNING DISABILITIES

Mean K-ABC global scale and subtest scores for several samples of children with learning disabilities (LDs) are shown in Table 9.2. An interesting trend appears in these data. In four of the five studies, a profile in which Simultaneous Processing scores were greater than Sequential Processing scores emerged at the global scale level. In these four studies, the average differences between the two scales ranged from 6 to 8 standard-score points. (In the fifth study, the Sequential Processing and Simultaneous Processing mean standard scores were almost identical.) Whether this trend toward different global scale scores is of practical utility is unknown because of the limited research at this time; however, because of its consistency, it cannot be ignored. The trend of Simultaneous Processing > Sequential Processing for children with LDs is reminiscent of the mild trend of Performance > Verbal for the Wechsler Intelligence Scale for Children—Revised (WISC-R) (Kavale & Forness, 1984).

Another pattern of note is that in four of the five studies, the average MPC was greater than the average Achievement scale

TABLE 9.2. K-ABC Global Scale and Subtest Standard Score Means for Samples of Children with Learning Disabilities

	Sample				
Scale of subtest	Naglieri, 1985b ($n = 34$)	Klanderman et al., 1985 ($n = 44$)	Smith, Lyon, Hunter, & Boyd, 1986 ($n = 32$)	Hooper & Hynd, 1985 ($n = 87$)	Fourqurean, 1987 ($n = 42$)
Global scales					
Sequential Processing	92.1	92.7	90.0	86.7	80.5
Simultaneous Processing	99.6	92.3	98.1	92.9	87.7
Mental Processing Composite	96.1	—	94.2	89.0	82.9
Achievement	86.2	87.8	89.8	89.5	67.7
Mental Processing subtests					
3. Hand Movements	8.6	—	—	7.5	6.8
4. Gestalt Closure	11.4	—	—	9.4	9.1
5. Number Recall	8.7	—	—	8.4	7.2
6. Triangles	9.9	—	—	9.6	7.6
7. Word Order	9.1	—	—	7.7	6.5
8. Matrix Analogies	8.5	—	—	7.7	8.2
9. Spatial Memory	9.9	—	—	9.3	8.5
10. Photo Series	10.5	—	—	9.8	7.5
Achievement subtests					
12. Faces and Places	91.6	—	—	89.3	72.8
13. Arithmetic	90.4	—	—	88.9	77.7
14. Riddles	96.9	—	—	96.0	74.0
15. Reading/Decoding	81.2	—	—	87.5	72.2
16. Reading/Understanding	80.8	—	—	93.1	66.4

Note. From Kamphaus and Reynolds (1987, p. 70). Copyright 1987 by American Guidance Service. Reprinted by permission.

score. (Note that Klanderman, Perney, & Kroeschell, 1985, did not present data on the MPC, but the MPC most certainly would be about 92, as opposed to about 88 for the Achievement standard score.) In only one study were the MPC and Achievement standard scores similar (89.0 and 89.5, respectively).

This pattern of MPC > Achievement is strongly reinforced by the results of the study by Fourqurean (1987) for a sample of Latino children with LDs. This group was also documented as having limited proficiency in English. With this group, it appears that the Achievement scale is adversely affected not only by problems with achievement, but also by cultural and/or linguistic differences. In addition, it is noteworthy that in this investigation the authors of the K-ABC met their goal of designing a test that to some extent was able to circumvent linguistic or cultural differences in or-

der to assess intelligence. The mean WISC-R Verbal IQ of 68.1 for these children, for example, was almost identical to their mean Achievement scale score on the K-ABC of 67.7. As a result, the MPC for this sample was considerably higher (82.9) than the Full Scale IQ (76.7). The K-ABC, because it has a separate Achievement scale, may indeed be valuable in those cases where a clinician is presented with the challenge of trying to differentiate among intellectual and cultural or linguistic influences on learning.

The data on the performance of children with LDs on the K-ABC subtests are so limited that any generalizations are tentative. In fact, a number of additional studies using the K-ABC with such children will have to be conducted in order to demonstrate the viability of even global scale profile analysis.

A few preliminary conclusions regarding the use of the K-ABC for children with LDs do seem to be in order. In general, these children's performance on the K-ABC is typically below the population mean. In addition, they are most likely to have their lowest scores on the Sequential Processing and Achievement global scales of the K-ABC.

A study from the Stanford–Binet Fourth Edition technical manual (Thorndike, Hagen, & Sattler, 1986) reinforces these findings. In this study, involving 30 students, the K-ABC MPC and Stanford–Binet Composite means were below average: 94.2 and 92.5, respectively. Furthermore, there was again a mild Simultaneous Processing (97.5) > Sequential Processing (91.9) pattern. Further replications of these findings will support the use of the Sequential and Simultaneous Processing scales to make differential diagnoses for nondisabled children and those with LDs.

The relationship of the K-ABC to neuropsychological measures for samples of public school children with LDs has also been studied. Two studies (Leark, Snyder, Grove, & Golden, 1983; Snyder, Leark, Golden, Grove, & Allison, 1983) have compared the K-ABC to the Luria–Nebraska Neuropsychological Battery—Children's Revision. In the first study (Snyder et al., 1983), the Luria–Nebraska scales were used as predictors of K-ABC composite scores for 46 children ages 8 to $12\frac{1}{2}$ who were referred for evaluation for various types of suspected LDs. The resulting multiple-regression analysis yielded very predictable results. For example, the best predictor of the K-ABC MPC and Sequential Processing, Simultaneous Processing, and Nonverbal scales was the Intelligence scale of the Luria–Nebraska. The best predictor of the K-ABC Achievement scale composite was the Arithmetic scale of the Luria–Nebraska.

In a second and very similar investigation, Leark and colleagues (1983) tested 65 children with LDs with both the K-ABC and the Luria–Nebraska. The obtained intercorrelations were again highly plausible, in that the Intelligence scale of the Luria–Nebraska had among the highest correlations with the K-ABC composite scores. The high correlates of the K-ABC Achievement scale included the Perceptive and Expressive Language, Reading, Arithmetic, and Memory scales of the Luria–Nebraska. There was also some evidence that the K-ABC composite scores may be sensitive indices of brain dysfunction because of the fact that the Pathognomic Signs scale of the Luria–Nebraska was significantly related (correlations ranging from .47 to .65) to *all* of the K-ABC composite scores.

Although the K-ABC correlated in a predictable fashion with the Luria–Nebraska, some less predictable nuances were found in a factor-analytic investigation of the K-ABC for a sample of 198 public school children identified as having LDs (Kaufman & McLean, 1986). In this unusual opportunity to factor-analyze the data for a large sample of such children, a factor structure emerged that showed a strong correspondence between K-ABC scales and WISC-R factors: K-ABC Achievement subtests loaded on the same factor as WISC-R Verbal tasks; K-ABC Simultaneous Processing and WISC-R Performance subtests formed a second factor; and K-ABC Sequential Processing and WISC-R Freedom from Distractibility subtests loaded together on a third factor.

Objective and clinical methods for determining the number of factors to rotate suggested that either three or four factors might be interpreted as meaningful. When four factors were rotated, a separate dyad composed of the two K-ABC reading subtests constituted the fourth factor. Considering that the group was composed of children with LDs, many of whom were identified because their reading ability did *not* correlate with their intelligence, the splitting off of the two reading tasks was an expected outcome. This type of split did *not* occur for a sample of 212 nondiagnosed children tested on both instruments (Kaufman & McLean, 1987). Which interpretation of the factors is correct—the K-ABC labels or the WISC-R labels? The four-factor solution for the sample with LDs suggests that the Wechsler labels might be more appropriate. The Verbal/Achievement dimension, for example, was defined primarily by verbal conceptual and reasoning tasks (WISC-R Vocabulary and Comprehension). In contrast, the three-factor solutions for both the nondiagnosed children and those with LDs seemed to favor a K-ABC approach to factor definition. For the group with LDs, the Verbal/Achievement factor was defined mostlyby factual and school-oriented subtests (WISC-R Information; K-ABC Reading/Understanding and

Riddles). The most sensible approach is to realize that there is no one answer to the question, but that test interpretation depends on understanding a test's constructs for the individual being assessed.

One practical limitation of the K-ABC in LD diagnosis is the lack of several needed academic measures on the K-ABC Achievement scale. In order to assess all possible areas of LDs, the K-ABC Achievement scale must be supplemented with measures of written spelling, mathematics calculation, phonemic awareness, and so on.

INTELLECTUALLY GIFTED CHILDREN

Global scale profiles for gifted children are difficult to discern from the results for the four samples of such children shown in Table 9.3. Two samples, for example, show a Simultaneous Processing > Sequential Pro-

cessing pattern; one shows just the opposite pattern; and the fourth shows no meaningful difference between Sequential Processing and Simultaneous Processing means. This diversity probably results from the many differences in the goals and selection criteria of programs for gifted children.

Some trends are identifiable at the subtest level. Gestalt Closure is one of the worst subtests for gifted children. Apparently, to some extent, the higher the general intelligence (g) loading of the subtest, the more likely it is that samples of gifted children will score higher. Triangles and Matrix Analogies are among the best subtests for these children.

What is most striking, however, in the findings for samples of gifted children is the fact that the K-ABC MPC is consistently lower than the Stanford–Binet and Wechsler IQs for these children. In the Naglieri and Anderson (1985) study, for example, the

TABLE 9.3. K-ABC Global Scale and Subtest Standard Score Means for Samples of Gifted Children

Scale of subtest	Mealor & Curtiss, 1985 (n = 40)	Barry, 1983 (n = 50)	McCallum, Karnes, & Edwards, 1984 (n = 41)	Naglieri & Anderson, 1985 (n = 38)
Global scales				
Sequential Processing	116.7	129.0	114.8	122.4
Simultaneous Processing	122.2	123.3	118.2	122.8
Mental Processing Composite	123.1	130.5	119.2	126.3
Achievement	122.3	126.5	120.2	124.4
Mental Processing subtests				
3. Hand Movements	11.7	13.2	11.9	—
4. Gestalt Closure	12.0	11.9	11.6	—
5. Number Recall	12.8	15.7	13.2	—
6. Triangles	13.6	13.7	12.9	—
7. Word Order	13.4	14.4	11.8	—
8. Matrix Analogies	14.1	14.3	13.7	—
9. Spatial Memory	13.0	13.3	12.6	—
10. Photo Series	12.9	13.1	12.1	—
Achievement subtests				
12. Faces and Places	115.9	118.8	116.9	—
13. Arithmetic	118.5	122.2	116.2	—
14. Riddles	123.4	126.2	116.9	—
15. Reading/Decoding	119.1	119.4	118.3	—
16. Reading/Understanding	115.8	122.6	116.2	—

Note. From Kamphaus and Reynolds (1987, p. 72). Copyright 1987 by American Guidance Service. Reprinted by permission.

K-ABC mean was 126.3, and the WISC-R mean was 134.3. Similar results occurred in other studies. In the McCallum, Karnes, and Edwards (1984) study, the mean Stanford–Binet IQ (1972 edition) was about 16.19 points higher than the mean K-ABC MPC. In the Barry (1983) study, the difference between the Stanford–Binet and K-ABC was about 6.8 points.

A number of factors may be involved in explaining this phenomenon, but two seem to loom largest: selection bias and different norming samples. Both the Naglieri and Anderson (1985) and the McCallum and colleagues (1984) samples were preselected as gifted by individually administered tests such as the 1972 Stanford–Binet and the WISC-R. In other words, individuals with relatively low scores on these tests were not allowed to participate in these studies; this biased the outcome. Linn (1983) and others (e.g., Kaufman, 1972) have written about this problem extensively, and these results exemplify the failure to correct for regression effects when using preselected samples. As can be seen from Figure 9.1, this bias

makes it virtually impossible to compare means in validity studies of this nature, because it artificially inflates the mean of the selection test (in this case, the WISC-R and the Stanford–Binet).

Figure 9.1 illustrates the problem by showing the scatter plot of the relationship (r = .61) between the Stanford–Binet and the K-ABC. Note that if the sample is preselected based on a cutoff score of 130 (as seen by the horizontal line), a number of low scores will be removed from the sample. This seems to eliminate low scores on the selection test (1972 Stanford–Binet; quadrants 3 and 4). As a result, the K-ABC mean is deflated and the 1972 Stanford–Binet mean is inflated. We can get a rough estimate of the magnitude of this problem by computing the amount of regression toward the mean, given the correlation between the K-ABC MPC and the 1972 Stanford–Binet IQ. The correlation between these two measures, as shown in Table 4.21 on page 117 of the K-ABC interpretive manual (Kaufman & Kaufman, 1983), was .61.

Using the mean Stanford–Binet IQ of

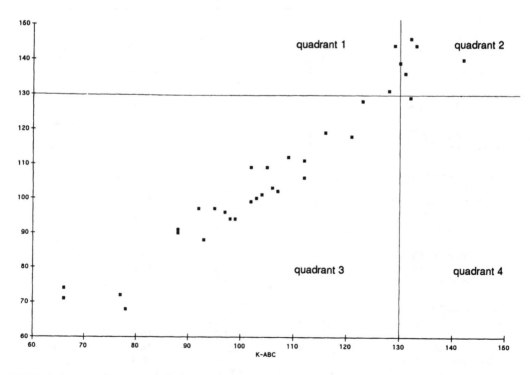

FIGURE 9.1. An illustration of selection bias where the Stanford–Binet is the selection test and the K-ABC is the new test under investigation. From Kamphaus and Reynolds (1987). Copyright 1987 by American Guidance Service. Reprinted by permission.

130.94 for the previously identified gifted sample tested by McCallum and colleagues (1984), and applying the procedure described by Hopkins and Glass (1978) based on the correlation between the two tests, we can obtain a predicted K-ABC MPC of 118.87. The MPC actually obtained for this sample, as shown in Table 9.3, was 119.24. Hence the K-ABC mean MPC can be fairly accurately predicted if we know the mean Stanford–Binet IQ and the correlation between the two tests.

It should be noted that for the Barry (1983) study shown in Table 9.3, the problem of selection bias was avoided by testing a referred sample of gifted children as opposed to an identified (preselected) sample of gifted children. As a result, the children who scored below 130 on the Stanford–Binet remained in the sample.

Even with this referral sample, however, the mean K-ABC MPC was still about 6.8 standard-score points lower than the mean Stanford–Binet IQ. The samples for the four studies cited in Table 9.3 were all children near the upper end of the K-ABC age range. Naglieri and Anderson (1985), using a sample with a mean age of about 11 years, 6 months, found considerable problems with a lack of difficulty on the K-ABC. They noted that perfect subtest scores were obtained 14 times on the WISC-R but 67 times on the K-ABC. This is probably to be expected, since the K-ABC age range goes only to $12\frac{1}{2}$. Examiners should probably use the same logic that they do when selecting other intelligence tests, and always keep the K-ABC age range and the referral questions clearly in mind. In effect, examiners are as likely to experience problems with a lack of difficulty for gifted children on the K-ABC at age 12 as on other tests near the upper end of their age range of application.

CHILDREN WITH EMOTIONAL DISTURBANCE

Pommer (1986) administered the K-ABC and the WISC-R to a group of 59 children with serious emotional disturbance. Individual subtest scores were not reported, but a clear difference was found between the Simultaneous Processing (mean = 82.52) and Sequential Processing (mean = 89.52) scales.

This trend did not emerge for the group of children with behavior disorders cited in the K-ABC interpretive manual (Kaufman & Kaufman, 1983). There are, however, several differences between the Pommer study and the one cited in the manual. In particular, it is interesting that the children in the Pommer study generally scored lower than the group cited in the K-ABC interpretive manual.

The results of the Pommer study have been replicated in other investigations. Hickman and Stark (1987) identified two groups of third and fourth graders as impulsive (n = 27) versus nonimpulsive (n = 18), using latency scores from the Matching Familiar Figures Test (Kagan & Salkind, 1965). They found that whereas nonimpulsive children differed from impulsive children by only 5 points on the Sequential Processing scale, they scored, on average, 11 points higher than the impulsive children on the Simultaneous Processing scale. Overall, impulsive children scored lower than nonimpulsive children on all of the K-ABC global scales, with Simultaneous Processing showing the most pronounced deficit.

A group of children with autism also showed a trend in favor of Simultaneous Processing (Freeman, Lucas, Forness, & Ritvo, 1985). This study involved 21 children ages 6 through 12 years. Although this sample obtained a 4-point advantage on the Sequential Processing scale (Simultaneous Processing mean = 98.2, Sequential Processing mean = 101.9), they performed relatively poorly on the Achievement scale (mean = 92.8).

These three early investigations indicate that perhaps many children with behavioral or emotional disturbance who are tested with the K-ABC can attend to the brief stimuli on the Sequential Processing scale, but have problems sustaining attention and concentration on the more involved Simultaneous Processing scale items. In any case, this finding requires replication, as it is still purely speculative.

CHILDREN WITH HEARING IMPAIRMENTS

At least three studies have evaluated the utility of the K-ABC Nonverbal scale with children who have severe hearing impairments (Ham, 1985; Porter & Kirby, 1986; Ulissi, Brice, & Gibbons, 1985). All of these studies found that these children, even residential populations, scored in the average range when a pantomimed administration of the K-ABC Nonverbal scale was used (see Table 9.4). The mean Nonverbal scale standard score for the Porter and Kirby (1986) sample was 98.8; for the Ham (1985) sample, 96.5; and for the Ulissi and colleagues (1985) sample, 100.7. Although the samples for these studies were relatively small, the trend is clear: Children with hearing impairments have relatively normal intelligence as assessed by the K-ABC Nonverbal scale.

The Porter and Kirby (1986) study also tested the utility of pantomimed versus sign language administrations of the K-ABC Nonverbal scale. The means for the pantomimed and sign language administration groups were 98.8 and 96.8, respectively. For this relatively small sample, this difference was not statistically significant. These results argue for using the K-ABC Nonverbal scale as it was originally designed, in pantomime.

CHILDREN WITH BRAIN INJURIES

A few investigations have examined the use of the K-ABC for children with brain injuries. Morris and Bigler (1985) investigated the relationship of the K-ABC and WISC-R to hemispheric functioning for 79 children seen at a neurology clinic. These children had received intensive neurological evaluations, including computed axial tomography (CAT) scans, electroencephalograms (EEGs), and neuropsychological evaluations with the Halstead–Reitan. Based on the neuropsychological test results, composite scores were computed for right- and left-hemisphere functioning, and these scores were correlated with Verbal and Performance scores from the WISC-R and Sequential and Simultaneous Processing scores from the K-ABC. The main conclusion from this study was that the K-ABC Sequential and Simultaneous Processing scales were more highly related to right-hemisphere (Simultaneous Processing) and left-hemisphere (Sequential Processing) functioning than the Wechsler scales. The authors concluded further that the main reason for this finding

TABLE 9.4. K-ABC Global Scale and Subtest Standard Score Means for Samples of Children with Hearing Impairments

	Sample		
Scale of subtest	Ullssi, Brice, & Gibbons, 1985 (n = 50)	Ham, 1985 (n = 17)	Porter & Kirby 1986 (n = 25)[a]
Global scales			
Sequential Processing	87.9	—	—
Simultaneous Processing	101.2	—	—
Mental Processing Composite	95.3	—	—
Nonverbal	100.7	96.5	98.8
Subtests			
3. Hand Movements	10.3	8.2	10.6
4. Gestalt Closure	10.7	—	—
5. Number Recall	7.1	—	—
6. Triangles	10.3	10.7	11.0
7. World Order	6.5	—	—
8. Matrix Analogies	10.2	11.0	9.3
9. Spatial Memory	9.3	9.1	9.1
10. Photo Series	10.1	8.6	9.4
12. Faces and Places	—	11.8	—

Note. From Kamphaus and Reynolds (1987, p. 75). Copyright 1987 by American Guidance Service. Reprinted by permission.
[a]These data are for the group in this study that received pantomimed as opposed to American Sign Language instructions.

was that the WISC-R was not able to diagnose right-hemisphere dysfunction at a significant level.

Similar findings resulted in a smaller scale investigation of 27 children with brain injuries by Shapiro and Dotan (1985). These investigators also used EEGs, CAT scans, and other measures to norm groups of children with focal right- and left-hemisphere damage. These authors corroborated the results of Morris and Bigler (1985) by finding a K-ABC Sequential Processing < Simultaneous Processing pattern for the majority of children with left-hemisphere findings, and a Simultaneous Processing < Sequential Processing pattern for the majority of children with right-hemisphere findings. The predicted patterns were even more accurate for right-handed boys. In direct contrast, the relationship of the WISC-R Verbal and Performance scales to hemispheric functioning was unclear. Shapiro and Dotan concluded that, as compared to K-ABC, the lack of relationship between WISC-R Verbal–Performance differences and neurological findings may reflect lack of homogeneity of function assessed by those scales.

These results for children with brain injuries suggested that the K-ABC's Sequential–Simultaneous Processing dichotomy may have an intuitive relationship to left- and right-hemisphere cognitive functions as defined by the split-brain research tradition. There is, however, a great need for research that will clarify this relationship, since moderator variables (such as gender and handedness) may confound the findings for an individual child. Even though there is some relationship between the K-ABC and localization of function, this does not make the K-ABC particularly useful for localizing damage. The K-ABC may, on the other hand, be useful for identifying analytic or holistic processing dysfunction.

AT-RISK PRESCHOOLERS

Several studies have evaluated the use of the K-ABC in the assessment of high-risk preschoolers. Lyon and Smith (1986) compared the performance of high-risk (n = 44) and low-risk (n = 49) preschoolers ranging in age from 45 to 70 months. In all cases, the mean K-ABC global scales were significantly lower for the high-risk than for the low-risk preschoolers. The mean K-ABC Sequential and Simultaneous Processing, MPC, and Achievement standard scores for the high-risk group ranged from 89.3 to 92.5, consistently below average.

In a concurrent validity study, Smith and Lyon (1987) administered the K-ABC and the McCarthy Scales of Children's Abilities to groups of repeating (n = 13) and nonrepeating (n = 27) preschoolers. The K-ABC and McCarthy Scales both discriminated between the group recommended for retention in a preschool program and the group recommended for advancement to kindergarten. The mean MPC for the repeating preschoolers was 76.2 and for the nonrepeating preschoolers was 91.4. Similarly, other K-ABC global scales were lower for the repeating group (Sequential Processing mean = 80.3, Simultaneous Processing mean = 77.5, Achievement mean = 80.5) than for the nonrepeating group (Sequential Processing mean = 91.3, Simultaneous Processing mean = 93.4, Achievement mean = 94.7).

Ricciardi and Voelker (1987) essentially cross-validated the findings of Smith and Lyon (1987) by testing four groups of preschoolers with the K-ABC: nondisabled children (n = 15), children with language impairments (n = 14), children with behavior problems (n = 17), and children with both types of problems (n = 13). Again, the K-ABC clearly discriminated between the nondisabled and disabled groups. The nondisabled children had a mean MPC of 104.0, while the means for the remaining groups were as follows: children with language impairments, 83.1; children with behavior problems, 95.3; and children with both types of problems, 77.0.

As I have noted elsewhere (Kamphaus, 2001), several characteristics of the K-ABC make it attractive for use with preschoolers. These include its relative brevity, attractive materials, simple examiner instructions, theoretical model, and sample and teaching items. On the other hand, the K-ABC has some weaknesses when used with preschoolers, including ceiling (too many perfect raw scores) and floor (too many raw scores of 0) effects, a lack of assessment of expressive language, and a lack of manipulatives.

K-ABC SHORT FORMS

Applegate and Kaufman (1988) developed short forms of the K-ABC, which may be useful when only general measures of mental processing and achievement that can be administered in relatively brief amounts of time are needed. Examples of uses of short forms include preschool screening for identification of "at-risk" or potentially gifted children, research, and certain clinical or educational circumstances. Although the administration of a short form can never replace the multiple scores and clinical evaluations obtained from administration of a complete battery, short forms of the K-ABC demonstrate excellent psychometric properties and offer useful estimates of functioning.

Extensive analysis of the reliability and validity of various combinations of subtests led to the selection of the following short forms for ages 4 through 12½ years. (Short forms were not developed for younger children, because the K-ABC is already relatively brief for these ages.)

Mental Processing Dyad: Triangles, Word Order

Mental Processing Triad: Triangles, Word Order, Matrix Analogies

Mental Processing Tetrad: Hand Movements, Triangles, Word Order, Matrix Analogies

Achievement Dyad: Riddles, Reading/Decoding

Mean reliability coefficients for the short forms are excellent, ranging from .88 to .93. Although the corrected validity coefficient between the Mental Processing Dyad and the complete K-ABC is a marginal .80, the remaining short forms demonstrate excellent validity, with corrected coefficients of .86 for the Mental Processing Triad, .88 for the Mental Processing Tetrad, and .93 for the Achievement Dyad. Applegate and Kaufman (1988) recommend using either the Mental Processing Triad or Tetrad along with the Achievement Dyad whenever a short form of the K-ABC is needed. Applegate and Kaufman provide equations for computing Estimated MPC and Achievement standard scores ($\overline{X} = 100$, $SD = 15$), based on the sum of subtest scaled or standard scores ($\overline{X}_c$). The word "Estimated" should be used whenever scores from short forms are reported.

CONCLUSIONS

Those seeking a more comprehensive overview of all aspects of the K-ABC are referred elsewhere (Kamphaus, 2001). The K-ABC, however, is likely to change substantially in the future as it undergoes a comprehensive revision. Given the known creativity of Alan and Nadeen Kaufman, one can expect numerous changes of interesting nature. These changes will merit careful consideration by the field of child intelligence testing.

REFERENCES

Anastasi, A. (1988). *Psychological testing* (6th ed.). New York: Macmillan.

Applegate, B., & Kaufman, A. S. (1988). Short form estimation of K-ABC Sequential and Simultaneous Processing for research and screening purposes. *Journal of Clinical Child Psychology, 17,* 359–360.

Barry, B. J. (1983). *Validity study of the Kaufman Assessment Battery for Children compared to the Stanford–Binet, Form L-M, in the identification of gifted nine- and ten-year-olds.* Unpublished master's thesis, National College of Education, Chicago.

Bauer, J. J., & Smith, D. K. (1988, April). *Stability of the K-ABC and S-B: 4 with preschool children.* Paper presented at the meeting of the National Association of School Psychologists, Chicago.

Binet, A., & Simon, T. (1905). Méthodes nouvelles pour le diagnostic du niveau intellectuel des anormaux. *L'Année Psychologique, 11,* 191–244.

Flanagan, R. (1995) The utility of the Kaufman Assessment Battery for Children (K-ABC) and the Wechsler intelligences scales for linguistically different children: Clinical considerations. *Psychology in the Schools, 32*(1), 5–11.

Fourqurean, J. M. (1987). A K-ABC and WISC-R comparison for Latino learning-disabled children of limited English proficiency. *Journal of School Psychology, 25,* 15–21.

Freeman, B. J., Lucas, J. C., Forness, S. R., & Ritvo, E. R. (1985). Cognitive processing of high-functioning autistic children: Comparing the K-ABC and the WISC-R. *Journal of Psychoeducational Assessment, 3,* 357–362.

Ham, S. J. (1985). *A validity study of recent intelligence tests on a deaf population.* (Available from the author, School Psychologist, North Dakota School for the Deaf, Devils Lake, ND 58301)

Hickman, J. A., & Stark, K. D. (1987, April). *Relationship between cognitive impulsivity and information* processing abilities in children: Implications for training programs. Paper presented at the meeting of the National Association of School Psychologists, New Orleans.

Hooper, J. R., & Hynd, G. W. (1985). Differential diagnosis of subtypes of developmental dyslexia with the Kaufman Assessment Battery for Children (K-ABC). *Journal of Clinical Child Psychology, 14,* 145–152.

Hopkins, K. D., & Glass, G. V. (1978). *Basic statistics for the behavioral sciences.* Englewood Cliffs, NJ: Prentice-Hall.

Kagan, J., & Salkind, N. J. (1965). *Matching Familiar Figures Test.* (Available from J. Kagan, Harvard University, 33 Kirkland Street, 1510 William James Hall, Cambridge, MA 02138)

Kamphaus, R. W. (2001). *Clinical assessment of children's intelligence* (2nd ed.). Needham Heights, MA: Allyn & Bacon.

Kamphaus, R. W., & Reynolds, C. R. (1987). *Clinical and research applications of the K-ABC.* Circle Pines, MN: American Guidance Service.

Kaufman, A. S. (1972, May). *Restriction of range: Questions and answers* (Test Service Bulletin No. 59). New York: Psychological Corporation.

Kaufman, A. S., & Kaufman, N. L. (1983). *Interpretive manual for the Kaufman Assessment Battery for Children.* Circle Pines, MN: American Guidance Service.

Kaufman, A. S., & McLean, J. E. (1986). K-ABC/WISC-R factor analysis for a learning disabled population. *Journal of Learning Disabilities, 19,* 145–153.

Kaufman, A. S., & McLean, J. E. (1987). Joint factor analysis of the K-ABC and WISC-R with normal children. *Journal of School Psychology, 25,* 105–118.

Kavale, K. A., & Forness, S. R. (1984). A meta-analysis of the validity of Wechsler scale profiles and recategorizations: Patterns or parodies. *Learning Disability Quarterly, 7,* 136–156.

Keith, T. Z., & Dunbar, S. B. (1984). Hierarchical factor analysis of the K-ABC: Testing alternate models. *Journal of Special Education, 18,* 367–375.

Klanderman, J. W., Perney, J., & Kroeschell, Z. B. (1985, April). *Comparisons of the K-ABC and WISC-R for LD children.* Paper presented at the meeting of the National Association of School Psychologists, Las Vegas, NV.

Leark, R. A., Snyder, T., Grove, T., & Golden, C. J. (1983, August). *Comparison of the K-ABC to standardized neuropsychological batteries: Preliminary results.* Paper presented at the meeting of the American Psychological Association, Anaheim, CA.

Linn, R. L. (1983). Pearson selection formulas: Implications for studies of predictive bias and estimates of educational effects in selected samples. *Journal of Educational Measurement, 20,* 1–15.

Lyon, M. A., & Smith, D. K. (1986). A comparison of at-risk preschool children's performance on the K-ABC, McCarthy Scales, and Stanford–Binet. *Journal of Psychoeducational Assessment, 4,* 35–43.

McCallum, R. S., Karnes, F. A., & Edwards, R. P. (1984), The test of choice for assessment of gifted

children: A comparison of the K-ABC, WISC-R, and Stanford–Binet. *Journal of Psychoeducational Assessment, 21,* 57–63.

Mealor, D. J., & Curtiss, D. J. (1985, April). *Comparative analysis of the K-ABC and WISC-R for selected minority students.* Paper presented at the meeting of the National Association of School Psychologists, Las Vegas, NV.

Morris, J. M., & Bigler, E. (1985, January). *An investigation of the Kaufman Assessment Battery for Children (K-ABC) with neurologically impaired children.* Paper presented at the meeting of the International Neuropsychological Society, San Diego, CA.

Naglieri, J. A. (1985a). Assessment of mentally retarded children with the Kaufman Assessment Battery for Children. *American Journal of Mental Deficiency, 89,* 367–371.

Naglieri, J. A. (1985b). Use of the WISC-R and K-ABC with learning disabled, borderline, mentally retarded, and normal children. *Psychology in the Schools, 22,* 133–141.

Naglieri, J. A., & Anderson, D. F. (1985). Comparison of the WISC-R and K-ABC with gifted students. *Journal of Psychoeducational Assessment, 3,* 175–179.

Nelson, R. B., Obrzut, A., & Cummings, J. (1984). *Construct and predictive validity of the K-ABC with EMR children.* (Available from R. Brett Nelson, Weld County School District #6, Greeley, CO 80631)

Obrzut, A., Nelson, R. B., & Obrzut, J. E. (1990). Construct validity of the K-ABC with mildly mentally retarded students. *American Journal of Mental Deficiency.*

Pommer, L. T. (1986). Seriously emotionally disturbed children's performance on the Kaufman Assessment Battery for Children: A concurrent validity study. *Journal of Psychoeducational Assessment, 4,* 155–162.

Porter, L. J., & Kirby, E. A. (1986). Effects of two instructional sets on the validity of the Kaufman Assessment Battery for Children—Nonverbal Scale with a group of severely hearing impaired children. *Psychology in the Schools, 23,* 1–6.

Reynolds, C. R. (1987). Playing IQ roulette with the Stanford–Binet, 4th edition. *Measurement and Evaluation in Counseling and Development, 20,* 139–141.

Reynolds, C. R., Kamphaus, R. W., & Rosenthal, B. (1988). Factor analysis of the Stanford–Binet Fourth Edition for ages 2 years through 23 years. *Movement and Evaluation in Counseling and Development, 21,* 52–63.

Ricciardi, P. W. R., & Volker, S. L. (1987, August). *Measuring cognitive skills of language impaired preschoolers with the K-ABC.* Paper presented at the annual meeting of the American Psychological Association, New York.

Shapiro, E. G., & Dotan, N. (1985, October). *Neurological findings and the Kaufman Assessment Battery for Children.* Paper presented at the meeting of the National Association of Neuropsychologists, Philadelphia.

Smith, D. K., & Lyon, M. A. (1987). *K-ABC/Mc-*

Carthy performance for repeating and nonrepeating preschoolers. Paper presented at the annual meeting of the National Association of School Psychologists, New Orleans. (ERIC Document Reproduction Service No. ED 280889)

Smith, D. K., Lyon, M. A., Hunter, E., & Boyd, R. (1986, April). *Relationships between the K-ABC and WISC-R for students referred for severe learning disabilities.* Paper presented at the meeting of the National Association of School Psychologists, Hollywood, FL.

Snyder, T. J., Leark, R. A., Golden, C. J., Grove, T., & Allison, R. (1983, March). *Correlations of the K-ABC, WISC-R, and Luria–Nebraska Children's Bat-tery for exceptional children.* Paper presented at the meeting of the National Association of School Psychologists, Detroit, MI.

Sparrow, S. S., Balla, D. A., & Cicchetti, D. V. (1984). *Vineland Adaptive Behavior Scales.* Circle Pines, MN: American Guidance Service.

Thorndike, R. L., Hagen, E. P., & Sattler, J. M. (1986). *Technical manual for the Stanford–Binet Intelligence Scale: Fourth Edition.* Chicago: Riverside.

Ulissi, S. M., Brice, P. J., & Gibbons, S. (1985, April). *The use of the Kaufman Assessment Battery for Children with the hearing impaired.* Paper presented at the meeting of the National Association of School Psychologists, Las Vegas, NV.

10

Stanford–Binet Intelligence Scale: Fourth Edition (SB4): Evaluating the Empirical Bases for Interpretations

ERIC A. YOUNGSTROM
JOSEPH J. GLUTTING
MARLEY W. WATKINS

The Stanford–Binet Intelligence Scale: Fourth Edition (SB4; Thorndike, Hagen, & Sattler, 1986b) is the most recent edition in a line of instruments going back almost a century (viz., Binet & Simon, 1905). The 1986 revision revitalized the Stanford–Binet by both maintaining links with previous editions of the scale and simultaneously incorporating more recent developments found in other popular tests of intelligence. The SB4 retains as much item content as possible from the Stanford–Binet Intelligence Scale: Form L-M (SB-LM; Thorndike, 1973). SB4 also respects tradition by covering approximately the same age range as SB-LM (ages 2–23); it incorporates familiar basal and ceiling levels during testing; and it provides an overall score that appraises general cognitive functioning. As this chapter is being written, the fifth edition of the Stanford–Binet (SB5) is beginning item tryouts in preparation for standardization. The plan for this newest edition also shares a commitment both to the Stanford–Binet tradition and to incorporating current theories about psychometrics (e.g., item response theory) and the structure of intelligence.

Despite these similarities, these revisions are substantially different from their predecessors. The SB4 eliminated the traditional age scale format. In its place are 15 subtests whose age-corrected scaled scores make it possible to interpret profile elevations and profile depressions. Four "area" scores, derived from theoretically based subtest groupings, are also new. These reformulations add to interpretative possibilities, and they attempt to broaden the coverage of cognitive ability over that offered by SB-LM. SB4 permits calculation of the Composite (overall IQ) for performances based on specific "abbreviated batteries," as well as for *any* combination of subtests psychologists wish to regroup—promoting flexibility in administration and interpretation.

This chapter familiarizes readers with the structure and content of SB4. It also evaluates selected aspects of the test's psychometric and technical properties. In addition, we hope to sensitize psychologists to factors pertinent to the administration of SB4 and to the interpretation of its test scores. The chapter aims to present a balanced treatment of strengths and limitations. The highest professional standards were applied throughout the development of SB4. Prior to publication, the authors and publisher dedicated over 8 years to development and 2 years to extensive data analyses of the final product. Thus, it is no surprise that we identify unique and praiseworthy features. Similarly, no test is without faults, and this thought should place the potential shortcomings of SB4 in context.

The first section of this chapter outlines the theoretical model underlying SB4. We turn then to a general description of the structure of SB4 and issues related to its test materials, administration, and scaling. Thereafter, we discuss the strengths and weaknesses associated with SB4's standardization, its reliability and validity, and factors related to the interpretation of its test scores. Finally, we take a look at the development of SB5.

THEORETICAL FOUNDATION

Perhaps the most fundamental change incorporated into SB4 is the expansion of its theoretical model. Figure 10.1 shows that SB4 has three levels, which serve both traditional and new Binet functions. At the apex is the Composite, or estimate of general ability, traditionally associated with Binet scales. The second level is new to SB4. It proposes three group factors: Crystallized Abilities, Fluid-Analytic Abilities, and Short-Term Memory. The first two dimensions originate from the Cattell–Horn theory of intelligence (Cattell, 1940; Horn, 1968; Horn & Cattell, 1966). These are shaded in the figure, because the published interpretive system for the SB4 does not emphasize the calculation of observed scores corresponding with these factors. The additional component, Short-Term Memory, is not contained in the Cattell–

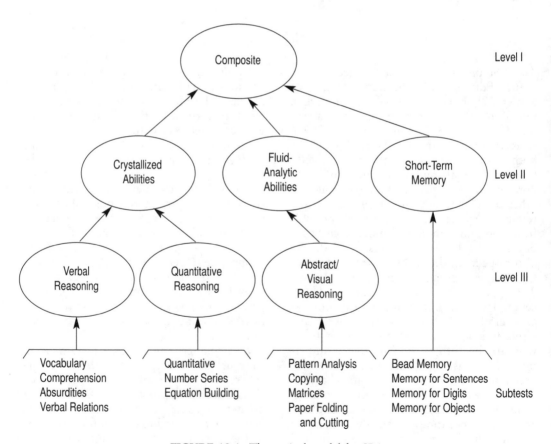

FIGURE 10.1. Theoretical model for SB4.

Horn theory. Its inclusion reflects the way in which psychologists used previous editions of the Binet (Thorndike, Hagen, & Sattler, 1986a); to some extent, it also reflects factor-analytic work with other intelligence tests, suggesting that short-term memory is related to long-term memory and to more complex learning and problem solving (Thorndike, Hagen, & Sattler, 1986c).

The third level illustrates another difference between the SB4 and earlier editions of the scale. Here, factors are identified in terms of three facets of reasoning: Verbal Reasoning, Quantitative Reasoning, and Abstract/Visual Reasoning. These components resemble the third level of Vernon's (1950) hierarchical model of intelligence, wherein well-known Verbal–Educational and Practical–Mechanical factors are subdivided to obtain even more homogeneous estimates of ability. Vernon, for example, splits the Verbal–Educational factor into the scholastic content of verbal fluency, numerical operations, and so on. SB4 follows this orientation by incorporating dimensions for the assessment of Verbal Reasoning and Quantitative Reasoning. Similarly, SB4's Abstract/Visual Reasoning dimension parallels the Practical–Mechanical component of the Vernon model.

The three group factors at the third level (Verbal Reasoning, Quantitative Reasoning, Abstract/Visual Reasoning), plus the Short-Term Memory factor at the second level, form the four "area" scores derived by SB4. The Abstract/Visual Reasoning score at the third level corresponds to the Fluid-Analytic Abilities dimension at the second level. No area score is readily available for the third dimension at the second level, Crystallized Abilities; nevertheless, scores for this broadband factor can be estimated by collapsing results across the remaining two of the four areas (Verbal Reasoning and Quantitative Reasoning).

Thus the SB4 model is an eclectic unification of multiple theories of intelligence. Such synthesis is not unique to SB4. The Kaufman Assessment Battery for Children (K-ABC; Kaufman & Kaufman, 1983) also accounts for test performance through interrelationships among theories (i.e., the Luria–Das and Cattell–Horn theories of ability). In addition, both tests share the desirable quality of using explicit theoretical frameworks as guides for item development and for the alignment of subtests within modeled hierarchies.

TEST STRUCTURE

Subtest Names and Content

SB4's subtests retain some reliable variance that is distinct from the score variation captured by area scores or the Composite. Because of this specificity within each subtest, the developers described the "unique abilities" evaluated by SB4's subtests. Profile analysis is a popular method for explicating an examinee's strengths and weaknesses on these abilities (see Delaney & Hopkins, 1987; Naglieri, 1988a, 1988b; Rosenthal & Kamphaus, 1988; Sattler, 1992; Spruill, 1988). Therefore, inasmuch as SB4 supports comparisons among subtest scores, it is worthwhile to understand the identity and composition of these measures.

Descriptions of the 15 SB4 subtests are provided in Table 10.1, organized according to the theoretical area each occupies in the scale.

Content Similarity with Other IQ Tests

SB4 items appear representative of the item content found in intelligence tests (see Jensen, 1980, for a detailed analysis of item types common among IQ tests). Visual inspection reveals that six SB4 subtests share core content with the Wechsler Intelligence Scale for Children—Third Edition (WISC-III; Wechsler, 1991). For example, both SB4 Vocabulary and WISC-III Vocabulary assess word knowledge. SB4 Comprehension and WISC-III Comprehension measure breadth of knowledge of social and interpersonal situations, and the visual-perceptual abilities evaluated by SB4 Pattern Analysis generally apply to WISC-III Block Design. Likewise, there are marked similarities between the SB4 Quantitative subtest and WISC-III Arithmetic, between SB4 Memory for Digits and WISC-III Digit Span, and between SB4 Verbal Relations and WISC-III Similarities. Resemblances in subtest content are also ap-

TABLE 10.1. SB4 Subtests: Age Range, Median Reliability, and Content

Area/subtest	Ages	Reliability	Content
Verbal Reasoning			
Vocabulary	2–23	.87	Examinees supply word definitions. The first 15 items tap receptive word knowledge (examinees name pictured objects), and items 16 through 46 are presented both orally and in writing vocabulary.
Comprehension	2–23	.89	Items 1 through 6 require the receptive identification of body parts. Items 7 through 42 elicit verbal responses associated with practical problem solving and social information.
Absurdities	2–14	.87	This subtest presents situations that are essentially false or contrary to common sense. Examinees point to the inaccurate picture among three alternatives (items 1 through 4), or they verbalize the absurdity in a single picture (items 5 through 32).
Verbal Relations	12–23	.91	Examinees state how three words, out of a four-word set, are similar. The fourth word in each item is always different from the three words preceding it.
Quantitative Reasoning			
Quantitative	2–23	.88	Examinees are required to count, add, seriate, or complete other numerical operations (e.g., count the number of blocks pictured; how many 12″ by 12″ tiles would be needed to cover a floor that is 7 feet by 9 feet?).
Number Series	7–23	.90	A row of four or more numbers is presented, and the task is to identify the principle underlying a series of four or more numbers and to apply that principle to generate the next two numbers in the series (e.g., 1, 3, 7, 15, __, __).
Equation Building	12–23	.91	Examinees resequence numerals and mathematical signs into a correct solution (e.g., 15, 12, 2, 25, =, +, −).
Abstract/Visual Reasoning			
Pattern Analysis	2–23	.92	Items 1 through 6 require examinees to complete formboards. Items 7 through 42 involve the replication of visual patterns through block manipulations.
Copying	2–13	.87	Examinees either reproduce block models (items 1 through 12) or draw geometric designs, such as lines, rectangles, and arcs, that are shown on cards (items 13 through 28).
Matrices	7–23	.90	Each item presents a matrix of figures in which one element is missing. The task is to identify the correct element among multiple-choice alternatives.
Paper Folding and Cutting	12–23	.94	Figures are presented in which a piece of paper has been folded and cut. Examinees chose among alternatives that show how the paper might look if it were unfolded.
Short-Term Memory			
Bead Memory	2–23	.87	Examinees recall the identity of one or two beads exposed briefly (items 1 through 10), or they reproduce bead models in a precise sequence (items 11 through 42).
Memory for Sentences	2–23	.89	Examinees are required to repeat each word in a sentence in the exact order of presentation.
Memory for Digits	7–23	.83	Examinees repeat digits either in the sequence they are presented, or in reverse order.
Memory for Objects	7–23	.73	Pictures of objects are viewed briefly. Examinees then identify the objects in correct order from a larger array.

parent between SB4 and the K-ABC. The four most striking parallels occur between (1) SB4 Pattern Analysis and K-ABC Triangles, (2) SB4 Matrices and K-ABC Matrix Analogies, (3) SB4 Memory for Digits and K-ABC Number Recall, and (4) SB4 Memory for Objects and K-ABC Word Order. These comparisons suggest that there exists a core set of subtests (generally including those with the highest *g* saturation) that are shared across commonly used measures of ability.

MATERIALS

Three manuals accompany SB4: the *Guide for Administering and Scoring* (Thorndike et al., 1986a), the *Technical Manual* (Thorndike et al., 1986c), and the supplementary *Examiner's Handbook* (Delaney & Hopkins, 1987). All three manuals are well written and informative. Chapters pertinent to test administration are especially well organized in the *Examiner's Handbook*. Psychologists new to SB4 are encouraged to read these sections of the handbook prior to reviewing the *Guide for Administering and Scoring*.

SB4 materials are attractive, well packaged, and suitable to the age groups for which they are applied. The Bead Memory subtest is a noteworthy exception. Directions for Bead Memory caution psychologists to **"BE SURE THAT EXAMINEES DO NOT PLAY WITH THE BEADS. THERE IS A DANGER THAT YOUNG EXAMINEES MAY TRY TO PUT THE BEADS IN THEIR MOUTHS"** (Thorndike et al., 1986b, p. 23; boldface capitals in original). This caution is insufficient for the danger presented. Two of the four bead types fit easily in a "choke tube"—an apparatus used to determine whether objects are sufficiently small that young children will gag or suffocate on them. Psychologists, therefore, should *never* allow young children to play with these objects.[1]

Publishers are increasingly adding color to test stimuli. Rich colors enhance the attractiveness of test stimuli, and they have the positive effect of making test materials more child-oriented (Husband & Hayden, 1996). Color helps to maintain children's interest during testing, and it augments the probability of obtaining valid test scores. However, sometimes color is not equally salient or perceptually unambiguous to examinees. Such a situation can arise when persons with color-blindness are being assessed. For these individuals, color represents an additional source of score variance that can reduce test validity. They are most likely to experience difficulty when confronted by the following color combinations: red–brown, green–orange, red–grey, blue–purple, and red–green (Coren, Ward, & Enns, 1999).

Two examples are presented where color may alter SB4 item difficulties. Item 1 of the Vocabulary subtest shows a red car on a brown background. This color combination makes it more difficult for some individuals with color-blindness to distinguish the important foreground stimulus (the car) from its background. Another example can be seen in the formboard items in Pattern Analysis. The red puzzle pieces and green background make the formboard more difficult for examinees with red–green color blindness. (See also Husband & Hayden, 1996, for an investigation of the effects of varying stimulus color on several SB4 subtests.) Fortunately, the problems associated with color stimuli can be corrected by simply *not* pairing these colors within test items. By adopting such changes, test publishers will be able to continue offering the benefits of color stimuli and simultaneously reduce the visual discrimination problems of examinees with color-blindness.

ADMINISTRATION

SB4 uses "adaptive testing" to economize on administration time. This format offers the added benefit of decreasing frustration, because examinees are exposed only to those test items most appropriate to their ability level. The Vocabulary subtest serves as a "routing" measure at the beginning of each assessment. Performance on the Vocabulary subtest, in conjunction with an examinee's chronological age, is used to determine the appropriate entry level for succeeding subtests. Entry levels are arranged hierarchically by item pairs (labeled "A" through "Q" on the test protocol). Basal and ceiling rules are then applied within subtests. A basal level is established when all items are passed at two consecutive levels. A ceiling is reached, and testing advances to the next subtest, when three failures (out of four possible) take place across adjacent levels. There is some concern that the entry levels may be too high for youths and adults with mental retardation (Sattler, 1992; Spruill, 1991). This routing system also can be confusing to examiners unfamiliar with the SB4 testing format (Vernon, 1987; Wersh & Thomas, 1990). Supervisors and instructors should make certain that trainees are comfortable navigating the routing system (Choi & Proctor, 1994), and trainees should be vigilant for possible difficulty at subtest entry points when testing children with suspected cognitive deficits.

SB4 deserves credit for its efficient testing format and for directions that are readable and straightforward. In contrast to SB-LM, SB4 administration is simpler due to such features as incorporating most of the directions, stimuli, and scoring criteria within the easel kits. The use of sample items helps familiarize examinees with directions and item formats prior to actual testing. In addition, SB4 is a "power" test (as opposed to a "speeded" test; Anastasi & Urbina, 1997). Pattern Analysis is the only subtest requiring mandatory time limits. Doing away with the need for accurate timekeeping coincidentally makes SB4's administration more convenient.

Administration times appear reasonable. The *Technical Manual* (Thorndike et al., 1986c) does not offer administration times by age level. Delaney and Hopkins (1987) provide administration times by entry level (A through M or higher), and we used this information to approximate testing times by age. Based on these estimates, testing would take between 30 and 40 minutes for preschool-age children; 60 minutes for children between the ages of 6 and 11; and between 70 and 90 minutes for those at higher age levels. These values may underestimate actual testing times. Sattler (1992) reports that the full battery is much too long to complete in most circumstances, and he indicates that it may take 2 hours to administer the entire test to an adolescent. The length of time required for the full battery has spurred the development of a plethora of short forms, which are discussed below.

One final area of concern is the developmental appropriateness of an instrument for use with young children. Preschoolers vary in their knowledge of basic concepts (e.g., "top," "behind," "same as"). As a result, basic concepts in test directions may hinder preschool children's understanding of what is expected of them. Kaufman (1978) examined this issue by comparing the number of basic concepts in the Boehm Test of Basic Concepts (BTBC; Boehm, 1971) to those found in the directions for several preschool-level ability tests, including the following: SB-LM; the McCarthy Scales of Children's Abilities (MSCA; McCarthy, 1972); and the Wechsler Preschool and Primary Scale of Intelligence (WPPSI; Wechsler, 1967). Results revealed that scores from SB-LM (5 basic concepts) were less susceptible to this influence than scores from the MSCA (7 basic concepts) or WPPSI (14 basic concepts).

We compared directions in SB4 to basic concepts in the BTBC.[2] In particular, directions were analyzed for the eight SB4 subtests routinely administered to preschoolers. Our findings show that SB4 assumes young children know eight BTBC basic concepts. Although this represents an increase over the number found for SB-LM, it compared favorably to the number of basic concepts in the MSCA, and it is fewer than that found for the WPPSI. Thus SB4 directions are at least as likely to be understood by preschoolers as those contained in other IQ tests.

SCALING

Raw SB4 scores are converted to standard age scores (SASs). SASs for the four areas and the Composite are synonymous with deviation IQs ($M = 100$, $SD = 16$, consistent with Binet tradition). Subtest SASs are normalized standard scores with $M = 50$ and $SD = 8$. This metric is highly unusual. We find no compelling reasoning for this choice, and we share Cronbach's (1987) criticism of SB4 that there is no advantage for choosing these units over conventional T-scores.

Percentile ranks are available for subtests, area scores, and the Composite. Although SB4 is no longer an age scale, age equivalents are supplied for the 15 subtests. Moreover, a conversion table is produced for professionals who wish to interpret area scores and the Composite in a metric identical to the Wechsler series ($M = 100$, $SD = 15$).

A historical advantage of Binet scales has been an extended floor for detecting moderate to severe mental retardation. Psychologists will be no doubt disappointed that this benefit is generally unavailable for young children on SB4 (Bradley-Johnson, 2001; Grunau, Whitfield, & Petrie, 2000; McCallum & Whitaker, 2000; Saylor, Boyce, Peagler, & Callahan, 2000). Table 10.2 presents minimum overall ability scores attainable for preschoolers on SB-LM, SB4, the WPPSI, and the K-ABC. Column 2 indicates that SB-LM was fully capable of diagnosing mild intellectual retardation by age 3, and moderate retardation by age 3 years, 6 months. In contrast, column 3 reveals that for all practical purposes, SB4's Composite is unable to diagnose mild intellectual deficits prior to age 4, and it shows no capacity for detecting moderate retardation until age 5.

Tests such as the WPPSI, WPPSI-R, and the K-ABC have been criticized for being insensitive to preschoolers who perform at the lower end of the ability continuum (Bracken, 1985; Olridge & Allison, 1968; Sattler, 1992). Column 5 in Table 10.2 shows that SB4 is somewhat more precise in this regard than the K-ABC. However, column 4 also reveals that SB4 is no more sensitive than the WPPSI-R. These comparisons, combined with existing views on the limitations

of the WPPSI-R and K-ABC, lead to the conclusion that SB4 provides an insufficient floor for testing young children suspected to perform at lower levels of ability (Flanagan & Alfonso, 1995). These findings are disappointing, since SB-LM was the only IQ test capable of diagnosing mental retardation with preschoolers between the ages of 2 years, 6 months (the upper age range of the Bayley Scales) and 4 years, 0 months.

Problems are compounded for younger preschoolers by the fact that area scores evidence even higher floors than the Composite. For example, the lowest SAS for Quantitative Reasoning between the ages of 2 years, 0 months and 4 years, 6 months is 72. This score is above the range for mental retardation, and the median lowest attainable SAS is 87 for children between these ages. With this instrument, it is impossible for younger preschoolers to show deficient or abnormal functioning in Quantitative Reasoning. Even more disturbing, the truncated floor makes it more probable that an artifactual "pattern" of strength in Quantitative Reasoning will emerge for any such preschooler whose Composite is in the gender range. Floor limitations dissipate by the age of kindergarten entry. SB4's Composite is able to identify both mild and moderate intellectual retardation at the age of 5 years, 0 months. Similarly, shortcomings noted for the Quantitative Reasoning area are resolved essentially by the age of 4 years, 6 months (cf. Grunau et al., 2000).

Table 10.3 illustrates SB4's facility to detect functioning at the upper extreme. By in-

TABLE 10.2. Preschoolers' Minimum Overall Ability Scores on SB-LM, SB4, the WPPSI-R, and the K-ABC

Age in years and months	SB4[a]	SB-LM	WPPSI-R	K-ABC
2 years, 0 months	94[b,c]	87[b,c]	—	—
2 years, 6 months	87[b,c]	69[c]	—	79[b,c]
3 years, 0 months	73[b,c]	57[c]	62[c]	70[b,c]
3 years, 6 months	66[c]	47	57[c]	60[c]
4 years, 0 months	55[c]	40	48	60[c]
4 years, 6 months	50	31	45	54
5 years, 0 months	44	27	43	58[c]
5 years, 6 months	41	24	42	55[c]

Note. $M = 100$, $SD = 16$ for SB-LM and SB4; $M = 100$, $SD = 15$ for the WPPSI and K-ABC.
[a]SB4 Composites are based on the assumption that a valid score (i.e., raw score > 1) is obtained on each subtest appropriate for administration at a given age level and ability level.
[b]Principal indicator is insensitive to performances more than two standard deviations below the test mean.
[c]Principal indicator is insensitive to performances more than three standard deviations below the test mean.

TABLE 10.3. **Maximum Overall Ability Scores for Select Age Groups on SB4, SB-LM, the Wechsler Scales, and the K-ABC**

Age in years and months	SB4[a]	SB-LM	Wechsler scale[b]	K-ABC
2 years, 0 months	164	162	—	—
4 years, 0 months	164	160	160	160
6 years, 0 months	164	159	160	160
8 years, 0 months	164	164	160	160
10 years, 0 months	164	160	160	160
12 years, 0 months	164	164	160	155
14years, 0 months	158	154	160	—
16 years, 0 months	152	138	155	—
18 years, 0 months	149	136	155	—
20 years, 0 months	149	—	155	—

Note. $M = 100$, $SD = 16$ for SB4 and SB-LM; $M = 100$, $SD = 15$ for all Wechsler scales and the K-ABC.
[a]For any given age level, SB4 Composites are based on the maximum number of subtests specified in Appendix F of the *Guide for Administering and Scoring* (Thorndike et al., 1986a).
[b]The WPPSI-R Full Scale IQ (FSIQ) is the principal Wechsler indicator at age 4 years, 0 months; the WISC-III FSIQ is used at ages 6 years, 0 months through 16 years, 0 months; and the WAIS-III FSIQ is used at ages 18 years, 0 months and 20 years, 0 months.

clusion of standard scores three or more standard deviations above the test mean, SB4 discriminates talent as adequately as SB-LM did at all age levels, and it possesses slightly higher ceilings at ages 16 and above (columns 2 and 3). The Composite also compares favorably to optimal performance on the Wechsler scales and the K-ABC (columns 4 and 5, although the latest revisions of the Wechsler scales have eliminated most of SB4's previous advantage in this area). These comparisons suggest that the SB4 would be a good choice for evaluations assessing potentially gifted youths, although it provides significantly higher scores than the more recent WISC-III (Simpson et al., 2002).

STANDARDIZATION

The goal in developing the standardization sample for the SB4 was to approximate the demographics of the United States based on the 1980 census (Thorndike et al., 1986c). There have been important demographic changes in the two decades since then. Most notable has been the increase in ethnic minority populations, particularly Spanish-speaking groups (Hernandez, 1997). Two interrelated issues must be considered in regard to the representativeness of SB4 norms. The first is the loss of randomness that resulted from the need to obtain examinees'

cooperation. The second is the weighting of test scores to compensate for discrepancies between the designated sampling plan for socioeconomic status (SES) and SES levels in the obtained sample.

Nonrandomness and General Referents

One popular view holds that the strength of an IQ test depends upon the degree to which its sample represents the general population. "Stratified random sampling" would be a relatively efficient method for obtaining such a representation. Many practitioners, as well as notable measurement specialists (e.g., Hopkins, 1988), assume that individually administered IQ tests are normed on stratified random samples. This, however, is never the case. Test developers must request examinees' cooperation. The net effect is a loss of randomness, because people who volunteer are rarely like those who do not (Jaeger, 1984).

The common alternative to stratified random sampling is to select examinees purposively through "quota sampling." The shortcoming of quota sampling is that its selections are likely to be biased, unless of course cooperation rates are high and uniform across strata (Hansen, Hurwitz, & Madow, 1953; Kish, 1965; Thorndike, 1982). SB4 was normed on 5,013 individuals arranged into 17 age groups (2 years, 0 months through 23 years, 11 months). Quota sampling was employed to approximate the U.S. population in terms of geographic region, community size, race, gender, and SES. Unfortunately, lower-SES examinees were underrepresented in the sample (10.6% vs. 29.2% of the U.S. population), and higher-SES examinees were overrepresented (43.1% vs. 19.0%, respectively).

It would be simplistic to discredit SB4 for sampling problems. The quota sampling in SB4, as well as the differential rates of cooperation, are common to *all* individually administered IQ tests, including the K-ABC, WISC-III, and the Woodcock–Johnson Psycho-Educational Battery—Revised (WJ-R) Tests of Cognitive Ability (Woodcock & Johnson, 1990a). The standardization samples of even the best available instruments are imperfect approximations of the general U.S. population at the time any given instrument was developed.

Nonrandomness and Other Referents

An alternative perspective is that it is not necessary for IQ tests to reference the general population. There are other legitimate referents to which test scores can be compared. Instruments such as SB4 are most often administered to two groups—namely, examinees who truly volunteer to be tested and examinees with suspected disabilities. Consequently, it is essential that IQ tests accurately reflect the capabilities of these two groups. Examinees who willingly consent to testing (self-referred individuals, those who may be gifted, certain segments of the population receiving special education) do not necessarily differ from the "volunteer" subjects in standardization samples. At least in this regard, IQ test norms should be appropriate for volunteers. The second group is more problematic. Individuals with disabilities are administered IQ tests for special purposes (e.g., assignment to special education categories, mandatory reevaluations). As such, most of these individuals cannot be truly regarded as volunteers. Clearly linked to this phenomenon is the need to consider persons with disabilities *systematically*—if not directly in test norms, then through special studies.

One proposal for test development is to sample individuals with disabilities in proportion to their presence in the general population. Such an approach assumes that prevalence rates are known for the various exceptionality subtypes. This assumption is problematic for such conditions as learning disabilities, for which there is no uniformly accepted rate of occurrence in the general population and for which diagnostic rates continue to escalate (see Ysseldyke & Stevens, 1986). The dilemma in such instances becomes this: "What is the appropriate percentage of individuals with learning disabilities to include in stadardization samples?"

Unsettling problems arise even when prevalences are known. A prevalence of 3% is the standard endorsed for mental retardation (Grossman, 1983). Yet it would be improper to systematically target individuals identified as having mental retardation to form 3% of a test's sample. Probability theory dictates that a percentage of the volunteers in the sample who are *not* thus identified will also have mental retardation. When the two groups are merged, individuals with mental retardation will be overrepresented. Counterintuitively, this overrepresentation increases the likelihood that test norms will be diagnostically insensitive to persons with mental retardation. The overrepresentation of low-scoring examinees (i.e., those with retardation) will affect the conversion of raw scores to normalized standard scores. As a result, a *lower* raw score will be needed to obtain an IQ in the range for mental retardation (i.e., an IQ < 70) than if such examinees had not been oversampled. The diagnostic result is that test norms will fail to qualify higher-functioning individuals with mental retardation for needed services.

One final issue is that either approach—whether including specific conditions in the standardization sample, or developing separate specialized samples—assumes that developers will include all potentially relevant diagnostic categories. Unfortunately, at present we have incomplete knowledge of the different exceptionalities that might influence performance on a cognitive ability battery. There is evidence that some psychiatric diagnoses, such as attention-deficit/hyperactivity disorder (e.g., Saklofske, Schwean, Yackulic, & Quinn, 1994; Schwean, Saklofske, Yackulic, & Quinn, 1993) or autism (Carpentieri & Morgan, 1994; Harris, Handleman, & Burton, 1990), may be associated with mean differences in performance on at least some aspects of ability. Currently it is unclear whether these group differences reflect changes in cognitive processing, or whether the effect is mediated by changes in motivation or test session behavior (Glutting, Youngstrom, Oakland, & Watkins, 1996).

Thus there are at least four links in the chain connecting knowledge to the design of an appropriate standardization sample: (1) awareness of all the conditions and exceptionalities that may influence performance on an ability test; (2) accurate data about the prevalence rate of these conditions in the population; (3) efficient and affordable ways of identifying potential participants meeting criteria for the conditions, either by doing so among the "volunteers" or by generating a special reference sample; and (4) a clear theoretical rationale about the appropriateness of developing a separate set of norms for a particular group (e.g., is it meaningful to know how the working memory performance of a youth with depression compares to other such youths, or only to other youths the same age, regardless of exceptionality?). Given these hurdles, the most practical solution for test developers will probably continue to be approximation of stratified sampling, with the hope that participation biases do not lead to serious underrepresentation of important conditions. A statistical alternative might be to explicitly model the selection process for participants, and then use estimates based on this model to correct observed values for "nonsampling bias" (see Wainer, 1999, for discussion and examples). Either way, it is important for test consumers and users to remain aware of these assumptions about the representativeness of the standardization sample.

Enhancing Diagnostic Utility

For the reasons discussed above, proportional sampling of individuals with disabilities is likely to create as many problems as it solves. A more practical response is to systematically oversample these individuals, but not necessarily to include them in test norms. Instead, special studies should be conducted to determine how the test behaves in these populations. Confirmatory factor analysis, for example, could identify whether test dimensions are similar for persons with and without disabilities (e.g., Keith & Witta, 1997). Comparisons based on item response theory (IRT; e.g., Hambleton, Swaminathan, & Rogers, 1991) could verify whether item difficulties are identical among exceptional and nonexceptional groups. IRT would also uncover whether item calibrations are sufficient for the maximum differentiation of low-scoring and high-scoring exceptionalities (Embretson, 1999). Multiple-regression slope comparisons (and not bivariate correlations) should supply information relevant to whether test scores predict equally for persons with and without disabilities (Jensen, 1980). Finally, univariate and multivariate contrasts could shed light on whether all possible test scores (e.g., overall IQs, factor scores, subtest scores) differ between the general sample and the various exceptionality subtypes (persons with mental retardation, learning disabilities, etc.).

Compared to these ideals, SB4 leaves room for improvement. This finding is disappointing, since sufficient data were gathered during SB4's development to complete many of the analyses identified above. SB4 is to be commended for verifying that its Composite and area scores (but not necessarily subtest scores) differ between exceptional and nonexceptional samples. Nevertheless, no attempt was made to determine whether SB4's items are unbiased for those with disabilities, or that its test dimensions are similar for individuals functioning normally and exceptionally. Likewise, although criterion-related validity is reported for those with disabilities, quantitative comparisons were not conducted for the relative accuracy of predictions between those with and without disabilities.

In fairness, no IQ test has met all of these standards at the time of its publication. However, the issue is not whether SB4 should be excused because it is no more deficient than other ability tests. Rather, the issue is why IQ tests are marketed without adequate evidence that they reflect the aptitudes of individuals with disabilities. We, as professionals responsible for the welfare of clients, must demand this information at the time of a test's publication. Otherwise, we must accept the fact that we are willing to apply tests whose diagnostic capabilities are unknown.

Elimination versus Weighting

There is often "slippage" between a test's sampling plan and the testing as executed (Thorndike, 1982). Two methods can bring a sample back into alignment with its sampling plan. The first option is to eliminate examinees randomly from oversampled strata. The second option is to *weight* scores from each stratum to their correct percentage of the population. Whereas both methods have their benefits, neither can fully compensate for a loss of randomness in the sampling process (Glutting & Kaplan, 1990).

Until SB4, norms for individually administered IQ tests were typically aligned by eliminating examinees from oversampled strata. The benefit of elimination is that there is no redundancy in subject-generated variance (i.e., an examinee is not counted as more, or less, than one case). Moreover, the practice is tidy. "Final" samples often align well with the population, in part, because test manuals provide little discussion of discarded cases. Therefore, had SB4 used elimination, it would have been easy to marvel at how well the sample approximated the general population on race, gender, SES, and so on. Instead, SB4 retained all 5,013 participants in the standardization sample, even though higher-SES families were more likely to provide informed consent and to participate than were lower-SES families. In an effort to correct for these sampling biases, the SES variables of occupation and education were weighted so that examinees' scores would conform to their correct percentages in the U.S. population. That is, "each child from an advantaged background was counted as only a fraction of a case (as little as 0.28), while each child from a less advantaged background was counted as more than one case" (Thorndike et al., 1986c, p. 24).

One advantage of weighting is that it accounts for all scores in the sample. Relatedly, it produces estimates of higher reliability than does elimination. A potential flaw is that weighted estimates are not based entirely on actual cases. Examinees in under-represented strata are counted *more than once* by multiplying the original sample variance upward to the desired population estimate. The process is dependent upon the assumption that examinees in the sample are representative of the *entire* population—including those individuals who, for whatever reason, were not sampled.

There is no guarantee that the scores of examinees already in the sample are similar to the scores of potential examinees who were not tested. However, this assumption becomes more plausible when the obtained sample has large numbers of examinees in each stratum who are representative of that particular population segment. SB4's standardization sample is quite large ($n = 5,013$), and its strata are probably of sufficient subject size for weighting. Moreover, weighting is an accepted procedure for standardizing group tests. Consequently, from this perspective, the weighting of test scores in SB4 appears as reasonable as the weighting used to norm group tests.

RELIABILITY

By and large, SB4's reliabilities are quite good. Internal consistency for the Composite is excellent, with Kuder–Richardson 20 coefficients ranging from .95 to .99 across age levels. Reliabilities for area scores are also substantial. Internal consistency for two-, three-, and four-subtest groupings vary from .86 to .97 for Verbal Reasoning (median $r = .95$). Coefficients for Abstract/Visual Reasoning range from .85 to .97 and show a median of .95. Similarly, estimates for Quantitative Reasoning vary from .80 to .97 (median $r = .94$), and internal consistency for Short-Term Memory ranges from .86 to .95 (median $r = .86$). It is worth noting that only the Composite achieves reliability coefficients consistently greater than Kelley's (1927) recommended threshold of .94 for making decisions about individuals. Most of the area scores attain the less conservative threshold (reliabilities $\geq .85$) proposed by Weiner and Stewart (1984) for individual classification.

Subtest internal consistencies are lower, as would be expected from their shorter test lengths. Nonetheless, with the exception of one subtest, median coefficients are reasonably high (range = .83 to .94 across age groups). The exceptional subtest (Memory for Objects) is located in the Short-Term Memory area, and it produces coefficients of marginal reliability (median r = .73). The subtest with the second lowest reliability is also in the Short-Term Memory area (Memory for Digits; median r = .83). As a result, psychologists should be alert that subtest scores from the Short-Term Memory area are likely to be less precise than subtest scores from other areas in SB4.

Standard errors of measurement (SEMs), and "confidence bands" derived from SEMs, are the reliability issues most likely to affect everyday practice. Confidence bands produce information relevant to the fallibility of test scores, and consequently help to clarify the relative verity and utility of test scores in decision making about individuals (Glutting, McDermott, & Stanley, 1987).

Memory for Objects provides the least precise scores in SB4 (i.e., the largest confidence bands). Its SEM shows a median of 4.15 points across age groups. The subtest with the second largest SEM is Memory for Digits (median = 3.25). However, the SEMs of these two subtests (and for all other more reliable subtests) are within reasonable limits. Also, as might be expected, greater precision in scores is found when interpretations are based on the four area scores. Median SEMs for Verbal Reasoning, Abstract/Visual Reasoning, Quantitative Reasoning, and Short-Term Memory are as follows: 3.9, 3.6, 3.8, and 4.8, respectively. Finally, the most precise score in SB4 is the Composite (median SEM = 2.3; all SEMs as reported in Sattler, 1992).

The *Technical Manual* (Thorndike et al., 1986c) calculates score stability for samples of preschoolers (5-year-olds) and children attending elementary school (8-year-olds). Preschoolers' test–retest coefficients are reasonable for the Composite (r = .91) and for area scores (range = .71 to .78). Less stability is evident for individual subtests, and in particular for Bead Memory (r = .56). The pattern of test–retest coefficients of elementary school children is similar to that found for preschoolers. Appreciable stability is present for the Composite (r = .90) and for the areas of Verbal Reasoning, Abstract/Visual Reasoning, and Short-Term Memory

(r's = .87, .67, and .81, respectively). However, somewhat lower stability is found for the Quantitative Reasoning area (r = .51).

Preschoolers' Composites will, on average, increase approximately 8.2 points from test to retest administrations. Similarly, Composites are likely to increase by 6.4 points for elementary school children who are tested twice across short intervals. SB4 offers no stability data for examinees of junior high or high school age, or for young adults, making it difficult to approximate the score increases that might be expected of these age groups.

VALIDITY

An impressive amount of validity information has been gathered in support of SB4. In particular, investigations have addressed developmental changes of raw scores by age; quantitative analyses of item fairness across gender and ethnic groups; correlations with other IQ tests, using samples of both normal and exceptional examinees; correlations with achievement tests; score differences between the standardization sample and special groups (individuals who are gifted, have learning disabilities, or have mental retardation); and the factor structure of SB4's test dimensions.

Concurrent Validity

Table 10.4 presents concurrent correlations between SB4 and other IQ tests administered to normal samples. This compilation was obtained from studies reported in the *Technical Manual* (Thorndike et al., 1986c) and in a review by Laurent, Swerdlik, and Ryburn (1992), as well as from studies conducted by independent investigators. Laurent and colleagues present validity data for exceptional samples, too. Results show substantial associations between SB4's Composite and overall scores on SB-LM, all Wechsler scales, the K-ABC, the WJ-R (Woodcock & Johnson, 1990a), and the Differential Ability Scales (DAS; Elliott, 1990). Correlations ranged from .53 to .91 (average r = .78 using Fisher's z' transformation). The consistency and magnitude of these relationships speak well for the Composite's construct validity.

Spearman's (1923) principle of the "indif-

TABLE 10.4. Score Characteristics and Correlations of SB4 with Other IQ Tests Administered to Nonexceptional Samples

Study	n	Mean age (years)	Mean SB4 Composite	Other IQ test	Other test mean IQ	IQ difference	Correlation
Elliott (1990)	55	9.9	109.8	DAS	106.3	3.5	.88
Thorndike, Hagen, & Sattler (1986c, Study 5)	175	7.0	112.7	K-ABC	112.3	0.4	.89
Hendershott, Searight, Hatfield, & Rogers (1990)	36	4	110.5	K-ABC	118.2	−7.7	.65
Krohn & Lamp (1989)[a,b]	89	4.9	93.4	K-ABC	96.0	−2.6	.86
Krohn & Lamp (1989)[a,b]	65	4	93.8	K-ABC	95.8	−2.0	—
Krohn & Lamp (1989)[a,b]	65	6	93.3	K-ABC	99.7	−6.4	—
Krohn & Lamp (1989)[a,b]	65	9	96.5	K-ABC	97.9	−1.4	—
Kaufman & Kaufman (1983)	121	School-age	116.5	K-ABC	114.5	+2.0	.61
Smith & Bauer (1989)	30	4.9	—	K-ABC	—	—	.57
Clark, Wortman, Warnock, & Swerdlik (1987)	47	—	—	SB-LM	—	—	.53
Hartwig, Sapp, & Clayton (1987)	30	11.3	113.1	SB-LM	114.4	−1.3	.72
Thorndike, Hagen, & Sattler (1986c, Study 1)	139	6.9	105.8	SB-LM	108.1	−2.3	.81
Krohn & Lamp (1989)[a,b]	89	4.9	93.4	SB-LM	—	—	.69
Lukens (1988)	31	16.75	44.8	SB-LM	46.7	−1.9	.86
Psychological Corporation (1997)	26	28.6	114.8	WAIS-III	113.3	+1.5	.88
Carvajal, Gerber, Hughes, & Weaver (1987)	32	18.0	100.9	WAIS-R	103.5	−2.6	.91
Thorndike, Hagen, & Sattler (1986c, Study 4)	47	19.4	98.7	WAIS-R	102.2	−3.5	.91
Lavin (1996)	40	10.6	108.0	WISC-III	107.0	+1.0	.82
Rust & Lindstrom (1996)	57	6–17	109.9	WISC-III	111.3	−1.4	.81
Rothlisberg (1987)	32	7.8	105.5	WISC-R	112.5	−7.0	.77
Thorndike, Hagen, & Sattler (1986c, Study 2)	205	9.4	102.4	WISC-R	105.2	−2.8	.83
Carvajal & Weyand (1986)	23	9.5	113.3	WISC-R	115.0	−1.7	.78
Greene, Sapp, & Chissom (1990)[c]	51	Grades 1–8	80.5	WISC-R	78.1	+2.4	.87
Wechsler (1991)	205	6–16	—	WISC-R	—	—	.83
Woodcock & Johnson (1990b, Study 1)	64	2.9	—	WJ-R	—	—	.69
Woodcock & Johnson (1990b, Study 2)	70	9.5	—	WJ-R	—	—	.69
Woodcock & Johnson (1990b, Study 3)	51	17.5	—	WJ-R	—	—	.65
Thorndike, Hagen, & Sattler (1986c, Study 3)	75	5.5	105.3	WPPSI	110.3	−5.0	.80
Carvajal, Hardy, Smith, & Weaver (1988)	20	5.5	114.4	WPPSI	115.6	−1.2	.59

(*continues*)

TABLE 10.4. *Continued*

Study	n	Mean age (years)	Mean SB4 Composite	Other IQ test	Other test mean IQ	IQ difference	Correlation
Carvajal, Parks, Bays, & Logan (1991)	51	5.7	103.0	WPPSI-R	109.5	−6.5	.61
McCrowell & Nagle (1994)	30	5.0	95.9	WPPSI-R	94.1	+1.8	.77
Wechsler (1989)	105	5.6	107.2	WPPSI-R	105.3	+1.9	.74

Note. DAS, Differential Ability Scales; K-ABC, Kaufman Assessment Battery for Children; SB-LM, Stanford–Binet, Form L-M; WAIS-R, Wechsler Adult Intelligence Scale—Revised; WAIS-III, Wechsler Adult Intelligence Scale—Third Edition; WISC-R, Wechsler Intelligence Scale for Children—Revised; WISC-III, Wechsler Intelligence Scale for Children—Third Edition; WPPSI, Wechsler Preschool and Primary Scale of Intelligence; WPPSI-R, Wechsler Preschool and Primary Scale of Intelligence—Revised; WJ-R, Woodcock–Johnson Psychoeducational Battery—Revised.
[a]Same sample appears multiple times in table, because participants completed multiple ability tests.
[b]Head Start sample, followed longitudinally.
[c]African American sample.

ference of the indicator" suggests that the specific item content in intelligence tests is unimportant to the evaluation of general ability (or g). The truly important phenomenon for g is that IQ tests measure inductive and deductive reasoning. Thus correlations between one IQ test and IQ tests with dissimilar content can help evaluate the extent to which the first test measures g. Based on the correlations in Table 10.4, at least 60.8% of the Composite's variance is accounted for by g. These data suggest that the Composite provides a reasonably trustworthy estimate of general intelligence.

Of applied interest are score differences that can be expected between SB4 and other IQ tests. Column 7 in Table 10.4 (labeled "IQ difference") shows that the Composite *averages* 2.5 points lower than the IQs from other intelligence tests published prior to SB4. Interestingly, scores on the SB4 also average 0.5 points *higher* than scores obtained on tests published after SB4 (i.e., the WPPSI-R, DAS, WJ-R, WISC-III, and WAIS-III). Individual comparisons are less precise because of the smaller number of studies between SB4 and any one test. With this caveat in mind, psychologists might expect SB4 to produce IQs that are about 2 points lower than those from SB-LM; 5 points lower than those from the WISC-R; 3 points lower than those from the Wechsler Adult Intelligence Scale—Revised (WAIS-R); 3 points lower than those from the WPPSI; and 2.5 lower than those from the K-ABC. Given the difference in times when these respective standardization samples were col-

lected, it is likely that the "Flynn effect" accounts for much of this variance in scores (Flynn, 1984, 1999). By virtue of the Flynn effect, which refers to apparent secular gains in average performance on ability tests, it is likely that SB4 scores would be about 3 points higher than scores derived from tests normed a decade later, such as the WAIS-III, the forthcoming revision of the K-ABC, and the new WJ-III.

Factor Structure

The most controversial aspect of SB4 concerns the interpretability of its area scores. That is, do the capabilities evaluated by SB4 actually conform to the four-factor model of intelligence that has been advanced for the test? This question of construct validity is open to empirical verification, and it is one that usually can be answered through factor analysis.

It is disconcerting that the authors of SB4 themselves disagree about the number of interpretable factors. Thorndike, for example, in light of his own factor-analytic results, offers no explanation for why the four-factor model should be applied to examinees younger than age 12. He "confirms" only two factors between ages 2 and 6 (Verbal, Abstract/Visual). His analyses then support a three-factor model between ages 7 and 11 (Verbal, Abstract/Visual, Memory). Most importantly, the proposed four-factor model does not emerge until ages 12 through 23.

Sattler (1992), on the other hand, eschews the SB4 model. He proposes a two-factor solution between ages 2 and 6 (Verbal Comprehension, Nonverbal Reasoning/Visualization) and a three-factor solution at ages 7 through 23 (Verbal Comprehension, Nonverbal Reasoning/Visualization, Memory). Conspicuously absent in Sattler's findings is the dimension of Quantitative Reasoning, and at no age level does he recommend the interpretation of all four area scores.

Perhaps because of this open disagreement, investigators have extensively reanalyzed the SB4 normative data as well as conducting independent replications. We found a dozen different published factor analyses of SB4. Four provided evidence consistent with the published four-factor structure (Boyle, 1989, 1990 [especially if one is willing to exclude certain subtests]; Keith, Cool, Novak, & White, 1988; Ownby & Carmin, 1988). Five studies challenge the four-factor structure, suggesting anywhere from one general ability factor (Reynolds, Kamphaus, & Rosenthal, 1988) to two or three factors, depending on age (Gridley & McIntosh, 1991; Kline, 1989; Molfese, Yaple, Helwig, & Harris, 1992; Sattler, 1992). The remaining studies are equivocal about the competing models (McCallum, Karnes, & Crowell, 1988; Thorndike et al., 1986c; Thorndike, 1990). There is a tendency to detect more factors in older age groups, with a two-factor structure describing preschool data, and three factors describing data for youths above 7 years of age. These differences in factor structure, if true, could reflect either developmental change or alterations in the subtest battery administered at each age. Older youths completed more subtests on average, increasing the likelihood of statistically recovering additional factors (if such additional dimensions of ability were measured by the subtests).[3]

Interestingly, we are not aware of any published study that has used either Horn's parallel analysis (Horn, 1965) or the method of minimum average partials (Velicer, 1976) as decision rules to determine the appropriate number of factors to retain for the SB4. Methodological evidence strongly suggests that these are the two techniques most likely to recover the accurate number of factors, and they tend to retain fewer factors than more commonly used procedures, such as the maximum-likelihood chi-square test or the Kaiser criterion (Zwick & Velicer, 1986). The common element in all this is that no single study has definitively substantiated the existence of *four* area factors. It therefore stands to reason that psychologists should refrain from interpreting area scores until more evidence is offered on their behalf.

It should be kept in mind that current inabilities to support a four-factor model may not necessarily represent a failure of SB4 per se. Rather, the difficulty may lie in the sensitivity of factor analysis to data-related issues in SB4. This is particularly true when confirmatory factor analysis is applied. The relationship between confirmatory factor analysis and SB4 was explored in detail by Glutting and Kaplan (1990).

SCORE INTERPRETATION

The SB4 can potentially support clinical interpretation at a variety of levels of analysis. The battery yields a single, global estimate of general cognitive ability, the Composite score, which represents the most general level of analysis available on the SB4. Beneath the Composite, the SB4 also theoretically could yield scores for Fluid and Crystallized cognitive ability, which are referred to as "Level II scores" in the SB4 manuals. SB4 also includes the Short-Term Memory factor score in Level II. Level III scores on the Binet include factor-based scores measuring the specific cognitive abilities of Verbal Reasoning, Quantitative Reasoning, and Abstract/Visual Reasoning. SB4, unlike SB-LM, also provides standardized age scores for specific subtests, enabling potential interpretation of subtest profiles. This exemplifies the most fine-grained level of clinical interpretation that would be considered in most cases (cf. Sattler, 1992, for discussion of attention to responses to specific items).

This structure for the SB4 is similar to the hierarchical structures adopted by most contemporary measures of cognitive ability, and this format lends itself readily to the "top-down" models of interpretation advocated by many assessment authorities (e.g., Aiken, 2000; Kamphaus, 1993; Kaufman, 1994; Sattler, 1992). It is important to consider the evidence supporting these different levels of interpretation; assessment practice is better driven by scientific evidence than by convention and appeals to authority.

The Level I score, the Composite, possesses good evidence of validity. The preponderance of research involving the SB4 and its predecessors has concentrated on the Composite score, so there is considerable accumulated evidence about the Composite score's convergent, criterion, and predictive validity for such constructs as academic achievement. The Composite score also has gained fairly consistent support from factor analyses of the SB4 subtests (which typically have indicated either several correlated factors or one general ability factor). Although some have questioned the treatment validity of even these most global scores from cognitive ability tests (Macmann & Barnett, 1997; McCallum et al., 1988), a good case can be made for using and interpreting these global scores (Neisser et al., 1996), particularly in terms of psychoeducational and vocational assessment.

Level II scores are less well supported. The SB4 as published provides an observed score for the Short-Term Memory area, but the Abstract/Visual Reasoning area score is the only potential indicator of Fluid-Analytic Abilities in the battery. This limits the construct validity of estimates of fluid ability derived from the SB4, inasmuch as fluid ability may involve processes beyond abstract/visual reasoning (Carroll, 1993; Horn & Noll, 1997). Furthermore, the SB4 manuals and interpretive aids do not formally present a way of calculating a summary score for Crystallized Abilities, although it is possible to estimate such a score by combining the Verbal and Quantitative Reasoning area scores. The proposed Level II structure of the SB4 has not consistently been confirmed by secondary analyses of the standardization data or independent samples. Perhaps most crucially, there is a dearth of research addressing the criterion validity of Level II scores from the SB4 (cf. Caruso, 2001). The paucity of research is probably largely related to the lack of emphasis on Level II interpretation in the SB4 materials, and it is possible that future research will demonstrate value in interpreting these more discrete ability estimates (e.g., Moffitt & Silva, 1987). At present, however, there is minimal literature to guide clinical hypothesis generation or interpretation of Level II scores, and there is

little guidance offered to the practitioner about how to calculate the Level II scores beyond Short-Term Memory. This level of analysis has not received much attention in practice, and it probably should not be emphasized until more evidence is available demonstrating clear incremental validity above and beyond the information derived from the Composite score.

Level III scores are also problematic, because of disagreement about factor structure as well as a lack of information about incremental validity. The purported structure of Verbal Reasoning, Quantitative Reasoning, and Abstract/Visual Reasoning as three distinct factors has not consistently emerged across the ages covered by SB4, or in analyses of independent samples (and not always in secondary analyses of the standardization data). Currently there is insufficient evidence to permit us to conclude whether the subtests on the SB4 adequately assess these three different dimensions of ability. More importantly from a practical perspective, at present there is no information about incremental validity for these area scores after the Composite score is interpreted. Although researchers have begun to explore the possibility that more discrete ability scores might provide additional clinical data about achievement or behavior problems not subsumed in a more global ability score (cf. Glutting, Youngstrom, Ward, Ward, & Hale, 1997; Youngstrom, Kogos, & Glutting, 1999), this work still needs to begin with the SB4. Area score interpretation imposes burdens on the practitioner and consumer in terms of longer tests, greater complexity of results, and potentially greater likelihood of diagnostic errors (Silverstein, 1993). In light of these costs, it would seem premature to emphasize Level III area scores in SB4 interpretations. The lack of consensus about the construct validity for these scores, based on factor analyses, further calls for caution.

Psychologists may be tempted to make "area" interpretations (e.g., Naglieri, 1988a), even though there is little justification for this practice. Indeed, Hopkins (1988) appears to believe that SB4's four area scores should be interpreted, and that practitioners need not "become emotionally involved in the 'great debate' regarding the theoretical structure of intelligence a determined by the factor analytic method" (p. 41). Hopkins's position is incorrect, because it implies that clinical necessity should supersede what can be supported empirically. However, the need to generate hypotheses about an examinee is *never* sufficient grounds for the interpretation of a test score. This is especially true in the case of SB4's four area scores, since claims for their construct validity have yet to be substantiated, in spite of a considerable amount of investigation. Even if this were accomplished, it would also be necessary to document criterion validity and incremental validity (above more parsimonious *g*-based models) before clinical interpretation of area scores could be justified.

The addition of standard age scores for subtests to the SB4 created the possibility of subtest profile interpretation, which has become a prevalent practice in the use of other major ability tests (e.g., Kaufman, 1994; Naglieri, 1988b; Sattler, 1992). Many clinicians and researchers welcomed this addition as an opportunity to improve the perceived clinical value of the SB4, hoping that more detailed attention to patterns of performance on subtests would lead to improved psychoeducational prescription (Lavin, 1995) or to identification of profiles characterizing the performance of specific diagnostic groups (e.g., Carpentieri & Morgan, 1994; Harris et al., 1990). Procedures and recommendations are available to promote this sort of analysis with the SB4 (Naglieri, 1988b; Rosenthal & Kamphaus, 1988; Spruill, 1988). Sattler (1992) also provides a detailed table (Table C-52) listing the abilities thought to be reflected in each subtest, background factors thought to affect subtest performance, possible implications of high and low scores on each subtest, and instructional implications of unusual performance on each subtest. Sattler's table is thorough. For example, Sattler lists from 3 to 18 distinct abilities for each of the 15 subtests ($M = 8.5$, $SD = 3.8$), and an average of five implications for every high or low score per subtest. This presentation clearly encourages the clinical interpretation of individual strengths and weaknesses at the subtest level. Although Sattler provides some cautionary statements about not interpreting a subtest score in isolation, such tables seem prone to abuse. The situation confronting the clinician is complex: Who can generate a hypothesis with any confidence when faced with an average of eight or nine different abilities and another three background factors that could contribute to performance on a specific subtest?

In addition, subtest analysis faces substantial psychometric challenges (Macmann & Barnett, 1997; McDermott, Fantuzzo, & Glutting, 1990; McDermott, Fantuzzo, Glutting, Watkins, & Baggaley, 1992) that make it unlikely to deliver on the promise of improved assessment or treatment planning. In fact, the studies available to date for the SB4 clearly indicate that there is no significant improvement in assessment when subtest interpretation is added to the analytic strategy (Kline, Snyder, Guilmette, & Castellanos, 1992, 1993). This is consistent with growing evidence from investigations with other tests, indicating that subtest analysis is problematic at best when applied to routine assessment goals such as predicting academic achievement or diagnosis (e.g., Watkins, 1996; Watkins, Kush, & Glutting, 1997). In short, it appears that the SB-LM was not missing much by failing to include subtest scores, and that practitioners would do well to avoid relying much on SB4 subtests as a distinct level of analysis in conducting evaluations.

SHORT FORMS

Cognitive assessment is a time-consuming enterprise (Meyer et al., 1998). This expense, combined with the lack of validity information supporting the clinical use of scores beyond the Composite as described above, strongly suggests the potential value of short forms of the SB4 that provide reliable estimates of general ability without entailing the costs of a complete administration. SB4 offers four short forms that result in a substantial savings of testing time: the six-subtest General Purpose Assessment Battery (GPAB; Vocabulary, Bead Memory, Quantitative, Memory for Sentences, Comprehension, and Pattern Analysis); the four-subtest Quick Screening Battery (Vocabulary, Bead Memory, Quantitative, and Pattern Analysis); the four- to six-subtest Battery for the Assessment of Students for Gifted Programs; and the six-subtest Battery for Students Having Problems Learning in School. Short forms with four or fewer subtests are intended for screening purposes, but batteries composed of at least six subtests can be used for placement decisions (Thorndike et al., 1986c, p. 50). This latter possibility makes it essential that test scores from six-subtest abbreviated batteries be psychometrically equivalent to those from the full test.

According to the data presented in the *Technical Manual* (Thorndike et al., 1986c), split-half reliabilities for two-, four-, and six-subtest short forms are fairly constant and appreciable for examinees of different ages. Correlations between Composites from short forms and the complete battery are also acceptable. However, the *Technical Manual* fails to present information about differences between estimated Composites and area scores from abbreviated batteries and actual scores on the full test. Since publication of the SB4, more than a dozen independent studies have investigated the psychometric properties of various abridged forms, using samples ranging from low to high ability and from preschool to college. The majority of these investigations concluded that the six-subtest GPAB was the most acceptable substitute for a complete administration (Atkinson, 1991; Carvajal & Gerber, 1987; DeLamatre & Hollinger, 1990; Kyle & Robertson, 1994; McCallum & Karnes, 1990; Prewett, 1992; Volker, Guarnaccia, & Scardapane, 1999), possessing both good correspondence with the full battery and good external validity with other measures of ability (Carvajal, Hayes, Lackey, & Rathke, 1993; Carvajal, McVey, Sellers, & Weyand, 1987). On the other hand, two investigations concluded that the four-subtest battery performs essentially as well as the six-subtest version, and argued that the four-subtest version is preferable for screening purposes in light of its brevity (Prewett, 1992; Volker et al., 1999). Finally, Nagle and Bell (1993) found that all of the short forms produced what they considered to be unacceptable levels of disagreement for individual classification purposes. Instead, these authors recommend the use of item reduction short forms rather than subtest reduction versions (Nagle & Bell, 1995). On the whole, these studies alleviate earlier

concerns that the short forms might show substantially lower external validity, in spite of correlating well with the full-battery composite (Levy, 1968; McCormick, 1956). It is less clear that short forms provide an adequate substitute for the full battery when individual classification decisions are required; in addition, the two-subtest battery clearly is suitable only for group research and not individual assessment.

In spite of the burgeoning literature examining SB4 short forms, important questions remain unanswered. One problem is that practitioners often may develop idiosyncratic short forms that have not been empirically validated. Norms tables in SB4 make it possible to calculate Composites from practically *any* combination of subtests. Thus practitioners can develop their own short forms by "picking and choosing" among favorite subtests. No matter how the particular combination is chosen, problems are likely to arise for short forms if the *administration sequence* of the subtests is disturbed.[4] Assume, for example, that a psychologist elects to administer a short form consisting of subtests 1, 3, 4, 5, 6, and 13. The psychologist in such an instance is operating under the belief that norms for subtest 13 (Paper Folding and cutting) will remain constant, regardless of the fact this subtest now occupies position 6 in the new battery. Thus the validity of the procedure is critically dependent on the assumption that norms and examinees' performances are independent of a subtest's location in the battery.

Such assumptions of independence are certainly open to question. Decreases in testing time may lessen an examinee's frustration and improve test scores on the shorter battery. Differences in the fatigue of the psychologist or examinee, or the fact that the full test offers more opportunities to gain experience in understanding test directions and familiarity with test materials, could also affect performance. Learning or "carryover" effects from one subtest to the next are particularly likely for measures that require examinees to manipulate objects (i.e., nonverbal/performance subtests). Finally, even if these assumptions were satisfied, the psychologist must consider whether the external validity of the shorter battery is the same as that of the full test (see Smith, McCarthy, & Anderson, 2000, for further recommendations about the development and evaluation of short forms). This limitation also applies to the majority of extant research with SB4 short forms: Researchers typically administer the full battery and then extract different short forms from that battery. Thus practice, fatigue, and motivation effects are based on a full administration, which would not be the case when a short form was administered clinically.

Without more information about the effects of subtest sequencing and battery length, as well as short-form external validity, it could be argued that psychologists should administer SB4 in its entirety (or possibly use the six-subtest GPAB) and should refrain from selectively administering alternative batteries. We acknowledge that this recommendation runs counter to current neuropsychological practice and "multibattery" approaches to assessment, both of which appropriate subtests from a variety of sources to construct idiosyncratic batteries intended to test clinical hypotheses and address specific referral needs. Our position is a conservative one, recognizing that multibattery approaches represent a departure from the standardized administration procedures used to develop test norms. An alternative would be to use brief ability tests that were designed for short administration and that have known reliability and validity when used in this manner (e.g., Glutting, Adams, & Sheslow, 2000; Psychological Corporation, 1999). Practitioners must be cautious about trading away the advantages inherent in following a standardized protocol in exchange for a briefer, more flexible, and allegedly more "focused" battery of unknown validity.

FUTURE DIRECTIONS: THE DEVELOPMENT OF SB5

As this chapter is being written, preliminary item tryouts are beginning for the development of the SB5, which is planned to be released in Spring 2003. There obviously may be substantial changes between the proposed version of the test and the final published edition, with actual data playing a substantial role in the translation from theo-

ry to the published incarnation. Even so, the theory and planning behind the SB5 deserve some comment.

The plans for the SB5 seek to honor the Binet tradition while also incorporating current methodology and theories of intelligence (J. Wasserman, personal communication, February 17, 2000). One major change is explicit adoption of the multi-level model of intelligence expounded by Cattell, Horn (see Horn & Noll, 1997), and Carroll (see Carroll, 1993). The goal in developing the SB5 is to include items that will adequately sample all eight hypothesized specific ability factors: fluid reasoning, general knowledge, quantitative reasoning, working memory (previously short-term memory), long-term memory, auditory processing, visual–spatial ability, and processing speed. The battery is also expected to include measures of procedural knowledge in an effort to measure Gc, or crystallized ability. If the data support the desired model, then the plan would be for SB5 to yield factor scores for each of these specific abilities. In a departure from tradition, the SB5 will probably express these standard scores in a metric with $M = 100$ and $SD = 15$ (not the $SD = 16$ of previous Stanford–Binet scales). The expectation is that the SB5 will also yield three superordinate scores: Verbal Ability, Nonverbal Ability, and a full-scale Composite score reflecting the single best estimate of psychometric g obtained from the test. Each of these constructs will also have an observed scaled score that practitioners will calculate as part of the standard scoring of the battery.

Current plans also include other features designed to make the test more appealing to clinicians. One is to utilize a balanced set of verbal and nonverbal indicators for each of the eight specific ability factors, addressing a historical criticism of the SB instruments as overemphasizing verbal abilities. A second feature is the plan to generate linking samples of youths completing the SB5 and either the Wechsler Individual Achievement Test—Second Edition or the Achievement tests from the WJ-III. This would substantially facilitate the analysis of IQ–achievement discrepancies when these popular measures of academic achievement are used. Perhaps most notable of all, the SB5 is expected to extend through adulthood, with new norms reaching ages 80–90. Extensive validity studies are also planned, comparing the SB5 with a variety of other measures of cognitive ability, as well as looking at performance on the SB5 within special populations (defined using independent research and diagnostic criteria). This would be an important contribution to the body of knowledge, in addition to being useful data for test interpretation, because such an approach would avoid the circular reasoning that plagues much research in this area. Too often researchers have used a test to define a diagnosis (e.g., mental retardation or learning disabilities), and then demonstrated that this group shows different performance on other measures of the same construct—without acknowledging the tautology of this approach (Glutting, McDermott, Watkins, Kush, & Konold, 1997).

Also under consideration is a return to the age scale format used in versions prior to SB4. This would eliminate individual subtest scores from the SB5 and make the factor scores the lowest level of analysis. This approach would be consistent with the goal of making SB5 developmentally sensitive, allowing a blending of items designed to measure the same construct across different ages, without requiring a formal change in subtest. Item-level factor analysis (or analysis of parcels developed using IRT) would guide the organization of items as indicators of the specific ability factors.

This return to an age scale format is likely to be controversial, given the amount of clinical lore surrounding the practice of subtest interpretation. However, this change is also consistent with the best evidence currently available, which shows that subtest interpretation is fraught with psychometric problems (Macmann & Barnett, 1997; McDermott et al., 1990, 1992) and generally has failed to deliver the promised improvements in interpretation, diagnosis, or intervention (Watkins & Kush, 1994). Because of their greater reliability and larger amount of variance attributable to an underlying cognitive ability (i.e., greater validity), factor scores are more likely to enable clinicians to make finer-grained analyses than simple interpretation of a global score. The planned format for the SB5 could do much to promote good clinical practice in this regard. Excluding the subtests would certainly discourage the scientifically unwarranted practice of interpreting them. At the same time, providing better measures of the specific ability constructs of the Cattell–Horn–Carroll model would equip practitioners to measure distinct cognitive abilities underlying g. It would still be necessary to demonstrate the treatment validity of the different factor scores (cf. Glutting, Youngstrom, et al., 1997; Youngstrom et al., 1999), but these scores would inherently possess better construct validity than subtest scores. We hope that the finished product for the SB5 achieves the goals its developers have set for this revision.

RECOMMENDATIONS

On the basis of this review, we offer the following general recommendations affecting use of the SB4. As with any recommendation or clinical practice, these are subject to change in light of new research findings.

1. Reasonable construct validity is present for the Composite, and the Composite also has accumulated the most evidence for external and criterion-related validity. This is a score that psychologists can interpret on the basis of psychometric principles, empirical evidence, and best practices.

2. SB4 area scores are problematic because of the continued controversy about SB4's factor structure, as well as the current lack of any data showing incremental validity of the area scores surpassing the interpretive value of the Composite. We have also advanced the position that current disagreement about the adequacy of a four-factor model may not necessarily represent a failure of SB4 per se. Nevertheless, until optimal methodological procedures are applied and empirical evidence supports four underlying factors, psychologists would do well to avoid comparing or interpreting these scores.

3. Subtest interpretation should be deemphasized or avoided, on both psychometric and scientific grounds. Subtest interpretation increases the possibility of Type I errors and complicates the assessment process. Most importantly, subtest analysis has yet to demonstrate incremental validity or treatment validity with the SB4 or other major tests of ability.

4. We believe we have amply demon-

strated the hazards psychologists face in constructing their own SB4 short forms. Cases could be made either for administering the test in its entirety, or for using one of the established and validated short forms. The two most documented and empirically supported short forms currently appear to be the four-subtest form (especially as a screener) and the six-subtest GPAB. Better documentation of the effects of subtest sequencing, as well as the establishment of short forms' the external validity, should remain high priorities on the research agenda. Though less glamorous than some investigations, this work would have important applications in an era focusing on efficiency and cost containment in the provision of psychological assessment.

5. SB4 should not be administered to preschoolers believed to have mental retardation. Because of floor effects, the test shows little capacity for detecting moderate to severe retardation at these age levels. Moreover, the WPPSI-R generally supports floors equal to or slightly lower than those of SB4.

6. SB4 provides a sufficient ceiling for the identification of examinees who may be gifted at any age. The breadth of constructs measured and its extended age range also increase the likelihood that SB4 will become a favored instrument for the assessment of giftedness (Laurent et al., 1992). However, it is worth noting that the revisions of the Wechsler scales published after the SB4 also extended their norms to 3.67 or 4 standard deviations (i.e., maximum standard scores of 155 to 160), essentially establishing parity with the SB4 in this respect.

7. We have argued that IQ tests should not be marketed without adequate evidence that they reflect the aptitudes of individuals with disabilities. However, we cannot reasonably hold SB4 to standards that have never been imposed on any IQ tests at the time of their publication. The SB4 clearly met the standard of practice in test development when it was published. It is this standard of practice itself that needs improvement. Currently marketed tests have yet to do an adequate job of documenting the appropriateness of the instrument for individuals with disabilities or other specific populations. In practical terms, the SB4 appears comparable to the other best tests available in technical adequacy in this area.

8. It is critical that examiners control test pieces when evaluating young children (especially the Bead Memory pieces, due to the potential choking hazard).

9. Examiners should inquire about color-blindness or family history of color-blindness, as well as remaining alert to this possibility in their clinical observations during testing. The prevalence of color-blindness is high enough that clinicians will encounter this issue with some frequency, and it can influence performance on some subtests of SB4.

CONCLUSION

At the beginning of this chapter, we stated that no test is entirely without fault or virtue. Perhaps SB4's greatest limitation is that it tries too hard to offer everything psychologists want in an IQ test. Nevertheless, SB4's potential for meeting the avowed purposes of IQ tests is great, and, as is far too rare in the field of test development, the positive features of this instrument outweigh its limitations.

ACKNOWLEDGMENTS

Special thanks to John Wasserman, project coordinator for the development of the Stanford–Binet Intelligence Scale: Fifth Edition (SB5), for discussing the planned revisions while the SB5 project was still in progress. Thanks also to Carla Kmett Danielson, Shoshana Kahana, and Erin McMullen for their help in tracking down references for the various tables.

NOTES

1. The problem of small test pieces extends beyond SB4. Several other tests administered to young children, including the Bayley Scales of Infant Development (Bayley, 1969), contain item pieces so small that they are dangerous. Of course, test publishers could argue that it is the responsibility of psychologists to exercise due caution with test materials. Such a position, however, ignores the likelihood that the publisher will be named in any lawsuit stemming from accidents with test materials. Superseding any financial considerations, it is in the best interest of *children* that test materials be safe.

2. Although the BTBC was replaced recently by

the Boehm Test of Basic Concepts—Revised (Boehm, 1986) the original BTBC (Boehm, 1971) was used so that current results would be comparable to those reported by Kaufman (1978).

3. Some of the best evidence for four-factor solutions relies on data using median subtest correlations collapsed across age ranges (e.g., Keith et al., 1988; Thorndike, 1990). Two considerations argue for caution in interpreting these solutions: (a) Using median correlations may hide developmental change (Sattler, 1992); and (b) such approaches have ignored the problem of missing data. Vastly different numbers of participants completed subtests within each age group. Tables B.1 to B.17 in the *Technical Manual* report the "pairwise" n's for each correlation, and numbers can fluctuate dramatically (e.g., n's from 38 to 314 for age 12; see Table B.11) within a given age group. These sampling problems are likely to contribute to technical difficulties in estimating factor structure, and they bias observed results in unknown ways.

4. The abbreviated batteries discussed earlier do not suffer from this problem, because they are composed of subtests 1 through 6 in SB4's administration sequence.

REFERENCES

Aiken, L. R. (2000). *Psychological testing and assessment*. Boston: Allyn & Bacon.

Anastasi, A., & Urbina, S. (1997). *Psychological testing* (7th ed.). New York: Macmillan.

Atkinson, L. (1991). Short forms of the Stanford–Binet Intelligence Scale, Fourth Edition, for children with low intelligence. *Journal of School Psychology, 29,* 177–181.

Bayley, N. (1969). *Bayley Scales of Infant Development: Birth to two years.* New York: Psychological Corporation.

Binet, A., & Simon, T. (1905). Méthodes nouvelles pour le diagnostic du niveau intellectual des anormaux. *L'Année Psychologique, 11,* 191–244.

Boehm, A. E. (1971). *Boehm Test of Basic Concepts: Manual.* New York: Psychological Corporation.

Boehm, A. E. (1986). *Boehm Test of Basic Concepts—Revised: Manual.* New York: Psychological Corporation.

Boyle, G. J. (1989). Confirmation of the structural dimensionality of the Stanford–Binet Intelligence Scale (Fourth Edition). *Personality and Individual Differences, 10,* 709–715.

Boyle, G. J. (1990). Stanford–Binet IV Intelligence Scale: Is its structure supported by LISREL congeneric factor analyses? *Personality and Individual Differences, 11,* 1175–1181.

Bracken, B. A. (1985). A critical review of the Kaufman Assessment Battery for Children (K-ABC). *School Psychology Review, 14,* 21–36.

Bradley-Johnson, S. (2001). Cognitive assessment for the youngest children: A critical review of tests. *Journal of Psychoeducational Assessment, 19,* 19–44.

Carpentieri, S. C., & Morgan, S. B. (1994). Brief report: A comparison of patterns of cognitive functioning of autistic and nonautistic retarded children on the Stanford–Binet—Fourth Edition. *Journal of Autism and Developmental Disorders, 24,* 215–223.

Carroll, J. B. (1993). *Human cognitive abilities: A survey of factor-analytic studies.* New York: Cambridge University Press.

Caruso, J. C. (2001). Reliable component analysis of the Stanford–Binet Fourth Edition for 2- to 6-year-olds. *Psychological Assessment, 13,* 261–266.

Carvajal, H. H., & Gerber, J. (1987). 1986 Stanford–Binet abbreviated forms. *Psychological Reports, 61,* 285–286.

Carvajal, H. H., Gerber, J., Hewes, P., & Weaver, K. A. (1987). Correlations between scores on Stanford–Binet IV and Wechsler Adult Intelligence Scale—Revised. *Psychological Reports, 61,* 83–86.

Carvajal, H. H., Hardy, K., Smith, K. L., & Weaver, K. A. (1988). Relationships between scores on Stanford–Binet IV and Wechsler Preschool and Primary Scale of Intelligence. *Psychology in the Schools, 25,* 129–131.

Carvajal, H. H., Hayes, J. E., Lackey, K. L., & Rathke, M. L. (1993). Correlations between scores on the Wechsler Intelligence Scale for Children—III and the General Purpose Abbreviated Battery of the Stanford–Binet IV. *Psychological Reports, 72,* 1167–1170.

Carvajal, H. H., McVey, S., Sellers, T., & Weyand, K. (1987). Relationships between scores on the General Purpose Abbreviated Battery of Stanford–Binet IV, Peabody Picture Vocabulary Test—Revised, Columbia Mental Maturity Scale, and Goodenough–Harris Drawing Test. *Psychological Record, 37,* 127–130.

Carvajal, H. H., Parks, J. P., Bays, K. J., & Logan, R. A. (1991). Relationships between scores on Wechsler Preschool and Primary Scale of Intelligence—Revised and Stanford–Binet IV. *Psychological Reports, 69,* 23–26.

Carvajal, H. H., & Weyand, K. (1986). Relationships between scores on Stanford–Binet IV and Wechsler Intelligence Scale for Children—Revised. *Psychological Reports, 59,* 963–966.

Cattell, R. B. (1940). A culture-free intelligence test, I. *Journal of Educational Psychology, 31,* 161–179.

Choi, H.-S., & Proctor, T. B. (1994). Error-prone subtests and error types in the administration of the Stanford–Binet Intelligence Scale: Fourth Edition. *Journal of Psychoeducational Assessment, 12,* 165–171.

Clark, R. D., Wortman, S., Warnock, S., & Swerdlik, M. (1987). A correlational study of Form L-M and the 4th edition of the Stanford–Binet with 3- to 6-year olds. *Diagnostique, 12,* 112–130.

Coren, S., Ward, L. M., & Enns, J. T. (1999). *Sensation and perception.* New York: Harcourt Brace Jovanovich.

Cronbach, L. J. (1987). *Review of the Stanford–Binet*

Intelligence Scale: Fourth Edition (1007–310). Lincoln, NE: Buros Institute of Mental Measurements.

DeLamatre, J. E., & Hollinger, C. L. (1990). Utility of the Stanford–Binet IV abbreviated form for placing exceptional children. *Psychological Reports, 67,* 973–974.

Delaney, E. A., & Hopkins, T. F. (1987). *Examiner's handbook: An expanded guide for Fourth Edition users.* Chicago: Riverside.

Elliott, C. D. (1990). *Differential Ability Scales: Introductory and technical handbook.* San Antonio, TX: Psychological Corporation.

Embretson, S. E. (1999). Issues in the measurement of cognitive abilities. In S. E. Embretson & S. L. Hershberger (Eds.), *The new rules of measurement: What every psychologist and educator should know* (pp. 1–16). Mahwah, NJ: Erlbaum.

Flanagan, D. P., & Alfonso, V. C. (1995). A critical review of the technical characteristics of new and recently revised intelligence tests for preschool children. *Journal of Psychoeducational Assessment, 13,* 66–90.

Flynn, J. R. (1984). IQ gains and the Binet decrements. *Journal of Educational Measurement, 21,* 283–290.

Flynn, J. R. (1999). Searching for justice: The discovery of IQ gains over time. *American Psychologist, 54,* 5–20.

Glutting, J. J., Adams, W., & Sheslow, D. (2000). *Wide Range Intelligence Test manual.* Wilmington, DE: Wide Range.

Glutting, J. J., & Kaplan, D. (1990). Stanford–Binet Intelligence Scale, Fourth Edition: Making the case for reasonable interpretations. In C. R. Reynolds & R. W. Kamphaus (Eds.), *Handbook of psychological and educational assessment of children: Intelligence and achievement* (pp. 277–295). New York: Guilford Press.

Glutting, J. J., McDermott, P. A., & Stanley, J. C. (1987). Resolving differences among methods of establishing confidence limits for test scores. *Educational and Psychological Measurement, 47,* 607–614.

Glutting, J. J., McDermott, P. A., Watkins, M. M., Kush, J. C., & Konold, T. R. (1997). The base rate problem and its consequences for interpreting children's ability profiles. *School Psychology Review, 26,* 176–188.

Glutting, J. J., Youngstrom, E. A., Oakland, T., & Watkins, M. (1996). Situational specificity and generality of test behaviors for samples of normal and referred children. *School Psychology Review, 25,* 94–107.

Glutting, J. J., Youngstrom, E. A., Ward, T., Ward, S., & Hale, R. (1997). Incremental efficacy of WISC-III factor scores in predicting achievement: What do they tell us? *Psychological Assessment, 9,* 295–301.

Greene, A. C., Sapp, G. L., & Chissom, B. (1990). Validation of the Stanford–Binet Intelligence Scale: Fourth Edition with exceptional black male students. *Psychology in the Schools, 27,* 35–41.

Gridley, B. E., & McIntosh, D. E. (1991). Confirmatory factor analysis of the Stanford–Binet: Fourth Edition for a normal sample. *Journal of School Psychology, 29,* 237–248.

Grossman, J. J. (Ed.). (1983). *Classification in mental retardation.* Washington, DC: American Association on Mental Deficiency.

Grunau, R. E., Whitfield, M. F., & Petrie, J. (2000). Predicting IQ of biologically "at risk" children from age 3 to school entry: Sensitivity and specificity of the Stanford–Binet Intelligence Scale IV. *Journal of Developmental and Behavioral Pediatrics, 21,* 401–407.

Hambleton, R. K., Swaminathan, H., & Rogers, H. J. (1991). *Fundamentals of item response theory.* Newbury Park, CA: Sage.

Hansen, M. H., Hurwitz, W. N., & Madow, W. G. (1953). *Sample survey methods and theory.* New York: Wiley.

Harris, S. L., Handleman, J. S., & Burton, J. L. (1990). The Stanford–Binet profiles of young children with autism. *Special Services in the Schools, 6,* 135–143.

Hartwig, S. S., Sapp, G. L., & Clayton, G. A. (1987). Comparison of the Stanford–Binet Intelligence Scale: Form L-M and the Stanford–Binet Intelligence Scale Fourth Edition. *Psychological Reports, 60,* 1215–1218.

Hendershott, J. L., Searight, H. R., Hatfield, J. L., & Rogers, B. J. (1990). Correlations between the Stanford–Binet, Fourth Edition and the Kaufman Assessment Battery for Children for a preschool sample. *Perceptual and Motor Skills, 71,* 819–825.

Hernandez, D. J. (1997). Child development and the social demography of childhood. *Child Development, 68,* 149–169.

Hopkins, T. F. (1988). Commentary: The Fourth Edition of the Stanford–Binet: Alfred Binet would be proud. . . . *Measurement and Evaluation in Counseling and Development, 21,* 40–41.

Horn, J. L. (1965). A rationale and test for the number of factors in factor analysis. *Psychometrika, 30,* 179–185.

Horn, J. L. (1968). Organization of abilities and the development of intelligence. *Psychological Review, 79,* 242–259.

Horn, J. L., & Cattell, R. B. (1966). Refinement and test of the theory of fluid and crystallized intelligence. *Journal of Educational Psychology, 57,* 253–270.

Horn, J. L., & Noll, J. (1997). Human cognitive capabilities: Gf-Gc theory. In D. P. Flanagan, J. L. Genshaft, & P. L. Harrison (Eds.), *Contemporary intellectual assessment: Theories, tests, and issues* (pp. 53–91). New York: Guilford Press.

Husband, T. H., & Hayden, D. C. (1996). Effects of the addition of color to assessment instruments. *Journal of Psychoeducational Assessment, 14,* 147–151.

Jaeger, R. M. (1984). Refinement and test of the theory of fluid and crystallized intelligence. *Journal of Educational Psychology, 57,* 253–270.

Jensen, A. R. (1980). *Bias in mental testing.* New York: Free Press.

Kamphaus, R. W. (1993). *Clinical assessment of children's intelligence.* Boston: Allyn & Bacon.

Kaufman, A. S. (1994). *Intelligent testing with the WISC-III.* New York: Wiley.

Kaufman, A. S. (1978). The importance of basic concepts in the individual assessment of preschool children. *Journal of School Psychology, 16,* 207–211.

Kaufman, A. S., & Kaufman, N. L. (1983). *K-ABC: Kaufman Assessment Battery for Children.* Circle Pines, MN: American Guidance Service.

Keith, T. Z., Cool, V. A., Novak, C. G., & White, L. J. (1988). Confirmatory factor analysis of the Stanford–Binet Fourth Edition: Testing the theory–test match. *Journal of School Psychology, 26,* 253–274.

Keith, T. Z., & Witta, E. L. (1997). Hierarchical and cross-age confirmatory factor analysis of the WISC-III: What does it measure? *School Psychology Quarterly, 12,* 89–107.

Kelley, T. L. (1927). *Interpretation of educational measurements.* Yonkers, NY: World Books.

Kish, L. (1965). *Survey sampling.* New York: Wiley.

Kline, R. B. (1989). Is the Fourth Edition Stanford–Binet a four-factor test?: Confirmatory factor analyses of alternative models for ages 2 through 23. *Journal of Psychoeducational Assessment, 7,* 4–13.

Kline, R. B., Snyder, J., Guilmette, S., & Castellanos, M. (1992). Relative usefulness of elevation, variability, and shape information from WISC-R, K-ABC, and Fourth Edition Stanford–Binet profiles in predicting achievement. *Psychological Assessment, 4,* 426–432.

Kline, R. B., Snyder, J., Guilmette, S., & Castellanos, M. (1993). External validity of the profile variability index for the K-ABC, Stanford–Binet, and WISC-R: Another cul-de-sac. *Journal of Learning Disabilities, 26,* 557–567.

Krohn, E. J., & Lamp, R. E. (1989). Concurrent validity of the Stanford–Binet Fourth Edition and K-ABC for Head Start children. *Journal of School Psychology, 27,* 59–67.

Krohn, E. J., & Lamp, R. E. (1999). Stability of the SB:FE and K-ABC for young children from low-income families: A 5-year longitudinal study. *Journal of School Psychology, 37,* 315–332.

Kyle, J. M., & Robertson, C. M. T. (1994). Evaluation of three abbreviated forms of the Stanford–Binet Intelligence Scale: Fourth Edition. *Canadian Journal of School Psychology, 10,* 147–154.

Laurent, J., Swerdlik, M., & Ryburn, M. (1992). Review of validity research on the Stanford–Binet Intelligence Scale: Fourth Edition. *Psychological Assessment, 4,* 102–112.

Lavin, C. (1995). Clinical applications of the Stanford–Binet Intelligence Scale: Fourth Edition to reading instruction of children with learning disabilities. *Psychology in the Schools, 32,* 255–263.

Lavin, C. (1996). The Wechsler Intelligence Scale for Children—Third Edition and the Stanford–Binet Intelligence Scale: Fourth Edition: A preliminary study of validity. *Psychological Reports, 78,* 491–496.

Levy, P. (1968). Short-form tests: A methodological review. *Psychological Bulletin, 69,* 410–416.

Lukens, J. (1988). Comparison of the Fourth Edition and the L-M edition of the Stanford–Binet used with mentally retarded persons. *Journal of School Psychology, 26,* 87–89.

Macmann, G. M., & Barnett, D. W. (1997). Myth of the master detective: Reliability of interpretations for Kaufman's "intelligent testing" approach to the WISC-III. *School Psychology Quarterly, 12,* 197–234.

McCallum, R. S., & Karnes, F. A. (1990). Use of a brief form of the Stanford–Binet Intelligence Scale (Fourth) for gifted children. *Journal of School Psychology, 28,* 279–283.

McCallum, R. S., Karnes, F. A., & Crowell, M. (1988). Factor structure of the Stanford–Binet Intelligence Scale (4th Ed.) for gifted children. *Contemporary Educational Psychology, 13,* 331–338.

McCallum, R. S., & Whitaker, D. P. (2000). The assessment of preschool children with the Stanford–Binet Intelligence Scale Fourth Edition. In B. A. Bracken (Ed.), *The psychoeducational assessment of preschool children* (3rd ed., pp. 76–102). New York: Grune & Stratton.

McCarthy, D. A. (1972). *Manual for the McCarthy Scale of Children's Abilities.* New York: Psychological Corporation.

McCormick, R. L. (1956). A criticism of studies comparing item-weighting methods. *Journal of Applied Psychology, 40,* 343–344.

McCrowell, K. L., & Nagle, R. J. (1994). Comparability of the WPPSI-R and the S-B:IV among preschool children. *Journal of Psychoeducational Assessment, 12,* 126–134.

McDermott, P. A., Fantuzzo, J. W., & Glutting, J. J. (1990). Just say no to subtest analysis: A critique on Wechsler theory and practice. *Journal of Psychoeducational Assessment, 8,* 290–302.

McDermott, P. A., Fantuzzo, J. W., Glutting, J. J., Watkins, M. W., & Baggaley, A. R. (1992). Illusions of meaning in the ipsative assessment of children's ability. *Journal of Special Education, 25,* 504–526.

Meyer, G. J., Finn, S. E., Eyde, L. D., Kay, G. G., Kubiszyn, T. W., Moreland, K. L., Eisman, E. J., & Dies, R. R. (1998). *Benefits and costs of psychological assessment in health care delivery: Report of the Board of Professional Affairs Psychological Assessment Workgroup, Part I.* Washington, DC: American Psychological Association.

Moffitt, T. E., & Silva, P. A. (1987). WISC-R Verbal and Performance IQ discrepancy in an unselected cohort: Clinical significance and longitudinal stability. *Journal of Consulting and Clinical Psychology, 55,* 768–774.

Molfese, V., Yaple, K., Helwig, S., & Harris, L. (1992). Stanford–Binet Intelligence Scale (Fourth Edition): Factor structure and verbal subscale scores for three-year-olds. *Journal of Psychoeducational Assessment, 10,* 47–58.

Nagle, R. J., & Bell, N. L. (1993). Validation of Stanford–Binet Intelligence Scale: Fourth Edition abbreviated batteries with college students. *Psychology in the Schools, 30,* 227–231.

Nagle, R. J., & Bell, N. L. (1995). Validation of an item-reduction short form of the Stanford–Binet Intelligence Scale: Fourth Edition with college students. *Journal of Clinical Psychology, 51,* 63–70.

Naglieri, J. A. (1988a). Interpreting area score variation on the fourth edition of the Stanford–Binet Scale of Intelligence. *Journal of Clinical Child Psychology, 17,* 225–228.

Naglieri, J. A. (1988b). Interpreting the subtest profile

on the fourth edition of the Stanford–Binet Scale of Intelligence. *Journal of Clinical Child Psychology*, *17*, 62–65.

Neisser, U., Boodoo, G., Bouchard, T. J., Jr., Boykin, A. W., Brody, N., Ceci, S. J., Halpern, D. F., Loehlin, J. C., Perloff, R., Sternberg, R. J., & Urbina, S. (1996). Intelligence: Knowns and unknowns. *American Psychologist*, *51*, 77–101.

Olridge, O. A., & Allison, E. E. (1968). Review of Wechsler Preschool and Primary Scale of Intelligence. *Journal of Educational Measurement*, *5*, 347–348.

Ownby, R. L., & Carmin, C. N. (1988). Confirmatory factor analyses of the Stanford–Binet Intelligence Scale, Fourth Edition. *Journal of Psychoeducational Assessment*, *6*, 331–340.

Prewett, P. N. (1992). Short forms of the Stanford–Binet Intelligence Scale: Fourth Edition. *Journal of Psychoeducational Assessment*, *10*, 257–264.

Psychological Corporation. (1997). *Wechsler Adult Intelligence Scale—Third Edition, Wechsler Memory Scale—Third Edition technical manual*. San Antonio, TX: Author.

Psychological Corporation. (1999). *Wechsler Abbreviated Scale of Intelligence manual*. San Antonio, TX: Author.

Reynolds, C. R., Kamphaus, R. W., & Rosenthal, B. L. (1988). Factor analysis of the Stanford–Binet Fourth Edition for ages 2 years through 23 years. *Measurement and Evaluation in Counseling and Development*, *21*, 52–63.

Rosenthal, B. L., & Kamphaus, R. W. (1988). Interpretive tables for test scatter on the Stanford–Binet Intelligence Scale: Fourth Edition. *Journal of Psychoeducational Assessment*, *6*, 359–370.

Rothlisberg, B. A. (1987). Comparing the Stanford–Binet, Fourth Edition to the WISC-R: A concurrent validity study. *Journal of School Psychology*, *25*, 193–196.

Rust, J. O., & Lindstrom, A. (1996). Concurrent validity of the WISC-III and Stanford–Binet IV. *Psychological Reports*, *79*, 618–620.

Saklofske, D. H., Schwean, V. L., Yackulic, R. A., & Quinn, D. (1994). WISC-III and SB:FE performance of children with attention deficit hyperactivity disorder. *Canadian Journal of School Psychology*, *10*, 167–171.

Sattler, J. (1992). *Assessment of children* (3rd ed.). San Diego, CA: Author.

Saylor, C. F., Boyce, G. C., Peagler, S. M., & Callahan, S. A. (2000). Brief report: Cautions against using the Stanford–Binet-IV to classify high-risk preschoolers. *Journal of Pediatric Psychology*, *25*, 179–183.

Schwean, V. L., Saklofske, D. H., Yackulic, R. A., & Quinn, D. (1993). WISC-III performance of ADHD children. *Journal of Psychoeducational Assessment (WISC-III Monograph)*, pp. 56–70.

Silverstein, A. B. (1993). Type I, Type II, and other types of errors in pattern analysis. *Psychological Assessment*, *5*, 72–74.

Simpson, M., Carone, D. A., Burns, W. J., Seidman, T., Montgomery, D., & Sellers, A. (2002). Assessing giftedness with the WISC-III and the SB4. *Psychology in the Schools*, *39*, 515–524.

Smith, D. K., & Bauer, J. J. (1989). *Relationship of the K-ABC and S-B:FE in a preschool sample*. Paper presented at the annual meeting of the National Association of School Psychologists, Boston.

Smith, G. T., McCarthy, D. M., & Anderson, K. G. (2000). On the sins of short-form development. *Psychological Assessment*, *12*, 102–111.

Spearman, C. (1923). *The nature of intelligence and the principles of cognition*. London: Macmillan.

Spruill, J. (1988). Two types of tables for use with the Stanford–Binet Intelligence Scale: Fourth Edition. *Journal of Psychoeducational Assessment*, *6*, 78–86.

Spruill, J. (1991). A comparison of the Wechsler Adult Intelligence Scale—Revised with the Stanford–Binet Intelligence Scale (4th Edition) for mentally retarded adults. *Psychological Assessment*, *3*, 133–135.

Thorndike, R. L. (1973). *Stanford–Binet Intelligence Scale: Form L-M, 1972 norms tables*. Boston: Houghton Mifflin.

Thorndike, R. L. (1990). Would the real factors of the Stanford–Binet Fourth Edition please come forward? *Journal of Psychoeducational Assessment*, *8*, 412–435.

Thorndike, R. L. (1982). *Applied psychometrics*. Boston: Houghton Mifflin.

Thorndike, R. L., Hagen, E. P., & Sattler, J. M. (1986a). *Guide for administering and scoring the Stanford–Binet Intelligence Scale: Fourth Edition*. Chicago: Riverside.

Thorndike, R. L., Hagen, E. P., & Sattler, J. M. (1986b). *Stanford–Binet Intelligence Scale: Fourth Edition*. Chicago: Riverside.

Thorndike, R. L., Hagen, E. P., & Sattler, J. M. (1986c). *Technical manual, Stanford–Binet Intelligence Scale: Fourth Edition*. Chicago: Riverside.

Velicer, W. F. (1976). Determining the number of components from the matrix of partial correlations. *Psychometrika*, *41*, 321–327.

Vernon, P. E. (1950). *The structure of human abilities*. London: Methuen.

Vernon, P. E. (1987). The demise of the Stanford–Binet Scale. *Canadian Psychology*, *28*, 251–258.

Volker, M. A., Guarnaccia, V., & Scardapane, J. R. (1999). Short forms of the Stanford–Binet Intelligence Scale: Fourth Edition for screening potentially gifted preschoolers. *Journal of Psychoeducational Assessment*, *17*, 226–235.

Wainer, H. (1999). The most dangerous profession: A note on nonsampling error. *Psychological Methods*, *4*, 250–256.

Watkins, M. W. (1996). Diagnostic utility of the WISC-III Developmental Index as a predictor of learning disabilities. *Journal of Learning Disabilities*, *29*, 305–312.

Watkins, M. W., & Kush, J. C. (1994). Wechsler subtest analysis: The right way, the wrong way, or no way? *School Psychology Review*, *23*, 640–651.

Watkins, M. W., Kush, J. C., & Glutting, J. J. (1997). Prevalence and diagnostic utility of the WISC-III SCAD profile among children with disabilities. *School Psychology Quarterly*, *12*, 235–248.

Wechsler, D. (1967). *Manual for the Wechsler Preschool and Primary Scale of Intelligence*. New York: Psychological Corporation.

Wechsler, D. (1989). *Wechsler Preschool and Primary Scale of Intelligence—Revised: Manual.* San Antonio, TX: Psychological Corporation.

Wechsler, D. (1991). *Manual for the Wechsler Intelligence Scale for Children—Third Edition.* San Antonio, TX: Psychological Corporation.

Weiner, E. A., & Stewart, B. J. (1984). *Assessing individuals.* Boston: Little, Brown.

Wersh, J., & Thomas, M. R. (1990). The Stanford–Binet Intelligence Scale—Fourth Edition: Observations, comments and concerns. *Canadian Psychology, 31,* 190–193.

Woodcock, R. W., & Johnson, M. B. (1990a). *Woodcock–Johnson Psychoeducational Battery—Revised Edition.* Allen, TX: DLM Teaching Resources.

Woodcock, R. W., & Johnson, M. B. (1990b). *Woodcock–Johnson Psychoeducational Battery—Revised Edition: Examiner's manual.* Allen, TX: DLM Teaching Resources.

Youngstrom, E. A., Kogos, J. L., & Glutting, J. J. (1999). Incremental efficacy of Differential Ability Scales factor scores in predicting individual achievement criteria. *School Psychology Quarterly, 14,* 26–39.

Ysseldyke, J. E., & Stevens, L. J. (1986) Specific learning deficits: The learning disabled. In R. T. Brown & c. R. Reynolds (Eds.), *Psychological perspectives on childhood exceptionality: A handbook* (pp. 381–422). New York: Wiley.

Zwick, W. R., & Velicer, W. F. (1986). Comparison of five rules for determining the number of components to retain. *Psychological Bulletin, 99,* 432–442.

11

Assessing Diverse Populations with Nonverbal Tests of General Intelligence

BRUCE A. BRACKEN
JACK A. NAGLIERI

Psychologists have long wrestled with the challenge of assessing the cognitive functioning of individuals who lack the language skills needed to demonstrate their ability. During the early 1800s, French clinicians were among the first to attempt methods to assess and remediate the intellectual abilities of children with limited language. In the celebrated case of Victor, the Wild Boy of Aveyron, Jean Itard sought to assess the cognitive abilities of the feral youth and to determine whether the boy could acquire functional language skills (Carrey, 1995; Itard, 1932). In addition to Itard, other historical figures have pursued the problem of assessing the intellectual abilities of children who could not or would not speak (e.g., Seguin, 1907). In this vein, Seguin is possibly best known for his development of unique instrumentation to aid in the assessment of children's cognitive abilities through nonverbal means. Seguin's instrument required the puzzle-like placement of common geometric shapes into inserts of the same shape. The instrument (and its many derivatives) has become widely used internationally and is known universally as the "Seguin Formboard."

During the early decades of the 20th century, the press for nonverbal assessment be-

came especially important in the United States as the armed forces sought methods to assess the abilities of foreign-born and illiterate military recruits, in addition to the typical literate, English-speaking recruits. To address this pressing need during World War I, the Committee on the Psychological Examination of Recruits was formed and included some of the most notable psychologists of the time (Thorndike & Lohman, 1990).

According to the examiner's guide for the Army Psychological Examination (U.S. Government Printing Office, 1918), military testing was deemed necessary to classify soldiers according to mental ability, to create organizational units of equal strength, to identify soldiers with potential problems, to assist in training and assignments, to identify potential officers, and to discover soldiers with special talents or skills. The Army Mental Tests resulted in Group Examination Alpha and Beta forms, described by Yoakum and Yerkes (1920). The Group Examination Alpha Test (Army Alpha) was administered to recruits who could read and respond to the written English version of the scale. Army Alpha was limited in its utility as a measure of ability when recruits had limited English proficiency or were insufficiently literate to read and respond reliably to verbal items. The Group Examination Beta Test portion of the Mental Tests (Army Beta) was developed as a nonverbal supplement to Army Alpha.

Army Beta was designed specifically for the assessment of illiterate recruits or those with limited ability to speak or read English. Yoakum and Yerkes (1920) stated, "Men who fail in alpha are set to beta in order that injustice by reason of relative unfamiliarity with English may be avoided" (p. 19). As a nonverbal group measure of ability, Army Beta served an important need, especially in a country with a population as diverse as the United States. It included a variety of performance tasks, many of which were to appear later in the widely used Wechsler scales (e.g., puzzles, cube constructions, digit symbols, mazes, picture completions, picture arrangements). Most if not all of these tasks originated in experimental procedures developed before the Army Group Exams; these procedures included some of the pioneer tests developed by Kohs (1919), Seguin (1907), Porteus (1915), Pintner and Patterson (1917), and others.

In the private sector, the need for nonverbal ability measures was developing in a parallel fashion. In 1924 and with a $5,000 grant, Arthur began work on the Point Scale of Performance Tests at the Amherst H. Wilder Child Guidance Clinic in St. Paul, Minnesota (Arthur, 1943, 1947). Development of the Point Scale began in 1917 under the guidance of Herbert Woodrow (Arthur, 1925; Arthur & Woodrow, 1919), but Arthur brought it to its completion. The Point Scale is important because it combined and modified a variety of existing performance tests, including a revision of the Knox Cube Test (Knox, 1914), the Seguin Formboard, the Arthur Stencil Design Test, the Porteus Maze Test (Porteus, 1915), and an adaptation of the Healy Picture Completion Test (Healy, 1914, 1918, 1921) into a battery. The Point Scale was intended for individuals with deafness or other hearing impairments, who were distinctly disadvantaged when administered language-loaded intelligence tests. In response to this press for a useful nonverbal battery, Arthur had sought to create a nonverbal battery that

collectively would "furnish an IQ comparable to that obtained with the Binet scales" (Arthur, 1947, p. 1).

In addition to nonverbal assessments for cross-cultural populations, nonverbal procedures were needed to assess the cognitive abilities of people with neurological impairments (e.g., traumatic brain injury), psychiatric conditions (e.g., selective/elective mutism, autism), speech and language disorders/learning disabilities, and other language-related conditions. Essentially, nonverbal assessment procedures have been needed for all individuals for whom traditional language-loaded intelligence tests do not provide an accurate representation of the individuals' true current level of intellectual functioning. In this sense, nonverbal tests of intelligence are designed to reduce the bias associated with influences of language in an assessment, when language is not the primary construct targeted for assessment. That is, when general intelligence is the construct of interest, the heavy verbal demands of intelligence tests like the Wechsler scales—the early versions of which were largely based on the Army Mental Tests (Kaufman & Lichtenberger, 1999; Naglieri, 1999)—can create unfair "construct-irrelevant" influences on examinees' performance (Brown, Reynolds, & Whitaker, 1999; Hilliard, 1984; Reynolds, Lowe, & Saenz, 1999). Just as all group-administered tests with written directions and content become primarily "reading tests" for individuals with poor reading skills, all tests with verbal directions and content become primarily "language tests" for individuals with limited language proficiency.

Recognizing the problems inherent in tests of general intelligence that contains verbal directions and items with verbal (e.g., Vocabulary, Information, Similarities subtests) and achievement (e.g., Arithmetic subtest) content, many professionals use the Wechsler tests' Performance scale as a "nonverbal" test of intelligence. The Wechsler Intelligence Scale for Children (WISC; Wechsler, 1949) and its later editions have regularly been employed whenever children's hearing or language skills were considered a confound or threat to the validity of assessment results. Importantly, each of the Wechsler Performance subtests has test directions that are heavily laden with wordy verbal instructions, including basic language concepts (Bracken, 1986; Kaufman, 1990, 1994); these make the Performance scale a tool of very limited utility as a nonverbal measure of general ability.

Three major factors—the recognition of the limitations of using Performance subtests to measure ability nonverbally; the increase in social awareness and heightened sensitivity among psychologists; and the recent trend in the settlement of immigrants into communities of all sizes and all regions throughout the United States—have resulted in a proliferation of nonverbal tests of intelligence during the 1990s and into the new century. Perhaps most influential has been the increase in the numbers of children who speak English as a second language (ESL) in the U.S. public schools (e.g., Pasco, 1994).

Traditionally, immigrants have resettled in large metropolitan areas on the Atlantic and Pacific seaboards, and psychologists who work in these coastal cities have learned to anticipate that many languages will be spoken by the children in their schools. More recently, the resettlement efforts of churches and social organizations have encouraged more immigrants to settle in nontraditional regions and locales (e.g., Midwestern regions, rural locations, Southern Gulf Coastal areas). For example, Vietnamese immigrants have settled in large numbers along the Texas and Louisiana Gulf Coast, where they have become active in the shrimp industry. Similarly, Cubans and Hmong have resettled in colder, rural locations, such as Wisconsin and Minnesota. The result of such geographic dispersion among immigrant groups has meant that many communities that were once fairly homogeneous in race, ethnicity, culture, and language are now multicultural, multilingual, multiethnic, and multiracial.

Although cities have always been considered the center of the U.S. melting pot, the actual numbers of immigrants and the diverse nationalities and languages spoken in our urban schools are truly staggering. For example, it has been reported that more than 200 languages are spoken by the children who attend the Chicago city schools (Pasco, 1994)! And Chicago is not unique. More than 1.4 million children who have limited English proficiency are estimated to reside in California (Puente, 1998), with

more than 140 languages represented in this population (Unz, 1997).

It would be anticipated that schools in the U.S. Southwest would have large populations of English- and Spanish-speaking children; however, somewhat surprising is the very large number of other languages that are also spoken throughout this region of the country. For example, 67 languages are spoken by the students in the Tempe, Arizona school system (Ulik, 1997), and more than 50 languages are spoken in the nearby community school district of Scottsdale (Steele, 1998). Also in the U.S. Southwest, the schools of Plano, Texas report having a student body that collectively speaks more than 60 languages (Power, 1996). There has long been a press for Spanish-speaking bilingual psychologists and Spanish-language tests throughout the Southwestern United States. However, there is also a less obvious but equally important need for multilingual psychologists to competently serve a population of school children who collectively speak scores of languages other than English or Spanish throughout this region.

Other regions of the country report similar trends in linguistic and cultural diversity among their student populations. For example, diverse student bodies are just as prevalent in the schools throughout the U.S. Southeast as in the Southwest. Recent reports claim that more than 80 languages are spoken in Palm Beach County (Florida) Schools ("Fast Fact," 1996); 54 languages are spoken in Broward County (Florida) schools (Donzelli, 1996); 48 languages are spoken in Prince William County (Virginia) schools (O'Hanlon, 1997); and 45 languages are spoken by Cobb County (Georgia) students (Stepp, 1997). The list of communities with similarly diverse school populations grows longer each year, with a continually increasing number of languages spoken in both urban and rural public schools throughout the country.

The difficulties associated with conducting psychoeducational assessments of children who collectively speak so many different languages is exacerbated by legislation mandating that children be assessed in their native language. Although high-quality test translations are both possible and available (e.g., Bracken, 1998b; Bracken et al., 1990;

Bracken & Fouad, 1987; Munoz-Sandoval, Cummins, Alvarado, & Ruef, 1998), test translations and subsequent norming and validation efforts are both costly and time-consuming for a single dominant language (e.g., Spanish)—let alone 200 or more low-incidence languages. Given the relative unavailability of high-quality translated tests and the very limited number of bilingual school psychologists, the primary alternative to testing children in their native languages is to remove language as a variable and employ nonverbal tests (Frisby, 1999).

Nonverbal tests of intelligence have been available for decades, but the 1990s have experienced a surge in the development and improvement of these instruments. Psychologists currently have several nonverbal tests of intelligence from which to choose, depending on their individual needs and the nature of their referrals. With increased professional interest in nonverbal assessment and nonverbal instrumentation, there has been a concomitant refinement of knowledge, procedures, and practices with these newer measures. This growing field has also experienced some necessary refinement in terminology and conceptualization of what is measured.

DEFINITION OF TERMS

Because terms such as "nonverbal assessment," "nonverbal intellectual assessment," and "nonverbal intelligence" have often been used loosely and frequently have different connotations among assessment specialists, these terms warrant definition.

Nonverbal Assessment

Bracken and McCallum (1998a) use the term "nonverbal assessment" to describe a test administration process in which no receptive or expressive language demands are placed on *either* the examinee or the examiner. That is, a nonverbal test administration should include no spoken test directions, and no spoken responses should be required of the examinee. Many test manuals for extant "nonverbal tests" claim that the tests are administered in a nonverbal manner, but most of these tests are actually administered with verbal directions. Most "nonverbal

tests" in fact are best described as language-reduced instruments with verbal directions—sometimes with lengthy and complex verbal directions. For example, the Wechsler tests' Performance scale, the Nonverbal Scales of the Kaufman Assessment Battery for Children (K-ABC; Kaufman & Kaufman, 1983), and the Differential Ability Scales (DAS; Elliott, 1990) are all presented with verbal directions. Each of these "nonverbal tests" requires that examinees understand spoken test directions before they can attempt the respective intellectual assessment tasks. It is important to note that simply calling a test "nonverbal" does not render it nonverbal. According to the operational definition given above, there are very few intelligence tests that are truly nonverbal. The Test of Nonverbal Intelligence (TONI) and its revisions (Brown, Sherbenou, & Johnsen, 1982, 1990, 1997), the Comprehensive Test of Nonverbal Intelligence (CTONI; Hammill, Pearson, & Wiederholt, 1996), and the Universal Nonverbal Intelligence Test (UNIT; Bracken & McCallum, 1998a) are all administered in a 100% nonverbal fashion. The Leiter International Performance Test—Revised (Leiter-R; Roid & Miller, 1997) is administered in a nonverbal manner, with the exception of a few subtests; it requires or advocates the use of verbal directions only rarely.

Nonverbal Intellectual Assessment

Bracken and McCallum (1998a) use the term "nonverbal intellectual assessment" to describe the *process* of assessing the construct of general intelligence in a nonverbal fashion. That is, ability (defined as general intelligence) is assessed with tests that do not require examinees to understand spoken language or express themselves verbally. This nonverbal approach to assessing general intelligence should not be confused with measuring nonverbal intelligence, which hypothetically is a different construct from general intelligence.

Nonverbal Intelligence or General Intelligence Measured Nonverbally

When Wechsler developed his individual tests of intelligence from the Army Alpha and Beta Tests, his assignment of IQs for the

Verbal and Performance scales set the stage for an implicit identification of two types of intelligence. It is important to recall, however, that this test was built on the concept of "general intelligence" developed during the early part of the 20th century. The vagueness of this concept is apparent in Wechsler's (1944) definition of intelligence as "the aggregate or global capacity of the individual to act purposefully, to think rationally, and to deal effectively with his environment" (p. 3). Note that there is no discussion of verbal and nonverbal intelligence in this definition; Wechsler's Verbal and Performance scales appear to have been intended as only two different methodologies designed to assess the same general construct. Moreover, the origin of the concept of general intelligence was described by Pintner (1925), who wrote that "we did not start with a clear definition of general intelligence . . . [but] borrowed from every-day life a vague term implying all-round ability and knowledge, and . . . we [are] still attempting to define it more sharply and endow it with a stricter scientific connotation" (p. 53). Thus there is little reason to assume that those who originated these tests of general ability conceptualized verbal and nonverbal types of intelligence. Rather, it is critical to understand that Wechsler's dichotomy was based on the Army Mental Tests, which contained verbal and nonverbal versions so that a wider variety of persons could be effectively assessed. The separation of tests by verbal–nonverbal content is an obvious and simple idea to address the problem of assessing persons from diverse cultural and linguistic populations. Thus the organization of tests into Verbal and Performance scales on the Wechsler tests is a reflection of a practical dichotomy rather than a representation of different types of intelligence.

Although some test authors describe the assessment of a construct called "nonverbal intelligence," "nonverbal reasoning," or "nonverbal abilities" (Brown et al., 1982, 1990, 1997; Hammill et al., 1996), Bracken and McCallum (1998a) suggest that the central construct assessed by most "nonverbal intelligence tests" is in fact general intelligence. This distinction in terminology is more than a matter of hair-splitting semantics; it has implications for how instruments are conceptualized and used with the many diverse populations for which they were intended. If intelligence tests that purportedly assess nonverbal intelligence (e.g., the TONI, the CTONI) do in fact assess a construct that is theoretically different from the construct assessed on traditional intelligence tests (i.e., general intelligence), then these tests would be inappropriate for drawing inferences about children's overall intellectual functioning. Such tests should not be used interchangeably with traditional intelligence tests in making decisions about eligibility for services. However, given the strong correlations and comparable mean scores between some nonverbal intelligence tests (e.g., the Leiter-R, the UNIT) and traditional language-loaded intelligence tests, one could conclude that these instruments do in fact assess the same construct as language-loaded intelligence tests, and that this construct is general intelligence.

VERBAL, NONVERBAL, AND GENERAL INTELLIGENCE

Our position that general intelligence tests with verbal content and nonverbal content measure essentially the same construct as general ability tests that are entirely nonverbal is based on our understanding of the origin and theoretical underpinnings of these instruments. We can evaluate this view by looking at the question logically, and we can test some of the ideas experimentally. For example, if it were true that a nonverbal test of general intelligence was less complete than a verbal and nonverbal test of general intelligence, then some evidence for that could be found in evaluating the validity of the instruments. Naglieri (1999) addressed this type of question when he looked at the correlations between various tests of intelligence and achievement. He found that the median correlation between the WISC-III (Wechsler, 1991) and the Wechsler Individual Achievement Test (Wechsler, 1992) was .59 for the sample of 1,284 children who were administered both measures. This correlation can be compared to validity data reported in the manual of the Naglieri Nonverbal Ability Test (NNAT; Naglieri, 1997), which is described later in this chapter. Naglieri (1997) found a median correlation of .61 between the NNAT, which is a nonverbal progressive matrix test, and Stanford Achievement Test—Ninth Edition (SAT-9) Reading, Mathematics, Language, Thinking Skills, and Complete Battery scores for 21,476 children in grades K–12. These data clearly show that a group-administered nonverbal test of general ability (the NNAT) consisting of one item type (a progressive matrix) was as effective for predicting academic achievement (the SAT-9 scores) as the individually administered Verbal and Performance scales of the WISC-III. The reason why these two tests correlate similarly with achievement is that, despite their different contents, they are both measures of general ability.

TYPES OF NONVERBAL TESTS OF GENERAL ABILITY

There are two basic types of nonverbal tests. Some such tests assess intelligence through the use of one method (e.g., progressive matrices), and others assess multiple facets of children's intelligence (e.g., memory, reasoning, attention) using a variety of methods. Although there are several progressive matrix tests available, there are only two comprehensive nonverbal tests of intelligence (i.e., the UNIT and the Leiter-R). Tests of the matrix solution type include the C-TONI, TONI-3, the Matrix Analogies Test (MAT; Naglieri, 1985a, 1985b), the NNAT (Naglieri, 1997), and the Raven's Progressive Matrices (RPM; Raven, Court, & Raven, 1986). The General Ability Measure for Adults (GAMA; Naglieri & Bardos, 1997) includes some items that are similar to progressive matrices and some that are not (this test is more fully described later in this chapter).

The choice of which of these various nonverbal tests to use should be determined by several issues, including the reason for testing, the characteristics of the examinee, and the administration format desired (group or individual). For example, if a professional is conducting an individual assessment of a child with no English-language skills, then instruments that use pantomime directions will be most beneficial. If, however, the child has limited English-language skills, then the list of possible nonverbal tests is larger. When fair assessment of a large number of children (e.g., identification of gifted children, especially gifted minority children) is desired, then a group nonverbal test or abbreviated versions of comprehensive scales (e.g., the UNIT Abbreviated Battery) should be considered. However, when a person is to be evaluated for purposes of diagnosis, determination of special-programming eligibility, or treatment planning, then these instruments will have to be augmented with others that are designed and validated for such purposes.

The remainder of this chapter presents and reviews two comprehensive nonverbal measures of intelligence (the Leiter-R and the UNIT) and several of the matrix analogy format tests suitable for use in the United States. In this discussion, the term "comprehensive" connotes the use of a group of subtests with different formats that assess multiple aspects of general intelligence. One test that purportedly assesses "nonverbal intelligence" per se (the CTONI) is also discussed.

COMPREHENSIVE NONVERBAL TESTS OF GENERAL INTELLIGENCE

Leiter International Performance Scale—Revised

The Leiter-R (Roid & Miller, 1997) is a 20-subtest battery that can be administered in $1\frac{1}{2}$ to 2 hours to individuals between the ages of $2\frac{1}{2}$ and 20 years. Administered largely through pantomimed instructions, the revised instrument, like its 1940s predecessor, is intended for use when language-loaded intelligence tests would be inappropriate. The Leiter-R is an updated version of its predecessor in design and presentation; the test still contains a myriad of colorful stimulus materials. Instead of the blocks found in the original test, the Leiter-R employs various colorful chips, cards, pictures, and stimulus easels, as well as a wide variety of assessment activities. The test allows for the comprehensive assessment of children's and adolescent's intellectual functioning. It also provides four optional rating scales that can be used to assess children's psychosocial behaviors in a third-party response format. This description and review of the Leiter-R is restricted to the cognitive portions of the test.

As a 20-subtest instrument, the Leiter-R is conveniently divided into two separate cognitive batteries, each with 10 subtests. The first battery, Visualization and Reasoning (VR), was designed for the assessment of examinees' fluid reasoning and visual–spatial abilities. The second battery, Attention and Memory (AM), was designed to assess examinee's attention, memory, and learning processes.

The VR Battery produces five composites, which include a Brief IQ Screener (ages 2–20), a Full Scale IQ (FSIQ, ages 2–20), Fundamental Visualization (ages 2–5), Fluid Reasoning (ages 2–20), and Spatial Visualization (ages 11–20). The AM Battery produces six composites, including a Memory Screener (ages 2–20), Recognition Memory (ages 2–10), Associative Memory (ages 6–20), Memory Span (ages 6–20), Attention (ages 6–20), and Memory Process (ages 6–20). The two batteries and their respective composites produce standard scores with means of 100 and standard deviations set at 15. Leiter-R subtests produce scaled scores with means set at 10 and standard deviations of 3.

A description of the Leiter-R subtests by battery follows.

VR Battery Subtests

1. *Figure Ground.* The Figure Ground subtest presents embedded figures on stimulus cards. The examinee is to identify the embedded figures within the more complex stimulus background presented on each stimulus plate. This subtest is appropriate for ages 2–21 years.

2. *Design Analogies.* Design Analogies is a subtest that presents abstract analogies in 2 × 2 and 2 × 4 matrix formats, as well as some matrices of more complexly designed formats. This subtest is appropriate for ages 6–21 years.

3. *Form Completion.* Form Completion is a puzzle-solving task; it requires the examinee to assemble fragmented puzzle pieces to form a whole. This subtest is appropriate for ages 2–21 years.

4. *Matching.* The Matching subtest requires examinees to discriminate and match visual stimuli that are presented on response cards with identical designs that are presented on a stimulus easel. It is appropriate for ages 2–10 years.

5. *Sequential Order.* Sequential Order presents pictorial or figural sequences, and the examinee is expected to identify from an array of options the appropriate designs that best complete the stimulus sequence. It is appropriate for ages 2–21 years.

6. *Repeated Patterns.* The Repeated Patterns subtest presents pictorial or figural objects that are repeated in stimulus patterns; the examinee is required to use stimulus cards to complete each incomplete repeated pattern. It is appropriate for ages 2–21.

7. *Picture Context.* Picture Context requires the examinee to identify the part of a picture that is missing within the context of the overall picture. It is designed for ages 2–5 years.

8. *Classification.* Classification is a subtest that requires the examinee to organize or classify materials according to their salient characteristics (e.g., shape, color, size). Classification is intended for ages 2–5.

9. *Paper Folding.* Paper Folding requires the examinee to identify from several options what a paper figure would look if it were folded. It is a timed visualization subtest for ages 6–21 years. The subtest requires the examiner to verbally "remind" the examinee of how much time remains to complete the task.

10. *Figure Rotation.* The Figure Rotation subtest presents two- or three-dimensional objects, which the examinee must recognize after "mental rotation." Figure Rotation is appropriate for examinees between the ages of 11 and 21 years.

AM Battery Subtests

11. *Associated Pairs.* One or more pairs of stimuli (e.g., colored shapes, single colored line drawings of objects) are presented for a 5- to 10-second exposure. After the brief exposure, examinees are required to select the correct stimuli to complete each pair shown previously. Associated Pairs is appropriate for ages 2–21 years.

12. *Immediate Recognition.* A stimulus array depicting a variety of stimuli is presented for 5 seconds. After the brief exposure, the stimulus page is turned, revealing a second page with aspects of the first page absent. The examinee selects from response cards the stimulus that correctly matches the initial stimulus arrangement. Immediate

Recognition is appropriate for ages 4–10 years.

13. *Forward Memory.* The examiner presents a number of stimuli to be recalled, along with additional foils that are to be ignored. The examiner points to each relevant stimulus in a specified sequence, and encourages the examinee to replicate the sequence by pointing to the stimuli in the same order as the examiner. Forward Memory is appropriate for ages 2–21 years.

14. *Attention Sustained.* Attention Sustained requires the examinee to identify and cross-out target stimuli embedded within rows of stimuli on a page including the target stimuli as well as several foils. It is appropriate for ages 2–21 years.

15. *Reverse Memory.* Using the same artwork as in Forward Memory, the examiner points to stimuli in a sequence. The examinee is required to point to the same stimuli in reverse order. Reverse Memory is appropriate for ages 6–21 years.

16. *Visual Coding.* Visual Coding presents pairs of stimuli within boxes arranged in an over-and-under design; that is, a target stimulus in the top row is paired with a second stimulus in the box below. Items are presented in rows with target stimuli in the top row, but the bottom row contains empty boxes. The examinee is to identify the proper stimulus that would appropriately be placed in each empty box to complete the stimulus pairs. Visual Coding is appropriate for ages 6–21 years.

17. *Spatial Memory.* Spatial Memory presents a stimulus plate that depicts a variety of pictured objects within an increasingly complex grid. After a 10-second exposure, the stimulus plate is removed from the examinee's view. The examinee is then directed to place response cards in the grid locations where each object originally had been presented. SM is appropriate for ages 6–21 years.

18. *Delayed Pairs.* After approximately a 30-minute delay, the examinee's recall of objects depicted on the Associated Pairs subtest is assessed. Although Associated Pairs is appropriate for the entire age range, the follow-up Delayed Pairs subtest is appropriate only for ages 6–21 years.

19. *Delayed Recognition.* After approximately a 30-minute delay, the examinee's recall of objects depicted on the Immediate

Recognition subtest is assessed. Like Immediate Recognition, Delayed Recognition is appropriate for ages 4–10 years.

20. *Attention Divided.* In Attention Divided, a controlled number of objects are exposed to the examinee through "windows" on a movable insert that slides through a cardboard sheath. The examinee points to the objects viewed in each trial exposure. In addition, the examinee is taught a numerical card sorting activity, which is intended to compete with the card identification task for the examinee's attention. Attention Divided is appropriate for ages 6–21 years.

Normative Sample

The Leiter-R has two somewhat different normative samples for its two batteries, with only about one-third of the examinees having been administered both complete batteries. The VR Battery was normed on a relatively small total sample of 1,719 children, adolescents, and adults; the AM Battery normative sample included an even smaller sample of 763 children, adolescents, and adults. All 763 examinees who were administered the AM Battery during the instrument's norming were also administered the entire VR Battery, which is all that exists to provide a normative linkage between the two batteries.

Overall, the VR norms were based on an average sample size of slightly fewer than 100 individuals per age level (i.e., 19 age levels, 1,719 examinees). Importantly, fewer than 300 subjects *total* were included in the 7-year age span between 14 through 20 years, with an average of only 41 subjects per age level. The AM Battery included fewer than 100 examinees at *every* age level across the entire age span, with samples that ranged from a low of 42 examinees at four age levels (i.e., 7, 8, 11, and 18–20 years) to a high of 86 children sampled at the 2-year age level. The test's authors justify these exceptionally small sample sizes by claiming that the Leiter-R norm samples compare "favorably to that of a prominent memory and neuropsychological instrument, the Wechsler Memory Scale—Revised (Wechsler, 1987), which was standardized on a total sample of 316 subjects" (Roid & Miller, 1997, p. 143). Despite this justification, norms based on small samples are problematic for tests that contribute to important diagnostic and placement decisions.

The Leiter-R normative sample was stratified on the basis of gender, race, socioeconomic status, community size, and geographic region—although the number and location of specific standardization sites were not reported in the Leiter-R examiner's manual (Roid & Miller, 1997). Representation of the standardization sample, as compared to the U.S. census percentages, shows a fairly close match for the entire VR normative sample on each of the stratification variables (i.e., within 2% match); however, at individual age levels the samples were under- or overrepresented by as much as 6%–8% for individual stratification variables. For example, the authors indicate that 68.4% of the U.S. population in the census data was European American, whereas only 60.2% of the 10-year-old sample was European American (i.e., –8.2%); 73.9% of the 18- to 20-year-old sample was European American (i.e., +5.5%). Even on those demographic variables that are typically easily accessed (e.g., gender), the match between the Leiter-R sample and the U.S. population was less accurate than it should have been. Across all the age levels, gender representation for the VR norms ranged from 46.7% male at ages 18–20 years to 54.8% male at age 10.

The AM sample, given its overall smaller size, had proportionately larger deviations from the U.S. population than does the larger VR sample. For example, the gender representation in the AM sample ranged from 39.6% male at ages 14–15 years to 64.6% male at age 3, with disparity from the population parameters by approximately 11%–15%. Over- and underrepresentation of the population on the remaining AM stratification variables also varied a bit more widely than for the VR sample across the age levels. For example, the examinee representation at the parental educational level "less than high school," ranged from 2.3% at age 6 to 26.7% at age 2; the national average was 19.8%. In general, the VR and AM samples matched the U.S. population parameters fairly well only at the total sample level; however, at individual age levels, the disparities between the normative sample and the population were frequently quite large.

Administration

The Leiter-R is administered almost completely nonverbally. It should be noted, however, that at least three subtests require the examiner to indicate verbally how much time remains during the timing of the subtests, and another subtest suggests that it "may require brief verbal supplementation" (Roid & Miller, 1997, p. 60). Possibly more problematic than the Leiter-R verbal directions is the vast—and sometimes vague and confusing—collection of pantomimed gestures used to demonstrate the various Leiter-R subtests. Rather than employing a standard set of gestures throughout all 20 subtests, the Leiter-R employs unique gestures for individual subtests. Having unique directions for each subtest limits the generalizations that examinees can make when progressing from subtest to subtest when taking the test. The examiner's manual often provides only general directions without specifying accompanying gestures, such as "Encourage the child to imitate you," "Indicate nonverbally that each pair goes together," "Indicate that the child should point to red apples only," or "Indicate nonverbally that the child should point to all orange speed limit 55 signs AND red road construction signs seen on picture plate."

When specific gestures are called for, they are sometimes too broad, often confusing, and occasionally even silly. For example, the directions for one Leiter-R subtest state that the examiner should do the following:

> Indicate that card is "mentally rotated" by touching your head and eyes and nodding "Yes." To demonstrate that cards should not be turned, begin to physically rotate card with your hand. Lightly tap that hand, with the other. Shake your finger back and forth to indicated [sic] "No" to turning the card. (Roid & Miller, 1997, p. 44)

The examiner's manual also provides general information about adapting the administration of the Leiter-R for exceptional populations, suggesting that "it may be necessary to create unusual methods by which the child can communicate . . . answers to test items" (p. 76). The authors recognize that test adaptation also affects the value of the norms, and caution that the Leiter-R norms may be radically changed in the adaptation process. The value of adapting the Leiter-R is unclear, as are the conditions under which adaptation would be justifiable.

Technical Properties

Average internal consistency (coefficient alpha) for the VR subtests across the age levels ranged from .75 to .90; average internal consistency for the AM subtests was generally lower and ranged from .67 to .87. Composite reliabilities for the Leiter-R VR Battery ranged from .88 to .93 (FSIQ = .91 to .93); composite reliabilities for the AM Battery also tended to be lower than the VR composites and ranged from .75 to .93.

Evidence for Leiter-R stability is presented in the examiner's manual for a sample of 163 children and adolescents (ages 2–20 years; median age 8 years, 11 months) for the VR Battery. The test–retest interval for the stability study was not identified. VR stability coefficients for the subtests across three broad age levels, as reported in the examiner's manual, ranged between .61 and .81 (ages 2–5), .70 and .83 (ages 6–10), and .65 and .90 (ages 11–20). VR composite stability coefficients ranged from .83 to .90 (ages 2–5), .83 to .91 (ages 6–10), and .86 to .96 (ages 11–20). It is important to note that these stability coefficients were inflated due to very significant expansion in the range of variability among examinees' test scores, and should be considered as extremely favorable estimates. In this stability study, all subtests and scales produced standard deviations that were significantly greater than their respective normative standard deviations. For example, the standard deviation for the VR FSIQ was 30.00 at ages 11–20 years, which is twice the magnitude of the normative standard deviation of 15. Only when one considers that the variability of the pretest FSIQ for this age level was also significantly expanded (i.e., $SD = 29.5$) can the degree of inflation in the resulting correlation coefficient be fully appreciated. It is also important to note that the *Standards for Educational and Psychological Testing* (American Educational Research Association [AERA], American Psychological Association [APA], & National Council on Measurement in Education [NCME], 1999) admonish test developers that whenever correlations are corrected for

attenuation or restriction in range, both the corrected and obtained correlations should be reported. The Leiter-R examiner's manual reports only corrected correlations.

In addition to the VR stability coefficients, the examiner's manual reports mean score differences for the VR Battery subtests and composites for the test–retest interval. Subtest gain scores varied considerably across the age levels and ranged from minor differences (e.g., 0.10 SD) to large, meaningful differences (e.g., 1.4 SD). The VR composites evinced similar gain scores, ranging from minor differences to gains of 0.33 to 0.5 SD across the age levels. It is difficult to evaluate the stability of the VR Battery subtests' and composites' correlations and mean gain scores, because the time interval between initial testing and posttesting is not reported in the examiner's manual.

An investigation of the stability of the AM Battery is also presented in the examiner's manual, although it included a sample of only 45 children and adolescents (ages 6–17 years; median age 10 years, 11 months). As for the VR stability study, no indication of the test–retest interval is given for the AM study. The AM Battery was generally less stable than the VR Battery, with corrected subtest coefficients ranging from .55 to .85 (median = .615). AM composite stability coefficients ranged from .61 to 85 (median = .745). The practice effects on the AM subtests and composites were also generally larger than those found on the VR Battery and were typically about 0.5 SD across the age span.

The Leiter-R examiner's manual reports 11 separate validity studies describing the instrument's ability to discriminate among special groups (i.e., children with speech/language impairments, hearing impairments, traumatic brain injury, motor delays, cognitive delays, attention-deficit/hyperactivity disorder, giftedness, nonverbal learning disabilities, verbal learning disabilities, ESL–Spanish, and ESL–Asian or other). Examining the mean scores for these various groups leads one to question the sampling procedures employed, however. The mean FSIQs for the various 6- to 20-year-old samples were generally lower than one would anticipate (i.e., every sample except the gifted sample earned a mean FSIQ that was less than the test's normative mean of 100).

Specifically, the gifted sample earned a mean FSIQ of 114.6 (i.e., < +1.0 *SD*), while all remaining groups earned mean FSIQs of less than 90, except the two ESL groups. That the samples performed at lower levels than would be anticipated is surprising. That is, there would be no apparent reason why children identified as having motor delays, hearing impairments, speech/language impairments, or learning disabilities would have earned mean IQs in the mid–70s and 80s on a measure of intelligence, especially when the measure is a non-verbal intelligence test.

Several concurrent validity studies are also reported in the Leiter-R examiner's manual. These include comparisons of the Leiter-R with other intelligence tests, such as the original Leiter, the WISC-III, and select subtests from the Stanford–Binet Intelligence Scale: Fourth Edition (Thorndike, Hagen, & Sattler, 1986). Although the correlation between the Leiter-R FSIQ and WISC-III FSIQ for a mixed sample (children with no exceptionalities, with cognitive delays, with giftedness, or with ESL–Spanish) is reported in the examiner's manual as .86, the standard deviations on both instruments employed in this study were between 23 and 26 IQ points. As with the Leiter-R stability studies, such a grossly expanded range of variability produced a highly inflated and misleading validity coefficient between these two instruments. Also similar to the stability study, the Leiter-R authors did not present obtained correlations in addition to corrected correlations.

A number of small-sample studies (i.e., 17–33 subjects) were conducted and reported in the Leiter-R examiner's manual, which compared the Leiter-R Brief IQ and FSIQs with aspects of various memory scales and achievement measures. The manual reports moderate to strong correlations (e.g., mostly .40s to .80s) between the Leiter-R Brief IQ and FSIQ, but the means and, most importantly, the standard deviations are not reported for these comparisons. Without the standard deviations, it is impossible to judge whether expansion of range was an issue with these studies, as it was with the Leiter-R stability and validity studies. Without means, it is impossible to discern whether two forms of differing lengths provide comparable results.

The authors *suggest* that the Leiter-R subtests fit the proposed underlying hierarchical *g* model that was used to design the instrument (p. 184). However, according to Kaufman's (1979, 1994) criteria for "good" (>.70), "fair" (.50 to .69), and "poor" loadings on the *g* factor, all of the Leiter-R subtests must be classified as either fair or poor measures of *g*, except two. At ages 2–5 years, the Leiter-R *g* loadings range from .26 to .66, with a median of .595; *g* loadings range from .26 to .65 at ages 6–10 years (median = .45); and at ages 11–20 years, the *g* loadings range from .24 to .70, with a median of .56 (Roid & Miller, 1997, p. 192). The two subtests qualifying as good *g* loaders (i.e., Sequential Order and Paper Folding) meet Kaufman's criterion at only one of the three broad age levels studied (i.e., ages 11–20 years); like the remaining 18 subtests, these two latter subtests must be classified as fair or poor measures of *g* at the remaining age levels.

Exploratory and confirmatory factor (LISREL and AMOS) analyses reported in the Leiter-R examiner's manual provide evidence for a reasonably good fit to a proposed four- or five-factor model. Given that the Leiter-R is founded on a two-battery model, one might reasonably anticipate a two-factor fit; however, such a parsimonious theoretical model and the data do not match. The model fit is fairly consistent across the age span, with support for a four-factor model at the younger age levels (i.e., ages 2–5 years) and a five-factor model from ages 6 through 20 years. The factors identified by the authors vary slightly in name and subtest composition across the age levels, but include such proposed abilities as Fluid Reasoning/Reasoning, Visualization/Visual Spatial, Attention, Recognition Memory, and Associative/Memory Span.

Summary

The Leiter-R is a colorful, multitask instrument for ages 2 through 20 years. The instrument's normative sample matches the U.S. population fairly well on important stratifying variables and at the total sample level, but the sample-to-population match varies considerably at individual age levels. Although the test is largely nonverbal in its administration, the Leiter-R requires some verbalization; it also includes an array of gestures and pantomimed instructions that are vast in number and that some examiners may find vague or confusing. The Leiter-R appears to have adequate reliability at the scale level for an instrument intended for important decision making (Bracken, 1987, 1988; Nunnally & Bernstein, 1994). Importantly, however, as a measure of general intelligence, the test is composed of subtests that are predominantly rated as only fair or poor measures of *g*. The instrument matches a proposed four- or five-factor theoretical model fairly well, with some minor model variation across the age levels. When the Leiter-R is used with individuals who have recently immigrated to the United States, practitioners should be aware that it contains stimulus materials that are heavily influenced by Western culture and specifically by the culture of the United States.

Universal Nonverbal Intelligence Test

The UNIT (Bracken & McCallum, 1998a) was developed to address psychologists' need to assess diverse populations of children and adolescents in a fair and language-free fashion. In addition to multicultural and multilingual populations, the UNIT was intended to be used with children who have sensory limitations (e.g., deafness or other hearing impairments), learning disabilities (e.g., nonverbal or expressive language disabilities), psychiatric conditions (e.g., elective mutism, autism, social phobia), and various language-impairing neurological disorders. UNIT materials include two-colored blocks, stimulus chips and cards, laminated response mats, and stand-alone stimulus easels.

As a comprehensive six-subtest instrument, the UNIT assesses general intelligence, as well as memory, reasoning, symbolic processing, and nonsymbolic processing, in an interlocking 2 × 2 model. Of the UNIT's six subtests, three subtests constitute each of two primary scales, Memory and Reasoning; three subtests also constitute each of two secondary scales, include Symbolic and Nonsymbolic cognitive processing. Memory and Reasoning are "primary" in the sense that they represent foundational intellectual abilities identified by historical and current theorists, such as Thurstone (1938) and Carroll (1993). The Symbolic and Nonsymbolic scales are considered "secondary" measures because they represent the inferred processes that underlie and facilitate task solution.

From the perspective of the primary scales, three subtests comprise the Memory scale (i.e., Symbolic Memory, Spatial Memory, and Object Memory), and three subtests make up the Reasoning scale (i.e., Cube Design, Analogic Reasoning, and Mazes). Of the six Memory and Reasoning subtests, three rely heavily on verbal mediation for task solution and contribute to the Symbolic scale (i.e., Symbolic Memory, Object Memory, and Analogic Reasoning). The three remaining subtests include content that is largely nonsymbolic in nature and contribute to the Nonsymbolic scale (i.e., Spatial Memory, Cube Design, and Mazes). Figure 11.1 illustrates the UNIT 2 × 2 theoretical model and the UNIT subtest composition.

The UNIT subtests can be combined to form three optional batteries, depending on

	Memory Subtests	Reasoning Subtests
Symbolic Subtests	Symbolic Memory Object Memory	Analogic Reasoning Cube Design
Nonsymbolic Subtests	Spatial Memory	Mazes

FIGURE 11.1 UNIT Subtests and Scale Assignment.

the examiner's needs and the referral problem. The initial Memory and Reasoning subtests (i.e., Symbolic Memory and Cube Design) together form a two-subtest 15-minute Abbreviated Battery intended for intellectual screening. The first two Memory and Reasoning subtests (i.e., Symbolic Memory, Cube Design, Spatial Memory, and Analogic Reasoning) constitute a 30-minute Standard Battery intended for making decisions about placement and eligibility. All six subtests are combined to form the Extended Battery, which requires about 45 minutes to administer and is intended for eligibility testing and the provision of additional diagnostic information.

A description of the six UNIT subtests follows.

1. *Symbolic Memory.* Symbolic Memory assesses examinees' sequential short-term memory of universal symbols that are printed in two colors (i.e., green and black) and represent the concepts of "baby," "girl," "boy," "woman," and "man." Sequenced arrays of between one and six symbols are presented during a 5-second exposure. After the stimulus plate is removed, the examinee moves the 1-square-inch plastic response chips in the tabletop workspace to replicate the pictured sequence. This subtest is a measure of both Memory and Symbolic processing.

2. *Cube Design.* The Cube Design task requires the examinee to construct designs from bicolored cubes to match the front, top, and right faces of complex three-dimensional designs pictured on a stimulus plate. The cube designs to be replicated range from a single block to nine block designs. Cube Design is a timed task, and it contributes to the Reasoning and Nonsymbolic scales.

3. *Spatial Memory.* Spatial Memory presents arrays of green and black disks on either a 3 × 3 or 4 × 4 grid for a 5-second exposure. After 5 seconds, the stimulus page is removed, and the examinee is required to move corresponding plastic green and black chips onto a response mat to match the stimulus arrangement. This subtest assesses both Memory and Nonsymbolic processing.

4. *Analogic Reasoning.* Analogic Reasoning presents pictorial and geometric (concrete and abstract, fluid and crystal-lized) analogies in a traditional matrix format. The matrices are solved from a left-to-right direction, never on the diagonal or from top to bottom. This subtest assesses Reasoning and Symbolic processing.

5. *Object Memory.* The Object Memory subtest presents an array of common objects on a stimulus page during a 5-second exposure. After the stimulus page has been removed, a second page is exposed upon which the original stimulus objects and additional foils are presented. Although the second page contains all of the original stimuli, the stimuli are presented in new locations. The examinee places black plastic discs on the objects presented on the first page. This subtest is a measure of Memory and Symbolic processing.

6. *Mazes.* The Mazes subtest presents a series of mazes ranging in difficulty from simple to complex. Simple mazes have a single starting point option and a single maze exit. Complex mazes present multiple possible starting paths (i.e., one true path and one or more foils) and two or more maze exits (i.e., one true exit and one or more foils). The examinee earns 1 point for each correct decision made as he or she progresses through the maze, until the first incorrect decision is made (e.g., entering into a blind alley). The total score for each item is the number of correct decisions made as the examinee progressed through the maze prior to the first error. Scoring is discontinued from the point of the examinee's last correct decision. The Mazes subtest is a timed measure of Reasoning and Nonsymbolic processing, as well as of planning (see later discussion).

Normative Sample

The UNIT was normed on a sample of 2,100 children and adolescents, ages 5 through 17 years, 11 months (175 examinees at each age level). An additional 1,765 students were tested for UNIT reliability, validity, and fairness studies. The UNIT normative sample was drawn from 108 sites in 38 states and all four regions of the United States. The norming sample was stratified on the basis of sex, race, Hispanic origin, region of the country, classroom placement, special education services, and parental education attainment. The match between the UNIT normative sample and the U.S. population parameters was close, and generally within 1 percentage point for the total sample on all stratifying variables. When the stratifying variables were compared within specific age levels, most ages included samples that match the U.S. population within 3–4 percentage points. For example, across the entire age span, the percentage of males ranged from 49.1% to 50.3% (i.e., ±1%); race was within 3% of the U.S. population at all ages; and geographic region and Hispanic origin were within 4% at all age levels. UNIT norms were also divided further (e.g., age × sex × parental education; age × sex × race), and each subsample's match with the population is reported in the examiner's manual. Even at these more precise levels of specificity, the norms remained uniformly within 4% of the U.S. population.

The inclusion of special populations in the UNIT normative sample was done to insure representation of those populations for whom the test was intended. Many authorities in cross-cultural or nonbiased assessment believe that test fairness is enhanced when normative samples include proportionate representation of students with various disabilities or cultural/linguistic backgrounds (e.g., Barona & Santos de Barona, 1987; Caterino, 1990; Cohen, Swerdlik, & Smith, 1992; Gonzales, 1982). In addition to nationally representative proportions of racial and ethnic groups, the UNIT normative sample included students with learning disabilities (5.6%), speech and language delays or disorders (2.3%), serious emotional disturbance (0.9%), mental retardation (1.2%), hearing impairments (1.8%), and giftedness (6.2%), as well as students speaking ESL (2.0%) or enrolled in bilingual education classes (1.8%).

Administration

The UNIT is administered in a 100% language-free manner, using eight standardized gestures and four distinct item types to insure that the examinee understands the demands of each task. The item types include Demonstration Items, Sample Items, follow-up Checkpoint Items, and traditional scored items. Demonstration Items require the examiner to demonstrate the nature of the task and show the examinee how the subtest is approached and how items are solved. After each Demonstration Item is completed, the examiner immediately demonstrates *why* the item was solved correctly (e.g., the examiner reexposes and compares stimuli and his or her responses). After the Demonstration Item is administered, the examiner administers one or more Sample Items, which allow the examinee an opportunity to attempt at least one item without penalty. Upon the examinee's completion of each Sample Item, the examiner either confirms the correctness of the examinee's response or corrects the examinee's response and illustrates how the item is solved correctly. Checkpoint Items are administered after Sample Items and serve as transitional items. These items are scored for accuracy, but they allow the examiner to correct the examinee's incorrect responses; however, the examiner takes no additional instructional action if the examinee's response is correct. The traditional scored items are scored for credit and allow no further guidance from the examiner.

UNIT administration is facilitated though the use of a consistent administration format for each of the six subtests (e.g., consistent subtest presentation format, consistent use of gestures, and consistent 5-second stimulus exposure on all memory items). The examiner's manual demonstrates how materials should be differentially presented for right-handed versus left-handed examinees (i.e., stimulus materials placed on the dominant side), and illustrates the eight standardized gestures (i.e., head nodding, head shaking, open-hand shrugging, palm rolling, pointing, hand waving, stop, and thumbs up).

A 22-minute training video (Bracken & McCallum, 1998b) was also developed to facilitate learning the administration of the test. In addition to presenting the theoretical orientation of the test, the video demonstrates the standardized gestures and shows how each subtest is administered to examinees. In addition to the detailed test directions in the examiner's manual, abbreviated directions are printed on a laminated "Administration at a Glance" card. This card presents abbreviated administration directions on one side and illustrations of the eight standardized UNIT gestures on the other side. Once examiners understand how the UNIT is administered, they need only refer to this $8\frac{1}{2}$″ × 11″ card to administer the test.

Technical Properties

Coefficient alpha reliabilities were calculated for the standardization sample, for a clinical/exceptional sample, and separately for African American and Hispanic examinees. Across the 5- to 17-year age span, average subtest reliabilities ranged from .64 to .91 for the standardization sample, .82 to .96 for the clinical/experimental sample, .81 to .96 for the African American sample, and .83 to .95 for the Hispanic sample.

For the entire standardization sample, average internal-consistency coefficients for the four UNIT scales ranged from .86 to .91 across the Standard and Extended Batteries. Scale reliabilities ranged from .95 to .97 for the clinical/exceptional sample, .93 to .96 for the African American sample, and .92 to .96 for the Hispanic sample. The average reliabilities of the Abbreviated, Standard, and Extended Battery FSIQs were .91, .93, and .93, respectively, for the standardization sample, and .96, .98, and .98, respectively, for the clinical/exceptional sample. Abbreviated, Standard, and Extended FSIQ reliabilities for the African American sample were .95, .97, and .96, respectively, and .94, .96, and .96 for the Hispanic sample.

In addition to the previously mentioned reliability figures, the UNIT examiner's manual reports local reliability coefficients for important decision-making score ranges (i.e., for identification of mental retardation, FSIQ = 70 ± 10; for identification of giftedness, FSIQ = 130 ± 10). Because the test was intended to contribute to the identification of these two conditions, it was deemed important to calculate reliabilities at these important cutoff levels. FSIQ reliability coefficients were identical for both levels, and were .97, .98, and .98 for the Abbreviated, Standard, and Extended Batteries, respectively.

UNIT stability was examined in a test–retest study that included 197 participants, with approximately 15 examinees in each age group between 5 and 17 years. The mean test–retest interval was 20.3 days, and the racial/ethnic composition of the sample

was as follows: 76.1% European American, 19.8% African American, 3% Asian, 1% Hispanic, and 1% "other" groups. The sample also was 49.2% male, and proportionately divided by parental educational attainment. Across the entire sample, average subtest stability coefficients, corrected for restriction in range of variability, ranged from .58 to .85 (uncorrected coefficients are also presented); average scale reliabilities ranged from .78 to .84; and average FSIQ reliabilities for the Abbreviated, Standard, and Extended Batteries were .83, .88, and .85, respectively. Stability coefficients varied slightly across the age groups, with the older age levels being generally more reliable than the younger age levels.

Gain scores due to practice effects varied more across the age span than by the different abilities assessed by the UNIT scales. That is, score gains were uniformly low (i.e., 3–5 points) for the 5–7 and 11–13 age groups across the four scales and three batteries. The greatest gains were found for the 8–10 year age group, with gains of 14–15 points across the four scales and three batteries—with the exception of the Memory and Reasoning scales in the Standard Battery, which evidenced about half as much gain as the remaining scales (i.e., about 7 points). It is unclear why this age level experienced greater retest gains than the other age levels.

The UNIT examiner's manual presents some additional information that is relatively unique by comparison with most intelligence test manuals. Consistent with the standards set by Bracken (1988) and first presented in the examiner's manual for the Bracken Basic Concept Scale (Bracken, 1984, 1998a), the UNIT examiner's manual presents tables that describe the adequacy of UNIT floors, ceilings, and item gradients for each of the subtests and FSIQs by age and battery. The UNIT manual reports "excellent" average subtest floors and ceilings at all ages for the Standard and Extended Batteries. For the Abbreviated Battery, the UNIT has "good" subtest floors at ages 5 years, 0 months to 5 years, 11 months, and "very good" floors from ages 6 years, 0 months to 6 years, 7 months. Beyond age 6 years, 7 months, the Abbreviated Battery has "excellent" subtest floors and "excellent" ceilings across the entire age range.

Similarly, the UNIT FSIQ has "excellent" ceilings at all ages for the Abbreviated, Standard, and Extended Batteries; it also has "excellent" floors for all ages on each of the batteries, except ages 5 years, 0 months to 5 years, 11 months on the Abbreviated Battery, where the total test floor is rated "very good." Across the age levels, the UNIT subtests evidence item gradients that are sufficiently sensitive that a change in raw score by the passing or failing of one item will not alter the subtest scaled score by more than 0.33 SD. This tabled information is especially useful when one is determining whether a test is appropriate for a referral.

The UNIT examiner's manual presents various studies that examined the convergent validity of the instrument. These studies included concurrent administration of the UNIT and the WISC-III, the Woodcock–Johnson Psychoeducational Battery—Revised (WJ-R; Woodcock & Johnson, 1990), the Bateria Woodcock–Munoz-Sandoval (1996), the Kaufman Brief Intelligence Test (K-BIT; Kaufman & Kaufman, 1990), the MAT (Naglieri, 1985a, 1985b), the Raven Standard Progressive Matrices (SPM; Raven, 1990), and the TONI-2 (Brown et al., 1990). Correlations between the UNIT and the comprehensive measures of intelligence (e.g., the WISC-III, the WJ-R) were conducted with a variety of samples (e.g., children with learning disabilities, mental retardation, and giftedness; Native American youths) and produced full scale correlations in the .65 to .88 range, with similar mean scores on the UNIT and the criterion tests.

Correlations between the UNIT and the Bateria, on the other hand, produced mostly low full scale correlations (e.g., .00 to .39), with a few moderate-level correlations (e.g., .55 to .72) for two samples of Spanish-speaking youths. The two instruments also produced sizable mean score differences, which suggest that the two instruments should not be used interchangeably. The reason for the differences between tests' mean scores and the low correlations seems to be related to the lack of Spanish proficiency among the "Spanish-speaking" samples, as their Bateria Broad Cognitive mean scores were generally 15–20 points lower than the UNIT mean scores.

The correlations between the UNIT and various matrix-related nonverbal tests (i.e., the MAT, TONI-2, and SPM) were slightly lower than those with the other comprehensive measures of intelligence and were generally in the moderate to high range (i.e., .56 to .82). The UNIT also produced comparable mean scores with these matrix-based screening instruments. Lower correlations were found with the SPM and TONI-2 (i.e., mid-.50s) than with the MAT (.82).

The UNIT was designed first and foremost to provide a strong measure of general intelligence, and exploratory factor analysis of the UNIT Standard Battery provided evidence for a strong g factor. In addition to g, the exploratory factor analyses provided evidence for the two primary factors (i.e., Reasoning and Memory). Analysis of the Extended Battery provided evidence for a strong g factor and three additional factors, with Mazes alone creating the third factor. All Extended Battery subtests except Mazes loaded on either a Reasoning or a Memory factor, as predicted. The unique factor created by Mazes appears to be related to planning, given the subtest's unique scoring system that rewards reflective, planful responding. According to Kaufman's (1979, 1994) classification for g loadings, five of the six UNIT subtests were rated as good measures of general intelligence, with loadings of .71 to .79 on the first unrotated factor. Mazes (on the Extended Battery) was the only subtest that was rated less favorably, with a g loading of .44 (i.e., poor). Although Mazes had a poor g rating, improvements made to this UNIT subtest appear to have enhanced its g loadings over the Mazes subtest on the WISC-III, which had a g loading of .30.

UNIT confirmatory factor analyses provide strong support for the entire UNIT theoretical model. That is, good model fits exist for a one-factor (g) model, a two-factor model that includes Reasoning and Memory, and a two-factor model that includes Symbolic and Nonsymbolic processing. A strikingly similar model fit exists for each of the three models and the four age levels studied.

Fairness

The UNIT was designed to provide a fair assessment of intelligence for minority children and children of poverty, who historically have been over- and underrepresented in programs for children with mental retardation and giftedness, respectively (Rycraft, 1990). This issue has become especially important, given the U.S. Office of Civil Rights interest in school systems that have had histories of gross over- and underrepresentation of minority students in these two types of programs (e.g., Ulik, 1997).

In its effort to address the issue of fair assessment for children, regardless of their gender, race, nation of origin, or exceptional condition, the UNIT authors have included a chapter dedicated to "fairness in testing" in the examiner's manual. This chapter addresses the manner in which fairness was a consideration throughout the UNIT's development. In an effort to achieve fair assessment for multilingual, multicultural, and multiracial peoples, the UNIT subtests are 100% nonverbal; they demonstrate good psychometric qualities, and in general are low in cultural content. Such subtest characteristics lead to fairer assessment of children for whom traditional language- and culture-loaded intelligence tests would be inappropriate (Frisby, 1999). In addition, every UNIT item was reviewed by a comprehensive and inclusive "sensitivity panel," and subjected to extensive differential item functioning (DIF) analyses as part of the test development process. Items identified as problematic by either the DIF analyses or the sensitivity panel were eliminated from the test. An independent DIF investigation (Maller, 2000) was also conducted for students with deafness, and compelling and favorable results were obtained (i.e., no UNIT items evidenced significant DIF for these students).

Differences in mean scores between groups (e.g., males and females, whites and blacks) are not an a priori indication of test bias (Jensen, 1980). However, large mean score differences between groups on intelligence tests and the implications of those differences are frequently discussed with concern in both professional and lay media. Fairness in psychological testing can also be defined in many varying ways. In a broad sense, "fairness" refers to the degree to which a test is free from test bias (i.e., elements that are construct-irrelevant and that systematically cause different levels or patterns of performance by members of various groups). However, according to Schmeiser (1992), "fairness relates to the equity of the uses made of a test rather than referring to the absence of bias. A test free of bias can be used unfairly" (p. 80).

To address this issue of the equitable use of tests, matched sample comparisons of European Americans, Hispanics, African Americans, Native Americans, Asians/Pacific Islanders, bilingual children, and children residing in Ecuador were conducted and reported in the UNIT examiner's manual. Also, a mean score comparison between a matched sample of children with and without deafness is reported in the manual. Sizable reductions in the "typical" mean score discrepancies reported in the literature were found between the various matched samples on the UNIT. These reduced mean score differences appear to be related to the minimization of cultural content and the removal of language from the UNIT assessment process. These reduced mean score differences also mean that the UNIT thereby creates a more equitable assessment for these various populations.

Summary

The UNIT is a comprehensive measure of intelligence with six subtests that are administered in a totally nonverbal fashion, via examiner demonstration and eight standardized gestures. The UNIT assesses general intelligence, reasoning, memory, symbolic processing, and nonsymbolic processing in an interlocking 2 × 2 design. The test can be administered as a two-subtest Abbreviated Battery (screening; 15 minutes); a four-subtest Standard Battery (eligibility decision making, 30 minutes); or a six-subtest Extended Battery (eligibility determination and diagnostic testing, 45 minutes). The UNIT includes a variety of tasks that allow for examinees' active participation and manipulation of objects (e.g., plastic blocks, chips, response cards). The test is administered through the systematic use of Demonstration Items, Sample Items, and Checkpoint Items to insure that the examinee understands the nature of each task before being assessed for credit on traditional scored items. The UNIT demonstrates acceptable levels of reliability for important decision making, and produces strong correlations with comprehensive measures of intelligence and achievement. Exploratory factor analyses reveal strong g loadings for five of the six UNIT subtests. Confirmatory factor analyses provide strong support for a one-factor model (i.e., g) and two separate two-factor models (e.g., Memory and Reasoning; Symbolic and Nonsymbolic processing). The examiner's manual includes a chapter dedicated to fairness in testing and addresses the topic through a wide variety of subjective and objective analyses.

Comprehensive Test of Nonverbal Intelligence

The CTONI (Hammill et al., 1996) is described as a comprehensive measure of nonverbal intelligence for children and adolescents (ages 6 years, 0 months through 18 years, 11 months). The test authors describe the CTONI as a battery of six subtests that measure different but interrelated nonverbal intellectual abilities based on the idea that abilities should be assessed in different contexts. The CTONI was designed to assess an aspect of intelligence that differs inherently from the general intellectual abilities assessed by the Leiter-R and UNIT. The CTONI examiner's manual describes the construct that the test measures as "nonverbal intelligence." Nonverbal intelligence is described as "those particular abilities that exist independently of language and that increase a person's capacity to function intelligently. These nonverbal capacities stand in contrast to those abilities that are inherently verbal" (Hammill et al., 1996, p. 1). The authors also state that the test title emphasizes "that the particular type of intelligence assessed is *nonverbal*" (p. 10; italics in original). In this sense, the CTONI differs both from traditional language-loaded intelligence tests and from many nonverbal tests of intelligence—tests that assess *general intelligence* in a nonverbal fashion.

The authors stated that "in developing the CTONI, we were not guided by any one theoretical perspective" (Hammill et al., 1996, p. 9), but instead used the concept that assessment of intelligence should include reference to both *abilities* and *contexts*. The assessment procedure employs item types that assess three "abilities" (i.e.,

analogical reasoning, categorical classifications, sequential reasoning) and two "contexts" (i.e., pictorial objects and geometric designs). Given this practical model, the six CTONI subtests include two measures each of analogical reasoning (i.e., Pictorial Analogies, Geometric Analogies), categorical classifications (i.e., Pictorial Categories, Geometric Categories), and sequential reasoning (i.e., Pictorial Sequences, Geometric Sequences). The six CTONI subtests combine to form a total test score (the Nonverbal Intelligence Composite), as well as two composite scores (the Pictorial Nonverbal Intelligence Composite and the Geometric Nonverbal Intelligence Composite). Each of the CTONI subtests produces normalized means of 10 and standard deviations of 3; the composites all produce standard scores with means of 100 and standard deviations of 15.

Normative Sample

The CTONI was normed on a sample of 2,129 children and adolescents in 23 states. The samples were stratified according to geographic region, gender, race, residence (i.e., urban, rural), ethnicity, family income, educational attainment of parents, and disability status. For the total sample, all stratifying variables matched the U.S. population parameters within 3%–4%. In addition to the 2,129 children and adolescents, the CTONI was also normed on 772 adults ages 19–89 who are described by region, gender, race, residence, ethnicity, and educational levels. The CTONI examiner's manual provides breakdowns of the sample only by age and a second variable (e.g., age × geographic region), so it is not possible to determine the extent to which more finite cells were accurately filled (e.g., age × ethnicity × geographic region). However, the variability between the CTONI two-item stratification variables and the U.S. population is generally within 3%–4%.

Administration

The CTONI examiner's manual indicates that the test can be administered either orally or through pantomimed instructions with six standardized gestures. Although having two administration options seems like an attractive option, the examiner's manual does not indicate whether this test was normed with oral (i.e., verbal) administration or pantomimed (i.e., nonverbal) administration. In either case, there are not separate norms for oral and pantomimed administrations. The justification for using either administration option and a single set of norms is absent from the CTONI examiner's manual, leaving examiners to determine how best to use the administration options and single set of norms. This shortcoming is especially serious, because the manual reports only one small-sample ($n = 63$) study that was limited because of the sample's age (33 students in grade 3 and 30 in grade 11) and geographic representation (i.e., Llano, TX), and because the test administration was not concurrent or counterbalanced. Rather, the two forms were administered with a 1-month delay and a set administration sequence.

The six CTONI subtests, their description, and administration formats follow.

• *Pictorial Analogies and Geometric Analogies.* Pictorial Analogies employs 2 × 2 matrix format that presents a pictorial analogy (e.g., "fork is to meat as spoon is to . . . soup"). The examiner points to the two elements in the first row of the matrix to highlight the relationship between the two variables, and then points to the first picture in the second row. The second element in the second row is an empty box, which is to be completed by one of the five options provided below. The examinee is "expected to understand that *this* is to *that* . . . as this is to what. . .?" (Hammill et al., 1996, p. 8). Geometric Analogies employs the same 2 × 2 matrix format, but uses geometric figures rather than pictorial stimuli.

• *Pictorial Categories and Geometric Categories.* Both Pictorial Categories and Geometric Categories employ "an association format to intuit relationships and to construct categories." (p. 8). The examinee is expected to select from within a matrix format which of five objects (i.e., pictured or geometric) is related to the stimulus objects presented. In Pictorial Categories, for example, two different chairs might be presented as stimulus objects, and the keyed response would be a chair selected from among five pieces of furniture. Geometric

Categories employs the same administration format, but uses geometric designs rather than concrete objects.

• *Pictorial Sequences and Geometric Sequences.* These two subtests present problem-solving tasks using objects or geometric designs; the solutions are reached through the identification of a progressive sequence. In Pictorial Sequences, for example, three stimulus pictures might depict a tall tree, a medium-sized tree, a smaller tree, and a blank box. Below the stimulus items are presented several trees of differing sizes, with only one tree being smaller than the last tree depicted in the stimulus sequence. Geometric Sequences uses the same administration format, but depicts geometric designs instead of pictured objects.

Technical Properties

Internal consistency (coefficient alpha) was calculated for subtests and composites for each age across the 13 age levels. The six CTONI subtests produced average subtest reliabilities ranging from .86 to .92. The Pictorial Nonverbal Intelligence Quotient (PNIQ) produced an average reliability of .93; the Geometric Nonverbal Intelligence Quotient (GNIQ) average alpha was .95; and the Nonverbal Intelligence Quotient (NIQ) has an average alpha of .97. As demonstrated in these alpha coefficients, the CTONI evidences strong internal consistency for the total sample. The authors also calculated alpha reliabilities for subsets of the standardization sample, including samples of so-called "Caucasoids," African Americans, Native Americans, Panamanians, Asians, and speakers of ESL; males and females; and children with learning disabilities and deafness. Each of these groups produced comparable subtest reliability coefficients to those obtained for the standardization sample, which suggests that the test is equally reliable for the various groups for whom it was intended.

The CTONI stability was investigated with a small sample of students (33 grade 3 students, 30 grade 11 students) from Llano, Texas, and a 1-month test–retest interval. As noted above, this study was unique in that the first administration of the test was conducted using the standardized pantomimed administration, whereas the second testing was conducted using an oral administration. The two administrations produced negligible mean score differences for the subtests and composites, with composites generally within 1 point of each other. Across the two groups of students, subtest "stability" (i.e., delayed alternate-form reliability) coefficients ranged from .79 to .89; the composite scores' stability coefficients ranged from .88 to .94. Importantly, again, this single study is all the evidence examiners have that the two administration formats (i.e., oral and pantomimed) produce comparable scores.

The CTONI examiner's manual reports overall reliability in a highly unusual manner. The authors averaged three forms of reliability (i.e., interrater, internal consistency, and stability) to provide one overall "average" reliability coefficient for each of the subtests and the IQs. Given the disparate nature of these three forms of reliability, there is no justification for averaging the coefficients. The "average" reliability reported in Table 7.5 of the CTONI examiner's manual defies measurement convention and interpretation.

Two criterion-related validity studies were conducted with the CTONI. The first study correlated the CTONI, the WISC-III, and the TONI-2 with 43 students who were identified as having learning disabilities and who lived in Dallas, Texas. After correcting correlations for attenuation due to imperfect reliability, the authors report concurrent validity coefficients of .64, .66, and .81 between the WISC-III FSIQ and the PNIQ, GNIQ, and NIQ, respectively. Given that all tests produce some error variance and there are no "error-free" instruments, correcting for attenuation was a very liberal and nonconventional approach to comparing the instruments in this validity study. Ironically, when the three CTONI composites were correlated with the WISC-III subscales, higher correlations were found with the WISC-III Verbal IQ (VIQ) than with Performance IQ (PIQ) (i.e., .59, .56, .76 versus .51, .55, .70). One possible explanation for these unusual results is that it is unstated whether the CTONI was administered in this study using pantomime (nonverbal) or oral (verbal) directions. In the same study, the CTONI "attenuation-corrected" correlations of the NIQ with the TONI-2 Quotient and the Peabody Picture Vocabulary Test—Revised (PPVT-R) total test score were .82 and .74, respectively. Uncorrected correlations were not presented in this study.

The second criterion-related study involved the administration of the WISC-III Performance Scale and the CTONI to 32 students with deafness from two cities in Texas. In this instance, the correlations were corrected for both restriction in range *and* attenuation; again, uncorrected correlations are not reported in the examiner's manual, as recommended by the *Standards for Educational and Psychological Testing* (AERA, APA, & NCME, 1985). In this study, the twice-corrected correlations between the CTONI PNIQ, GNIQ, and NIQ and the WISC-III PIQ were .87, .85, and .90, respectively. Unfortunately, the authors do not provide the means or standard deviations for either the predictor or criterion measures in either study. Therefore, it is not possible to determine from the information reported in the examiner's manual whether the CTONI produces scores that are comparable in magnitude with those of the other ability tests. Also, the examiner's manual does not indicate which administration format (i.e., oral or pantomime) was used in either study.

As partial evidence of validity, the CTONI examiner's manual provides data describing the correlation between subtest scores and examinees' chronological age. Correlations between .45 and .66 are reported across the 13 age groups; however, the tabled data also reveal that the CTONI reflected virtually no growth in adolescents' ability after age 13. From ages 13 through 18, as few as one and three items separated the respective group mean scores. As an example, the mean raw score for 13-year-olds on the Pictorial Sequences subtest is 15; the average score for 14- through 18-year-olds was either 15 or 16. An exploratory factor analysis was conducted on the CTONI standardization sample, as well as for a variety of demographically different subgroups (e.g., males, females, Hispanics, Native Americans) and a one-factor solution was reported in all cases. Factor loadings on the *g* factor for the standardization sample were mostly in the moderate range (i.e., fair *g* loadings), with only one subtest earning

Kaufman's (1979) rating of "good." Other than Geometric Sequences, which had a *g* loading of .71, the remaining subtests' *g* loadings ranged from .50 to .68.

Fairness

The CTONI examiner's manual reports the results of DIF studies by gender, race/ethnicity/language (e.g., African Americans, Native Americans, speakers of ESL), and disability (e.g., students with learning disabilities, deafness, and mental retardation). In each of these samples, a small number of items were found to be biased within the test, with a range of one to five biased items per sample studied. Mean score differences across a broad spectrum of students were small and evidenced minor score variation from the standardization mean of 100 for most groups studied, except where anticipated (e.g., the sample with mental retardation). For example, as compared to the national normative mean of 100, both Hispanics and African Americans earned a mean NIQ of 97. Students with deafness, however, earned a mean NIQ that was a full 10 points lower than the normative mean (i.e., NIQ = 90), and the mean NIQ for students with ESL was a full 8 points below the normative mean of 100.

There are several problems with these group comparisons, however. First, the samples that were compared were not matched on any demographic or stratifying variables. Therefore, the comparisons between groups were not controlled in any meaningful way. This being the case, it is impossible to discern the extent to which samples were equivalent or in what ways they may have been dissimilar in terms of important characteristics (e.g., socioeconomic status, parental education). Second, and more importantly, the students who represented the "special samples" were in fact included in *both* comparison groups. That is, students with learning disabilities, for example, comprised the comparison sample for that disability type *and* were included in the standardization sample. Such double inclusion seriously confounds the analyses and inferences that can be made from these nonindependent results. The problem becomes more serious when one considers that the various "special samples" were not even independent among themselves. For example, there were special comparison groups for males, "Caucasoids," and children with learning disabilities; however, any child falling into all of these categories would have been included in each of the three special comparison groups *and* the standardization group. In addition, it was not clear whether these studies were conducted under pantomime or oral test administration conditions. Therefore, the CTONI special-sample comparisons should be considered only minimally useful, and judgment about the utility of the CTONI with special populations should be suspended until appropriately designed matched sample comparison studies are conducted.

Summary

According to the test authors, the CTONI assesses a construct called "nonverbal intelligence" by means of six subtests, each of which is presented in either a pictorial or a geometric matrix format. The CTONI can be administered via either oral or pantomimed directions; however, there is only a single set of norms, regardless of which administration procedure is used. Importantly, it is unclear whether the CTONI norms were based on an oral or a pantomimed administration. CTONI evidences strong internal consistency (i.e., alpha) and 1-month stability (actually, delayed alternate-form reliability). That is, the "stability" coefficients were generated from a first testing conducted with pantomimed directions and a second administration conducted with oral directions. In addition to moderate to strong "stability" coefficients, minor mean score differences were produced by this unconventional alternate-forms administration. CTONI validity was demonstrated in a number of ways, ranging from age x raw score correlations to concurrent validity studies with the WISC-III. The concurrent validity coefficients, corrected both for attenuation due to imperfect reliability and restriction in range, were moderate in magnitude, with higher correlations paradoxically existing between the CTONI and the WISC-III VIQ than between the CTONI and the WISC-III PIQ. Neither means and standard deviations nor uncorrected correlations were reported for the validity studies; hence the extent to which the two tests are similar and produce comparable mean scores is unknown. It is also not known whether the validity studies were conducted using pantomime or oral administrations. Special-sample comparisons with the CTONI are confounded by the samples' lack of independence and should be considered cautiously. The CTONI evidences a very limited ceiling at upper age levels, with very limited cognitive growth evident between ages 13 and 18.

MATRIX OR MATRIX-LIKE NONVERBAL TESTS

Raven's Progressive Matrices

The RPM (Raven et al., 1986) is a nonverbal test of reasoning that employs visual stimuli that are presented in a matrix format. The Raven scales were envisioned as "tests of observation and clear thinking" (Raven et al., 1986, p. G2) to contribute to J. C. Raven's "study of the genetic and social origins of mental defect" (Raven, 1990, p. 72). Since their publication, the multiple forms of the RPM have been employed internationally as brief, practical "nonverbal" measures of general ability.

The RPM is published in three forms: the Standard form, mentioned earlier (SPM; Raven, Raven, & Court, 1998c), the Coloured Progressive Matrices (CPM; Raven, Raven, & Court, 1998b), and the Advanced Progressive Matrices (APM; Raven, Raven, & Court, 1998a). The SPM was designed to sample a general range of ability, which proved less than useful for clinical applications (i.e., it had limited ceilings and floors). Therefore, the CPM and APM were created to extend the SPM's upper and lower ranges of ability. SPM is generally used for the typical school-age range, 6–17 years; however, adult norms are also available. The SPM is divided into five sets of 12 items, for a total of 60 items. The CPM includes three sets of 12 items, for a total of 36 items, and is appropriate for children ages 5–11 years. The APM consists of two sets; Set I includes only 12 items, and Set II includes 36 items. APM was designed for individuals with advanced intellectual ability and is intended for adolescents and adults.

Normative Sample

The RPM was originally published in 1938, but in 1986 Raven and colleagues published an updated supplement that included values that could be used to obtain standard scores based on data collected in the United States; a 1998 publication (Raven et al., 1998a) also provides U.S. norms from an adult 1993 standardization sample in Des Moines, Iowa. The authors did not, however, provide a U.S. normative sample in the 1986 publication, but rather referred examiners to the *Research Supplement No. 3* (Raven, 1990), which wasn't published for another few years. The 1986 published raw-score-to-standard-score conversion tables, and the 1993 Des Moines adult sample referred to in the 1998 publication, were intended to render the test more appropriate for use throughout the United States.

The U.S. samples that were used as norm groups were severely limited in quality, because they were largely samples of convenience. The U.S. sample was not collected in a stratified manner to represent the nation and all of its ethnic groups, regions, socioeconomic strata, or other important demographic characteristics. To create the "U.S. norms" (which actually include two Canadian communities), the SPM was administered in Des Moines, Iowa; Holt and Westland, Michigan; Omaha, Nebraska; Decatur, Alabama; Montgomery County, Maryland; Sequatchie County, Tennessee; Woodlin, Colorado; St. John's and Corner Brook, Newfoundland; and a western U.S. town fictitiously named "Westown." As can be seen from the list of standardization sites, the Midwestern regions of the United States were grossly overrepresented, the Western region was underrepresented, and the Northeast and Northwest regions were not represented at all. The Midwestern and Southern regions were overrepresented to the same degree that the other regions were underrepresented. Given the demographic characteristics of the various U.S. regions (e.g., socioeconomic status, race/ethnic composition, educational attainment), such misrepresentation of the population resulted in norms of very questionable utility. Similar normative samples were gathered for the CPM.

Determining the exact nature of RPM norms is made more difficult by the haphazard manner in which the RPM manuals and supplements have been assembled over the years, with frequent cross-references between the various sources and the lack of references for citations made in the respective manuals. What the RPM lacks most is one comprehensive examiner's manual that includes one concisely written description and treatment of the various RPM normative samples. As it stands, the RPM is poorly normed for virtually every country, and the extant norms for most countries are seriously outdated. For example, the 1986 U.S. norms are already well over a decade old, which suggests that the resulting scores obtained from these norms would be significantly inflated (Flynn, 1984, 1987, 1999).

The authors' only justification for creating norms based on the samples of convenience is that the alternative—a nationally representative stratified random sample—is much more difficult to organize and very much more expensive (Raven, 1990). Couldn't the same be said for the difficulty of norming any current intelligence test in any country? Claims of excessive cost and inconvenience are not made by modern test publishers and would not be accepted as legitimate by practicing psychologists. Why would the RPM publisher make such an outrageous claim, and why would psychologists accept such a claim as legitimate?

It is fair to say that if the RPM had not been published originally in an era when careful sampling was not typical, and if the instrument had not made significant inroads as a pioneer scale, current psychologists would not find the instrument acceptable. The RPM is deferred to and continues to be widely used largely because of its historical contributions—not because it provides a well-written, comprehensive examiner's manual; sound and representative normative samples; recent and updated stimulus materials; or a clinically and diagnostically useful and descriptive system for reporting test scores (i.e., percentile ranks). It is amazing that the test continues to be used despite all these limitations. As is true for other pioneering tests (e.g., the Stanford–Binet, the Wechsler scales, the Vineland Adaptive Behavior Scales, the PPVT), the RPM should no longer be accepted as a useful tool only

because of its historical stature, especially given that excellent alternatives for nonverbal assessment are currently available (e.g., the Leiter-R, the NNAT, the UNIT). The RPM is in dire need of a careful and thoughtful revision. Its wide use is sufficient justification for a comprehensive and representative renorming in *all* the countries in which it is being used. And the RPM, and its users, deserve one comprehensive, coherent, and concise examiner's manual that stands alone as the sole RPM information source.

Administration

Throughout the three scales (i.e., the SPM, CPM, and APM), RPM items are presented on individual stimulus pages within test booklets. Each stimulus plate resembles a unique wallpaper pattern—a pattern in which a small, bullet-shaped section has been cut away. Below the stimulus plate, six response options are presented, from which the examinee selects the one option that best completes the abstract visual stimulus design.

Technical Properties

Each of the three forms provides raw scores that can be converted to percentile ranks. The percentile ranks can be further converted to standard scores ($M = 100$, $SD = 15$). Regarding the U.S. normative data, the research supplement states:

> Summary US norms for the Standard Progressive Matrices are shown in the context of British data in Table RS3SPM4 and in the form in which they will be of most value to readers in Table RS3SPM5. Detailed norms are given in Table RS3SPM6. A table to convert these to deviation-IQs and Standard Scores will be found inside the back cover. (Raven, 1990, p. 11)

However, upon examination of Table RS3SPM6 (which provides percentile ranks for ages $6\frac{1}{2}$ to $16\frac{1}{2}$ years) and the conversion table that allows the creation of IQs, a footnote prominently notes that that "RPM scores should not be converted to deviation IQs" (p. 98). Given that the test authors recommend not using the RPM to generate IQs for the American sample, it is apparent that the RPM is seriously limited in its clinical use in the United States.

Because the RPM are homogeneous measures of ability, one would anticipate high internal consistency. Raven and colleagues (1986) cite a number of reliability studies conducted by others throughout the world. Cited, but not referenced, studies reportedly conducted within the United States between 1952 and 1979 list reliability "values" of .89 to .97 for adults; .89 and .93 for junior high and senior high students, respectively; and .90 for 6- to 10-year-old students and .92 for 11- to 15-year-old students with deafness. Although it is unclear how large these samples were, what their demographic characteristics were, or what form of internal consistency was employed, the SPM appeared at least through the 1970s to produce highly reliable scores. A better description of these samples is needed to determine their applicability, and studies with more recent populations are needed to determine the continued utility of these values.

Although test–retest data are presented in the *Manual for Raven's Progressive Matrices and Vocabulary Scales* (Raven et al., 1986), no data are presented for the U.S. normative sample. The only study is clearly identified as a U.S. sample. In this unreferenced citation (Tully, 1967, cited in Raven et al., 1986), the manual reports that 1-year stability for white and black American high school students on the SPM ranged from .55 to .84.

As with the RPM reliability studies, the 1986 manual reports a variety of validity studies conducted by other individuals. These studies, which date from the 1940s through the 1970s, are cited but are not referenced in the manual. Validity coefficients between the RPM and other intelligence tests mostly range from the .50s to .70s; however, none of these studies were conducted with current-generation intelligence tests (e.g., the present versions of the Wechsler scales or the Stanford–Binet), and most of them were conducted in other countries. Correlations between the RPM and measures of achievement for a variety of samples range from the low .20s to low .80s, with most correlations in the .40 to .70 range. The studies reported in the 1986

manual date mostly to the 1950s and 1960s.

Summary

The three forms of the RPM—the SPM, CPM, and APM—have been used widely for several decades. The psychological community has accepted these instruments as sound measures of general ability, and the scales have been employed in many countries. In many independent studies, the RPM has demonstrated generally good internal consistency and stability, with split-half and test–retest correlations that are consistently in the moderate to high levels. Likewise, validity coefficients, with tests of both intelligence and achievement, have demonstrated good concurrent and predictive validity. The principal limitations of the RPM, however, outweigh the strengths of the instrument. The RPM continues to employ outdated materials; outdated norms based generally on samples of convenience; and a compilation of research supplements and brief test manuals that lack the care, thoughtfulness, and sophistication of current tests of intelligence. The RPM sorely needs a full revision, careful standardization, and a thorough and concisely written examiner's manual. Given the test's outdated U.S. norms, which have never been representative of the population, the RPM is of very little use for *any* application in the United States. The norms and percentile-rank-score reporting system are far too crude to be useful in clinical decision making or for educational screening.

Matrix Analogies Test

The MAT has two forms. The Expanded Form (MAT-EF; Naglieri, 1985a) is a 64-item test that was designed as a general nonverbal measure of ability for children and adolescents between the ages of 5 years and 17 years, 11 months. A briefer, 34-item Short Form (MAT-SF; Naglieri, 1985b) also exists for individual and group screening purposes. The MAT-EF employs a consistent matrix format for item presentation throughout the test, with four different abstract design types embedded within the various test items. The four item types are

Pattern Completion, Reasoning by Analogy, Serial Reasoning, and Spatial Reasoning, with 16 items of each type in the test. These item types are not intended to represent different kinds of ability, but rather four ways to measure general ability nonverbally. All of the MAT-EF items are printed in yellow, white, black, and blue, to reduce the effects of impaired color vision on examinees' test performance. Naglieri (1985a) indicates that some of the MAT-EF items were influenced by the factors that underpinning the RPM, and that some were new to the field (e.g., Spatial Reasoning items). The MAT-EF produces a total test standard score with a mean of 100 and standard deviations set at 15. The four-item groups produce scaled scores with means of 10 and standard deviations of 3.

Normative Sample

The MAT-EF was normed in two phases, according to the examiner's manual (Naglieri, 1985a). Phase 1 involved the administration of 34 items to a sample of 4,468 students in class-sized groups. Phase 2 involved the individual administration of all 64 items to a sample of 1,250 students. In combination, phases 1 and 2 of the norming process allowed for equating the MAT-SF and MAT-EF norms. Naglieri recommends that due to the equating of the MAT-SF with its group norms and the MAT-EF with its individual norms, the reader should consider the larger group sample as reflecting the true norms of both forms of the test. The stratifying variables used in the norming of both forms of the MAT included age, sex, geographic region, and ethnic group. "Community size and socioeconomic status were also considered" (p. 7). Sample sizes across the 13 age levels (i.e., ages 5 through 17 years) were generally large and varied from a low of 259 in the 5-year-old group to 431 in the 10-year-old group.

The match between the group-administered sample and the U.S. population was generally within 4 or 5 percentage points on stratifying variables. For example, the MAT total sample's (n = 4,468) match with the population on geographic representation ranged from an approximate 4% underrep-

resentation of the North Central region to an approximate 4% overrepresentation of the Western region. Whereas the match between the MAT total sample and the population was within 1 point for gender, the match was more variable for race and Spanish origin. For example, although 82.6% of the U.S. population is white, 86.5% of the MAT sample was white (i.e., 4% overrepresentation), which left blacks and Hispanics underrepresented by approximately 6% and 3%, respectively. However, such underrepresentation is of less importance than would normally be the case, given the overall large normative sample size.

The individually administered sample of 1,250 students varied across the age range from a low of 60 in the 5-year-old group to 151 in the 10-year-old group. The match between the individually administered normative sample and the U.S. population was less precise than for the group-administered sample. To use the North Central region again as an example, 46.0% of the total individual sample resided in the North Central region of the country, as compared to 26.4% of the U.S. population. Overrepresentation of this region by approximately 20% meant that other U.S. regions were concomitantly misrepresented (i.e., Northeast, –17%; South, –2%; West, +0.4%). However, because this sample was equated to the larger, more representative one, this is less problematic than it would seem.

Administration

The MAT-EF is administered with brief verbal directions. The four item types, each with 16 corresponding items, are administered beginning with item one. Each of the four groups of items has a time allowance of 12 minutes, for a total maximum administration time of 48 minutes for the test. Each item group is discontinued after the examinee has failed four consecutive items, thereby shortening the administration time of the test in direct proportion to the examinee's level of success. Although the MAT-EF provides no demonstration or sample items, the examiner acknowledges correct responses on the first two items within each of the four item groups. If the examinee fails either or both of the first two items within each group, the examiner corrects the examinee's response on the failed items.

Technical Properties

Internal consistency (coefficient alpha) was calculated and reported for each of the 13 age levels for the MAT-EF individual normative sample of 1,250 students. Alpha coefficients for the total test were strong and ranged from a low of .88 to a high of .95 (median = .93) across the ages for the total test score. Alpha coefficients for the four item groups were more variable, but were generally strong (ranging from .35 to .92, with the majority of the coefficients in the middle to high .80s).

Stability of the MAT-EF was evaluated for a sample of 65 fifth-grade students over a 4-week test–retest interval. The sample included 30 males and 35 females; there were 52 white, 10 black, and 2 other-race students; and the average age was 10 years, 3 months. The MAT-EF total test stability coefficient was .77, with a 5-point gain score across the test–retest interval. The 4-week stability of the four item groups ranged from .40 to .67, with gain scores of approximately 0.33 SD for each item type.

Exploration of the MAT-EF's validity included a variety of procedures, including correlation of the MAT-EF raw scores and the students' chronological ages for each of the item groups. In these age differentiation analyses, raw score × age correlations ranged from .58 to .64 for the item types. Factor analysis at the item level for grades 2 through 5 provided moderate support for three of the four item types upon which the test was founded, with most Pattern Completion and Spatial Reasoning items loading significantly on the item group to which they were assigned. There were instances, however, especially in the Reasoning by Analogy and Serial Reasoning item types, in which items evidenced significant loadings on the same factor. Factor analysis for grades 6 through 9 also produced three discernible factors. However, factor analysis at this age level produced a factor structure that was less consistent across item types, with many items having significant loadings on two or more factors. The issue of factorial support for the item groups must be considered in light of the fact that the test is a single-format measure of general ability, using items that vary only slightly on the basis of how they were constructed. The item types are not considered to represent different types of intelligence, but instead all similar methods of measuring the same construct—general ability—nonverbally.

In a concurrent validity study of the MAT-EF and WISC-R for 82 normal students, the MAT produced a total test mean score that was 11 points lower than the WISC-R FSIQ, 10 points lower than the PIQ, and 8 points lower than the VIQ. Correlations between the MAT-EF and WISC-R VIQ, PIQ, and FSIQ were .37, .41, and .52, respectively. A separate concurrent validity study compared the MAT-EF and the Raven CPM for a sample of 200 normal children. The two matrix-based instruments correlated .71 and produced total test mean scores that were approximately 8 points discrepant, with the MAT-EF producing the lower mean score.

Given the age of the MAT-EF norms, it would be anticipated that the instrument would produce higher scores than when the test was originally normed in the mid–1980s. Considering that IQs tend to change cross-sectionally at a rate of 3 points per decade (Flynn, 1984, 1987, 1999), the MAT-EF norms could be expected to produce scores that are approximately 5 points higher than when the test was published. In a comparison between the MAT-EF and the UNIT (Bracken & McCallum, 1998a, 1998b), the older MAT-EF produced a total test mean score ($M = 98.37$) that was about 7 points higher than the UNIT Extended Battery FSIQ ($M = 91.03$). Thus it appears that the older MAT-EF norms may have produced inflated scores relative to tests with current norms.

Fairness

Naglieri (1985a) conducted studies examining the differential performance of different racial/ethnic groups. The first study compared 55 black and 55 white students, matched on the basis of testing site, socioeconomic status, age, and gender. The mean scores for these two samples differed by only 0.6 standard score points (i.e., 90.6 for white students versus 90.0 for black students). Differences of such a small magnitude suggest that the MAT-EF can be expected to be very useful for the assessment of minority students in the average range of intelligence.

A second study compared 114 Native American students' performance on the MAT-EF, the Raven CPM, and the WISC-R PIQ. For this sample of 57 males and 57 females, the MAT-EF produced at total test mean score (88.1) that was lower than both the CPM mean (96.3) and the PIQ (97.7). As anticipated, the MAT-EF correlated more strongly with the CPM (.64) than with the PIQ (.43).

Summary

The MAT-EF is a 64-item measure of nonverbal reasoning, with four separate item types presented in yellow, blue, white, and black abstract designs. The MAT-EF norming was conducted in two phases, with a 34-item group administered to over 4,000 students and all 64 items individually administered to approximately 1,100 students; final norms were then created through an equating process. The test evidences strong internal consistency and moderate levels of stability. Concurrent validity studies with the WISC-R and the Raven CPM produced moderate-level correlations and MAT-EF mean scores that were approximately 0.66 SD lower than the other instruments studied. The MAT-EF produced a very small mean score difference between black students and a matched sample of white students.

Naglieri Nonverbal Ability Test

The NNAT (Naglieri, 1997) is a group-administered revision and extension of the MAT-SF (Naglieri, 1985b). The NNAT employs the same four abstract matrix item types (i.e., Pattern Completion, Reasoning by Analogy, Serial Reasoning, and Spatial Reasoning), an identical standard-score metric ($M = 100$, $SD = 15$), and similar administration procedures (i.e., very brief verbal directions). It is also intended for the same age range: The NNAT, like the MAT-SF and MAT-EF, was normed for children ages 5 years through 17 years, 11 months. The main difference between these tests is that the NNAT comprises seven levels, each

of which contains items tailored to children's ability by grade. The seven overlapping item levels consist of 38 items apiece, and each item level can be administered in approximately 30 minutes.

Normative Sample

The NNAT was normed on a very large sample of 22,600 children in grades K–12 tested for development of the fall norms, and 67,000 children in grades K–12 tested for the spring norms. The total sample of approximately 89,600 children and adolescents was stratified by geographic region, socioeconomic status, urban–rural setting, ethnicity, and type of school attended. The sample included children in special educational settings, such as those with emotional disturbance, learning disabilities, hearing and visual impairments, and mental retardation. Children with limited English proficiency were also included in the standardization sample. The two samples closely approximated the U.S. population on these variables.

Technical Properties

The NNAT evidences high total test (i.e., Nonverbal Ability Index) reliabilities, ranging from .82 to .87 across the seven levels. The test also demonstrates strong correlations with academic achievement, correlating .63, .54, and .64 with SAT-9 Complete Battery, Reading, and Mathematics scores, respectively (see Naglieri, 1997, Table 10). A median correlation of .75 ($n = 3,032$) between the NNAT and the MAT-SF for samples of children in grades K, 1, 2, 5, 7, and 10 was reported by Naglieri (1997), thus demonstrating the continuity between these two instruments. These data illustrate that the NNAT and MAT-SF are highly related; also, based on the information provided in the original MAT-SF as well as the NNAT manuals, there is strong evidence that these tests are strongly related to academic achievement.

Fairness

Naglieri and Ronning (2000) provided a detailed study of mean score differences between matched samples of white ($n = 2,306$)

and black (n = 2,306); white (n = 1,176) and Hispanic (n = 1,176); and white (n = 466) and Asian (n = 466) children on the NNAT. The groups were carefully selected from a larger sample of children included in the NNAT standardization sample and were matched on the demographic characteristics of the U.S. population, including geographic region, socioeconomic status, ethnicity, and type of school setting (public or private). Only small differences were found between the NNAT scores for the white and black samples (Cohen's d ratio = .25, or about 4 standard score points). Minimal differences between the white and Hispanic (d ratio = .17, or about 3 standard score points), as well as the white and Asian (d ratio = .02, less than 1 standard score point), groups were reported.

In addition, the correlations between NNAT and academic achievement were similar for the white and minority groups. The small mean score differences and the strong correlations strongly suggest that the NNAT has utility for fair assessment of white and minority children.

Naglieri and Ford (2003) reported further evidence that the NNAT is useful as a fair measure of general ability for minority children. They studied the percentages of white, black, and Hispanic children who earned scores high enough to be used as one criterion for placement in classes for gifted students. Naglieri and Ford found that 5.6% of the white (n = 14,141), 5.1% of the black (n = 2,863), and 4.4% of the Hispanic (n = 1,991) children earned an NNAT standard score of 125 (95th percentile rank) or higher. The authors suggest that the NNAT is effective at identifying diverse students for gifted education services, and thus may help address the persistent problem of the underrepresentation of diverse students in gifted education.

Summary

The NNAT is a revision and expansion of the MAT-SF (Naglieri, 1985b); it consists of seven levels, which contain 38 progressive matrix items. The group-administered test assesses general intelligence for children 5 through 17 years of age and was normed on an extremely large standardization sample (n = 89,600). The NNAT has acceptable levels of internal reliability and is strongly related to achievement, as are the previous versions of the test. Research on race differences has shown that the test yields small differences in mean scores for whites, blacks, and Hispanics, and yet predicts achievement similarly for these groups. In addition, researchers have found that the NNAT identified very similar percentages of whites, blacks, and Hispanics with scores of 125 and above, suggesting that the test has utility for fair identification of gifted children.

General Ability Measure for Adults

The GAMA (Naglieri & Bardos, 1997) is a test that "evaluates an individual's overall general ability with items that require the application of reasoning and logic to solve problems that exclusively use abstract designs and shapes" (Naglieri & Bardos, 1997, p. 1). The 66 GAMA items are presented in the same blue, yellow, white, and black designs as the MAT (Naglieri, 1985a, 1985b). One difference between the GAMA and the MAT is that whereas the MAT directions are presented orally, the GAMA instructions may be read by examinees. The GAMA instructions are written at a grade 2.4 level, according to Naglieri and Bardos (1997), which renders the directions readable for many adults who are only semiliterate. Another major differences between the two tests is that the GAMA is intended for adults between the ages 18 and 96 years, whereas the MAT is designed for ages 5 through 17 years. Finally, the GAMA differs from the MAT in the types of items that are included and the way in which the items are presented. Both tests provide a nonverbal measure of general ability. Like the MAT, the GAMA produces a standard score for the total test (GAMA IQ) with a mean of 100 and standard deviations of 15. Subtest scaled scores on both tests have means of 10 and standard deviations of 3.

Normative Sample

The GAMA was normed on a national sample of 2,360 adults. Stratifying variables for the normative sample included age, gender, race/ethnic group, educational level, and geographic region. Standardization testing occurred in 80 cities and 23 states across the United States; representation of the four geographic regions of the country matched the U.S. population within 1% for the total sample and at most age levels. The oldest age level (i.e., 75 years and older) was the only sampled age group that experienced significant deviation from the national population in terms of U.S. regions, with some discrepancies of approximately 8%. Gender, race/ethnicity, and education level also had a fairly good match to the U.S. population at independent age levels, with only minor (2%–5%) discrepancies.

Administration

There are four sets of directions for administering the GAMA, depending on whether the test is administered on an individual or group basis and whether the examiner uses a self-scoring or scannable record form. Despite these four administration options, the actual test administration is essentially the same in each situation. Differences in the test directions are basically differences in what the examiner must do to prepare the materials, not what the examinee hears or reads. The test begins with four sample items that present each of the four item types. After completing the sample items, examinees are given 25 minutes to complete the items presented in the stimulus book.

Technical Properties

Reliability coefficients (split-half) were calculated for the four item types and the total test score (GAMA IQ) for the entire standardization sample. Reliabilities for the GAMA IQ across the 11 age levels ranged from .79 to .94, with 7 of the age levels reporting reliabilities at or above .90. The average GAMA IQ split-half reliability was .90 across all age levels. Average reliabilities for the four item types were .65, .66, .79, and .81 for the Construction, Matching, Sequences, and Analogies items, respectively.

Test–retest reliability was investigated using a sample of 86 adults that, while not representative of the U.S. population, was broadly represented according to gender, race/ethnicity, and educational level. With a mean test–retest interval of 25 days, the GAMA IQ score produced a stability coeffi-

cient of .67. The four item types produced test–retest correlations that ranged from .38 (Construction) to .74 (Sequences). Gain scores of slightly less than 0.33 SD were consistent across the item types and GAMA IQ.

Given that the GAMA was created for adults, and that the developmental pattern for adults is to show diminished intellectual abilities over time (especially in visual–spatial reasoning skills), it is not surprising that the GAMA IQ and item types all correlated moderately and negatively with chronological age. Correlations between raw score and chronological age were between –.43 and –.56 for the four item types and –.59 for the GAMA IQ score.

Concurrent validity studies with the GAMA included comparisons with the Wechsler Adult Intelligence Scale—Revised (WAIS-R; Wechsler, 1981) and the K-BIT (Kaufman & Kaufman, 1990) for a sample of 194 individuals between the ages of 25 and 74 years. The total sample correlation of the GAMA IQ with the WAIS-R FSIQ was .75, and it was .70 with the K-BIT IQ. All three instruments produced mean total test scores that were within 2 standard-score points of each other, thus evidencing high correlations and similar mean scores. Similar results were reported in the GAMA Manual for adult ability tests, such as the Wonderlic Personnel Test and the Shipley Institute of Living Scale.

Various special population studies (e.g., matched sample comparisons, concurrent validity) are also reported in the GAMA manual. These studies include separate samples of adults with learning disabilities ($n = 34$), traumatic brain injury ($n = 50$), mental retardation ($n = 41$), and deafness ($n = 49$), as well as adults residing in nursing homes ($n = 43$). Each of these studies provided reasonable evidence for the criterion-related validity of the GAMA, with moderate-level correlations and comparable total test scores between the GAMA and the WAIS-R or K-BIT. One exception to this trend was the comparison of the GAMA and K-BIT for adults with mental retardation. In this study the two tests produced comparable total test mean scores, but the correlation between the GAMA IQ and the WAIS-R FSIQ was low (.36). In this instance, however, the correlation was significantly reduced due to uncorrected restriction in range.

Summary

The GAMA is a brief, convenient measure of general ability for adults. The test evidences strong internal consistency and stability for the total test score (i.e., GAMA IQ) and, with some variability, for the four item types. Strong evidence of construct and criterion-related validity are also apparent: The GAMA shows moderate to high correlations with the WAIS-R and K-BIT, and comparable total test means. The GAMA is easily administered in either individual or group formats, and requires limited reading skills (i.e., second grade). The GAMA, like the MAT and NNAT, has nonverbal test content, but is administered with minimal verbal directions.

CONCLUSIONS

In this chapter, we have attempted to elucidate the nonverbal assessment of general ability from a conceptual basis, and to provide some practical information about some nonverbal tests practitioners may wish to consider. Importantly, we have stressed that nonverbal tests of general ability may use items that have different formats (e.g., the UNIT and Leiter-R) or use very similar items (e.g., the RPM and NNAT), but they all measure general cognitive ability. These tests reflect theoretical orientations or methodology present in instruments developed during the early part of the 1900s, when the concept of measuring general intelligence via verbal and nonverbal tests was developed. The value of a nonverbal test of general ability is that it allows for more accurate assessment of diverse populations than a verbal test does. Despite the similarities of these various nonverbal tests, they differ primarily along two dimensions. First, as noted above, the diversity of item content may be large as that found in the UNIT and Leiter-R, or the test may contain items that use the same item type (e.g., the RPM and NNAT). Second, some of the tests are carefully developed and very well standardized, and others reflect less than optimal standards. Professionals should consider closely the technical characteristics and validity evidence for each of these nonverbal measures of general ability, and should carefully consider their own the goals and reasons for assessment, before selecting tests for different uses and applications.

REFERENCES

American Educational Research Association (AERA), American Psychological Association (APA), & National Council on Measurement in Education (NCME). (1985). *Standards for educational and psychological testing.* Washington, DC: Authors.

Arthur, G. (1925). A new point performance scale. *Journal of Applied Psychology, 9,* 390–416.

Arthur, G. (1943). *A Point Scale of Performance Tests: Clinical manual.* New York: Commonwealth Fund.

Arthur, G. (1947). *Point Scale of Performance Tests: Form II* (rev.). New York: Psychological Corporation.

Arthur, G., & Woodrow, H. (1919). An absolute intelligence scale: A study in method. *Journal of Applied Psychology, 3,* 118–137.

Barona, A., & Santos de Barona, M. (1987). A model for the assessment for limited English proficient students referred for special education services. In S. H. Fradd & W. J. Tikunoff (Eds.), *Bilingual education and bilingual special education* (pp. 183–209). Austin, TX: Pro-Ed.

Bracken, B. A. (1984). *Bracken Basic Concept Scale.* San Antonio, TX: Psychological Corporation.

Bracken, B. A. (1986). Incidence of basic concepts in the directions of five commonly used American tests of intelligence. *School Psychology International, 7,* 1–10.

Bracken, B. A. (1987). Limitations of preschool instruments and standards for minimal levels of technical adequacy. *Journal of Psychoeducational Assessment, 5,* 313–326.

Bracken, B. A. (1988). Ten psychometric reasons why similar tests produce dissimilar results. *Journal of School Psychology, 26,* 155–166.

Bracken, B. A. (1998a). *Bracken Basic Concept Scale—Revised.* San Antonio, TX: Psychological Corporation.

Bracken, B. A. (1998b). *Bracken Basic Concept Scale—Revised: Spanish Form.* San Antonio, TX: Psychological Corporation.

Bracken, B. A., Barona, A., Bauermeister, J. J., Howell, K. K., Poggioli, L., & Puente, A. (1990). Multinational validation of the Spanish Bracken Basic Concept Scale for cross-cultural assessment. *Journal of School Psychology, 28,* 325–341.

Bracken, B. A., & Fouad, N. (1987). Spanish translation and validation of the Bracken Basic Concept Scale. *School Psychology Review, 16,* 94–102.

Bracken, B. A., & McCallum, R. S. (1998a). *Universal Nonverbal Intelligence Test.* Itasca, IL: Riverside.

Bracken, B. A., & McCallum, R. S. (1998b). *Universal Nonverbal Intelligence Test: Training video* [Videotape]. Itasca, IL: Riverside.

Brown, L., Sherberou, R. J., & Johnsen, S. (1982). *Test of Nonverbal Intelligence.* Austin, TX: Pro-Ed.

Brown, L., Sherberou, R. J., & Johnsen, S. (1990). *Test of Nonverbal Intelligence—2.* Austin, TX: Pro-Ed.

Brown, L., Sherbenou, R. J., & Johnsen, S. K. (1997). *Test of Nonverbal Intelligence—3rd Edition.* Austin, TX: Pro-Ed.

Brown, R. T., Reynolds, C. R., & Whitaker, J. S. (1999). Bias in mental testing since *Bias in mental testing. School Psychology Quarterly, 14,* 208–238.

Carrey, N. J. (1995). Itard's 1828 memoire on "mutism caused by a lesion of the intellectual functions": A historical analysis. *Journal of the American Academy of Child and Adolescent Psychiatry, 341,* 655–1661.

Carroll, J. B. (1993). *Human cognitive abilities: A survey of factor-analytic studies.* Cambridge, England: Cambridge University Press.

Caterino, L. C. (1990). Step-by-step procedure for the assessment of language-minority children. In A. Barona & E. E. Garcia (Eds.), *Children at risk: Poverty, minority status, and other issues of educational equity* (pp. 269–282). Washington, DC: National Association of School Psychologists.

Cohen, R. J., Swerdlik, M. E., & Smith, D. K. (1992) *Psychological testing and assessment.* Mountain View, CA: Mayfield.

Donzelli, J. (1996, September 11). How do you say "milk" in 54 different ways? *Sun-Sentinel* [Fort Lauderdale, FL], East Broward Edition, Community Close-Up section, p. 11.

Elliott, C. D. (1990). *Differential Ability Scales.* San Antonio, TX: Psychological Corporation.

Fast Fact. (1996, December 5). *Sun-Sentinel* [Fort Lauderdale, FL], Palm Beach Edition, Local section, p. 1B.

Flynn, J. R. (1984). The mean IQ of Americans: Massive gains 1932 to 1978. *Psychological Bulletin, 95,* 29–51.

Flynn, J. R. (1987). Massive gains in 14 nations: What IQ tests really measure. *Psychological Bulletin, 101,* 171–191.

Flynn, J. R. (1999). Searching for justice: The discovery of IQ gains over time. *American Psychologist, 54*(1), 5–20.

Frisby, C. L. (1999). Straight talk about cognitive assessment and diversity. *School Psychology Quarterly, 14,* 195–207.

Gonzales, E. (1982). Issues in assessment of minorities. In H. L. Swanson & B. L. Watson (Eds.), *Educational and psychological assessment of exceptional children* (pp. 375–389). St. Louis, MO: Mosby.

Hammill, D. D., Pearson, N. A., & Wiederholt, J. L. (1996). *Comprehensive Test of Nonverbal Intelligence.* Austin, TX: Pro-Ed.

Healy, W. L. (1914). A Pictorial Completion Test. *Psychological Review, 20,* 189–203.

Healy, W. L. (1918). *Pictorial Completion Test II.* Chicago: Stoelting.

Healy, W. L. (1921). Pictorial Completion Test II. *Journal of Applied Psychology, 5,* 232–233.

Hilliard, A. G., III. (1984). IQ testing as the emperor's new clothes: A critique of Jensen's *Bias in mental testing.* In C. R. Reynolds & R. T. Brown (Eds.), *Perspectives on bias in mental testing* (pp. 139–169). New York: Plenum Press.

Itard, J. M. G. (1932). *The wild boy of Aveyron.* New York: Appleton-Century-Crofts.

Jensen, A. R. (1980). *Bias in mental testing.* New York: Free Press.

Kaufman, A. S. (1979). *Intelligent testing with the WISC-R.* New York: Wiley.

Kaufman, A. S. (1990). *Assessing adolescent and adult intelligence.* Boston: Allyn & Bacon.

Kaufman, A. S. (1994). *Intelligent testing with the WISC-III.* New York: Wiley.

Kaufman, A. S., & Kaufman, N. L. (1983). *Kaufman Assessment Battery for children.* Circle Pines, MN: American Guidance Service.

Kaufman, A. S., & Kaufman, N. L. (1990). *Kaufman Brief Intelligence Test.* Circle Pines, MN: American Guidance Service.

Kaufman, A. S., & Lichtenberger, E. O. (1999). *Essentials of WAIS-III Assessment.* New York: Wiley.

Knox, H. A. (1914). A scale based on the work at Ellis Island for estimating mental defect. *Journal of the American Medical Association, 62,* 741–747.

Kohs, S. C. (1919). *Intelligence measurement.* New York: Macmillan.

Maller, S. (2000). Item invariance in four subtests of the Universal Nonverbal Intelligence Test across groups of deaf and hearing children. *Journal of Psychoeducational Assessment, 18,* 240–254.

Munoz-Sandoval, A. E., Cummins, J., Alvarado, C. G., & Ruef, M. L. (1998). *Bilingual Verbal Ability Tests.* Itasca, IL: Riverside.

Naglieri, J. A. (1985a). *Matrix Analogies Test—Expanded Form.* San Antonio, TX: Psychological Corporation.

Naglieri, J. A. (1985b). *Matrix Analogies Test—Short Form.* San Antonio, TX: Psychological Corporation.

Naglieri, J. A. (1997). *Naglieri Nonverbal Ability Test.* San Antonio, TX: Psychological Corporation.

Naglieri, J. A. (1999). *Essentials of CAS assessment.* New York: Wiley.

Naglieri, J. A., & Bardos, A. N. (1997). *General Ability Measure for Adults.* Minneapolis, MN: NCS Assessments.

Naglieri, J. A., & Ford, D. (2003). Addressing underrepresentation of gifted minority children using the Naglieri Nonverbal Ability Test (NNAT). *Gifted Child Quarterly, 47,* 155–160.

Naglieri, J. A., & Ronning, M. E. (2000). Comparison of white, African American, Hispanic, and Asian children on the Naglieri Nonverbal Ability Test. *Psychological Assessment, 12,* 328–334.

Nunnally, J., & Bernstein, I. H. (1994). *Psychometric theory* (3rd ed.). New York: McGraw-Hill.

O'Hanlon, A. (1997, May 11). Non-English speakers are testing schools. *The Washington Post,* Prince William Extra section, p. V01.

Pasco, J. R. (1994). Chicago—Don't miss it. *Communiqué, 23*(4), 2.

Pintner, R. (1925). *Intelligence testing.* New York: Holt.

Pintner, R., & Patterson, D. G. (1917). *A scale of performance tests.* New York: Appleton.

Porteus, S. D. (1915). Mental tests for the feebleminded: A new series. *Journal of Psycho-Asthenics, 19,* 200–213.

Power, S. (1996, May 9). Panel suggests school clerks

learn Spanish: Board takes no action on report. *The Dallas Morning News,* Plano section, p. 1F.

Puente, M. (1998, May 27). Californians likely to end bilingual ed. *USA Today,* News section, p. 4A.

Raven, J. (1990). *Manual for Raven's Progressive Matrices and Vocabulary Scales: Research Supplement No. 3. American and international norms, neuropsychological uses.* Oxford: Oxford Psychologists Press.

Raven, J., Raven, J. C., & Court, J. H. (1998a). *Advanced Progressive Matrices.* Oxford: Oxford Psychologists Press.

Raven, J., Raven, J. C., & Court, J. H. (1998b). *Coloured Progressive Matrices.* Oxford: Oxford Psychologists Press.

Raven, J., Raven, J. C., & Court, J. H. (1998c). *Standard Progressive Matrices.* Oxford: Oxford Psychologists Press.

Raven, J. C., Court, J. H., & Raven, J. (1986). *Manual for Raven's Progressive Matrices and Vocabulary Scales* (1986 edition, with U.S. norms). London: H. K. Lewis.

Reynolds, C. R., Lowe, P. A., & Saenz, A. L. (1999). The problem of bias in psychological assessment. In C. R. Reynolds & T. B. Gutkin (Eds.), *Handbook of school psychology* (3rd ed., pp. 549–595). New York: Wiley.

Roid, G. H., & Miller, L. J. (1997). *Leiter International Performance Scale—Revised.* Wood Dale, IL: Stoelting.

Rycraft, J. R. (1990). Behind the walls of poverty: Economically disadvantaged gifted and talented children. *Early Child Development and Care, 63,* 139–147.

Schmeiser, C. B. (1992). Reactions to technical and societal issues in testing Hispanics. In K. F. Geisinger (Ed.), *Psychological testing of Hispanics* (pp. 79–85). Washington, DC: American Psychological Association.

Seguin, E. (1907). *Idiocy and its treatment by the physiological method.* New York: Teachers College, Columbia University.

Steele, M. (1998, January 23). Bilingual education program an expensive failure. *The Arizona Republic,* Northeast Phoenix Community section, p. 2.

Stepp, D. (1997, November 20). School watch: As demographics change, language programs grow; transition help: The International Welcome Center helps non-English-speaking students adjust. *The Atlanta Journal and Constitution,* Extra section, p. 2g.

Thorndike, R. L., Hagen, E. P., & Sattler, J. M. (1986). *Stanford–Binet Intelligence Scale: Fourth Edition.* Itasca, IL: Riverside.

Thorndike, R. M., & Lohman, D. F. (1990). *A century of ability testing.* Chicago: Riverside.

Thurstone, L. L. (1938). Primary mental abilities. *Psychometric Monographs,* No. 1.

Ulik, C. (1997, January 6). Civil rights officials check Tempe schools; limited-English programs studied. *The Arizona Republic/The Phoenix Gazette,* Tempe Community Section, p. 1.

Unz, R. (1997, October 19). Perspective on education: Bilingual is a damaging myth; a system that ensures failure is kept alive by the flow of federal dollars. A 1998 initiative would bring change. *Los Angeles Times,* Opinion section, Part M, p. 5.

U.S. Government Printing Office. (1918). *Examiner's guide for psychological examining in the Army.* Washington, DC: Author.

Wechsler, D. (1944). *The measurement of adult intelligence* (3rd ed.). Baltimore: Williams & Wilkins.

Wechsler, D. (1949). *Wechsler Intelligence Scale for Children.* New York: Psychological Corporation.

Wechsler, D. (1981). *Wechsler Adult Intelligence Scale—Revised.* New York: Psychological Corporation.

Wechsler, D. (1987). *Wechsler Memory Scale—Revised.* San Antonio, TX: Psychological Corporation.

Wechsler, D. (1991). *Wechsler Intelligence Scale for Children—Third Edition manual.* San Antonio, TX: Psychological Corporation.

Wechsler, D. (1992). *Wechsler Individual Achievement Test.* San Antonio, TX: Psychological Corporation.

Woodcock, R. W., & Johnson, M. B. (1990). *Woodcock–Johnson Revised Tests of Cognitive Ability: Standard and Supplemental Batteries.* Chicago: Riverside.

Woodcock, R. W., & Munoz-Sandoval, A. F. (1996). *Bateria Woodcock–Munoz-Revisada.* Itasca, IL: Riverside.

Yoakum, C. S., & Yerkes, R. M. (1920). *Army mental tests.* New York: Holt.

12

Comprehensive Assessment of Child and Adolescent Memory: The Wide Range Assessment of Memory and Learning, the Test of Memory and Learning, and the California Verbal Learning Test—Children's Version[1]

MICHAEL J. MILLER
ERIN D. BIGLER
WAYNE V. ADAMS

Memory, across all of its heuristic divisions, is the conduit that makes higher cognitive functioning possible. For example, aspects of executive abilities are dependent on working memory; expressive language requires retrieval of words from memory stores; certain spatial abilities may be contingent on cognitive maps; and sophisticated processes such as judgment may require the retrieval of context-specific memories. Although there are cases when memory is affected and other cognitive abilities may remain intact, the functional ramifications of the memory disturbance alone may be considerable. Such was the case with H. M., a 27-year-old man who underwent a bilateral resection of the medial temporal lobe for intractable epilepsy. Despite H. M.'s preserved intelligence, he was unable to care for himself because of a severe anterograde amnesia, which prevented the formation of new memories. Although he could carry on an intelligent conversation, H. M. had to be reminded to shave, read magazines over and over again, was only vaguely aware (years

after the fact) that his father had died, and was only capable of doing vocational work designed for persons with mental retardation (Kolb & Whishaw, 1996). H. M. appeared to be perpetually disoriented, as he could not remember events that had recently transpired. His comment, "Every day is alone in itself, whatever enjoyment I've had, and whatever sorrow I've had" (Kolb & Whishaw, 1996, p. 359) underscores that his experience from moment to moment was encapsulated, with no connection to the past or present. Memory may therefore provide a context for the self. As Mesulam (2000) recently wrote, "memory is the glue that holds together our thoughts, impressions, and experiences. Without it, past and future would lose their meaning and self-awareness would be lost as well" (p. 257). These observations suggest that memory is the core of what makes us uniquely human. The case of H. M. is important not only because of what it teaches about the profound implications of circumscribed memory disturbance, but also because of its central role in delineating the functions of the medial temporal lobe structures in memory processes (reviewed below).

In light of the broad neural distribution of cortical and subcortical brain regions associated with memory, and the diverse cognitive, behavioral, and emotional processes dependent on these substrates, it is not surprising that many neurological and neuropsychiatric disorders disrupt memory and associated functions (Baron, Fennell, & Voeller, 1995; Cullum, Kuck, & Ruff, 1990; Cytowic, 1996; Gillberg, 1995; Knight, 1992; Lezak, 1995; Mapou & Spector, 1995; Reeves & Wedding, 1994). Indeed, memory assessment is critical because of its relevance in evaluating the overall functional and physiological integrity of the brain (Cowan, 1997; Parkin, 1993). In fact, in cases of traumatic brain injury (TBI), memory disturbances are the most common of patient complaints (Cronwall, Wrightson, & Waddell, 1990; Golden, Zillmer, & Spiers, 1992; Reeves & Wedding, 1994). Because of the prevalence of TBI in children (Goldstein & Levin, 1990), assessment of memory disorder in children who have experienced TBI has become a particular focus for pediatric neuropsychologists and other clinicians involved in the assessment of children. In addition, memory deficits, which often accompany learning disorders, are among the most common referrals for chil-

dren requiring psychological assessment (Bull & Johnston, 1997; de Jong, 1998; Lorsbach, Wilson, & Reimer, 1996; Nation, Adams, Bowyer-Crain, & Snowling, 1999; Swanson, Ashbacker, & Lee, 1996). In the rehabilitation setting, memory disorders are also the most common therapeutic focus in cognitive rehabilitation (Prigatano, 1990). Given that the probability of positive outcomes for individuals with memory impairment is dependent on the identification of highly specific deficits that can only be determined through comprehensive assessment, it is surprising that inclusive memory batteries have not been available for children until recently. Table 12.1 lists the most common childhood disorders in which memory and learning are affected.

Although formal memory batteries for children are a relatively recent phenomenon, it appears that assessment of memory in children and adolescents was considered to be of some importance, as the earliest of modern intelligence tests (the 1907 Binet and the early Wechsler scales) incorporated brief assessments of immediate recall. Evidence of early attention to the import of memory assessment can also be found in one subtest of the McCarthy Scales of Children's Abilities (McCarthy, 1972) and in the more detailed four-subtest Visual–Aural Digit Span Test (Koppitz, 1977). Although 80% of a sample of clinicians interviewed in

TABLE 12.1. Most Frequent Childhood Disorders in Which Memory and Learning Are Likely to Be Compromised

Attention-deficit/hyperactivity disorder (ADHD)	*In utero* toxic exposure (e.g., cocaine, alcohol)	Neurofibromatosis
Autism and other developmental disorders	Juvenile Huntington's disease	Prader–Willi syndrome
Cancer (especially brain tumors, lung cancer, parathyroid tumors, leukemia, and lymphoma)	Juvenile parkinsonism	Rett's syndrome
	Kidney disease/transplant	Schizophrenia
	Learning disability	Seizure disorders
	Lesch–Nyhan disease	Tourette's syndrome
Cerebral palsy	Major depressive disorder	Toxic exposure (e.g., lead, mercury, carbon monoxide)
Down's syndrome	Meningitis	Traumatic brain injury (TBI)
Endocrine disorders	Mental retardation	Turner's syndrome
Extremely low birth weight	Myotonic dystrophy	XXY syndrome
Fragile-X sydrome	Neurodevelopmental abnormalities affecting brain development (e.g., anencephaly, microcephaly, callosal dysgenesis)	XYY syndrome
Hydrocephalus		
Hypoxic–ischemic injury		
Inborn errors of metabolism (e.g., phenylketonuria, galactosemia)		

1987 cited memory as a core component of cognitive assessment (Snyderman & Rothman, 1987), the major child neuropsychology texts of the 1970s and 1980s (e.g., Hynd & Obrzut, 1981; Rourke, Bakker, Fisk, & Strang, 1983) made little reference to memory assessment. Not until the 1990s was this gap between theory and practice addressed (e.g., Baron et al., 1995; Gillberg, 1995). The increasing focus on assessment of memory is now also evident in the major works of child neuropsychology (Pennington, 1991; Rourke, 1991; Tramontana & Hooper, 1988).

The Wide Range Assessment of Memory and Learning (WRAML; Sheslow & Adams, 1990) represented the first effort to develop an inclusive memory battery for children and adolescents. The Test of Memory and Learning (TOMAL; Reynolds & Bigler, 1994b) and the California Verbal Learning Test—Children's Version (CVLT-C; Delis, Kramer, Kaplan, & Ober, 1994) are additional batteries specifically designed for the assessment of childhood memory. All three batteries are reviewed below, following a discussion of the basic neurobiology of memory.

A PRIMER ON THE NEUROBIOLOGY OF MEMORY

Although a comprehensive review of the neurobiology of memory is beyond the scope of this chapter, a brief discussion of the neural substrates of memory systems is provided as a critical foundation for discussing the assessment of memory. For a more in-depth discussion of this topic, excellent reviews are provided by Bauer, Tobias, and Valenstein (1993), Cohen (1993), Diamond (1990), and Scheibel (1990). It should be emphasized that the current primer is cursory because of space limitations. We hope that readers will seek a further grounding in the basic neurobiology of memory, given the importance of this background for clinical assessment.

For memories to be formed, an individual must experience a single sensation or multiple sensations in combination. These sensations can emanate from the environment or can be produced internally. The manner in which sensory processing occurs lays the

foundation for the modality (i.e., auditory, verbal, olfactory, gustatory, or somatosensory) in which learning occurs. A recent memory that is common to virtually all Americans may illustrate this point. For example, most Americans first learned of the events of September 11, 2001, through horrific images viewed on television, over the Internet, or in newspapers of a commercial aircraft plowing through the North Tower of the World Trade Center, followed by a second aircraft 10 minutes later that banked left and crashed into the South Tower. Others may have first heard of the tragedy on the radio or been told the news by another person. People who were working near the World Trade Center may recall the smell of the burning steel in the towers; others who were very close to "Ground Zero" may recall the taste of the clouds of smoke that filled the streets; still others may recall their awareness of their physical reaction (e.g., racing heart, goose bumps, feeling faint, etc.). Regardless of the modality in which an event is processed, memories are formed and often recalled via the sensory channel(s) in which they were experienced. Although memories can be formed and retrieved within each of these modalities, the visual and auditory senses are dominant in most individuals. Assessment of memory has therefore focused on these modalities, although a greater emphasis has been placed on verbal processing. As will be discussed further below, the verbal–visual distinction provides an important heuristic for the clinician, as the left hemisphere is more oriented toward language-based memory and the right toward visual–spatial memory (Bigler & Clement, 1997).

Regardless of the sensory modality, several critical brain structures—including the hippocampus, amygdala, fornix, mammillary bodies, diverse thalamic nuclei, and distributed regions of the neocortex—are involved in the development of memories (see Figure 12.1). Briefly, from the sensory stimulus, neural impulses travel from the sensory organs, primary cortex, and association neocortex (attention/working memory) to the hippocampus via pathways that course through the medial-inferior aspect of the temporal lobe en route to the hippocampus (see Figure 12.1). The hippocampus and associated limbic structures represent a "way

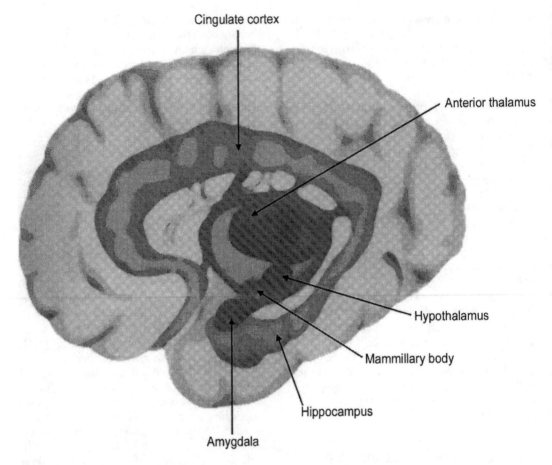

FIGURE 12.1. Schematic of the brain highlighting the limbic system, particularly the hippocampus. The hippocampus is located in the temporal lobe and is critical in the process of memory function. From Banich (1997). Copyright 1997 by Houghton-Mifflin. Reprinted by permission.

station" of sorts, in which a stimulus is either attended to for further processing or ignored. Once the stimulus is experienced as relevant, further processing, including binding, occurs in the medial temporal lobe structures. "Binding" is the process wherein associations are formed between a new, relevant stimulus and previously processed information. Following damage to the hippocampus or its efferent projections (i.e., the fornix, mammillary bodies, and anterior thalamus), short-term or working memory may remain intact, and the patient may be able to recall a brief stimulus (e.g., a list of two or three words or numbers). However, for retention of information beyond immediate or short-term memory span (greater than several seconds), additional processing subsumed by hippocampal and associated limbic structures must occur. Following processing of information in the hippocampal circuit, long-term storage occurs in the distributed neural networks of the cerebral cortex, where memories receive the most extensive processing and are the least vulnerable to injury. In fact, the recall of well-established memories tends to be one of the most robust of neural functions, whereas sustained attention, concentration, and the formation of new memories tend to be the most fragile.[2]

The World Trade Center example is also useful in illustrating the emotional processing that is critical to memory. In addition to the above-mentioned limbic circuit involved in memory processes, a second limbic circuit exists that includes the amygdala and related structures. This circuit is responsible for processing emotional material and "coloring" memories with feeling. Why would it be important that memories are given an emotional hue? In short, the emotion associated with a memory brings greater richness and dimensionality to the experience recalled from memory. If we return to the example of the World Trade Center disaster, it is likely that the very mention of "September 11" or "9/11" evokes strong emotions tied to memories of the tragedy. Before these events, "September 11" for most persons was a neutral stimulus that bore no particular meaning. However, in light of the horrific events the world experienced on September 11, 2001, the mention of the month and day may now for many people be inextricably bound to the emotions associated with those events. Indeed, strong emotions associated with memories cause people to pay attention and may therefore contribute to their survival. Americans (and citizens of other countries) have developed a new awareness of terrorism and are consequently more likely to react to suspicious behavior. On an individual basis, many people have debated when (or even whether) they will resume their lives as they were before September 11. Thus a previously meaningless date is now fraught with meaning that has caused billions of people to reconsider their very existence. Although this example is extreme, the binding of emotion to memory is an ongoing part of consciousness; disruption of this process may manifest clinically as an inability to recognize facial expressions indicating fear or threat (Phelps et al., 2001), as well as verbal and nonverbal memory deficits (Buchanan, Denburg, Tranel, & Adolphs, 2001).

Two additional concepts, which have important implications for the assessment of memory disorders, deserve brief discussion. First, as mentioned earlier, lateralization of brain function (Stark & McGregor, 1997) provides a useful heuristic for the clinician. That is, in most individuals, the left hemisphere of the brain is more dedicated to language-based functions and the right hemisphere to visual–spatial processes. Lateralization of functions provides useful generalizations for assessing differences in memory processes, based on whether the information is language-based or visual–spatial in nature. Therefore, damage to the left hemisphere (particularly the left temporal lobe) may result in verbal memory deficits, while visual–spatial abilities are likely to be spared. The converse is true with damage to the right hemisphere (particularly the right temporal lobe), which is more involved in visual–spatial aspects of memory.

Finally, it is important to recognize that learning and memory are dependent on attention. Making distinctions between attention and memory processes has proven to be one of the most difficult challenges for neuropsychologists. Although the reticular activating system and diffuse thalamic projecting systems have been recognized as essential to arousal, there is no specific neuroanatomical mapping of the construct of attention. From the neuropsychological perspective, "attention" is probably a nonlocalized neural process with major contributions from frontal and temporal lobe regions. However, it is also well known that damage to diverse regions of the cerebral cortex has the potential to cause attentional deficits. Thus, at the most basic level, attention may be considered a function of the integrated brain—one that is vulnerable when the integrity of the brain as a whole is threatened. The clinician must become adept at distinguishing attentional deficits from impairment in memory functions during the early stages of information processing (e.g., attention vs. encoding). Presently there are "attention" components of memory batteries as well as independent measures of attention, but due to the inherent difficulty in distinguishing between attentional deficits and memory processing deficits, these measures are far from perfect. The assessment of attention in relation to memory thus requires the integration of formal assessment, careful observation, and data collected from the patient and his or her family.

WIDE RANGE ASSESSMENT OF MEMORY AND LEARNING

Structure

The WRAML (Sheslow & Adams, 1990) was the first inclusive memory battery for children and adolescents. Prior to the WRAML's inception, clinicians interested in assessing child and adolescent memory had to rely upon measures from various independent sources, as no cohesive memory battery designed specifically for children existed. The norms associated with these tests of memory varied in quality, and were often based on different samples of children, thus limiting their usefulness. These shortcomings were addressed with the introduction of the WRAML, which provided clinicians and researchers with a comprehensive sampling of memory tasks based on a common normative group; this permitted meaningful intertask comparisons.

The WRAML is normed for children 5 through 17 years of age. Administration ranges from 45 to 60 minutes, depending on the child's age and response rate as well as the experience of the examiner. An Examiner Record Form and an Examinee Response Form are utilized in the standard administration.

Figure 12.2 illustrates the structure and hierarchical organization of the WRAML. Combined performance in the Verbal Memory, Visual Memory, and Learning domains determines the composite General Memory Index. The first two domains evaluate verbal and visual modalities, the principal information-processing modalities of memory for children and adolescents. The third WRAML domain assesses memory acquired across consecutive learning opportunities. These opportunities occur across trials involving visual, verbal, and dual-modality (visual with verbal) tasks, and allow for the assessment of learning gradients.

The Verbal Memory and Visual Memory domains are organized according to a simi-lar rationale. As subtests from each domain progress, the information to be immediately recalled is increased. Tasks within these domains vary from rote memory tasks with little meaningful content to tasks with significantly greater meaning. The examiner thus has the opportunity to observe a child's immediate memory ability across varied modalities and degrees of meaningfulness. "Meaning" refers both to the complexity of the task and the relevance to everyday functioning. This concept will become clearer as we discuss the individual subtests below.

Each of the WRAML's three domains is composed of three subtests. Each subtest produces a scaled score ($M = 10$, $SD = 3$), and each domain produces a standard score ($M = 100$, $SD = 15$). The scaled scores of all nine subtests are combined to produce the General Memory Index ($M = 100$, $SD = 15$). These familiar metrics are intuitive for the examiner and allow for comparison with the results of other cognitive measures, such as intelligence and achievement tests.

In addition to the nine primary subtests composing the three major domains, there are "optional" Delayed Recall components associated with each of the learning across trials subtests. One of the Verbal Memory subtests (Story Memory) also provides both a Delayed Recall and a Recognition option.

Description, Rationale, and Clinical Applications of Subtests

Table 12.2 provides a description of the subtests within each domain. The rationale for each subtest is discussed below, as well

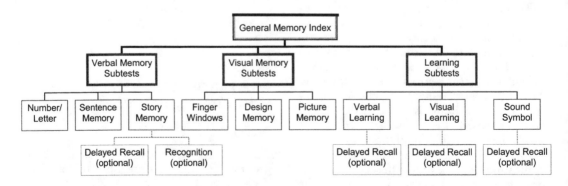

FIGURE 12.2. Schematic of the Index and Subtest Structure of the Wide Range Assessment of Memory and Learning (WRAML).

TABLE 12.2. Description of Subtests Associated with Each WRAML Domain

Domain/Subtest name	Subtest description
Verbal Memory	
Number/Letter	The child is asked to repeat a series of both numbers and letters verbally presented at the rate of one per second. The subtest begins with an item two units in length (e.g., "1-A") and proceeds until the "discontinue" rule is satisfied.
Sentence Memory	The child is asked to repeat meaningful sentences. Starting with a three-word sentence, the child attempts to repeat progressively longer sentences until the "discontinue" rule is satisfied.
Story Memory	The child is read and then asked to retell a one- or two-paragraph story. A second story is then read and again the child is asked to retell the story. The examiner records both exact and "gist" recalled information for scoring.
Visual Memory	
Finger Windows	The child indicates his or her memory of a rote visual pattern by sequentially placing a finger into "windows," or holes, in a plastic card, attempting to reproduce a sequence demonstrated by the examiner. Starting with a sequence of two holes, the child continues until the "discontinue" rule is satisfied.
Design Memory	A card with geometric shapes is shown to the child for 5 seconds. Following a 10-second delay, the child is asked to draw what was seen. A blank card with spatial demarcations is provided for the child's drawing. Four different cards are presented in this fashion.
Picture Memory	The child is shown a meaningful scene with people and objects for 10 seconds. The child is then asked to look at a second, similar scene. Memory of the original picture is indicated by the child's marking elements that have been altered or added in the second picture. This procedure is repeated with three additional cards.
Learning	
Verbal Learning	The child is read a list of common single-syllable words and is provided a free-recall opportunity. Three additional learning trials are administered in a similar fashion. A delayed-recall trial is available following an interference task.
Visual Learning	After initially seeing all locations, the child is asked to indicate the specific location of 12 or 14 (depending on age) visual stimuli nested within a 4×4 array. Correction of errors occurs. Three additional learning trials follow. A delayed-recall trial is also available.
Sound Symbol	The child is presented a paired-associate task requiring him or her to recall which sound is associated with which abstract and unfamiliar symbol shape. Four separate learning trials are administered, and a delayed-recall trial is also available.

as clinical uses and interpretations of testing patterns.

Verbal Memory Scale

The subtests that encompass the Verbal Memory scale provide an opportunity for the examiner to assess the child's capabilities on rote auditory memory tasks and to contrast this performance with tasks placing greater language demands on the child. This comparison allows the examiner to generate hypotheses about whether the child utilizes language as an aid or whether it is a hindrance in remembering. The three subtests (i.e., Number/Letter, Sentence Memory, and Story Memory) can be conceptualized as placing increasing demands on language processing. This allows the clinician to assess language deficits, which may confound memory assessment within the Verbal Memory domain. The three subtests constituting the Verbal Memory scale are as follows.

Number/Letter

The format of the Number/Letter subtest may be familiar to most clinicians; however, only a "forward" trial of recall is required in this subtest. This distinction was made because evidence suggests that backward recall taps different cognitive skills than forward recall (Lezak, 1995).

Sentence Memory

The units of information presented for recall on the Sentence Memory task are more sophisticated than those in the Number/Letter subtest because of the "mental glue" that language affords (see Howes, Bigler, Burlingame, & Lawson, 2003). In clinical terms, since this task requires the ability to remember one or two sentences, this task is believed to tap the kind of memory skills that may carry functional significance for a child (e.g., following oral directions at home or at school).

Story Memory

Two stories are read to the child, which differ in developmental level of interest and linguistic complexity. Using two stories permits better sampling than using a single story. It is then reasonable to assume that a greater-than-chance difference between the child's recollections of the first and second stories suggests lower verbal intellectual ability, a language disorder, or an inefficient or inconsistent ability to attend to oral information.

Similarly, a child who retells a story in an erratic sequence may have sequencing or organizational problems. By comparing sequencing in Number/Letter and Sentence Memory with that in Story Memory, the clinician can begin to distinguish among sequencing, organizational, and language deficits. Because of the importance of memory in classroom and social functioning, the clinician may wish to examine whether a child performing poorly on Story Memory recognizes the material but fails to produce it in a free-recall format. The Recognition option for the Story Memory subtest affords

this opportunity by presenting 15 questions related to the harder story, using a multiple-choice format to help determine whether the child is experiencing a deficit in retention or retrieval.

Comparison of performance on the Sentence Memory and Story Memory subtests can also be of utility in making predictions about a child's functioning. For example, if performance on Sentence Memory is relatively poor, the child may experience difficulties understanding directions. In contrast, relatively better performance on Story Memory would support the hypothesis that the child may be able to understand the "essence" of the orally delivered directions (or lecture), despite difficulties in remembering rote details.

Visual Memory Scale

Similar to the Verbal Memory subtests, the Visual Memory subtests vary from rote memory to more complex memory demands. The three Visual Memory subtests are as follows.

Finger Windows

The Finger Windows subtest is analogous to the Number/Letter subtest within the Verbal Memory domain, as discrete and relatively nonmeaningful units of information are presented at a rate of one per second, and immediate recall is required. This task taps the ability to retain a visual trace in a sequence.

Design Memory

The Design Memory subtest introduces a greater degree of meaningfulness than Finger Windows, as the child is instructed to copy a display of common shapes (e.g., circles, dots, straight lines, rectangles, and triangles). There is a 5-second exposure, followed by a 10-second delay before the child begins drawing. For a youngster who may struggle to reproduce such shapes because of perceptual–motor difficulties, an optional copy task is first administered, so that the child's reproduction of each shape becomes the criterion for scoring in the recall phase. The design is scored on both the inclusion and placement of design components. Poor placement may indicate spatial memory deficits, whereas shape omission may indicate impaired memory for visual detail. The relatively brief 5-second exposure allowed for each stimulus card is intended to minimize the use of verbal strategies to aid in completion of the task. Everyday tasks such as copying from a classroom chalkboard, or remembering visual details of a room after leaving, are included to maximize ecological validity.

Picture Memory

Building upon the Design Memory subtest (which includes rote and configural memory tasks), the Picture Memory subtest adds increased meaning, as each of four stimulus pictures depicts a scene that most children will find familiar. Children possessing "photographic" memory abilities may excel on this subtest, since task expectations demand storage of a visually presented scene to be compared with memory from a similar scene in which 20%–40% of the visual details have been altered in some manner.

Clinically, it should be noted that children with attention-deficit/hyperactivity disorder (ADHD) may score as well as or better than nonreferred children on the Picture Memory subtest because of a confound in the scoring procedure (Adams, Hyde, & deLancey, 1995). The subtest's directions indicate that the examiner is to instruct the child to identify perceived changes in each scene with a marker, "marking the things you are sure of." The examiner is instructed to discourage guessing (but not to penalize guessing), and to give credit only for correct responses in the scoring. Because of their impulsivity, children with ADHD may mark some correct details by chance, resulting in a spuriously inflated score. We have observed that children with ADHD between the ages of 5 and 8 typically make three incorrect selections per picture, compared to one incorrect selection per picture made by their age-matched counterparts in the standardization sample. It is noteworthy that although the errors-per-picture ratio drops from 3:1 to 2:1 for older children with ADHD, the effect remains statistically significant.

Learning Scale

The three Learning subtests are as follows.

Verbal Learning

The Verbal Learning subtest was adapted from Rey (1958) to assess learning across trials. In this procedure, the child is read a list of either 13 or 16 (depending on the child's age) common words, immediately followed by instructions to recall as many words as possible. The procedure is then repeated three times. The procedure in the WRAML differs in two ways. First, in contrast to Rey's (1958) procedure, four rather than five learning trials are administered; the WRAML prestandardization data demonstrated, similar to Rey's own findings, that a fifth trial contributes little additional information. Second, an interference trial following the final list recall trial is not included on the WRAML, as learning in everyday life is usually not followed by an almost identical activity serving as interference. Thus, to reduce the time of administration and the potential frustration that some children may experience, the Story Memory subtest follows the Verbal Learning subtest and serves as the interference task. Approximately 5 minutes later, a delay trial of the Verbal Learning task is administered.

Children will on occasion produce words not on the list during recall tasks. Such errors, termed "intrusion errors," occurred once or twice over the four trials among the standardization sample, especially with younger children. However, children with ADHD often average four to five intrusion errors over the four trials (Adams, Robins, Sheslow, & Hyde, 2002). The nature of the intrusion error may be relevant. For instance, semantic errors (e.g., responding with "eye" instead of "ear") may suggest expressive language difficulties, while phonetic errors (e.g., responding with "bake" instead of "lake") may suggest phonological or auditory processing difficulties.

Visual Learning

Analogous to its verbal counterpart, the Visual Learning task asks the child to learn a set number of stimuli presented across four trials. Visual designs are presented in a specific position on a "game" board, and the child is asked to recall the spatial location related to each design. Immediate feedback for item correctness is provided to promote learning. As with the Verbal Learning subtest, a delayed-recall trial may be administered following the Sound Symbol subtest, which may in turn serve as an "interference" task.

Sound Symbol

The phonological and visual symbolic requirements of the cross-modal Sound Symbol task approach the demands of early reading mastery. The child is asked to remember a sound that goes with a printed "nonsense" symbol. In a paired-associate format, shapes are presented and the child is asked to produce the corresponding sound, across four "sound–shape" learning trials. A delayed-recall trial is also available.

Although it has not been established empirically, substantial anecdotal evidence suggests that children who produce responses resembling few of the sounds associated within the subtest (typically on the third and fourth trials), may experience considerable difficulty learning phonics in their early elementary school years. Should this assertion be empirically demonstrated, one form of a reading disorder might be conceptualized as a selective memory disorder affecting processes involved in remembering units of sound associated with symbols.

Screening Form

A short form of the WRAML, called the Screening Form, was developed to aid the examiner in determining whether a more in-depth assessment is indicated. Preliminary research identified four subtests that are varied in content but highly correlated with the General Memory Index ($r = .84$). The four subtests that constitute the Screening Form—Picture Memory, Design Memory, Verbal Learning, and Story Memory—are consequently ordered first in the WRAML. Thus the Screening Form samples aspects of visual and verbal memory, and verbal learning, while maintaining a reasonable portion of the utility of the General Memory Index. The Screening Form requires approximately 10–15 minutes to administer. The psychometric integrity of the norms associated with the Screening Form is commensurate with that of the full WRAML, as the complete standardization sample was utilized to

derive the norms. In practice, the General Memory Index estimated from the Screening Form version averages about 4 points higher than the General Memory Index generated from the entire battery (Kennedy & Guilmette, 1997).

Standardization

The WRAML was standardized on a population-proportionate sample stratified by age, gender, ethnicity, socioeconomic status, geographic region, and community size. The sample consisted of 2,363 children ranging in age from 5 to 17 years. Details of the standardization procedure and stratification data are provided in the test manual (Sheslow & Adams, 1990).

Reliability

The WRAML subtests and composite Indexes show high internal-consistency reliability, as indicated by the following statistics. Item separation statistics ranged from .99 to 1.00. Person separation statistics ranged from .70 to .94. Coefficient alphas ranged from .78 to .90 for the nine individual subtests. Median coefficients alphas for the Verbal Memory Index, the Visual Memory Index, and the Learning Index were .93, .90, and .91, respectively. The General Memory Index coefficient alpha was .96.

A test–retest study was conducted with a subgroup of the standardization sample ($n = 153$). Because memory and learning tasks are vulnerable to practice effects, an analysis of the incremental effect of readministration was performed. On average, a 1-point increase in scores on the Verbal Memory and Visual Memory Memory subtests, and a 2-point increase in scores on the Learning subtests, were observed. Across a 3- to 6-month interval, no correlation existed between the number of days elapsed and the initial incremental increase in score, within the time interval assessed. That is, the slight incremental increase in WRAML subtest performance appears to be consistently maintained over a 3- to 6-month posttest interval.

Validity

In light of the considerable and varied demands of memory in the school setting, memory ability would be expected to relate to academic achievement. Moreover, as children progress in school, verbal memory would be expected to become more predictive than visual memory of academic achievement. Table 12.3 illustrates that the first expectation is borne out, as WRAML Indexes are correlated with measures of reading, spelling, and arithmetic. The second expectation is likewise supported, when the upper and lower portions of Table 12.3 are compared. That is, verbal memory appears to play only a minimal role for children in early elementary school; visual memory and especially learning over trials play a more dominant role in early scholastic achievement. In high school the pattern appears to reverse, suggesting that these differences may be associated with content demands. For example, learning to visually identify letters, numbers, and words, and learning to write, are major tasks in first and second grades. Conversely, traditional high school curricula (such as history, science, literature, and mathematics courses) require greater verbal memory demands relative to those of visual memory and rote learning across trials.

Factor Structure

Three-factor principal-components analyses were conducted on the nine WRAML subtests, using the complete standardization sample of 2,363 children and adolescents. Separate factors were derived from two age groups of children, determined by the test's age division (there were negligible differences in administration between the two age groups). The results are reported in Tables 12.4 and 12.5.

As Table 12.4 indicates, the Visual factor for younger children was composed of Picture Memory, Design Memory, and Finger Windows, as expected. Visual Learning, however, also loaded on this same factor. Further counterintuitive findings included the clustering of Sentence Memory and Number/Letter with the Verbal factor, but not Story Memory. Verbal Learning and Sound Symbol loaded according to theoretical expectations (i.e., on the Learning factor), but as previously mentioned, Visual Learning did not load on the same predicted factor.

A similar pattern was evident within the older sample (see Table 12.5), again casting doubt on the validity of the Learning construct. Several investigators have reported similar factor-analytic results with the WRAML, using both nonreferred and clinical samples (Aylward, Gioia, Verhulst, & Bell, 1995; Burton, Donders, & Mittenberg, 1996; Burton, Mittenberg, Gold, & Drabman, 1999; Dewey, Kaplan, & Crawford, 1997; Gioia, 1998; Phelps, 1995). Gioia (1998) has suggested, based upon some of the inconsistent factor-analytic results of the WRAML Index scores, that the subtest scores may be a more appropriate level of analysis. Others have asserted that this recommendation may be somewhat extreme,

TABLE 12.3. Correlations of WRAML Index Scores and Wide Range Achievement Test—Revised (WRAT-R) Subtests

	Verbal Memory Index	Visual Memory Index	Learning Index	General Index
	Ages 6 years, 0 months–8 years, 11 months			
Reading	.18	.26*	.40*	.35*
Spelling	.22	.32*	.42*	.39*
Arithmetic	.24	.46*	.40*	.46*
	Ages 16 years, 0 months–17 years, 11 months			
Reading	.41*	.14	.05	.23
Spelling	.40*	.09	.24	.30
Arithmetic	.34*	.26	.34*	.38*

Note. *p < .05.

TABLE 12.4. Results of Principal-Components Analysis with Varimax Rotation of WRAML Subtests (Completed on Children 5 Years, 0 Months through 8 Years, 11 Months of Age)

	Factor		
	Visual	Verbal	Learning
Picture Memory	.569	−.148	.320
Design Memory	.669	.078	.259
Finger Windows	.655	.382	−.160
Story Memory	.285	.222	.585
Sentence Memory	.159	.800	.320
Number/Letter	.082	.859	.113
Verbal Learning	.311	.111	.615
Visual Learning	.605	.158	.157
Sound Symbol	−.004	.125	.749

Note. Shading connotes that the subtest loaded on the predicted factor.

as only two of nine subtests (Story Memory and Visual Learning) loaded inconsistently. It should be kept in mind that the Learning factor clearly consists of visual and verbal memory components, contributing non-orthogonality to the analyses.

Another manner in which to approach these inconsistencies is to retain the Visual factor, rename the Learning factor "Verbal," and substitute "Attention" for the original Verbal factor designation. The re-

sults of this relatively minor alteration are illustrated in Tables 12.6 and 12.7. This conceptual organization continues to group the highly intercorrelated subtests of Sentence Memory and Number/Letter together, but as measures of attention/concentration rather than of verbal memory. Clinically, this is relevant to the research reported below, which suggests that children with attention problems consistently perform poorly on these two subtests as well as Finger

TABLE 12.5. Results of Principal-Components Analysis with Varimax Rotation of WRAML Subtests (Completed on Children 9 Years, 0 Months through 17 Years, 11 Months of Age)

	Factor		
	Visual	Verbal	Learning
Picture Memory	.674	.012	.221
Design Memory	.720	.023	.277
Finger Windows	.584	.585	−.145
Story Memory	.216	.196	.695
Sentence Memory	.017	.749	.441
Number/Letter	.005	.837	.215
Verbal Learning	.239	.091	.648
Visual Learning	.583	.076	.401
Sound Symbol	.214	.240	.638

Note. Shading connotes that the subtest loaded on the predicted factor.

TABLE 12.6. Alternative Interpretation of the Principal-Components Analysis of
WRAML Subtests (Completed on Children 5 Years, 0 Months through 8 Years, 11
Months of Age)

	Factor		
	Visual	Attention	Learning
Picture Memory	.569	−.148	.320
Design Memory	.669	.078	.259
Finger Windows	.655	.382	−.160
Story Memory	.285	.222	.585
Sentence Memory	.159	.800	.320
Number/Letter	.082	.859	.113
Verbal Learning	.311	.111	.615
Visual Learning	.605	.158	.157
Sound Symbol	−.004	.125	.749

Note. Shading connotes that the subtest loaded on the predicted factor.

Windows. With regard to older children, Finger Windows loads on the renamed Attention factor and the Visual factor almost equally, suggesting that both visual memory skills and attention are required to succeed on this subtest. This reorganization would then leave Verbal and Visual factors, but add the factor of Attention. Such a reconceptualization avoids the apparent shared variance of the Learning subtests, and provides a conceptual organization for all WRAML subtests within the new empirically derived factors.

WRAML Performance in Children with Reading Disability and ADHD

Adams and colleagues (2002) administered the WRAML to children with common referral diagnoses, including reading disability (RD) and ADHD, combined type. A total of four groups were examined: one with RD, one with ADHD, one with both RD and ADHD, and a nonclinical comparison group. Children with RD were those with Wechsler Intelligence Scale for Children—Third Edition (WISC-III) Full Scale IQs ≥

TABLE 12.7. Alternative Interpretation of the Principal-Components Analysis of
WRAML Subtests (Completed on Children 9 Years, 0 Months through 17 Years, 11
Months of Age)

	Factor		
	Visual	Attention	Verbal
Picture Memory	.674	.012	.221
Design Memory	.720	.023	.277
Finger Windows	.584	.585	−.145
Story Memory	.216	.196	.695
Sentence Memory	.017	.749	.441
Number/Letter	.005	.837	.215
Verbal Learning	.239	.091	.648
Visual Learning	.583	.076	.401
Sound Symbol	.214	.240	.638

Note. Shading connotes that the subtest loaded on the predicted factor.

85, but arithmetic achievement scores that were not statistically different from their Full Scale IQs, and reading achievement scores at least 15 points below their Verbal IQs. The second group consisted of children diagnosed with ADHD. Each child was diagnosed through a hospital-based ADHD clinic, and most scored at least 2 standard deviations above average (indicating impairment) on a standard attention rating scale both at home and at school. To be included, children in the ADHD group also had to have Full Scale IQs $\geq$ 85 and reading, spelling, and math achievement scores that were not statistically different from their Full Scale IQs. The third group met criteria for both clinical conditions. The mean age of children in each group was approximately 10 years; no subjects had a history of neurological disorder (e.g., seizures, head injury, etc.) or significant comorbid psychiatric diagnoses. Finally, the nonclinical comparison group was culled from the standardization sample, which allowed matching by age, gender, geographic region, urban/rural, and socioeconomic status.

Each child was administered the WRAML. A discriminant function analysis was completed on the WRAML's nine subtest scores. The results showed that WRAML scores discriminated between groups: Wilks's lambda = .560, χ^2 = 115.2, df (27), p < .001. The two significant functions, in succession, accounted for 73.5%

and 26.5% of the between-group variability.

The group centroids shown in Table 12.8 reveal that the first function (discussed below) best distinguished the clinical groups (i.e., those with ADHD, RD, and RD/ADHD) from the nonreferred cohort. The second function (discussed below) best differentiated children with RD from those with ADHD and those who were nonreferred. The pattern of correlations (in Table 12.8) indicates that the first function was defined by appreciable contributions from the Number/Letter, Sound Symbol, Sentence Memory, and Finger Windows subtests. Data from the group centroid comparisons, as well as from the discriminant-function variable correlations, suggest that the construct of rote, short-term memory best distinguishes children with ADHD and RD from those without documented symptomatology. Support for this assertion comes from a recent study (Howes et al., 1999, 2003), which also showed that subjects with RD performed the most poorly on TOMAL subtests requiring rote oral recall (reciting digits or letters forward, as well as backward).

The Verbal Learning subtest represents the second function, which distinguished the group with RD from the other three groups. A univariate analysis of this subtest showed that the RD scaled-score group mean (M = 8.8) was statistically lower than that of the other groups, with the

TABLE 12.8. Canonical Discriminant Functions Using WRAML Subtest Performance

Subtest	Canonical loadings	
	Function I	Function II
Number/Letter	.75	−.08
Sound Symbol	.60	.31
Sentence Memory	.51	.33
Finger Windows	.50	−.09
Verbal Learning	.22	.64

Group	Canonical discriminant functions (group centroids)	
	Function I	Function II
ADHD	−.5935	.3655
RD	−.6407	−.4762
Nonreferred	.6785	.0087
RD/ADHD	−.8462	.4191

Note. Data from Adams et al. (2002) and Sheslow & Adams (1990).

RD/ADHD group mean (9.3) only trending toward significance ($p < .10$), compared to the ADHD ($M = 10.5$) and nonreferred ($M = 10.4$) group means.

We can conclude from these results that children with average intelligence who perform poorly on Number/Letter, Sound Symbol, Sentence Memory, and Finger Windows (but perform reasonably well on the remaining WRAML subtests) are likely to have *some* kind of psychopathology. Low Verbal Learning scores in such children increases the probability that the diagnosis is RD. It should be noted that children with dual diagnoses (RD and ADHD) could not be adequately distinguished from those children with a single diagnosis.

From a methodological standpoint, the diagnostic diversity in this study was critical. For example, if just children with ADHD (or only children with RD) had been compared to the nonreferred sample, it might have been falsely concluded that lower scores on Number/Letter, Sound Symbol, Sentence Memory, and Finger Windows represent a "cluster" useful in diagnosing ADHD (or RD). It is of interest that initial findings from a study of depressed children are also demonstrating lower scores on the "pathology" cluster composed of the four WRAML subtests (Whitney, 1996). Including diverse diagnostic groups may therefore be especially important in cognitive investigations, to reduce the potential that erroneous conclusions will be drawn about findings appearing to be "specific" to a given clinical population.

Clinical Applications of the WRAML: TBI and Other Central Nervous System Disorders

A recent investigation (Duis, 1998) demonstrated that children who had experienced moderate or severe TBI showed deficits on all WRAML subtests following a period of rehabilitation and recovery. Table 12.9 shows WRAML subtest means and standard deviations for groups with ADHD, RD, and TBI. The WRAML subtest scores of the children with TBI were approximately 1 standard deviation below average, and the scores of the children with RD and ADHD were approximately 0.5 standard deviations below average. Farmer and colleagues (1999) reported similar degrees of memory impairment in children who had experienced severe TBI. Research utilizing the WRAML Screening Form has shown significant correlations with length of coma, which rival similar correlations reported with the WISC Performance IQ (Woodward & Donders, 1998). Moreover, children who had incurred severe TBI exhibited significantly lower Screening Form Indexes than did children with mild or moderate injuries, suggesting that the WRAML Screening Form may be useful in delineating memory impairments associated with varying degrees of TBI severity.

In contrast to the WRAML subtest pattern demonstrated by children with ADHD, RD, or TBI, children with seizure disorders performed at a slightly higher level as a group than the children with TBI did. How-

TABLE 12.9. WRAML Subtest Means and Standard Deviations (in Parentheses) for Children with ADHD, RD, and TBI

Subtests	Groups			
	ADHD	RD	TBI	Nonreferred
Number/Letter	7.3 (2.5)	7.8 (2.5)	7.1 (2.8)	10.1 (2.4)
Sound Symbol	8.5 (3.1)	7.6 (2.1)	7.6 (3.0)	10.3 (2.9)
Sentence Memory	9.1 (2.8)	8.1 (2.9)	7.1 (3.4)	10.6 (3.2)
Finger Windows	8.3 (2.5)	8.7 (3.0)	7.5 (3.2)	10.1 (2.6)
Verbal Learning	10.5 (2.9)	8.8 (2.9)	8.2 (3.1)	10.5 (2.9)
Story Memory	10.1 (2.7)	9.7 (2.8)	7.2 (3.7)	10.1 (2.6)
Design Memory	7.9 (3.1)	9.5 (2.8)	7.2 (3.5)	9.8 (2.9)
Picture Memory	10.1 (2.6)	9.8 (2.3)	8.7 (3.4)	10.1 (3.0)
Visual Learning	9.4 (3.1)	9.7 (3.0)	8.5 (3.1)	10.1 (3.2)

Note. Adapted from Duis (1998).

ever, these patients also showed greater subtest variability than the children with ADHD, RD, or TBI (Williams & Haut, 1995). Child survivors of lymphoblastic leukemia who were treated with intrathecal chemotherapy exhibited mild but consistent residual deficits on most WRAML Visual Memory and Verbal Memory subtests, as well on as the Visual Learning subtest. These results correspond to lower IQ scores in the same sample of children, compared to healthy, matched controls (Hill, Ciesielski, Sethre-Hofstad, Duncan, & Lorenzi, 1997).

Case Study

Name: George Smith
Age: 9 years, 4 months
Sex: M
Education: 3rd grade
Medications: None

Background and Presenting Problem

George Smith was referred by his mother and teacher for evaluation of an attention disorder. George is reported to have begun struggling academically around the middle of first grade and has become worse each grade thereafter. George's behavior is described as "restless, especially in the morning," but no overt behavior difficulties characterize his classroom behavior. There is no history of learning difficulties in the immediate family, including attention disorders, although little is known of his biological father. There is an older maternal cousin who experienced some reading difficulties early on, but those seem to have been corrected by the time she entered junior high school and she is now doing relatively well academically. George's history is also noncontributory with respect to developmental delay, neurological disease, and medical history. George's mother finished high school and is currently employed full time as a secretary/receptionist at a local manufacturing company. George's brother, age 6, is in first grade and is reportedly doing well academically and is behaviorally. No prior psychological testing was available for this young man.

Behavioral Observations

George was a pleasant and cooperative young man throughout the evaluation; rapport was easily established from the outset. He did become visibly restless while completing a page of arithmetic computation items, but otherwise his ability to sustain his attention throughout our 3 hours of assessment was admirable.

Summary of Test Results

Test Interpretation

George's overall performance on a traditional test of intellectual ability (WISC-III) places him well within the average range when compared to agemates (see Table 12.10). His verbal and spatial reasoning abilities are consistent with the overall IQ estimate. However, the Freedom from Distractibility Index is significantly lower than would be predicted by chance. Further examination of this finding revealed that the two contributing subtests (Arithmetic and Digit Span) were performed poorly compared to other WISC-III subtests. Although attention is required on each of these WISC-III subtests, tasks requiring sustained attention on the WRAML were performed well, with the exception of a task in which numbers are utilized for short-term memory evaluation. Therefore, it seems that rather than an attention or short-term memory problem, George's difficulty is linked to struggles processing information containing numbers. Further support for this contention is provided by George's performance on the WRAT-3 subtest requiring arithmetic calculation; on this subtest George performed at a mid-first grade level. In contrast, the mechanics of reading and spelling are progressing at a rate predicted by his overall IQ estimate. His ability on short-term memory tasks, devoid of numerical content, was also found to be within age-appropriate levels.

Weak performance on the WISC-III Coding subtest could also be explained by its numerical content, especially when assessment of visual motor abilities, also task requirements of the Coding subtest, were found to be at or above George's agemate's skill levels.

TABLE 12.10. WRAML Case Study Data

	Standard/ scaled scores	Percentile	.95 confidence interval
Wechsler Intelligence Scale for Children—Third Edition			
Verbal IQ	105	63rd	99–111
Performance IQ	104	61st	106–122
VCI =	111	77th	104–112
POI =	109	73rd	100–116
FDI =	81	10th	74–93
Information	11		
Similarities	13		
Arithmetic	06		
Vocabulary	12		
Comprehension	12		
Digit Span	07		
Picture Completion	10		
Coding	08		
Picture Arrangement	12		
Block Design	11		
Object Assembly	12		
Wide Range Achievement Test			
Reading	110		
Spelling	102		
Arithmetic	81		
Wide Range Assessment of Visual–Motor Integration			
Fine-Motor Skills	116		
Visual–Spatial Skills	n/a		
Visual–Motor Integration	107		
Wide Range Assessment of Memory and Learning			
Verbal Memory	106		
Number/Letter	8		
Sentence Memory	12		
Story Memory	13		
Visual Memory	107		
Finger Windows	11		
Design Memory	12		
Picture Memory	10		
Learning			
Verbal Learning	12		
Visual Learning	12		
Sound Symbol	n/a		
Delay Recall			
Verbal Learning	average		
Story Memory	average		

Note. n/a = not administered

It is interesting to note that the first subject of George's day is math. It may be that he is made anxious during this class because of his math disability, and is responsible for what is perceived as restless and inattentive behavior for this and ensuing classes. This notion is supported by the report of his afternoon reading teacher who does not note any attention or behavior difficulties.

Clinical Impressions/Diagnosis

The results of the assessment do not support a diagnosis of ADHD, but rather indicate a learning disability in mathematics of moderate severity. This young man has a number of cognitive strengths that may prove helpful in developing effective compensatory skills for his struggles with math.

Recommendations

1. Those responsible for programming for George's math skills should meet and perform a careful analysis of his abilities. This may require further testing by an educational diagnostician. Today's results suggest that George's addition and subtraction skills beyond single integers are not consistently correct. Therefore, it does not seem reasonable for him to continue in his current math class, which is starting to learn multiplication. Use of computer software written to provide game-like math drills probably deserves a trial to see how effectively they can supplement special educational instruction during his math class.
2. Because he is able in many other academic and athletic areas, it will be important for his mother and teachers to affirm George's strengths. With respect to his understanding of his struggles in math, it may prove helpful for the school counselor to meet with George and his mother to explain that a math disability is a challenge faced by many other children and that it is no indication of his overall intelligence and abilities. Supplementing that discussion with some appropriate take-home material may also be helpful, and might include the book *Mucking-Up My Math,* a supportive and explanatory book especially written for a parent to read with their child experiencing a math disability.

WRAML Commentary

In this case, the WRAML was used for an assessment of memory, following the administration of a measure of intelligence. The WISC-III subtest results could legitimately be interpreted as suggestive of a short-term memory problem. The WRAML results do not support such a hypothesis because of strong verbal and spatial memory skills in a variety of contexts. However, low scores on the one WRAML subtest having numerical content, along with the low WRAT Arithmetic result, is strong evidence for a math disability and not a disability based on attention or short-term memory deficits.

TEST OF MEMORY AND LEARNING

Structure

The TOMAL (Reynolds & Bigler, 1994a, 1994b) is a comprehensive battery of 14 tasks assessing learning and memory for children and adolescents ranging in age from 5 years, 0 months to 19 years, 11 months (see Table 12.11). Ten primary subtests are divided into the Verbal Memory and Nonverbal Memory domains, which can be combined to form a Composite Memory Index. The Delayed Recall Index is composed of repeat recall trials of the first four subtests.

As previously noted, the pattern of overall memory functioning for a particular individual may be singular and variable and in such cases content approaches to memory may be limited. Therefore, the TOMAL provides alternative groupings of the subtests into five Supplementary Indexes: Sequential Recall, Free Recall, Associative Recall, Learning, and Attention and Concentration. The Supplementary Indexes were organized by "expert" neuropsychologists who were asked to arrange the 14 TOMAL subtests into categories with face validity (Reynolds & Bigler, 1994a). In addition, four empirically derived Factor Indexes representing Complex Memory, Sequential Recall, Backward Recall, and Spatial Memory were provided to provide greater flexibility to the clinician (Reynolds & Bigler, 1996).

Table 12.11 lists each of the subtests/Indexes and their respective standardized

TABLE 12.11. Core and Supplementary Subtests and Indexes Available for the TOMAL

	M	SD
Core subtests		
Verbal Memory		
Memory for Stories	10	3
Word Selective Reminding	10	3
Object Recall	10	3
Digits Forward	10	3
Paired Recall	10	3
Nonverbal Memory		
Facial Memory	10	3
Visual Selective Reminding	10	3
Abstract Visual Memory	10	3
Visual Sequential Memory	10	3
Memory for Location	10	3
Supplementary subtests		
Verbal		
Letters Forward	10	3
Digits Backward	10	3
Letters Backward	10	3
Nonverbal		
Manual Imitation	10	3
Summary scores		
Core Indexes		
Verbal Memory Index	100	15
Nonverbal Memory Index	100	15
Composite Memory Index	100	15
Delayed Recall Index	100	15
Supplementary Indexes (expert-derived)		
Sequential Recall Index	100	15
Free Recall Index	100	15
Associative Recall Index	100	15
Learning Index	100	15
Attention and Concentration Index	100	15
Factor Indexes (empirically derived)		
Complex Memory Index	100	15
Sequential Recall Index	100	15
Backward Recall Index	100	15
Spatial Memory Index	100	15

means and standard deviations. Each TOMAL subtest is scaled according to the often-used mean value of 10 and standard deviation of 3. Each Index is similarly scaled to the common mean of 100 and standard deviation of 15. Scaling was accomplished through the rolling weighted averages method described in detail by Reynolds and Bigler (1994a).

Subtests of the TOMAL

The 10 core subtests, the 4 supplementary subtests, and the delayed-recall trials of the TOMAL take approximately 60 minutes for the experienced examiner to administer. The subtests are named and briefly described in Table 12.12.

The administration of the TOMAL sub-

TABLE 12.12. Description of TOMAL Subtests

Subtest	Description
Core subtests	
Memory for Stories	A verbal subtest requiring recall of a short story read to the examinee. Provides a measure of meaningful and semantic recall, and is also related to sequential recall in some instances.
Facial Memory	A nonverbal subtest requiring recognition and identification from a set of distractors: black-and-white photos of various ages, males and females, and various ethnic backgrounds. Assesses nonverbal meaningful memory in a practical fashion and has been extensively researched. Sequencing of responses is unimportant.
Word Selective Reminding	A verbal free-recall task in which the examinee learns a word list and repeats it only to be reminded of words left out in each case; tests learning and immediate-recall functions in verbal memory. Trials continue until mastery is achieved or until eight trials have been attempted; sequence of recall is unimportant.
Visual Selective Reminding	A nonverbal analogue to Word Selective Reminding, where examinees point to specified dots on a card, following a demonstration of the examiner, and are reminded only of items recalled incorrectly. As with Word Selective Reminding, trials continue until mastery is achieved or until eight trials have been attempted.
Object Recall	The examiner presents a series of pictures, names them, has the examinee recall them, and repeats this process across four trials. Verbal and nonverbal stimuli are thus paired, and recall is entirely verbal; this creates a situation found to interfere with recall for many children with learning disabilities, but to be neutral or facilitative for children without disabilities.
Abstract Visual Memory	A nonverbal task that assesses immediate recall for meaningless figures when order is unimportant. The examinee is presented with a standard stimulus and is required to distinguish the standard from any of six distractors.
Digits Forward	A standard verbal number recall task; it measures low-level rote recall of a sequence of numbers
Visual Sequential Memory	A nonverbal task requiring recall of the sequence of a series of meaningless geometric designs. The designs are shown in a standard order, followed by a presentation in a different order, and the examinee indicates the order in which they originally appeared.
Paired Recall	A verbal paired-associate learning task. Easy and hard pairs, and measures of immediate associative recall and learning, are provided.
Memory for Location	A nonverbal task that assesses spatial memory. The examinee is presented with a set of large dots distributed on a page, and is asked to recall the locations of the dots in order.
Supplementary subtests	
Manual Imitation	A psychomotor, visually based assessment of sequential memory, in which the examinee is required to reproduce a set of ordered hand movements in the same sequence as presented by the examiner.
Letters Forward	A language-related analogue to the Digits Forward task, using letters as the stimuli in place of numbers.
Digits Backward	This is the same basic task as Digits Forward, except the examinee recalls the numbers in reverse order.
Letters Backward	A language-related analogue to the Digits Backward task, using letters as the stimuli instead of numbers.

tests is varied, so that verbal, visual, and motor modalities, plus combinations of these, are sampled from alternating presentation and response formats. Learning and acquisition curves are made possible by multiple "trials to a criterion," which are included on several tasks. For example, multiple trials are included on the Word and Visual Selective Reminding subtests to allow for a "depth-of-processing" analysis (Kaplan, 1996). In the selective reminding format (in which examinees are reminded of omitted words), if items that were correctly recalled are not recalled on subsequent trials, it may be inferred that there is a deficit in transfer of information from immediate/working memory to long-term storage. At the end of selected subtests, cuing is allowed so that depth of processing can be further explored. For instance, differences between cued recall and free recall may be associated with certain neurological disorders, and therefore may serve as a diagnostic aid.

Traditional memory tasks (e.g., Memory for Stories) that are associated with academic learning are also included. In addition, memory tasks more common to experimental neuropsychology that have high (e.g., Facial Memory) and low (e.g., Visual Selective Reminding) ecological validity are included in the TOMAL. Similarly, subtests vary in meaningfulness. For example, Memory for Stories is high in meaning compared to Abstract Visual Memory, which requires abstract visual processing (i.e., analysis of complex geometric forms).

The TOMAL's comprehensive review of multiple memory functions allows for a relatively fine-grained and inclusive assessment of potential memory deficits. It cannot be emphasized enough that "memory" is a complex construct, and that the most effective batteries will be those assessing a wide range of well-defined functions that are clinically relevant and ecologically valid. The TOMAL succeeds on these grounds because of its breadth, which provides an opportunity for detailed analysis of diverse memory processes within the information-processing paradigm.

Standardization

The TOMAL was standardized on a population-proportionate sample of children throughout the United States, stratified by age, gender, ethnicity, socioeconomic status, region of residence, and community size. Standardization and norming were conducted for children and adolescents ages 5 to 20. Details of the standardization and specific statistics on the sample are provided by Reynolds and Bigler (1994a).

Reliability

The TOMAL subtests and summary Indexes exhibit excellent internal-consistency reliability. Reynolds and Bigler (1994a) report coefficient alpha reliability estimates that often exceed .90 for individual subtests and .95 for composite scores. Stability coefficients are typically in the .80 range.

Validity

The TOMAL scores show correlations of approximately .50 with standard measures of intelligence and achievement—indicating that the TOMAL shares variance with intelligence and achievement measures, but also that it taps unique constructs (Reynolds & Bigler, 1994a). The specificity of the TOMAL in relation to intellectual measures is bolstered by the observation that measures of intelligence characteristically exhibit intersubtest correlations of approximately .75 to .85. This is true to a lesser extent with the achievement measures, which typically show subtest correlations of approximately .55 to .65. Similarly, the Word Selective Reminding subtest correlates positively with a previously accepted standard test of verbal memory, the Rey Auditory Verbal Learning Test. Likewise, for adolescents (16–20 years), the Memory for Stories subtest correlates highly with a similar subtest from the well-established Wechsler Memory Scale—Revised (see Reynolds & Bigler, 1997).

The nonverbal sections of the TOMAL are relatively orthogonal to existing nonverbal memory tests (see Reynolds & Bigler, 1997). In contrast to other tests of visual and nonverbal memory (which do not attempt to prevent verbally mediated strategies for encoding and recall of to-be-remembered stimuli), the TOMAL, by virtue of its design, reduces the opportunities for such attempts and thus may be a "purer" measure of visual/nonverbal memory. Thus examiners using visual and verbal tasks on traditional memory batteries should expect larger scatter across tests than on verbal memory measures.

Factor Structure

Detailed analyses of the factor structure and Indexes of the TOMAL, based on a normative sample of 1,342 children, have been extensively reviewed by Reynolds and Bigler (1996, 1997). Briefly, in a principal-factors analysis with varimax and promax rotations, the correlation matrix for all 14 TOMAL subtests was examined. Factors were extracted and found to be consistent across children/adolescents ages 5–8, 9–12, and 13–18. It is noteworthy that the analyses discussed below are based on normal, nonreferred children, and that the factor analyses will not demonstrate the same consistency in clinic-referred subjects, particularly children with central nervous system dysfunction (see review material by Kamphaus & Reynolds, 1987).

The two-factor solutions for the TOMAL did not support the verbal–nonverbal dichotomy. The factor structure of the TOMAL is clearly more multifaceted than is represented by the verbal–nonverbal groupings. Nevertheless, Reynolds and Bigler (1994b) preserved the verbal–nonverbal construct because of its clinical utility. A general factor was evident, similar in concept to the intelligence factor g, but weaker in magnitude. This factor nonetheless supports the use of a composite score such as the Composite Memory Index with nonclinical populations. Exploratory factor analyses were also conducted; a four-factor solution appeared to best characterize the clinical organization of the TOMAL, as outlined below (Reynolds & Bigler, 1997):

1. Complex Memory = Memory for Stories + Word Selective Reminding + Object Recall + Paired Recall + Visual Selective Reminding + Facial Memory
2. Sequential Recall = Digits Forward + Letters Forward + Visual Sequential Memory + Manual Imitation
3. Backward Recall = Digits Backward + Letters Backward
4. Spatial Memory = Abstract Visual Memory + Memory for Location

The first and most robust factor derived from the promax solution appeared to be a general factor, reflective of overall memory skills subsuming multiple modalities and memory processes. The second factor seemed to represent sequential recall and attention processes. The third factor was composed of Digits Backward and Letters Backward, suggesting that backward and forward memory span tasks should be separately scaled. Backward digit recall is known to be a more highly g-loaded task than forward digit recall and places more information-processing demands on the examinee (e.g., see Jensen & Figueroa, 1975). The fourth factor consisted of Abstract Visual Memory and Memory for Location, which appeared to represent a nonverbal factor. This factor appeared to capture spatial memory more strongly than other tasks. The four-factor varimax solution resulted in similar findings.

At 1-year age intervals, internal-consistency reliability data for the four TOMAL Factor Indexes were above .90, with the exception of the Spatial Memory Index at 5 years of age (reliability coefficient = .85). It is noteworthy that the values of the other three factors fell between .94 and .99, with median values of .95 for the Complex Memory Index and .94 for the Spatial Memory Index. The reliability coefficients of the empirically derived Factor Indexes are therefore comparable to those of the Core Indexes and Supplementary Indexes described in the TOMAL manual (Reynolds & Bigler, 1994a).

The strong psychometrics of the four Factor Indexes support constructs representing useful tools that the clinician can use to better understand individual cases. The TOMAL factor structure suggests that the aspects of memory assessed in this instrument may be more process-driven than content-driven. Although the verbal–nonverbal memory distinction is clinically useful, particularly for patients with TBI or with hemispherically distinct lesions, process appears to be more relevant than content or presentation modality in healthy individuals.

Subtest Specificities

Variance specific to each subtest can be derived from factor analysis, which represents the proportion of variance for a particular subtest that is specific to the subtest and that is not shared with other factors. That is, a particular subtest may inform the clinician about aspects of an examinee's performance that are independent of those revealed by other subtests (i.e., construct validity). A specificity value of .25 has been considered appropriate to support interpretation of an individual subtest score (e.g., see Kaufman, 1979). The values reported by Reynolds and Bigler (1994a, 1994b, 1996) represent rather respectable specificity compared to measures of intelligence and achievement, which often show more highly interrelated subtests. Indeed, each of the TOMAL subtests shows specificity values ≥ .40, and each specificity value exceeds the error variance of the subtest. Such sound psychometrics allow the clinician to be confident with respect to interpretation of component subtests. Direction in generating such hypotheses from clinical observation is included in the TOMAL manual (Reynolds & Bigler, 1994a), as well as through automated software designed for the TOMAL (Stanton, Reynolds, & Bigler, 1995).

Cross-Ethnic Stability of Factor Indexes

Normative data for the TOMAL were standardized on an ethnically diverse population. This is a particular strength of the TOMAL, as little research has been conducted with regard to neuropsychological measures and the cultural test bias hypothesis, particularly by comparison with the large body of such research on intelligence tests (e.g., see Reynolds, 1995). Preliminary analyses suggest consistency of the factor structures of the TOMAL across race for African American and European American subjects (see Mayfield & Reynolds, 1997; Reynolds & Bigler, 1994a, 1996). These findings, although preliminary, suggest that African Americans and European Americans perceive the stimuli of the TOMAL in a highly comparable manner. Although changes in interpretation as a function of race do not appear to be warranted based on current results, further research is needed to validate this finding, as well as to explore comparisons between other ethnicities.

Forward versus Backward Recall of Digits

As mentioned earlier in this chapter, assessment of recall of digits in the forward and reverse directions has been a staple in cognitive assessment. It has also been the tradition on many tests to sum the number of digits recalled in the forward direction with those recalled in the reverse direction, to form a total score of "digit span." As previous research has suggested that digits-forward and digits-backward tasks demand different although overlapping abilities (Ramsey & Reynolds, 1995; Reynolds, 1997), the TOMAL normed each of these subtests separately. It appears that forward digit span has strong attentional and sequential components, and that backward digit span appears to have spatial and/or integrative elements that are not prominent in forward digit span. Current evidence and clinical observation suggest that a digits-forward task carries fewer cognitive demands and may be more verbally oriented, requiring sequential memory abilities. In contrast, a digits-backward task appears to tap more complex processes, requiring cognitive manipulations that are not necessary with a digits-forward task. For instance, backward recall may also require visual–spatial imaging processes (for some individuals); this may even be true when ostensibly verbal materials (e.g., letters), rather than digits, are being recalled. Because of these distinctions between forward and backward recall and the clinical implications for differences in performance, the tasks are presented and interpreted separately on the TOMAL.

Delayed Recall

Delayed recall has been another mainstay in the area of memory assessment. On the TOMAL, the examinee is asked to recall stimuli from the first four subtests administered (two verbal, two nonverbal), 30 minutes after testing has begun. The Delayed Recall Index serves in essence as a measure of forgetting. Most examinees will score within about 10 points of their Composite Memory Index on the Delayed Recall Index. The TOMAL manual contains values for evaluating differences between these two Indexes. The TOMAL's computerized scoring program will also provide an analysis of Index comparisons.

A Delayed Recall Index significantly lower than the Composite Memory Index is often an indication of a memory disturbance with an organic basis, although several neuropsychiatric disorders with varied etiology can produce memory deficits (e.g., Grossman, Kaufman, Mednitsky, Scharff, & Dennis, 1994). The Delayed Recall Index provides the clinician with a useful tool to explore hypotheses about processing depth, forgetting, and motivation.

Interpretation

Kaufman's (1979, 1994) "top-down" interpretive strategy, which requires a systematic integration of history and other test data, is reviewed in the TOMAL manual. Reynolds and Bigler (1994a) provide further considerations for interpretation, including data on within-test variability and on the relationship between the TOMAL and intellectual and achievement measures.

An example of the clinical usefulness of the TOMAL was provided by Lajiness-O'Neill (1996), who examined the performance of children with varying severities of

TBI (see Table 12.13). In this study, memory disturbance increased as a function of TBI severity.

Case Study

Name: Mary
Age: 10
Sex: F
Education: 5th grade
Medications: None
Date of injury: 11/16/93
Date of evaluation: 10/10/02

Background and Presenting Problem

At the age of 15 months, Mary sustained a skull fracture associated with a fall on a cement floor. Imaging studies at the time of injury demonstrated a nondisplaced linear left occipital skull fracture. Acutely, Mary exhibited signs of concussion including nausea and vomiting. Although her course of recovery was generally uncomplicated, her parents have had ongoing concerns regarding residual difficulties with reading, retention, and comprehension. Mary's mother also reported that Mary has problems with attention/concentration, nervousness, and that

TABLE 12.13. Means and Standard Deviations by Group for TOMAL Indices, WRAT-3 and PPVT Scaled Scores, and FSIQ Score

	Control	Mild	Moderate	Severe
TOMAL				
VMI	102 (8)*	95 (12)*	96 (12)*	86 (16)*[a,b,c]
NMI	104 (11)*	97 (11)	92 (19)*[a]	89 (14)*[a]
CMI	103 (8)*	96 (10)*	94 (15)*[a]	87 (14)*[a,b]
DRI	104 (7) *	99 (7)*	96 (9)*[a]	92 (13)*[a,b]
WRAT-3				
ASS	103 (12)*	94 (13)	94 (17)	93 (21)*[a]
RSS	104 (11)*	98 (11)	87 (14)*[a]	92 (18)*[a]
SSS	103 (12)*	96 (22)	88 (16)*[a]	91 (15)*[a]
PPVT-R	106 (12)*	99 (14)	98 (21)	94 (18)*[a]
FSIQ	105 (12)*	99 (13)	95 (15)	94 (18)*[a]

Note. TOMAL, Test of Memory and Learning; VMI, Verbal Memory Index; NMI, Nonverbal Memory Index; CMI, Composite Memory Index; DRI, Delayed Recall Index; WRAT-3, Wide Range Achievement Test-3; ASS, Arithmetic Scale Score; RSS, Reading Scaled Score; SSS, Spelling Scaled Score; PPVT-R, Peabody Picture Vocabulary Test—Revised; FSIQ, Wechsler Full Scale IQ.
*$p < .05$ as examined by post-hoc Tukey's HSD procedure.
[a]Reliably different from control group.
[b]Reliably different from mild brain injury group.
[c]Reliably different from moderate brain injury group.

she has a "roller coaster personality." Mary is reportedly in good health but it is noteworthy that she had experienced a hypoxic episode perinatally for approximately 4 hours.

Behavioral Observations

Mary was oriented to person, place, and time. Her affect was appropriate for the context. During testing she showed average motivation and was very cooperative but showed some attentional problems. The examiner noted that she required considerable prodding to stay on task. Overall, the results of the test are believed to be valid.

Summary of Test Results

Mary's performance on the Wechsler Abbreviated Scale of Intelligence (WASI) showed significant VIQ–PIQ difference (VIQ = 91, PIQ = 110), suggesting below average–aver-

TABLE 12.14. TOMAL Case Study Data

Wechsler Abbreviated Scale of Intelligence	
Verbal IQ	91
Performance IQ	110
Vocabulary	44
Similarities	45
Block Design	57
Matrix Reasoning	57

Wide Range Achievement Test-3	
	SS
Reading	86
Spelling	82
Arithmetic	85

Peabody Picture Vocabulary Test—Revised	
Standard Score	96

Test of Memory and Learning	
Verbal Memory Index	82
Nonverbal Memory Index	105
Composite Memory Index	94
Delayed Recall Index	95
Attention and Concentration Index	89
Sequential Recall Index	95
Free Recall Index	97
Associative Recall Index	91
Learning Index	85

age verbal intelligence and average–above average performance intelligence. Her performance on the Peabody Picture Vocabulary Test—Revised (standard score = 96) was also nearly one standard deviation below her PIQ index score on the WASI.

The impact of Mary's learning difficulties was evident in a screen of academic achievement. In particular, her standard scores on Reading, Spelling, and Mathematics on the WRAT-3 were 86, 82, and 85, respectively. These results suggest that on average her academic achievement is approximately 1 standard deviation below her intellectual abilities (FIQ = 101).

Memory

Mary's scaled score on the Verbal Memory Index was nearly 1.5 standard deviations below her scaled score on the Non-Verbal Memory Index (p = .01). This difference generally mirrored the VIQ–PIQ pattern shown on the WASI. Within the subtests composing the Verbal Memory Index, Mary's performance ranged from low average (Word-Selective Reminding, Object Selective Reminding, Paired Recall, Letters Forward, and Digits Backward) to average (Memory for Stories, Letters Backward, and Digits Forward). Intrascale comparisons of the subtests composing the Verbal Memory Index showed that compared to the average of Mary's scores on all of the Verbal Memory subtests, she showed a relative strength for Memory for Stories (p = .05). This strength suggests that she may remember verbal information presented in a sequential narrative form better than other verbal tasks that are less contextual. Mary's performance on the Non-Verbal Memory Index was more consistent than on the Verbal Memory Index, with all subtests reflecting average performance. A comparative analysis of the Non-Verbal subtests showed that Mary had a weakness for Memory for Location (p = .05) compared to the mean of all of the Non-Verbal Memory tests. This relative weakness suggests that compared to her overall performance on nonverbal memory tasks, she may have difficulties with visual–spatial memory, which requires reliance on right-hemisphere-mediated cognitive maps. It should be noted, however, that this relative weakness is not clinically significant and falls within the average range.

Although there were no significant differences between the Attention/Concentration Index and the Composite Memory Index, the Attention/Concentration Index was somewhat lower than the Composite Memory Index and the test conditions may have differed qualitatively from those of Mary's everyday life. In particular, to the extent that the examiner had to prod Mary to stay on task, the results of the Attention/Concentration Index may lack ecological validity, as it is unlikely that such prompts are present when she is in a large classroom or studying alone. Thus, because of the attention problems observed by the examiner and Mary's mother, attention remains an area that may require further assessment. Mary's score on the Learning Index was 1 standard deviation below the mean of the normative sample of children her age, suggesting that she may not profit from experience at a level commensurate with her peers. The scaled scores of the Delayed Recall Index and Composite Memory indices were highly similar, suggesting that processes underlying consolidation and retrieval from long-term memory stores are intact.

Conclusions and Recommendations

In conceptualizing Mary's learning difficulties, it may be important to consider the many levels at which her learning process may break down. First, Mary's lability and nervousness may interfere with her ability to learn. A consultation with a psychiatrist or psychologist is recommended to evaluate the extent to which these symptoms may be impacting her scholastic performance. Similarly, professional observation of Mary's classroom may help to determine obstacles that hinder Mary's learning and accommodations can be made accordingly. Second, as previously noted, her attentional difficulties observed by others may impact her ability to process information and a formal assessment of attention is indicated.

Third, although it is probable that psychiatric and/or attentional problems may contribute to Mary's overall functioning and that these areas may need to be the focus of clinical attention, clearly Mary demonstrates a verbal intellectual and memory deficit that is consistent with left-hemisphere brain injury. Moreover, this deficit may be discrepant with her overall intellectual abilities and appears to be impacting her academic achievement. The data of the present assessment suggest that Mary may benefit from efforts to build her vocabulary as well as associative learning strategies. Her relative strength for processing sequentially presented verbal information should also be capitalized upon, as the results suggest that she can process and retrieve such information (e.g., verbal instructions), provided that she is attending to the task. Efforts to help Mary to increase the efficiency of her learning process may be directed toward helping her to remind herself of what she has learned from previous experience and to apply this information to increasingly complex problems. This is both an executive task and an exercise in forming associations from previous experience that is relevant to the task at hand. One-on-one tutoring may also help Mary to stay on task as well as build compensatory strategies (e.g., note taking, tape recording lectures, etc).

CALIFORNIA VERBAL LEARNING TEST— CHILDREN'S VERSION

Structure

The CVLT-C (Delis et al., 1994) is a measure of auditory verbal learning and recall that was adapted from its adult counterpart, the California Verbal Learning Test (CVLT; Delis, Kramer, Kaplan, & Kaplan, 1987). It also shares characteristics with the Rey Auditory Verbal Learning Test (Rey, 1964) and the Verbal Learning subtest of the WRAML (Sheslow & Adams, 1990). The CVLT-C was designed for children ranging in age from 5 to 16 years. The primary task is designed with respect to everyday memory tasks; it includes two lists of familiar and categorized words presented as "shopping lists." In particular, the child is read a list of 15 words, and then is asked to recall as many words as possible in a free-recall format. Four additional recall trials are then administered to evaluate learning across trials. Although strategies are not given to the child, the words are such that they can be sorted into three semantic categories (clothes, fruits, and toys), with an equal number of words in each category.

Following this administration of the first list of words, the second "shopping list" is then read aloud to the child. The second list, which is also composed of 15 different words, can be sorted into the semantic groupings of furniture, fruits, and desserts. After a learning/recall trial with the second list, the child is instructed to recall the first shopping list. The child is then given the three categories in which the words of the first list may be grouped. With this strategy offered, recall for each category is repeated.

A 20-minute delay period is then introduced, during which other nonverbal testing may be completed. After 20 minutes, the child is again administered a free-recall trial of the first list, followed by a cued-recall trial. Finally, the child is asked to listen to a list of words that include items from both learning lists as well as distractor words. The child is then asked to identify those words from the first shopping list. The entire procedure requires approximately 30 minutes to complete, not including the 20-minute delay.

Great care was taken in selecting the items for the CVLT-C. For instance, words chosen for the shopping lists were selected based on their frequency in the English language, as well as by how often they were reported by children. To avoid the potential confound in which children would simply respond with the most common words in a given category rather than a word from the list, the three most commonly used words for each category were excluded.

Standardization

The CVLT-C standardization was stratified by age, gender, ethnicity, geographic region, and parental education, based on the 1988 U.S. census. Details of the standardization procedures, including sampling statistics, can be found in the CVLT-C manual (Delis et al., 1994).

Reliability

Reliability estimates for the CVLT-C are reported as measures of internal consistency, as well as test–retest reliability. Across the five trials for the first shopping list, the average internal-consistency correlations ranged from .84 to .91, with a mean of .88. Reliability across categories yielded an average internal-consistency coefficient of .72 for all age groups. Test–retest measures were obtained across average test–retest intervals of 28 days. Recall performance on the second CVLT-C administration increased by 5, 6, and 9 words for the 8-, 12-, and 16-year-old age groups, respectively. Reliability coefficients based on the first and second administration scores ranged from .31 to .90, which the authors considered acceptable, based on the auditory–verbal–memory nature of the CVLT-C.

Clinical Utility of the CVLT-C

The CVLT-C is relatively brief, is simple to administer, and provides useful information for the clinician. For instance, perseverations and intrusions are recorded; these allow for inferences about inhibition, as well as expressive and phonological language impairment. Various process scores can also be calculated to provide an empirical basis for more qualitative analyses of memory. These process scores answer questions such as the following: Does the child tend to learn things in categories or randomly? Does the child benefit from greater intervals between presentations of stimuli? Answers to such questions may carry implications for treatment recommendations. For example, in the case of a child who shows difficulty with learning tasks that are presented too closely together, it may be recommended that academic subjects with similar content should be separated throughout the child's day/week, to avoid interference effects from previously learned material. Software program for the CVLT-C is available that provides computation and multilevel interpretive analyses.

CONCLUSION

In the present chapter we have briefly reviewed the neurobiology of memory, child neurological and neuropsychiatric disorders that impact memory functioning, and the history of assessment of memory in pediatric populations. Within this context, the psychometrics, structure, and clinical utility of three commonly used batteries used to assess memory in children and adolescents were discussed in detail. This review illustrates that although each battery assesses overlapping constructs, clearly the tests discussed also tap unique aspects of memory functioning. For example, the WRAML divides its verbal memory tasks into a hierarchy that varies as a function of increasing language-processing demands, the TOMAL is noted for its breadth of assessment, including several unique indices (e.g., Sequential Recall Index, Associative Recall Index, Complex Memory Index, and Attention Concentration Index), and the CVLT-C provides information about encoding strategies. Because of these distinctive qualities, the neuropsychologist must be well versed in the properties of each battery as well as contextual variables that may guide the choice of a battery or combination of tests. For instance, a particular test may be more sensitive to deficits in a defined population or, based on the judgment of the assessor, more ecologically valid than another given the context of the patient and the demands of his or her environment. Although it is understandable that neuropsychologists often use preferred tests of memory, a flexible approach utilizing the strengths of the available batteries may be the most useful. It is suggested that this chapter is a starting point to understanding the use of popular methods of child memory assessment, but clinicians must also stay abreast with the growing literature, which will provide a more rich empirical grounding for the application of current assessment tools to diverse clinical populations. Future research directions include investigations of tasks that may better discriminate between memory and attentional processes as well as a general focus on developing measures with the most ecological validity.

NOTES

1. This chapter is based on a previous work by Bigler and Adams (2001) and is printed with the permission of Cambridge University Press.
2. The scientific debate over memory terminology (Fuster, 1995) is not discussed in this chapter. We acknowledge differences between "immediate" and "short-term" memory, but for simplicity of presentation, have maintained the older taxonomy rather than the more recent "declarative" (or "explicit"), and "nondeclarative" (or "implicit" or "procedural") memory. Other memory terms, such as "episodic" and "semantic" memory, are also not discussed, as the older classification of memory is in step with how the general clinician approaches the pragmatic conceptualization as well as the assessment of memory. For instance, when a clinician is providing feedback to parents, teachers, and school counselors, terminology that extends beyond "immediate," "short-term," and "long-term" may become confusing.

REFERENCES

Adams, W. V., Hyde, C. L., & deLancey, E. R. (1995). *Use of the Wide Range Assessment of Memory and Learning in diagnosing ADHD in children.* Paper presented at the Child Health Psychology Conference, Gainesville, FL.

Adams, W. V., Robins, P. R., Sheslow, D. V., & Hyde, C. L. (2002). *Performance of children with ADHD and/or reading disabilities on the Wide Range Assessment of Memory and Learning.* Manuscript submitted for publication.

Aylward, G. P., Gioia, G., Verhulst, S. J., & Bell, S. (1995). Factor structure of the Wide Range Assessment of Memory and Learning in a clinical population. *Assessment, 13,* 132–142.

Banich, M. T. (1997). *Neuropsychology: The neural bases of mental function.* Boston: Houghton-Mifflin.

Baron, I. S., Fennell, E. B., & Voeller, K. K. S. (1995). *Pediatric neuropsychology in the medical setting.* London: Oxford University Press.

Bauer, R. M., Tobias, B. A., & Valenstein, E. (1993). Amnestic disorders. In K. M. Heilman & E. Valenstein (Eds.), *Clinical neuropsychology* (pp. 523–602). New York: Oxford University Press.

Bigler, E. D., & Adams, W. V. (2001). Clinical neuropsychological assessment of child and adolescent memory with the WRAML, TOMAL, and CVLT-C. In A. S. Kaufman & N. L. Kaufman (Eds.), *Specific learning disabilities in children and adolescents* (pp. 387–429). Cambridge, UK: Cambridge University Press.

Buchanan, T. W., Denburg, N. L., Tranel, D., & Adolphs, R. (2001). Verbal and nonverbal emotional memory following unilateral amygdala damage. *Learn and Memory, 8*(6), 326–335.

Bull, R., & Johnston, R. S. (1997). Children's arithmetical difficulties: Contributions from processing speed, item identification, and short-term memory. *Journal of Experimental Child Psychology, 65,* 1–24.

Burton, D. B., Donders, J., & Mittenberg, W. (1996). A structural equation analysis of the Wide Range Assessment of Memory and Learning in the standardization sample. *Child Neuropsychology, 2,* 39–47.

Burton, D. B., Mittenberg, W., Gold, S., & Drabman, R. (1999). A structural equation analysis of the Wide Range Assessment of Memory and Learning in a clinical sample. *Child Neuropsychology, 5,* 34–40.

Cohen, R. A. (1993). *The neuropsychology of attention.* New York: Plenum Press.

Cowan, N. (1997). *The development of memory in childhood.* Hove, England: Psychology Press.

Cronwall, D., Wrightson, P., & Waddell, P. (1990). *Head injury: The facts.* London: Oxford University Press.

Cullum, M., Kuck, J., & Ruff, R. M. (1990). Neuropsychological assessment of traumatic brain injury in adults. In E. D. Bigler (Ed.), *Traumatic brain injury* (pp. 129–163). Austin, TX: Pro-Ed.

Cytowic, R. E. (1996). *The neurological side of neuropsychology.* Cambridge, MA: MIT Press.

de Jong, P. F. (1998). Working memory deficits of reading disabled children. *Journal of Experimental Child Psychology, 70,* 75–96.

Delis, D. C., Kramer, J. H., Kaplan, E., & Ober, B. A. (1994). *California Verbal Learning Test—Children's Version.* San Antonio, TX: Psychological Corporation.

Delis, D. C., Kramer, J. H., Kaplan, J. H., & Kaplan, E. (1987). *California Verbal Learning Test.* San Antonio, TX: Psychological Corporation.

Dewey, D., Kaplan, B. J., & Crawford, S. G. (1997). Factor structure of the WRAML in children with ADHD or reading disabilities: Further evidence of an attention/concentration factor. *Developmental Neuropsychology, 13,* 501–506.

Diamond, M. C. (1990). Morphological cortical changes as a consequence of learning and experience. In A. B. Schiebel & A. Wechsler (Eds.), *Neurobiology of higher cognitive function* (pp. 1–12). New York: Guilford Press.

Duis, S. S. (1998). Differential performances on the wide range assessment of memory and learning of children diagnosed with reading disorder, attention-deficit/hyperactivity disorder, and traumatic brain injury. *Dissertation Abstracts International, 58*(7-B), 3919.

Farmer, J. E., Haut, J. S., Williams, J., Kapila, C., Johnstone, B., & Kirk, K. S. (1999). Comprehensive assessment of memory functioning following traumatic brain injury in children. *Developmental Neuropsychology, 15,* 269–289.

Fuster, J. M. (1995). *Memory in the cerebral cortex: An empirical approach to neural networks in the human and nonhuman primates.* Cambridge, MA: MIT Press.

Gillberg, C. (1995). *Clinical child neuropsychiatry.* Cambridge, England: Cambridge University Press.

Gioia, G. A. (1998). Re-examining the factor structure of the Wide Range Assessment of Memory and Learning: Implications for clinical interpretation. *Assessment, 5,* 127–139.

Golden, C. J., Zillmer, E., & Spiers, M. (1992). *Neuropsychological assessment and intervention.* Springfield, IL: Thomas.

Goldstein, F. C., & Levin, H. S. (1990). Epidemiology of traumatic brain injury: Incidence, clinical characteristics, and risk factors. In E. D. Bigler (Ed.), *Traumatic brain injury* (pp. 51–67). Austin, TX: Pro-Ed.

Grossman, I., Kaufman, A. S., Mednitsky, S., Scharff, L., & Dennis, B. (1994). Neurocognitive abilities for a clinically depressed sample versus a matched control group of normal individuals. *Psychiatry Research, 51,* 231–244.

Hill, D. E., Ciesielski, K. T., Sethre-Hofstad, L., Duncan, M. H., & Lorenzi, M. (1997). Visual and verbal short-term memory deficits in childhood leukemia survivors after intrathecal chemotherapy. *Journal of Pediatric Psychology, 22,* 861–870.

Howes, N. L., Bigler, E. D., Burlingame, G. M., & Lawson, J. S. (in press). Memory performance of children with dyslexia: A comparative analysis of theoretical perspectives. *Journal of Learning Disabilities.*

Howes, N. L., Bigler, E. D., Lawson, J. S., & Burlingame, G. M. (1999). Reading disability subtypes and the Test of Memory and Learning. *Archives of Clinical Neuropsychology, 14*(3), 317–339.

Hynd, G., & Obrzut, J. (1981). *Neuropsychological assessment of the school-aged child: Issues and procedures.* New York: Grune & Stratton.

Jensen, A. R., & Figueroa, R. (1975). Forward and backward digit span interaction with race and IQ: Predictions from Jensen's theory. *Journal of Educational Psychology, 67,* 882–893.

Kamphaus, R. W., & Reynolds, C. R. (1987). *Clinical and research application of the K-ABC.* Circle Pines, MN: American Guidance Service.

Kaplan, E. (1988). A process approach to neuropsychological assessment. In T. Boll & B. K. Bryant (Eds.), *Clinical neuropsychology and brain function: Research, measurement, and practice* (pp. 129–167). Washington, DC: American Psychological Association.

Kaufman, A. S. (1979). *Intelligent testing with the WISC-R.* New York: Wiley–Interscience.

Kaufman, A. S. (1994). *Intelligent testing with the WISC-III.* New York: Wiley–Interscience.

Kennedy, M. L., & Guilmette, T. J. (1997). The relationship between the WRAML Memory Screening and General Memory Indices in a clinical population. *Assessment, 4,* 69–72.

Knight, R. G. (1992). *The neuropsychology of degenerative brain diseases.* Hillsdale, NJ: Erlbaum.

Kolb, B., & Whishaw, I. Q. (1996). *Fundamentals of human neuropsychology* (4th ed.). New York: Freeman.

Koppitz, E. M. (1977). *The Visual–Aural Digit Span Test.* New York: Grune & Stratton.

Lajiness-O'Neill, R. (1996). *Age at injury as predictor of memory performance in children with traumatic brain injury.* Unpublished doctoral dissertation, Department of Psychology, Brigham Young University.

Lezak, M. D. (1995). *Neuropsychological assessment* (3rd ed.). New York: Oxford University Press.

Lorsbach, T. C., Wilson, S., & Reimer, J. F. (1996). Memory for relevant and irrelevant information: Evidence for deficient inhibitory processes in language/learning disabled children. *Contemporary Educational Psychology, 21,* 447–466.

Mapou, R. L., & Spector, J. (Eds.). (1995). *Clinical neuropsychological assessment*. New York: Plenum Press.

Mayfield, J. W., & Reynolds, C. R. (1997). Black–white differences in memory test performance among children and adolescents. *Archives of Clinical Neuropsychology, 12,* 111–122.

McCarthy, D. (1972). *McCarthy Scales of Children's Abilities*. New York: Psychological Corporation.

Mesulam, M. M. (2000). *Principles of behavioral and cognitive neurology*. Oxford University Press.

Nation, K., Adams, J. W., Bowyer-Crain, A., & Snowling, M. J. (1999). Working memory deficits in poor comprehenders reflect underlying language impairments. *Journal of Experimental Child Psychology, 73,* 139–158.

Parkin, A. J. (1993). *Memory: Phenomena, experiment and theory*. Oxford: Blackwell.

Pennington, B. F. (1991). *Diagnosing learning disorders: A neuropsychological framework*. New York: Guilford Press.

Phelps, L. (1995). Exploratory factor analysis of the WRAML with academically at-risk students. *Journal of Psychoeducational Assessment, 13,* 384–390.

Phelps, E. A., O'Connor, K. J., Gatenby, J. C., Grillon, C., Gore, J. C., & Davis, M. (2001). Activation of the human amygdala to a cognitive representation of fear. *Nature Neuroscience, 4,* 437–441.

Prigatano, G. P. (1990). Recovery and cognitive retraining after cognitive brain injury. In E. D. Bigler (Ed.), *Traumatic brain injury* (pp. 273–295). Austin, TX: Pro-Ed.

Ramsey, M. C., & Reynolds, C. R. (1995). Separate digit tests: A brief history, a literature review, and a reexamination of the factor structure of the Test of Memory and Learning (TOMAL). *Neuropsychology Review, 5,* 151–171.

Reeves, D., & Wedding, D. (1994). *The clinical assessment of memory*. Berlin: Springer-Verlag.

Rey, A. (1958). *L'examen clinique en psychologie*. Paris: Presses Universitaires de France.

Rey, A. (1964). *L'examen clinique en psychologie* (2nd ed.). Paris: Presses Universitaires de France.

Reynolds, C. R. (1995). Test bias and the assessment of intelligence and personality. In D. Saklofske & M. Zeidner (Eds.), *International handbook of personality and intelligence* (pp. 545–573). New York: Plenum Press.

Reynolds, C. R. (1997). Forward and backward memory span should not be combined for clinical analysis. *Archives of Clinical Neuropsychology, 12,* 29–40.

Reynolds, C. R., & Bigler, E. D. (1994a). *Manual for the Test of Memory and Learning*. Austin, TX: Pro-Ed.

Reynolds, C. R., & Bigler, E. D. (1994b). *Test of Memory and Learning*. Austin, TX: Pro-Ed.

Reynolds, C. R., & Bigler, E. D. (1996). Factor structure, factor indexes, and other useful statistics for interpretation of the Test of Memory and Learning (TOMAL). *Archives of Clinical Neuropsychology, 11*(1), 29–43.

Reynolds, C. R., & Bigler, E. D. (1997). Clinical neuropsychological assessment of child and adolescent memory with the Test of Memory and Learning. In C. R. Reynolds & E. Fletcher-Janzen (Eds.), *Handbook of clinical child neuropsychology* (2nd ed., pp. 296–319). New York: Plenum Press.

Rourke, B. P. (Ed.). (1991). *Neuropsychological validation of learning disability subtypes*. New York: Guilford Press.

Rourke, B. P., Bakker, D. J., Fisk, J. L., & Strang, J. D. (1983). *Child neuropsychology*. New York: Guilford Press.

Scheibel, A. B. (1990). Dendritic correlates of higher cognitive function. In A. B. Scheibel & A. Wechsler (Eds.), *Neurobiology of higher cognitive function* (pp. 239–270). New York: Guilford Press.

Sheslow, D., & Adams, W. (1990). *Wide Range Assessment of Memory and Learning*. Wilmington, DE: Jastak Associates.

Snyderman, M., & Rothman, S. (1987). Survey of expert opinion on intelligence and aptitude testing. *American Psychologist, 42,* 137–144.

Stanton, H. C., Reynolds, C. R., & Bigler, E. D. (1995). *PRO-SCORE: Computer Scoring System for the Test of Memory and Learning*. Austin, TX: Pro-Ed.

Stark, R. E., & McGregor, K. K. (1997). Follow-up study of a right- and left-hemispherectomized child: Implications for localization and impairment of language in children. *Brain and Language, 60,* 222–242.

Swanson, H. L., Ashbacker, M. H., & Lee, C. (1996). Learning-disabled readers' working memory as a function of processing demands. *Journal of Experimental Child Psychology, 61,* 242–275.

Tramontana, M. G., & Hooper, S. R. (1988). *Assessment issues in child neuropsychology*. New York: Plenum Press.

Whitney, S. J. (1996). *The performance of children who are depressed on the Wide Range Assessment of Memory and Learning*. Unpublished manuscript, Rutgers University.

Williams, J., & Haut, J. S. (1995). Differential performances on the WRAML in children and adolescents diagnosed with epilepsy, head injury, and substance abuse. *Developmental Neuropsychology, 11*(2), 201–213.

Woodward, H., & Donders, J. (1998). The performance of children with traumatic head injury on the Wide Range Assessment of Memory and Learning—Screening. *Applied Neuropsychology, 5,* 113–119.

13

Neuropsychological Perspectives on the Assessment of Children

CYNTHIA A. RICCIO
MONICA E. WOLFE

The neuropsychological approach to assessment and case conceptualization incorporates information from various behavioral domains believed to be related to functional neurological systems. The major premise of neuropsychological assessment is that different behaviors involve differing neurological structures or functional systems (Luria, 1980). Based on the individual's performance across a variety of domains, inferences are made about brain integrity. Thus neuropsychological assessment samples behaviors known to depend on the integrity of the central nervous system (CNS) through the use of various measures that correlate with cognitive, sensory–motor, and emotional functioning (Dean & Gray, 1990). In this way, the clinical neuropsychologist is able to apply the understanding of brain–behavior relations to the conceptualization of clinical cases (Stuss & Levine, 2002).

Historically, the neuropsychological assessment of children and youths has been based on a downward extension of what was known about neuropsychological functioning of adults. There has been significant research activity, however, in the area of neuropsychological assessment of children in the past few decades (Franzen, 2000). As a result of this growing interest in pediatric neuropsychology, the available knowledge base about the developing brain has increased dramatically since the 1980s (e.g., Ardila & Roselli, 1994; Halperin, McKay, Matier, & Sharma, 1994; Miller & Vernon, 1996; Molfese, 1995). With this increased knowledge, the application of neuropsychology to children and adolescents has yielded several positive outcomes. First, the range of diagnostic techniques available has been extended, in turn extending the range of behaviors that can be sampled via standardized techniques. The wider range of behavioral domains sampled facilitates differential diagnosis among disorders with similar symptom presentations (Morris, 1994; Rourke, 1994). At the same time, neuropsychological perspectives provide a foundation for better integration of behavioral data (Dean, 1986; Gray & Dean, 1990), which leads to a more unified or holistic picture of a child's functioning (Rothlisberg & D'Amato, 1988).

Neuropsychological assessment of children has provided a better understanding of the ways in which neurological conditions affect behavior, and has facilitated the translation of this knowledge into educationally relevant information (Allen, 1989). The neuropsychological perspective leads to better understanding of underlying causes of learning and behavior problems; this in turn results in an increased ability to develop appropriate interventions or circumvent future problems (Boll & Stanford, 1997; D'Amato, Rothlisberg, & Rhodes, 1997). Neuropsychological techniques have been used in the assessment of children for special education (Haak, 1989; Hynd, 1981), and have resulted in improved understanding of learning disabilities (Feagans, Short, & Meltzer, 1991; Riccio, Gonzalez, & Hynd, 1994; Riccio & Hynd, 1996) as well as traumatic brain injury (TBI; Snow & Hooper, 1994).

Research consistently demonstrates that adjustment and behavioral problems are associated with children who have neurodevelopmental deficits secondary to, if not as a direct result of, their neurological impairments (Dean, 1986; Hooper & Tramontana, 1997; Tramontana & Hooper, 1997). Various models (e.g., Gray, 1982; Kinsbourne, 1989; Nussbaum et al., 1988; Rourke, 1989) have been proposed to explain the interface between brain function and behaviors associated with childhood psychopathology. Neuropsychological perspectives have improved the understanding of autism (e.g., Shields, Varley, Broks, & Simpson, 1996), attention-deficit/hyperactivity disorder (see Riccio, Hynd, & Cohen, 1996, for a review), and conduct disorder (Moffitt, 1993). Furthermore, many components of neuropsychological assessment can be helpful in documenting changes in behavior and development over time (Hynd & Willis, 1988).

The purpose of this chapter is to provide a framework for the neuropsychological assessment of children and youths. As such, the chapter includes an overview of the neurodevelopmental issues that need to be considered in the neuropsychological assessment of children and youths, components of neuropsychological assessment, inferential processes, and the linkages between assessment and intervention.

NEURODEVELOPMENTAL ISSUES

As noted earlier, the assessment measures and processes traditionally used with children and youths were modifications of existing neuropsychological batteries and other measures used for adults (Hartlage & Long, 1997). This approach was based on an underlying assumption that tasks used with adults would measure the same constructs in the same ways when used with children. Although it is tempting to assume that neuropsychological findings from adults will be useful with children, this has not been shown to be a valid assumption. Unfortunately, many of the measures that have clinical efficacy when used with adults do not have the sensitivity necessary to reflect developmental issues; as a result, the utility of procedures used with adults in the neuropsychological assessment of children has multiple pitfalls and has been questioned (e.g., Cohen, Branch, Willis, Weyandt, & Hynd, 1992; Fletcher & Taylor, 1984).

When neuropsychological theory is applied to children and adolescents, the premise that behavior can be used to make inferences about brain functioning and integrity has to be modified to include consideration of neurodevelopmental differences existing as a function of the youngsters' age (Hooper & Tramontana, 1997; Riccio & Reynolds, 1998). Applying adult inferences/hypotheses directly to children ignores what is known about changes in the functional organization of the brain as children mature (Cohen et al., 1992; Fletcher & Taylor, 1984). Because of these neurodevelopmental changes, it is also not possible to view brain dysfunction on a continuum, as behavioral deficits may change or emerge over time (Fletcher & Taylor, 1984).

Neurodevelopment follows a predictable course. Only the primary cortical zones are generally mature by birth (Luria, 1980); all other cortical areas continue to develop postnatally, and some cortical areas do so through adolescence. These later-developing cortical areas include the integrative systems involved in higher-order functions of learning, memory, attention, emotion, cognition, and language, as well as the association areas (Goldman & Lewis, 1978; Goldman-Rakic, 1987). Not only is there continued development of cortical areas throughout childhood, but the interaction of cortical areas is likely to change over the course of development (Merola & Leiderman, 1985; Rutter, 1981).

Despite our growing knowledge of typical neurodevelopmental processes, the theoretical bases and practice of neuropsychology are based on observations and informal assessment of individuals with identified brain damage (Reynolds, 1997b). Research regarding typical neurodevelopment (particularly in relation to higher-order cognitive skills) is limited, and the changing organization of brain function in children over time is only beginning to be understood (Hynd & Willis, 1988). There are still many unanswered questions regarding the developmental progression of many functional systems, particularly at the associative and integrative levels. Furthermore, how the neurodevelopmental progression maps onto cognitive functioning is not fully understood.

In addition to neurodevelopmental courses that need to be considered, there are complex differences between children and adults in the mechanisms and progression of brain pathology that lead to neuropsychological and behavioral/affective problems (Fennell & Bauer, 1997; Fletcher & Taylor, 1984). Course and outcome do not necessarily follow a similar progression in children and in adults. For acquired disorders such as TBI, the impact of neurological insult is influenced by age as well as location and nature of injury, gender, socioeconomic status, level of emotional adjustment and coping, and the individual's own adaptive skills (Bolter & Long, 1985). The theory of neural plasticity (Harris, 1957) has been used to explain the potential for recovery of function in children that is not evidenced in adults. It has since been suggested that what is termed "recovery" may in fact reflect "reorganization" of brain function (Satz & Fletcher, 1981). This "recovery" or "reorganization" is more likely to occur following a focal lesion than following a more diffuse injury, and is also more likely in younger children who experience a closed head injury (Brink, Garrett, Hale, Woo-Sam, & Nickel, 1970). Reorganization may alter the development of functional systems and the corresponding behavioral domains. For this reason, it has been argued that age of injury is an important factor to be considered in neuropsychological assessment (Fletcher-Janzen & Kade, 1997).

DOMAINS FOR NEUROPSYCHOLOGICAL ASSESSMENT

Regardless of the reason for referral, neuropsychological assessment of children needs to be focused more on analysis of the functional systems and overall integrity of the CNS than on the identification of a single neurological disorder (Riccio & Reynolds, 1998). In order to establish global neuropsychological functioning, evaluation of a majority of cognitive and higher-order processes is necessary. On the level of more specific abilities, neuropsychological assessment generally includes the evaluation of a number of functional domains that are, based on clinical evidence, associated with functional systems of the brain. Each component of the assessment process and each functional domain assessed are taken together to form an integrated view of the individual; these domains are listed in Table 13.1. All of these domains are considered important for case conceptualization, as well as in the formulation of treatment goals and the generation of potential interventions (Hartlage & Telzrow, 1986; Whitten, D'Amato, & Chitooran, 1992).

Developmental and Social History

The assessment itself should be organized in such a manner that the majority of areas of functioning, as well as the various contexts in which the child is expected to function, are considered (Riccio & Reynolds, 1998). Obtaining a comprehensive history is an important component of neuropsychological

TABLE 13.1. Domains of Neuropsychological Assessment of Children

General neuropsychological functioning
Sensory perception (auditory, visual, tactile)
Motor functioning (gross and fine)
Auditory/linguistic functioning
Visual–spatial functioning
Learning/memory
Attention/concentration
Executive functions (problem solving, etc.)
Academic skills
Behavior and personality

assessment. A complete history provides information that is useful in differentiating chronic deficits or neurodevelopmental disorders from new, acute problems. Developmental and social history also provide information on the supports available within the family system. A number of developmental and social history forms exist for this purpose. Most of these forms can be completed either in interview format or independently by the parents. The Structured Developmental History (SDH) form of the Behavior Assessment System for Children (BASC; Reynolds & Kamphaus, 1992) is one example of a developmental history questionnaire. The SDH form solicits information specific to prenatal, perinatal, postnatal, and early childhood development; medical problems and concerns; exposure to formal education; progress in school; and so on. It also asks for information specific to the child's family situation, living quarters, preferred leisure and other activities, and so on, which may be helpful in case conceptualization and intervention planning (Riccio & Reynolds, 1998).

Cognitive Functioning

The domains of cognition and achievement are assessed as part of a general psychological evaluation and are part of the neuropsychological evaluation as well. Assessment of the child's cognitive skills will generally include an assessment of general intellectual ability (g), using a standardized measure such as the Wechsler Intelligence Scale for Children—Third Edition (Wechsler, 1991). Assessment of cognition with a reliable measure is essential in providing a baseline for the interpretation of other aspects of the child's functioning (Riccio & Reynolds, 1998). The major measures of cognition are reviewed elsewhere in this volume and in other volumes (e.g., Kamphaus, 2001).

Academic Functioning

Given that school is a major context in which children must function, assessment of basic academic skills (including reading, written language, and mathematics) is also important in order to determine the need for classroom modifications or remediation efforts. Use of a standardized battery such

as the Woodcock–Johnson Psychoeducational Battery—Third Edition Tests of Achievement (Woodcock, McGrew, & Mather, 2001) can provide information on the child's current functioning in basic academic areas. The use of a fluency-based measure as part of academic assessment is considered important, given that slow processing or difficulty in retrieving information needed for responding may be one effect of some neurological disorders (Chadwick, Rutter, Brown, Shaffer, & Traub, 1981; Shaw & Yingst, 1992). This reduced rate of processing can have cumulative effects on long-term educational progress (Chadwick et al., 1981).

Integrity of Brain Functioning

The history and results from the combination of cognitive and achievement measures provide some standard information about a child. A neuropsychological evaluation provides for consideration of a wider array of functions than is addressed in a typical psychological or psychoeducational evaluation (Dean & Gray, 1990; Reynolds & Mayfield, 1999; Riccio, Hynd, & Cohen, 1993; Riccio & Reynolds, 1998). The need to assess a wider range of higher cortical functions is supported by research findings that neurological disorders are seldom expressed as a single dysfunction (Dean & Gray, 1990). As stated earlier, one goal of the neuropsychological evaluation is to obtain a global picture of the integrity of the CNS or general neuropsychological functioning. Many cognitive tasks (e.g., those requiring concept formation or reasoning) provide a general sense of CNS integrity. To make a determination of overall functioning, however, it is important to insure that the results obtained allow for evaluation of the four major quadrants of the neocortex (left, right, anterior, posterior). As such, it is important that the assessment sample the relative efficiency of the right and left hemispheres. This is important in that, to some extent, differing brain systems are involved in each hemisphere. Lateralization of dysfunctional and intact systems can have implications for treatment. Similarly, the anterior region of the brain is generally viewed as subserving differing functions (e.g., regulatory functions) from those of the posterior region (e.g., receptivity). Just as lateralization of dysfunction is important, anterior–posterior comparisons can provide important information for treatment planning. Even in a diffuse injury, it is possible to find greater impact on one area of the brain than on others, and cognitive measures do not necessarily tap all four quadrants.

To insure comprehensive evaluation of the CNS, neuropsychological evaluation includes the assessment of multiple domains that are not usually covered in a standard psychoeducational battery. These include sensory, motor, auditory/linguistic, and visual–spatial areas, as well as learning and memory, attention, and the so-called "executive functions" of planning, organization, and problem solving (e.g., Dean & Gray, 1990; Shurtleff, Fay, Abbot, & Berninger, 1988). Problems with memory, learning new information, and attention are the most common of all complaints following any type of CNS compromise and are often subtle (Gillberg, 1995; Reynolds & Bigler, 1997). Finally, behavioral and personality factors that may be secondary to the neurological dysfunction or that may impede intervention efforts need to be explored. Each of these domains is discussed further.

Sensory Functioning

The somatosensory system is the first to develop prenatally (Zillmer & Spiers, 2002). Most often, not only is performance on tactile, auditory, and visual tasks assessed, but performance differences (right to left) are considered. For tactile tasks, this usually involves determining the ability of the individual to identify where he or she has been touched, to identify the nature of a symbol drawn on a finger or to recognize a shape or object by touch. For auditory perception, dichotic listening tasks that examine accuracy of responses for each ear (ear advantage) or other auditory-perceptual tasks have been used (Cohen, Riccio, & Hynd, 1999). Visual tracking tasks or presentation of items to left or right visual fields may be included to assess visual perception. (Some of these visual tasks may overlap with those used to assess visual–spatial functioning; see below.) Notably, the tasks included in the neuropsychological battery should not be viewed as a substitute for, or an equivalent

to, a formal vision or audiological evaluation that assesses acuity.

Motor Functioning

Motor functioning is generally assessed at the level of fine motor tasks, with less direct assessment of gross motor ability. As with sensory areas, not only are the overall motor capabilities considered, but left–right differences are examined as well. Tasks may include imitation of hand positions; rapid alternation of hand movements; finger-tapping tasks; or tasks that require the child to place an object into a board of some time as quickly as possible, similar to the Animal Pegs subtest on the Wechsler Preschool and Primary Scale of Intelligence—Revised (Wechsler, 1989). Although direct assessment of gross motor coordination is not typically included, observational data on gait and balance may provide qualitative information on the child's neurodevelopmental status; observations may also indicate the need for more intensive occupational or physical therapy evaluation.

Auditory/Linguistic Functioning

Difficulties in language areas are not infrequent among children or youths with neurological disorders; in fact, language disorders are among the most common disorders of higher cerebral functioning in children (Tomblin et al., 1999). Regardless of the measure used for assessment of cognitive functioning, neuropsychological assessment supplements cognitive testing with additional language measures. In particular, additional measures may look at naming skills, understanding of language, expressive language characteristics, and pragmatic aspects of language. More specific measures of language provide for assessment of anterior (expressive language) and posterior (receptive language) brain functions. Often language deficits are interpreted as representing left-hemisphere (language-dominant) functions (Restrepo, Swisher, Plante, & Vance, 1992; Trauner, Ballantyne, Chase, & Tallal, 1993). Left-hemisphere posterior systems are also associated with the presence of developmental dyslexia in conjunction with language deficits (Brunswick, McCrory, Price, Frith, & Frith, 1999; Pugh et al., 2000).

Visual–Spatial Functioning

Whereas auditory/linguistic abilities are generally presumed to reflect left-hemisphere function, performance on visual–spatial (or visual-perceptual; see above) tasks is often interpreted as reflecting right-hemisphere (non-language-dominant) function. Specific spatial deficits may include right–left confusion, figure–ground confusion, inability to complete mental rotation tasks, impaired performance on maze tasks, and so on. Specific visual-perceptual deficits may include the inability to understand facial expressions or other nonverbal social cues, which is often associated with nonverbal learning disability (Rourke, 1989). Visualization abilities and orientation in space are of importance as well, but often are not assessed directly; however, parents or teachers may report behaviors that reflect these problems. A frequent method of assessing visual–spatial (and visual-perceptual) abilities is through the use of various constructional or drawing tasks (Kolb & Whishaw, 1996). In assessing these abilities, it is important to insure that not all tasks require a motor response; it is best to include both motor-dependent and motor-free tasks, in order to account for potential confounds of motor impairment.

Learning and Memory

Research across neurological disorders points to the importance of assessing memory in order to evaluate brain integrity effectively (Reynolds & Bigler, 1997). Children with neurological disorders may have difficulty in encoding, storage, or retrieval of information that is necessary for learning (Ewing-Cobbs, Fletcher, & Levin, 1986; Lezak, 1986; Ryan, LaMarche, Barth, & Boll, 1996). With memory involving a number of interconnections throughout the brain, damage to one or more of the structures involved in memory can have an impact on the formation (encoding) or the retrieval process; memory deficits can be expansive or more specific and subtle.

Historically, the assessment of memory in children was derived from specific subtests of the various cognitive batteries (e.g.,

Branch, Cohen, & Hynd, 1995; Nussbaum et al., 1988), particularly the Digit Span subtest from the Wechsler scales. A number of problems with the reliance on Digit Span or similar subtests have been described in the literature (e.g., Reynolds, 1997a; Talley, 1986); particular concern has been noted about combining forward and backward digits (Ramsey & Reynolds, 1995; Reynolds, 1997a). Because of these concerns, children's norms for adult measures of memory have been obtained (e.g., Delis, Kramer, Kaplan, & Ober, 1994). The use of adult measures of memory with children is perceived as inappropriate by some practitioners, however (Riccio & Reynolds, 1998). Optimally, given the need for educational relevance in the assessment of children, it may be appropriate for assessment of memory to include tasks more similar to everyday tasks and list learning, so that a learning slope can be determined (which may be more useful in assessing learning and memory). In an attempt to address the collective concerns with existing measures, several measures for the assessment of memory and learning have been developed and are described in detail elsewhere (see Riccio & Reynolds, 1998; see also Miller, Bigler, & Adams, Chapter 12, this volume).

Attention

The most frequent symptoms associated with childhood neuropsychological disorders include problems with attention/concentration, difficulties with self-regulation, and emotional/behavioral problems. "Attention" is a multidimensional construct including alertness, selective attention, sustained attention or vigilance, and so on (Barkley, 1998). Attention affects memory and learning, in that the neural traces left by attention are the likely roots of memory. There are multiple measures of attention; however, the best is still direct observation in naturalistic settings (Barkley, 1998).

One of the most frequently employed measures of attention is often some version of a continuous-performance test (CPT) (Halperin, 1991). The basic paradigm for all CPTs involves selective attention or vigilance for an infrequently occurring stimulus (Eliason & Richman, 1987). CPTs involve the rapid presentation of continuously changing stimuli with a designated "target" stimulus or "target" pattern. A comprehensive review of studies using a variety of CPTs provides consistent evidence that CPTs are sensitive to brain damage or dysfunction across multiple disorders but lack specificity (Riccio, Reynolds, & Lowe, 2001).

A number of other tasks are used for the assessment of attention as well. For example, cancellation tasks often are used to assess attentional abilities, with specific note made of neglect of any visual field. Consistent with the idea of multimodal assessment, it may be best to insure that assessment of attentional processes includes both auditory and visual modalities as well as multiple methods.

Executive Functions

The domain of "executive functions" has been defined in multiple ways and often is presumed to include those higher-order processes associated with planning, organization, and problem solving (judgment). More precisely, those behaviors believed to constitute executive functions include the ability to maintain an appropriate problem-solving set for attainment of a goal (Luria, 1980; Zelazo, Carter, Reznick, & Frye, 1997), mental representation of a task (Luria, 1980), planning and self-monitoring of behavior (e.g., Zelazo et al., 1997), and the ability to use environmental cues effectively (Passler, Isaac, & Hynd, 1985). The domain of executive functions thus incorporates a variety of constructs (e.g., attention, self-regulation, working memory), but the processes generally focus on effortful and flexible organization, strategic planning, and proactive reasoning (Denckla, 1994).

The predominant neural substrates of executive processes are believed to be located in the frontal and prefrontal areas. Developmentally, since the frontal and prefrontal areas continue to mature through adolescence, the ability to assess differing aspects of executive functions in children is problematic. Tasks need to have sufficient items across the continuum of difficulty level in order to measure the developmental trajectory. Myelination of the frontal regions of the cortex is believed to continue through adolescence, with increased efficiency associated with maturity. As such, for those aspects of executive functions that normally develop later, deficits may not be evident until the skills do not develop.

Many measures of executive functions used with children are downward extensions of adult measures and may lack sensitivity to developmental differences that are of importance in the assessment of children. Furthermore, many "executive function" measures actually tap or are determined in part by other abilities. For example, measures of executive functions have been found to be related to intelligence (Chelune & Thompson, 1987; Riccio, Hall, et al., 1994) as well as internalized language (Denckla, 1994). Two of the most frequently used measures of executive functions are the Wisconsin Card Sorting Test (Heaton, 1981) and the Children's Category Test (Boll, 1993). However, child-centered, developmentally sensitive measures of executive processing that are more directly linked to the development of interventions are needed. Recently, a battery of measures similar to traditional adult measures of executive function has been developed by Delis, Kramer, and Kaplan (2001) for use with children. At this time there is limited research specific to this measure, its sensitivity to developmental differences, and its overall usefulness in the neuropsychological assessment of children and youths.

Behavior and Personality

Given the potential for adjustment/behavioral difficulties in conjunction with neurological disorders, the use of a transactional/reciprocal framework has been advocated (Batchelor, 1996b; D'Amato & Rothlisberg, 1996; Teeter, 1997; Teeter & Semrud-Clikeman, 1997). A transactional model takes into consideration the reciprocal interactions of the child, home and family members, teacher and peers, and other social environments in which the child functions. As such, assessment incorporates information from a variety of sources (e.g., parents, teachers, physicians, medical records, school records, etc.). In this way, the neuropsychological assessment process not only incorporates a more complete review of information regarding the child, but attempts to integrate this information with an understanding of brain–behavior relations and environmental factors (Batchelor, 1996a; Taylor & Fletcher, 1990).

The most common approach to emotional/behavioral assessment relies on published rating scales, of which there are many. A multifaceted approach that includes parent and teacher rating scales, self-report measures, direct observation, and clinical interviews provides the most comprehensive and broad-based view of the child's emotional and behavioral status (Kamphaus & Frick, 2002; Semrud-Clikeman, Kamphaus, Teeter, & Vaughn, 1997). For example, the BASC (Reynolds & Kamphaus, 1992) includes not only teacher and parent forms, but also a structured observation system (SOS) and, for children over age 9, a self-report measure that can be used to assess emotional and behavioral status effectively. Another advantage to the BASC (rating scales and SOS) is the inclusion of positive adaptive behaviors (e.g., social skills, adaptability to change in the environment), in addition to the more common maladaptive skills included on many rating scales. When children's adaptive behavior is an identified concern, completion of a more comprehensive adaptive behavior scale may be helpful for intervention planning.

TEST SELECTION

Issues Involved in Selecting Tests

There is no single method of selecting measures for inclusion in a neuropsychological assessment that is used across settings or individuals. Many practitioners continue to include naturalistic observation and informal assessment, while others have adopted more actuarial approaches; still others combine observation, informal methods, and actuarial approaches (Reynolds, 1997b). A more qualitative approach using experimental/informal measures and nonquantitative interpretation may provide additional information or insight into how a child approaches and processes tasks, as in the Boston "process approach" (see Kaplan, 1988, 1990). However, most clinicians prefer a combination of quantitative and qualitative measures, as a strictly qualitative approach does not allow for verification of

diagnostic accuracy, is not easily replicated, and does not allow for formal evaluation of treatment methods (Rourke, 1994).

Regardless of the approach taken to selecting standardized measures, the behavioral domains to be addressed as part of the neuropsychological assessment process, as well as the psychometric issues involved, remain the same. In choosing measures, it is important to attend to the psychometric properties and limitations of available measures instruments; however, clinical child neuropsychology is often criticized for its failure to incorporate psychometric advances in test use and construction (e.g., Cicchetti, 1994; Parsons & Prigatano, 1978; Ris & Noll, 1994). One major concern relates to the extent and nature of normative data for many measures used in the neuropsychological assessment of children. Although it has been argued that sound normative data provide a necessary backdrop against which to evaluate clinical insight (Reynolds, 1997b), the systematic development and presentation of normative data across the lifespan for many measures used in neuropsychological assessment have not received sufficient attention, and more work in this area is needed (Reynolds, 1986b). Because of the need for adequate normative data, some clinicians advocate the interpretation of traditional measures of cognitive ability (e.g., the Wechsler scales) from a neuropsychological perspective. Concerns and criticisms of the recategorization of subtests from standardized measures that were not developed based on neuropsychological theory and have not been validated for this purpose are evident in the literature, however (Kamphaus, 2001; Lezak, 1995). The availability of normative data is one argument for using traditional cognitive measures despite the lack of a theoretical foundation.

A second concern is that all too often, neuropsychologists overlook the psychometric concepts of reliability and validity, making interpretations based on the "clinical" nature of the tasks. The need for the establishment of reliability and validity of scores, as well as the interpretation, given to neuropsychological test performance has been a frequent issue in the literature (e.g., Parsons & Prigatano, 1978; Reynolds, 1982; Riccio & Reynolds, 1998). Reliability of test scores is critical, as it relates to the amount of variance that is systematic and related to true inter- and intraindividual differences. Reliability is also the foundation of a measure's validity (Reynolds, 1986a).

A third concern relates to the sensitivity and appropriateness of measures with children. Not only does neuropsychological assessment of children and adolescents require tests/measures with sufficient empirical support for the inferences being made, but it is important to document the measures' sensitivity to neurobehavioral and neurodevelopmental functioning in children (Cohen et al., 1992; Fletcher & Taylor, 1984). Thus, in addition to selecting tests based on psychometric properties, it has been suggested that measures used in the neuropsychological assessment process need to vary along a continuum of difficulty, to include both rote and novel tasks, and to include variations with regard to processing and response requirements within modalities (Rourke, 1994).

Neuropsychological Batteries for Children

The influences of child psychology, school psychology, and education are evident in the composition of neuropsychological assessment batteries, procedures, and measures used with children, and these influences contribute to the variations in methods used (Batchelor, 1996a). Some clinical child neuropsychologists adopt a more idiographic approach and tailor the selection of measures to a child's presenting problems and the child's actual performance on initial measures (Christensen, 1975; Luria, 1973). This type of approach is based on the intention to isolate those mechanisms that are contributing to a specific, identified problem, as opposed to providing a comprehensive view of the child. Although it may be more cost-effective (Goldstein, 1997), the emphasis is clearly on understanding deficit systems and not identifying intact functional systems. In addition, the more idiographic approach may fail to assess domains that are of importance and that subsequently have an impact on rehabilitation efforts (Riccio & Reynolds, 1998).

In practice, many clinicians use a predetermined battery of tests for neuropsychological assessment of children (Fennell, 1994); this is often referred to as the "fixed-battery" approach. Specific neuropsychological batteries, such as the Halstead–Reitan Neuropsychological Test Battery (HRNB; Reitan & Davison, 1974), the Reitan–Indiana Neuropsychological Battery (RINB; Reitan, 1969), and the Luria–Nebraska Neuropsychological Battery—Children's Revision (LNNB-CR; Golden, 1984), are often used in neuropsychological assessment in conjunction with intelligence tests, achievement tests, and measures of behavior and personality. The neuropsychological batteries provide a sampling of sensory and motor functions, as well as additional information relating to hemispheric (left–right) differences and anterior–posterior differences. More recently, Korkman and colleagues have developed the Developmental Neuropsychological Assessment (NEPSY; Korkman, Kirk, & Kemp, 1998). A comparison of domains tapped by these measures is provided in Table 13.2. As can be seen from the table, regardless of the fixed battery, comprehensive assessment of all domains requires the addition of supplemental measures.

The Halstead–Reitan Neuropsychological Battery and the Reitan–Indiana Neuropsychological Battery

The HRNB and the RINB are both downward extensions of the original adult version of the Halstead–Reitan battery, and are considered to be the most widely used in clinical practice (Howieson & Lezak, 1992; Nussbaum & Bigler, 1997). The RINB is intended for children through age 8 years; the HRNB is used for children ages 9–14 years. These batteries contain numerous measures that are considered necessary for understanding brain–behavior relationships. Areas of functioning tapped by these batteries include concept formation, sensory abilities, attention/concentration, motor speed and dexterity, verbal abilities, and memory. (For a more detailed description of tasks, see Reitan & Wolfson, 1985; Riccio & Reynolds, 1998, 1999.)

Both the HRNB and the RINB incorporate a multiple-inferential approach to interpretation that includes examination of level of performance, pathognomonic signs, patterns of performance, and right–left differences (Reitan, 1986, 1987). More recently,

TABLE 13.2. Comparison of Domain Coverage for Fixed Batteries

Domain	HRNB[a] subtest(s)	LNNB-CR[b] subtest(s)	NEPSY[c] subtest(s)
General neuropsychological functioning	Category Test Seashore Rhythm Test Trail Making Test	C11 (Intellectual)	
Auditory/linguistic functioning	Aphasia Screening Test Speech Sounds Perception	C5 (Receptive Speech) C6 (Expressive Speech) C7 (Writing) C10 (Memory)	Auditory Attention and Response Set Phonological Processing Comprehension of Instructions Oromotor Sequences
Motor functioning	Finger Oscillation Test Grip Strength Test	C1 (Motor) C7 (Writing)	Finger Tapping Imitating Hand Positions Visuomotor Precision Manual Motor Sequences Design Copy Oromotor Sequences
Visual–spatial functioning		C4 (Visual)	Design Copy Arrows Block Construction Route Finding
Sensory perception (tactile, auditory, visual)	Sensory Perceptual Examination Tactual Performance Test Tactile Form Recognition Finger-Tip Number Writing		Finger Discrimination Design Copy
Attention/ concentration	Speech Sounds Perception Seashore Rhythm Test Tactile Form Recognition		Auditory Attention and Response Set Visual Attention Statue
Learning/memory	Tactual Performance Test	C10 (Memory)	Memory for Faces Memory for Names Narrative Memory Sentence Repetition List Learning
Executive functions (problem solving, etc.)	Category Test Trail Making Test		Tower Statue Design Fluency Knock and Tap
Academic skills		C7 (Writing) C8 (Reading) C9 (Arithmetic)	
Behavior and personality			

[a]For ages 9–14 years; domains identified were based on Nussbaum and Bigler (1997) and Reitan and Wolfson (1985, 1988).
[b]Domains identified were based on Golden (1997).
[c]Domains identified were based on Korkman et al. (1998) and Kemp, Kirk, and Korkman (2001).

extensive efforts have been made to establish normative data for measures on the HRNB as well (e.g., Mitrushina, Boone, & D'Elia, 1999). Both the RINB and the HRNB have been found to be sensitive to brain damage even when the damage is not evident through neuroradiological methods (Nussbaum & Bigler, 1997). Furthermore, the addition of the HRNB to the traditional psychoeducational battery has been found to increase the extent to which variability in school achievement can be accounted for (Strom, Gray, Dean, & Fischer, 1987). However, research on the HRNB's usefulness in the differential diagnosis of learning disabilities is equivocal (e.g., Arffa, Fitzhugh-Bell, & Black, 1989; Batchelor, Kixmiller, & Dean, 1990). A noted concern with both the RINB and the HRNB is that they do not fully reflect the developmental continuum (Cohen et al., 1992). As can be noted from Table 13.2, although visual processing abilities are tapped somewhat by specific tasks, the domain of visual–spatial (or visual-perceptual) abilities is not assessed directly by the HRNB.

The Luria–Nebraska Neuropsychological Battery—Children's Revision

The neurodevelopmental stages of the child provide the basis for the LNNB-CR, which is intended for use with children ages 8–12 years (Golden, 1981, 1997). The most recently developed version of the scale combines the child and adult forms, for an age range of 5 years to adulthood; however, there is little research on the LNNB–3 with children (Golden, 1997). The various tasks of the LNNB-CR provide information specific to motor, rhythm, tactile, visual, verbal (receptive and expressive), and memory functions. (For a more detailed description, see Golden, 1997; Riccio & Reynolds, 1998.)

Interpretation of the LNNB-CR focuses predominantly on scale pattern (intraindividual) differences, as opposed to levels of performance or pathognomonic signs; however, there is a pathognomonic scale available. The LNNB-CR has been found to be sensitive to deficits in language and rhythm, as well as in reading and writing (Geary & Gilger, 1984). It has also been found to be more sensitive than either cognitive or

achievement measures to improvement in functioning following medical intervention (Torkelson, Liebrook, Gustavson, & Sundell, 1985). Research findings suggest that the LNNB-CR provides useful information for understanding learning problems (Tramontana, Hooper, Curley, & Nardolillo, 1990). The specificity of the LNNB-CR, however, has been questioned (e.g., Morgan & Brown, 1988; Snow & Hynd, 1985).

The Developmental Neuropsychological Assessment

The NEPSY is a flexible battery used to assess neuropsychological functioning of children ages 3–12 years. Korkman and colleagues (1998) based the NEPSY on Luria's (1980) approach to neuropsychological assessment, as well on current procedures of child assessment. The NEPSY assesses the five basic domains of attention/executive functions, language, visual–spatial ability, sensory–motor ability, and memory. These domains were theoretically designed to represent Luria's three functional and interactional brain systems (Korkman et al., 1998). Korkman and colleagues identified four purposes for the NEPSY: (1) the detection of subtle differences in neuropsychological functioning, (2) increased understanding of the effects of brain damage, (3) monitoring of long-term effects of brain damage, and (4) improved understanding of the development of children.

Interpretation of the NEPSY is based on standard and scaled scores derived from normative data on a sample of 1,000 children stratified by age, gender, ethnicity, geographic region, and level of parental education. Comparisons between domains and of scores within domains are used to identify primary and secondary deficits, as well as to identify intact functional systems. In addition, the NEPSY includes methods for recording and comparing base rates for qualitative observations (e.g., pencil grip maturity, the presence of tremors, the frequency of off-task behaviors, and presence of posturing and mirroring).

Since the NEPSY is a relatively new assessment battery, there is limited research regarding the validity and reliability of the results obtained. Available evidence suggests sensitivity to age effects across domains (Klenberg, Korkman, & Lahti-Nuuttila, 2001; Korkman, Kirk, & Kemp, 2001), learning disabilities, pervasive developmental disorders, fetal alcohol syndrome, and TBI (Korkman et al., 1998). The Finnish version of the NEPSY was published prior to the English version and was found to be sensitive to language delays (Korkman & Häkkinen-Rihu, 1994). Concurrent validity has been demonstrated with various other measures of neuropsychological function (Korkman et al., 1998). Subtest specificity was found to be adequate; however, confirmatory factor analysis on the standardization sample did not support the use of domain scores (Stinnett, Oehler-Stinnett, Fuqua, & Palmer, 2002). Although more research is needed to determine the usefulness of the NEPSY in clinical practice, the development of a comprehensive battery, with adequate normative data, is a step in the direction of improved psychometric properties for neuropsychological measures.

FROM INTERPRETATION TO INTERVENTION

As noted earlier, a child's cumulative performances on neuropsychological measures are seen as behavioral indicators of brain functioning (Fennell & Bauer, 1997); the data generated from the assessment process are used to make inferences about the integrity of the various functional systems of the brain. Inferences related to brain function require evaluation that is analogous to all four quadrants (right–left hemispheres, anterior–posterior regions) of the brain (Riccio & Reynolds, 1998). Based on all of the data generated in the evaluation process, specific hypotheses concerning how and why the child processes information are generated (D'Amato, 1990; Dean, 1986; Whitten et al., 1992). However, inferences are based not only on the child's performance on the measures themselves, but also on the clinician's theoretical perspective.

There are various paradigms for understanding and interpreting neuropsychological data (e.g., Batchelor, 1996a; Luria, 1980; Nussbaum & Bigler, 1997; Reynolds, 1981). For example, interpretation may be based on overall performance level across tasks (e.g., Reitan, 1986, 1987). With this model, conclusions are based on a comparison of the child's overall level of performance to normative data. There are multiple problems with this model, including variability among typically developing children; insensitivity for individuals with higher cognitive abilities; and a tendency to yield a high number of false positives, due to the potential impact of fatigue and motivation to affect performance (Nussbaum & Bigler, 1997; Reitan & Wolfson, 1985). Another model examines performance patterns across tasks (e.g., Reitan, 1986, 1987) as a means of differentiating functional from dysfunctional neural systems. This model allows for identification of strengths as well as weaknesses; emphasis on a strengths-based model for intervention planning is viewed as more efficacious than focusing only on deficits (Reynolds, Kamphaus, Rosenthal, & Hiemenz, 1997).

Another model of examining intraindividual differences involves examining asymmetry or lateralization of function (e.g., Reitan, 1986, 1987). As stated earlier, it is important to consider left–right hemisphere differences; however, exclusive reliance on left–right differences ignores the role of hemispheric interaction (e.g., Efron, 1990; Hiscock & Kinsbourne, 1987) and presumes hemispheric dominance for specific functions in children from adult data (Riccio & Reynolds, 1998). Still another model is to qualitatively assess the error patterns for the presence of pathognomonic signs (e.g., Kaplan, 1988; Lezak, 1995; Reitan, 1986, 1987). Although this method has been used reliably with adult populations, the reliability of this approach with children has not been demonstrated (Batchelor, 1996b). In practice, clinicians use any one or some combination of these features (Reitan, 1986, 1987; Riccio & Reynolds, 1998) in the process of making inferences and interpreting the results obtained. As such, there are considerable differences in the ways in which assessment results are used for making inferences and generating treatment recommendations. Although no one paradigm is necessarily always the best, it is important that the theoretical model used for interpretation lead to accurate predictions about the child's ability to function in multiple contexts and to benefit from various intervention programs (Reynolds et al., 1997; Riccio & Reynolds, 1998).

One component of the interpretation process is the identification of the child's specific deficits. Given that it may not be plausible or effective to address all identified deficits simultaneously, it may be necessary to prioritize these in terms of importance in the settings (home and school) in which the child is expected to function. The specific goals and objectives to be addressed should thus reflect not only the deficits themselves, but the information obtained regarding the home and school settings, the expectations for the child in these settings, and the supports and resources available for the child in the various contexts.

There is often a tendency to focus on identifying deficits; again, however, it is imperative to the development of effective treatment programs that the child's strengths and intact systems also be identified. Because the brain functions as a series of interdependent interactional processes, identifying both strengths and weaknesses provides more in-depth understanding of the types of accommodations or modifications that may be appropriate. With a focus on intact functional systems, rehabilitation and remediation programs based on strengths can then be implemented (see Reynolds, 1986b; Reynolds & Hickman, 1987). At the same time, the intact systems that have been identified can be used to develop compensatory behaviors as part of the rehabilitation program. Furthermore, identification of intact systems suggests a more positive outcome to parents as well as teachers, and thus increases the likelihood of motivated support systems for the child (Riccio & Reynolds, 1998).

Inferences are made not only regarding the specific behaviors that are assessed, but also about skills that have not been evaluated. This is done through the use of information about how various skills correlate in the developmental process. Ultimately, data generated from the neuropsychological assessment process are used to develop recommendations regarding whether the individual would profit from compensatory strategies, remedial instruction, or a combination (Gaddes & Edgell, 1994). Moreover, by clarifying the neurological correlates of these skills and of instructional methods,

neuropsychological assessment can assist in the formulation of hypotheses regarding potential instructional methods/materials for a particular child (Reynolds et al., 1997).

The second component of interpretation, also based on both quantitative and qualitative data, consists of inferences made regarding treatment. This inferential process needs to take into consideration not only the type(s) and the number of functional system(s) impaired, but also the nature, extent, and characteristics of the impairments (Reynolds & Mayfield, 1999; Riccio & Reynolds, 1998). This information is then integrated with similar information regarding the type(s), number, nature, and characteristics of the functional system(s) that remain intact. For example, intraindividual strengths or weaknesses in planning and concept formation skills, as well as other areas, will have an important impact on the long-term prognosis, in addition to providing important information for selecting intervention options (Reynolds & Mayfield, 1999).

The third component of the interpretive process is the report preparation. As noted by others (e.g., Kamphaus, 2001; Riccio & Reynolds, 1998), reports should be written in language that is easily understood by nonmedical persons; where jargon is unavoidable, concrete examples or explanations should be provided. The purpose of the report is to communicate the results to the child's parents, teachers, and others, as well as to provide information needed for the development of an appropriate program. The focus of the report should be on the child and the child's level of functioning, as opposed to tests. Results need to clearly address any academic, learning, or behavioral concerns and to reflect the child's instructional level. The report should provide a summation and integration of all the data presented and include any diagnostic conclusions. Finally, treatment implications should be provided by the neuropsychologist. Although the recommendations provided in the neuropsychological report relating to intervention programming may not be exhaustive, enough information should be provided to assist in developing appropriate interventions to meet the needs of the individual child.

SPECIAL CASE: TRAUMATIC BRAIN INJURY

For children with TBI, neuropsychological assessment is particularly important. Such children need a comprehensive evaluation of brain functioning that takes into consideration discrete impairment as well as more diffuse impairment, and that is sensitive to change over time (Ryan et al., 1996). The consequences of TBI in children are often underidentified and cannot be predicted well from the standard neurological examination (Boll, 1983). Ylvisaker (1985) made similar comments regarding the lack of recognition of deficits associated with TBI. The neuropsychological perspective allows for understanding of the connections between strengths and weaknesses, as well as the extent to which any given pattern is likely to remain stable or is subject to change over the course of development (Fletcher & Taylor, 1984; Temple, 1997). Many of the neuropsychological tests have been found to be sensitive to the subtle deficits associated with TBI (Ryan et al., 1996), and thus have much to offer in terms of informing rehabilitation planning. Diffuse impairment is also less likely to be evidenced on standard measures of cognitive ability or achievement, but it may have an impact on more complex cognitive functions (e.g., problem solving in novel situations), as well as on processing speed, ability to concentrate, and overall cognitive efficiency. Although more subtle than discrete deficits, these generalized deficits not only affect the child's immediate functioning level, but may also affect later development and the acquisition of new skills (Ryan et al., 1996).

Both the diffuse and generalized effects of TBI vary across individuals in terms of the number, nature, and severity of the deficits. This variability in deficit presentation precludes the use of a single measure for assessment or a single method for treatment. The interaction of a child's neuropsychological profile and the environments in which the child is required to function may have an impact on symptom presentation and chronicity. As with all children, neuropsychological assessment is useful in the identification of deficits as well as intact functional systems.

As pointed out by Ryan and colleagues (1996), the timing of the neuropsychological assessment needs to be considered in treatment planning. For children with TBI, the neuropsychological assessment optimally should be conducted prior to their reentry into the school setting, in order to assess strengths and identify areas of immediate need. For children with mild TBI who return to the school setting, even a standard psychoeducational evaluation may not be completed in a "timely" manner, due to the nature of the special education process. Anecdotally, the general practice in many school districts is to wait until a child with TBI is failing or in danger of failing (or, alternatively, the child's behavior has been problematic over time) prior to commencing the referral process; this is the course of events with other disability categories. Special education regulations require that the school district document the implementation of interventions within the regular education process over a period of time. It is only after various interventions have been implemented in the school setting without success that a child is referred for assessment. This can delay the assessment process for a child with TBI for an extended period of time, and the gap in time between the injury and the assessment can ultimately result in a misinterpretation of the results (Riccio & Reynolds, 1999). For example, it has been found that a number of children with TBI are subsequently classified as having a learning disability or other disorder (Ewing-Cobbs et al., 1986).

For these reasons, it has been recommended that whenever possible, the neuropsychological assessment be conducted efficiently and coordinated with a child's school district. It may be appropriate, for example, for school personnel (e.g., a school psychologist, a speech/language pathologist) to participate in the assessment process, thus reducing the financial strain on the school system. This type of collaborative effort can facilitate program planning for the child in the school setting. Early notification to the school district of the child's projected discharge date and timely assessment also allow the school district to prepare for the child's return to the school setting. This also facilitates necessary arrangements for any school-based direct or indirect service delivery for the child, as well as appropriate inservice programming for teachers and other school personnel if needed.

The fluctuation or variability in symptom presentation that is evident in children with TBI does not occur in most other disorders. Thus, for a child with TBI, the primary issue is not one of differential diagnosis or classification, but one of establishing postinjury baseline data and continually identifying strengths and weaknesses in neurocognitive as well as behavioral/emotional areas over time, in order to address the child's changing profile most appropriately. With repeated neuropsychological assessment, progress can be monitored, intervention methods can be evaluated, and changes in the pattern of symptomatology can be detected. The same methods can be used through adolescence to monitor the appropriate development of skills and abilities, based on the typical neurodevelopmental trajectory.

Unlike plans for children with other disabilities, the rehabilitation/treatment plan or individual educational plan for a child with TBI needs to be reassessed more frequently as a result of repeated evaluations (formal or informal) of the child's progress in previously identified deficit areas, as well as identification of additional areas of concern (Ball & Zinner, 1994; Ewing-Cobbs et al., 1986). Due to potentially rapid changes in brain function in children with TBI, it has been recommended that reassessment occur at least every 6–12 months (Boll & Stanford, 1997). Overall, neuropsychological assessment of children with TBI provides for the identification of strengths and weaknesses at a given point in the recovery and rehabilitation process, and the short-term assessment of treatment effects through careful psychometric monitoring of changes in neurocognition and behavior; it also allows for the long-term monitoring of expected neurodevelopmental progression and development of subsequent skills (Riccio & Reynolds, 1999).

SUMMARY

Neuropsychological assessment and the field of clinical child neuropsychology in general have much to offer in the way of understanding the learning and behavior problems of children and youths. Child neuropsychology provides a foundation for understanding the functional systems of the brain and the mechanisms involved in the learning and self-regulation process. The identification of patterns of strengths and weaknesses, the relationships between these strengths and weaknesses, and the extent to which these patterns may remain stable or are subject to change over time can be used to identify areas that may create difficulty for a child in the future, as well as compensatory strategies or methods to circumvent these difficulties (Fletcher & Taylor, 1984; Temple, 1997).

There are, however, continued problems with the application of neuropsychological practices and perspectives to child assessment. Historically, neuropsychological assessment of children has taken its lead from research and practice with adults (predominantly adults with acquired brain damage). Issues relating to neurodevelopmental trajectory, manifestation of developmental disorders over time, the varying contexts in which children function, and so on, render this continued approach inappropriate. Existing theoretical models are often used without consideration of developmental issues (Riccio & Reynolds, 1998). Further study of the linkage between neuropsychological assessment of children and the provision of information that is educationally relevant rather than medically focused for intervention planning is needed.

Continued methodological and measurement problems in the research that serves as a foundation for interpretation of neuropsychological data impede progress in the field of clinical child neuropsychology and detract from the accuracy of diagnosis (Riccio & Reynolds, 1998). Lack of attention to standard psychometric methods within the field of clinical child neuropsychology poses serious limitations to clinical practice (Reynolds, 1986b, 1997b). There is a need for continued research and attention to the psychometric properties of measures used in the neuropsychological assessment of children and youths.

REFERENCES

Allen, C. (1989). Why use neuropsychology in the schools? *The Neuro-Transmitter, 1,* 1–2.

Ardila, A., & Roselli, M. (1994). Development of language, memory, and visuospatial abilities in 5- to 12-year old children using a neuropsychological battery. *Developmental Neuropsychology, 10,* 97–120.

Arffa, S., Fitzhugh-Bell, K., & Black, F. W. (1989). Neuropsychological profiles of children with learning disabilities and children with documented brain damage. *Journal of Learning Disabilities, 22,* 635–640.

Ball, J. D., & Zinner, E. S. (1994). Pediatric brain injury: Psychoeducation for parents and teachers. *Advances in Medical Psychotherapy, 7,* 39–50.

Barkley, R. A. (1998). *Attention-deficit hyperactivity disorder* (2nd ed.). New York: Guilford Press.

Batchelor, E. S., Jr. (1996a). Introduction. In E. S. Batchelor, Jr., & R. S. Dean (Eds.), *Pediatric neuropsychology: Interfacing assessment and treatment for rehabilitation* (pp. 1–8). Boston: Allyn & Bacon.

Batchelor, E. S., Jr. (1996b). Neuropsychological assessment of children. In E. S. Batchelor, Jr., & R. S. Dean (Eds.), *Pediatric neuropsychology: Interfacing assessment and treatment for rehabilitation* (pp. 9–26). Boston: Allyn & Bacon.

Batchelor, E. S., Jr., Kixmiller, J. S., & Dean, R. S. (1990). Neuropsychological aspects of reading and spelling performance in children with learning disabilities. *Developmental Neuropsychology, 3,* 275–298.

Boll, T. J. (1983). Minor head injury in children—out of sight, but not out of mind. *Journal of Clinical Child Psychology, 12,* 74–80.

Boll, T. J. (1993). *The Children's Category Test.* San Antonio, TX: Psychological Corporation.

Boll, T. J., & Stanford, L. D. (1997). Pediatric brain injury: Brain mechanisms and amelioration. In C. R. Reynolds & E. Fletcher-Janzen (Eds.), *Handbook of clinical child neuropsychology* (2nd ed., pp. 140–156). New York: Plenum Press.

Bolter, J. F., & Long, C. J. (1985). Methodological issues in research in developmental neuropsychology. In L. Hartlage & C. Telzrow (Eds.), *The neuropsychology of individual differences* (pp. 42–60). New York: Plenum Press.

Branch, W. B., Cohen, M. J., & Hynd, G. W. (1995). Academic achievement and attention-deficit/hyperactivity disorder in children with left- or right-hemisphere dysfunction. *Journal of Learning Disabilities, 28,* 35–43.

Brink, J. D., Garrett, A. L., Hale, W. R., Woo-Sam, J., & Nickel, V. C. (1970). Recovery of motor and intellectual function in children sustaining severe head injuries. *Developmental Medicine and Child Neurology, 12,* 545–571.

Brunswick, N., McCrory, E., Price, C., Frith, C. D., & Frith, U. (1999). Explicit and implicit processing of words by adult developmental dyslexics: A search for Wernicke's *Wortschatz? Brain, 122,* 1901–1917.

Chadwick, O., Rutter, M., Brown, G., Shaffer, D., & Traub, M. (1981). A prospective study of children with head injuries: II. Cognitive sequelae. *Psychological Medicine, 11,* 49–61.

Chelune, G. J., & Thompson, L. L. (1987). Evaluation of the general sensitivity of the Wisconsin Card Sorting Test among younger and older children. *Developmental Neuropsychology, 3,* 81–89.

Christensen, A. L. (1975). *Luria's neuropsychological investigation.* New York: Spectrum.

Cicchetti, D. V. (1994). Multiple comparison methods: Establishing guidelines for their valid application in neuropsychological research. *Journal of Clinical and Experimental Neuropsychology, 16,* 155–161.

Cohen, M. J., Branch, W. B., Willis, W. G., Weyandt, L. L., & Hynd, G. W. (1992). Childhood. In A. E. Puente & R. J. McCaffrey (Eds.), *Handbook of neuropsychological assessment* (pp. 49–79). New York: Plenum Press.

Cohen, M. J., Riccio, C. A., & Hynd, G. W. (1999). Children with specific language impairment: Quantitative and qualitative analysis of dichotic listening performance. *Developmental Neuropsychology, 16,* 243–252.

D'Amato, R. C. (1990). A neuropsychological approach to school psychology. *School Psychology Quarterly, 5,* 141–160.

D'Amato, R. C., & Rothlisberg, B. A. (1996). How education should respond to students with traumatic brain injuries. *Journal of Learning Disabilities, 29,* 670–683.

D'Amato, R. C., Rothlisberg, B. A., & Rhodes, R. L. (1997). Utilizing neuropsychological paradigms for understanding common educational and psychological tests. In C. R. Reynolds & E. Fletcher-Janzen (Eds.), *Handbook of clinical child neuropsychology* (2nd ed., pp. 270–295). New York: Plenum Press.

Dean, R. S. (1986). Lateralization of cerebral functions. In D. Wedding, A. M. Horton, & J. S. Webster (Eds.), *The neuropsychology handbook: Behavioral and clinical perspectives* (pp. 80–102). Berlin: Springer-Verlag.

Dean, R. S., & Gray, J. W. (1990). Traditional approaches to neuropsychological assessment. In C. R. Reynolds & R. W. Kamphaus (Eds.), *Handbook of psychological and educational assessment of children: Intelligence and achievement* (pp. 317–388). New York: Guilford Press.

Delis, D. C., Kramer, J. H., & Kaplan, E. (2001). *Delis–Kaplan Executive Function System: technical manual.* San Antonio, TX: Psychological Corporation.

Delis, D. C., Kramer, J. H., Kaplan, E., & Ober, B. A. (1994). *CVLT-C (Children's California Verbal Learning Test): Manual.* San Antonio, TX: Psychological Corporation.

Denckla, M. B. (1994). Measurement of executive function. In G. R. Lyon (Ed.), *Frames of reference for the assessment of learning disabilities: New views on measurement* (pp. 117–142). Baltimore: Brookes.

Efron, R. (1990). *The decline and fall of hemispheric specialization.* Hillsdale, NJ: Erlbaum.

Eliason, M. J., & Richman, L. C. (1987). The continuous performance test in learning disabled and nondisabled children. *Journal of Learning Disabilities, 20,* 614–619.

Ewing-Cobbs, L., Fletcher, J. M., & Levin, H. S. (1986). Neurobehavioral sequelae following head injury in children: Educational implications. *Journal of Head Trauma Rehabilitation, 1*(4), 57–65.

Feagans, L. V., Short, E. J., & Meltzer, L. J. (1991). Subtypes of learning disabilities: Theoretical perspectives and research. Hillsdale, NJ: Erlbaum.

Fennell, E. B. (1994). Issues in child neuropsychological assessment. In R. Venderploeg (Ed.), *Clinician's* guide to neuropsychological assessment (pp. 165–184). Hillsdale, NJ: Erlbaum.

Fennell, E. B., & Bauer, R. M. (1997). Models of inference in evaluating brain–behavior relationships in children. In C. R. Reynolds & E. Fletcher-Janzen (Eds.), Handbook of clinical child neuropsychology (2nd ed., pp. 204–215). New York: Plenum Press.

Fletcher, J. M., & Taylor, H. G. (1984). Neuropsychological approaches to children: Toward a developmental neuropsychology. Journal of Clinical Neuropsychology, 6, 139–156.

Fletcher-Janzen, E., & Kade, H. D. (1997). Pediatric brain injury rehabilitation in a neurodevelopmental milieu. In C. R. Reynolds & E. Fletcher-Janzen (Eds.), Handbook of clinical child neuropsychology (pp. 452–481). New York: Plenum Press.

Franzen, M. (2000). Reliability and validity in neuropsychological assessment (2nd ed.). New York: Kluwer.

Gaddes, W. H., & Edgell, D. (1994). Learning disabilities and brain function: A neurodevelopmental approach. New York: Springer-Verlag.

Geary, D. C., & Gilger, J. W. (1984). The Luria–Nebraska Neuropsychological Battery—Children's Revision: Comparison of learning disabled and normal children matched on Full Scale IQ. Perceptual and Motor Skills, 58, 115–118.

Gillberg, C. (1995). Clinical child neuropsychiatry. Cambridge, England: Cambridge University Press.

Golden, C. J. (1981). The Luria–Nebraska children's battery: Theory and formulation. In G. W. Hynd & J. E. Obrzut (Eds.), Neuropsychological assessment and the school-age child: Issues and procedures (pp. 277–302). New York: Grune & Stratton.

Golden, C. J. (1984). Luria–Nebraska Neuropsychological Battery: Children's Revision. Los Angeles, CA: Western Psychological Services.

Golden, C. J. (1997). The Nebraska Neuropsychological Children's Battery. In C. R. Reynolds & E. Fletcher-Janzen (Eds.), Handbook of clinical child neuropsychology (2nd ed., pp. 237–251). New York: Plenum Press.

Goldman, P. S., & Lewis, M. E. (1978). Developmental biology of brain damage and experience. In C. W. Cotman (Ed.), Neuronal plasticity. New York: Raven Press.

Goldman-Rakic, P. S. (1987). Development of cortical circuitry and cognitive function. Child Development, 58, 601–622.

Goldstein, G. (1997). The clinical utility of standardized or flexible battery approaches to neuropsychological assessment. In G. Goldstein & T. M. Incagnoli (Eds.), Contemporary approaches to neuropsychological assessment (pp. 67–92). New York: Plenum Press.

Gray, J. A. (1982). The neuropsychology of anxiety: An enquiry into the functions of the septo-hippocampal system. Oxford: Oxford University Press.

Gray, J. W., & Dean, R. S. (1990). Implications of neuropsychological research for school psychology. In T. B. Gutkin & C. R. Reynolds (Eds.), The handbook of school psychology (pp. 269–288). New York: Wiley.

Haak, R. A. (1989). Establishing neuropsychology in a school setting: Organization, problems, and benefits. In C. R. Reynolds & E. Fletcher-Janzen (Eds.), Handbook of clinical child neuropsychology (pp. 489–502). New York: Plenum Press.

Halperin, J. M. (1991). The clinical assessment of attention. International Journal of Neuroscience, 58, 171–182.

Halperin, J. M., McKay, K. E., Matier, K., & Sharma, V. (1994). Attention, response inhibition, and activity level in children: Developmental neuropsychological perspectives. In M. G. Tramontana & S. R. Hooper (Eds.), Advances in child neuropsychology (Vol. 2, pp. 1–54). New York: Springer-Verlag.

Harris, P. (1957). Head injuries in childhood. Archives of Disease in Childhood, 6, 488–491.

Hartlage, L. C., & Long, C. J. (1997). Development of neuropsychology as a professional specialty: History, training, and credentialing. In C. R. Reynolds & E. Fletcher-Janzen (Eds.), Handbook of clinical child neuropsychology (2nd ed., pp. 3–16). New York: Plenum Press.

Hartlage, L. C., & Telzrow, C. F. (1983). The neuropsychological basis of educational intervention. Journal of Learning Disabilities, 16, 521–528.

Heaton, R. K. (1981). A manual for the Wisconsin Card Sorting Test. Odessa, FL: Psychological Assessment Resources.

Hiscock, M., & Kinsbourne, M. (1987). Specialization of the cerebral hemispheres: Implications for learning. Journal of Learning Disabilities, 20, 130–143.

Hooper, S. R., & Tramontana, M. G. (1997). Advances in neuropsychological bases of child and adolescent psychopathology: Proposed models, findings, and on-going issues. Advances in Clinical Child Psychology, 19, 133–175.

Howieson, D. B., & Lezak, M. D. (1992). The neuropsychological evaluation. In S. C. Yudofsky & R. E. Hales (Eds.), The American Psychiatric Press textbook of neuropsychiatry (2nd ed., pp. 127–150). Washington, DC: American Psychiatric Press.

Hynd, G. W. (1981). Neuropsychology in the schools. School Psychology Review, 10, 480–486.

Hynd, G. W., & Willis, W. G. (1988). Pediatric neuropsychology. New York: Grune & Stratton.

Kamphaus, R. W. (2001). Clinical assessment of children's intelligence (2nd ed.). Boston: Allyn & Bacon.

Kamphaus, R. W., & Frick, P. J. (2002). Clinical assessment of child and adolescent personality and behavior (2nd ed.). Boston: Allyn & Bacon.

Kaplan, E. (1988). A process approach to neuropsychological assessment. In T. Boll & B. K. Bryant (Eds.), Clinical neuropsychology and brain function (pp. 125–167). Washington, DC: American Psychological Association.

Kaplan, E. (1990). The process approach to neuropsychological assessment of psychiatric patients. Journal of Neuropsychiatry, 2(1), 72–87.

Kinsbourne, M. (1989). A model of adaptive behavior related to cerebral participation in emotional control. In G. Gainotti & C. Caltagirone (Eds.), Emotions and the dual brain (pp. 248–260). New York: Springer-Verlag.

Kemp, S. L., Kirk, U., & Korkman, M. (2001). Essentials of NEPSY assessment. New York: Wiley.

Klenberg, L., Korkman, M., & Lahti-Nuuttila, P. (2001). Differential development of attention and excutive functions in 3- to 12-year old Finnish children. *Developmental Neuropsychology, 20,* 407–428.

Kolb, B., & Whishaw, I. Q. (1996). *Fundamentals of human neuropsychology* (4th ed.). New York: Freeman.

Korkman, M., & Häkkinen-Rihu, P. (1994). A new classification of developmental language disorders. *Brain and Language, 47*(1), 96–116.

Korkman, M., Kirk, U., & Kemp, S. (1998). *NEPSY: A developmental neuropsychological assessment.* San Antonio, TX: Psychological Corporation.

Korkman, M., Kirk, U., & Kemp, S. (2001). Effects of age on neurocognitive measures of children ages 5 to 12: A cross-sectional study on 800 children from the United States. *Developmental Neuropsychology, 20,* 331–354.

Lezak, M. D. (1986). Psychological implications of traumatic brain damage for the patient's family. *Rehabilitation Psychology, 31,* 241–250.

Lezak, M. D. (1995). *Neuropsychological assessment* (3rd ed.). New York: Oxford University Press.

Luria, A. R. (1973). *The working brain.* New York: Basic Books.

Luria, A. R. (1980). *Higher cortical functions in man* (2nd ed.). New York: Basic Books.

Merola, J. L., & Leiderman, J. (1985). The effect of task difficulty upon the extent to which performance benefits from between hemisphere division of inputs. *International Journal of Neuroscience, 51,* 35–44.

Miller, L. T., & Vernon, P. A. (1996). Intelligence, reaction time, and working memory in 4- to 6-year-old children. *Intelligence, 22,* 155–190.

Mitrushina, M. N., Boone, K. B., & D'Elia, L. F. (1999). *Handbook of normative data for neuropsychological assessment.* New York: Oxford University Press.

Moffitt, T. E. (1993). The neuropsychology of conduct disorder. *Developmental Psychopathology, 5,* 135–151.

Molfese, D. L. (1995). Electrophysiological responses obtained during infancy and their relation to later language development: Further findings. In M. G. Tramontana & S. R. Hooper (Eds.), *Advances in child neuropsychology* (Vol. 3, pp. 1–11). New York: Springer-Verlag.

Morgan, S. B., & Brown, T. L. (1988). Luria–Nebraska Neuropsychological Battery—Children's Revision: Concurrent validity with three learning disability subtypes. *Journal of Consulting and Clinical Psychology, 56,* 463–466.

Morris, R. (1994). Multidimensional neuropsychological assessment models. In G. R. Lyon (Ed.), *Frames of reference for the assessment of learning disabilities: New views on measurement* (pp. 515–522). Baltimore: Brookes.

Nussbaum, N. L., & Bigler, E. D. (1997). Halstead–Reitan Neuropsychological Test Batteries for Children. In C. R. Reynolds & E. Fletcher-Janzen (Eds.), *Handbook of clinical child neuropsychology* (2nd ed., pp. 219–236). New York: Plenum Press.

Nussbaum, N. L., Bigler, E. D., Koch, W. R., Ingram, J. W., Rosa, L., & Massman, P. (1988). Personality/behavioral characteristics in children: Differential effects of putative anterior versus posterior cerebral asymmetry. *Archives of Clinical Neuropsychology, 3,* 127–135.

Parsons, O. A., & Prigatano, G. P. (1978). Methodological considerations in clinical neuropsychological research. *Journal of Consulting and Clinical Psychology, 46,* 608–619.

Passler, M., Isaac, W., & Hynd, G. W. (1985). Neuropsychological development of behavior attributed to frontal lobe functioning in children. *Developmental Neuropsychology, 1,* 349–370.

Pugh, K., Mencl, W., Shaywitz, B., Shaywitz, S., Fulbright, R., Constable, R., Skudlarksi, P., Marchione, K., Jenner, A., Fletcher, J., Liberman, A., Shankweiler, D., Katz, L., Lacadie, C., & Gore, J. (2000). The angular gyrus in developmental dyslexia: Task specific differences in functional connectivity within the posterior cortex. *Psychological Science, 11,* 51–56.

Ramsey, M. C., & Reynolds, C. R. (1995). Separate digits tests: A brief history, a literature review, and re-examination of the factor structure of the Test of Memory and Learning (TOMAL). *Neuropsychology Review, 5,* 151–171.

Reitan, R. M. (1969). *Manual for the administration of neuropsychological test batteries for adults and children.* Indianapolis, IN: Author.

Reitan, R. M. (1986). *Theoretical and methodological bases of the Halstead–Reitan Neuropsychological Test Battery.* Tucson, AZ: Neuropsychological Press.

Reitan, R. M. (1987). *Neuropsychological evaluation of children.* Tucson, AZ: Neuropsychological Press.

Reitan, R. M., & Davison, L. A. (Eds.). (1974). *Clinical neuropsychology: Current status and applications.* New York: Wiley.

Reitan, R. M., & Wolfson, D. (1985). *The Halstead–Reitan Neuropsychological Battery: Theory and clinical interpretation.* Tucson, AZ: Neuropsychological Press.

Reitan, R. M., & Wolfson, D. (1988). The Halstead–Reitan Neuropsychological Test Battery and REHABIT: A model for integrating evaluation and remediation of cognitive impairment. *Cognitive Rehabilitation, 6,* 10–17.

Restrepo, M. A., Swisher, L., Plante, E., & Vance, R. (1992). Relations among verbal and nonverbal cognitive skills in normal language and specifically language impaired children. *Journal of Communication Disorders, 25,* 205–220.

Reynolds, C. R. (1981). The neuropsychological basis of intelligence. In G. W. Hynd & J. E. Obrzut (Eds.), *Neuropsychological assessment and the school-aged child: Issues and procedures* (pp. 87–124). New York: Grune & Stratton.

Reynolds, C. R. (1982). The importance of norms and other traditional psychometric concepts to assessment in clinical neuropsychology. In R. N. Malathesha & L. C. Hartlage (Eds.), *Neuropsychology and cognition* (Vol. 3, pp. 55–76). The Hague: Nijhoff.

Reynolds, C. R. (1986a). Clinical acumen but psychometric naivete in neuropsychological assessment of educational disorders. *Archives of Clinical Neuropsychology, 1*(2), 121–137.

Reynolds, C. R. (1986b). Transactional models of intellectual development, yes. Deficit models of process remediation, no. *School Psychology Review, 15,* 256–260.

Reynolds, C. R. (1997a). Forward and backward memory span should not be combined for clinical analysis. *Archives of Clinical Neuropsychology, 12,* 29–40.

Reynolds, C. R. (1997b). Measurement and statistical problems in neuropsychological assessment of children. In C. R. Reynolds & E. Fletcher-Janzen (Eds.), *Handbook of clinical child neuropsychology* (2nd ed., pp. 180–203). New York: Plenum Press.

Reynolds, C. R., & Bigler, E. D. (1997). Clinical neuropsychological assessment of child and adolescent memory with the Test of Memory and Learning. In C. R. Reynolds & E. Fletcher-Janzen (Eds.), *Handbook of clinical child neuropsychology* (2nd ed., pp. 296–319). New York: Plenum Press.

Reynolds, C. R., & Hickman, J. A. (1987). Remediation: Deficit-centered models. In C. R. Reynolds & L. Mann (Eds.), *Encyclopedia of special education* (pp. 1339–1342). New York: Wiley–Interscience.

Reynolds, C. R., & Kamphaus, R. W. (1992). *Behavior Assessment System for Children.* Circle Pines, MN: American Guidance Service.

Reynolds, C. R., Kamphaus, R. W., Rosenthal, B. L., & Hiemenz, J. R. (1997). Application of the Kaufman Assessment Battery for Children (K-ABC) in neuropsychological assessment. In C. R. Reynolds & E. Fletcher-Janzen (Eds.), *Handbook of clinical child neuropsychology* (2nd ed., pp. 252–269). New York: Plenum Press.

Reynolds, C. R., & Mayfield, J. W. (1999). Neuropsychological assessment in genetically linked neurodevelopmental disorders. In S. Goldstein & C. R. Reynolds (Eds.), *Handbook of neurodevelopmental and genetic disorders in children.* New York: Guilford Press.

Riccio, C. A., Gonzalez, J. J., & Hynd, G. W. (1994). Attention-deficit hyperactivity disorder (ADHD) and learning disabilities. *Learning Disability Quarterly, 17,* 311–322.

Riccio, C. A., Hall, J., Morgan, A., Hynd, G. W., Gonzalez, J. J., & Marshall, R. M. (1994). Executive function and the Wisconsin Card Sorting Test: Relationship with behavioral ratings and cognitive ability. *Developmental Neuropsychology, 10,* 215–229.

Riccio, C. A., & Hynd, G. W. (1996). Neuroanatomical and neurophysiological aspects of dyslexia. *Topics in Language Disorders, 16*(2), 1–13.

Riccio, C. A., Hynd, G. W., & Cohen, M. J. (1993). Neuropsychology in the schools: Does it belong? *School Psychology International, 14,* 291–315.

Riccio, C. A., Hynd, G. W., & Cohen, M. J. (1996). Etiology and neurobiology of attention-deficit hyperactivity disorder. In W. Bender (Ed.), *Understanding ADHD: A practical guide for teachers and parents* (pp. 23–44). Columbus, OH: Merrill.

Riccio, C. R., & Reynolds, C. R. (1998). Neuropsychological assessment of children. In M. Hersen &

A. Bellack (Series Eds.) & C. R. Reynolds (Vol. Ed.), *Comprehensive clinical psychology: Vol. 4. Assessment* (pp. 267–301). New York: Elsevier.

Riccio, C. A., & Reynolds, C. R. (1999). Assessment of traumatic brain injury in children for neuropsychological rehabilitation. In M. Raymond, T. L. Bennett, L. Hartlage, & C. M. Cullum (Eds.), *Mild brain injury: A clinician's guide* (pp. 77–116). Austin, TX: Pro-Ed.

Riccio, C. R., Reynolds, C. R., & Lowe, P. A. (2001). *Clinical applications of continuous performance tests: Measuring attention and impulsive responding in children and adults.* New York: Wiley.

Ris, M. D., & Noll, R. B. (1994). Long-term neurobehavioral outcome in pediatric brain-tumor patients: Review and methodological critique. *Journal of Clinical and Experimental Neuropsychology, 16,* 21–42.

Rothlisberg, B. A., & D'Amato, R. C. (1988). Increased neuropsychological understanding seen as important for school psychologists. *Communique, 17*(2), 4–5.

Rourke, B. P. (1989). *Nonverbal learning disabilities: The syndrome and the model.* New York: Guilford Press.

Rourke, B. P. (1994). Neuropsychological assessment of children with learning disabilities: Measurement issues. In G. R. Lyon (Ed.), *Frames of reference for the assessment of learning disabilities: New views on measurement issues* (pp. 475–514). Baltimore: Brookes.

Rutter, M. (1981). Psychological sequelae of brain damage in children. *American Journal of Clinical Neuropsychology, 138,* 1533–1544.

Ryan, T. V., LaMarche, J. A., Barth, J. T., & Boll, T. J. (1996). Neuropsychological consequences and treatment of pediatric head trauma. In E. S. Batchelor, Jr., & R. S. Dean (Eds.), *Pediatric neuropsychology: Interfacing assessment and treatment for rehabilitation* (pp. 117–137). Boston: Allyn & Bacon.

Satz, P., & Fletcher, J. M. (1981). Emergent trends in neuropsychology: An overview. *Journal of Consulting and Clinical Psychology, 49,* 851–865.

Semrud-Clikeman, M., Kamphaus, R. W., Teeter, P. A., & Vaughn, M. (1997). Assessment of behavior and personality in neuropsychological diagnosis of children. In C. R. Reynolds & E. Fletcher-Janzen (Eds.) *Handbook of clinical child neuropsychology* (2nd ed., pp. 320–341). New York: Plenum Press.

Shaw, S. R., & Yingst, C. A. (1992). Assessing children with traumatic brain injuries: Integrating educational and medical issues. *Diagnostique, 17,* 255–265.

Shields, J., Varley, R., Broks, P., & Simpson, A. (1996). Hemisphere function in developmental language disorders and high level autism. *Developmental Medicine and Child Neurology, 38,* 473–486.

Shurtleff, H. A., Fay, G. E., Abbott, R. D., & Berninger, V. W. (1988). Cognitive and neuropsychological correlates of academic achievement: A levels of analysis assessment model. *Journal of Psychoeducational Assessment, 6,* 298–308.

Snow, J. H., & Hooper, S. R. (1994). *Pediatric traumatic brain injury.* Thousand Oaks, CA: Sage.

Snow, J. H., & Hynd, G. W. (1985). A multivariate investigation of the Luria–Nebraska Neuropsychological Battery—Children's Revision with learning disabled children. *Journal of Psychoeducational Assessment, 2,* 23–28.

Stinnett, T. A., Oehler-Stinnett, J., Fuqua, S. R., & Palmer, L. S. (2002). Examination of the underlying structure of the NEPSY: A developmental neuropsychological assessment. *Journal of Psychoeducational Assessment, 20,* 66–82.

Strom, D. A., Gray, J. W., Dean, R. S., & Fischer, W. E. (1987). Incremental validity of the Halstead–Reitan Neuropsychological Battery in predicting achievement for learning disabled children. *Journal of Psychoeducational Assessment, 5,* 157–165.

Stuss, D. T., & Levine, B. (2002). Adult clinical neuropsychology: Lessons from studies of the frontal lobes. *Annual Review of Psychology, 53,* 401–433.

Talley, J. L. (1986). Memory in learning disabled children: Digit span and the Rey Auditory Verbal Learning Test. *Archives of Clinical Neuropsychology, 1,* 315–322.

Taylor, H. G., & Fletcher, J. M. (1990). Neuropsychological assessment of children. In G. Goldstein & M. Hersen (Eds.), *Handbook of neuropsychological assessment* (pp. 228–255). New York: Plenum Press.

Teeter, P. A. (1997). Neurocognitive interventions for childhood and adolescent disorders: A transactional model. In C. R. Reynolds & E. Fletcher-Janzen (Eds.), *Handbook of clinical child neuropsychology* (2nd ed., pp. 387–417). New York: Plenum Press.

Teeter, P. A., & Semrud-Clikeman, M. (1997). *Child neuropsychology: Assessment and interventions for neurodevelopmental disorders.* Boston: Allyn & Bacon.

Temple, C. M. (1997). Cognitive neuropsychology and its application to children. *Journal of Child Psychology and Psychiatry, 38,* 27–52.

Tomblin, J. B., Records, N. L., Buckwalter, P., Zhang, X., Smith, E., & O'Brien, M. (1997). Prevalence of specific language impairment in kindergarten children. *Journal of Speech, Language, and Hearing Research, 40,* 1245–1260.

Torkelson, R. D., Leibrook, L. G., Gustavson, J. L., & Sundell, R. R. (1985). Neurological and neuropsy-chological effects of cerebral spinal fluid shunting in children with assumed arrested ("normal pressure") hydrocephalus. *Journal of Neurology, Neurosurgery and Psychiatry, 48,* 799–806.

Tramontana, M., & Hooper, S. (1997). Neuropsychology of child psychopathology. In C. R. Reynolds & E. Fletcher-Janzen (Eds.), *Handbook of clinical child neuropsychology* (2nd ed., pp. 120–139). New York: Plenum Press.

Tramontana, M., Hooper, S. R., Curley, A. S., & Nardolillo, E. M. (1990). Determinants of academic achievement in children with psychiatric disorders. *Journal of the American Academy of Child and Adolescent Psychiatry, 29,* 265–268.

Trauner, D. A., Ballantyne, A., Chase, C., & Tallal, P. (1993). Comprehension and expression of affect in language-impaired children. *Journal of Psycholinguistic Research, 22,* 445–452.

Wechsler, D. (1989). *The Wechsler Preschool and Primary Scale of Intelligence—Revised.* San Antonio, TX: Psychological Corporation.

Wechsler, D. (1991). *The Wechsler Intelligence Scale for Children—Third Edition.* San Antonio, TX: Psychological Corporation.

Whitten, C. J., D'Amato, R. C., & Chitooran, M. M. (1992). The neuropsychological approach to interventions. In R. C. D'Amato & B. A Rothlisberg (Eds.), *Psychological perspectives on intervention: A case study approach to prescriptions for change* (pp. 112–136). New York: Longman.

Woodcock, R. W., McGrew, K. S., & Mather, N. (2001). *Woodcock–Johnson Third Edition: Tests of Achievement.* Itasca, IL: Riverside.

Ylvisaker, M. (1985). *Head injury rehabilitation: Children and adolescents.* San Diego, CA: College Hill Press.

Zelazo, P. D., Carter, A., Reznick, J. S., & Frye, D. (1997). Early development of executive functions: A problem-solving framework. *Review of General Psychology, 1*(2), 198–226.

Zillmer, E. A., & Spiers, M. V. (2002). *Principles of neuropsychology.* Belmont, CA: Wadsworth/Thomson Learning.

14

Biological Approaches to the Assessment of Human Intelligence

GILLES E. GIGNAC
PHILIP A. VERNON

Although intelligence testing is one of psychology's most lucrative enterprises, the construct itself remains one of the most controversial (e.g., Herrnstein & Murray, 1994) and hotly debated (Eysenck, 1981). This appears true in regard not only to its predictive utility, but also to attempts to define the construct. Eysenck (1993) argued that "research into the biological foundations of intelligence is a prerequisite for the scientific acceptance of the concept" (p. 8). From a neuroscientific perspective, 100% of behavior is regarded to be mediated by the nervous system 100% of the time (Kandel, 1998). Thus, if one can infer a subject's completion of an intelligence test as behavior, one would have to conclude that the behavior was neurophysiologically mediated. It is therefore likely that the "biological foundations" mentioned by Eysenck reside in the nervous system.

Several parameters of the nervous system have been studied as possible mediators of intelligence (Vernon, 1993). The most extensively studied are brain size, neuroelectricity, nerve conduction velocity, and metabolic activity. By reviewing and discussing the literature, we hope to make it apparent that the area of neurophysiology and intelligence can make a substantial contribution to the understanding of intelligence and may very well help define it.

BRAIN VOLUME AND IQ

The human has the largest brain (in relation to body size) among all species. Averaging 1,450 g at age 25 (Ho, Roessmann, Straumfjord, & Monroe, 1980), it is three times larger than an average chimpanzee brain (Haug, 1987). Considering this conspicuous difference, it should come as no surprise that the first stream of research in the biology of intelligence attempted to establish a relationship between head perimeter and cognitive ability. According to Vernon, Wickett, Bazana, and Stelmack's (2000) review of the literature, a correlation of .20 exists between head size and intelligence. As has been noted by others (e.g., Peters, 1993), head size as a proxy of brain volume has its limitations. For instance, the correlation between head size and intelligence is only approximately .70 (Wickett, 1997). This limitation, among others, has been overcome by the advent of magnetic resonance imaging (MRI) technology, which has allowed for precise *in vivo* quantification of brain volume and estimation of IQ within a short period of time before or after brain imaging.

Our search of the literature revealed 11 studies of total brain volume (MRI) and IQ that have been conducted on neurologically normal individuals (see Table 14.1). These 11 studies exclude research based on psychiatric patients or persons with mental retardation, as well as studies that did not use a well-established standardized measure of intelligence. With one exception (Tramo et al., 1998), all have found statistically significant positive correlations between brain volume and IQ, suggesting convincingly that individuals with larger brains tend also to be more intelligent.

Willerman, Schultz, Rutledge, and Bigler (1991) were the first to test the hypothesis that there would be a positive relationship between brain volume and IQ in normal individuals. They strategically selected their sample (*n* = 40) to include a group with above-average IQs (>130) and a group with average IQs (<103), based on the Wechsler Adult Intelligence Scale—Revised (WAIS-R). They obtained a corrected-for-extreme-groups positive correlation of .35 between brain volume and Full Scale IQ (FSIQ). Once the researchers controlled for gender, there were no statistically significant correlations between weight or height and brain volume.

Furthermore, the correlation between brain size and IQ did not change appreciably when body size was controlled for.

In the study by Raz and colleagues (1993), 29 adults had their brain volume estimated, as well as their IQ assessed (via the Culture Fair Intelligence Test, or CFIT). Total brain volume correlated with IQ at .43. Furthermore, the residual from subtracting the right-hemisphere volume from the left correlated with IQ at .46. This correlation remained significant after age, sex, and head size (correlates of brain size) were controlled for—a finding suggesting that brain size and hemispheric asymmetry are independent correlates of IQ. Unfortunately, no specific multiple *R* was estimated with brain volume and hemispheric asymmetry as predictors of IQ; however, there is an indication that brain volume asymmetry may be a unique correlate of IQ, possibly indicating hemispheric specialization, since handedness has been correlated with cerebellar volume asymmetry (Snyder, Bilder, Wu, Bodgerts, & Lieberman, 1995).

In a sample of 48 healthy adults, Egan and colleagues (1994) found a correlation of .32 between brain volume and IQ (WAIS-R). When corrected for restriction in range, the correlation rose to .48 (Egan, Wickett, & Vernon, 1995). A serendipitous correlation of .40 was found between amount of cerebrospinal fluid (CSF) volume and IQ;

TABLE 14.1. Studies of Brain Volume and IQ, Using Neurologically Normal Subjects and Established Psychometric Tests

Study	*n*	Age characteristics	IQ test[a]	*r*[b]
Willerman et al. (1991)	40	Mean = 18.9 (*SD* = 0.6)	WAIS-R	.35
Andreason et al. (1993)	67	Mean = 38 (*SD* = 16)	WAIS-R	.38
Raz et al. (1993)	29	Mean = 43.8 (*SD* = 21.5)	CFIT	.43
Egan et al. (1994)	48	Mean = 22.5 (*SD* = 5)	WAIS-R	.32 (.48)
Wickett et al. (1994)	40	Range = 20–30	MAB	.40 (.54)
Reiss et al. (1996)	69	Range = 5–17	WISC-R[c]	.40
Flashman et al. (1998)	90	Mean = 27 (*SD* = 10)	WAIS-R	.25 (.31)[d]
Tramo et al. (1998)	20	Median = 34 (24–43)	WAIS-R	−.05
Gur et al. (1999)	80	Mean = 26 (*SD* = 5.5)	Various	.41
Tan et al. (1999)	103	Range = 18–26	CFIT	.40
Wickett & Vernon (2000)	68	Range = 20–35	MAB	.35 (.51)

Note. Total *n* = 654; unweighted mean *r* = .33 (.38) for all studies; *n*-weighted mean *r* = .35 (.40) for all studies.
[a]WAIS-R, Wechsler Adult Intelligence Scale—Revised; CFIT, Culture Free Intelligence Test; MAB, Multidimensional Aptitude Battery; WISC-R, Wechsler Intelligence Scale for Children—Revised.
[b]Correlations in parantheses are corrected for restriction in IQ score range.
[c]Reiss (personal communication, 2000).
[d]Corrected for restriction in IQ score range by Gignac, according to Guilford and Fruchter (1978).

this correlation rose to .58 when corrected for restriction in range (Egan et al., 1995). Furthermore, brain volume and CSF were found to be largely independent, correlating at only .30. The possible implication of this result will be discussed below.

The correlation between brain volume and IQ does not appear limited to adults. In Reiss, Abrams, Singer, Ross, and Denckla's (1996) study, children ages 5–17 had their brain volumes and IQs estimated (n = 69). Reiss and colleagues found a correlation of .40 between brain volume and IQ, once they controlled for gender and age. Age did not have an appreciable effect on the correlation, because there was no correlation between age and brain size. A lack of a correlation between brain volume and age in this sample should come as no surprise, since 92% of adult brain weight is achieved by age 6 (Ho et al., 1980). The fact that children and adults possess brain volumes of a similar magnitude is important, because it stresses that brain size is only one neurophysiological substrate of intelligence. That is, although 6-year-olds possess brains 92% the size of adults', they do not possess the intellectual capacity of healthy adults. Reiss and colleagues did find, however, a negative correlation of –.44 between age and grey matter volume, and a positive correlation of .40 between age and white matter volume. Perhaps there is an optimal ratio of grey to white matter volume that is most conducive to intellectual functioning. This optimal ratio may be achieved between the ages of 20 to 29—when adults perform best on IQ tests (Wechsler, 1997), and when their brain weight is known to be largely stable (Ho et al., 1980). It is known that after the age of 30, brain weight decreases at a rate of approximately 2 g a year (Ho et al., 1980), largely due to grey matter atrophy; this coincides with a corresponding decrease in IQ (Wechsler, 1997).

The only study (Tramo et al., 1998) not to find a relationship between brain volume and IQ in healthy subjects probably suffered from a lack of statistical power. This study was based on a sample of 20 subjects, but the sample size should be regarded as closer to 10, because the sample was made up of 10 monozygotic twin pairs.

The remarkable consistency of the correlations between brain volume and IQ is probably attributable to the small amount of measurement error involved in estimating brain volume with MRI and estimating IQ with an established psychometric test. Future directions in research may concentrate on establishing a valid method of estimating cortical surface area, rather than simply measuring brain volume. Although humans' brains are three times larger than those of chimpanzees, they have four times the cortical surface area (Haug, 1987). Moreover, the correlation between brain volume and cortical surface area within humans has been estimated to be as low as .59 (Haug, 1987). A possible explanation for Egan and colleagues' (1994) finding of a positive correlation between CSF and IQ is that CSF may be considered a proxy of cortical surface area, because the CSF within the subarachnoid space envelopes the brain's sulci and gyri (Egan et al., 1995).

THE ELECTROENCEPHALOGRAM AND IQ

The electroencephalogram (EEG) allows for the estimation of the sum of excitatory and inhibitory postsynaptic potentiation from a cluster of neurons, particularly those residing in the neocortex (Martin, 1991). The neuroelectrical activity is detected by either one or many electrodes placed on the subject's scalp. There are two primary methods of measuring neuroelectrical activity: (1) spontaneous activity, consisting of quantifying the frequency or amplitude of the oscillatory activity within a particular band (e.g, alpha [8–13 Hz]); and (2) evoked potentials (EPs), consisting of averaging the brain's neuroelectrical response to briefly presented stimuli.

The first alpha frequency study (Mundy-Castle, 1958) to use neurologically normal adult subjects and an established IQ test (n = 34) found a correlation of .51 between alpha frequency and FSIQ (Wechsler–Bellevue Adult Intelligence Test). The correlations with Verbal IQ (VIQ) and Performance IQ (PIQ) were of similar magnitude at .42 and .40, respectively. The mean age of the subjects was 24 (SD = 6), thus the vast majority were adults. This indicates that developmental maturation would not be a plausible explanation for the effect, since alpha frequency is known to be positively correlated with age in samples of children. Furthermore, only 2 of the 11 subtests, Conprehension (.59) and Vocabulary (.36), were significantly correlated with age. Finally, no statistically significant correlation was found between age and alpha frequency. Thus the obtained correlation of .51 between FSIQ and alpha frequency should not be discounted by maturational processes. These results were replicated in a follow-up study (Mundy-Castle & Nelson, 1960).

In a more recent and sophisticated study (Lutzenberg, Birbaumer, Flor, Rockstroh, & Elbert, 1992), it was hypothesized that a positive correlation would exist between the dimensionality (complexity) of the EEG pattern and IQ. This study was novel because the EEG data were analyzed using nonlinear dynamics, as opposed to linear dynamics, which are based on deterministic chaos theories (Lutzenberg et al., 1992). Effectively, the application of nonlinear dynamics is considered a means of quantifying competition among neural assemblies. Competition among the neural assemblies is associated with an EEG pattern of greater complexity. The subjects' EEG patterns were measured under two conditions: resting and imagery scenes. A correlation of .48 was found between dimensional complexity and IQ during the resting condition, indicating more neural competition among neurons in individuals with higher IQs. No relationship was found during the imagination condition. The authors replicated this effect in a second study reported in the same article. These results were interpreted to suggest that the neurons of persons with lower IQs tend to be activated in a more synchronous manner during rest, whereas the neurons of people with higher IQs manifest greater neural variability (i.e., neural activity). It is interesting to note that during the imagination task, the group with lower IQs showed a large increase in dimensional complexity, while the group with higher IQs showed a trend toward a decrease in dimensional complexity. Would this trend continue, such that the subjects with lower IQs would manifest greater neural activity during an intellectual problem-solving task (as opposed to simply imagining), in comparison to the subjects with higher IQs? Indirect support for this hypothesis has been provided by a study (Jausovec, 1996) comparing

intellectually gifted and average subjects during ill- and well-defined problem-solving tasks. During the later portion of the tasks (i.e., the actual problem solving), the gifted subjects manifested greater alpha power (ill-defined = 27%, well-defined = 18%) than the subjects with average IQs. Greater alpha power was interpreted to suggest lesser mental effort. Thus the results of these studies combined suggest that there is a negative relationship between neural assembly competition and degree of mental "stress" in individuals with higher IQs, whereas the opposite relationship appears to hold true for individuals with lower IQs. This interaction effect based on ability has been found in other EEG studies, particularly those studying cerebral asymmetry (see below). The extent to which this interaction pervades the literature on spontaneous EEG activity and IQ is probably not minimal and may explain the inconsistent results.

The first study of EPs and IQ consisted of the presentation of brief flashes of light at random intervals to adults whose IQs ranged from superior to mentally retarded (Chalke & Ertl, 1965). It was found that the group with superior IQs displayed shorter latencies in the later components of the EP (>200 milliseconds) than the group with average IQs. Furthermore, the group with average IQs also displayed shorter latencies in the later components of the EP than the group with mental retardation. Thus the weight of the effect was not due to the inclusion of the adults with mental retardation; rather, a linear trend from low to high IQ appeared to exist between EP latency and IQ. In a follow-up study (Ertl & Schafer, 1969), a correlation of −.35 was found between EP latency and IQ (Otis) in a sample of primary school children ($n = 573$). These effects were interpreted to suggest that intelligence is positively associated with the speed with which a person can process information. A shorter latency period may indicate faster processing capacity.

A resurgence of research interest in EPs and intelligence was initiated by Hendrickson and Hendrickson (1980), who proposed a new method of calibrating an EP: the "string measure." In a sample of 61 male and 32 female students, auditory EPs (AEPs) were induced by brief tones at three intensity levels (60, 80, and 100 dB) and at three randomly selected interstimulus intervals (4, 6, and 8 seconds). The latencies of the AEPs tended to correlate at about −.35, indicating that shorter latencies were associated with higher intelligence (e.g., AH4 Group Test of Intelligence and Digit Span from the WAIS). Amplitude of the AEPs was positively correlated with IQ at approximately the same strength, suggesting that higher amplitudes were associated with greater IQ. The second part of the study consisted of measuring the length of the EPs presented graphically in Ertl and Schafer's (1969) publication. The method used to quantify the complexity of an EP (the "string measure") consisted of "sticking pins in an enlarged copy of the published waveforms, and carefully drawing a thread between the pins so that it superimposed the waveforms" (Hendrickson & Hendrickson, 1980, p. 30). The thread was then measured after having been cut and straightened. A correlation of .77 was found between string length and Wechsler Intelligence Scale for Children (WISC) FSIQ.

This study was followed up by Blinkhorn and Hendrickson (1982). In a sample of 33 adult subjects, AEPs were obtained via a stimulus presentation sequence similar to Hendrickson and Hendrickson's (1980) procedure. On average, a correlation of .45 was obtained between various string length measures and IQ. When corrected for restriction in range in IQ scores, the average correlation increased to .71.

In the last string measure study by this group (Blinkhorn & Hendrickson, 1982), a diverse and large sample (n = 219) was tested, using virtually the same procedure as above. One notable exception was that a "variance measure" was also calculated. The variance measure corresponded roughly to the standard deviation in EP amplitude from stimulus to stimulus within the same trial in one individual. The string measure correlated with IQ at .72, whereas the variance measure correlated with IQ at −.72. These two measures were not measuring the same phenomenon, correlating with each other imperfectly (r = .53). Subtracting the string measure from the variance measure produced a composite score that correlated with IQ at −.83.

Although researchers continue to use the string measure (e.g., Bates, Stough, Man-gan, & Pellet, 1995), it has been criticized severely. Vetterli and Furedy (1985) note that there is a great deal of arbitrariness in determining the string length of a particular EP. Specifically, the magnitude of the correlation between string length and IQ is contingent upon the ratio of the ordinate (amplitude)-to-abscissa (time) axial length of the Cartesian graph the EP is plotted on. Applying the revised string length measure (Blinkhorn & Hendrickson, 1982) and the latency of the third peak to previously published data, Vetterli and Furedy provide a compelling argument for discounting the string measure as a valid measure of IQ. That is, the revised string length measure either did not correlate consistently with IQ, or it did so in the opposite direction that error theory would predict. The latency measure, however, did correlate consistently in the predicted direction, but much more modestly (r = −.30) than in the Blinkhorn and Hendrickson (1982) report.

In a recent review of the literature on the string measure and IQ, Burns, Nettlebeck, & Cooper (1997) report that five studies have found evidence in favor of correlations in the predicted direction; seven studies obtained near-zero correlations; and one study found a strong correlation in the opposite direction. Their review of the studies on EP amplitude and IQ presents this research as equally inconsistent. The authors also report that the string length measure and EP amplitude are correlated substantially. The consequence of this, they argue, is that the string measure is an invalid construct, because EP amplitude is affected seriously by skull thickness—a physical parameter no study of EEG and IQ ever controlled for. Thus the great amount of inconsistency in the string measure and EP amplitude studies can probably be attributed to using an invalid measure. No rebuttals have yet been put forward in defence of the string or EP amplitude measures. In fact, experimental research (Leissner, Lindholm, & Petersen, 1970) suggests a large positive correlation (r = .95) between degree of amplitude attenuation and the transmitting properties (blood, CSF, dura, skull bone, and scalp) enveloping the parenchyma (brain proper). Individual differences in these transmitting properties exist, and because none of the EEG-and-IQ studies accounted for this, it appears that much (but not all) of the research on the EEG and intelligence may be invalid.

The most valid EEG-and-IQ studies appear to be those that used a within-subject analysis approach, thereby controlling for individual differences in skull thickness. An example of this research is that conducted by Schafer, who proposed the "neural adaptability" (NA) theory (Schafer, 1982), which is now discussed.

A large amount of research has indicated that the amplitude of an EP can be modulated by attention. In one study (Schrechter & Buchsbaum, 1973), it was found that the amplitude of visual EPs (VEPs) underwent a 34% reduction from a no-task condition ("relax and watch the lights") to a mental arithmetic task ("subtract sevens serially from 2,000"). This was interpreted to suggest that during the mental arithmetic task, the subjects attended to the screen less, even though they remained facing it with their eyes open. The expectancy of a stimulus is also known to modulate the magnitude of an EP, with infrequently presented stimuli producing larger-amplitude EPs than repetitive stimuli do (Friedman, Hakerem, Sutton, & Fleiss, 1973). Based on these and other findings, Schafer (1984) contended that "cognitive neural adaptability manifests itself as the tendency of normal humans to produce cortical EPs with large amplitude to unexpected or attended inputs and small amplitude to inputs whose nature or timing the person foreknows" (p. 184). Schafer suggested that there must be an evolutionary advantage for an organism not to attend to a meaningless or known (not dangerous) stimulus, in favor of responding to novel and potentially dangerous stimuli. Furthermore, it appeared reasonable to hypothesize that individual differences would exist in this capacity to reduce attention spontaneously (EP amplitude response decrement), and that these individual differences would correlate with behavioral intelligence.

Schafer's first study conducted to support the notion of NA as a correlate of intelligence was published in 1973 (Schafer & Marcus, 1973). The subjects were selected to create three groups: persons with mental retardation ($n = 9$), technicians with average IQs ($n = 10$), and scientists with PhDs ($n = 13$). Both AEPs (the stimuli for these were 1-millisecond, 80-dB clicks) and VEPs

(these were responses to a "frosted window transilluminated by bright photic stimuli of 10 microsec duration") were derived during separate trials. There were also three different stimulation conditions: (1) self-stimulation, (2) machine stimulation, and (3) periodic stimulation. Self-stimulation consisted of a subject's initiating randomly the click or flash by pressing a handled microswitch. Machine stimulation consisted of a playback (recording) of the pattern of stimuli produced by the subject during condition 1. Periodic stimulation consisted of clicks or flashes produced regularly, once every 2 seconds.

Results revealed that the self-stimulation condition produced EPs with the smallest amplitudes; the machine stimulation condition produced EPs with the largest amplitudes; and the EPs produced by the periodic stimulation condition were in the middle ground. This effect was found only for the later components of the EP (e.g., P300), in contrast to the earlier ones (e.g., P100). Thus the degree of foreknowledge tends to attenuate the amplitude of an EP, particularly in the P300 region, which is known to be associated with cognition (Kutas, McCarthy, & Donchin, 1977). Next, a self-stimulation score was devised to estimate the "brain voltage saved" when subjects were responding to the self-stimulation condition. This was calculated as "the percentage of difference between the total integrated voltage of vertex potentials evoked by 50 self-delivered and 50 machine delivered click stimuli at a sound level of 80 dB" (p. 176). The PhD scientists had a larger self-stimulation score than the technicians ($\eta^2 = .25$). As well, the technicians had a larger self-stimulation score than the subjects with mental retardation ($\eta^2 = .38$).

In a follow-up study (Schafer, 1979), it was found that adults with normal IQs ($n = 10$) produced 24% smaller EPs during the self-delivered condition, in comparison to the average amplitude of the EPs over all three conditions. Adults with mental retardation ($n = 53$), however, did not produce EPs of a different magnitude during the self-stimulation condition. A correlation of .66 (corrected for restricted range = .82) was found between random ratios (the ratios of random EP amplitude to average EP amplitude) and WAIS FSIQ (range = 98–135).

Thus individuals who tended to produce larger-than-average EPs to unanticipated stimuli and smaller-than-average EPs to anticipated stimuli tended also to have higher IQs.

In a study of 54 adults with severe mental retardation (mean IQ = 39.11, SD = 14.39), Jensen, Schafer, and Crinella (1981) administered reaction time (RT) tests and also estimated NA. The RT and movement time (MT) composite score correlated −.54 with g, while NA correlated at .31 with g. The correlation between NA and the RT + MT composite score was −.33, suggesting that although the two constructs were related, they were also substantially independent. In fact, a multiple regression, using the two variables as predictors of g, produced a multiple R of .65.

In Schafer's (1984) final study, a simpler method to estimate NA was used. Only one trial of 50 click stimuli was presented to normal adult subjects (n = 47), at a fixed interstimulus interval of 2 seconds. Two EPs were derived: one from the first 25 stimuli, and the other from the second 25 stimuli. By calculating the percentage difference between the amplitude of the N1-P2-N2 portion of the two EPs, Schafer determined an estimate of NA. That is, the subject would consider the first half of the trial as less anticipated than the second half, and thus the EP from the first half would be larger than the EP from the second half; the larger the discrepancy, the higher the individual's IQ would be predicted to be. A correlation of .59 was found between NA and FSIQ (WAIS), which rose to .73 when corrected for restricted range.

There appear to be only two other studies ever conducted specifically hypothesizing individual differences in NA (Dustman & Callner, 1979; Shucard & Horn, 1973). Both obtained results supporting Schafer's work.

The other within-subject analysis approach that overcomes the confound of skull thickness involves the measurement of the hemispheric difference (right minus left) in a particular parameter of EEG activity. This is true because one assumes a strong correlation between the skull thickness of the two hemispheres within individuals. Only a small amount of the past EEG-and-IQ research consists of studies emphasising

the possible relationship between EP or band power asymmetry and IQ. This is puzzling, considering the magnitude and consistency of the effects that have been reported to date. The theory that seems to account for these results is based on hemispheric specialization. That is, it is an advantage to have one hemisphere processing and executing a task, without having to compete with or be interrupted by concomitantly related activity in the other hemisphere. The evidence presented below supports the notion that the greater the discrepancy in hemispheric EEG activity, the greater the cognitive ability.

An accumulation of neurological evidence has established the left temporo-parietal area as responsible for mediating verbal processing, and the right temporo-parietal area as responsible for mediating visual–spatial processing (Kolb & Whishaw, 1996). Electrophysiological research has been in accord with these findings. For instance, McLeod and Peacock (1977) recorded alpha activity over both hemispheres during two different mental tasks: a verbal task, consisting of covertly composing a letter or poem; and a spatial task, consisting of covertly completing six items from the Modified Minnesota Paper Form Board Test. A larger left-hemisphere reduction in alpha power (increased activity) was found during the verbal task. In contrast, a larger right-hemispheric decrease in alpha power during the spatial task was observed. Other studies have found similar results (e.g., Galin & Ornstein, 1972). Thus asymmetric electrocortical activity between the two cerebral hemispheres has been established.

In a study (Richlin, Weisinger, Weinstein, Giannini, & Morganstern, 1971) that measured VEPs from both hemispheres of subjects with normal IQs (n = 6) and subjects with mental retardation (n = 8) (mean age = 13.8), it was hypothesized that there would be greater hemispheric differences in the VEPs of the first group than in those of the second group. A significant effect was found for both amplitude and latency. For the subjects with normal IQs, the average amplitudes in microvolts for the right and left hemispheres were 24.9 and 16.1, respectively (a difference of 8.8). For the subjects with mental retardation, the right and left hemispheres produced amplitudes of 16.8 and

20.2, respectively (a difference of −3.4). The analysis of the P200 latencies of the VEPs revealed that for subjects with normal IQs, the P200 latencies were significantly longer in the left hemisphere than the right, whereas subjects with mental retardation did not manifest any interhemispheric differences. These results were interpreted in light of the notion that hemispheric specialization is a cognitive advantage. More specifically, the visual stimuli were nonverbal in nature, but the brains of those with mental retardation failed to distinguish this, whereas the left hemispheres of those with normal IQs "deferred" processing to their right hemispheres (hence the larger amplitudes). It is especially interesting to note that only 50% of the subjects with mental retardation were considered right-handed, whereas 83% of the normal-IQ subjects were considered right-handed.

Since it is well known that the right hemisphere is specialized for visual–spatial tasks, it was hypothesized (Furst, 1976) that subjects with greater right- than left-hemispheric activation would tend to perform better on a spatial ability task. To test this hypothesis, Furst (1976) measured the alpha-band activity (8–12 Hz) from both hemispheres (occipito-parietal area) during the performance of a mental rotation task by 16 males. Hemispheric differential deactivation was computed by dividing the alpha activity from the right hemisphere by the alpha activity in the left hemisphere (right-to-left ratios). A correlation of .55 was determined, indicating that greater right- than left-hemispheric activation was associated with better performance on the cognitive task. Although it seems reasonable to regard this estimate (.55) as a conservative one because of restriction in range (a university population), a peculiar interaction based on ability and gender has been observed.

Furst's (1976) study, which included only males with high IQs, was followed up by Ray, Newcombe, Semon, and Cole (1981). From a sample base of 110 introductory psychology students (62 males and 48 females), seven subjects were strategically selected for placement into four categories (thus total $n = 28$): "high-ability" males, "low-ability" males, "high-ability" females, and "low-ability" females. Active electrodes were placed over the left and right parietal lobes. In contrast to Furst, a somewhat different computation was used to calculate the right–left difference score: $(R − L)/(R + L)$. Consistent with Furst, a correlation of −.71 was found between differential hemispheric activation and spatial ability for the high-ability males. Thus greater right-hemispheric deactivation was associated with higher ability. For the low-ability males, however, the opposite association was found ($r = .77$); that is, greater left-hemispheric activity was associated with higher spatial ability. Within the female portion of the sample, no obvious trends could be determined. Thus, although Furst's results were replicated, an interaction based on gender and ability was found.

In a sample (9 males and 9 females) of graduate students and professionals (i.e., high-ability individuals), Corsi-Cabrera, Herrera, and Malvido (1989) recorded baseline EEG activity (alpha, beta, and theta) while the subjects were in a relaxed state and had their eyes closed. Electrodes were derived from C_3, C_4, T_3, T_4, P_3, P_4, O_1, and O_2, allowing for interhemispheric analyses. Intelligence was measured with the Differential Aptitude Test (DAT). In the male portion of the sample, interhemispheric activity correlated at −.75, −.83, and −.91 with DAT Abstract, Spatial, and Verbal ability, respectively. Thus lesser synchrony between the two hemispheres was associated with greater IQ. For the female portion of the sample, however, the correlations were in the opposite direction. Interhemispheric synchrony correlated positively at .87, .72, and .03 (n.s.) with Abstract, Spatial and Verbal ability. Thus the greater synchrony between the two hemispheres was an advantage. These interactions based on gender and ability have been replicated (Corsi-Cabrera, Arce, Ramos & Guevera, 1997).

VEP cerebral asymmetries have also been related to IQ. In one study (Tan, Akgun, Komsuoglu, & Telatar, 1993), the standard checkerboard pattern reversal stimulus was used to induce VEPs that were recorded from the left and right occipital lobes. The latency of the N1 and P1 waves from the right hemisphere were correlated at −.81 and −.88 with IQ (Cattell's CFIT). In contrast, the latency of the N1 and P1 waves from the left hemisphere was not found to be correlated with IQ. Virtually the same effect was found when the amplitude of the EPs was analyzed. The N1-P1 amplitude from the right hemisphere was negatively correlated with IQ at −.80. No relationship was found between amplitude and IQ for the left hemisphere. Thus individuals with higher IQs tended to produce EPs of smaller amplitude. The largest effect ($r = .−93$) was found when the right-hemisphere N1-P1 amplitude was subtracted from the left-hemisphere N1-P1 amplitude. That is, the smaller the amplitude was from the right and the larger the amplitude was from the left, the higher the subject's IQ tended to be. These findings not only support Schafer's NA theory (the checkerboard pattern reversed at a constant rate), but show clear evidence in support of cerebral specialization and cognitive ability.

The history of EEG-and-IQ studies has been evaluated frequently as inconsistent (e.g., Barrett & Eysenck, 1992). It has been argued above that this may be due to issues of validity regarding some of the EEG measures. Because of the EEG's relative inexpensiveness and the temporal resolution it offers, research in this area will probably continue. In the interest of a fruitful future, such research should employ a within-subject approach and should pay attention to the apparent interactions based on gender and ability.

NERVE CONDUCTION VELOCITY AND IQ

In humans, information (sequences of action potentials) travels along bundles of axons (Persinger, 1995). Bundles of axons within the central nervous system are called "tracks," whereas bundles of axons within the peripheral nervous system are called "nerves" (Kolb & Whishaw, 1996). The speed with which information travels along nerves and tracks in the nervous system is referred to as "conduction velocity" (Martin & Jessell, 1991). Reed (1984) hypothesized that conduction velocity may be at least a partial neurophysiological substrate of intelligence, because both are known to be substantially heritable.

The typical method used to estimate conduction time in a study of nerve conduction velocity (NCV) and IQ consists of stimulating briefly (e.g., 0.2 milliseconds) and supramaximally (above sensory threshold) various areas of the lower arm (the median nerve) via electrode, repeatedly (e.g., one stimulation per second), in order to obtain a clear average EP as measured by an electromyelograph (Martin & Jessell, 1991). The latency of the EP is then calibrated. The elapsed period between stimulation time and a particular peak of the EP is then estimated, which allows the determination of NCV.

Vernon and Mori (1989) were the first to put the hypothesis to the test. They estimated the NCV of the median nerve in 85 neurologically normal adults (45 females, 40 males). They also administered various RT tests, in order to determine whether NCV could be considered the basis of the well-established negative correlation between RT and IQ. A correlation of −.42 was found between NCV and intelligence (Multidimensional Aptitude Battery, or MAB), indicating that NCV tended to be faster in individuals with higher IQs. RT was negatively correlated with IQ in the expected range (−.44), and NCV and RT were correlated in the expected direction, although the correlation was much smaller than anticipated (−.29). This suggested that both RT and NCV were largely independent correlates of IQ. In fact, a multiple regression using RT and NCV as predictors and IQ as the criterion revealed a shrunken multiple R of .53. Using very similar methods, Vernon and Mori (1992) were successful at replicating their first study. NCV correlated with IQ at −.48. RT correlated with IQ at −.45. Again, although NCV did correlate with RT in the expected direction, the correlation was small at −.18. A multiple regression using RT and NCV as predictors and IQ as the criterion revealed a shrunken multiple R of .57, which was virtually identical to the R value (.53) obtained in the first study.

In Barrett, Daum, and Eysenck's (1990) study, absolute NCV was not found to be correlated with IQ (as assessed by Raven's Advanced Progressive Matrices, or RAPM) in a sample of 44 mixed-gender subjects; however, variability in NCV was found to correlate −.44 with IQ. Thus individuals who tended to produce NCVs with a smaller standard deviation tended to have higher IQs than those who produced NCVs with greater variability in speed from trial to trial. This finding is in accord with the contention that the basis of the RT-and-IQ correlation is due, at least in part, to individual differences in response variability (Jensen, 1992). That is, it is known that people with lower IQs can produce RTs of equal speed to those of people with higher IQs, but they manifest these fast RTs only infrequently, producing a lower mean in RT. It is interesting to note that variability in axonal width within the same axon also exists (Sakai & Woody, 1988). It is possible that individual differences exist in the amount of this variability, and that these individual differences are also mediating the variability in RTs. Stated alternatively, more homogenously layered axons may be less likely to produce errors in information transmission, and as a consequence, more likely to produce relatively fast RTs with greater consistency as well.

In a sample of 38 females, Wickett and Vernon (1994) attempted to replicate the Vernon and Mori (1989, 1992) studies. No statistically significant correlations were found either between NCV and IQ or NCV and RT. Because this study used females only, while the first two used both males and females, Wickett and Vernon were prompted to reexamine the Vernon and Mori studies to evaluate the possibility of an interaction based on gender. An interaction was in fact found, with the male portion of the sample yielding much larger correlations with IQ than the female portions (males, .62 and .54; females, .28 and .37). In a mixed sample of males ($n = 45$) and females (37), Tan (1996) also found a gender-based interaction. Correlations between NCV and IQ (as assessed with the CFIT) were of similar magnitudes for both males and females, but in opposite directions. NCV correlated with IQ at .63 for the males, indicating that faster conduction time was associated with greater cognitive ability. In contrast, NCV correlated with IQ at −.67 for the females, indicating that slower conduction time was associated with greater IQ.

In an original study, Reed and Jensen (1989, 1992) measured the latencies of the VEP N70 trough and P100 peak, as well as head length, in 147 adult males. It was rea-

soned that by dividing the N70 trough and P100 peak by head length (a proxy of brain length), a conduction velocity estimate of the visual pathway could be determined. This was reported as the first attempt to calibrate track conduction velocity (TCV)—that is, speed of information processing within the brain, as opposed to within the peripheral nervous system. Intelligence was estimated with Raven's Progressive Matrices (RPM). The uncorrected N70 latency did not correlate with IQ (−.12 n.s.), but the uncorrected P100 latency did at −.21. When these latencies were divided by head length (i.e., corrected), both coefficients rose: The VEP N70 latency component correlated at .18, and the VEP P100 component correlated at .26, with IQ. Corrected for restriction in IQ range, the VEP P100 latency correlated with IQ at .37. Thus, based on the results of this study, correcting for brain length by dividing the latencies by head length appears to have some validity. In a follow-up study, Reed and Jensen (1991) failed to find a relationship between TCV and IQ, using the same methods as in Reed and Jensen (1989), in a large sample of 190 students. They also estimated NCV (median nerve) and administered a series of RT tests. No significant correlations or trends were obtained between any of the variables. The authors interpreted their results as "puzzling."

In a second part of the first Reed and Jensen (1989, 1992) study, the subjects underwent a series of RT tests, in order to determine the possible relationship between RT and TCV (Reed & Jensen, 1993). RT correlated with IQ in the expected range, but none of the RT scores were related to TCV. Thus Reed and Jensen (1993) failed to determine TCV of the visual pathway as the neurophysiological substrate of the well-established RT-and-IQ correlation, just as Vernon and Mori's (1992) study failed to find a relationship between conduction velocity of the peripheral nervous system and RT. Reed and Jensen (1993) subsequently obtained a multiple R of .49, using RT and TCV as predictors of IQ. This result is remarkably similar to the multiple R's of .53 and .57 obtained by Vernon and Mori (1989, 1992), using RT and NCV as predictors of IQ.

The results of the three most recent NCV-and-IQ studies have been disappointing. Rijsdijk, Boomsma, and Vernon (1995) did not find a significant relationship between NCV and IQ in a sample of 156 twin pairs, although both IQ and NCV were found to be heritable (65% and 77%, respectively). Two years later (Rijsdijk & Boomsma, 1997), the same twin pairs underwent NCV testing again and were administered the WAIS-R. A small correlation of .15 was found between NCV and IQ, indicating that faster conduction time was associated with higher IQ scores. This correlation was determined to be mediated completely by common genetic factors. In accordance with the previous study, IQ and NCV were estimated to be 81% and 66% heritable, respectively. In order to explain why the first study may not have found an association between NCV and IQ, the authors suggested that genetically mediated changes in maturation may have to take place before a correlation between the two variables can be found. Lastly, in a sample of 58 males, Wickett (1997) also failed to find any consistent results between NCV and IQ.

The balance of the NCV-and-IQ evidence is very inconsistent. There is the suggestion of a possible relationship in males, on the order of approximately .50. However, there are just as many studies that found positive results as not. The analyses conducted on females are even more disappointing, suggesting that there is in fact no relationship, or that there is a major confound in measurement (possibly hormonal). The combined possible effects of hormones on both performance and NCV may be substantial. For instance, the substance myelin is composed largely of cholesterol, which is considered a steroid (Goodrum, 1991). Testosterone, which has shown a positive relationship with IQ (Tan, 1992), is also a steroid. The effects of the menstrual cycle or the use of estrogen/progestorone as a prophylactic may disrupt attempts to quantify a female's naturally occurring NCV. It should be noted also that the NCV studies described above did not estimate the synaptic transmission time that Reed (1984) discusses, because the area of the median nerve that these studies focused upon is composed of axons only, with no synapses.

A far more problematic confound in NCV-and-IQ research is that fact that efferent nerves ("muscle nerves") are substantially interwoven within the afferent (sensory) nerves (Parent, 1996). In experimental research, it is necessary to sever the efferent components of the median nerve to estimate NCV accurately (Martin & Jessell, 1991). This is not likely to take place in human IQ studies, given the ethical implications. Until a method is proposed to circumvent the problem of efferent activity (e.g., individual differences in the stretch reflex), simply estimating NCV in an intact median nerve may have to be considered an invalid procedure. The TCV work of Reed and Jensen seems to be far more promising. First, there are no efferent connections within the visual track pathway; second, there are synapses, which allow for indirect estimation of "transmission time" along with conduction velocity. However, there remains the issue of controlling for brain length. Measuring head length may not be adequate, given the small correlation of approximately .40 between head length and brain length (Wickett, 1997). MRI would allow for very accurate estimates of brain length; thus studies that combine MRI and TCV may prove to be very promising.

REGIONAL CEREBRAL METABOLIC RATE OF GLUCOSE UTILIZATION AND IQ

The human brain is known to consume 20% of the body's glucose, even though it accounts for only 2% of an average person's body weight (Armstrong, 1990). Individual differences in regional cerebral metabolic rate of glucose utilization (rCMRglc) have been hypothesized to be correlated with IQ. The neural efficiency theory submits that more intelligent individuals should use less glucose to perform a task. The glucose uptake studies in the area of neurophysiology and intelligence have all used a technique called positron emission tomography (PET). PET research consists of first introducing a radioactive isotope into the subject intravenously, then allowing some time to pass (typically about 30 minutes) before brain scanning is performed. This allows normal blood flow to carry the radioactive isotope to the brain. Neural activity is estimated from the amount of isotope that is detected by the PET scanner (Orrison, Lewine, Sanders, & Hartshorne, 1995).

There are two methods in this line of research: "resting state" and "activation" (Boivin et al., 1992). In the resting-state method, the radioactive isotope is injected into the subject, 30 minutes prior to being scanned. During the intervening 30 minutes, the subject is often put into a partially sensory-deprived state, including having his or her eyes covered and ears blocked. In contrast, the activation method consists of having the subject perform a cognitive task (e.g., the RAPM) during the intervening 30 minutes between injection and scanning. Thus the activation method allows for the direct estimation of cerebral glucose consumption during intellectual functioning.

Resting State

In the first study to attempt to establish a relationship between cognitive performance and cortical metabolic activity (Chase et al., 1984), 17 patients with Alzheimer's disease and five normal controls underwent PET scanning and were subsequently administered the WAIS. Substantial positive correlations were found between total cortical metabolic activity and FSIQ (.68), VIQ (.61), and PIQ (.56). Haier (1993) interpreted this positive association between glucose utilization and IQ, which was contrary to the efficiency theory, as due to the neuropathology of Alzheimer's disease. Analyses using the five normal control subjects and the five least cognitively impaired patients, however, were reported to have revealed similar positive correlations between glucose uptake and IQ.

In another study (Berent et al., 1988), 15 patients diagnosed with Huntington's disease and 14 neurologically normal adults underwent PET scanning. Scores on the Wechsler Memory Scale and the WAIS-R were also determined. Among the patients, greater performance was associated with greater resting metabolic activity in the area of .50 to .60, which was in accord with Chase and colleagues' (1984) findings. In contrast, the trend of the correlations was negative in the normal controls. Thus better cognitive performance was associated with more metabolic activity in the diseased brains, whereas better cognitive performance was associated with lesser amounts of metabolic activity in the nondiseased

brains. The negative association found in the normal controls was opposite to that found in the Chase and colleagues study and in accord with the neural efficiency theory.

The only study to measure rCMRglc and cognitive ability at rest in neurologically normal subjects (n = 33) was a study by Boivin and colleagues (1992). On the same day that the subjects underwent PET scanning, the subjects engaged in a verbal fluency (VF) task, which consisted of producing as many words starting with a particular letter as they could in 1 minute. A positive correlation of .56 was found between relative left inferior temporal cortex metabolic activity and VF score. Conversely, negative correlations of –.44 and –.59 were obtained between relative metabolic activity in the left and right frontal cortices and VF. Although regarding VF as an estimate of IQ may be questionable, the findings in this study suggest that it may be more appropriate to analyze rCMRglc in particular areas of the brain, as opposed to simply estimating rCMRglc from the whole brain. Given the known complex interplay of excitation and inhibition throughout the cerebrum, the whole-brain approach may be too simplistic, particularly in healthy subjects.

Activation

Parks and colleagues (1988) administered the same VF test as Boivin and colleagues (1992) during the 30-minute radioactive isotope uptake period, preceding brain scanning. They found correlations in the area of –.50 for the frontal, temporal, and parietal regions. Thus higher VF scores were associated with lower amounts of glucose utilization. The magnitude of this effect was virtually identical to that found in the Boivin and colleagues study, but was in the opposite direction. Again, this suggests an interaction based not only on particular areas of the brain, but on activation versus resting-state PET procedures.

In a regional cerebral blood flow (rCBF) study of neurologically normal adults (Gur et al., 1988), a positive correlation of .41 was obtained between rCBF and a verbal analogies test administered during tracer uptake. Thus, in contrast to the findings of Parks and colleagues (1988), greater cerebral activity during the cognitive task was associated with greater ability. Although rCBF and rCMRglc both use PET technology, they are somewhat different in terms of how neural activity is inferred. This may have mediated the conflicting results.

In another study (Haier et al., 1988), the subjects engaged in one of three forms of activation: (1) solving problems on the RAPM; (2) taking a continuous-performance test (CPT), involving the visual presentation of numbers (the subjects were required to press a button each time the number 0 appeared); or (3) viewing the same visual presentation of numbers as in the second task, but not being required to attend to any number in particular. An average correlation of –.75 was found between cortical absolute metabolic rate and RAPM score. In contrast, the trend of the correlations between cortical absolute metabolic rate and CPT score was positive, but only one brain image slice in the infraventricular area was statistically significant (.58). Thus the more intelligent subjects utilized less glucose during intelligence testing, suggesting that (1) glucose was used more efficiently, or (2) they did not find the task as difficult and consequently used less glucose. To test these two hypotheses, Larson, Haier, LaCasse, and Hazen (1995) divided subjects into groups with high ($n = 14$) and average ($n = 14$) ability, based on their previous performance on the RAPM. There were two PET scanning sessions, which involved (1) solving relatively easy backward digit span items, and (2) solving relatively difficult backward digit span items. A marginally significant ($p = .07$) analysis of variance showed that the high-ability group used more glucose during both sessions, contrary to the neural efficiency theory. That is, according to the neural efficiency theory, the high-ability individuals should have expended less energy to recall the digits, particularly during the relatively easy session. A subsequent analysis revealed a significant group × condition interaction: The average-ability group manifested a decrease in cortical metabolic rate from the easy to the more difficult condition, whereas the high-ability group showed an increase from one condition to the other. Furthermore, it was discovered that the high-ability group displayed greater hemispheric asymmetry in

glucose uptake during the difficult task than did the average-ability group. More specifically, the right hemisphere was more highly activated than the left. Thus, just as research on the EEG correlates of IQ has shown, there appears to be an interaction based on ability and cerebral hemisphere.

In another study (Haier, Siegel, Tang, Abel, & Buchsbaum, 1992), eight normal adults played the computer game Tetris during the radioactive isotope uptake period on two occasions: (1) when the subjects were naïve to the game, and (2) after several weeks of 30- to 45-minute practice sessions. The RAPM was administered to each subject between the first and second PET scans. The correlation between whole-brain glucose metabolic rate (GMR) and RAPM during the session when the subjects were playing Tetris for the first time was .77, indicating that larger amounts of glucose uptake were associated with greater intelligence. No statistically significant correlation was found for the practiced condition (.09). Subtracting the amount of GMR during the practiced session from that during the naive session, and correlating the residual with RAPM, resulted in a correlation of –.68. This indicated that the subjects with higher IQs tended to evidence a larger reduction in the amount of GMR from one session to the next, in line with neural efficiency theory

In an enlightening and original study (Haier et al., 1995) both brain volume (MRI) and GMR were estimated. During the 30-minute uptake of the tracer, the subjects engaged in the same CPT described above. Three groups of subjects were included in the study: adults with Down's syndrome ($n = 7$), adults with mild mental retardation ($n = 9$), and normal controls ($n = 10$). Each subject was administered the WAIS-R. The correlation between GMR and IQ was –.58. This result was in the opposite direction to the correlation obtained by Haier and colleagues (1988) between rCMRglc and IQ. A notable difference is that this study's sample was markedly heterogeneous, with 16 out of 26 subjects suffering from mental retardation. Furthermore, the correlation between brain size and IQ was .65. Interestingly, the correlation between brain size and GMR was –.69. This is very similar to the correlation of

−.75 that Hatawa, Brooks, Di Chiro, and Bacharach (1987) found between brain volume and resting metabolic rate in a group of 23 normal adults. In fact, it has been established that smaller brains have greater neural density, as well as greater glucose utilization per unit volume. Whether PET detects smaller human brains as utilizing more glucose because they in fact do, or because it is simply a pixel-parameter-setting artifact, has yet to be determined.

All studies of rCMRglc and cognitive ability have found moderate to substantial effects (see Table 14.2). The fact that the results are inconsistent, in terms of the direction of the coefficients, suggests the possible effect of interactions. Resting versus activation, whole brain versus particular region, and varying degrees of intelligence have been suggested as interacting factors here,

as well as neural density. Once these variables can be accounted for, more consistent results are likely to be obtained. In additon, functional MRI—a less expensive and more accurate technology (Orrison et al., 1995)—will possibly be the technology used in future research in this area.

BIOCHEMICAL CORRELATES OF IQ

Previous research investigating the biochemical correlates of information processing was largely experimental; it involved administering various drugs (e.g., nicotine) to subjects and measuring their resulting systematic effects on RTs or EPs (Naylor, Callway, & Halliday, 1993). A resurgence of clinical interest in magnetic resonance spectroscopy (MRS) appears to be the impetus

TABLE 14.2. Studies of Cerebral Metabolic Rates of Glucose Utilization and Cognitive Ability

Source	Subjects[a]	Task[b]	Brain region	Cognitive measure[b]	r
		Resting state			
Chase et al. (1988)	17 with AD,	—	Left temporal lobe	VIQ	.76
	5 NL	—	Right parietal lobe	PIQ	.70
Berent et al. (1988)	15 with HD	—	Caudate	Digit Symbol	.85
Berent et al. (1988)	14 NL	—	Putamen	Digit Symbol	−.68
Boivin et al. (1992)	33 NL	—	Left inferior temporal	VF	.56
		—	Left frontal	VF	−.44
		—	Right frontal	VF	−.59
Gur et al. (1988)	26 NL	—	Whole brain	VA	.25
		Active state			
Parks et al. (1988)	14 NL	VF	Frontal	VF	−.54
		VF	Temporal	VF	−.50
		VF	Parietal	VF	−.54
Gur et al. (1988)	26 NL	VA	Whole brain	VA	.41
Haier et al. (1988)	13 NL	CPT	Whole brain	CPT	.47
Haier et al. (1988)	8 NL	RAPM	Whole brain	RAPM	−.75
Larson et al. (1995)	28 NL	Digit Span	Right hemisphere	RAPM	.43
Haier et al. (1992)	8 NL	Tetris/naive	Whole brain	RAPM	.77
		Tetris/practiced	Whole brain	RAPM	.09
Haier et al. (1995)	7 with DS, 9 with MR, 10 NL	CPT	Whole brain	WAIS-R	−.58

[a]AD, Alzheimer's disease; HD, Huntington's disease; NL, normal; DS, Down's syndrome; MR, mild mental retardation.
[b]VIQ, Verbal IQ; PIQ, Performance IQ; VF, verbal fluency task; VA, verbal analogies task; CPT, continuous-performance task; RAPM, Raven's Advanced Progressive Matrices.

behind some original and very promising research on individual differences in brain chemistry and intelligence. The principles of operation underlying MRS are the same as those underlying MRI (Orrison et al., 1995). Effectively, the difference is that the signal derived and analyzed by MRS produces a frequency spectrum that allows researchers to quantify *in vivo* concentrations of particular neurometabolites in a particular area of the brain.

The first study to use MRS in intelligence research with neurologically normal subjects (Rae et al., 1996), estimated occipitoparietal white matter intracellular pH levels in a sample of 42 boys (mean age = 10). pH was estimated by "using the difference in chemical shift between phosphocreatine resonance and inorganic phosphate" (Rae et al., 1996, p. 1061). The WISC-III was administered to determine the subjects' IQs. A correlation of .52 was found between pH level and FSIQ, indicating that a higher pH level was associated with greater measured intelligence. The effect of pH levels on the nervous system is far-ranging. For instance, experimental *in vitro* research on rats (Elis, 1969) has shown a very close correspondence between pH level and nerve action potential amplitude (.92) and conduction time (−.86). Consequently, Rae and colleagues (1996) interpreted their result in light of the neural efficiency theory, implicating higher IQ as associated with faster conductivity and transmission.

In another MRS study (Jung et al., 1999), levels of N-acetylaspartate (NAA) and choline (Cho) were measured in 26 male and female college students. The authors chose NAA, because it has been shown to be positively related to neuronal injury and death. Furthermore, the authors report that levels of Cho appear to be related positively to demyelination, as increased levels have been observed in stroke and multiple sclerosis. Intelligence was assessed with the WAIS-III. NAA and Cho correlated with FSIQ at .52 and −.32, respectively. A multiple R of .67 was obtained by a multiple regression using NAA and Cho as predictors of IQ. As future research accumulates delineating the role of these neurometabolites in brain functioning, a clearer understanding of their role in intellectual functioning is likely.

CONCLUSION

What is most noteworthy about the discipline of neuropshysiology and intelligence is not only that it has established various correlates of intelligence, but that the area is progressing rapidly. Although only a little over a decade has passed since the first edition of this volume was published, the whole of this chapter has had to be rewritten to accommodate the major advances in the field: brain size (MRI); metabolic activity (PET); NCV/TCV; a possible reorientation in EEG research (within-subject analyses, nonlinear dynamics); and biochemical correlates (MRS). Unquestionably, these advances have been made in large part because of advances in technology. As the accuracy, resolution, versatility, and accessibility of these technologies continue to increase, there is little doubt that our understanding of the neurophysiological substrates of intelligence will improve.

Many but not all of the neurophysiological and biochemical correlates of IQ presented here appear to be intercorrelated. Future studies that combine technologies (MRI, PET, MRS, EEG) will have the capacity to estimate multiple correlates of IQ, which will allow for the direct appraisal of each variable as a potentially unique contributor to IQ. Should uniqueness be established for even a few, the prospect of estimating an individual's IQ without administering an IQ test is likely to become an imminent reality, however impractical it may currently seem.

REFERENCES

Andreason, N. C., Flaum, M., Swayze, V., O'Leary, D. S., Alliger, R., Cohen, G., Ehrhardt, J., & Yuh, W. T. C. (1993). Intelligence and brain structure in normal individuals. *American Journal of Psychiatry, 150*(1), 130–134.

Armstrong, E. (1990). Brains, bodies and metabolism. *Brain, Behavior and Evolution, 36,* 166–176.

Barrett, P. T., Daum, I., & Eysenck, H. J. (1990). Sensory nerve conduction and intelligence: A methodological study. *Journal of Psychophysiology, 4,* 1–13.

Barrett, P. T., & Eysenck, H. J. (1992). Brain electrical potentials and intelligence. In A. Gale & M. W. Eysecnck (Eds), *Handbook of individual differences: Biological perspectives* (pp. 255–285). New York: Wiley.

Bates, T., Stough, C., Mangan, G., & Pellet, O. (1995). Intelligence and complexity of the averaged evoked potential: An attentional theory. *Intelligence, 20,* 27–39.

Berent, S., Giordani, B., Lehtinen, S., Markel, D., Penney, J. B., Buchtel, H. A., Starosta-Rubinstein, S., Hichwa, R., & Young, A. B. (1988). Positron emission tomography scan investigations of Huntington's disease: Cerebral metabolic correlates of cognitive function. *Annals of Neurology, 23,* 541–546.

Blinkhorn, S. F., & Hendrickson, D. E. (1982). Averaged evoked responses and psychometric intelligence. *Nature, 295,* 596–597.

Boivin, M. J., Giordani, B., Berent, S., Amato, D. A., Lehtinen, S., Koeppe, R. A., Buchtel, H. A., Foster, N. L., & Kuhl, D. E. (1992). Verbal fluency and positron emission tomogrpahy mapping of regional cerebral glucose metabolism. *Cortex, 28,* 231–239.

Burns, N. R., Nettlebeck, T., & Cooper, C. J. (1997). The string measure of the ERP: What does it measure? *International Journal of Psychophysiology, 27,* 43–53.

Chalke, F. C. R., & Ertl, J. (1965). Evoked potentials and intelligence. *Life Sciences, 4,* 1319–1322.

Chase, T. N., Fedio, P., Foster, N. L., Brooks, R., Di Chiro, G., & Mansi, L. (1984). Wechsler Adult Intelligence Scale performance: Cortical localization by fluorodeoxyglucose F–18-positron emission tomogrpahy. *Archives of Neurology, 41,* 1244–1247.

Corsi-Cabrera, M., Arce, C., Ramos, J., & Guevara, M. A. (1997). Effect of spatial ability and sex on inter- and intrahemispheric correlation of EEG activity. *Electroencephalography and Clinical Neurophysiology, 102,* 5–11.

Corsi-Cabrera, M., Herrera, P., & Malvido, M. (1989). Correlation between EEG and cognitive abilities: Sex differences. *International Journal of Neuroscience, 45,* 133–141.

Dustman, R. E., & Callner, D. A. (1979). Cortical evoked responses and response decrement in nonretarded and Down's syndrome individuals. *American Journal of Mental Deficiency, 83*(4), 391–397.

Egan, V., Chiswick, A., Santosh, C., Naidu, K., Rimmington, J. E., & Best, J. J. K. (1994). Size isn't everything: A study of brain volume, intelligence and auditory evoked potentials. *Personality and Individual Differences, 17*(3), 357–367.

Egan, V., Wickett, J. C., & Vernon, P. A. (1995). Brain size and intelligence: erratum, addendum, and correction. *Personality and Individual Differences, 19*(1), 113–115.

Elis, F. R. (1969). Some effects of PCO_2 and pH on nerve tissue. *British Journal of Pharmacology, 35,* 197–201.

Ertl, J., & Schafer, E. (1969). Brain response correlates of chometric intelligence. *Nature, 223,* 421–422.

Eysenck, H. J. (1981). *The intelligence controversy.* New York:Wiley.

Eysenck, H. J. (1993). The biological basis of intelligence. In P. A. Vernon (Ed.), *Biological approaches to the study of human intelligence* (pp. 1–32). Norwood, NJ: Ablex.

Flashman, L. A., Andreasen, N. C., Flaum, M., & Swayze, V. W. (1998). Intelligence and regional brain volumes in normal controls. *Intelligence, 25*(3), 149–160.

Friedman, D., Hakerem, G., Sutton, S., & Fleiss, J. L. (1973). Effect of stimulus uncertainty on the pupillary dilation response and the vertex evoked potential. *Electroencephalography and Clinical Neurophysiology, 34,* 475–484.

Furst, C. J. (1976). EEG alpha asymmetry and visuospatial performance. *Nature, 260,* 224–225.

Galin, D., & Ornstein, R. (1972). Lateral specialization of cognitive mode: An EEG study. *Psychophysiology, 9,* 412–418.

Goodrum, J. F. (1991). Cholesterol from degenerating nerve myelin becomes associated with lipoproteins containing apolipoprotein E. *Journal of Neurochemistry, 56*(6), 2082–2086.

Guilford, J. P., & Fruchter, B. (1978). *Fundamental statistics in psychology and education.* New York: McGraw-Hill.

Gur, R. C., Gur, R. E., Skolnick, B. E., Resnick, S. M., Silver, F. L., Chalwluk, J., Muenz, L., Obrist, W. D., & Reivich, M. (1988). Effects of task difficulty on regional cerebral blood flow: Relationships with anxiety and performance. *Psychophysiology, 25*(4), 392–399.

Gur, R. C., Turetsky, B. I., Matsui, M., Yan, M., Bilker, W., Hughett, P., & Gur, R. E. (1999). Sex differences in brain grey and white matter in healthy young adults: Correlations with cognitive performance. *Journal of Neuroscience, 19*(10), 4065–4072.

Haier, R. J. (1993). Cerebral glucose metabolism and intelligence. In P. A. Vernon (Ed.), *Biological approaches to the study of human intelligence* (pp. 317–332). Norwood, NJ: Ablex.

Haier, R. J., Chueh, D., Touchette, P., Lott, I., Buchsbaum, M., Macmillan, D., Sandman, C., Lacasse, L., & Sosa, E. (1995). Brain size and cerebral glucose metabolic rate in nonspecific mental retardation and Down syndrome. *Intelligence, 20,* 191–210.

Haier, R. J., Siegel, B. V., Nuechterlein, K. H., Hazlett, E., Wu, J. C., Paek, J., Browning, H. L., & Buchsbaum, M. S. (1988). Cortical glucose metabolic rate correlated of abstract reasoning and attention studied with positron emission tomography. *Intelligence, 12,* 199–217.

Haier, R. J., Siegel, B., Tang, C., Abel, L., & Buchsbaum, M. S. (1992). Intelligence and changes in regional cerebral glucose metabolic rate following learning. *Intelligence, 16,* 415–426.

Hatawa, J., Brooks, R. A., Di Chiro, G., & Bacharach, S. L. (1987). Glucose utilization rate versus brain size in humans. *Neurology, 37,* 583–588.

Haug, H. (1987). Brain sizes, surfaces, and neuronal sizes of the cortex cerebri: A stereological investigation of man and his variability and a comparison with some mammals (primates, whales, marsupials, insectivores, and one elephant). *American Journal of Anatomy, 180,* 126–142.

Hendrickson, D. E., & Hendrickson, A. E. (1980). The biological basis of individual differences in intelligence. *Personality and Individual Differences, 1,* 3–33.

Herrnstein, R. J., & Murray, C. (1994). *The bell curve:*

Intelligence and class structure in American life. New York: Free Press.

Ho, K.-C., Roessmann, U., Straumfjord, J. V., & Monroe, G. (1980). Analysis of brain weight. I. Adult brain weight in relation to sex, race, and age. *Archives of Pathology and Laboratory Medicine, 104,* 635–645.

Jausovec, N. (1996). Differences in EEG alpha activity related to giftedness. *Intelligence, 23,* 159–173.

Jensen, A. R. (1992). The importance of intraindividual variation in reaction time. *Personality and Individual Differences, 13*(8), 869–881.

Jensen, A. R., Schafer, E. W. P., & Crinella, F. M. (1981). Reaction time, evoked brain potentials, and psychometric *g* in the severely retarded. *Intelligence, 5,* 179–197.

Jung, R. E., Brooks, W. M., Yeo, R. A., Chiulli, S. J., Weers, D. C., & Sibbit, W. L. (1999). Biochemical markers of intelligence: A proton MR spectroscopy study of normal human brain. *Proceedings of the Royal Society of London B, 266,* 1375–1379.

Kandel, E. R. (1998). A new intellectual framework for psychiatry. *American Journal of Psychiatry, 155*(4), 457–469.

Kolb, B., & Whishaw, I. Q. (1996). *Fundamentals of human neuropsychology.* New York: Freeman.

Kutas, M., McCarthy, G., & Donchin, E. (1977). Augmenting mental chronometry: The P300 as a measure of stimulus evaluation time. *Science, 197,* 792–795.

Larson, G. E., Haier, R. J., LaCasse, L., & Hazen, K. (1995). Evaluation of a "mental effort" hypothesis for correlations between cortical metabolism and intelligence. *Intelligence, 21,* 267–278.

Leissner, P., Lindholm, L. E., & Petersen, I. (1970). Alpha amplitude dependence on skull thickness as measured by ultrasound technique. *Electroencephalography and Clinical Neurophsyiology, 29*(4), 392–399.

Lutzenberger, W., Birbaumer, N., Flor, H., Rockstroh, B., & Elbert, T. (1992). Dimensional analysis of the human EEG and intelligence. *Neuroscience Letters, 143,* 10–14.

Martin, J. H. (1991). The collective electrical behavior of cortical neurons: The electroencephalogram and the mechanisms of epilepsy. In E. Kandel, J. Schwartz, & T. Jessel (Eds.), *Principles of neural science* (pp. 777–791). Norwalk, CT: Appleton & Lange.

Martin, J. H., & Jessell, T. M. (1991). Modality coding in the somatic sensory system. In E. Kandel, J. Schwartz, & T. Jessel (Eds.), *Principles of neural science* (pp. 341–352). Norwalk, CT: Appleton & Lange.

McLeod, S., & Peacock, L. J. (1977). Task-related EEG asymmetry: Effects of age and ability. *Psychophysiology, 14*(3), 308–311.

Mundy-Castle, A. C. (1958). Electrophysiological correlates of intelligence. *Journal of Personality, 26,* 184–199.

Mundy-Castle, A. C., & Nelson, G. K. (1960). Intelligence, personality and brain rhythms in a socially isolated community. *Nature, 185,* 484–485.

Naylor, H., Callway, E., & Halliday, R. (1993). Bio-

chemical correlates of human information processing. In P. A. Vernon (Ed.), *Biological approaches to the study of human intelligence* (pp. 333–373). Norwood, NJ: Ablex.

Orrison, W. W., Lewine, J. D., Sanders, J. A., & Hartshorne, M. F. (1995). *Functional brain imaging.* St. Louis, MO: Mosby.

Parent, A. (1996). *Carpenter's human neuroanatomy.* Baltimore: Williams & Wilkins.

Parks, R. W., Loewenstein, D. A., Dodrill, K. L., Barker, W. W., Yoshii, F., Chang, J. Y., Emran, A., Apicella, A., Sheramata, W. A., & Duara, R. (1988). Cerebral metabolic effects of a verbal fluency test: A PET scan study. *Journal of Clinical and Experimental Neuropsychology, 10*(5), 565–575.

Persinger, M. A. (1995). Neursopsychological *principia brevita*: an application to traumatic (acquired) brain injury. *Psychological Reports, 77,* 707–724.

Peters, M. (1993). Still no convincing evidence of a relation between brain size and intelligence in humans. *Canadian Journal of Experimental Psychology, 47,* 751–756.

Rae, C., Scott, R. B., Thompson, C. H., Kemp, G. J., Dumughn, I., Styles, P., Tracey, I., & Radda, G. K. (1996). Is pH a biochemical marker of IQ? *Proceedings of the Royal Society of London B, 263,* 1061–1064.

Ray, W. J., Newcombe, N., Semon, J., & Cole, P. M. (1981). Spatial abilities, sex differences and EEG functioning. *Neuropsychologia, 19*(5), 719–722.

Raz, N., Torres, I. J., Spencer, W. D., Millman, D., Baertschi, J. C., & Sarpel, G. (1993). Neuroanatomical correlates of age-sensitive and age-invariant cognitive abilities: An *in vivo* MRI investigation. *Intelligence, 17,* 407–422.

Reed, T. E. (1984). Mechanism for heritability of intelligence. *Nature, 311,* 417.

Reed, T. E., & Jensen, A. R. (1989). Short latency visual evoked potentials, visual tract speed, and intelligence: Significant correlations [Abstract]. *Behavior Genetics, 19,* 772–773.

Reed, T. E., & Jensen, A. R. (1991). Arm nerve conduction velocity (NCV), brain NCV, reaction time, and intelligence. *Intelligence, 15,* 33–47.

Reed, T. E., & Jensen, A. R. (1992). Conduction velocity in a brain nerve pathway of normal adults correlates with intelligence level. *Intelligence, 16,* 259–272.

Reed, T. E., & Jensen, A. R. (1993). Choice reaction time and visual pathway nerve conduction velocity both correlate with intelligence but appear not to correlate with each other: Implications for information processing. *Intelligence, 17,* 191–203.

Reiss, A. L., Abrams, M. T., Singer, H. S., Ross, J. L., & Denckla, M. B. (1996). Brain development, gender and IQ in children. *Brain, 119,* 1763–1774.

Richlin, M., Weisinger, M., Weinstein, S., Giannini, R., & Morganstern, M. (1971). Interhemispheric asymmetries of evoked cortical responses in retarded and normal children. *Cortex, 7*(1), 98–105.

Rijsdijk, F. V., & Boomsma, D. I. (1997). Genetic mediation of the correlation between peripheral nerve conduction velocity and IQ. *Behavior Genetics, 27*(2), 87–98.

Rijsdijk, F. V., Boomsma, D. I., & Vernon, P. A. (1995). Genetic analysis of peripheral nerve conduction velocity in twins. *Behavior Genetics, 25*(4), 341–348.

Sakai, H., & Woody, C. D. (1988). Relationships between axonal diameter, soma size, and axonal conduction velocity of HRP-filled, pyramidal tract cells of awake cats. *Brain Research, 460,* 1–7.

Schafer, E. W. P. (1979). Cognitive neural adaptability: A biological basis for individual differences in intelligence. *Psychophysiology, 16,* 199.

Schafer, E. W. P. (1982). Neural adaptability: A biological determinant of behavioral intelligence. *International Journal of Neuroscience, 17,* 183–191.

Schafer, E. W. P. (1984). Habituation of evoked cortical potentials correlates with intelligence. *Psychophysiology, 21*(5), 597.

Schafer, E. W. P., & Marcus, M. (1973). Self-stimulation alters human sensory brain responses. *Science, 181,* 175–177.

Schrechter, G., & Buchsbaum, M. (1973). The effects of attention, stimulus intensity, and individual differences on the average evoked response. *Psychophysiology, 10*(4), 392–400.

Shucard, D. W., & Horn, J. L. (1973). Evoked potential amplitude change related to intelligence and arousal. *Psychophysiology, 10*(5), 445–452.

Snyder, P. J., Bilder, R. M., Wu, H., Bodgerts, B., & Lieberman, J. A. (1995). Cerebellar volume asymmetries are related to handedness: a quantitative MRI study. *Neuropsychologia, 33*(4), 407–419.

Tan, U. (1992). There is a direct relationship between nonverbal intelligence and serum testosterone level in young men. *International Journal of Neuroscience, 64,* 213–216.

Tan, U. (1996). Correlations between nonverbal intelligence and peripheral nerve conduction velocity in right-handed subjects: Sex-related differences. *International Journal of Psychophysiology, 22,* 123–128.

Tan, U., Akgun, A., Komsuoglu, S., & Telatar, M. (1993). Inverse relationship between intelligence and the parameters of pattern reversal visual evoked potentials in left-handed male subjects: importance of right brain and testosterone. *International Journal of Neuroscience, 71,* 189–200.

Tan, U., Tan, M., Polat, P., Ceylan, Y., Suma, S., & Okur, A. (1999). Magnetic resonance imaging brain size/IQ relations in Turkish university students. *Intelligence, 27*(1), 83–92.

Tramo, M. J., Loftus, W. C., Stukel, T. A., Green, R. L., Weaver, J. B., & Gazzaniga. (1998). Brain size, head size, and intelligence quotient in monozygotic twins. *Neurology, 50,* 1246–1252.

Vernon, P. A. (Ed.). (1993). *Biological approaches to the study of human intelligence.* Norwood, NJ: Ablex.

Vernon, P. A., & Mori, M. (1989). Intelligence, reaction times, and nerve conduction velocity [Abstract]. *Behavior Genetics, 19,* 779.

Vernon, P. A., & Mori, M. (1992). Intelligence, reaction times, and peripheral nerve conduction velocity. *Intelligence, 16,* 273–288.

Vernon, P. A., Wickett, J. C., Bazana, P. G., & Stelmack, R. (2000). The neuropsychology an neurophysiology of human intelligence. In R. J. Sternberg (Ed.), *Handbook of intelligence* (pp. 245–264). Cambridge, England: Cambridge University Press.

Vetterli, C. F., & Furedy, J. J. (1985). Evoked potential correlates of intelligence: some problems with Hendrickson's string measure of evoked potential complexity and error theory of intelligence. *International Journal of Psychophysiology, 3,* 1–3.

Wechsler, D. (1997). *WAIS-II administration and Scoring Manual.* San Antonio, TX: Psychological Corporation.

Wickett, J. C. (1997). *The biological basis of general intelligence.* Unpublished doctoral dissertation, University of Western Ontario.

Wickett, J. C., & Vernon, P. A. (1994). Peripheral nerve conduction velocity, reaction time, and intelligence: An attempt to replicate Vernon and Mori (1992). *Intelligence, 18,* 127–131.

Wickett, J. C., & Vernon, P. A. (2000). Relationships between factors of intelligence and brain volume. *Personality and Individual Differences, 29*(6), 1095–1122.

Wickett, J. C., Vernon, P. A., & Lee, D. H. (1994). In vivo brain size, head perimeter, and intelligence in a sample of healthy adult females. *Personality and Individual Differences, 16*(6), 831–838.

Willerman, L., Schultz, R., Rutledge, J. N., & Bigler, E. D. (1991). *In vivo* brain size and intelligence. *Intelligence, 15,* 223–228.

15

Multifactored and Cross-Battery Ability Assessments: Are They Worth the Effort?

JOSEPH J. GLUTTING
MARLEY W. WATKINS
ERIC A. YOUNGSTROM

The practical merit of intelligence tests has been debated extensively. In the mid-1990s, as a consequence of the controversy surrounding Herrnstein and Murray's (1994) book *The Bell Curve: Intelligence and Class Structure in American Life,* the American Psychological Association formed a task force charged with developing a scientific report on the known meaning and efficacy of scores from tests of intelligence. The final report was published in the *American Psychologist* (Neisser et al., 1996). This account is especially intriguing in the context of a chapter examining the utility of multifactor ability assessments, because it offered no evidence that would support either the diagnostic or prescriptive relevance of subtest scores, factor scores, or other derived indices. Instead, IQ tests were defended solely on the basis of the more parsimonious construct coverage provided by global, or *g*-based, measures of intelligence (Neisser et al., 1996).

Psychologists today expend considerable effort administering and scoring the many subtests within most instruments that are intended to assess cognitive ability. Such an investment is presumably made in order to garner clinically useful information not available from interpretation of the single, global score. Accordingly, the trend among publishers of individually administered intelligence tests has been toward creating longer instruments that provide an ever-increasing diversity of discrete subtest scores and factor indices. A partial listing of some instruments introduced in recent years illustrates this trend.

Compared to the 10 mandatory (and 2 supplementary) subtests in the Wechsler Intelligence Scale for Children—Revised (WISC-R; Wechsler, 1974), the updated Wechsler Intelligence Scale for Children—Third Edition (WISC-III; Wechsler, 1991) is slightly longer, having added a new subtest. The Wechsler Adult Intelligence Scale—Third Edition (WAIS-III; Wechsler, 1997) contains 14 subtests versus the 11 subtests of its predecessor (Wechsler, 1981), a 27% increase in overall length. The Differential Ability Scales (DAS; Elliott, 1990) consists of 14 cognitive subtests. The revised Woodcock–Johnson Psycho-educational Battery (WJ-R; Woodcock & Johnson, 1989), including both ability and achievement subtests, allowed for the administration of 29 separate measures, while the new Woodcock–Johnson Psycho-educational Battery—

Third Edition (WJ-III; Woodcock & Johnson, 2000) includes 43 subtests!

Furthermore, in an attempt to capture all major components from Carroll's (1993) three-stratum model of intelligence, clinicians are now encouraged to move beyond the boundaries of specific, individually administered tests of intelligence. In their place, they are directed to employ multifactored, cross-battery assessments (Flanagan & McGrew, 1997; McGrew & Flanagan, 1998).

This chapter examines the relative efficacy of multifaceted abilities. The chapter is divided into five main sections. The first of these sections serves as a foundation; it establishes the amount and quality of validity evidence supporting the interpretation of global measures of intelligence. The second section reports on a series of empirical studies that assess continuing utility claims for the myriad specific abilities evaluated by subtest profiles. The third section moves away from subtest analysis and discusses research that has evaluated the validity of factor scores from individually administered tests of intelligence. The fourth section presents several troubling conceptual and practical issues associated with the interpretation of factor scores. The fifth section then scrutinizes evidence concerning the interpretation of scores (factor and subtest) obtained from cross-battery assessments.

WHAT g PREDICTS AND DEFINES

Validity Issues

As will be demonstrated shortly, utility is well established for global ability. This simple fact permits g-based estimates of intelligence to serve as a contrast for comparing the relative truth and value of multiple ability components. An even more important point—and one generally overlooked in the ability-testing literature—is that preference for interpretation should be given to g-based scores over other, more elaborate interpretative schemes. The reason is simply that global intelligence satisfies a foundational law of science: the law of parsimony. The common interpretation of parsimony is "Keep it simple." More formally, the law of parsimony (also known as "Occam's Razor") states that

"what can be explained by fewer principles is explained needlessly by more" (Jones, 1952, p. 620). Because the number of subtest and factor scores interpreted during an ability assessment is usually large, it therefore becomes imperative that this added information offer practical, diagnostic, or treatment benefits for the individual being assessed, and that these benefits extend *above and beyond* the level of help afforded by interpretation of a single, g-based score (Brody, 1985; Reschly, 1997; Reschly & Grimes, 1990). Should the analysis of subtest or factor scores fail to fulfill these promises, their relevance becomes moot.

Treatment versus Predictive Validity

Multiple sources of evidence can be used to validate interpretations of test scores (Messick, 1989). However, in diagnostic assessment, two types of validity evidence are primary. Diagnostic, score-based interpretations become valid to the extent that they (1) are associated with a viable *treatment* for individuals experiencing a particular psychological problem/disorder, or (2) accurately *predict* (either concurrently or in the future) with a high probability that a given person will develop a problem/disorder (Cromwell, Blashfield, & Strauss, 1975; Glutting, McDermott, Konold, Snelbaker, & Watkins, 1998; Gough, 1971).

Psychologists have come to believe that treatment validity is the most important validity evidence for psychological tests, IQ and otherwise. This belief is unfortunate, because it occurs at the expense of prediction. Prediction is valuable in its own right, because we may never be able to remediate all of the negative circumstances that can influence a person's growth and well-being.

Presented below are several common outcomes *predicted* by g-based IQs. The presentation is representative of variables associated with general intelligence, but is not meant to be exhaustive. Such treatment is beyond the scope of this chapter, and readers are referred to the accompanying citations for more thorough discussions.

Scholastic Achievement

The substantial relationship between general intelligence and school achievement is perhaps the best-documented finding in psychology and education (Brody, 1997; Neisser et al., 1996). Broadly speaking, g-based IQs correlate approximately .70 with standardized measures of scholastic achievement and .50 with grades in elementary school (Brody, 1985; Jensen, 1998). These correlations are somewhat higher than those obtained in the later school years; because of range restrictions, the correlations decrease progressively as individuals advance through the educational system. The typical correlation between g and standardized high school achievement is between .50 and .60; for college, coefficients vary between .40 and .50; for graduate school, correlations range between .30 and .40.

Jensen (1998) has indicated that g-based IQs predict academic achievement better than any other measurable variable. The reason he cites for the strong association is that school learning itself is g-demanding. Thorndike (1984) similarly concluded that 80%–90% of the *predicted* variance in scholastic performance is accounted for by g-based IQs, with only 10%–20% accounted for by *all* other scores in IQ tests. Thus the available evidence strongly suggests that global ability is the most important variable for estimating a person's academic achievement.

Years of Education

General intelligence is correlated with the number of years of a person's formal education and training. For instance, Jensen (1998) showed that, on average, years of education correlate .60 to .70 with g-based IQs. Jencks (1972) found longitudinal correlations above .50 between the IQs of preadolescents and the final grade level they completed. Likewise, in a review of 16 studies, Ceci (1991) reported correlations of .50 to .90 between measures of overall intelligence and an individual's years of education. Thus research results reveal a strong positive association between overall ability levels and years of education.

Job Training and Work Performance

Because of their strong correlation, there is much debate in the literature regarding whether intelligence or educational level is the variable more directly related to one's level of job performance (Ceci & Williams, 1997; Wagner, 1997; Williams & Ceci, 1997). Regardless of the interrelationship, some basic findings emerge. The average validity coefficient ranges between .20 and .30 for ability tests high in g and job performance (Hartigan & Wigdor, 1989). The coefficients rise to .50 when corrected for range restrictions and sources of measurement error (Hunter & Hunter, 1984; Ree & Earles, 1993).

Consequently, general ability provides surprisingly good prediction of job performance, and does so across a variety of occupations. Although the size of the correlations may not appear to be very high, the most impressive point to remember is that tests of general ability have a higher rate of predicting job performance than variables commonly employed to make such decisions, including class rank, grade point average, previous job experience, results from interviews, and performance on occupational interest inventories (Jensen, 1998).

Social Correlates

Global intelligence shows significant, but more moderate, criterion validity for personality and social dispositions. Typically, the independent contribution of IQ to any given social variable is small (a correlation of approximately .20; Glutting, Youngstrom, Oakland, & Watkins, 1996). At the same time, even such small correlations can have a striking impact in certain segments of the ability continuum. For example, adolescents with IQs of 90 and lower are more likely to have conduct disorder and to be arrested for juvenile delinquency than those with average or better IQs (Kazdin, 1995; Moffitt, Gabrielli, Mednick, & Schulsinger, 1981). Similarly, individuals with IQs of 80 or below experience an increased incidence of various social misfortunes, such as becoming disabled on the job or divorcing within the first 5 years of marriage (Jensen, 1998).

Summary of g-Based Interpretations

There is a tendency among some professionals to dismiss global intelligence as having mere historical value, and thereafter to tout the merits of viewing intelligence as a multi-differentiated construct. However, an extensive body of empirical evidence demonstrates the practical, prognostic utility of g-based IQs. This literature supports the notion that the g-based IQ is among the most dominant and enduring of influences associated with many consequential outcomes within our culture. To those who would dismiss the import of global ability because it does not also serve to remedy what it predicts, we would urge that the inherent value of predictors be appreciated. There are countless predictors of life's vicissitudes, including predictors of the weather, of accident risk, of AIDS infection, and of future achievements. We would hate to see them all ignored because they fail to fix what they forecast.

INTERPRETATION OF COGNITIVE SUBTESTS

Reliance upon subtests to hypothesize about children's cognitive strengths and weaknesses is endemic in psychological training and practice (Aiken, 1996; Alfonso, Oakland, LaRocca, & Spanakos, 2000; Blumberg,

1995; Bracken, McCallum, & Crain, 1993; Gregory, 1999; Groth-Marnat, 1997; Kamphaus, 1993; Kaufman, 1994; Kaufman & Lichtenberger, 2000; Kellerman & Burry, 1997; Prifitera, Weiss, & Saklofske, 1998; Sattler, 1992; Truch, 1993). Interpretation of individual subtests is a vestigial practice, but recommendations that rely essentially upon one or two subtests can still be found (Banas, 1993). This is especially true for neuropsychological assessment (Lezak, 1995). More commonly, however, interpretation of individual subtests is eschewed (Kamphaus, 1993). For example, Kaufman and Lichtenberger (2000) concluded that "the key to accurately characterizing a child's strong and weak areas of functioning is to examine his or her performance across several subtests, not individual subtest scores in isolation" (p. 81). In support of Kaufman and Lichtenberger's conclusion, Table 15.1 illustrates that only 3 of the 12 WISC-III subtests contributing to the WISC-III's four factors meet the reliability coefficient criterion of ≥.85 recommended by Hansen (1999) for making decisions about individuals, and that none meet the more stringent criterion of ≥.90 (Hopkins, 1998; Salvia & Ysseldyke, 1998). Furthermore, the increased error generated by the use of

TABLE 15.1. Reliability of the WISC-III

Subtest or index	Internal consistency[a]	Short-term test–retest[a]	Long-term test–retest[b]
Information	.84	.85	.73
Similarities	.81	.81	.68
Arithmetic	.78	.74	.67
Vocabulary	.87	.89	.75
Comprehension	.77	.73	.68
Digit Span	.85	.73	.65
Picture Completion	.77	.81	.66
Coding	.79	.77	.63
Picture Arrangement	.76	.64	.68
Block Design	.87	.77	.78
Object Assembly	.69	.66	.68
Symbol Search	.76	.74	.55
Verbal IQ	.95	.94	.87
Performance IQ	.91	.87	.87
Verbal Comprehension	.94	.93	.85
Perceptual Organization	.90	.87	.87
Freedom from Distractibility	.87	.82	.75
Processing Speed	.85	.84	.62
Full Scale IQ	.96	.94	.91

[a]Data from Wechsler (1991).
[b]Data from Canivez and Watkins (1998).

difference scores makes even the best sub-test-to-subtest comparison unreliable (e.g., the reliability of the difference between Block Design and Vocabulary is .76).

Elaborate interpretative systems (Kaufman, 1994; Kamphaus, 1993; Sattler, 1992) have been developed to identify specific cognitive subtest patterns that are assumed to reflect neurological dysfunction (Arizona Department of Education, 1992; Drebing, Satz, Van Gorp, Chervinsky, & Uchiyama, 1994; Ivnik, Smith, Malec, Kokmen, & Tangalos, 1994), to be related to learning disabilities (LDs) (Banas, 1993; Kellerman & Burry, 1997; Mayes, Calhoun, & Crowell, 1998; McLean, Reynolds, & Kaufman, 1990), and/or to be prognostic of emotional and behavioral impairments (Blumberg, 1995; Campbell & McCord, 1999). In fact, more than 75 patterns of subtest variation have been identified for the Wechsler scales alone (McDermott, Fantuzzo, & Glutting, 1990).

Diagnostic Efficiency Statistics

Identification of pathognomonic cognitive subtest profiles has generally been based upon statistically significant group differences. That is, the mean subtest score of a group of children with a particular disorder (e.g., LDs) is compared to the mean subtest score of a group of children without the problem. Statistically significant subtest score differences between the two groups are subsequently interpreted as evidence that the profile is diagnostically effective.

However, mean-score difference methods are inadequate to reach this conclusion. Almost 50 years ago, Meehl and Rosen (1955) made it clear that efficient diagnosis depends on the psychometric instruments employed *and* on a consideration of base rates (i.e., prevalence) of the criterion condition in both nondisabled and clinical populations. More recently, Elwood (1993) asserted that "significance alone does *not* reflect the size of the group differences nor does it imply the test can discriminate subjects with sufficient accuracy for clinical use" (p. 409; emphasis in original). As outlined in Table 15.2, Kessel and Zimmerman (1993) listed several diagnostic efficiency indices that allow a test's accuracy to be analyzed in relation to two pervasive alternative interpretations: base rate and chance (Cohen, 1990; Rosnow & Rosenthal, 1989).

An extension of the diagnostic efficiency statistics in Table 15.2 was originally developed in engineering as a way to tell how well a radar operator is able to distinguish signal from noise (Hanley & McNeil,

TABLE 15.2. Diagnostic Efficiency Statistics

Statistic	Description
Sensitivity	True-positive rate. Proportion of participants with a disorder who are identified by a positive test result.
Specificity	True-negative rate. Proportion of participants free of a disorder who are correctly identified by a negative test result.
Positive predictive power	Proportion of participants identified by a positive test result who truly have the target disorder.
Negative predictive power	Proportion of participants identified by a negative test result who truly do *not* have the target disorder.
False-positive rate	Proportion of participants identified by a positive test result who truly do *not* have the target disorder.
False-negative rate	Proportion of participants identified by a negative test result who truly have the target disorder.
Hit rate	Proportion of participants with *and* without the target disorder who were correctly classified by the test.
Kappa	Proportion of agreement between the test and actual condition of the participants (disordered vs. nondisordered) beyond that accounted for by chance alone.

1982). The methodology was then adapted and reformulated for biostatistical applications (Kraemer, 1988; Murphy et al., 1987; Swets, 1988), and it was recently recommended for use with psychological assessment data (McFall & Treat, 1999). Designated the "receiver operating characteristic" (ROC), this procedure entails plotting the balance between the sensitivity and specificity of a diagnostic test while systematically moving the cut score across its full range of values. As illustrated in Figure 16.1, the diagonal dashed line is the "random ROC," which reflects a test with zero discriminating power. The more clearly a test is able to discriminate between individuals with and without the target disorder, the farther its ROC curve will deviate toward the upper left corner of the graph.

The accuracy of an ROC can be quantified by calculating the area under its curve (AUC). Chance diagnostic performance cor-responds to an AUC of .50, whereas perfect diagnostic performance equates to 1.00. The AUC is independent of cut score and does not assume that the underlying score distributions are normal. It is interpreted in terms of two children: one drawn randomly from the distribution of children with the target disorder, and one selected randomly from the population of children without the problem. The AUC is the probability of the test's correctly rank-ordering the children into their appropriate diagnostic groups. According to Swets (1988), AUCs between .50 and .70 are characterized as showing low accuracy; those between .70 and .90 represent medium accuracy; and those between .90 and 1.00 denote high accuracy. Diagnostic utility statistics, including the ROC and its AUC, should be applied when subtest profiles are hypothesized as being able to distinguish between children with and without disorders.

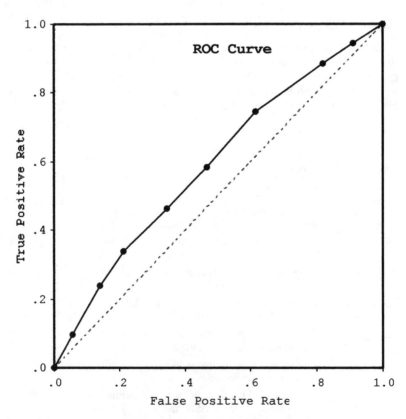

FIGURE 15.1. Receiver operating characteristic (ROC) of Wechsler Development Index (WDI), used to distinguish between participants with and without learning disabilities.

Diagnosis of Neurological Dysfunction

Wechsler's (1958) Deterioration Index (WDI) was originally developed as an indicator of cognitive impairment that was hypothesized to be sensitive to brain injury in adults. Conceptually, the WDI was composed of two groups of Wechsler subtest scores: (1) "hold" subtests, which were considered insensitive to brain injury (Vocabulary, Information, Object Assembly, and Picture Completion); and (2) "don't hold" subtests, which were judged vulnerable to intellectual decline (Digit Span, Similarities, Coding, and Block Design).

Application of the WDI with children was suggested by Bowers and colleagues (1992), given that neuropsychological deficits have often been hypothesized to account for LDs and attentional difficulties (Accardo & Whitman, 1991; Goodyear & Hynd, 1992). Bowers and colleagues recommended that the WDI be renamed the Wechsler *Developmental* Index, because children's cognitive skills are not deteriorating; rather, they are assumed to be developing unevenly. Klein and Fisher (1994) applied the WDI to children in LD programs and found that they scored significantly higher on the WDI (i.e., showed more problems) than children in regular education programs. Based on these statistically significant group differences, Klein and Fisher concluded that the WDI is useful for predicting which students would be found eligible for LD services.

However, mean-difference statistics cannot be used to justify this conclusion. Watkins (1996) replicated the Klein and Fisher (1994) study, but also applied more appropriate diagnostic efficiency procedures. Results revealed that the WDI performed at near-chance levels when distinguishing students diagnosed with LDs (*n* = 611) from those diagnosed with emotional disabilities (*n* = 80) or mental retardation (*n* = 33), as well as from randomly simulated, normal cases (*n* = 2,200). Based upon formulas provided by Hsiao, Bartko, and Potter (1989), the AUC for this study (see Figure 15.1) summed to .57 (compared with a chance rate of .50 for AUCs and a low accuracy rate of between .50 and .70). It was concluded that mean group differences were insufficient to determine diagnostic efficacy, and that the WDI must be definitively validated before it can be applied in actual practice.

Diagnosis of LDs

The ACID Profile

Several subtest profiles have long, storied histories in the field of psychodiagnosis. The most venerable is the "ACID" profile, characterized by low scores on Wechsler Arithmetic, Coding, Information, and Digit Span subtests. With development of the most recent revision of the Wechsler, the WISC-III, diagnostic merit of the ACID profile has once again been advanced (Groth-Marnat, 1997). Prifitera and Dersh (1993) compared percentages of children showing WISC-III ACID profiles in samples with LDs and attention-deficit/hyperactivity disorder (ADHD) to percentages showing the ACID profile in the WISC-III standardization sample. Their findings uncovered a greater incidence of ACID profiles in the clinical samples, with approximately 5% of the children with LDs and 12% of the children with ADHD showing the ACID profile, while such a configuration occurred in only 1% of the cases from the WISC-III standardization sample. Based upon this data, Prifitera and Dersh concluded that ACID profiles "are useful for diagnostic purposes" because "the presence of a pattern or patterns would suggest strongly that the disorder is present" (pp. 50–51). Ward, Ward, Hatt, Young, and Mollner (1995) investigated the prevalence of the WISC-III ACID profile among children with LDs (*n* = 382) and found a prevalence rate of 4.7% (vs. the expected rate of 1%). Likewise, upon achieving similar ACID results for a sample of children with LDs (*n* = 165), Daley and Nagle (1996) suggested practitioners that "investigate the possibility of a learning disability" (p. 330) when confronted by an ACID profile.

Watkins, Kush, and Glutting (1997a) evaluated the discriminative and predictive validity of the WISC-III ACID profile among children with LDs. As in previous research (Kaufman, 1994), ACID profiles were more prevalent among children with

LDs (n = 612) than among children without LDs (n = 2,158). However, when ACID profiles were used to classify students into groups with and without LDs, they operated with considerable error. At best, only 51% of the children identified by a positive ACID profile were previously diagnosed as having LDs. These data indicated that a randomly selected child with an LD had a more severe ACID profile than a randomly selected child without an LD about 60% of the time (AUC = .60). Although marginally better than chance, the degree of accuracy was quite low (cf. classificatory criteria presented by Swets, 1988).

The SCAD Profile

Preliminary empirical support was provided by Prifitera and Dersh (1993) for another subtest configuration hypothesized to be indicative of LDs. They combined subtests from the WISC-III Freedom from Distractibility and Processing Speed factors to create a new profile. This profile was more common in a sample of children with LDs (n = 99) and in another sample of children with ADHD (n = 65) than within the WISC-III standardization sample. Using the outcomes as guidance, Prifitera and Dersh suggested that the subtest configuration would be "useful in the diagnosis of LD and ADHD" (p. 53).

Kaufman (1994) coined an acronym for this new profile: "SCAD" (for the Symbol Search, Coding, Arithmetic, and Digit Span subtests). He recommended that the SCAD index be subtracted from the sum of Picture Completion, Picture Arrangement, Block Design, and Object Assembly to create a comparison between SCAD and the Perceptual Organization factor. Kaufman opined that Arithmetic, Coding, and Digit Span have "been quite effective at identifying exceptional groups from normal ones, and . . . are like a land mine that explodes on a diversity of abnormal populations but leaves most normal samples unscathed" (p. 213). Kaufman concluded that the SCAD profile is "an important piece of evidence for diagnosing a possible abnormality" (p. 221), which "won't identify the type of exceptionality, but [the profile is] likely to be valuable for making a presence–absence decision and

helping to pinpoint specific areas of deficiency" (p. 214).

The foregoing claims were tested by Watkins, Kush, and Glutting (1997b) with children who were enrolled in LD and emotional disability programs (n = 365). When these children were compared to the WISC-III standardization sample via diagnostic utility statistics, an AUC of .59 was generated. This finding suggests that the SCAD profile is not substantially more useful in making this diagnostic decision than any randomly chosen, irrelevant variable (McFall & Treat, 1999). Thus, contrary to Kaufman's (1994) assertion, SCAD subtest scores were not found to be important evidence for diagnosing exceptionalities.

Subtest Variability

Heterogeneous variability among subtest scores is a traditional diagnostic indicator of LDs. Subtest variability can be quantified in three ways (Schinka, Vanderploeg, & Curtiss, 1997). The first method examines the range (i.e., difference between an examinee's highest and lowest subtest scaled scores). The second method involves evaluating variances, using the variance formula applicable to the subtest scores of an individual examinee. Finally, researchers look at the number of subtests differing from the individual examinee's mean score by ±3 points.

The diagnostic utility of all three variability metrics was tested by Watkins (1999) and Watkins and Worrell (2000). Children from the WISC-III standardization effort were compared to children enrolled in LD programs (n = 684). Results included AUCs ranging from .50 to .54. Thus WISC-III subtest variability exhibited low diagnostic utility in distinguishing children with LDs from those without identified problems from the WISC-III standardization sample.

Diagnosis of Emotional and Behavioral Disorders

Despite long-standing assumptions, subtest profiles have consistently failed to demonstrate utility in predicting students' social and behavioral functioning (Beebe, Pfiffner, & McBurnett, 2000; Dumont, Farr, Willis, & Whelley, 1998; Glutting et al., 1998;

Glutting, McGrath, Kamphaus, & McDermott, 1992; Kramer, Henning-Stout, Ullman, & Schellenberg, 1987; Lipsitz, Dworkin, & Erlenmeyer-Kimling, 1993; McDermott & Glutting, 1997; Piedmont, Sokolove, & Fleming, 1989; Reinecke, Beebe, & Stein, 1999; Riccio, Cohen, Hall, & Ross, 1997; Rispens et al., 1997) and have been discounted as valid indicators of children's mental health. Thus Teeter and Korducki (1998) concluded that "in general there appears to be a consensus in the literature that there are no distinctive Wechsler [subtest] patterns that can provide reliable, discriminative information about a child's behavior or emotional condition" (p. 124). In contrast, instruments designed specifically to assess child behavior, such as teacher- and parent-completed rating scales, have produced highly accurate differential diagnoses (i.e., AUCs > .90; Chen, Faraone, Biederman, & Tsuang, 1994).

Hypothesis Generation

Although cognitive subtest profiles are not accurate in diagnosing childhood psychopathology, profile interpretation is frequently relied upon to identify distinctive abilities useful for hypothesis generation (Gregory, 1999). This practice implicitly assumes that cognitive subtest profiles are predictive of performance in important endeavors, such as children's academic achievement and/or their classroom conduct. For example, Kaufman (1994) asserted that "insightful subtest interpretation" (p. 32) allows an examiner to understand why a student experiences learning difficulties and how to remediate them.

As illustrated earlier in this chapter, global intelligence has a well-documented, robust relationship with academic achievement. However, the excellent predictive validity of the g-based IQ cannot be assumed to generalize to subtest profiles. One way to test the utility and validity of subtest scores is to decompose profiles into their elemental components. The unique, incremental predictive validity of each component can then be analyzed separately to determine what aspect(s), if any, of the subtest profile can be used to estimate academic performance.

To this end, Cronbach and Gleser (1953)

reported that subtest profiles contain only three types of information: "elevation," "scatter," and "shape." Elevation information is represented by a person's aggregate performance (i.e., mean, normative score) across subtests. Profile scatter is defined by how widely scores in a profile diverge from its mean; scatter is typically operationalized by the standard deviation of the subtest scores in a profile. Finally, shape information reflects where "ups and downs" occur in a profile. Even if two profiles have the same elevation and scatter, their high and low points may be different. Shape is thus defined by the rank order of scores for each person (Nunnally & Bernstein, 1994).

Watkins and Glutting (2000) tested the incremental validity of WISC-III subtest profile level, scatter, and shape in forecasting academic performance. WISC-III subtest profiles were decomposed into the three elements just described and sequentially regressed onto reading and mathematics achievement scores for nonexceptional (n = 1,118) and exceptional (n = 538) children. Profile elevation was statistically and practically significant for both nonexceptional (R = .72 to .75) and exceptional (R = .36 to .61) children. Profile scatter did not aid in the prediction of achievement. Profile shape accounted for an additional 5%–8% of the variance in achievement measures: One pattern of relatively high verbal scores positively predicted both reading and mathematics achievement, and a pattern of relatively low scores on the WISC-III Arithmetic subtest was negatively related to mathematics. Beyond these two somewhat intuitive patterns, profile shape information had inconsequential incremental validity for both nonexceptional and exceptional children. In other words, it was the averaged, norm-referenced information (i.e., elevation) contained in subtest profiles that best predicted achievement. This information is essentially redundant to the prognostic efficacy available from omnibus intelligence scores (i.e., Verbal IQ [VIQ], Performance IQ [PIQ]) and global ability (i.e., the Full Scale IQ [FSIQ]) and is consistent with outcomes obtained in previous studies (Glutting et al., 1992, 1998; Hale & Saxe, 1983; Kline, Snyder, Guilmette, & Castellanos, 1993). From these findings, it was concluded that subtest scatter and shape offer minimal assistance for generating hypotheses about children's academic performance.

Methodological Issues

Subtest analysis has also undergone serious methodological challenges. Specifically, within the last 15 years several methodological problems have been identified that operate to negate, or equivocate, essentially all research into children's ability profiles (Glutting et al., 1998; McDermott et al., 1990; McDermott, Fantuzzo, Glutting, Watkins, & Baggaley, 1992; Watkins & Kush, 1994).

Circular Reasoning and Selection Bias

Prominent among the methodological problems identified is the circular use of ability profiles for *both* the initial formation of diagnostic groups *and* the subsequent search for profiles that might inherently define or distinguish those groups. This problem is one of self-selection. The consequence is that self-selection unduly increases the probability of discovering group differences. Another factor affecting outcomes is the nearly exclusive use of children previously classified or those referred for psychoeducational assessments. Both classified and referral samples (the majority of whom are subsequently classified) are unrepresentative of the population as a whole and subject to selection bias (Rutter, 1989).

Solutions to Methodological Problems

It is possible to overcome the problems of circular reasoning and selection bias (Glutting, McDermott, Watkins, Kush, & Konold, 1997; Glutting et al., 1998; Sines, 1966; Wiggins, 1973). Three steps are necessary. First, rather than concentrating exclusively on exceptional or referral samples, researchers should use epidemiological samples from the general population (i.e., large, unselected cohorts), because such samples are representative of the child population as a whole. Second, the epidemiological samples should be further divided on the basis of their score configurations, rather than according to whether children fit predetermined diagnostic categories (e.g., "children

with LDs," "normal children," and the like). In other words, the epidemiological sample should be used to identify groups with unusual versus common ability score profiles. The identification of "unusual" profiles can be accomplished with a variety of methods. Examples include the traditional approaches of whether or not statistically significant normative or ipsative score differences are present. Alternatively, more current univariate–normative and univariate–ipsative base rate approaches could be used (e.g., a prevalence/base rate occurring in less than 5% of the child population), as well as multivariate prevalence approaches (cf. Glutting et al., 1998). Third, once classified on observed score configurations (e.g., groups with unusual vs. common ability profiles), the groups should subsequently be compared across a variety of important criteria, external to the ability test itself.

When we took *all* of the methodological factors described above into account, we were able to locate only a single investigation within the last 15 years that supported the interpretation of subtest scores (Prifitera & Dersch, 1993). By contrast, a substantial number of studies satisfying the dual criteria failed to find relationships between unusual subtest configurations on such tests as the WISC-III, the DAS, and the Kaufman Assessment Battery for Children (K-ABC; Kaufman & Kaufman, 1983) and performance on meaningful external criteria (Glutting et al., 1992, 1998; Glutting, McDermott, et al., 1997; McDermott et al., 1990, 1992; McDermott & Glutting, 1997; Watkins & Glutting, 2000; Watkins et al., 1997b).

Ipsative Assessment

Evidence reported in previous sections of this chapter suggests that subtest profiles are invalid indicators of childhood psychopathology, and that most of the predictive power carried by subtests resides in their level (i.e., their role as a vehicle of *g*) rather than in their shape or scatter. One psychometric source of this invalidity was described by McDermott and colleagues (1990, 1992) and later by McDermott and Glutting (1997). In essence, the operationalization of a large number of current interpretative systems moves away from normative measurement, and instead rests upon ipsative interpretation of test scores (Cattell, 1944). As described by Kaufman (1994), ipsative measurement is concerned with how a child's subtest scores relate to his or her personalized, average performance and discounts the influence of global intelligence. Thus Kaufman suggested that "it is of greater interest and potential benefit to know what children can do well, relative to their own level of ability, than to know how well they did [normatively]" (p. 8).

Ipsative measurement is operationalized by taking an individual's subtest scores and averaging them. Then each subtest score is subtracted from the child's personal grand mean. Subtest scores that deviate negatively from the personalized mean are considered to reflect cognitive weaknesses, and those that deviate positively are assumed to represent cognitive strengths. As Silverstein (1993) has cautioned, however, these repeated subtest versus grand-mean comparisons entail repeated statistical comparisons that produce excessive Type I and Type II error rates, for which there is no satisfactory solution.

More importantly, after employing a large number of statistical techniques across multiple samples (both large epidemiological samples and cohorts of exceptional children), McDermott and colleagues (1990, 1992) and McDermott and Glutting (1997) concluded:

> Ipsative measures have insufficient reliability for educational decisions, are significantly less reliable than normative measures, and are relatively insensitive to sources of individual variation that characterize omnibus ability measures. Further, any argument in favor of ipsatized assessment certainly is vitiated by the fact that such approaches fail to predict outcomes as well as normative approaches. And, were all of this not the case, we would still be left with uncertainty about the meaning of ipsative constructs and their limited utility for either group or individual studies. (McDermott et al., 1992, p. 521)

The preceding findings prompted Silverstein to observe that "the assumption of clinical meaningfulness [of subtest deviations around a personalized mean] may ultimately prove to be the fundamental error in pattern analysis" (1993, p. 73).

INTERPRETATION OF FACTOR SCORES FROM INDIVIDUALLY ADMINISTERED TESTS OF INTELLIGENCE

Factor scores are stronger candidates for interpretation than subtest profiles. Factor scores have better reliabilities than subtest scores (as per the Spearman–Brown prophecy; Traub, 1991), as illustrated in Table 15.1. And, because they theoretically represent phenomena beyond the sum of subtest specificity and measurement error, factor scores potentially escape the psychometric weaknesses that undermine analyses of conjoint subtest patterns. Factor score interpretation is also consistent with standards for good assessment practice, such as the "top-down" hierarchical approach recommended by authorities on intelligence testing (cf. Kamphaus, 1993; Kaufman, 1994; Sattler, 1992). Therefore, it is possible that ability constructs measured by factor deviation quotients (i.e., factor score IQs) from such tests as the WISC-III and DAS might show strong associations with important achievement, emotional, and/or behavioral criteria.

Criterion-Related Validity

Despite their psychometric advantages, the utility of factor scores has not been well researched. A major issue that remains is to demonstrate the validity of factor scores—and, specifically, to determine whether factor scores provide substantial improvements in predicting important criteria above and beyond levels afforded by general ability. Glutting, Youngstrom, Ward, Ward, and Hale (1997) assessed the ability of the four factors underlying the WISC-III (Verbal Comprehension, Perceptual Organization, Freedom from Distractibility, and Processing Speed), relative to the FSIQ, to predict performance in four areas of achievement (reading, mathematics, language, and writing). Two groups were examined: a nationally representative epidemiological sample ($n = 283$) and a sample of children referred for psychoeducational assessments ($n = 636$). In general, the four factor scores did not show any substantial increase in the prediction of achievement criteria after the FSIQ was partialed out. The Freedom from Distractibility factor showed the largest correlations after the FSIQ was controlled for, but it only uniquely accounted for between 1.4% and 5.2% of the variance in the various achievement measures. Results showed that the FSIQ was the most parsimonious and powerful predictor of academic achievement obtainable from the WISC-III. Using factor scores to estimate achievement levels, even in specific content areas, led to more complex models (and more laborious calculations for the practitioner) that provided either no or meager dividends. This relationship held true for both nonreferred and referred samples.

The research described above addressed only the inability of factor scores from the WISC-III to inform academic achievement. It is possible that factor scores from other IQ tests might yet tell something relevant about children's academic performance. Youngstrom, Kogos, and Glutting (1999) examined this issue. The incremental validity of the DAS's three factors (Verbal, Nonverbal, and Spatial Ability), relative to the test's General Conceptual Ability (GCA) score, was investigated in terms of predicting standardized achievement in three areas (word reading, basic number skills, and spelling). Results with an epidemiological sample ($n = 1,185$) showed that even when factor scores provided a statistically significant increment above the GCA score, the improvement was too small to be of clinical significance. Consequently, the outcomes extended prior findings with the WISC-III: that the more differentiated ability estimates provided by factor scores has not yet been found to better predict achievement than g.

Reversing the Hierarchical Order of Predictors

It could be argued that it is inappropriate to partial global ability (the FSIQ or GCA) prior to letting the ability factors predict achievement. In other words, in the two aforementioned studies, the hierarchical strategy should have been reversed (i.e., partialing the effect of the factor scores and then letting the FSIQ or GCA predict achievement). This strategy has some intuitive appeal. However, as noted at the beginning of this chapter, to sustain such logic, psychologists would have to repeal the law

of parsimony. We would have to accept the novel notion that when many things essentially account for no more, or only marginally more, predictive variance in academic achievement than that accounted for by merely one thing (global ability), we should adopt the less parsimonious system.

Obviously, in the preceding analyses, there was a high degree of multicollinearity (i.e., redundancy) among the predictors as a consequence of global ability's being drawn in large part (but not entirely) from the underlying factor scores. However, in situations where variables are all highly interrelated, more things (such as factor scores) will nearly always predict as well as, or even *marginally* better than, one thing (global ability)—but that is exactly why such multicollinearity is a violation of parsimony and not a virtue. Therefore, it is incumbent among advocates of factor score interpretation to present convincing empirical support in their favor—support that clearly extends above and beyond the contribution provided by the parsimonious g variable.

Validity of Processing Speed Factors

The role and function of specific factor scores have also been investigated. One such factor is processing speed. The construct of "processing speed" has received considerable scholarly attention through the information-processing theories of cognitive psychology (see Kranzler, 1997, for a review). Likewise, the discovery of a processing speed factor on the DAS (Keith, 1990) and the inclusion of a processing speed factor on the WISC-III make it likely that clinicians will interpret this dimension during routine clinical assessments. Oh and Glutting (1999) investigated the utility of processing speed factors from the DAS and WISC-III, respectively. An epidemiological sample was employed. From the cohort, groups with unusual strengths and weaknesses in processing speed were identified according to a rarity criterion (i.e., the strengths or weaknesses occurred in ≤5% of the child population). The group with these strengths and weaknesses were then matched to a control group on the demographic variables of race, gender, and parents' educational levels, as well as on overall ability level. The group and its control were compared across multiple, norm-referenced measures of achievement (and, in the DAS study, also across six teacher-rated indices of behavioral adjustment). In both studies, children with unusual strengths and weaknesses in processing speed were found to exhibit no significant differences in achievement or classroom adjustment from their respective controls. Consequently, these results suggested that measures of processing speed provide psychologists with no diagnostic help.

Factor Scores versus g

All of the foregoing results should come as no surprise. Kranzler (1997) summarized the evidence on general versus specific factors by noting:

> On IQ tests with at least several subtests measuring different abilities, g constitutes by far the single largest independent component of variance (e.g., Jensen, 1980). In fact, psychometric g usually explains more variance than all group factors *combined*. . . . Furthermore, the predictive validity of tests in education and vocational settings is overwhelmingly a function of g. (p. 152; emphasis in original)

Lubinski and Benbow (2000) concurred that general intelligence is the most potent predictor of academic performance for students in grades K–12, and attributed this ubiquitous finding to the fact that the K–12 educational curriculum is relatively uniform for most students. They hypothesized that specific mathematical, spatial, and verbal reasoning factors should become more important predictors of educational–vocational criteria as people begin to pursue more specialized educational and vocational training in young adulthood. According to their theory, this cognitive differentiation should be most apparent for students with high ability. Jensen (1998) also suggested that abilities are more differentiated at the upper end of the intelligence range, and supplied the analogy that rich people spend their money on a greater variety of things than do poor people. It would be worthwhile to test this hypothesis with jointly standardized cognitive and achievement tests that span the broad age and cognitive ability ranges specified by Lubinski and Benbow (2000).

Results from Structural Equation Modeling

Several authors recently contested the overwhelming research evidence in favor of general ability and suggested that specific factors have important effects beyond g (McGrew, Keith, Flanagan, & Underwood, 1997). Evidence presented to support these claims was based upon complex structural equation modeling (SEM) applied to the WJ-R (Keith, 1999). Researchers' conclusions seem to have moved from scientific caution to clinical certainty in only 2 years and two studies. For example, in the first study, McGrew and colleagues (1997) indicated that "the current results only suggest that *some* specific Gf-Gc abilities may be important for understanding *some* academic skills at *some* developmental levels" (p. 205, emphasis in original); by 1999, however, Keith concluded that "psychologists and educators who wish to understand students' reading and mathematics learning will gain more complete understanding of those skills for groups and individuals via the assessment of these specific abilities" (p. 257).

The conclusions must be tempered by several considerations. First, all of the studies cited just above used the WJ-R to formulate both general and specific intellectual factors. Flanagan, McGrew, and Ortiz (2000) report an unpublished study that apparently included the WISC-R and another that applied the WISC-III, but provided insufficient information to permit the evaluation of methods and results. Beyond the unknown generalizability to other intelligence tests, there is some danger that WJ-R cognitive and academic scales are confounded. In terms of generalizability, the WJ-R processing speed factor was related to math achievement (Keith, 1999; McGrew et al., 1997); however, the WISC-III and DAS processing speed factors, as noted earlier, demonstrated little incremental validity in predicting achievement and behavior (Glutting, Youngstrom, et al., 1997; Oh & Glutting, 1999; Youngstrom et al., 1999; Youngstrom & Glutting, 2000). When considering shared method variance, Keith (1999) and McGrew and colleagues (1997) both reported that the WJ-R Auditory Processing factor (Ga) was related to the WJ-R Letter–Word Identification and Word Attack subtests. The WJ-R Ga factor is composed of two subtests: Incomplete Words and Sound Blending. McGrew and colleagues equated this auditory processing factor to "phonological awareness (*Ga*) in reading" (p. 196). However, phonological awareness is usually considered to be an important component of reading itself (Adams, 1990; Stahl & Murray, 1994), is often included as a skill in the reading curriculum (Carnine, Silbert, & Kameenui, 1997), and can be developed through instruction with subsequent enhancement of children's' reading skills (Bus & van Uzendoorn, 1999; Ehri et al., 2001). Thus the "cognitive" subtests appear to be inexorably confounded with their contrasting "academic" subtests.

Second, the aforementioned studies based their conclusions solely on SEM, which is a multivariate correlational technique designed to identify relationships among *latent* variables (i.e., constructs). Thus the methodology provides results that are best interpreted as relationships between pure constructs measured without error. SEM is, of course, an excellent method for testing theory, but it can be less than satisfactory for direct diagnostic applications. The observed test scores employed by psychologists are not latent variables, and they clearly contain measurement error (i.e., reliability coefficients less than 1.00). Basing diagnostic decisions on theoretically pure constructs is impossible in practice. Even approximating true scores would require clinicians to perform complex, tedious calculations for which no published algorithms yet exist. For example, attempting to employ SEM to describe the association between a cognitive ability and achievement would demand both (1) a known, quantifiable relationship between the measured variables and the latent variable, and (2) a way of correcting the individual's scores on predictor and criterion to approximate the true scores. In practical terms, this would involve using the factor loadings from the measurement model as regression coefficients to predict the individual's factor score based on the observed subtest scores. Not only is this more complicated than current practice, but the estimated factor loadings will change depending on the reference sample (unless it is a large, representative, epi-

demiological sample) and on the combination of subtests used to measure the factor.

A careful parsing of published claims reveals a subtle distinction between what can be inferred from SEM results and what can be accomplished during day-to-day assessments. For example, McGrew (1997) suggested that research finding negligible effects for specific ability factors after considering general ability (e.g., Glutting, Youngstrom, et al., 1997; Youngstrom et al., 1999) was predictive in nature, but that

> to translate specific ability research into practice, to use it to develop meaningful interventions for students with learning problems, an *explanatory* approach is needed. That is, it is not enough to know simply that ability 'x' *predicts* reading comprehension; to translate research into practice it is necessary to know whether or not ability 'x' *affects* reading comprehension. (p. 197; emphasis in original)

Likewise, Keith (1999) proposed that a more complete "understanding" (p. 257) of academic skills could be obtained via assessment of specific cognitive factors. From a theoretical perspective, science seeks the simplest explanations of complex facts and uses those explanations to craft hypotheses that are capable of being disproved (Platt, 1964). Testing of hypotheses typically involves prediction of one kind or another (Ziskin, 1995). Thus, accurate prediction should flow from explanation and understanding of natural phenomena, but understanding without prediction is an inherently weak scientific proof. In clinical practice, an approach which "involves not confusing the ability to *explain* with the ability to *predict*" (Tracey & Rounds, 1999, p. 125; emphasis in original) is recommended to reduce bias and errors in clinical judgment (Garb, 1998). Thus both theory and practice suggest an approach that emphasizes prediction.

Multiple Regression versus SEM

An advantage of the multiple-regression analyses used by certain researchers (e.g., Glutting et al., 1997; Youngstrom et al., 1999) is that they rely on the same measured factor indices clinicians employ in practice. Factor index scores are imperfect, and this measurement error is present both in the regression analyses and in clinical practice. The advantage of SEM is that it provides estimates of the "true" relationship between such constructs as ability and achievement, with the measurement model removing the effects of measurement error.

The critical issue for both the regression and SEM approaches is to demonstrate effects sufficiently large to have meaningful consequences. In other words, when factor scores are considered to be clinically interpretable (i.e., to show statistically significant or rare strengths or weaknesses), it is still necessary to demonstrate their consequences for individual decision making. For example, Youngstrom and Glutting (2000) found that unusual discrepancies between Verbal Ability and Spatial Ability on the DAS provided a statistically significant improvement ($p < .00005$) to the prediction of reading achievement, above and beyond levels produced by general ability. However, the significant regression coefficient (.21) was then translated to show its consequence for clinical decisions. The comparison revealed that for every 5-point increase in the difference between a child's Verbal Ability and Spatial Ability scores, there was a 1-point change in reading. Even when children showed unusually large Verbal Ability versus Spatial Ability discrepancies (i.e., $\geq$ 29 points), which occured in less than 5% of the DAS standardization sample, the difference translated into a 6-point change in predicted word knowledge. This amount of predicted change possesses only limited clinical relevance, because it barely exceeds the *standard error of measurement* of the reading measure (i.e., 4 points)!

CONCEPTUAL AND PRACTICAL PROBLEMS WITH INTERPRETING FACTOR SCORES

Besides the lack of incremental, criterion-related validity, there are several troubling conceptual and practical issues associated with the interpretation of factor scores. We now discuss four of these issues, and provide an alternative recommendation addressing the proper diagnostic application of IQ tests.

Contemporary Pressures for Increased Productivity Are Strong

The inclusion of more subtests (and factors) in an ability battery extends administration time. Unfortunately, most psychologists are increasingly confronted with growing caseloads as a consequence of pressures generated from commercial mental health insurance carriers and recent federal regulations that affect school caseloads. At the same time, the Centers for Medicare and Medicaid Services federal guidelines stipulate that Medicaid will not pay for time spent scoring, interpreting, or writing assessment reports. Instead, only the "face-to-face" time spent on test administration will be reimbursed. This policy is significant, because these federal standards are often imitated by other third-party payers—particularly when adoption of the standards offers the possibility of decreased reimbursement.

Similarly, managed care organizations have begun to constrain psychological assessment reimbursement rates (Groth-Marnat, 1999). For example, one national managed care organization only allows 1 hour for administering, scoring, and interpreting a WAIS-III or WISC-III (Eisman et al., 1998), even though published data indicate that these tests require more than twice as long on average (e.g., median values are 75 minutes to administer, 20 minutes to score, and 20 minutes to interpret; Ball, Archer, & Imhof, 1994; Camara, Nathan, & Puente, 1998). The net effect of longer ability tests in these times is that psychologists are caught between societal demands for higher efficiency and a new generation of longer, more time-consuming ability tests.

It is possible to quantify the impact that changes in test administration and interpretation could have in terms of cost. For example, published estimates are available that document the number of practicing school psychologists and their median salary, the median number of assessments completed in a year, and the length of time typically spent in giving and scoring tests. Using these estimates, we find that a 1-hour change in the length of the average evaluation yields a more than $55 million change in costs to educational systems each year! Specifically, the following equation shows:

1-hour change × $33.33 × 72 assessments
in assessment   per hour   per year

  × 23,000   = $55,194,480
   practitioners   per year

The hourly rate is based on the median salary and work hours reported in Thomas (2000). The median number of assessments per year is based on remarkably similar figures from two independent surveys: Curtis, Hunley, and Baker (1996) found a median of 72, and Thomas obtained a median of 73. The number of practitioners is based on the report by Lund, Reschly, and Martin (1998).

The $55 million figure is only an estimate, but it is a conservative one for several reasons. One is that the numbers constitute median, not mean, values; therefore, they are less influenced by extreme cases with unusually large salaries or caseloads. In a broader sense, this result is a substantial underestimate of the cumulative effect of a change in assessment practice, because the example only considers school psychologists. There are other large practicing constituencies that spend substantial time in assessment activities (see Camara et al., 1998, for details about the assessment practices of clinical psychologists and neuropsychologists). Clearly, the addition of clinical psychologists, counseling psychologists, and neuropsychologists to the formula can only increase the estimated fiscal impact of changes in assessment practices.

Surveys suggest that there is room for streamlining current assessment-related activity, and that test administration time and scoring contribute substantially to the length of the assessment process (Brown, Swigart, Bolen, Hall, & Webster, 1998; Camara et al., 1998). Based on a review of 271 records from 59 school psychologists, the average time spent on an assessment case was 12.3 hours (median = 11.7, SD = 4.1), with test administration consuming the most time (M = 2.9 hours, SD = 1.2) and the combination of administration and scoring lasting an average of 6.3 hours (SD = 2.4; Lichtenstein & Fischetti, 1998).

The reality in most settings is that the demand for evaluation and services far outstrips capacity, with school psychologists spending the majority of their time in assessment-driven activities, and relatively little time in consultation, counseling, or other service delivery roles (Reschly & Wilson, 1997). The time savings offered by adoption of shorter assessment batteries could be viewed as a potential transfer of resources. Each hour not spent in assessment or interpretation is an hour available to provide support services and consultation, or at least to assess a child on a waiting list sooner. As the gross estimates above show, small changes in the assessment procedure (e.g., 1 hour is 8.1% of the average assessment cycle) can yield resource reallocations involving tens to hundreds of millions of dollars each year within the psychoeducational system alone.

Longer Tests May be No Better Diagnostically

The second issue has both theoretical and practical implications. As established at the outset of this chapter, the trend in intelligence testing has been toward developing longer IQ tests that provide psychologists with a wide variety of specific abilities, as reflected by the presence of more subtest scores and factor indices. Practically speaking, no test can hope to evaluate all specific abilities (Horn, 1988). One could imagine an assessment using the "breadth of specificity" created by administering nonredundant subtest measures found among the 14 cognitive subtests from the DAS, the 13 from the WISC-III, and the 21 cognitive subtests from the WJ-R. Such a combined ability measure is not typical of current evaluations, and it would probably be unappealing both to the psychologist and certainly to the individual being tested. Moreover, while such a battery would measure many specific abilities, such an extensive (and time-consuming) assessment would still fail to capture all of the specific abilities identified or proposed for the realm of intelligence (cf. Gardner, 1983; Guilford, 1967; Sternberg, 1988).

Some Variables Beyond g are Important

Third, as demonstrated earlier, it has not yet been proven whether the proliferation of factor and subtest scores found in longer IQ tests actually make a meaningful contribution to differential diagnosis and treatment planning. Most psychologists would agree that at least some abilities beyond g are clinically relevant. Examples are the verbal–nonverbal dichotomy in Wechsler's tests and the crystallized–fluid distinctions in the WJ-III, the Stanford–Binet Intelligence Scale: Fourth Edition (SB4; Thorndike, Hagen, & Sattler, 1986), and the Kaufman Adolescent and Adult Intelligence Test (KAIT; Kaufman & Kaufman, 1993).

There is substantial factor-analytic support for both verbal–visual and crystallized–fluid abilities (Carroll, 1993; Keith & Witta, 1997; McGrew, 1997; McGrew et al., 1997; Roid, Prifitera, & Weiss, 1993). More importantly, the external, diagnostic relevance of visual/fluid constructs is evident when psychologists evaluate (1) children and adults with hearing impairments, (2) those with language disorders, (3) individuals whose dominant language is not English, and (4) those with inadequate exposure to formal academic training. In each instance, a verbal/crystallized score is *not* likely to reflect a person's true ability. Similarly, a nonverbal/fluid score is *not* likely to represent the ability of those with (1) visual impairments, (2) physical limitations, or (3) certain forms of acute brain injury. Therefore, both components seem necessary to capture a more accurate estimate than one global score.

Several writers have reviewed the literature regarding the incremental efficacy of verbal versus visual dimensions relative to g-based IQs. Jensen (1998) indicates that visual–spatial abilities (along with visual–motor abilities) provide the greatest incremental validity of any second-order ability over and above the criterion variance predicted by g. Hunt (1995) found that visual–spatial reasoning is an important part of understanding mathematics. Children with depressed verbal/crystallized IQs relative to their visual/fluid IQs show more reading problems than normally would be expected (Moffitt & Silva, 1987; Watkins & Glutting, 2000; Youngstrom & Glutting, 2000). Finally, depressed verbal IQs are also more common among children and adolescents with conduct disorder (Kazdin, 1995; Moffitt et al., 1981).

The review above demonstrates that there is an empirical basis for hypotheses generated from discrepancies between verbal/crystallized and visual/fluid abilities. That is, certain outcomes can be predicted with greater precision than that which would result from g-based IQs alone. Psychologists therefore must pay careful attention to variation between an individual's verbal/crystallized and visual/fluid IQs.

The Number of Meaningful Variables beyond g Appears to Be Small

Fourth, the simple fact that a specific ability can be measured does not necessarily mean that the ability has diagnostic merit (Briggs & Cheek, 1986). As demonstrated in previous sections of this chapter (and elsewhere), a case in point is the well-known Wechsler Freedom from Distractibility factor. The diagnostic and treatment validity of the Freedom from Distractibility factor remains as conjectural today as it was over 40 years ago when Cohen (1959) first discovered the dimension. Indeed, more recent treatment reviews and analyses of diagnostic data raise serious concerns about the importance and utility of deviation IQs based on the Freedom from Distractibility factor (Barkley, 1998; Cohen, Becker, & Campbell, 1990; Kavale & Forness, 1984; Riccio et al., 1997; Wielkiewicz, 1990).

The assessments of factors for other specific abilities or groups of abilities, such as processing speed, sequential and simultaneous processing, Bannatyne categories, deterioration indexes, and the like, are also of theoretical interest. The problem is that their diagnostic and treatment validity is even less well investigated than that of the Freedom from Distractibility factor. Moreover, what little empirical information is available for these abilities is discouraging. Therefore, while a quest for more specific ability constructs is tempting, the amount of empirical support for using most newer constructs advanced over the past 25 years is disappointingly meager. At least for now, those involved in applied clinical assessment would have difficulty empirically justifying the utilization of more assessment tasks than those available in much shorter measures.

Alternative Recommendation

Groth-Marnat (1999) noted that "selection of instruments is a crucial cost consideration especially in cost containment efforts," and hypothesized that it "may be that simpler, briefer tests can make comparable predictions (p. 819). Rather than emphasizing the identification of new or different discrete abilities, taking a different tack might be more useful. An alternative to longer IQ tests would be to develop instruments whose subtests are chosen to possess high loadings on g. These measures could possibly be designed to be shorter than, and yet to assess theoretical g nearly as well as, longer ability tests. At the same time, these tests could concentrate on the identification of ability dimensions beyond g whose diagnostic validities are well established. Examples of this alternative trend are the verbal/crystallized and visual/fluid abilities measured by compact instruments such as the four-subtest Wide Range Intelligence Test (WRIT; Glutting, Adams, & Sheslow, 2000) and the four-subtest Wechsler Abbreviated Scale of Intelligence (WASI; Psychological Corporation, 1999).

CROSS-BATTERY ASSESSMENTS

Interpretation of cognitive test performance has traditionally been based upon subtests contained in a single instrument. Thus the interpretation of subtest profiles has generally been restricted to the individual cognitive test from which the subtests were derived. Recently, however, expansion of profile interpretation to subtests extracted from a variety of cognitive tests has been suggested (Flanagan & McGrew, 1997). Energized by the factor-analytic work of Carroll (1993), and relying upon newer theories about the structure of intelligence (Horn & Noll, 1997), Flanagan and McGrew (1997) have advocated a cross-battery approach to assessing and interpreting intelligence.

Flanagan and McGrew (1997) have asserted that a "synthesized Carroll and Horn–Cattell Gf-Gc model of human cognitive abilities . . . is the most comprehensive and empirically supported model of the structure of cognitive abilities" (p. 316). Operating from this foundation, they have

hypothesized that human cognitive abilities can be classified at two levels of hierarchical generality: (1) approximately 70 narrow abilities, which are in turn subsumed by (2) 10 broad abilities. This formulation omits general intelligence. The reason cited for doing so is that g

> has little practical relevance to cross-battery assessment and interpretation. That is, the cross-battery approach was designed to improve psychoeducational assessment practice by describing the unique *Gf-Gc pattern of abilities* of individuals that in turn can be related to important occupational and achievement outcomes and other human traits. (McGrew & Flanagan, 1998, p. 14; emphasis in original)

As explained by McGrew and Flanagan, "a global composite intelligence test score is at odds with the underlying Gf-Gc cross-battery philosophy" (p. 382), which "uncovers the individual skills and abilities that are more diagnostic of learning and problem-solving processes than a global IQ score" (p. 383).

Given the large number of abilities identified in the Gf-Gc model, all existing intelligence tests are considered to be "incomplete because they measure between three and five cognitive abilities [i.e., factors], reflecting only a subset of known broad cognitive abilities" (McGrew & Flanagan, 1998, p. 5). To conduct a compete cognitive assessment, therefore, an intelligence test should be augmented with "the most psychometrically sound and theoretically pure tests (according to ITDR [*Intelligence Test Desk Reference*] criteria . . . so that a broader, more complete range of Gf-Gc abilities can be assessed" (McGrew & Flanagan, 1998, p. 357).

McGrew (1997) and McGrew and Flanagan (1998) have published the procedures necessary to operationalize their cross-battery approach. First, subtests from all major intelligence tests have been characterized according to the 10 broad cognitive domains specified in Gf-Gc theory. Calling upon these subtest classifications, the second step in cross-battery assessment entails the examiner's selecting at least two subtests from existing intelligence tests to adequately represent each of the 10 broad cognitive abilities. Then mean scores from each pairing are calculated to form a factor, and are compared to other factors, to determine whether the abilities are significantly different.

The cross-battery approach is well articulated and noteworthy in many respects. Nonetheless, many theoretical and psychometric issues have not been adequately addressed with respect to cross-battery assessments. We now elucidate and discuss nine prominent concerns: (1) comparability of subtest scores obtained from different instruments, (2) effects associated with modifying the presentation order of subtests, (3) sampling and norming issues, (4) procedures used to group subtests into factors, (5) use of ipsative score interpretation, (6) extent of established external validity, (7) relative efficiency and economy of the assessment process, (8) vulnerability to misuse, and (9) determining the correct number of factors to examine and retain.

Comparability of Scores from Different Tests

All cross-battery comparisons implicitly assume that subtest scores are free from extraneous influences. Regrettably, a host of variables beyond those contributed by differentiated, cross-battery ability constructs could be responsible for score differences. Bracken (1988) identified 10 psychometric reasons why tests measuring similar constructs produce dissimilar results. Among the problems identified are errors introduced by differences in floor effects, ceiling effects, item gradients, and so forth. Similarly, Flynn (1999) has demonstrated that individuals invariably score lower on newer than on older ability tests (i.e., the well-documented "Flynn effect"), and has reported that IQ *subtests* show differential changes across time that are not normally distributed. McGrew and Flanagan (1998) confess that

> scores yielded by cross-battery assessments, taken together, represent an unsystematic aggregate of standardized tests. That is, cross-battery assessments employ tests that were developed at different times, in different places, on different samples, with different scoring procedures, and for different purposes. (p. 402)

Flanagan and colleagues (2000) have since asserted that "the potential error introduced

due to cross norm groups is likely negligible" (p. 223), but have provided no evidence to support this claim. However, in light of Bracken's and Flynn's work, it seems reasonable to conclude that subtest scores from cross-battery assessments are likely to be profoundly influenced by extraneous, contaminating influences—variables that subsequently can result in erroneous decisions about children's cognitive strengths and weaknesses.

Order Effects

Another uncontrolled influence inherent in cross-battery assessments is that subtests are administered out of their normative sequence. An example will help to clarify the problem. Let us assume, for instance, that the WISC-III Block Design subtest was administered out of order following administration of the WJ-R battery. A logical question in such circumstances is this: Would the child's Block Design score be lower than, higher than, or unchanged from what it would have been had Block Design been administered within the standard WISC-III test order?

Flanagan (2000) has asserted that "within the context of the cross-battery approach, order of subtests is a trivial matter" (p. 10). However, this statement is not based on data regarding subtest order effects, but rather upon an assumption regarding cross-battery assessment procedures. Namely, if a subtest score is unduly affected by administration order, it is assumed that it will deviate from the other subtests within its broad ability cluster and thus require supplemental subtests to be administered. Under this assumption, the "true" ability measures would cluster together and reveal the discrepant subtest score as spurious. However, this presupposes that erroneous subtest scores always deviate from the remainder of the subtests in their ability cluster, and it ignores the possibility that subtests could be spuriously affected in the direction of other subtests in their ability cluster. For example, let us assume that the WISC-III Block Design subtest is paired with the K-ABC Triangles subtest as constituents of the Visual Processing ability cluster. Let us further assume that the "true" Block Design score is 10, but that an out-of-order effect has caused it to drop to 8. If the hypothetical examinee's "true" and obtained Triangles scores is 6, then it would appear that the Visual Processing subtests are not significantly discrepant (i.e., 6 vs. 8). However, the Block Design "true" score of 10 is significantly different from the Triangles score; according to cross-battery procedures, another subtest should be administered to measure the Visual Processing cluster more adequately. Thus Flanagan's assumption that cross-battery procedures will correct out-of-order testing effects is faulty. There simply are no data on this issue. Anecdotal reports are available, however, which suggest that subtest scores change according to their administration position (Daniel, 1999). Furthermore, documented order effects are established for the administration of structured interview modules (Jensen, Watanabe, & Richters, 1999).

Practice effects are known to be substantial, especially for nonverbal subtests (Glutting & McDermott, 1990a, 1990b), and pose a related threat to cross-battery validity because the cross-battery approach requires the administration of multiple, similar subtests that were not co-normed. Let us consider yet another scenario: A child is administered Block Design in two different orderings. In one, Block Design is the first subtest administered, followed by Triangles (from the K-ABC) and then Diamonds (a chip construction task from the WRIT). In the second sequence, a child receives Block Design as the third subtest behind Diamonds and Triangles.

There is likely to be a substantial practice effect between the two hypothetical Block Design scores. In the first sequence, the child would not have had the benefit of exposure and practice with similar tasks (triangles, chips constructed of varying numbers of diamonds, and then blocks); in the second sequence, the child would have received such benefits. Test norms used to convert children's raw scores into standard scores are all based on the assumption that the tasks are novel, or at least that no children receive varying exposure to similar measures. Consequently, concerns about order effects and practice effects lead us to conclude that cross-battery procedures are likely to distort performance in an incalcu-

lable manner. Thereby, it is incumbent on cross-battery advocates to demonstrate that these effects pose no threat to valid interpretation of test scores.

Sampling and Norming Issues: Size and Representativeness

Ideally, cross-battery factor identification would be accomplished by factor analyses of large, nationally representative samples of children who were administered multiple intelligence tests. This, however, was not done with the cross-battery model. Instead, several small, unrepresentative samples of children completing a small number of intelligence tests were simultaneously analyzed (Flanagan & McGrew, 1998; McGhee, 1993; Woodcock, 1990). In terms of factor analyses, most used by McGrew (1997) as the basis for his categorization system came from the WJ-R concurrent validity samples summarized by Woodcock (1990). One data set included WJ-R and WISC-R scores from 89 third graders. A second included scores from 70 children age 9 on the WJ-R, WISC-R, K-ABC, and SB4. A third involved scores from 53 adolescents age 17 on the WJ-R, WAIS-R, and SB4. Children and adolescents participating in all three studies were from schools in the Dallas–Fort Worth area. Finally, a fourth study included WJ-R and WISC-R scores from 167 children in grades 3 and 5, from schools in Anoka County, Minnesota. Woodcock indicated that each study was analyzed via confirmatory factor analyses. Unfortunately, the sample sizes were simply too small for proper analysis, given the number of variables and parameters involved (Marsh, Hau, Balla, & Grayson, 1998). Furthermore, the samples were all grossly unrepresentative of the national population.

Another study cited by McGrew (1997) included 114 minority children (85 African American and 29 Hispanic) in sixth through eighth grade who were administered 16 WJ-R subtests, 10 KAIT subtests, and one WISC-III subtest. In addition to inadequate sample size and representativeness, analyses were marred by excessive respecification of models based on statistical criteria (Kline, 1998). As noted by Gorsuch (1988), "this procedure has the worst [characteristics] of both exploratory and confirmatory factor analysis and cannot be recommended" (p.

235). Even after capitalizing on sample characteristics with respecifications, model fit statistics did not meet commonly accepted levels necessary to claim plausibility (i.e., goodness-of-fit index (GFI) fit for the final model did not exceed .80, although fit statistics of ≥.90 are recommended; Kline, 1998). Thus the empirical foundation for subtest classifications reported in McGrew (1997) and McGrew and Flanagan (1998) seems weak.

Procedures Employed to Categorize Subtests

Theory should play a prominent role in the selection and organization of subtests. Therefore, it is laudable that proponents of cross-battery assessment have explicitly described their underlying rationale and worked to integrate theory into the structure of assessments. To identify candidate subtests and arrange them into a multifactored battery, the empirical data described above were supplemented by subjective ratings from 10 scholars. As explained by McGrew (1997), "these individuals were asked to logically classify the tests contained in one or more of the intelligence batteries according to the narrow ability factor definitions" (p. 160). However, McGrew reported that "no interrater reliability figures were calculated," and that "when noticeable differences were observed, I made a decision based on a detailed review of Carroll's narrow ability definitions and my task analysis of the test" (p. 160). Thus there is no evidence that experts demonstrated good agreement in assigning subtests into higher-order categories. Although there certainly is a place for the rational derivation of scales in measurement, the approach documented by McGrew did not achieve acceptable standards for constructing a typology of subtests (Bailey, 1994). In addition, the test categorizations originally provided by McGrew were modified by McGrew and Flanagan (1998) and again by Flanagan and colleagues (2000) based upon unspecified logical analyses. When considered together with the weak factor-analytic results, it seems fair to surmise that placement of subtests within cross-battery factors was more a matter of speculative deduction than of demonstrable fact.

Ipsative Interpretation

McGrew and Flanagan (1998) explicitly agreed with extant criticisms of ipsative score interpretation (McDermott et al., 1990, 1992). That is, they accepted that ipsative assessment of subtests from a single cognitive test (i.e., intratest interpretation) "is inherently flawed" (p. 415) due to the unreliability of subtests, the narrow conceptualization of intelligence expressed by subtest scores, and their lack of external validity. However, McGrew and Flanagan concluded that "*some* of the limitations of the ipsative approach to interpretation can be circumvented" (p. 415; emphasis in original) by cross-battery assessment, because it is based upon clusters of subtests that are more reliable and based upon current theories of the structure of intelligence. "Thus, most ipsative test interpretation practice and research have not benefited from being grounded in a well-validated structure of human cognitive abilities" (p. 415). At the same time, McGrew and Flanagan expressed caution regarding complete acceptance of ipsative methods, and suggested that "when significant intra-individual differences are found using Gf-Gc cross-battery data, they should be corroborated by other sources of data" (p. 417).

In essence, then, McGrew and Flanagan (1998) have maintained that the use of cross-battery ability clusters and the Gf-Gc theoretical foundation of their work make ipsative assessment less problematic for cross-battery assessments. However, no empirical data have been advanced in support of this claim. The ipsative interpretive system advocated by Flanagan and colleagues (2000) differs from other popular ipsative systems (e.g., Kaufman, 1994) *only* in its use of factor scores (calculated as the average of at least two subtests) instead of subtest scores. Thus cross-battery ipsative measurement is operationalized by taking factor scores, calculating their grand mean for a given child, and then comparing each factor to the child's personalized mean. Factor scores will nearly always be more reliable than individual subtests. Even so, all other problems elucidated by McDermott and colleagues (1990, 1992) and McDermott and Glutting (1997) remain unsolved. Consequently, it is not apparent how ipsatization within the cross-battery framework serves to reduce the mathematical and psychometric weaknesses inherent in the interpretation of ipsatized profiles!

External Validity

Floyd and Widaman (1995) noted that "the ultimate criterion for the usefulness of a factor solution is whether the obtained factor scores provide information beyond that obtained from the global score for the entire scale" (p. 296). Briggs and Cheek (1986) suggested that "factor analysis is not an end in itself but a prelude to programmatic research on a particular psychological construct" (p. 137). As explained by McGrew and Flanagan (1998), a foundational assumption of cross-battery assessment is that "individual skills and abilities . . . are more diagnostic of learning and problem-solving processes than a global IQ score" (p. 383); they asserted that "the cross-battery approach was developed as a means of potentially improving aptitude–treatment interaction (ATI) research" (p. 374). Flanagan and colleagues (2000) proclaimed that "The cross-battery approach defined here provides a systematic means for practitioners to make valid, *up-to-date* interpretations of the Wechsler Intelligence Scales, in particular, and to augment them in a way consistent with the empirically supported *Gf-Gc* theoretical model" (p. 209; emphais in original); asserted that the measurement of Gf-Gc factors "via Wechsler-based cross-battery assessment, supercedes global IQ in the evaluation of learning and problem-solving capabilities"; and stated that the "intracognitive data gleaned from Wechsler-based cross-battery assessments can be translated into educational recommendations" (p. 209).

These claims are sweeping, given the previously reviewed research on specific versus general cognitive factors and the historic failure of aptitude profiles to inform treatments. Reliance on ATI effects is, of course, optimistic, considering the historically unfavorable research literature (Cronbach & Snow, 1977; Gresham & Witt, 1997). Especially strong is the claim that the cross-battery approach leads to the "valid" interpretation of Wechsler scales. However, no new data have been offered to support this

broad assertion (Flanagan et al., 2000). Perhaps most telling is a conclusion Flanagan and colleagues (2000) reach themselves: "the diagnostic and treatment validity of the *Gf-Gc* cross-battery approach, like traditional assessment approaches, is not yet available" (p. 288).

Efficiency and Economy

Cross-battery methodology increases test length and complexity at several decision points. For instance, the examiner must determine how many of the 10 postulated broad abilities to measure. Each broad ability area must then be measured by at least two subtests, so if all 10 are selected, then at least 20 subtests would be required. Finally, if the two subtests that measure a specific broad ability are statistically discrepant, then an additional subtest should be administered to clarify the composition of that broad ability cluster.

For the sake of argument, let us compare a 20-subtest cross-battery assessment to the typical WISC-III administration. Most practitioners use the 10 mandatory subtests, rarely administering the optional subtests (Symbol Search and Digit Span) and almost never giving Mazes (cf. Glutting, Youngstrom, et al., 1997). Thus the cross-battery protocol would be roughly twice as long as the modal WISC-III administration. In addition, given the lack of published scoring software or conversion tables, cross-battery approaches are likely to take longer to score. Even assuming that this method adds only 70 minutes to administration and 45 minutes to scoring and interpretation (both estimates are based on the median length of time reported for the WISC-III by practicing clinical psychologists and neuropsychologists; Camara et al., 1998), in practical terms the 20-subtest cross-battery assessment would yield an increased expense of well over $100 million per year within the psychoeducational realm alone (based on our estimates provided earlier in this chapter).

In contrast, McGrew and Flanagan (1998) asserted that the increase in test administration time associated with the cross-battery approach is "negligible" (p. 387), because only portions of complete IQ batteries are used. However, McGrew and

Flanagan and Flanagan and colleagues (2000) have presented model case studies that seem to contradict this conclusion. In the McGrew and Flanagan case study, 14 WJ-R and WISC-III subtests that represented seven broad cognitive areas were first administered. Two broad cognitive areas contained statistically discrepant subtest scores, so at least two more subtests should have been administered to better define these two broad factors (see the Gf-Gc flowchart, p. 405). However, this decision rule was ignored, and only one additional subtest was administered. Thus this cross-battery model case study required 15–16 subtests, depending on adherence to cross-battery decision rules. In the Flanagan and colleagues case study, 14 subtests representing seven cognitive areas were first administered. It was then noted that subtests within three of the seven areas were significantly different. According to their flowchart (p. 267), this should have resulted in administration of at least three more subtests for a minimum of 17 subtests. However, through a complex series of rationalizations, it was determined that two of these cognitive areas should not be further explored while two other cognitive areas should receive detailed attention. This resulted in the administration of a total of 18 subtests. Making a very conservative estimate that each additional subtest beyond the standard 10-subtest battery would require only 6 minutes to administer, score, interpret, and report, cross-battery assessments would increase the length of each cognitive assessment by about 30–48 minutes. Based upon previous presented financial estimates, cross-battery assessment as modeled in McGrew and Flanagan and Flanagan and colleagues would increase yearly psychoeducational assessment expenses by roughly $27.5 to $44.1 million.

The admittedly rough estimates offered here do not include a variety of hidden costs associated with the cross-battery approach. For example, this procedure is likely to require increases in the time spent writing reports. The cross-battery approach also necessitates the purchase of multiple tests and expensive protocols. Furthermore, in many instances the cross-battery approach will incur increased costs for training in the various instruments, or else practitioners run the risk of increased error in administration and scoring. Such expenses could certainly be justified if the new interpretive practices resulted in more worthwhile predictions or educational programming; as shown throughout our presentation on cross-battery assessments, however, the issue of added validity is suspect and certainly open to debate.

Vulnerability to Misuse

Gf-Gc theory, although supported by considerable research as a theory of the structure of intelligence, is still only a theory and not fact (Sternberg, 1996). Even its advocates acknowledge that "there is still much work to do in the factorial study of cognitive abilities. The time is not yet ripe for closing the curtains on this field, as some have suggested" (Carroll, 1995, p. 430). For example, there is no general factor in the Gf-Gc model, whereas factor analyses of intelligence tests persist in finding a robust general factor (Jensen, 1998). With the WISC-III, for example, Keith and Witta (1997) concluded that "the test is first and foremost a measure of general intelligence, or g" (p. 105). In addition, there is no widely accepted explanation as to why the correlation between the Gf factor and the g factor is often so close to unity as to suggest only one construct (Gustafsson & Undheim, 1996).

Cross-battery methods have not been validated simply because they are based on Gf-Gc theory. In particular, as previously noted, no evidence to date has conclusively demonstrated that cross-battery assessments are reliable and valid. Repeated statements that cross-battery approaches are based on contemporary, current, modern, or comprehensive theory do not constitute evidence. However, school psychologists and school districts may be prematurely operationalizing cross-battery methods. For example, the Learning Disabilities Assessment Model of the Washington Elementary School District in Phoenix, Arizona (n.d.) utilizes a cross-battery ipsative procedure as one step in the diagnosis of an LD. Seven Gf-Gc factors are delineated and ipsatively compared, but there is no consideration of the theoretical relationships between these factors and various academic achievement dimensions; nor is there any discrimination among factors regarding importance or scope. In addition, cognitive strengths and weaknesses identified in this manner are not considered in a normative framework. This appears to be directly contrary to a statement by Flanagan and colleagues (2000): "In the absence of empirical evidence that supports the practice of intraindividual or ipsative analysis, it is recommended that ipsative intracognitive analysis be de-emphasized or that it be used in conjunction with interindividual analysis" (p. 284).

Determining the Number of Factors Underlying a Group of Subtests

In factor analysis, one of the most important decisions is determining the appropriate number of dimensions necessary to describe the structure of the data adequately. Various different statistical algorithms have been offered as potential determinants of the number of factors or components to retain in an analysis (see Gorsuch, 1988, for a review). Five of these techniques deserve mention here, although there are other heuristics available.

The "Kaiser criterion" is one of the most widely adopted decision rules, and it is the default criterion employed by exploratory factor analysis procedures in popular statistical software, such as SPSS (SPSS, 1999) and SAS (SAS Institute, Inc., 1990). According to this criterion, components or factors are retained if they possess eigenvalues greater than or equal to 1.0. There is some intuitive appeal to this rule, because it maintains that a component or factor must explain at least as much variance as any single variable contributing to the analysis. Put more simply, a component should be "larger" than a variable in terms of the variance explained.

A second popular procedure is Cattell's scree test, in which the eigenvalues of successive components are plotted and printed. The analyst then takes a straight edge and draws a best-fit line through the "scree" of small eigenvalues. The first point that clearly falls above this line is interpreted as being the smallest component that should be retained for subsequent analyses. The scree test is not as popular as some other alternatives, because it involves subjective judg-

ment in plotting the line (Zwick & Velicer, 1986).

The third approach has begun to supplant the previous two rules in many literatures, including cognitive ability testing. The trend now is to use a chi-square "goodness-of-fit" test, fitting an unrestricted solution to the data. This procedure uses maximum-likelihood (ML) procedures to iteratively estimate the population parameter values that would be most likely to produce the observed data if the specified model were true. The goodness-of-fit test compares the predicted covariances between variables to the actually observed covariances, weighting the discrepancies by sample size. The resulting statistic has a chi-square distribution (if the assumptions of multivariate normality and large sample size are met), with significant values indicating that there is a reliable discrepancy between the model and the observed data. The chi-square technique has gained popularity rapidly, probably both because the statistical software needed to perform these analyses is increasingly available, and also because the approach forms a bridge between exploratory factor analysis (EFA) and confirmatory factor analysis (CFA). Whereas other types of EFA determine the number of factors via post hoc criteria, analysts using ML EFA can specify the number of factors a priori, and then determine the goodness of fit of a model containing that number of factors. ML EFA is more liberal and less theory-driven than CFA, in that it does not require a priori specification of which variables load on which factors (Kline, 1998). In practice, investigators have typically used ML EFA to test the adequacy of several models specifying different numbers of factors. The most parsimonious model producing the lowest chi-square statistic becomes the accepted model in this approach (see Table 6.7 in the WISC-III manual for an example of this sort of application; Wechsler, 1991, p. 195).

The other two procedures—Horn's parallel analysis (HPA; Horn, 1965) and the method of minimum average partials (MAP)—have been available for decades, but have not been incorporated into popular statistical software (Zwick & Velicer, 1986). The omission has hindered widespread adoption of these procedures. Both approaches have intuitively meaningful interpretations. HPA addresses the fact that principal-components analysis (PCA) summarizes observed variance, even though it may be the product of measurement or sampling error. In theory, if k uncorrelated variables were submitted to PCA, the analysis should produce k components, each with eigenvalues of 1.0. In practice, analyzing a set of variables uncorrelated in the population will yield a first principal component with an eigenvalue somewhat larger than 1.0. How much larger depends on the number of variables (more variables will result in larger first components, all else being equal) and the number of cases (fewer cases lead to less precise estimates, and therefore larger estimated first components when the true population eigenvalue would be 1.0). HPA involves generating artificial data sets with numbers of cases and variables identical to those found in the actual, observed data. The artificial variables are created randomly, implying that the random variables should be uncorrelated in the population. Both the actual and the artificial data are submitted to separate PCAs, and then eigenvalues are compared. Factors (components) are retained only when eigenvalues in an actual data set exceed those in the artificial data. Put another way, components are only considered interpretable if they are larger than what one might observe by chance in analyzing data where the variables are known not to correlate in the population.

The MAP method (Velicer, 1976) relies on the conceptual definition of a factor as a dimension summarizing the correlation between variables. To perform MAP, the investigator submits the data to PCA and saves all component scores. Then the investigator examines partial correlations between the indicator variables, after controlling for the first principal component (in SPSS, this could be achieved using the PARTIAL CORR procedure, specifying the saved principal-component score as a covariate). Next, the investigator calculates the partial-correlation matrix—controlling for the first and second components; then the first, second, and third components; and so on. The average magnitude of the partial correlations will decrease as each factor is removed, until the indicators have been conditioned on all the real factors. When additional components are partialed out, the partial correlations will not decrease further and may even increase. Thus the appropriate number of components is indicated when the smallest, or minimum, average partial correlation is observed.

Until recently, there were no clear advantages to any one of these approaches for identifying the correct number of factors in a data set. Consequently, the choice of which criterion to use was largely a matter of convention or convenience. Factor analyses conducted with most ability tests employed several decision rules, typically adopting the Kaiser criterion, Cattell's scree test, and ML goodness-of-fit tests as the standards (e.g., Thorndike et al., 1986; Wechsler, 1991, 1997; Woodcock & Johnson, 1989). However, Monte Carlo studies conducted over the last 15 years convincingly demonstrate that MAP and HPA perform much better than the alternatives in recovering the correct number of factors (Velicer, Eaton, & Fava, 2000; Zwick & Velicer, 1986). The Kaiser criterion and ML goodness-of-fit test both tend to overestimate the number of factors. Cattell's scree test appears fairly accurate, but still less so than MAP or HPA.

The methodological findings in the preceding paragraph imply that published ability tests have probably overestimated the number of dimensions assessed by each battery. For example, the WISC-III purportedly measures four cognitive abilities, according to analyses published in the technical manual (Wechsler, 1991). However, other authorities dispute whether or not the Freedom from Distractibility factor emerges (e.g., Sattler, 1992). No published analysis to date has used HPA or MAP—the procedures that possess the best methodological support. When HPA is applied to the median correlations published in the WISC-III manual, results using all 13 subtests suggest that only two components should be interpreted, clearly corresponding to the Verbal Comprehension and Perceptual Organization Indexes (see Table 15.3). If only the 10 mandatory subtests are administered, then the WISC-III only measures one factor sufficiently to meet the HPA criterion.

The preceding analyses should not be interpreted as indicating that the Freedom from Distractibility and Processing Speed

TABLE 15.3. Horn's Parallel Analysis (HPA) of the WISC-III Median Correlations: Eigenvalues Listed by Component Number (n = 2,200)

Component	13 subtests		10 subtests	
	Observed	Avg. random	Observed	Avg. random
1	5.63	1.12	4.97	1.10
2	1.25	1.10	1.01	1.08
3	1.04	1.07	0.89	1.05
4	0.84	1.06	0.67	1.03
5	0.76	1.03	0.56	1.01

Note. "Avg. random" values based on the average of five random data sets. **Boldface** numbers exceed comparable eigenvalue for random data, thus meeting HPA criterion for retention.

factors do not exist. Instead, the outcomes make it reasonable to conclude that the WISC-III does not contain a sufficient number of subtests to adequately satisfy statistical criteria for interpretation of the Freedom from Distractibility and Processing Speed factors. The addition of subtests that identify these specific dimensions could increase the amount of covariance attributable to each factor (thus increasing the eigenvalue, leading to the retention of the factor when the augmented battery is used). However, results clearly indicate that the WISC-III is not long enough (i.e., does not contain a sufficient number of subtests) to meet statistical criteria for retaining more than one or two factors.

Similar to that for the WISC-III, the cross-battery approach has not applied either of the two optimal algorithms for determining the appropriate number of factors to retain. Without using these types of decision rule in an empirical analysis, the risk is that investigators will interpret factors that have not adequately been measured by the battery of indicators. Experts agree that overfactoring is less problematic than underfactoring (i.e., retaining too few dimensions), but that neither is desirable (Wood, Tataryn, & Gorsuch, 1996). In a clinical context, overfactoring leads practitioners to interpret aggregates of subtests as if they measured a more general construct—when in fact the communality between the subtests is not sufficient to measure the purported factor in large groups, let alone individuals. The HPA analysis of the WISC-III shows that it has been overfactored. The poor measurement of the Freedom from Distractibility and Processing Speed dimen-

sions has probably contributed to the difficulty in establishing incremental validity for these constructs.

In summary, cross-battery approaches should carefully document which combinations of subtests are adequate to measure broad cognitive abilities. These analyses should rely on decision rules such as MAP or HPA, and not traditional criteria, because there are clear methodological advantages to these newer approaches. MAP or HPA analyses of the WISC-III suggest that it actually may be difficult to measure an ability adequately with only a pair of subtests (both the Freedom from Distractibility and Processing Speed factors contain only two subtests as indicators). Consequently, it becomes more crucial for advocates of cross-battery approaches to determine what subtest constellations are sufficient to measure each construct.

CONCLUSION

Cross-battery cognitive assessment is explicitly based upon the theories of Horn and Noll (1997) and Carroll (1993), and sees 10 broad second-order factors as more important for diagnosis and treatment than the higher order g factor. Since no single intelligence test adequately measures all ten broad cognitive factors hypothesized within the cross-battery model, subtests are extracted from a variety of cognitive tests and combined to create measures of the Gf-Gc factors. However, a number of theoretical and psychometric issues underlying cross-battery assessments have not been adequately addressed. Many of these technical impediments to the cross-battery approach derive from measurement issues created by pulling subtests from their standardized protocols and forming conglomerates of subtests with different reference groups. Many of these pitfalls could be avoided by standardizing subtests measuring the various Gf-Gc broad cognitive ability factors all within one test and sample. This is planned for the Stanford–Binet Intelligence Scales: Fifth Edition (measuring nine factors; see Youngstrom, Glutting, & Watkins, Chapter 10, this volume) and has been done for the WJ-III (measuring nine factors using 46 subtests).

However, even if these tests possess the desired factor structure and the same excellent psychometric qualities that have distinguished earlier editions of these instruments, important issues will still remain before multifactor assessment will be ready to contribute to clinical and psychoeducational assessment. First, the law of parsimony will require demonstrations that specific ability factors substantially outperform predictions based on omnibus, full-scale scores alone. Second, ipsative interpretation methods used with factors must be empirically demonstrated to be reliable and valid. Finally, the incremental validity of factor scores must translate into improved treatment, diagnosis, or educational interventions. These gains must be judged large enough—by policy makers and consumers, as well as practitioners—to justify the increased time and expense required for thorough multifactor assessment. Although research on assessment, including cross-battery methods, should continue, it should not prematurely be applied to make high-stakes diagnostic decisions about children.

REFERENCES

Accardo, P. J., & Whitman, B. Y. (1991). The misdiagnosis of the hyperactive child. In P. J. Accardo, T. A. Blondis, & B. Y. Whitman (Eds.), *Attention deficit disorders and hyperactivity in children* (pp. 1–21). New York: Marcel Dekker.

Adams, M. J. (1990). *Beginning to read: Thinking and learning about print.* Cambridge, MA: MIT Press.

Aiken, L. R. (1996). *Assessment of intellectual functioning.* New York: Plenum Press.

Alfonso, V. C., Oakland, T. D., LaRocca, R., & Spanakos, A. (2000). The course on individual cognitive assessment. *School Psychology Review, 29,* 52–64.

Arizona Department of Education. (1992). *Standard reporting format for psychoeducational evaluation.* Phoenix: Author.

Bailey, K. D. (1994). *Typologies and taxonomies: An introduction to classification techniques* (Vol. 102). Thousand Oaks, CA: Sage.

Ball, J. D., Archer, R. P., & Imhof, E. A. (1994). Time requirements of psychological testing: A survey of practitioners. *Journal of Personality Assessment, 63,* 239–249.

Banas, N. (1993). *WISC-III prescriptions: How to work creatively with individual learning styles.* Novato, CA: Academic Therapy.

Barkley, R. A. (1998). *Attention-deficit hyperactivity disorder: A handbook for diagnosis and treatment* (2nd ed.). New York: Guilford Press.

Beebe, D. W., Pfiffner, L. J., & McBurnett, K. (2000). Evaluation of the validity of the Wechsler Intelligence Scale for Children—Third Edition Comprehension and Picture Arrangement subtests as measures of social intelligence. *Psychological Assessment, 12,* 97–101.

Blumberg, T. A. (1995). A practitioner's view of the WISC-III. *Journal of School Psychology, 33,* 95–97.

Bowers, T. G., Risser, M. G., Suchanec, J. F., Tinker, D. E., Ramer, J. C., & Domoto, M. (1992). A developmental index using the Wechsler Intelligence Scale for Children: Implications for the diagnosis and nature of ADHD. *Journal of Learning Disabilities, 25,* 179–185.

Bracken, B. A. (1988). Ten psychometric reasons why similar tests produce dissimilar results. *Journal of School Psychology, 26,* 155–166.

Bracken, B. A., McCallum, R. S., & Crain, R. M. (1993). WISC-III subtest composite reliabilities and specificities: Interpretive aids. *Journal of Psychoeducational Assessment Monograph Series,* 22–34.

Briggs, S. R., & Cheek, J. M. (1986). The role of factor analysis in the development and evaluation of personality scales. *Journal of Personality, 51,* 106–148.

Brody, N. (1985). The validity of tests of intelligence. In B. Wolman (Ed.), *Handbook of intelligence: Theories, measurements, and applications* (pp. 353–389). New York: Wiley.

Brody, N. (1997). Intelligence, schooling, and society. *American Psychologist, 52,* 1046–1050.

Brown, M. B., Swigart, M. L., Bolen, L. M., Hall, C. W., & Webster, R. T. (1998). Doctoral and nondoctoral practicing school psychologists: Are there differences? *Psychology in the Schools, 35,* 347–354.

Bus, A. G., & van Uzendoorn, M. H. (1999). Phonological awareness and early reading: A meta-analysis of experimental training studies. *Journal of Educational Psychology, 91,* 403–413.

Camara, W., Nathan, J., & Puente, A. (1998). *Psychological test usage in professional psychology: Report of the APA practice and science directorates.* Washington, DC: American Psychological Association.

Campbell, J. M., & McCord, D. M. (1999). Measuring social competence with the Wechsler Picture Arrangement and Comprehension subtests. *Assessment, 6,* 215–223.

Canivez, G. L., & Watkins, M. W. (1998). Long-term stability of the Wechsler Intelligence Scale for Children—Third Edition. *Psychological Assessment, 10,* 285–291.

Carnine, D. W., Silbert, J., & Kameenui, E. J. (1997). *Direct instruction reading* (3rd ed.). Upper Saddle River, NJ: Merrill.

Carroll, J. B. (1993). *Human cognitive abilities: A survey of factor-analytic studies.* New York: Cambridge University Press.

Carroll, J. B. (1995). On methodology in the study of cognitive abilities. *Multivariate Behavioral Research, 30,* 429–452.

Cattell, R. B. (1944). Psychological measurement: Normative, ipsative, interactive. *Psychological Review, 51,* 292–303.

Ceci, S. J. (1991). How much does schooling influence general intelligence and its cognitive components?: A reassessment of the evidence. *Developmental Psychology, 27,* 703–722.

Ceci, S. J., & Williams, W. M. (1997). Schooling, intelligence, and income. *American Psychologist, 52,* 1051–1058.

Chen, W. J., Faraone, S. V., Biederman, J., & Tsuang, M. T. (1994). Diagnostic accuracy of the Child Behavior Checklist scales for attention-deficit hyperactivity disorder: A receiver-operating characteristic analysis. *Journal of Consulting and Clinical Psychology, 62,* 1017–1025.

Cohen, J. (1959). The factorial structure of the WISC at ages 7–6, 10–6, and 13–6. *Journal of Consulting and Clinical Psychology, 23,* 285–299.

Cohen, J. (1990). Things I have learned (so far). *American Psychologist, 45,* 1304–1312.

Cohen, M., Becker, M. G., & Campbell, R. (1990). Relationships among four methods of assessment of children with attention deficit-hyperactivity disorder. *Journal of School Psychology, 28,* 189–202.

Cromwell, R. L., Blashfield, R. K., & Strauss, J. S. (1975). Criteria for classification systems. In N. Hobbs (Ed.), *Issues in the classification of children* (Vol. 1, pp. 4–25). San Francisco: Jossey-Bass.

Cronbach, L. J., & Gleser, G. C. (1953). Assessing similarity between profiles. *Psychological Bulletin, 50,* 456–473.

Cronbach, L. J., & Snow, R. E. (1977). *Aptitudes and instructional methods.* New York: Irvington.

Curtis, M. J., Hunley, S. A., & Baker, A. C. (1996, March). *Demographics and professional practices in school psychology: A national perspective.* Paper presented at the annual meeting of the National Association of School Psychologists, Atlanta, GA.

Daley, C. E., & Nagle, R. J. (1996). Relevance of WISC-III indicators for assessment of learning disabilities. *Journal of Psychoeducational Assessment, 14,* 320–333.

Daniel, M. (1999, September). *Subtest order* [Online]. Available: http://www.home.att.net

Drebing, C., Satz, P., Van Gorp, W., Chervinsky, A., & Uchiyama, C. (1994). WAIS-R intersubtest scatter in patients with dementia of Alzheimer's type. *Journal of Clinical Psychology, 50,* 753–758.

Dumont, R., Farr, L. P., Willis, J. O., & Whelley, P. (1998). 30-second interval performance on the Coding subtest of the WISC-III: Further evidence of WISC folklore? *Psychology in the Schools, 35,* 111–117.

Ehri, L. C., Nunes, S. R., Willows, D. M., Schuster, B. V., Yaghoub-Zadeh, Z., & Shanahan, T. (2001). Phonemic awareness instruction helps children learn to read: Evidence from the National Reading Panel's meta-analysis. *Reading Research Quarterly, 36,* 250–287.

Eisman, E. J., Dies, R. R., Finn, S. E., Eyde, L. D., Kay, G. G., Kubiszyn, T. W., Meyer, G. J., & Moreland, K. L. (1998). *Problems and limitations in the use of psychological assessment in contemporary health care delivery: Report of the Board of Professional Affairs Psychological Assessment Workgroup, Part II.* Washington, DC: American Psychological Association.

Elliott, C. D. (1990). *Differential Ability Scales.* San Antonio, TX: Psychological Corporation.

Elwood, R. W. (1993). Psychological tests and clinical discriminations: Beginning to address the base rate problem. *Clinical Psychology Review, 13,* 409–419.

Flanagan, D. P. (2000). *Giving subtests out of the framework of the standardization procedure* [Online]. Available: http://www.home.att.net

Flanagan, D. P., & McGrew, K. S. (1997). A cross-battery approach to assessing and interpreting cognitive abilities: Narrowing the gap between practice and cognitive science. In D. P. Flanagan, J. L. Genshaft, & P. L. Harrison (Eds.), *Contemporary intellectual assessment: Theories, tests and issues* (pp. 314–325). New York: Guilford Press.

Flanagan, D. P., & McGrew, K. S. (1998). Interpreting intelligence tests from contemporary Gf-Gc theory: Joint confirmatory factor analysis of the WJ-R and KAIT in a non-white sample. *Journal of School Psychology, 36,* 151–182.

Flanagan, D. P., McGrew, K. S., & Ortiz, S. O. (2000). *The Wechsler intelligence scales and Gf-Gc theory: A contemporary approach to interpretation.* Boston: Allyn & Bacon.

Floyd, F. J., & Widaman, K. F. (1995). Factor analysis in the development and refinement of clinical assessment instruments. *Psychological Assessment, 7,* 286–299.

Flynn, J. R. (1999). Evidence against Rushton: The genetic loading of WISC-R subtests and the causes of between group IQ differences. *Personality and Individual Differences, 26,* 373–379.

Garb, H. N. (1998). *Studying the clinician.* Washington, DC: American Psychological Association.

Gardner, H. (1983). *Frames of mind: The theory of multiple intelligences.* New York: Basic Books.

Glutting, J. J., Adams, W., & Sheslow, D. (2000). *Wide Range Intelligence Test Manual.* Wilmington, DE: Wide Range.

Glutting, J. J., & McDermott, P. A. (1990a). Childhood learning potential as an alternative to traditional ability measures. *Psychological Assessment: A Journal of Consulting and Clinical Psychology, 2,* 398–403.

Glutting, J. J., & McDermott, P. A. (1990b). Principles and problems in learning potential. In C. R. Reynolds & R. W. Kamphaus (Eds.), *Handbook of psychological and educational assessment: Vol. 1. Intelligence and achievement* (pp. 296–347). New York: Guilford Press.

Glutting, J. J., McDermott, P. A., Konold, T. R., Snel-baker, A. J., & Watkins, M. W. (1998). More ups and downs of subtest analysis: Criterion validity of the DAS with an unselected cohort. *School Psychology Review, 27,* 599–612.

Glutting, J. J., McDermott, P. A., Watkins, M. W., Kush, J. C., & Konold, T. R. (1997). The base rate problem and its consequences for interpreting children's ability profiles. *School Psychology Review, 26,* 176–188.

Glutting, J. J., McGrath, E. A., Kamphaus, R. W., & McDermott, P. A. (1992). Taxonomy and validity of subtest profiles on the Kaufman Assessment Battery for Children. *Journal of Special Education, 26,* 85–115.

Glutting, J. J., Youngstrom, E. A., & McDermott, P. A. (2000). *Validity of the WISC-III processing speed factor in identifying children's achievement problems: An epidemiological study using the WISC-III/WIAT linking sample.* Manuscript submitted for publication.

Glutting, J. J., Youngstrom, E. A., Oakland, T., & Watkins, M. (1996). Situational specificity and generality of test behaviors for samples of normal and referred children. *School Psychology Review, 25,* 94–107.

Glutting, J. J., Youngstrom, E. A., Ward, T., Ward, S., & Hale, R. (1997). Incremental efficacy of WISC-III factor scores in predicting achievement: What do they tell us? *Psychological Assessment, 9,* 295–301.

Goodyear, P., & Hynd, G. W. (1992). Attention-deficit disorder with (ADD/H) and without (ADD/WO) hyperactivity: Behavioral and neuropsychological differentiation. *Journal of Clinical Child Psychology, 21,* 273–305.

Gorsuch, R. L. (1988). Exploratory factor analysis. In J. R. Nesselroade & R. B. Cattell (Eds.), *Handbook of multivariate experimental research* (2nd ed., pp. 231–258). New York: Plenum Press.

Gough, H. (1971). Some reflections on the meaning of psychodiagnosis. *American Psychologist, 26,* 106–187.

Gregory, R. J. (1999). *Foundations of intellectual assessment: The WAIS-III and other tests in clinical practice.* Boston: Allyn & Bacon.

Gresham, F. M., & Witt, J. C. (1997). Utility of intelligence tests for treatment planning, classification, and placement decisions: Recent empirical findings and future directions. *School Psychology Review, 12,* 249–267.

Groth-Marnat, G. (1997). *Handbook of psychological assessment* (3rd ed.). New York: Wiley.

Groth-Marnat, G. (1999). Financial efficacy of clinical assessment: Rational guidelines and issues for future research. *Journal of Clinical Psychology, 55,* 813–824.

Guilford, J. P. (1967). *The nature of human intelligence.* New York: McGraw-Hill.

Gustafsson, J.-E., & Undheim, J. O. (1996). Individual differences in cognitive functions. In D. C. Berliner & R. C. Calfee (Eds.), *Handbook of educational psychology* (pp. 186–242). New York: Macmillan.

Hale, R. L., & Saxe, J. E. (1983). Profile analysis of the Wechsler Intelligence Scale for Children—Revised. *Journal of Psychoeducational Assessment, 1,* 155–162.

Hanley, J. A., & McNeil, B. J. (1982). The meaning and use of the area under a receiver operating characteristic (ROC) curve. *Radiology, 143,* 29–36.

Hansen, J. C. (1999). Test psychometrics. In J. W. Lichtenberg & R. K. Goodyear (Eds.), *Scientist–practitioner perspectives on test interpretation* (pp. 15–30). Boston: Allyn & Bacon.

Hartigan, J. A., & Wigdor, A. K. (1989). *Fairness in employment testing.* Washington, DC: National Academy Press.

Herrnstein, R. J., & Murray, C. (1994). *The bell curve: Intelligence and class structure in American life.* New York: Free Press.

Hopkins, K. D. (1998). *Educational and psychological measurement and evaluation* (8th ed.). Needham Heights, MA: Allyn & Bacon.

Horn, J. L. (1965). A rationale and test for the number of factors in factor analysis. *Psychometrika, 30,* 179–185.

Horn, J. L. (1988). Thinking abut human abilities. In J. R. Nesselroade & R. B. Cattell (Eds.), *Handbook of multivariate experimental psychology* (2nd ed., pp. 645–685). New York: Plenum Press.

Horn, J. L., & Noll, J. (1997). Human cognitive capabilities: Gf-Gc theory. In D. P. Flanagan, J. L. Genshaft, & P. L. Harrison (Eds.), *Contemporary intellectual assessment: Theories, tests and issues* (pp. 53–91). New York: Guilford Press.

Hsiao, J. K., Bartko, J. J., & Potter, W. Z. (1989). Diagnosing diagnoses. *Archives of General Psychiatry, 46,* 664–667.

Hunt, E. (1995). The role of intelligence in modern society. *American Scientist, 83,* 356–368.

Hunter, J. E., & Hunter, R. F. (1984). Validity and utility of alternative predictions of job performance. *Psychological Bulletin, 96,* 72–98.

Ivnik, R. J., Smith, G. E., Malec, J. F., Kokmen, E., & Tangalos, E. G. (1994). Mayo cognitive factor scales: Distinguishing normal and clinical samples by profile variability. *Neuropsychology, 8,* 203–209.

Jencks, C. (1972). *Inequality: A reassessment of the effect of family and schooling in America.* New York: Basic Books.

Jensen, A. R. (1980). *Bias in mental testing.* New York: Free Press.

Jensen, A. R. (1998). *The g factor: The science of mental ability.* Westport, CT: Praeger.

Jensen, P. S., Watanabe, H. K., & Richters, J. E. (1999). Who's up first?: Testing for order effects in structured interviews using a counterbalanced experimental design. *Journal of Abnormal Child Psychology, 27,* 439–445.

Jones, W. T. (1952). *A history of Western philosophy.* New York: Harcourt, Brace.

Kamphaus, R. W. (1993). *Clinical assessment of children's intelligence.* Boston: Allyn & Bacon.

Kaufman, A. S. (1994). *Intelligent testing with the WISC-III.* New York: Wiley.

Kaufman, A. S., & Kaufman, N. L. (1983). *K-ABC: Kaufman Assessment Battery for Children.* Circle Pines, MN: American Guidance Service.

Kaufman, A. S., & Kaufman, N. L. (1993). *The Kaufman Adolescent and Adult Intelligence Test manual.* Circle Pines, MN: American Guidance Service.

Kaufman, A. S., & Lichtenberger, E. O. (2000). *Essentials of WISC-III and WPPSI-R assessment.* New York: Wiley.

Kavale, K. A., & Forness, S. R. (1984). A meta-analysis of the validity of Wechsler scale profiles and recategorizations: Patterns or parodies? *Learning Disabilities Quarterly, 7,* 136–156.

Kazdin, A. E. (1995). *Conduct disorders in childhood and adolescence* (2nd ed.). Thousand Oaks, CA: Sage.

Keith, T. Z. (1990). Confirmatory and hierarchical confirmatory analysis of the Differential Ability Scales. *Journal of Psychoeducational Assessment, 8,* 391–405.

Keith, T. Z. (1999). Effects of general and specific abilities on student achievement: Similarities and differences across ethnic groups. *School Psychology Quarterly, 14,* 239–262.

Keith, T. Z., & Witta, E. L. (1997). Hierarchical and cross-age confirmatory factor analysis of the WISC-III: What does it measure? *School Psychology Quarterly, 12,* 89–107.

Kellerman, H., & Burry, A. (1997). *Handbook of psychodiagnostic testing: Analysis of personality in the psychological report* (3rd ed.). Boston: Allyn & Bacon.

Kessel, J. B., & Zimmerman, M. (1993). Reporting errors in studies of the diagnostic performance of self-administered questionnaires: Extent of the problem, recommendations for standardized presentation of results, and implications for the peer review process. *Psychological Assessment, 5,* 395–399.

Klein, E. S., & Fisher, G. S. (1994, March). *The usefulness of the Wechsler Deterioration Index as a predictor of learning disabilities in children.* Paper presented at the annual meeting of the National Association of School Psychologists, Seattle, WA.

Kline, R. B. (1998). *Principles and practice of structural equation modeling.* New York: Guilford Press.

Kline, R. B., Snyder, J., Guilmette, S., & Castellanos, M. (1993). External validity of the profile variability index for the K-ABC, Stanford–Binet, and WISC-R: Another cul-de-sac. *Journal of Learning Disabilities, 26,* 557–567.

Kraemer, H. C. (1988). Assessment of 2 × 2 associations: Generalization of signal-detection methodology. *American Statistician, 42,* 37–49.

Kramer, J. J., Henning-Stout, M., Ullman, D. P., & Schellenberg, R. P. (1987). The viability of scatter analysis on the WISC-R and the SBIS: Examining a vestige. *Journal of Psychoeducational Assessment, 5,* 37–47.

Kranzler, J. H. (1997). What does the WISC-III measure?: Comments on the relationship between intelligence, working memory capacity, and information processing speed and efficiency. *School Psychology Quarterly, 12,* 110–116.

Lezak, M. D. (1995). *Neuropsychological assessment* (3rd ed.). New York: Oxford University Press.

Lichtenstein, R., & Fischetti, B. A. (1998). How long does a psychoeducational evaluation take?: An urban Connecticut study. *Professional Psychology: Research and Practice, 29,* 144–148.

Lipsitz, J. D., Dworkin, R. H., & Erlenmeyer-Kimling, L. (1993). Wechsler Comprehension and Picture Arrangement subtests and social adjustment. *Psychological Assessment, 5,* 430–437.

Lubinski, D., & Benbow, C. P. (2000). States of excellence. *American Psychologist, 55,* 137–150.

Lund, A. R., Reschly, D. J., & Martin, L. M. C. (1998). School psychology personnel needs: Correlates of current patterns and historical trends. *School Psychology Review, 27,* 106–120.

Marsh, H. W., Hau, K. T., Balla, J. R., & Grayson, D. (1998). Is more ever too much?: The number of indicators per factor in confirmatory factor analysis. *Multivariate Behavioral Research, 33,* 181–220.

Mayes, S. D., Calhoun, S. L., & Crowell, E. W. (1998). WISC-III profiles for children with and without learning disabilities. *Psychology in the Schools, 35,* 309–316.

McDermott, P. A., Fantuzzo, J. W., & Glutting, J. J. (1990). Just say no to subtest analysis: A critique on Wechsler theory and practice. *Journal of Psychoeducational Assessment, 8,* 290–302.

McDermott, P. A., Fantuzzo, J. W., Glutting, J. J., Watkins, M. W., & Baggaley, R. A. (1992). Illusion of meaning in the ipsative assessment of children's ability. *Journal of Special Education, 25,* 504–526.

McDermott, P. A., & Glutting, J. J. (1997). Informing stylistic learning behavior, disposition, and achievement through ability subtests—or, more illusions of meaning? *School Psychology Review, 26,* 163–175.

McFall, R. M., & Treat, T. A. (1999). Quantifying the information value of clinical assessments with signal detection theory. *Annual Review of Psychology, 50,* 215–241.

McGhee, R. (1993). Fluid and crystallized intelligence: Confirmatory factor analysis of the Differential Ability Scales, Detroit Tests of Learning Aptitude—3, and Woodcock–Johnson Psycho-Educational Battery—Revised. *Journal of Psychoeducational Assessment Monograph Series,* 20–38.

McGrew, K. S. (1997). Analysis of the major intelligence batteries according to a proposed comprehensive Gf-Gc framework. In D. P. Flanagan, J. L. Genshaft, & P. L. Harrison (Eds.), *Contemporary intellectual assessment: Theories, tests and issues* (pp. 151–179). New York: Guilford Press.

McGrew, K. S., & Flanagan, D. P. (1998). *The intelligence test desk reference (ITDR): Gf-Gc cross-battery assessment.* Boston: Allyn & Bacon.

McGrew, K. S., Keith, T. Z., Flanagan, D. P., & Underwood, M. (1997). Beyond g: The impact of Gf-Gc specific cognitive ability research on the future use and interpretation of intelligence tests in the schools. *School Psychology Review, 26,* 189–201.

McLean, J. E., Reynolds, C. R., & Kaufman, A. S. (1990). WAIS-R subtest scatter using the profile variability index. *Psychological Assessment: A Journal of Consulting and Clinical Psychology, 2,* 289–292.

Meehl, P. E., & Rosen, A. (1955). Antecedent probability and the efficiency of psychometric signs, patterns, or cutting scores. *Psychological Bulletin, 52,* 194–216.

Messick, S. (1989). Validity. In R. L. Linn (Ed.), *Educational measurement* (pp. 13–103). New York: Macmillan.

Moffitt, T. E., Gabrielli, W. F., Mednick, S. A., & Schulsinger, F. (1981). Socioeconomic status, IQ, and delinquency. *Journal of Abnormal Psychology, 90,* 152–156.

Moffitt, T. E., & Silva, P. A. (1987). WISC-R Verbal and Performance IQ discrepancy in an unselected cohort: Clinical significance and longitudinal stability. *Journal of Consulting and Clinical Psychology, 55,* 768–774.

Murphy, J. M., Berwick, D. M., Weinstein, M. C., Borus, J. F., Budman, S. H., & Klerman, G. L. (1987). Performance on screening and diagnostic tests. *Archives of General Psychiatry, 44,* 550–555.

Neisser, U., Boodoo, G., Bouchard, T. J., Boykin, A. W., Brody, N., Ceci, S. J., Halpern, D. F., Loehlin, J. C., Perloff, R., Sternberg, R. J., & Urbina, S. (1996). Intelligence: Knowns and unknowns. *American Psychologist, 51,* 77–101.

Nunnally, J. C., & Bernstein, I. H. (1994). *Psychometric theory* (3rd ed.). New York: McGraw-Hill.

Oh, H. J., & Glutting, J. J. (1999). An epidemiological-cohort study of the DAS process speed factor: How well does it identify concurrent achievement and behavior problems? *Journal of Psychoeducational Assessment, 17,* 362–275.

Piedmont, R. L., Sokolove, R. L., & Fleming, M. Z. (1989). An examination of some diagnostic strategies involving the Wechsler intelligence scales. *Psychological Assessment, 1,* 181–185.

Platt, J. R. (1964). Strong inference. *Science, 146,* 347–352.

Prifitera, A., & Dersh, J. (1993). Base rates of WISC-III diagnostic subtest patterns among normal, learning-disabled, and ADHD samples. *Journal of Psychoeducational Assessment Monograph Series,* 43–55.

Prifitera, A., Weiss, L. G., & Saklofske, D. H. (1998). The WISC-III in context. In A. Prifitera & D. H. Saklofske (Eds.), *WISC-III clinical use and interpretation: Scientist–practitioner perspectives* (pp. 1–39). New York: Academic Press.

Psychological Corporation. (1999). *Wechsler Abbreviated Scale of Intelligence Manual.* San Antonio, TX: Author.

Ree, M. J., & Earles, J. A. (1993). Intelligence is the best predictor of job performance. *Current Directions in Psychological Science, 1,* 86–89.

Reinecke, M. A., Beebe, D. W., & Stein, M. A. (1999). The third factor of the WISC-III: It's (probably) not freedom from distractibility. *Journal of the American Academy of Child and Adolescent Psychiatry, 38,* 322–328.

Reschly, D. J. (1997). Diagnostic and treatment validity of intelligence tests. In D. P. Flanagan, J. L. Genshaft, & P. L. Harrison (Eds.), *Contemporary intellectual assessment: Theories, tests and issues* (pp. 437–456). New York: Guilford Press.

Reschly, D. J., & Grimes, J. P. (1990). Best practices in intellectual assessment. In A. Thomas & J. Grimes (Eds.), *Best practices in school psychology II* (pp. 425–439). Washington, DC: National Association of School Psychologists.

Reschly, D. J., & Wilson, M. S. (1997). Characteristics of school psychology graduate education: Implications for the entry-level discussion and doctoral-level specialty definition. *School Psychology Review, 26,* 74–92.

Riccio, C. A., Cohen, M. J., Hall, J., & Ross, C. M. (1997). The third and fourth factors of the WISC-III: What they don't measure. *Journal of Psychoeducational Assessment, 15,* 27–39.

Rispens, J., Swaab, H., van den Oord, E. J. , Cohen-Kettenis, P., van Engeland, H., & van Yperen, T. (1997). WISC profiles in child psychiatric diagnosis: Sense or nonsense? *Journal of the American Academy of Child and Adolescent Psychiatry, 36,* 1587–1594.

Roid, G. H., Prifitera, A., & Weiss, L. G. (1993). Replication of the WISC-III factor structure in an independent sample. *Journal of Psychoeducational Assessment Monograph Series,*

Rosnow, R. L., & Rosenthal, R. (1989). Statistical procedures and the justification of knowledge in psychological science. *American Psychologist, 44,* 1276–1284.

Rutter, M. (1989). Isle of Wight revisited: Twenty-five years of child psychiatric epidemiology. *Journal of the American Academy of Child and Adolescent Psychiatry, 28,* 833–653.

Salvia, J., & Ysseldyke, J. E. (1998). *Assessment* (5th ed.). Boston: Houghton Mifflin.

SAS Institute, Inc. (1990). *SAS/STAT User's Guide: Version 6, Fourth Edition, Volume 1, ACECLUS-FREQ.* Cary, NC: Author.

Sattler, J. M. (1992). *Assessment of children: Revised and updated third edition.* San Diego, CA: Author.

Schinka, J. A., Vanderploeg, R. D., & Curtiss, G. (1997). WISC-III subtest scatter as a function of highest subtest scaled score. *Psychological Assessment, 9,* 83–88.

Silverstein, A. B. (1993). Type I, Type II, and other types of errors in pattern analysis. *Psychological Assessment, 5,* 72–74.

Sines, J. O. (1966). Actuarial methods in personality assessment. In B. A. Maher (Ed.), *Progress in experimental personality research* (pp. 133–193). New York: Academic Press.

SPSS. (1999). *SPSS Base 9.0 Applications Guide* (Version 9.0). Chicago: Author.

Stahl, S. A., & Murray, B. A. (1994). Defining phonological awareness and its relationship to early reading. *Journal of Educational Psychology, 86,* 221–234.

Sternberg, R. J. (1988). *The triarchic mind: A new theory of human intelligence.* New York: Viking Press.

Sternberg, R. J. (1996). Myths, countermyths, and truths about intelligence. *Educational Researcher, 25,* 11–16.

Swets, J. A. (1988). Measuring the accuracy of diagnostic systems. *Science, 240,* 1285–1293.

Teeter, P. A., & Korducki, R. (1998). Assessment of emotionally disturbed children with the WISC-III. In A. Prifitera & D. H. Saklofske (Eds.), *WISC-III clinical use and interpretation: Scientist–practitioner perspectives* (pp. 119–138). New York: Academic Press.

Thomas, A. (2000). School psychology 2000: Salaries. *Communique, 28,* 32.

Thorndike, R. L. (1984). *Intelligence as information processing: The mind and computer.* Bloomington, IN: Center on Evaluation, Development, and Research.

Thorndike, R. L., Hagen, E. P., & Sattler, J. M. (1986). *Stanford–Binet Intelligence Scale: Fourth Edition.* Chicago: Riverside.

Tracey, T. J., & Rounds, J. (1999). Inference and attribution errors in test interpretation. In J. W. Lichtenberg & R. K. Goodyear (Eds.), *Scientist–practitioner perspectives on test interpretation* (pp. 113–131). Boston: Allyn & Bacon.

Traub, R. E. (1991). *Reliability for the social sciences.* Newbury Park, CA: Sage.

Truch, S. (1993). *The WISC-III companion: A guide to interpretation and educational intervention.* Austin, TX: Pro-Ed.

Velicer, W. F. (1976). Determining the number of components from the matrix of partial correlations. *Psychometrika, 41,* 321–327.

Velicer, W. F., Eaton, C. A., & Fava, J. L. (2000). Construct explication through factor or component analysis: A review and evaluation of alternative procedures for determining the number of factors or components. In R. D. Goffin & E. Helmes (Eds.), *Problems and solutions in human assessment: A festschrift to Douglas Jackson at seventy* (pp. 1–89). Mahwah, NJ: Erlbaum.

Wagner, R. K. (1997). Intelligence, training, and employment. *American Psychologist, 52,* 1059–1069.

Ward, S. B., Ward, T. J., Hatt, C. V., Young, D. L., & Mollner, N. R. (1995). The incidence and utility of the ACID, ACIDS, and SCAD profiles in a referred population. *Psychology in the Schools, 32,* 267–276.

Washington Elementary School District. (n.d.). *Learning disabilities assessment model.* Phoenix, AZ: Author.

Watkins, M. W. (1996). Diagnostic utility of the WISC-III Developmental Index as a predictor of learning disabilities. *Journal of Learning Disabilities, 29,* 305–312.

Watkins, M. W. (1999). Diagnostic utility of WISC-III subtest variability among students with learning disabilities. *Canadian Journal of School Psychology, 15,* 11–20.

Watkins, M. W., & Glutting, J. J. (2000). Incremental validity of WISC-III profile elevation, scatter, and shape information for predicting reading and math achievement. *Psychological Assessment, 12,* 402–408.

Watkins, M. W., & Kush, J. C. (1994). WISC-R subtest analysis of variance: The right way, the wrong way, or no way? *School Psychology Review, 23,* 640–651.

Watkins, M. W., Kush, J. C., & Glutting, J. J. (1997a). Discriminant and predictive validity of the WISC-III ACID profile among children with learning disabilities. *Psychology in the Schools, 34,* 309–319.

Watkins, M. W., Kush, J. C., & Glutting, J. J. (1997b). Prevalence and diagnostic utility of the WISC-III SCAD profile among children with disabilities. *School Psychology Quarterly, 12,* 235–248.

Watkins, M. W., & Worrell, F. C. (2000). Diagnostic utility of the number of WISC-III subtests deviating from mean performance among students with learning disabilities. *Psychology in the Schools, 37.*

Wechsler, D. (1958). *The measurement and appraisal of adult intelligence* (4th ed.). Baltimore: Williams & Wilkins.

Wechsler, D. (1974). *Wechsler Intelligence Scale for Children—revised.* New York: Psychological Corporation.

Wechsler, D. (1981). *Wechsler Adult Intelligence Scale—Revised.* New York: Psychological Corporation.

Wechsler, D. (1991). *Wechsler Intelligence Scale for Children—Third Edition.* San Antonio, TX: Psychological Corporation.

Wechsler, D. (1997). *Wechsler Adult Intelligence Scale—Third Edition.* San Antonio, TX: Psychological Corporation.

Wielkiewicz, R. M. (1990). Interpreting low scores on the WISC-R third factor: It's more than distractibility. *Psychological Assessment, 2,* 91–97.

Wiggins, J. S. (1973). *Personality and prediction: Principles of personality assessment.* Reading, MA: Addison-Wesley.

Williams, W. M., & Ceci, S. J. (1997). Are Americans becoming more or less alike?: Trends in race, class, and ability differences in intelligence. *American Psychologist, 52,* 1226–1235.

Wood, J. M., Tataryn, D. J., & Gorsuch, R. L. (1996). Effects of under- and overextraction on principal axis factor analysis with varimax rotation. *Psychological Methods, 1,* 354–365.

Woodcock, R. W. (1990). Theoretical foundations of the WJ-R measures of cognitive ability. *Journal of Psychoeducational Assessment, 8,* 231–258.

Woodcock, R. W., & Johnson, M. B. (1989). *Woodcock–Johnson Tests of Cognitive Ability—Revised.* Chicago: Riverside.

Woodcock, R. W., & Johnson, M. B. (2000). *Woodcock–Johnson Tests of Cognitive Ability—Third Edition.* Itasca, IL: Riverside.

Youngstrom, E. A., & Glutting, J. J. (2000). *Individual strengths and weaknesses on factor scores from the Differential Ability Scales: Validity in predicting concurrent achievement and behavioral criteria.* Manuscript submitted for publication.

Youngstrom, E. A., Kogos, J. L., & Glutting, J. J. (1999). Incremental efficacy of Differential Ability Scales factors in predicting individual achievement criteria. *School Psychology Quarterly, 14,* 26–39.

Ziskin, J. (1995). *Coping with psychiatric and psychological testimony* (5th ed.). Los Angeles, CA: Law and Psychology Press.

Zwick, W. R., & Velicer, W. F. (1986). Comparison of five rules for determining the number of components to retain. *Psychological Bulletin, 99,* 432–442.

PART III

ASSESSMENT OF ACADEMIC SKILLS

16

Advances in Criterion-Referenced Testing Methods and Practices

RONALD K. HAMBLETON
APRIL ZENISKY

Criterion-referenced tests (CRTs) are constructed to provide information about the level of an examinee's performance in relation to a clearly defined domain of content and/or behaviors (Popham, 1978b). Normally, performance standards are set on the test score scale so that examinees' scores on a CRT can be sorted or classified into performance categories, such as "failing," "basic," "proficient," and "advanced." Today extensive use is being made of CRTs, and students' scores from these tests are often sorted into three (e.g., New Jersey), four (e.g., Massachusetts), or even five (e.g., Florida) performance levels or categories on state proficiency tests. With still other CRTs (e.g., state achievement tests required for high school graduation, credentialing exams), test scores are combined into a single "pass" or "fail" score.

Today CRTs are widely used in education, credentialing, the armed services, and industry. They are used by state departments of education to monitor the educational progress of students and groups of students (e.g., blacks, Hispanics, and whites), as well as to assist in state educational accountability of students and schools (Linn, 2000). These tests are an integral part of the standards-based educational reform movement

in place around the country, as well as of the recently signed No Child Left Behind Act of 2001 (Public Law [PL] 107-110). This new legislation requires the reporting of student performance in relation to state curriculum goals and objectives (often called "content standards"). Special educators use CRTs with individual education programs to monitor student progress and achievements. Classroom teachers use CRTs both in their day-to-day management of student progress, and in their evaluation of instructional approaches. In credentialing, CRTs are used to identify persons who have met the test performance requirements for a license or certificate to practice in a profession (e.g., medical practice, nursing, teaching, and accountancy). Over 1,000 agencies today are involved in the credentialing process. In the armed services and industry, CRTs are used to identify the training needs of individuals, to judge people's job competence, and to determine whether or not trainees have successfully completed training programs (e.g., continuing education programs in the securities industry).

Basically, a CRT can be a valuable assessment instrument when the focus of interest is a candidate's performance in relation to a body or domain of content and/or behaviors. For example, perhaps the goal is to determine how much of a grade 10 mathematics curriculum students have mastered, or to evaluate the writing skills of fourth graders. At other times, the focus of assessment might be examinees' mastery of a set of learning objectives in a reading curriculum. CRTs can be contrasted with norm-referenced tests (NRTs), which are constructed to provide information that is used to compare or to rank-order examinees on the construct being measured.

Today, CRTs are called by many names—"domain-referenced tests," "competency tests," "objectives-referenced tests," "basic skills tests," "mastery tests," "performance assessments," "authentic tests," "proficiency tests," "standards-based tests," "licensure exams," and "certification exams," to give many of the more common terms. The choice of name depends on the context in which a test is used. For example, in school contexts, the terms "mastery testing" or "performance assessment" are common. When CRTs are developed to model classroom activities or exercises, the term "authentic test" is sometimes preferred. In its purest form, an authentic test is one where the student is in complete control (i.e., picks the topic, allocates time to complete the topic, and chooses the pace for topic completion). When CRTs consist of performance tasks—as, for example, the Maryland School Performance Assessment Program does—the terms "performance test" or "performance assessment" are preferred (see, e.g., Yen & Ferrara, 1997).

CRTs today typically use a wide array of item types for providing valid information about examinee proficiency; therefore, every item type from multiple-choice test items and true–false test items to essays to complex performance tasks and simulations will be used (Zenisky & Sireci, 2002). New item types permit the assessment of a wider array of skills than is possible with multiple-choice test items. These tests may even be administered and scored via computer (see, e.g., Drasgow & Olson-Buchanan, 1999; Mills, Potenza, Fremer, & Ward, 2002). And with more use of computers in test administration, and the need to measure higher-level cognitive skills, the addition of more new item types to enhance assessment can be expected.

The goal of this chapter is to provide readers with an up-to-date description of CRTs, which have undergone major advances since the concept of criterion-referenced measurement was introduced by Glaser (1963) and Popham and Husek (1969). Debates about their merits and value have subsided. More item types are being used, especially those of the "constructed-response" type; new approaches for setting performance standards are now in place; emphasis has shifted from the assessment of basic skills and minimum competencies in the 1970s to the assessment of higher-level cognitive skills today; the number of performance categories has increased from two to typically three or four; there is less emphasis on the measurement of particular objectives, and more emphasis on the assessment of broader domains of content; and computers are now being used in test administration. Clearly, CRTs are very different today than in the early 1970s.

The chapter is divided into five main sections. First, the differences between NRTs and CRTs are addressed. Failure to understand these main areas of difference has caused problems for many educators and school psychologists in the past and has led to many less than adequate tests and test applications. For one, all too often the assumption is made that the two types of tests can be constructed using the same approaches to test development and evaluation. As we describe later in the chapter, this assumption is incorrect. Second, 12 steps for constructing CRTs are highlighted. Several of these steps are similar to steps used in constructing NRTs, but several others are different. Third, methodological information about CRTs is provided, including new item types, the setting of performance standards, and the assessment of reliability and validity. Fourth, the topics of reporting and using CRT scores are described, including some thoughts about the potential role of NRTs for making criterion-referenced interpretations. Finally, some thoughts about the future of CRTs are presented.

DIFFERENCES BETWEEN CRTs AND NRTs

CRT scores and NRT scores serve very different purposes, and so it should not be surprising to anyone that approaches to test development, test evaluation, and test score interpretation for these two types of tests differ considerably. There are four primary differences between CRTs and NRTs. Hambleton (1998) categorizes these differences as (1) test purpose, (2) contents specificity, (3) test development and evaluation, and (4) test score generalizability. The difference in purpose between NRTs and CRTs can be characterized as "the basic distinction" (Popham & Husek, 1969). An NRT is designed and constructed to provide a basis for making comparisons among examinees in the content area or areas measured by the test. Test score norms are generally used as the standard of comparison. A CRT, by contrast, is constructed to facilitate a sharper interpretation of examinee performance in relation to the content covered in the test. CRTs are intended to provide scores that can be used to (1) describe the level of examinees' performance, (2) make performance classifications, and (3) evaluate instructional program effectiveness or provide information for educational accountability. Just as criterion-referenced interpretations can be made on the basis of NRTs (test items can nearly always be linked to objectives they measure, and inferences about examinees' mastery can be made from their performance on these items), norm-referenced interpretations can be made from CRTs. However, comparisons among examinees using CRT scores are problematic when test scores are relatively homogeneous, and this is often the case with CRTs, since they are not constructed to ensure test score variability (as is the case with NRTs).

The second difference is concerned with test construction. Construction of both NRTs and CRTs begins with the development of test blueprints or specifications that define the content, characteristics, and intent of the tests. Although NRTs can utilize objectives to define and limit the intended content domain, often the expectations for domain clarity are higher for CRTs because of the way the scores are used. Popham (1984) suggested that one way to rigorously define the content domain for each major component of a curriculum (i.e., the content standards) to be assessed would involve specifying four aspects: (1) description, (2) sample test item, (3) content description, and (4) response description. Stringent adherence to

domain or item specifications would be ideal for constructing CRTs, because the resulting scores are referenced back to the item specifications at the interpretation stage. Clear "targets" for test score interpretations are essential with CRTs. Practically speaking, however, content domains are not usually spelled out as clearly as is desirable to achieve Popham's description of the ideal situation. Still, it would be accurate to note that the requirements for detailed content specifications are higher for CRTs than for NRTs, because of the intended uses of the information from each test.

The third difference between NRTs and CRTs is in the area of test development and evaluation. NRTs are designed, by definition, to "spread examinees out" so as to increase the stability of the examinees' rankings by test scores. To accomplish this, NRT score variance must be increased; this is accomplished by selecting items or tasks of moderate difficulty (item difficulty levels of .30 to .70) and high discriminating power (correlations between item or task score and total test scores of over .30), subject to content specifications as well as other test design constraints that may be imposed (e.g., meeting any test specifications about the balance of item formats, specifications about the number of graphics, etc.). In general, the increased score variability from NRTs will improve test score validity and reliability, but can also result in tests' failing to contain items that "tap" the central concepts of a particular area of achievement (Popham, 1984). For a full review of NRT development methods, readers are referred to Linn (1989).

CRT interpretations, on the other hand, do not depend on score comparisons among examinees. Content considerations are essential. CRT scores are interpreted "directly" by referencing scores to the appropriate domains of content and the associated performance standards (Hambleton, 1998). A valid test item bank is constructed in relation to the content standards, curriculum frameworks, job analysis, and so on. Items or tasks that do not meet the content specifications, that are poorly written, or that are identified as flawed from any field tests are removed from the bank. From that point onward, assessment material from the bank can be used to construct tests, and scores can be used to make criterion-referenced interpretations. Item statistics are typically less important than content considerations in item selection. Exceptions occur when CRTs are being constructed to maximize the tests' discriminating power in the region of the performance standards (see Hambleton, Swaminathan, & Rogers, 1991).

Test evaluations follow from the intended uses of tests. With NRTs, all of the well-known classical statistics are of interest: test–retest reliability, parallel-form reliability, internal-consistency reliability, content validity, construct validity, and so on. With CRTs, focus is shifted to new statistics such as item–objective congruence or item validity (do the item or task, and its associated scoring rubric, measure the construct of interest?) and the consistency and accuracy of classifications made with the test scores. Construct validity evidence remains critical because of the desire to interpret scores in relation to constructs rather than in relation to norms groups. The matter of test evaluation is discussed in more detail later in this chapter, but it remains one of the main differences between NRTs and CRTs.

The fourth major difference is score generalizability. Norm-referenced performance is interpreted best in relation to a "norm" group. Generalizations of examinees' performance to a body of content are rarely justified, because of the way in which test items and tasks are selected for inclusion in an NRT. By contrast, test score generalization is a valuable attribute of criterion-referenced measurement, at least in concept. Sometimes the actual implementation comes up short. Because examinees' performance on a specific set of test items or tasks is rarely of interest, and because items or tasks can be matched to domains of content, test score generalizations beyond the specific items on a CRT can be made to the larger domains of content measuring each objective, standard, or outcome assessed by the test. For example, the criterion-referenced performance of a student who can successfully identify the main idea of paragraphs taken from a fourth-grade basal reader can be generalized to the student's ability to identify the main idea in all other material covered by the item specifications that define the item pool for the objective.

At the same time, NRTs and CRTs are not mutually exclusive concepts. Both types of tests use (1) similar test directions and item types (e.g., multiple-choice test items are common to both), (2) standardized test administrations, and (3) similar scoring procedures. For further discussion of the differences between NRTs and CRTs, see Ebel (1978), Popham (1978a), Popham and Husek (1969), or Hambleton (1998); for further discussion of definitions of CRTs, see Nitko (1980).

CONSTRUCTING CRTs

When CRTs were introduced by Glaser (1963) and Popham and Husek (1969), the goal was to assess examinees' performance in relation to a set of behavioral objectives. Over the years, it became clear that behavioral objectives did not have the specificity needed to guide instruction or to serve as targets for test development and test score interpretation (Popham, 1978b). Numerous attempts were made to increase the clarity of behavioral objectives, including the development of detailed domain specifications that included a clearly written objective, a sample test item or two, detailed specifications for appropriate content, and details on the construction of relevant assessment materials (see Hambleton, 1998). Domain specifications seemed to meet the demand for clearer statements of the intended targets for assessment, but they were very time-consuming to write, and often the level of detail needed for good assessment was impossible to achieve for higher-order cognitive skills; thus test developers found domain specifications to be limiting. An example is provided in Figure 16.1.

More recently, the trend in CRT practices has been to write objectives focused on the more important educational outcomes (fewer instructional and assessment targets seem to be preferable) and then to offer a couple of sample assessments—preferably samples showing the diversity of approaches that might be used for assessment (Popham, 2000). Coupled with these looser specifications of the objectives is an intensive effort to demonstrate the validity of any assessments that are constructed. These detailed specifications provide item writers with clearer guidelines for both writing assessment mate-

General description

Examinee will be able to apply Ohm's law in various word problems.

Directions and sample test item

Directions: Read the word problem below and answer it by circling the correct answer. All the answer choices have been
rounded to the first decimal place.

Test item: A current of 4.2 amperes flows through a coil whose resistance is 1.4 ohms. What is the potential difference
applied at the ends of the coil?

a. 0.3 volts   b. 3.0 volts   c. 5.6 volts   d. 5.9 volts

Content limits

1. All problems will be similar to but different from the ones presented in classroom instruction.
2. Examinees will not be told in the directions to use Ohm's law, nor given the mathematical formula.
3. The directions will specify how the answers have been rounded off.
4. Examinee can be asked to calculate *any* of the variables in Ohm's law.
5. The variables given in the word problem will always have correct units and contain a decimal form (e.g., 2.5 volts, not $2\frac{1}{2}$).

Response limits

1. Answer choices will be placed in a numerical sequence from smallest to largest number.
2. The incorrect answer choices will be of the correct unit and in a decimal form.
3. The answer choices will include the correct answer and three plausible distractors.

Calculating current

Correct answer: $\dfrac{\text{voltage}}{\text{resistance}}$

Plausible distractors: $\dfrac{\text{resistance}}{\text{voltage}}$, resistance × voltage, resistance + voltage

Calculating voltage

Correct answer: current × resistance

Plausible distractors: $\dfrac{\text{current}}{\text{resistance}}$, $\dfrac{\text{resistance}}{\text{current}}$, resistance + current

Calculating resistance

Correct answer: $\dfrac{\text{voltage}}{\text{current}}$

Plausible distractors: $\dfrac{\text{current}}{\text{voltage}}$, current × voltage, current + voltage

FIGURE 16.1. A sample item domain specification to assess Ohm's law. This objective would be found
in a high school physics course.

rial and judging its quality than might be available from simply a statement of some desired outcome. They are also helpful in interpreting the test scores themselves, since the intent of the objective is clearer. An example is provided in Figure 16.2.

Twelve steps for preparing a CRT are now offered. The intended purposes of the test and resulting test scores dictate the degree of attention to detail and thoroughness with which these steps are carried out. A classroom or special education teacher de-

Content Strand: Number Sense
Objective: Numbers and Numeration

Demonstrates an understanding of and uses the symbolic representations of real numbers; explains the magnitude of numbers by comparing and ordering real numbers.

Item Characteristics:

- Multiple-choice and short-answer items can be used to test this learning target.
- Items will assess symbolic representations of real numbers, including the forms of fractions, decimals, percents, integers, positive integer exponents (negative exponents may be used only as part of scientific notation), absolute value, the number line, geometric representations, and pictorial models.
- Test items that ask for understanding of place value by comparing, sequencing, and ordering real numbers will include numbers from the hundred billions place to the sixth decimal place. (Exponents and scientific notation may be used in ordering numbers.)
- In comparing, sequencing, and ordering fractions, students should know how to express fractions in their lowest terms and understand how to convert improper fractions to mixed numbers and vice versa (fractions should be reasonable).
- Students may be asked to illustrate and compare mixed numbers and improper fractions.
- Students should be able to find equivalents between common fractions, decimals, and percents, and between decimals and scientific notation. (Reasonable numbers should be used.)
- Items may have students show or describe relationships between the different forms of real numbers using words or pictures.
- Test items may have students compare, sequence, and order any combination of forms of real numbers.

Stimulus Attributes:

- For whole numbers, test items may include illustrations of number lines and other pictorial models.
- For fractions, decimals, or fractional parts of sets, test items may include illustrations of real-life objects or geometric shapes.

Vocabulary/Mathematical and Terms:

- Terms that can be used: base, common denominator, convert, decimal form, equivalent, exponent, improper fraction, mixed number, negative, numerator, percent, place value, power, scientific notation, simplify

FIGURE 16.2. An example of an item specification from the Washington Assessment of Student Learning (this is an excellent example of a currently popular way to describe a domain of content matched to an objective).

veloping a test to assess students' acquisition of multiplication facts may complete only several of the steps and may need only one or two objectives. On the other hand, a state department of education preparing high school graduation tests, or a certifying board preparing an exam, will complete *all* of the steps with considerable attention to detail.

The steps are as follows:

1. Preliminary considerations
   a. Specify test purposes, and describe domain of content and/or behaviors that are of interest.
   b. Specify groups of examinees to be measured, and any special testing re-

quirements resulting from examinees' age, race, gender, socioeconomic status, linguistic differences, disabilities, and so on.
   c. Determine time and financial resources available (or specify them, if not given) for constructing and validating the test.
   d. Identify and select qualified staff members (note any individual strengths and their role in test development).
   e. Specify an initial estimate of test length (include number of test items and/or tasks, as well as approximate time requirements for their development), and set a schedule for com-

pleting steps in the test development and validation process.

2. Review of content domain/behaviors of interest (or prepare, if not available)
   a. Review the descriptions of the content standards/objectives to determine their acceptability for inclusion in the test.
   b. Select final group of objectives (i.e., finalize the content standards) to be included in the test.
   c. Prepare item specifications for each objective (or something equivalent, to lay out the content clearly) and review them for completeness, accuracy, clarity, and practicality.

3. Item/task writing and preparation of any scoring rubrics that are needed
   a. Draft a sufficient number of items and/or tasks for field testing.
   b. Carry out item/task editing, and review scoring rubrics.

4. Assessment of content validity
   a. Identify a pool of judges and measurement specialists.
   b. Review the test items and tasks to determine their match to the objectives, their representativeness, and their freedom from stereotyping and potential bias (items/tasks show potential bias when aspects of the assessment appear to place one group at a disadvantage—perhaps because of choice of language or situation).
   c. Review the test items and/or tasks to determine their technical adequacy (does the assessment material measure the content standards of interest?).

5. Revisions to test items/tasks
   a. Based upon data from steps 4b and 4c, revise test items/tasks (when possible and necessary) or delete them.
   b. Write additional test items/tasks (if needed), and repeat step 4.

6. Field test administration (sometimes carried out within the context of an ongoing test administration)
   a. Organize the test items/tasks into forms for field testing.
   b. Administer the test forms to appropriately chosen groups of examinees (i.e., groups like those for whom the final test is intended).
   c. Conduct item analyses and item bias

studies (usually called "studies to identify differentially functioning test items").
   d. If statistical linking or equating of forms is needed, this step might be done here. (See below for more information about statistical linking or equating of tests.)

7. Revisions to test items/tasks
   a. Revise test items/tasks when necessary or delete them, using the results from step 6c. Also, check scoring rubrics for any performance tasks being field-tested.

8. Test assembly
   a. Determine the test length, the number of forms needed, and the number of items/tasks per objective.
   b. Select test items/tasks from available pool of valid test material.
   c. Prepare test directions, practice questions (when necessary), test booklet layout, scoring keys, answer sheets, and so on.
   d. Specify modifications to instructions, medium of presentation or examinees' responses, and time requirements that may be necessary for examinees with special needs.
   e. Include anchor test items if the test is being statistically linked to a previous test or tests.

9. Selection of performance standards
   a. Determine whether performance standards are needed to accomplish the test purpose (usually they are).
   b. Initiate (and document) a process to determine the performance standards for separating examinees into performance categories. Compile procedural, internal, and external validity evidence to support the performance standards (Cizek, 2001).
   c. Specify considerations that may affect the performance standards when they are applied to examinees with special needs (i.e., alternative administration or other modifications to accommodate such examinees).
   d. Identify "alternative" test score interpretations for examinees requiring alternative administration or other modifications.

10. Pilot test administration (if possible, and if relevant—sometimes this step is

replaced with the actual test administration)

    a. Design the test administration to collect score reliability and validity information.

    b. Administer the test form(s) to appropriately chosen groups of examinees.

    c. Identify and evaluate alternative administration/other modifications to meet individual special needs that may affect validity and reliability of the test or forms of the test.

    d. Evaluate the test administration procedures, test items/tasks, and score reliability and validity.

    e. Make final revisions to the test or forms of the test based on the available technical data.

11. Preparation of manuals

    a. Prepare a test administrator's manual.

    b. Prepare a technical manual.

12. Additional technical data collection

    a. Conduct reliability and validity investigations on a continuing basis.

With many of the state-mandated tests and credentialing exams, the new tests need to be statistically linked or equated to tests administered previously. This step insures that scores across tests are comparable, so that previously established performance standards can be used with the new tests and any growth or change can be identified. This statistical equating activity is complicated and is typically done by using some "anchor test items" and then "statistically equating" any new test or tests to those given in the past. This means trying to find scores from one test that are comparable to scores on another. (Other methods for linking tests are available, but are not discussed here.) Anchor items (sometimes called "common items") are items administered in the current version of a test that were included in a previous version. (Normally, anchor items are chosen to match the content of the tests being linked and to be of comparable difficulty.) Comparing performance on these anchor or common items/tasks on the two occasions makes it possible to disentangle any differences over time due to ability shifts, and any differences due to the use of nonequivalent tests. For more information on how states, test publishers, and credentialing agencies statistically equate tests, see Hambleton and colleagues (1991).

The process is straightforward if large samples of examinees are used and the amount of common or anchor material is not too small. (Normally, 1,000 or more examinees with 10–15 common test items are sufficient to statistically equate two tests; obviously, though, the larger the sample of examinees and number of common items, the better.) When tests are statistically equated, fairness can be achieved, the same performance standards can be used over time, and progress in achievement over time can be monitored.

A few remarks on each of the test development steps follow.

1. Step 1 insures that a test development project is well organized. The early articulation of test purpose(s) and factors that might affect test quality will help manage resources. Also, identifying special groups (e.g., examinees with disabilities) insures that when the test is administered, it will measure examinees' achievement rather than reflecting their special needs.

2. Domain specifications or equivalent ways to articulate content standards are invaluable to item writers. Considerable time and money can be saved later in revising test items/tasks if item/task writers are clear about the appropriate knowledge and skills to measure.

3. Some training of item/task writers in the proper use of domain (or item) specifications and in the principles of item/task writing is often desirable, particularly if novel item types are to be prepared. Most testing agencies today have prepared training procedures and manuals to guide the item/task development process. Also, new and more mechanical methods (and even computer software) are now being developed for producing test items from item shells. An "item shell" is a test item with key elements removed. When these key elements are substituted, new test items are generated. Suppose a set of test items is needed to assess computation of statistics to measure central tendency. In the test item "Find the mean of the numbers 5, 10, 15, and 20," one key element is the statistical concept "mean." If "median" or "mode" is substituted, new test items are generated.

The numbers themselves are a key element; if they are changed, a new test item is generated. In fact, the numbers can be changed many times to generate many more test items. The result of using item shells (sometimes called "item facets" or "item models") is the production of more good-quality test items at a faster rate than they can be produced by item writers (for a review, see Pitoniak, 2002).

4. Step 4 is essential. Items/tasks are evaluated by reviewers to assess their technical quality, and to confirm the absence of bias and stereotyping. Early identification of problems can save time, money, and embarrassment to the testing agency. It has become routine, for example, for agencies constructing tests to establish content review and item sensitivity review committees.

5. Any necessary revisions to test items/tasks can be made at step 5; when additional test items/tasks are needed, they can be written, and step 4 is then repeated.

6. The test items/tasks are organized into booklets and administered to a sample of examinees like those for whom the test is intended. (The desirable sample size will depend on the importance of the test; a few hundred examinees are normally sufficient to identify flawed items and obtain stable item/task statistics.) Necessary revisions to test items/tasks can be made at this stage. Item/task statistics that reflect level of difficulty and discriminating power are used to identify assessment material in need of revision. The same statistics are used at a later point in constructing parallel forms of tests.

7. Whenever possible, malfunctioning test items/tasks can be revised and added to the pools of acceptable test items/tasks. When substantial revisions are made to an item/task, it should be placed again at step 4. In this way, its effectiveness can be investigated, and new item/task statistics can be produced.

8. Final test booklets are compiled at step 8. When parallel forms are required, and especially if the tests are short, item/task statistics should be used to insure that matched forms are produced.

9. A standard-setting procedure must be selected, implemented, and documented. Specifications for an appropriate panel are made and panelists are selected; a method is chosen (e.g., the Angoff method for multiple-choice items, the booklet classification method for performance tasks); training materials for the method are developed; the process is implemented with the panel; and performance standards are finally set. With important CRTs, it is also important to field-test the standard-setting method. If standard setting is handled poorly, the validity of any test use is suspect. For an excellent discussion of standard setting, see Cizek (2001). If a description of examinees' performance is used in place of or as a supplement to performance standards, its interpretability and relation to the test's purpose should be explained.

10. Test directions must be evaluated; scoring keys must be checked; and the reliability and validity of scores and decisions must be assessed.

11. For important tests, such as those used for awarding high school diplomas or credentials, a test administration manual and a technical manual should be prepared. The test administration manual will be especially useful in standardizing the test administration conditions.

12. No matter how carefully a test is constructed or evaluated initially, reliability and validity studies must be carried out on a continuing basis.

The development of CRTs can be time-consuming and expensive. For example, the setting of performance standards, just one step in the process, may require 20–30 persons (perhaps 10–20 persons with credentialing exams) to come together for 2 days or so. Considerable preparation is involved, along with technical assistance during and after the meeting to analyze data, set the performance standards, and compile a report. Also, content review and item sensitivity review committees may consist of more than 10 or so members, and may meet several times a year.

Not covered in the 12 CRT development and validation steps are the critically important tasks of identifying audiences to receive test scores, preparing and field-testing test score reports, and ultimately finalizing these score reports. In the case of CRTs used in education, these audiences might include students and their parents, teachers and school administrators, policy makers, and the public. Usually CRT score reporting in other contexts (such as credentialing exams) is easier to finalize, but not without more problems. For example, questions such as these often arise: On what numerical scale should scores be reported? Should scores be reported along with pass–fail decisions? How should the concept of error be communicated? Is diagnostic information for failing candidates necessary? The topic of score reporting is discussed in some detail later in this chapter.

PSYCHOMETRIC ADVANCES

In this section, several psychometric advances are considered: emerging item types, the setting of performance standards, and the assessment of reliability and validity. The first topic is relevant for both NRTs and CRTs; the second is specific to CRTs; and the third is also relevant for both NRTs and CRTs, though the actual approaches are quite different because of the different uses of NRT and CRT scores.

Emerging Item Types

The production of valid test items—that is, test items that provide a psychometrically sound basis for assessing examinees' level of proficiency or performance—requires (1) well-trained item writers, (2) item reviews, (3) field testing, and often (4) the use of multiple item types. Well-trained item writers are persons who have had experience with the intended population of examinees, know the intended curricula, and have experience writing test items/tasks in a variety of formats. Test companies will often hire teachers, curriculum specialists, and other persons who think they have the skills to write items/tasks. Some training is provided, and writing assisgnments are made. Those who can meet deadlines and produce high-quality work are then encouraged to stay on and write more items/tasks.

Assessment review often involves checking test items/tasks for their validity in measuring the intended objectives, their technical adequacy (i.e., their consistency with the best item/task-writing practices), and their freedom from bias and stereotyping. Field testing must be carried out on samples large enough to provide stable statistical information and to be representative of the intended population of examinees. Unstable and/or biased item statistical information only complicates the test development process and threatens its validity. And, finally, one of the most important changes today in testing is the introduction of new item types— item types that permit the assessment of higher-level cognitive skills (see Zenisky & Sireci, 2002).

In the preceding section, we have described some of the ways in which CRTs are developed. We turn in this section of the chapter to one important way in which CRTs are evolving: in terms of the kinds of item types that appear on these and other such tests.

With regard to the kinds of item types in the psychometric literature, the list is long (Hambleton, 1996; Osterlind, 1989, 1998; Zenisky & Sireci, 2002). Traditionally, the item types used in educational testing have been objectively classified as either "selected-response" or "constructed-response," with multiple-choice items being the most prevalent example of the selected-response variety and written responses (either short-answer or extended-length essays) epitomizing common constructed-response items.

However, while the selected- versus constructed-response approach to grouping item types remains a useful dichotomy on a general level, an alternative classification scheme suggested by Bennett and colleagues (1990) involves somewhat finer gradations of the specific nature of examinees' responses for different item types. Table 16.1 provides this latter classification scheme. This approach permits consideration of assessment tasks with respect to cognitive features such as answer format and response constraint; it is particularly useful for conceptualizing and categorizing many familiar and emerging assessment tasks that are increasingly being used (and studied for use) in different testing contexts, including various applications of the criterion-referenced model. As seen in Table 16.1, Bennett and colleagues' classification framework describes seven discrete categories for item types based on differences in the nature and extent of responses for different item types. Movement from category to category through the framework corresponds to key

TABLE 16.1. Several Examples of Possible Item Types for Use in CRTs

Response type	Description	Example 1: *Familiar task or implementation strategy*	Example 2: *Innovative task or implementation strategy*
Multiple-choice	Task is to select one of a limited set of possible response alternatives.	Text only, still graphics, or with external stimulus such as audio or video administered in group.	Text only, still graphics, audio, and video all possible; individualized pacing with external stimuli is more feasible.
Selection/ identification	Examinees choose a response from presented alternatives with number of options typically large enough to limit possible effects of guessing.	*Multiple selection:* Upon presentation of stimulus, examinees choose best answer from extended list (each answer may be used more than once).	*Highlighting text:* Examinees choose a sentence from a passage displayed on screen that best fits selection criteria given in item stem.
Reordering/ rearrangement	Task is defined by placing items from stimulus array in correct sequence (or in one of several possible correct alternatives).	*Ordering sentences:* Examinees arrange series of sentences to form a coherent written passage.	*Build, list, and reorder:* Examinees are asked to build answer list from items in list of answer choices and then arrange the items in specified order.
Substitution/ correction	Examinees must replace what is presented to them with a correct alternative.	*Correcting spelling:* Examinees identify the misspelled word and provide correct alternative spelling.	*Editing tasks:* As used for computer programmers, examinees find mistakes in programs and must revise them to make them work.
Completion	Task is to supply a correct response to an incomplete stimulus.	*Cloze:* Examinees provide the appropriate word to complete a sentence.	*Formulating hypotheses:* Given situation, examinees generate several possible explanatory theories.
Construction	The task requires the entire unit to be constructed.	*Essay:* Examinees are presented with a topic and hand-write a response of a set length.	*Essay:* Examinees are presented with a topic and write a response of a set length; on computer, may incorporate spell-checks, cut-and-paste, and other editing tools.
Presentation	Physical presentation or performance delivered under real or simulated conditions; object is in some substantial part the manner of performance and not simply its result.	*Laboratory experiment:* Examinees carry out an experiment within prescribed parameters; final product may be written, graphically represented, or orally presented.	*Dynamic problem solving:* Online situation adapts and evolves as examinees enter response actions into the computer.

changes in the range of response possibilities.

To provide a sampling of what sorts of assessment tasks correspond to each of the seven categories in Table 16.1, for each category two practical examples are presented and described. For each category, example 1 is defined to be a familiar assessment task (one that is likely to be commonly implemented in current CRT programs). Example 2 is intended as an illustration of the sorts of innovations in item types that are emerging in the psychometric literature. Such novel item types are very much related to expanded use of computers and computing technology, as using computers to administer tests to examinees is becoming an attractive possibility for more and more large-scale testing programs. Although this is not yet an everyday occurrence for most testing programs, it is an exciting prospect in terms of standards-based assessment, and these examples are given to demonstrate the potential for such technology to influence measurement practices.

At one end of the category framework in Table 16.1 are traditional "multiple-choice" items, where examinees are presented with an item stem (either a phrase or a question) and must select one of several presented alternative responses (either the single correct answer or the best answer of the choices provided). Large-scale school assessments in practice have long made especial use of the multiple-choice item type, as there are both measurement and practical benefits associated with such items. For example, many multiple-choice items can be administered in a relatively short time (thereby supporting efforts toward satisfactory domain coverage), and the format is highly familiar to item writers, so that it is a fairly straightforward procedure to train writers to produce such items on a large scale. Multiple-choice items have, however, been the subject of much criticism over the years (see Boodoo, 1993), as people have suggested that they encourage and assess mere memorization skills, although research by Traub (1993) documented a number of studies in which multiple-choice items were found to be equivalent in information value to other kinds of item types for some constructs (see also Bennett et al., 1990; Bennett, Rock, & Wang, 1991; Hambleton & Murphy, 1992).

Furthermore, as Martinez (1999) has mentioned, multiple-choice items can be written to assess higher-level cognitive skills beyond rote memorization.

However, there are many distinctive variations in the vein of selected-response items, and these become clearer through consideration of the category structure of Table 16.1. In the "selection/identification" category, the notion of selecting among presented alternatives remains, but item types that fit into in that category typically have many more than the three to five response options common to standard multiple-choice items. Similarly, "reordering/rearrangement" items ask examinees to organize presented items according to a predetermined scheme (alphabetical, size, theme, etc.). "Substitution/correction" items involve both identification of error (selection) and self-generation of more appropriate responses (construction). This category of items therefore occupies the position of bridge between the two familiar groupings of selected- and constructed-response items: The three previous categories all generally fall under the broad heading of selected-response items, and the next three categories correspond to different levels of complexity for examinees in generating a unique answer. In "completion" items, examinees respond to an incomplete stimulus, while "construction" items necessitate a more involved level of response generation. "Presentation" items are defined by evaluation of not just product but also process; that is, the manner of going about the task is as relevant as the object of the task. This last category of items also includes assessment methods that are commonly referred to as "performance assessments," which are defined by Rudner and Boston (1994) as testing methods that ask examinees to create an answer or product that presents ability or skill in the prescribed domain. As with presentation items in the Bennett and colleagues (1990) scheme, the emphasis for these item types is on "doing"; the degree of realism or fidelity to the construct should be high; and there may be no or many more than one "correct" answer (Hambleton, 1996).

The seven categories of item types within the Bennett and colleagues (1990) framework reflect a broad range of approaches to measurement, and contained within those categories are many, many specific item types for use in assessment instruments. Operationally speaking, however, implementation of the different item types varies greatly with the purpose and measurement needs of different testing programs. Although many large-scale NRTs use items of the selected-response variety (primarily the multiple-choice item type), numerous state-level CRTs are integrating different forms of constructed-response items, including short-answer items and extended-length essays. Massachusetts (among other states, of course) is one notable example of this, in that more then half of the points on those tests are associated with constructed-response items. The state of Maryland introduced an entirely performance-based testing program in the early 1990s, where students were assessed with a series of problem-solving situations. In large-scale admissions tests, multiple-choice items predominate, although essays are increasingly being used as well (as in the Medical College Admissions Test and the Graduate Management Admissions Test).

In many respects, testing for professional credentialing and licensure has taken the lead in terms of innovations in item types. Many assessments in such fields as medicine (the U.S. Medical Licensing Examination), architecture (Architecture Registration Examination), and information/technology (Microsoft, Novell) now use computer-based testing infrastructure to create and administer exams that are very different from traditional assessment methods in form and substance. Innovations in that area of testing has relevance for CRTs in the schools, however, in that there are currently many possibilities for using computers in schools during instruction and evaluation, particularly in diagnostic applications. The National Assessment of Educational Progress (NAEP) is one testing program that is formally exploring the possibility of technology-based assessment (National Center for Education Statistics, 2002). Testing by computer greatly facilitates use of such media as still graphics, audio, and video, and each student can work at his or her own pace. As illustrated by the innovative task or implementation strategy examples in Table 16.1, items administered via computer can take advantage of the potential to manipulate on-screen images and data in innovative ways.

In light of the computer-based advances in item types, as well as more widespread use of constructed-response items in paper-and-pencil assessment, issues related to data management and scoring have taken on greater prominence. Many developers of CRTs desire the measurement and content coverage benefits of such formats, although one historical limitation of constructed-response item types (particularly items that prompt examinees for longer and/or less constrained answers) has been developing ways to grade such responses efficiently and reliably. Examinees like to get immediate feedback, and such item types have not been associated with quick score turnaround. However, computer scanners that electronically code and store student constructed-response data now allow student responses to be displayed on the computer screens of trained scorers (thus doing away with the need to handle, sort, and pass around thousands of paper sheets). In some testing programs, the possibility even exists for raters in remote locations to view examinee responses in this electronic form over the Internet, thereby reducing or eliminating the logistics of bringing raters together in a centralized site.

Furthermore, at the cutting edge of testing technology are computer algorithms that can process and grade text, such as the Educational Testing Service's E-rater (Burstein, Kukich, Wolff, Lu, & Chodorow, 1998), Project Essay Grade (Page, 1994; Page & Peterson, 1995), and latent semantic analysis (Landauer, Foltz, & Laham, 1998). Although neither computerized text readers nor other computer technologies replace the need for humans to be involved with every step of test development and scoring, they can and do facilitate use of assessment methods beyond traditional, objective, one-answer-correct item types.

The move toward more varied assessment methods and expanded use of open-ended item types is a positive change for criterion-referenced measurement. Indeed, the kinds of items examinees are encountering on many CRTs today are in many cases very different from those seen by their parents a generation ago. Such changes in approaches to assessment in CRTs are reasonable, given the evolution to date of testing technologies, and can only be expected to continue as research into assessment methods carries on.

In exploring different methods to provide information about a construct or constructs of interest, the potential exists for test developers to provide test users with a broader picture of what examinees (both at the individual level and in the aggregate) know and are able to do. However, a number of measurement hurdles remain. The efficiency of many constructed-response tasks remains in question, given that relatively few such items can be administered to examinees in the same time as it would take to present many more selected-response items; both the nature and type of information are qualitatively different, though, and so perhaps different standards for evaluating such information are necessary. In other words, testing programs looking to use such items must present a comprehensive validity case to support decisions about item types, and must reckon with choices about how much structure of the steps in complex tasks to include. Some questions for future research associated with implementation of computerization include the costs related to equipping testing sites (schools or other centralized testing centers) with specific minimum capabilities in terms of computer hardware and software; the need to install and maintain secure data networks; the desire to avoid testing only computer proficiency; and issues of verifying the identities of examinees.

Clearly, the choice among different item types is a validity issue, as some item types are more appropriate for some domains of knowledge or skill than for others. Ultimately, the decisions made about item types in the process of developing CRTs can significantly shape the quality of the inferences to be made on the basis of test scores.

The Setting of Performance Standards

Perhaps the most difficult and certainly the most controversial step in the CRT development process is the setting of performance standards. Ultimately, this process is judgmental, regardless of the method selected; thus the goal of any standard-setting method is to create a framework in which judgments provided by panelists lead to reliable and valid ratings, and ultimately to reliable and valid performance standards (see, e.g., Hambleton, 2001).

Many aspects of the standard-setting process have changed over the years. First, more emphasis today is given to the selection and training of panelists to set the performance standards. Panelists need to be representative of the appropriate stakeholder groups, and to be thoroughly trained in the method being implemented. Second, detailed descriptions of the performance categories are established early in the process. These are needed to provide the framework for panelists to make meaningful judgments about the performance standards. Here, for example, are the performance descriptors used in Massachusetts at the 10th-grade level in mathematics:

- *Basic.* A student at this level demonstrates partial understanding of the numeration system; performs some calculations and estimations; identifies examples of basic math concepts; reads and constructs graphs, tables, and charts; applies learned procedures to solve routine problems; and applies some reasoning methods to solve simple problems.
- *Proficient.* A student at this level demonstrates solid understanding of the numeration system; performs most calculations and estimations; defines concepts and generates examples and counterexamples of concepts; represents data and mathematical relationships in multiple forms (e.g., equations, graphs); applies learned procedures and mathematical concepts to solve a variety of problems, including multistep problems; and uses a variety of reasoning methods to solve problems and to explain steps and procedures.
- *Advanced.* A student at this level connects concepts from various areas of mathematics, and uses concepts to develop generalizations; performs complex calculations and estimations; selects the best representation for a given set of data and purpose; generates unique strategies and procedures to solve nonroutine problems; and uses multiple reasoning methods to solve complex problems and to justify strategies and solutions.

Descriptors like those above are used by standard-setting panelists to decide the number of test score points an examinee needs to reach each level. Often these descriptors are developed by a committee that is separate from the standard-setting committee, though not always.

Third, several new methods for standard setting have emerged for use with CRTs, but research remains to be done to determine the most valid ways in which these methods can be implemented. Contributors to Cizek's (2001) volume describe a number of these new methods, including the bookmark method, the body-of-work method, the analytic judgment method, and more. Probably four categories of methods are available today: those that involve a review of test items/tasks and scoring rubrics by panelists (e.g., the Angoff, Ebel, and Nedelsky methods, the bookmark method); those that involve judgments of examinees independent of their test scores (e.g., contrasting group, borderline group); those that involve a review of the actual work of examinees—that is, their answers to the test items/tasks (e.g., the booklet classification method, the item cluster method); and those that involve judgments about examinees based upon a review of their score profiles (e.g., the dominant-score profile method). For example, with the booklet classification method (see the third category above), panelists are asked to consider actual examinee responses to the test items/tasks on the test and to identify those examinees demonstrating performance at the various levels—below basic, basic, proficient, and advanced. From these classifications, it is possible to identify performance standards on the test score scale that result in assignments of examinees' work (i.e., their answers to the test items/tasks) to performance categories that are in the closest possible agreement with the classifications of the panelists. Research suggests that the booklet classification method is popular with panelists, because they prefer making judgments of examinees' actual work (something they are familiar with) to making judgments about examinees' performance based upon reviews of items/tasks (a fairly abstract task compared to classifying actual work). All of these methods and others are described in Cizek (2001) and Hambleton, Jaeger, Plake, and Mills (2000).

Fourth, the topic of feedback to panelists has become very important. How much and what kind of information do panelists need to set valid performance standards? Do they need information about their own consistency over items and over rounds of ratings; their agreement with other panelists; and/or their consistency with empirical evidence about the test items and the examinees?

Finally, in recent years, the topic of validation of performance standards has become extremely important. Validation begins with a full documentation of the process—everything from how the composition of the panel was decided and how panelists were actually selected, to training, implementation of the method, and detailed analyses of the results. It is common today to ask panelists questions about the method: Was training of the method effective? Were the discussions among panelists meaningful? Did they have confidence in the method, and do they have confidence in the resulting performance standards? Is there evidence of performance standards' being consistent over panels? Also, evidence for the interpanelist and intrapanelist consistency of ratings is investigated. Finally, external evidence for the validity of the performance standards is investigated. For example, are the pass rates consistent with other evidence that may be available? Readers are referred to Cizek (2001) for more details on emerging issues and practices for setting performance standards.

The Assessment of Reliability and Validity

Traditions for reporting test score reliability for NRTs are well known. It is routine to report in a test manual evidence pertaining to the stability of test scores over short periods of time (i.e., test–retest reliability) and consistency of test scores over parallel forms (i.e., parallel-form reliability). Because reliability designs involving a single group of examinees taking two forms of a test or even a single test a second time are often not realistic, single-administration estimates of reliability are very common. For example, it is routine to report corrected split-half reliability estimates and/or coefficient alpha. Both can be obtained from a single test administration. But all of these approaches to reliability estimation are focused on test scores and their consistency over time, over parallel forms, or over items within the test. CRTs are not focused on scores; rather, they are focused on performance categories and classifications.

CRT scores are used to assign examinees to performance categories. It is obvious, then, that the reliability of test scores is less important than the reliability of the classifications of examinees into performance categories. This point is well accepted in the CRT field (see Hambleton, 1998). But it is difficult, if not impossible, in practice to administer parallel forms (or even a retest) of a CRT to assess the consistency with which examinees are assigned to performance categories. What have evolved over the years, therefore, are the following: (1) single-administration estimates of decision consistency for CRTs when items are scored 0–1 and there are two performance categories (Hambleton, 1998); and (2) single-administration estimates of decision consistency when items are polytomously scored (i.e., more than two score categories are used per test item) (see, e.g., Livingston & Lewis, 1995; Subkoviak, 1976). Both statistical procedures for obtaining single-administration estimates of decision consistency involve strong true-score modeling of the available data to obtain the estimates.

Table 16.2 provides a typical example of the way the reliability of performance classifications is being reported (this example comes from one of the state CRT technical manuals). In this case, as in most cases, it is impossible actually to determine the consistency of classifications over parallel forms or two administrations of the same test; either the second form does not actually exist, or if it did exist, it is unlikely in practice that examinees would take the second form.

However, with reasonable assumptions (for dichotomously scored data, see Subkoviak, 1976; for polytomously scored data, see Livingston & Lewis, 1995), it is possible to estimate the consistency of classifications, much as reliability is estimated from a single administration of an NRT. (Recall that the single test is split into two halves; scores on the half tests are calculated; the correlation between scores on the two halves is calculated to obtain the "split-half" reliability estimate; and then the "split-half" correlation is stepped up via the Spearman–Brown formula to obtain an estimate of the parallel-form reliability for the full-length test.)

In Table 16.2, .262 is shaded. This is the proportion of students in the total sample who were classified into the "basic" category on both administrations (of course, the second administration is only hypothetical). Obviously, these examinees were consistently classified on the two administrations. The consistency of classifications of students into four performance categories is .702 (.083 + .262 + .339 + .018). The row and column totals provide information about the proportion of the total sample of examinees in each performance category (below basic = 11.3%, basic = 36.9%, proficient = 45.8%, advanced = 6.0%). With some CRTs, examinees may be sorted into four performance categories, but the distinction between failing and passing (i.e., examinees' being identified as basic, proficient, or advanced) is the most important one. From the information available in Table 16.2, it can easily be seen that the consistency of pass–fail decisions would be .94. Of course, this value is only an estimate, but research has shown that it is a very good estimate (Livingston & Lewis, 1995). The level of decision consistency needed in practice will

TABLE 16.2. Grade 4 English Language Arts Decision Consistency Results

Status on test form taken	Status on parallel form				
	Failing	Basic	Proficient	Advanced	Total
Failing	.083	.030	0	0	.113
Basic	.030	.262	.077	.001	.369
Proficient	0	.077	.339	.042	.458
Advanced	0	.001	.042	.018	.060
Total	.113	.369	.458	.060	1

Note. From Massachusetts Department of Education (2001d).

depend on the intended uses of the CRT and the number of performance categories.

There have been two additional developments in the reporting of reliability results for CRTs. First, it is common to adjust decision consistency and decision accuracy results (to be defined below) for the amount of agreement that might be due to chance agreement only. This adjusted statistic is referred to as the "kappa statistic"; it is often reported in test manuals; and it basically provides information about agreement in performance classifications, after correcting for any agreement due to chance. Second, it is common today to report the measurement error associated with test scores at each of the performance standards (this is called "conditional error" and can be calculated by many different formulas). This is a more accurate estimate of measurement error than is provided by the standard error of measurement for the test, and it is of considerable interest because it indicates the size of the measurement error for examinees close to each performance standard.

Validity assessment might focus on the relationship between classifications made on the basis of the test scores and classifications or performance ratings provided externally to the test (e.g., teacher ratings or job performance ratings). Table 16.3 shows some real data for a grade 4 English Language Arts test. Here the cross-tabulation is between student classifications based on the test and classifications based on the examinees' true scores. An examinee's true score is considered to be the examinee's expected score on the test at the time he or she takes the test. It is the examinee's score without any measurement error due to improper sampling of test questions, flawed test items, problems with the test administra-

tion, or the like. The shaded parts of the table highlight the proportion of examinees correctly classified—failing students (based on true scores) who actually fail, basic students (based on their true scores) who actually are classified as basic, and so on. In Table 16.3, it can be seen that the accuracy with which students are classified—that is, the decision accuracy—is .788 (.087 + .299 + .402 + .000).

If the levels of decision consistency and decision accuracy fall short of expectations, test developers have several options. (1) The most obvious solution would be to lengthen the test; adding more test items/tasks will increase both statistics. (2) A less obvious solution might be to use fewer performance categories. Finally, (3) the developers could redesign the test so that the test has more measurement precision in the regions of the performance standards. Regarding possibility 2, with fewer performance categories, examinees can be more consistently and accurately classified. Possibility 3 is more complicated and would require complex test design procedures based on item response theory (Hambleton et al., 1991). Such strategies are often implemented in practice.

Other evidence to support the score inferences from a CRT can come from the compilation of content, criterion-related, and construct validity evidence. For example, the detailed match between test content and content specifications provides evidence about content validity. For CRTs, this type of evidence is especially important. Sometimes evidence relating classifications made from the test with classifications based on an external criterion (e.g., teacher ratings) is possible. See, for example, the extensive validity work carried out by American College Testing in

TABLE 16.3. Grade 4 English Language Arts Decision Accuracy Results

True-score status	Test score status				
	Failing	Basic	Proficient	Advanced	Total
Failing	.087	.016	0	0	.103
Basic	.026	.299	.056	0	.382
Proficient	0	.054	.402	.060	.515
Advanced	0	0	0	0	0
Total	.113	.369	.458	.059	1

Note. From Massachusetts Department of Education (2001d).

validating performance standards set on the NAEP. This type of study was carried out though the study was expensive, and many possible interpretations exist for why agreement in the classifications might not be high. For example, one possibility for a low level of agreement might be that teachers classify students' performance based upon a different content domain than the one covered by the test. Another problem might be that teachers' ratings are based on everyday classroom performance. NAEP assesses something different. With new forms of assessment, evidence of construct validity is especially important. It needs to be established that these new approaches to assessment, including the scoring rubrics, are producing scores consistent with the intended interpretations. (For an excellent review of methods for scoring performance assessments, see Clauser, 2000.) Factor analysis and structural equation modeling are methodological tools being used to establish construct validity. Evidence that test items/tasks are free of bias is also compiled and used to address questions about score validity. Finally, validity evidence today is being extended to address consequences of the testing and test scores. Consequential validity evidence might include evidence about whether the CRT is affecting how candidates are preparing for a test, or whether it is affecting what actually is being taught or studied in preparation for the test. For more structured approaches to compiling validity evidence in support of an intended use, readers are referred to Kane (1992).

Documenting the Technical Adequacy of a CRT

The American Educational Research Association (AERA), the American Psychological Association (APA), and the National Council for Measurement in Education (NCME) *Standards for Educational and Psychological Testing* (AERA, APA, & NCME, 1999) make it very clear that a test developer's job is not completed with the administration of his or her CRT (or any test). A major initiative is needed to compile the relevant procedural and technical information to document the usefulness of the test for achieving particular purposes. To quote the AERA and colleagues (1999) volume, "Test docu-

ments need to include enough information to allow test users and reviewers to determine the appropriateness of the test for its intended purposes" (p. 67).

SCORE REPORTING

As standards-based school testing has taken root at the state and national levels, and as high-stakes decisions have come to be associated with scores from CRTs, one topic that has taken on great prominence is the issue of reporting student test results. The No Child Left Behind Act of 2001 not only requires CRT score reporting, but mandates that the reporting be understandable to parents. Clearly, the stakes for test score reporting have been raised.

Reporting Scores Themselves

To start, test scores themselves can take many forms. The most straightforward score that an examinee can receive in any testing context is a "raw score" (also referred to as a "number-correct score"), and related to these are "percent-correct scores." Although raw scores hold obvious intrinsic appeal in terms of ease of explanation, they can be limited in their usefulness for large-scale testing when the testing program needs to make comparisons among examinees across test forms if such forms are not strictly parallel.

In fact, creating a new and unique scale for a test allows the testing program to define performance independently of other assessments. Such distinctiveness, in terms of score scales, means that test developers must exert extra effort to supply contextual information to assist in interpretation, but one advantage is a decreased likelihood of test users bringing preconceived notions about score levels to the process of understanding test scores to all tests. For example, perhaps the most familiar test score scale in use today is the 200–800 score range of the Scholastic Assessment Tests, which is unlike the score scales of most other tests currently in use. Scores such as 200, 500, and 800 have meaning unique to this test. Directly relating such scores to high school grades and scores on state- and district-level achievement tests, however, is not so easy.

In terms of CRTs, raw scores on the Massachusetts Comprehensive Assessment System tests are transformed to a scale that ranges from 200 to 280 (with 220 as the passing score each year), while the Florida Comprehensive Assessment Test uses a 100—500 scale. Though these different scales may seem arbitrary, they are designed to provide unique contexts for each test to facilitate particular score interpretations, as they can be constructed to reflect differing levels of precision depending on the needs of the testing program. Other possible numerical score types that could be reported to test takers are z-scores, percentile ranks, stanine scores, and normal curve equivalents. These four examples of scores, however, are all associated with NRTs.

Documenting Context for Scores

Documenting the context for test results is of fundamental importance (AERA et al., 1999; Lyman, 1998). Therefore, in addition to reporting simple numerical scores (in the form of any of the options described above), more and more CRT programs are developing other ways to communicate results to a variety of audiences. Oftentimes, well-defined performance standards are also indicated on reports for each individual test taker. For one example, see Figure 16.3. Furthermore, in reporting CRT results about individual students to parents and classroom teachers, the level of information is often highly detailed and can serve a diagnostic purpose. For these examples, see Figures 16.4 and 16.5.

Some additional test-based sources of context for results include providing examples of what student work looks like at various score levels; providing samples of test questions across the difficulty continuum; informing people about the content of the tests (including details about subject matter, the kinds of test questions [open-ended, selected-response], etc.); indicating whether scoring is objective or subjective; and defining the performance expectations of students, districts, or states. For these examples, see Figures 16.6 and 16.7. For example, in regard to CRTs with high stakes for individual students (e.g., high school graduation tests), test users are very interested in understanding the qualities associated with persons whose scores are near the passing score. What is it that makes someone who barely passes different from someone who fails (but is a point or two away from passing)?

After context, the *means* of communication is critical. "Means" here refers to how the reporting data are organized, what kinds of score-reporting materials are produced, and how such materials are actually disseminated to interest groups. Text, tables, graphs, charts, and/or figures are some common ways to organize information in a clear and readable way. Some suggestions in this regard from the National Education Goals Panel (1998) include using pictures and graphics in reports, using large print for the text and labels, defining terms clearly, and avoiding psychometric jargon.

Indeed, at every level of large-scale testing (international, national, state, and district), there are many different audiences who are interested in how students are doing. These include the students themselves, educators, their families, politicians, the business community, and the public at large. Each of these groups has different levels of understanding of technical test data, as well as different needs for such information. For different testing purposes, the physical means most appropriate to display test score information may vary widely, given audience considerations. In the context of large-scale school assessment, fact sheets, local report card prototypes, "frequently asked questions" flyers, manuals of technical definitions, tips for teachers on providing information to parents, video, television, radio, billboards, a telephone hotline, workshops, and Web sites all represent unique methods for presenting test score data. The key here is providing multiple modes of distribution to insure that all people who are interested in test results have access to the information they seek.

By and large, states are working to communicate school assessment results more effectively, and this effort is especially reflected in the development of materials supplementary to the formal score reports to explain what the scores mean. For example, the Connecticut State Board of Education provides examples and detailed descriptions of many of its official reporting documents online, including its *2001 Interpretive Guide* (Connecticut State Board of

Massachusetts Department of Education
MCAS TESTS OF SPRING 2001
Parent/Guardian Report for
Smith, Jane

SCHOOL: Elm Middle School

DISTRICT: Anytown, MA

GRADE: 8

DATE OF BIRTH: 4/23/1986

I. How did ___ do on these tests?

SUBJECT AREA	PERFORMANCE LEVEL	SCALED SCORE	DISPLAY OF SCORE AND PROBABLE RANGE OF SCORES			
			Warning	Needs Improvement	Proficient	Advanced
English Language Arts	Proficient	252			⊞	
Mathematics	Needs Improvement	224		⊞		
History and Social Science	Needs Improvement	220		⊞		

200   220   240   260   280

II. Score Ranges by Performance Level

PERFORMANCE LEVEL	SCORE RANGE
Advanced	260 – 280
Proficient	240 – 259
Needs Improvement	220 – 239
Warning	200 – 219

III. Comments about your child's writing performance

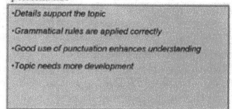

- Details support the topic
- Grammatical rules are applied correctly
- Good use of punctuation enhances understanding
- Topic needs more development

IV. How did your child's score compare to school, district, and state average scores?

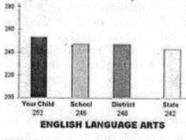

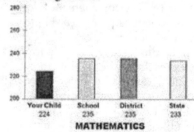

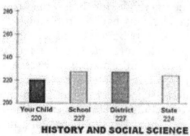

FIGURE 16.3. Sample individual report for state-level criterion-referenced assessments. From Massachusetts Department of Education (2001b).

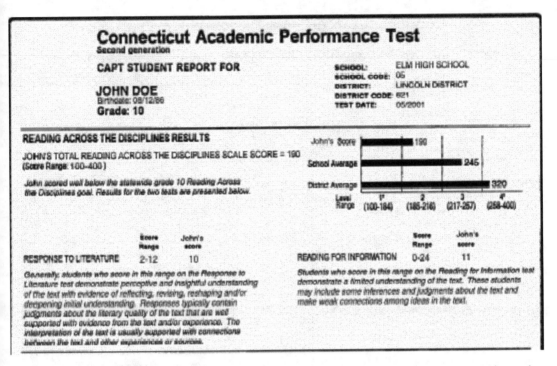

FIGURE 16.4. Sample of individual student report relating student performance to specific goals across disciplines. From Connecticut State Board of Education (2001).

Education, 2001). This document includes clearly written descriptions of not only the content of the tests, but also the scores that students receive and explicit details about a number of the official score reports produced by the department (at the individual level, as well as by school and district). Documents such as this are also being issued by other states, including Maryland (Maryland State Board of Education, 2001) and Massachusetts (Massachusetts Department of Education, 2001a). This sort of approach to reporting acknowledges both the complexity of test data in large-scale school assessments, and the importance of promoting understanding of test results.

Ultimately, reporting test scores is a complex process, and it too often occurs as an afterthought to other aspects of test development. However, it is critical that more testing agencies commit resources to promoting understanding of their CRTs.

CRT Score Reporting of NRT Score Results

Because CRTs are created to measure a designated domain of content (e.g., a curriculum in a subject area) and to assess student achievement in this domain of content, the reporting of results from CRTs is expressed at the level of such skills for individuals and often for groups. In contrast, since NRTs are designed with a different purpose in mind (i.e., to rank individuals with respect to the achievement of others, often with an emphasis on differentiating between high- and low-performing individuals), these test scores have traditionally been represented as percentiles, grade equivalents, or stanine scores, which are computed in reference to established norm groups (Bond, 1996; Popham, 1975).

However, as states and local districts look to find multiple uses of test information, and specifically to increase the diagnostic information from tests, more and more testing programs that create and administer large-scale NRTs for use in schools are developing methods to use such test results in terms of achievement in more specific skill areas (Hoover, 2002). The Metropolitan Achievement Test and the Stanford Achievement Test (both from Harcourt Educational Measurement), as well as the Iowa Tests of

Connecticut Academic Performance Test
Second generation

CMT/CAPT SKILLS CHECKLIST PROFILE FOR

JOHN DOE
Birthdate: 06/12/86

GRADE 10

SCHOOL: LINCOLN HIGH SCHOOL
SCHOOL CODE: 60
DISTRICT: LINCOLN DISTRICT
DISTRICT CODE: 201
TEST DATE: 06/2001

Quantitative Scale Results

The rating that John received for each quantitative scale indicator is reflected by a +
For more information about this profile, contact John's teacher.

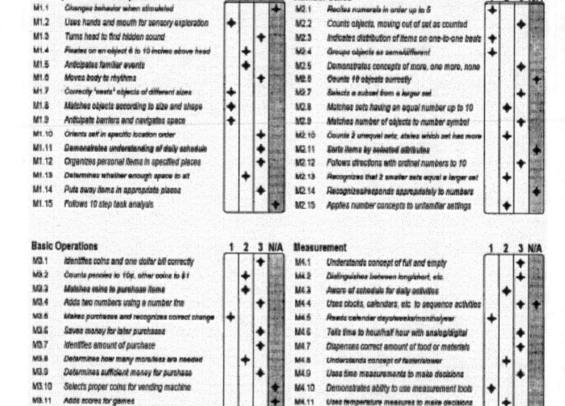

KEY: 1 = does not demonstrate skill
2 = demonstrates inconsistently or only with support
3 = demonstrates independently and consistently
N/A = skill may be inappropriate for student

B = Blank Response
M = Multiple Marks

Copy 01

Process No. 16650000-8999999-0000-05240-1

Copyright © 2001 by the Connecticut State Board of Education in the name of the Secretary of the State of Connecticut.

FIGURE 16.5. Sample skills checklist profile for an individual student. From Connecticut State Board of Education (2001).

Open Response Question 39

In 1775 and 1776, people living in the American colonies were arguing about whether or not the colonies should be independent from Great Britain.

    a. Describe TWO reasons why some colonists were in favor of independence.

    b. Describe TWO reasons why some colonists were against independence.

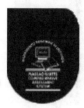

Massachusetts Comprehensive Assessment System

2001 MCAS Sample Student Work:

Grade 5 History and Social Science
Question 39; Score Point 4

    a. Two reason that some colonists wanted independence from England were that the king was taxing them and they couldn't vote on what the money was going to be used for. The second reason was because they thought that if they helped England fight in the Seven Years War they would be able to move past the Apalation Mountains. After the war the king said they couldn't move and it angered the colonists.

    b. Two reasons why some colonists were against independence from England because some colonists still liked England and had relatives in England. The other reason could be because they were afraid that if they helped gain independence and the British won they were afraid they would be killed.

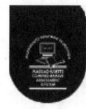

Massachusetts Comprehensive Assessment System

2001 MCAS Sample Student Work:

Grade 5 History and Social Science
Question 39; Score Point 1

    One reason people were in favor of independence was because they wanted to be free from Great Britan. Another reason is that their dream was to be free from Great Britan.

    One reason people were against independence was because they wanted to be with Great Britan, because some of them might have been British. Another reason is that if they stayed with Great Britan that they would be with family in Great Britan. That is what I think.

FIGURE 16.6. Sample of examinee work on an open-response question included in the 2001 Massachusetts Comprehensive Assessment System's Grade 5 History and Social Studies Test. In the top example, the student received a score of 4 (the highest possible score). The bottom example is a response that was rated as 1. The score scale for this item ranged from 0 to 4. From Massachusetts Department of Education (2001c).

Florida Department of Education
Charlie Crist, Commissioner
www.firn.edu/doe

GRADING FLORIDA PUBLIC SCHOOLS 2000-2001

A
- Meet Higher Performing Criteria in reading, writing and math for current year
- Test at least 95% of eligible students[1]
- Maintain or improve reading scores of lowest performing students[2]
- Demonstrate substantial improvement in reading and no substantial decline in math or writing[3]
- Meet criteria for "other" data[4]

B
- Meet Higher Performing Criteria in reading, writing and math for current year
- Test at least 90% of eligible students[1]
- Maintain or improve reading scores of lowest performing students[2]
- Meet criteria for "other" data[4]

C
- Meet Minimum Criteria in reading, writing and math for current year
- Test at least 90% of eligible students[1]
- Meet criteria for "other" data[4]

D
- Below Minimum Criteria in reading or writing or math for current year
- Test at least 90% of eligible students[1]

F
- Below Minimum Criteria in reading and writing and math for current year OR
- Meet "D" performance criteria, but test less than 90% of eligible students[1] without reasonable explanation

PROCESS: Schools are evaluated primarily on the basis of performance data. However, the initial grade may be reduced by one level if the percent of eligible students tested is below 90% after all extenuating circumstances have been considered.

Higher Performing Criteria for A and B

FCAT	Reading	Math	Writing
Elementary	50% score Level 3 & above	50% score Level 3 & above	67% score 3 & above
Middle	50% score Level 3 & above	50% score Level 3 & above	75% score 3 & above
High	50% score Level 3 & above	50% score Level 3 & above	80% score 3 & above

Minimum Criteria for C, D and F

FCAT	Reading	Math	Writing
Elementary	60% score Level 2 & above	60% score Level 2 & above	50% score 3 & above
Middle	60% score Level 2 & above	60% score Level 2 & above	67% score 3 & above
High	60% score Level 2 & above	60% score Level 2 & above	75% score 3 & above

[1]Eligible students also include speech impaired, gifted, hospital/homebound, and Limited English Proficient with more than two years in ESOL.

[2]The percent of students scoring in the lowest 25% in the state in reading (FCAT Level 1) must decrease or remain within two percentage points from the previous year. If a school has fewer than 30 students in Level 1, then the cumulative number of students scoring in Level 1 and Level 2 in reading must decrease or remain within two percentage points. If there are fewer than 30 students in Levels 1 and 2, this requirement will not apply.

[3]Substantial improvement in reading means more than two percentage points increase in students scoring FCAT Level 3 and above. If a school has 75% or more scoring Level 3 and above and not more than two percentage points decrease from the previous year, then substantial improvement is waived.

Substantial decline means five or more percentage points decrease in students scoring Level 3 and above in math or writing.

[4]"Other" data for 2000-2001 includes 1999-2000 high school dropout rate. High schools must have a dropout rate no higher than one standard deviation above the 1999-2000 state average or show improvement from the previous year.

NOTE: School participation rates and test results are based only on eligible students enrolled in both the October and February FTE surveys at the same school.

(05/04/01)

FIGURE 16.7. Sample of definition of performance expectations for schools. From Florida Department of Education (2001).

Basic Skills from Riverside Publishing and the TerraNova Test Battery from CTB/McGraw-Hill, are some examples of familiar NRTs that offer test users score reports allowing for criterion-referenced interpretations. As with CRTs, this is generally being done in two ways: first, at the level of performance standards for an entire content area; and second, in terms of performance on specific instructional objectives within the content area. For one example, see the display in Figure 16.8. Specific approaches to reporting NRTs in criterion-referenced ways include reports of individual profiles that describe results with respect to both objectives and norms (CTB/McGraw-Hill, 2001); the linking of reading achievement test scores to books that correspond to those reading levels (Harcourt Educational Measurement, 2001); and narrative reports profiling student performance (University of Iowa, 1999a).

With NRTs, the reporting of performance standards and specific skill results is possible; however, there are a number of challenges associated with reporting NRTs in this way, particularly with regard to subcontent areas and specific skills within a content domain. Test users must work to define the content area and to identify and set standards for criterion levels of performance to make such comparisons (University of Iowa, 1999b). Furthermore, NRTs are not aligned with any particular curriculum and cover a wide range of content or skills. This means that making high-quality criterion-referenced inferences from an NRT is difficult, because on each form of the test only a few items may assess each skill. Of course, this too can be a limitation of state proficiency tests.

FUTURE PERSPECTIVES AND CONCLUSIONS

CRTs have a central role in testing practices today—in the United States and around the world, and in literally every aspect of education (see Hambleton, 1994, for a summary of the impact of CRTs on assessment practices). These tests are being used in (1) the diagnosis of individual skills, (2) the evaluation of learning and achievement, (3) program evaluation, and (4) credentialing. At

the same time, CRTs look quite different today from their predecessors of even 20 years ago, and are likely to be different again in another 20 years. Today, more attention is being directed to the definition and clarification of constructs that need to be measured. If these constructs are to be taught and assessed, clarity and relevance are of the utmost importance. Domain/item specifications like the example in Figure 16.1 proved to be cumbersome to write, especially for the assessment of cognitively complex skills. New strategies for writing content standards are now in place (see Figure 16.2), and other strategies can be anticipated in the coming years. The targets of instruction and assessment must be clear for CRT methodology to be implemented successfully, and for CRTs to be a positive force in education.

Also, multiple-choice test items are not the only item types being used today in CRTs. New item types increase the likelihood of being able to assess higher-level cognitive skills and increase the fidelity of assessments. At the same time, questions remain about the validity of these new assessments. How should they be produced and scored to insure test score validity? What knowledge and skills are actually being measured? More item types can be anticipated in the future, especially as more CRTs are moved to computer administrations. At the same time, more efforts to validate these new forms of assessment will be necessary to insure that CRTs are not all face validity and "sizzle," with little substance and relevance. Item/task development and validation remain are two of the most important steps in the CRT development process.

Standard setting has been in the past, and can be expected to be in the future, one of the most troublesome aspects of CRT use. It is also another of the most important steps. Standard-setting methods have been developed for use with new item types. These new methods are responses to criticisms directed at some of the older approaches to standard setting, and responses to the recognized need for methods that can be applied successfully to new forms of testing such as performance assessments. At the same time, considerably more research will be needed to determine the most appropriate ways to apply these new methods and validate the

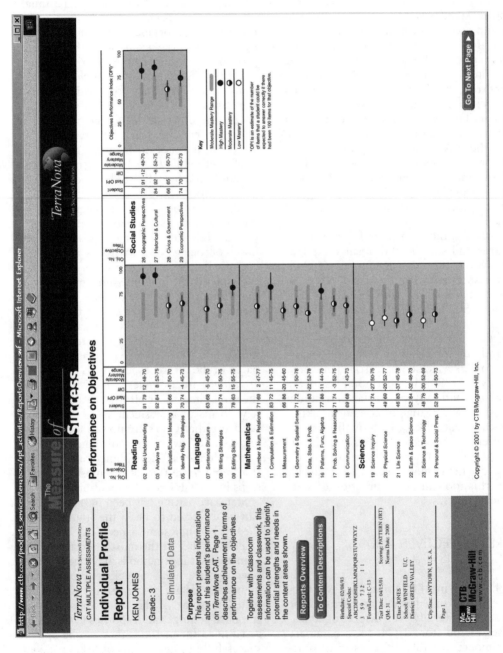

FIGURE 16.8. Example of criterion-referenced reporting with an NRT. From CTB/McGraw-Hill (2001). Copyright 2001 by CTB/McGraw-Hill, Inc.

results. More new methods in the coming years can be expected as researchers search for more defensible ways to set performance standards.

Finally, probably the biggest change to CRTs in the future is expected to be in the area of CRT score reporting. To date, only limited research on the topic exists. There are few findings to guide the practice of score reporting. More attention to the intended audiences for the test results and their informational needs should result in more user-friendly and informative test score reports. This problem must be resolved if CRTs are to achieve their full potential.

REFERENCES

American Educational Research Association (AERA), American Psychological Association (APA), and National Council on Measurement in Education (NCME). (1999). *Standards for educational and psychological testing.* Washington, DC: Authors.

Bennett, R. E., Rock, D. A., Braun, H. I., Frye, D., Spohrer, J. C., & Soloway, E. (1990). The relationship of constrained free-response to multiple-choice and open-ended items. *Applied Psychological Measurement, 14*(2), 151–162.

Bennett, R. E., Rock, D.A., & Wang, M. (1991). Equivalence of free-response and multiple-choice items. *Journal of Educational Measurement, 28*(1), 77–92.

Bond, L. A. (1996). Norm- and criterion-referenced testing. *Practical Assessment, Research and Evaluation, 5*(2) [Online]. Available: http://www.ericae.net/pare/getvn.asp?v=5&n=2

Boodoo, G. M. (1993). Performance assessment or multiple choice? *Educational Horizons, 72,* 50–56.

Burstein, J., Kukich, K., Wolff, S., Lu, C., & Chodorow, M. (1998, April). *Computer analysis of essays.* Paper presented at the annual meeting of the National Council on Measurement in Education, San Diego, CA.

Cizek, G. (Ed.). (2001). *Setting performance standards: Concepts, methods, and perspectives.* Mahwah, NJ: Erlbaum.

Clauser, B. E. (2000). Recurrent issues and recent advances in scoring performance assessments. *Applied Psychological Measurement, 24*(4), 310–324.

Connecticut State Board of Education. (2001). *CAPT: Connecticut Academic Performance Test Second Generation 2001 interpretive guide* [Online]. Available: http://www.csde.state.ct.us/public/der/s-t/testing/capt/interpretive_guide_2001_reports.pdf [2002, April 5].

CTB/McGraw-Hill. (2001). *TerraNova: The second edition reports* [Online]. Available: http://www.ctb.com/products_services/terranova/rpt_activities/flash_reports.shtml [2002, February 19].

Drasgow, F., & Olson-Buchanan, J. B. (1999). *Innovations in computerized assessment.* Mahwah, NJ: Erlbaum.

Ebel, R. L. (1978). The case for norm-referenced measurements. *Educational Researcher, 7,* 3–5.

Florida Department of Education. (2001). *FCAT briefing book* [Online]. Available: http://www.firn.edu/doe/sas/fcat/pdf/fcat_brief.pdf [2002, April 5].

Glaser, R. (1963). Instructional technology and the measurement of learning outcomes. *American Psychologist, 18,* 519–521.

Hambleton, R. K. (1994). The rise and fall of criterion-referenced measurement? *Educational Measurement: Issues and Practice, 13,* 21–26.

Hambleton, R. K. (1996). Advances in assessment models, methods, and practices. In D. C. Berliner & R. C. Calfee (Eds.), *Handbook of educational psychology* (pp. 899–925). New York: Simon & Schuster Macmillan.

Hambleton, R. K. (1998). Criterion-referenced testing principles, technical advances, and evaluation guidelines. In C. Reynolds & T. Gutkin (Eds.), *Handbook of school psychology* (3rd ed., pp. 409–434). New York: Wiley.

Hambleton, R. K. (2001). Setting performance standards on educational assessments and criteria for evaluating the process. In G. Cizek (Ed.), *Setting performance standards: Concepts, methods, and perspectives* (pp. 89–116). Mahwah, NJ: Erlbaum.

Hambleton, R. K., Jaeger, R. M., Plake, B. S., & Mills, C. N. (2000). Setting performance standards on complex educational assessments. *Applied Psychological Measurement, 24*(4), 355–366.

Hambleton, R. K., & Murphy E. (1992). A psychometric perspective on authentic measurement. *Applied Measurement in Education, 5*(1), 1–16.

Hambleton, R. K., Swaminathan, H., & Rogers, H. J. (1991). *Fundamentals of item response theory.* Newbury Park, CA: Sage.

Harcourt Educational Measurement. (2001). *Metropolitan Achievement Tests—Eighth Edition: Score reports and technical information* [Online]. Available: http://www.hemweb.com/trophy/achvtest/mat8srti.htm [2002, February 19].

Hoover, H. D. (2002, April). *Some common misperceptions about tests and testing.* Presidential address at the annual meeting of the National Council on Measurement in Education, New Orleans, LA.

Kane, M. (1992). An argument-based approach to validation. *Psychological Bulletin, 112,* 527–535.

Landauer, T. K., Foltz, P. W., & Laham, D. (1998). An introduction to latent semantic analysis. *Discourse Processes, 25*(2–3), 259–284.

Linn, R. L. (Ed.). (1989). *Educational measurement* (3rd ed.). New York: Macmillan.

Linn, R. L. (2000). Assessments and accountability. *Educational Reseacher, 29*(2), 4–16.

Livingston, S., & Lewis, C. (1995). Estimating the consistency and accuracy of classifications based on test scores. *Journal of Educational Measurement, 32,* 179–197.

Lyman, H. B. (1998). *Test scores and what they mean.* Boston: Allyn & Bacon.

Martinez, M. E. (1999). Cognition and the question of test item format. *Educational Psychologist, 34*(4), 207–218.

Maryland State Board of Education. (2001). *Introduction to 2001 hard copy report card* [Online]. Available: http://msp.msde.state.md.us/pdfdownloads/42834_StofMD.pdf [2002, February 20].

Massachusetts Department of Education. (2001a). *Guide to interpreting the spring 2001 reports for schools and districts* [Online]. Available: http://www.doe.mass.edu/mcas/2001/interpretive_guides/full.pdf [2002, February 20].

Massachusetts Department of Education. (2001b). *MCAS sample parent/guardian report* [Online]. Available: http://www.doe.mass.edu/mcas/2001/pgreport/g8elamhss.jpg [2002, April 5].

Massachusetts Department of Education. (2001c). *MCAS student work: Grade 5 history and social science* [Online]. Available: http://www.doe.mass.edu/mcas/student/2001/g5hist.html [2002, April 5].

Massachusetts Department of Education. (2001d). *2001 Massachusetts MCAS technical manual.* Malden, MA: Author.

Mills, C. N., Potenza, M. T., Fremer, J. J., & Ward, W. C. (Eds.). (2002). *Computer-based testing: Building the foundation for future assessments.* Mahwah, NJ: Erlbaum.

National Center for Education Statistics. (2002). *Technology-based assessment project* [Online]. Available: http://nces.ed.gov/nationsreportcard/studies/tbaproject.asp [2002, April 11].

National Education Goals Panel. (1998). *Talking about tests: An idea book for state leaders.* Washington, DC: U.S. Government Printing Office.

Nitko, A. J. (1980). Distinguishing the many varieties of criterion-referenced tests. *Review of Educational Research, 50,* 461–485.

Osterlind, S. J. (1989). *Constructing test items.* Boston: Kluwer Academic.

Osterlind, S. J. (1998). *Constructing test items: Multiple-choice, constructed-response, performance, and other formats* (2nd ed.). Boston: Kluwer Academic.

Page, E. B. (1994). Computer grading of student prose, using modern concepts and software. *Journal of Experimental Education, 62*(2), 27–142.

Page, B. P., & Peterson, N. S. (1995). The computer moves into essay grading: Updating the ancient test. *Phi Delta Kappan, 76*(7), 561–565.

Pitoniak, M. J. (2002). *Automatic item generation methodology in theory and practice* (Center for Educational Assessment Research Report No. 444).

Amherst: University of Massachusetts, School of Education.

Popham, J. W. (1975). *Educational evaluation.* Englewood Cliffs, NJ: Prentice-Hall.

Popham, W. J. (1978a). The case for criterion-referenced measurement. *Educational Researcher, 7,* 6–10.

Popham, W. J. (1978b). *Criterion-referenced measurement.* Englewood Cliffs, NJ: Prentice-Hall.

Popham, W. J. (1984). Specifying the domain of content or behaviors. In R. A. Berk (Ed.), *A guide to criterion-referenced test construction* (pp. 29–48). Baltimore: Johns Hopkins University Press.

Popham, W. J. (2000, June). *Assessments that illuminate instructional decisions.* Paper presented at the 30th Annual Conference on Large-Scale Assessment, Council of Chief State School Officers, Snowbird, UT.

Popham, W. J., & Husek, T. R. (1969). Implications of criterion-referenced measurement. *Journal of Educational Measurement, 6,* 1–9.

Rudner, L. M., & Boston, C. (1994). Performance assessment. *ERIC Review, 3*(1), 2–12.

Subkoviak, M. (1976). Estimating reliability from a single administration of a criterion-referenced test. *Journal of Educational Measurement, 13,* 265–275.

Traub, R. E. (1993). On the equivalence of the traits assessed by multiple-choice and constructed-response tests. In R. E. Bennett & W. C. Ward (Eds.), *Construction versus choice in cognitive measurement: Issues in constructed response, performance testing, and portfolio assessment* (pp. 29–44). Mahwah, NJ: Erlbaum.

University of Iowa. (1999a). *Iowa Testing Programs—Basic Skills: Interpreting the tests. Description of ITBS scoring services* [Online]. Available: http://www.uiowa.edu/~itp/bs-interpret-scr.htm [2002, February 19].

University of Iowa. (1999b). *Iowa Testing Programs—Basic Skills: Interpreting the tests. Interpreting test scores* [Online]. Available: http://www.uiowa.edu/~itp/bs-interpret-rept.htm [2002, February 19].

Yen, W. M., & Ferrara, S. (1997). The Maryland School Performance Assessment Program: Performance assessment with psychometric quality suitable for high stakes usage. *Educational and Psychological Measurement, 57*(1), 60–84.

Zenisky, A. L., & Sireci, S. G. (2002). Technological innovations in large-scale assessment. *Applied Measurement in Education, 15*(4), 337–362.

17

Diagnostic Achievement Testing in Reading

JEANNE S. CHALL
MARY E. CURTIS

Our purpose in this chapter is twofold: to describe the process of diagnostic testing in reading, and to illustrate how it is used to design instructional programs. We begin by discussing some general characteristics of this kind of testing and the procedures involved. We then describe the particular approach to diagnosis that we have used (both in the Harvard Reading Laboratory and at the Boys Town Reading Center), focusing on the theory underlying the approach and the ways in which the theory is translated into practice. Finally, we present examples of how results from diagnostic testing can be used to guide the design of instructional programs.

AN OVERVIEW OF DIAGNOSTIC TESTING IN READING

Diagnostic achievement testing involves identifying the relationships among an individual's strengths and needs in reading, so that steps toward improvement can be taken. As such, it differs from the survey achievement testing of a more general nature done in schools, as well as from the di-

agnostic testing done in hospital settings (Chall & Curtis, 1992).

Survey achievement tests are used to establish how well students read, and are often given to satisfy educational accountability requirements imposed by school districts, state departments of education, or state legislatures (Popham, 1999). Diagnostic achievement testing, on the other hand, is used to discover areas of strengths and needs in students who have already been identified as not reading as well as they should. Because of this, diagnostic achievement testing tends to be more extensive than survey testing, consisting of several different tasks at different levels of difficulty.

Diagnostic testing in a hospital setting is designed to clarify the relationship between a reading difficulty and specific medical/neurological and psychological (behavioral) variables (e.g., see Bernstein, Kammerer, Prather, & Rey-Casserly, 1998). Diagnostic achievement testing is focused more on establishing instructional solutions than on describing underlying causes. In both kinds of diagnostic testing, however, special training and expertise are required.

Components Assessed in Diagnostic Achievement Testing

To identify the relationships among a student's strengths and needs in reading, the reading specialist must assess the student's knowledge and skill in different areas, or components, of reading. In this section we describe some of the components that the specialist will assess, focusing on published tests and assessment tools. Later we discuss how a more informal approach to evaluating a student's abilities plays an essential role as well.

Phonemic Awareness, Word Analysis, and Word Recognition

For more than 75 years, it has been recognized that one of the most reliable indicators of a reading problem is difficulty in dealing with words (Orton, 1925). More recently, however, syntheses of the research have renewed appreciation for the significance of the role that word-level processing plays in reading development (Lyon, 1995; National Reading Panel, 2000; Snow, Burns, & Griffin, 1998). Tests of reading vary in the extent to which they make apparent students' knowledge and skills in the following areas: mapping sounds onto letters (phonemic awareness), using letter–sound relationships to decode words (word analysis), and identifying words by sight (word recognition).

Some group-administered norm-referenced tests assess students' ability to recognize words by asking them to match words with pictures (e.g., the Gates–MacGinitie Reading Tests; MacGinitie, MacGinitie, Maria, & Dreyer, 2000). On tests like these, performance can always be affected by other factors, such as knowledge of word meanings. Other group-administered tests attempt to assess students' facility at the word level more directly. For example, on the Stanford Diagnostic Reading Test (Karlsen & Gardner, 1995), students are asked to match up the sound made by the letters in one word (e.g., the " ie" in " tie") with a word that contains the same sound ("fly").

The most direct measure of students' word-level knowledge and skills, however, is provided by tests in which students are asked to read aloud items of increasing difficulty. Often the specialist will begin by assessing students' performance on isolated words and word parts. Students may be asked to read aloud lists composed of high-frequency words that need to be recognized as wholes, as well as words that can be identified through word analysis. Testing continues until a student reaches a point in the list where the words are too difficult for him or her to continue (e.g., the Ekwall/Shanker Reading Inventory; Ekwall & Shanker, 1993). Or a student may be asked to pronounce the individual sounds in words (e.g., the Yopp–Singer Test of Phoneme Segmentation; Yopp, 1995) or to delete sounds from words and blend sounds together to make words (e.g., the Phonological Awareness Test; Robertson & Salter, 1997).

Usually the specialist will choose tests that allow him or her to assess phonemic awareness, word analysis, and word recognition skills separately. A few tests, like the Roswell–Chall Diagnostic Reading Test of Word Analysis Skills (Roswell & Chall, 1978), are designed to provide information about all three areas. Knowledge of the sounds of single consonants, consonant blends, short- and long-vowel sounds, the rule of "silent e," and so on is assessed, in addition to a student's ability to read a graded list of sight words.

Although many tests use actual words to assess word analysis, nonsense words are sometimes used as well. The Woodcock Reading Mastery Tests—Revised (Woodcock, 1987) battery is an example of an instrument that does this. Nonsense words can help to identify students who rely on whole-word recognition strategies or use of context because of a gap in their knowledge about symbol–sound correspondences (Johnson, 1973; Share & Stanovich, 1995). Nonsense words can also assist in distinguishing difficulties in word recognition that stem from decoding problems from those that stem from limitation in vocabulary knowledge. However, nonsense words can also confuse students who expect that a string of letters will correspond to a meaningful unit. For instance, a child may say "brake" in response to "brate" simply because the former is a word while the latter is not. Moreover, with use of nonsense words, great care must be taken to insure that the test is a test of letter patterns that occur frequently in the language. Otherwise, students' performances will have little or no generalizability to their skill in dealing with real words.

Spelling tests are another way in which reading specialists examine students' knowledge and skills at the level of isolated words; examples include the Test of Written Spelling—3 (Larsen & Hammill, 1994) and the Spelling subtest of the Wide Range Achievement Test—3 (Wilkinson, 1993). Correct and incorrect spellings reveal much about a student's facility with particular letter–sound relationships (Ganske, 2000), as well as his or her overall approach for dealing with print (i.e., visual vs. phonetic).

Since reading requires identification of words in context, the diagnostic assessment of reading achievement will always involve asking students to read text aloud. On such tests as the Diagnostic Assessments of Reading (Roswell & Chall, 1992) or the Gray Oral Reading Tests (Wiederholt & Bryant, 2001), students are asked to read a series of passages increasing in level of difficulty. The examiner records the kinds of words read correctly and those missed, as well as the level at which reading aloud becomes too difficult for a student. A comparison will then be made between the student's performance on word identification in context and his or her performance on words in isolation. Often it will be the case that when a student's word identification in context is better than in isolation, the student is relying on context as a way to compensate for poor word analysis and/or word recognition skills (Perfetti, 1985; Spear-Swerling & Sternberg, 1996; Stanovich, 1986).

Fluency in Word Identification

Beginning with the work of Huey (1908), psychologists have understood that a significant aspect of developing students' skills in reading involves lessening their dependence on the need to sound out every word. When readers must devote attention to the process of decoding words, less attention is available for understanding what they read.

In a diagnostic assessment of a student's reading ability, the specialist usually estimates the degree of fluency in two ways. The first way involves measuring the rate at which a student is able to complete tasks accurately (Good & Kaminski, 2002). For example, using an oral reading test like one of those mentioned above, the examiner records the amount of time it takes the student to read each passage aloud. Reading time is then combined with the information about oral reading accuracy to establish students' independent and instructional fluency levels. Rate in reading words in isolation is also usually assessed. For instance, the examiner might use a tool like the Test of Word Reading Efficiency (Torgesen, Wagner, & Rashotte, 1999), counting the number of real printed words that the student reads accurately within 45 seconds, along with the number of pronounceable printed nonsense words that can be decoded within the same time period.

Fluency is also assessed by listening to students while they read aloud. Failure to pause at phrases or sentence boundaries, or difficulty in identifying "signal words" such as "when," "then," "through," and "although," indicates that students are expending more effort than they should be on processing at the word level—effort that could be better directed toward understanding the meaning of what is being read. Errors that are based more on the context of what is being read than on the actual words on the page also suggests to the specialist that a student has a fluency problem (i.e., guessing at the words is easier than trying to read them). The running record, one of the tasks in An Observation Survey of Early Literacy Achievement (Clay, 1993), is a popular procedure for recording and analyzing a student's behaviors as he or she is reading aloud.

Increasingly, in addition to assessing the nature and rate of students' reading behaviors, the specialist will also include one or more naming-speed tasks in the diagnostic session (e.g., the Comprehensive Test of Phonological Processing; Wagner, Torgesen, & Rashotte, 1999). A large body of evidence now shows that children with dyslexia are significantly slower than their nondisabled peers in naming the most basic and familiar visual symbols, such as digits, letters, and colors (Denckla & Rudel, 1976; Wolf, 1991).

Knowledge of Word Meanings and Background Information

Because reading is a major avenue for acquiring knowledge, students who are not reading as well as they should will usually have needs related to vocabulary knowledge. Reading specialists have a variety of tests available for obtaining information about these needs.

Most reading inventories tend not to test vocabulary separately, adhering instead to a philosophy that literacy assessment should be "authentic"—that is, arranged so that students are applying their knowledge and skills to actual reading tasks (Paris et al., 1992). On tests like the Classroom Reading Inventory (Silvaroli, 1997), students read a passage aloud and then are asked some comprehension questions, one of which assesses their knowledge of the meaning of a word from the passage. On the Analytic Reading Inventory (Woods & Moe, 1999), before students are asked to read each passage, they are asked about their knowledge of the topic and their predictions about the passage content.

Although we agree that authentic assessment has its advantages, when a student does not perform well on these kinds of items, the examiner ends up having more questions than answers, and additional testing needs to be done.

Another way in which to gain information about vocabulary knowledge is through tests that require recognition of word meanings (e.g., the Stanford Diagnostic Reading Test). By assessing students' ability to recognize synonyms, reading specialists can make inferences about the breadth or extent of students' vocabulary knowledge (Curtis, 1987). Because such tests usually require reading, however, they measure skill in word identification as well as knowledge of word meanings. When word identification skills are weak, misreading of a test item or answer alternative (rather than lack of vocabulary knowledge) can cause an incorrect response.

For a truer measure of students' vocabulary knowledge, tests that require no reading are preferable. The Diagnostic Assessments of Reading test battery is an example. On its Word Meaning subtest, students are asked to define the meanings of increasingly difficult words that are read aloud to them. Similar to the Vocabulary subtests on the Stanford–Binet Intelligence Scale: Fourth Edition (Thorndike, Hagen, & Sattler, 1986) and the Wechsler Intelligence Scales

for Children—Third Edition (WISC-III; Wechsler, 1991), the Diagnostic Assessments of Reading can be used as an approximation of a student's verbal ability.

Analogies, classification tasks, cloze procedures, and sentence-writing tasks are still other ways in which vocabulary knowledge is assessed by standardized tests and informal measures. Instruments with such tasks include the Test of Reading Comprehension (Brown, Hammill, & Wiederholt, 1995) and the Test of Written Language (Hammill & Larsen, 1996). In general, students who know the meanings of many words usually have deep knowledge about the words they know and are able to use context to derive meanings for words they do not know. Therefore, performances on various vocabulary item types are highly interrelated (see Curtis, 1987; Davis, 1972). However, for purposes of making instructional decisions for students who do not know many word meanings, use of different kinds of vocabulary formats can provide valuable information.

Constructing Meaning from Print

In assessing a student's strengths and needs in comprehension, a reading specialist may use either a process measure, a product measure, or both (Chang, 1983; Harris & Sipay, 1990). Process measures are intended to provide information about comprehension as it takes place; product measures are intended to provide information about what the student is able to comprehend from reading.

Most norm-referenced standardized tests rely on product measures—multiple-choice items, true–false items, and open-ended response questions. At the lowest grade levels, students may be asked to select from a set of pictures the one that is best described by a sentence. At higher grade levels, students may be asked to determine the main idea of a passage, to identify an author's purpose in writing a selection, to recognize particular kinds of text (e.g., a fable or a legend), and so on. As grade level increases, reading passages become more difficult (both conceptually and structurally), and the responses required from the reader become more varied and complex.

Informal reading inventories usually rely on both process and product measurement.

Miscue analysis—an analysis of the frequency and kinds of reading errors a student makes—is the process measure most often used. Passage retelling and use of questions/answers are the most common product measures.

Because they provide both process and product measures, informal reading inventories are preferred by many specialists over norm-referenced tests. However, for some students, the constraint of reading words aloud (a prerequisite for miscue analysis) makes comprehension more difficult for them than it would have been if they had been allowed to read silently. For other students, the knowledge that they will be required to retell a story or answer questions about it after reading aloud can make their oral reading less accurate than it would have been if the product measure had not been used. In either case, testing comprehension after oral reading can result in less information than would have been gained from a product measure alone.

In assessing a student's ability to construct meaning from text, a reading specialist will often compare the student's reading performance with what he or she is able to understand from a listening task. From research on the relationship between reading and listening (e.g., see Sticht & James, 1984), we know that listening comprehension is generally better than reading comprehension throughout the elementary grades. During high school, reading and listening comprehension are about equal. By comparing comprehension performances on reading and listening tasks, therefore, a reading specialist is better able to distinguish between comprehension problems that stem from more general language-based needs and those that stem from reading difficulties. The Analytic Reading Inventory is one instrument that is designed to compare listening and reading comprehension levels.

Summary

Up to this point, we have discussed diagnostic achievement testing in terms of different components of reading, emphasizing the options available to reading specialists for assessing each. Decisions about which tests to use and which components are the most essential to assess depend on the characteristics of the students being tested (particularly their level of reading development), along with a specialist's theoretical orientation. The model of reading to which an examiner subscribes (e.g., the extent to which skills, content knowledge or strategies are emphasized), as well as the way in which the model gets translated into practice, determine the diagnostic assessment process he or she uses.

Independent of decisions about which components to assess and which tests and measures to use, however, are some general issues related to diagnosis. We discuss these in the next section.

Issues in Diagnostic Assessment

General issues in diagnostic achievement testing are related to test administration; conversion of test scores; establishing patterns of strengths and needs; and awareness of linguistic and cultural differences.

Test Administration

Choosing the correct level of difficulty of a test is of vital importance in achieving a valid measure of a student's strengths and needs. In the case of more general, survey-type achievement testing, the appropriate level of difficulty is determined by the student's grade level in school. However, for students known to be experiencing difficulty, such a practice can often yield very little information; students miss the majority of items, making inferences about their strengths and needs impossible. Because of this, in diagnostic achievement testing a reading specialist tries to choose the level of test difficulty that reflects a student's reading ability, rather than his or her grade placement in school. This practice has been referred to as "out-of-level testing" (see Harris & Sipay, 1990). When the student is known to the examiner, the current reading level is used as a guide. When the student's current functioning level is not known, the specialist will use a score from a word recognition or oral reading assessment to select the correct levels for additional tests.

During testing, the specialist notes evidence of interest, strain, "carelessness," the ways in which problems are attacked, the student's reactions when items become too difficult (e.g., erasing, talking), and so on. Spontaneous verbalizations can often give interesting insights. In addition, between tests the reading specialist will engage the student in an informal discussion of his or her interests in and out of school, school subjects that are liked best and least, subjects that are easy and difficult, books that have been read recently, and so on. The student is also asked about his or her perceived strengths and needs in reading. Specifically, what is hard? Where does the student think the difficulty lies? Why? What kind of assistance has the student had with this difficulty? Although published instruments are available for gathering this kind of information (e.g., the Motivation to Read Profile; Gambrell, Palmer, Codling, & Mazzoni, 1996), we have found that using a more casual approach, interspersed with the more formal testing, produces excellent results.

For some students, the standard time limits are not sufficient for them to complete the test. When a student is still getting most of the items correct at the point when time is up, an examiner will often make a note of where the student is and suggest that he or she continue working until the items become too difficult. At the end of the test, the specialist notes the additional time that was taken and calculates a score based on the untimed performance, as well as one based on the last item completed within the standard time limit. Conversely, when students reach a point of difficulty where it is obvious that answers are being marked randomly, the examiner will generally stop the test, even if the full time allowed in the test manual has not been reached.

Conversion of Test Scores

Following the selection and administration of tests, a student's scores on the various tests must be converted into comparable units, so that the scores can be interpreted. Information from criterion-referenced tests varies as a function of the way that each test calibrates its findings into age, grade level, or mastery of the specific knowledge or skills tested. Most norm-referenced tests offer three types of conversions: grade equivalents, percentile ranks, and scale scores (Popham, 1999).

The grade equivalent score is a conversion of the raw score into the school grade (year and month) typical of students who achieve it. For instance, when a seventh grader gets a score of 4.5 on a vocabulary test, our estimate is that his or her knowledge about the word meanings sampled on the test is roughly the same as that of an average fourth grader at midyear. Percentiles indicate the relative rank of students on a test. A 25th-percentile ranking, for example, means that a student did better on the test than 25% of the students in the group with whom the student is being compared. Scale scores result from a conversion of a raw score to a new score based on a new scale.

All three types of scores have advantages and disadvantages. Grade equivalents and percentiles are more useful for understanding the relative performance of students than are scale scores. Scale scores and grade equivalents are better for tracking progress than are percentiles. Of the three, the grade equivalent score has been the source of the most controversy, due to the fact that it is the easiest one to misunderstand. As noted by the International Reading Association (1982), the use of grade equivalents can lead to the mistaken assumption that "a grade equivalent of 5.0 on a reading test means that the test taker will be able to read fifth grade material" (p. 464).

In spite of such criticism, however, reading specialists often find the grade equivalent measure to be the most useful for diagnostic purposes. Even in cases where differences exist between students' grade equivalents and the actual difficulty levels of the material from which they are able to learn, the very robust correlations that exist between grade equivalents and instructional levels (from .80 to .90) make these equivalents the most useful scores. And, since most reading materials tested by readability formulas also use grade equivalent scores, converting test scores to grade equivalents facilitates the process of selecting appropriate materials for instruction.

Patterns of Strengths and Needs

Once a student's scores have been converted into comparable units, the specialist then examines them in order to identify a "pattern"—one that helps to explain the nature of the causes and consequences of the student's reading ability. Patterns emerge from the different ways in which the components tested seem to be affecting one another.

To illustrate, consider the profiles in Table 17.1 for two 13-year-olds, both of whom scored about one grade level below their grade placement in school on a survey-type reading achievement test. Student A appears to be experiencing difficulty in many aspects of reading, although comprehension is a clear strength. Student B, on the other hand, seems to be experiencing difficulty only in the area of comprehension. Word identification, oral reading, and word meaning are all strengths.

Analyses of profiles are guided by the specialist's knowledge of what reading involves and how it develops. Based on these analyses, the specialist is able to make recommendations for remediating students' reading difficulties. Consider again student A. From the test scores, we know that this student has needs in terms of accuracy and fluency in identifying words, both in context and in isolation, along with significant gaps in knowledge of word meanings. From our knowledge of reading theory (Chall, 1983), though, we also know that inaccuracy in word identification is the primary cause of the reading problem, while the other areas are consequences. Hence, as specialists, we would recommend a program that uses direct instruction to remediate the cause of the problem.

Because of the importance of profile analysis and its dependence on the view of reading and reading development to which a specialist adheres, we provide a more complete description of the approach we have found to be successful. Before turning to that, however, we need to raise one final general issue related to diagnostic assessment.

Linguistic and Cultural Differences

The diversity of the population in the United States is ever-increasing. Estimates are that in 50 years, almost half of the U.S. population will be of Hispanic, African American, Native American, or Asian/Pacific descent (Council of Economic Advisors, 1998). Many educators believe that prob-

TABLE 17.1. Reading Profiles for Two 13-Year-Olds

Component	Student A	Student B
Chronological age	13	13
School grade placement	7	8
Total reading score	6.2	7.0
Word identification score	3.0	7.8
Oral reading score	4.8	8.4
Word meaning score	4.6	9.8
Comprehension score	7.1	4.9

Note. Test scores have been converted to grade equivalents.

lems exist now in recognition, understanding, and valuing of different cultural, social, and/or linguistic characteristics of students (Kea & Utley, 1998). And disproportionate representation of culturally and linguistically diverse students in special education has become a major concern for the U.S. Office of Special Education Programs and for the U.S. Office for Civil Rights (Burnette, 1998).

Distinguishing language difference from language delay and disorder can be difficult (Menyuk, 1999). Test scores from norm-referenced tests for students who have not had the opportunity to achieve proficiency in English for at least 5–7 years can be misleading (Cummins, 1981). Nor is it appropriate to use the norms when these tests are administered in a language other than English. At present, the best solution is to gather data about students' reading from more informal situations, recognizing the many ways in which students can differ in how they use language.

PROCEDURES FOR TESTING IN READING

The particular approach to diagnostic testing that we describe in this section is one that was developed at the Harvard Reading Laboratory and adapted for use at the Boys Town Reading Center.

The Harvard Reading Laboratory was established in 1966 by Jeanne Chall as an integral part of the graduate programs in reading, language, and learning disabilities. Under her direction until 1991, graduate students enrolled in courses worked with children and adults referred to the laboratory for reading problems. The work consisted of testing and identifying a student's reading problem; developing a plan for remediation based on the diagnosis; teaching twice weekly for 1-hour sessions; assessing the student's progress at the end of each semester; and preparing reports for the laboratory, the student's school, and the student's parents (in the case of a child). The laboratory served about 30 teacher–student pairs each semester, and all of the work was closely supervised by the laboratory directors and teaching assistants.

The Boys Town Reading Center was founded in 1990 by Mary E. Curtis to help adolescents to improve their reading skills and to disseminate instructional programs found effective in Boys Town schools to schools around the country. Girls and Boys Town (as it is now known) is a residential and educational facility providing care and treatment for older adolescents who are emotionally and socially at risk because of such factors as school failure, broken homes, chronic neglect or abuse, and illegal/antisocial behaviors. Annually, about 850 youths are in residence, with 300 or so new youths arriving each year.

Two assumptions formed the basis for assessment that was conducted at both the Harvard Reading Laboratory and the Boys Town Reading Center. The first is that reading is best conceived as a set of interrelated components, consisting of processes, content, knowledge, and strategies (Perfetti & Curtis, 1987); the second is that the relationship among these components changes as reading ability develops (Chall, 1983). Thus, as we illustrate next, the age, grade placement, and reading level of the student all suggest the most critical aspects of reading to assess.

Lower Reading Levels (First through Third Grades)

Reading at the lower grade levels consists of two different stages: first, learning to associate combinations of letters with their spoken equivalents; and second, learning to use knowledge about letter–sound redundancies to gain accuracy and fluency in reading (Chall, 1983). As a consequence, the most useful information at lower reading levels will usually be obtained from assessments of the skills and knowledge related to word identification and oral reading of connected text.

For word identification, in addition to obtaining grade-level information, we look closely at a student's correct and incorrect responses. How proficient is the student on the most common high-frequency words? When he or she makes errors, are the errors real words? Which letter–sound correspondences has the student mastered? Which ones is he or she still having difficulty with? Making a comparison between a student's reading and spelling grade levels, as well as reading and spelling errors, provides us with important supplementary information about how well the student is able to deal with the way words look and sound.

Oral reading of connected text provides all sorts of useful information, such as the level of difficulty a student can read accurately, the kinds of errors he or she makes, the extent to which the student is able to use context, and the level of text he or she is able to read fluently. When we are assessing oral reading, if students make gross errors in reading (e.g., saying "duck" for "dog"), we tell them the correct word after noting the error. We have found that when this is not done, students will often misread other words in a text in order to make sense out of the original error. We also compute an additional score based on oral reading performance—a "criterion grade-level score," developed by Chall, which is useful for selecting materials at the appropriate difficulty level for instruction. The criterion grade-level score is based on the number of "real errors" (errors that will interfere with comprehension) made on passages at varying levels of readability. Real errors include such things as nonrecognitions, mispronunciations, insertions of other words, and so on. Not included as real errors are those that seem to be temporary or careless and not detrimental to students' understanding. The criterion grade-level score is estimated by the readability level of the most difficult passage on which a student makes 3%–5% real errors.

At lower reading grade levels, tests of reading vocabulary and comprehension are often not as critical for diagnostic purposes as they are at higher grade levels. This is because at lower levels, the content of what students are being asked to read is often familiar to them and contains words that they already use in their speech. However, results from vocabulary and comprehension assessments can help in designing instruction for students who may lack experience with frequently occurring concepts and linguistic structures (e.g., students who speak a language other than English at home). Thus, when time and circumstances permit, we administer vocabulary and comprehension tests for those reading at the lower levels.

We always undertake a "trial teaching session" to obtain information on the methods and materials that are suitable and acceptable to each student. Trial lessons also serve a further function: They confirm for the student that he or she *can* learn.

For those students encountering difficulties with sight word recognition, we use the trial lessons suggested by Chall and Roswell (1998). Three major approaches to word identification are tried—visual, phonic, and visual–motor—and if none of these is effective, a kinesthetic approach may be used. The method indicated is always viewed as an initial approach that will change as the student progresses and as other approaches are needed to further his or her reading development.

The visual approach involves learning words by picture clues. An unknown word is paired with a picture depicting it. The teacher points to the picture and word while pronouncing it, and then asks the student to say the word. After this procedure is repeated several times, the student is then tested on the word without the picture.

For a phonic approach, we first see whether the student is able to do auditory blending (e.g., the teacher produces slowly and distinctly the sounds of a word, such as "c-a-t," and the student is asked to say the word). For students who cannot yet do this, we try a "word families" approach (e.g., teaching "at," "sat," and "bat," then making other words by changing the initial consonant and asking the student to read them). If a student is able to do auditory blending, we teach several consonant sounds and one vowel, asking him or her to sound out and blend them. Following that, one of the consonants is changed, and the student is asked to read the word.

The visual–motor approach is particularly useful when a student is having difficulty with words that are not spelled regularly. The teacher selects an unknown word, prints it on a card, and tells the student what the word is. The student then closes his or her eyes, tries to visualize the word, names the letters (taking more looks if necessary), and then writes it from memory.

The kinesthetic method involves teaching words by having the student trace them over and over and then write them several times. Although it is the most time-consuming of the teaching approaches to use, the kinesthetic method has been successful with students who have had long histories of reading failure (Chall & Roswell, 1998).

For students at first- to third-grade reading levels, we also try out story materials for oral reading at levels suggested by the published test results. Materials on lower and higher levels are also tried, and students are asked about which level they find "easy," "hard," and "just right." We also ask about which types of content they find interesting, helping us to determine the materials that are most likely to be effective.

Intermediate Reading Levels (Fourth through Eighth Grades)

At the lower reading levels, a student's task is to master the medium (i.e., the printed words and sounds); at the intermediate levels, the task begins to become one of mastering the meanings, concepts, information and ideas that make up the message (Chall, 1983). As a result, the most essential components to assess at these levels are word meaning and comprehension.

For word meaning, we often begin by administering a published test of vocabulary knowledge (such as the Gates–MacGinitie Reading Tests). If vocabulary seems to be a need, we then use more informal measures. For example, we might use an oral format to determine whether students are able to define more difficult words than they are able to do when the testing format requires reading. This tells us whether word recognition (rather than word meaning) is the source of difficulty. (Published tests like the Diagnostic Assessments of Reading [Roswell & Chall, 1992] and the Peabody Picture Vocabulary Test—3 [Dunn & Dunn,

1997] have a similar goal: assessing receptive or listening vocabulary.)

We also consider the precision with which students define words. When definitions are tied to specific contexts in which words can occur, students will experience difficulties when encountering the words in new contexts, even when the contexts differ only slightly from the more familiar ones (see Curtis, 1987). We also look at what students do when they encounter words whose meanings are unfamiliar to them. Do they skip them? Or do they try to use context to figure them out? If they attempt to use context, how successful are they?

For students who test low on meaning vocabulary, trial lessons are used to establish whether one method will work best for them. Methods we try include a direct method, in which definitions of unknown words are given, sentence contexts are provided, and learning is assessed by recall and production tasks; an indirect method, in which unknown words are presented in context and learning is assessed by students' ability to derive their meanings; and a structural method, in which meanings of unknown words are discussed in terms of word parts (such as prefixes, suffixes, root words, and morphemes) and the student is asked to supply definitions for different combinations of parts (see Longo, 1997).

In establishing both the breadth and depth of students' reading and listening vocabularies, graded word lists can be invaluable. Sources we consult include Biemiller (1999), Chall and Dale (1995), and Johnson and Moe (1983).

For assessment of comprehension, we usually begin with a published test in order to get an overall estimate of a student's strength on this component compared to the others. If comprehension is identified as a need, we then give students different content area materials at various levels of difficulty to read. Through brief and informal discussions after reading, we look to see whether a student's difficulties lie primarily in (1) lack of knowledge about the concepts and ideas in particular subject areas; (2) limited understanding of the organizational aspects of text (e.g., topic sentences, examples, details, etc.); (3) difficulties in summarizing, drawing inferences, or predicting what will come next; or (4) dealing with the

demands of print (i.e., word recognition and word analysis) while comprehending. Listening comprehension ability may be assessed informally as well.

Trial lessons for students with difficulties in comprehension help us to determine the teaching strategies and materials that will be most appropriate. Among the possibilities that we consider are wide and varied reading; use of such techniques as reciprocal teaching (Palinscar & Brown, 1984) and strategy training (Deshler & Schumaker, 1986); and use of writing (Curtis & Longo, 1999). We also use trial lessons as a way of "trying materials on" for fit to determine the level of difficulty most appropriate for a student as well as his or her reaction to content and style. We have found that at the fourth- through eighth-grade reading levels, it is particularly important to identify both the level that is appropriate with teacher assistance (i.e., a challenging level) and a more comfortable, independent level (see Vygotsky, 1978).

LINKS BETWEEN DIAGNOSIS AND REMEDIATION

To illustrate the links between diagnosis and remediation, we begin by presenting diagnostic and remedial information for two adolescents experiencing difficulties in reading (whose cases have previously been described in Curtis & Longo, 1999). Following the presentation of these cases, we conclude with a more general discussion of how patterns in assessment data are used to design programs of instruction.

Ted

Ted was placed in residential care by a social service agency because of academic failure and behavior problems. He was 14 years old at the time.

On a test of word identification, Ted began having difficulty reading words at the third-grade level. Substitutions were his most frequent kind of error (e.g., he said "another" for "although"). When reading aloud from text, he was accurate but slow on third-grade-level materials. He stopped frequently to reread words and phrases, and when he encountered unfamiliar words, he most often would skip them. His definitions for the words whose meanings he knew were clear and concise; however, he knew the meanings of very few words beyond the fourth-grade level. Comprehension was a relative strength for Ted. On a multiple-choice test, he was able to answer questions correctly on fifth-grade-level material; when asked to summarize text at that level, he also did fairly well. Beyond the fifth-grade level, though, he reported that he understood very little of what he was asked to read.

Like many of the students with whom we have worked, Ted found it easier to guess at words or just to skip them than to attempt to read them. The first step in improving his reading was to help him to apply the phonics knowledge that he already had, and to teach him the word analysis skills and knowledge he had yet to learn.

With Ted, direct instruction in phonics via spelling worked well, as did reading aloud from materials beginning at the fourth-grade level. During oral reading, the emphasis was on getting Ted to take risks in applying what he was learning about words and word parts in order to help him to identify unfamiliar words.

Oliver

Oliver's teachers thought that, like many ninth graders, he was not applying himself to the task of reading. To them he appeared to be quite proficient, demonstrating the ability to decode 11th-grade-level texts with ease. He remembered very little information from what he read, however, causing his teachers to question his motivation as well as his strategic reading skills. When administered a published comprehension test, Oliver scored at the sixth-grade level, confirming his teachers' observations. But it was when his meaning vocabulary was assessed that a key finding emerged. Oliver had very little knowledge about the meanings of words beyond a fourth-grade level, and for many of the words that he knew, his knowledge was based more on aural than on written exposures.

Oliver's reading improved as a result of direct instruction in vocabulary, where each word was presented in a variety of contexts and he was given multiple opportunities to

learn the new meanings. Emphasis was placed on his ability to use words as well as to recognize their meanings, and his awareness of words and their uses increased significantly (Curtis & Longo, 2001).

The Design of Remediation

As illustrated above, diagnostic information allows the examiner to see differences in the strengths and needs between two students, as well as differences in the same student at different times. These patterns, along with information from observations during testing and the results of informal tests, are used to plan successful instructional programs. We find it useful to think in terms of three broad categories in these patterns (see also Carroll, 1977):

1. *Skills and abilities that are unique to reading and assessed by tests of single-word recognition, phonics knowledge and skills, spelling, and accuracy/fluency in oral reading of connected text (without reference to comprehension).* Reading rate is also important here, and although it is not always assessed directly, it can be inferred from other test performances.

2. *Factors such as language, cognition, and background knowledge, which are not reading-specific but ultimately determine the extent of an individual's literacy development.* These are used to estimate reading potential at any point, regardless of reading skills; they are measured by such tests as the WISC-III, the Stanford–Binet, the Peabody, and tests of listening vocabulary and comprehension.

3. *Aspects that reflect the interaction of the language/cognitive factors with reading skills.* These are frequently assessed by standardized reading achievement tests of vocabulary and reading comprehension.

Like Ted, most children who fall behind in first through third grades will score lower in reading skills than in language and cognition. Other patterns occur, particularly in the intermediate and upper grades. For instance, in Oliver's case we saw strengths in word recognition and word analysis, and needs in word meanings, cognition, and background knowledge (see also Chall & Curtis, 2003).

Once patterns in strengths and needs have been identified, recommendations for instruction can be made. Care must be taken to insure that a well-rounded instructional program is designed—one that will develop the full range of a student's reading ability, building on strengths as well as addressing needs. Attention must also be given to the student's interests and preferences, in an effort to maximize the pleasure that he or she will gain from reading.

Although instructional recommendations will vary according to the student's level of reading development and pattern of test scores, we have found that the following guidelines help in the design of a successful program (Chall & Curtis, 1987):

1. *Each session is divided into a number of different activities that address different components.* Even when a student needs a great deal of help with a particular component (e.g., phonics), that component is not the focus of the entire session. Instead, only a part of the lesson is devoted to it, and sometimes a game later in the session is used to reinforce and review.

2. *Teachers participate in activities with students.* For example, when oral reading is used as a way to improve accuracy or fluency of word identification, a teacher will take turns with a student in reading portions of the text. Collaboration not only helps to provide a model and shares the burden with the student; it also creates a relaxed and friendly environment that is more conducive to learning.

3. *In general, the lower the reading level and the younger the student, the more direct the instruction should be.* Students reading at higher levels are more able to learn on their own, but they too require a program that provides guidance and instructional activities tailored to their needs.

4. *The level of difficulty of the instructional materials should be above what students are able to achieve on their own.* With encouragement and support from their teachers, we find that students make the most progress when they are challenged.

In summary, the view of diagnostic achievement testing in reading that we have presented is based on assessing various reading components and on viewing reading as a developmental process. The procedures discussed are those developed at the Harvard Reading Laboratory and adapted for use at the Boys Town Reading Center. The goal of the diagnostic process we have described is to assess students' strengths and needs in reading and related areas, for the purpose of designing instruction that will bring students' reading achievement up to their potential.

REFERENCES

Bernstein, J. H., Kammerer, B., Prather, P., & Rey-Casserly, C. (1998). Developmental neuropsychological assessment. In G. P. Koocher, J. C. Norcross, & S. S. Hill (Eds.), *Psychologists' desk reference* (pp. 34–38). New York: Oxford University Press.

Biemiller, A. (1999). *Language and reading success.* Cambridge, MA: Brookline Books.

Brown, V. L., Hammill, D. D., & Wiederholt, J. L. (1995). *Test of Reading Comprehension* (3rd ed.). Austin, TX: Pro-Ed.

Burnette, J. (1998). *Reducing the disproportionate representation of minority students in special education.* (ERIC/OSP Digest #E566; ERIC Document Reproduction Service No. ED 417501 98)

Carroll, J. B. (1977). Developmental parameters in reading comprehension. In J. T. Guthrie (Ed.), *Cognition, curriculum, and comprehension* (pp. 1–15). Newark, DE: International Reading Association.

Chall, J. S. (1983). *Stages of reading development.* New York: McGraw-Hill.

Chall, J. S., & Curtis, M. E. (1987). What clinical diagnosis tells us about children's reading. *The Reading Teacher, 40,* 784–788.

Chall, J. S., & Curtis, M. E. (1992). Teaching the disabled or below-average reader. In S. J. Samuels & A. E. Farstrup (Eds.), *What research has to say about reading instruction* (pp. 253–276). Newark, DE: International Reading Association.

Chall, J. S., & Curtis, M. E. (2003). Children with reading difficulties. In J. Flood, D. Lapp, J. Jensen, & J. R. Squire (Eds.), *Handbook of research on teaching English language arts* (2nd ed., pp. 413–420). Mahwah, NJ: Erlbaum.

Chall, J. S., & Dale, E. (1995). *Readability revisited.* Cambridge, MA: Brookline Books.

Chall, J. S., & Roswell, F. G. (1998). *Reading difficulties.* Elizabethtown, PA: Continental Press.

Chang, F. R. (1983). Mental processes in reading: A methodological review. *Reading Research Quarterly, 18,* 216–230.

Clay, M. M. (1993). *An Observation Survey of Early Literacy Achievement.* Portsmouth, NH: Heinemann.

Council of Economic Advisors for the President's Initiative on Race. (1998). *Changing America: Indicators of social and economic well-being by race and*

Hispanic origin. Washington, DC: U.S. Government Printing Office. (ERIC Document Reproduction Service No. ED 424 344)

Cummins, J. (1981). Empirical and theoretical underpinnings of bilingual education. *Journal of Education, 163,* 16–29.

Curtis, M. E. (1987). Vocabulary testing and vocabulary instruction. In M. G. McKeown & M. E. Curtis (Eds.), *The nature of vocabulary acquisition* (pp. 37–51). Hillsdale, NJ: Erlbaum.

Curtis, M. E., & Longo, A. M. (1999). *When adolescents can't read: Methods and materials that work.* Cambridge, MA: Brookline Books.

Curtis, M. E., & Longo, A. M. (2001). Teaching vocabulary to adolescents to improve comprehension. *Reading Online* [Online]. Available: www.reading online.org

Davis, F. B. (1972). Psychometric research on comprehension in reading. *Reading Research Quarterly, 7,* 628–678.

Denckla, M. B., & Rudel, R. G. (1976). Rapid automatized naming (R.A.N.): Dyslexia differentiated from other learning disabilities. *Neuropsychologia, 14,* 471–479.

Deshler, D. D., & Schumaker, J. B. (1986). Learning strategies: An instructional alternative for low-achieving adolescents. *Exceptional Children, 52,* 583–590.

Dunn, L. M., & Dunn, L. M. (1997). *Peabody Picture Vocabulary Test* (3rd ed.). Circle Pines, MN: American Guidance Service.

Ekwall, E. E., & Shanker, J. L. (1993). *Ekwall/Shanker Reading Inventory* (3rd ed.). Boston: Allyn & Bacon.

Gambrell, L. B., Palmer, B. M., Codling, R. M., & Mazzoni, S. A. (1996). Assessing motivation to read. *The Reading Teacher, 49,* 518–533.

Ganske, K. (2000). *Word journeys: Assessment-guided phonics, spelling, and vocabulary instruction.* New York: Guilford Press.

Good, R. H., & Kaminski, R. A. (Eds.). (2002). *Dynamic indicators of basic early literacy skills* (6th ed.). Eugene, OR: Institute for the Development of Educational Achievement.

Hammill, D. D., & Larsen, S. C. (1996). *Test of Written Language* (3rd ed.). Austin, TX: Pro-Ed.

Harris, A. J., & Sipay, E. R. (1990). *How to increase reading ability: A guide to developmental and remedial methods* (9th ed.). New York: Longman.

Huey, E. B. (1908). *The psychology and pedagogy of reading.* Cambridge, MA: MIT Press.

International Reading Association. (1982). Misuse of grade equivalents. *The Reading Teacher, 35,* 464.

Johnson, D. D. (1973). Guidelines for evaluating word attack skills in the primary grades. In W. H. MacGinitie (Ed.), *Assessment problems in reading* (pp. 21–26). Newark, DE: International Reading Association.

Johnson, D. D., & Moe, A. J. (1983). *The Ginn word book for teachers.* Lexington, MA: Ginn.

Karlsen, B., & Gardner, E. F. (1995). *Stanford Diagnostic Reading Test* (4th ed.). San Antonio, TX: Psychological Corporation.

Kea, C. D., & Utley, C. A. (1998). To teach me is to know me. *Journal of Special Education, 32,* 44–47.

Larsen, S. C., & Hammill, D. D. (1994). *Test of Written Spelling—3.* Austin, TX: Pro-Ed.

Longo, A. M. (1997). Trial lessons in reading: A dynamic assessment approach. In L. R. Putnam (Ed.), *Readings on language and literacy* (pp. 211–233). Cambridge, MA: Brookline Books.

Lyon, G. R. (1995). Research initiatives in learning disabilities: Contributions from scientists supported by the National Institute of Child Health and Human Development. *Journal of Child Neurology, 10,* 120–126.

MacGinitie, W. H., MacGinitie, R. K., Maria, K., & Dreyer, L. G. (2000). *Gates–MacGinitie Reading Tests* (4th ed.). Itasca, IL: Riverside.

Menyuk, P. (1999). *Reading and linguistic development.* Cambridge, MA: Brookline Books.

National Reading Panel. (2000). *Teaching children to read: An evidence-based assessment of the scientific research literature on reading and its implications for reading instruction.* Bethesda, MD: National Institute of Child Health and Human Development.

Orton, S. T. (1925). "Word blindness" in school-children. *Archives of Neurological Psychology, 14,* 581–615.

Palinscar, A. S., & Brown, A. L. (1984). Reciprocal teaching of comprehension-fostering and comprehension-monitoring activities. *Cognition and Instruction, 1,* 117–175.

Paris, S. G., Calfee, R. C., Filby, N., Hiebert, E. H., Pearson, P. D., Valencia, S. W., & Wolf, K. P. (1992). A framework for authentic literacy assessment. *The Reading Teacher, 46,* 88–98.

Perfetti, C. A. (1985). *Reading ability.* New York: Oxford University Press.

Perfetti, C. A., & Curtis, M. E. (1987). Reading. In R. F. Dillon & R. J. Sternberg (Eds.), *Cognition and instruction* (pp. 13–57). New York: Academic Press.

Popham, W. J. (1999). *Classroom assessment: What teachers need to know.* Boston: Allyn & Bacon.

Robertson, C., & Salter, W. (1997). *The Phonological Awareness Test.* East Moline, IL: LinguiSystems.

Roswell, F. G., & Chall, J. S. (1978). *Roswell–Chall Diagnostic Reading Test of Word Analysis Skills* (Revised and extended). La Jolla, CA: Essay.

Roswell, F. G., & Chall, J. S. (1992). *Diagnostic Assessments of Reading.* Chicago: Riverside.

Share, D. L., & Stanovich, K. E. (1995). Cognitive processes in early reading development: A model of acquisition and individual differences. *Issues in Education: Contributions from Educational Psychology, 1,* 1–57.

Silvaroli, N. J. (1997). *Classroom Reading Inventory* (8th ed.). New York: McGraw-Hill.

Snow, C., Burns, S., & Griffin, P. (Eds.). (1998). *Preventing reading difficulties in young children.* Washington, DC: National Academy Press.

Spear-Swerling, L., & Sternberg, R. J. (1996). *Off track: When poor readers become "learning disabled."* Boulder, CO: Westview Press.

Stanovich, K. E. (1986). Matthew effects in reading: Some consequences of individual differences in the acquisition of literacy. *Reading Research Quarterly, 21,* 360–407.

Sticht, T. G., & James, J. H. (1984). Listening and

reading. In P. D. Pearson (Ed.), *Handbook of reading research* (pp. 293–317). New York: Longman.

Thorndike, R. L., Hagen, E., & Sattler, J. (1986). *Stanford–Binet Intelligence Scale: Fourth Edition.* Chicago: Riverside.

Torgesen, J., Wagner, R., & Rashotte, C. (1999). *Test of Word Reading Efficiency.* Austin, TX: Pro-Ed.

Vygotsky, L. S. (1978). *Mind in society.* Cambridge, MA: Harvard University Press.

Wagner, R. K., Torgesen, J. K., & Rashotte, C. A. (1999). *Comprehensive Test of Phonological Processing.* Austin, TX: Pro-Ed.

Wechsler, D. (1991). *Wechsler Intelligence Scale for Children—Third Edition.* San Antonio, TX: Psychological Corporation.

Wilkinson, G. S. (1993). *Wide Range Achievement Test–3.* Wilmington, DE: Jastak.

Wiederholt, J. L., & Bryant, B. R. (2001). *Gray Oral Reading Tests* (4th ed.). Austin, TX: Pro-Ed.

Wolf, M. (1991). Naming speed and reading: The contribution of the cognitive neurosciences. *Reading Research Quarterly, 26,* 123–141.

Woods, M. L., & Moe, A. J. (1999). *Analytic Reading Inventory* (6th ed.) New York: Macmillan.

Woodcock, R. W. (1987). *Woodcock Reading Mastery Tests–Revised.* Circle Pines, MN: American Guidance Service.

Yopp, H. K. (1995). A test for assessing phonemic awareness in young children. *The Reading Teacher, 49,* 20–29.

18

Assessing the Writing Abilities and Instructional Needs of Students

BRIAN R. BRYANT

DIANE PEDROTTY BRYANT

The 20th century saw an incredible rise in the number of tests that were created and made available for consumer purchase (Bryant & Rivera, 1997). As would be expected, these tests either were devoted entirely to writing or had a writing component as part of an overall achievement measure. This chapter examines writing assessment in two ways. First, we provide a brief historical overview of the development of writing assessment. Second, we examine a sampling of currently available standardized tests, and present various ways to supplement standardized test data by informal means.

HISTORICAL OVERVIEW OF WRITING ASSESSMENT

It is illuminating to study the history of assessment in general, and writing assessment in particular, for two reasons. First, it provides us with a frame of reference within which we can view current practices. Second, it provides us with a sense of perspective. That is, by studying what early assessors have contributed to our field, we realize that "new assessment advances" either have their roots in the early 20th century or are

actually replicates of long-held practices. Put simply, the means to assess written expression have been available for almost 100 years; current test writers simply elaborate on past practices. That said, we provide readers with an overview of assessment history.

We have previously borrowed from the work of Thorndike and Hagen (1955) to discuss the history of psychological and educational measurement, and to divide assessment history into three periods: the Pioneering Period (1845–1915), the Proliferation Period (1916–1940), and the Refinement Period (post-1940) (Bryant & Rivera, 1997). We discuss writing assessment accordingly, using those periods as guides.

Pioneering Period

Greene, Jorgenson, and Gerberich (1953) provided an excellent overview of early academic testing. In their review, these researchers discussed the landmark 1845 decision by the Boston school system to revise its assessment practices drastically. Up to that time, assessments were conducted via one-on-one interviews with students. Because of the increasing number of students and the resultant strain on assessment resources, the interviews were replaced with a written evaluation system. The new assessment policy was scrutinized by the secretary of the Massachusetts Board of Education, Horace Mann, who cogently commented on the new practice (as summarized in Greene et al., 1953, p. 23):

1. It is impartial.
2. It is just to the pupil.
3. It is more thorough than older forms of examination.
4. It prevents "official interference" of the teacher.
5. It "determines, beyond appeal or gainsaying, whether pupils have been faithfully and competently taught."
6. It takes away "all possibility of favoritism."
7. It makes the information obtained available to all.
8. It enables all to appraise the ease or difficulty of the questions.

Greene and colleagues (1953) gave credit to the Reverand George Fisher, an English schoolteacher, for creating and using the first achievement test in 1864. His "scale books," as they were called, assessed student performance in a variety of skill areas, including the writing skills of handwriting, spelling, grammar, and composition.

In 1894, Dr. J. M. Rice provided the first objective test of writing when he conducted a national survey of elementary school students' spelling abilities using two scales—one in list form and the other using sentences (Ruch & Stoddard, 1927). It is interesting to note that Rice's work was initially criticized, because his research dictated that those who studied spelling for 40 minutes a day fared no better than those who studied spelling for 10 minutes a day (Smith & Wright, 1928). Rice's critics argued that spelling was taught not simply to improve spelling, but to develop pupils' minds (Greene et al., 1953). Later, Rice's work was praised, and his efforts are now generally regarded as "the beginning of work in educational measurement" (Gilliland & Jordan, 1924, p. 55).

Edward L. Thorndike, a pioneer in educational and psychological measurement, made an early contribution to assessment when he published the first text on mental and educational measurement, *An Introduction to the Theory of Mental and Social Measurements* (Thorndike, 1904). Six years later, he published the *Thorndike Scale for Handwriting of Children* (Thorndike, 1910), which began a 6-year period that brought forth several scales for assessing English composition, spelling, and handwriting (Jordan, 1953). Clearly, the groundwork had been laid for the increased focus on pupil measurement of academic skills, but few could have foretold the vast numbers of tests that would be written and published over the course of the following 25 years.

Of particular interest to this chapter are the works of Freeman (1914) in handwriting assessment and Hillegas (1912) in writing composition assessment. Freeman created a measure of handwriting that involved examination of the following areas: uniformity of slant, quality of line, letter formation, and kinds of spacing. Freeman's scale was the first attempt at providing teachers a means to identify strengths and weaknesses across these handwriting dimensions, and also to plan remedial efforts to correct identified weaknesses.

Hillegas pioneered composition assessment in 1912 by soliciting a set of children's writings using such prompts as "What I Should Like to Do Next Saturday" and "The Most Exciting Experience of My Life." The resulting essays were examined by a team of writing experts, and 10 samples were selected and given ratings from 0 to 9, based on the general quality of the passage. Teachers could then obtain writing samples from their students, compare the products to the samples, and make a holistic judgments as to how the students compared to the 0–9 standard.

By 1913, the use of district-wide standardized achievement testing that included writing subtests had been documented in the School Survey of New York City (Smith & Wright, 1928). As a result of successful use of tests to document pupils' progress, opposition to standardized testing diminished shortly thereafter. Such an atmosphere of acceptance led to the development of many new tests during the Proliferation Period.

Proliferation Period

By 1915, testing had become a popular fixture in psychology and education; throughout the next 25 years, dozens of tests were written to measure various dimensions of academic achievement. In describing the rapid growth of testing that occurred in the early years of the Proliferation Period, Tiegs (1931) made the following observation:

> Once the [testing] movement took root, many became interested. There was an orgy of test making. No definite philosophy and method of validation had yet been developed. The origin of many of these tests is shrouded in mystery; no data are available. For this reason, many tests, presumably carefully validated, were next to useless. (p. 75)

Good or bad, tests were being published with increasing frequency. In the 10-year period between 1915 and 1925, Gilliland and Jordan (1924) reported that over 40 tests were published, including many that assessed various dimensions of writing. Three early developments occurred that encouraged the development of standardized tests during the Proliferation Period:

(1) The numerous important studies of the accuracy of school marks, revealing the fact that they are highly subjective and inaccurate, demonstrated the need for instruments that would yield more accurate measures of achievement.
(2) The surveys of certain of the larger school systems both stimulated the construction and use of tests and were influenced by the development of more objective devices for measuring the abilities of pupils.
(3) The development of educational measurement in research bureaus organized in many of the larger school systems, universities, and state departments of public instruction was influential in popularizing the use of educational tests. Although the pioneer and most of the early standardized tests were for use in the elementary school, it was not many years until the high school and even the college were well provided with such instruments. (Gilliland & Jordan, 1924, p. 25)

Several events occurred in the 1920s that aided test construction. In 1921, Thorndike published his classic text *The Teacher's Word Book,* in which he provided teachers with a listing of 10,000 words that could be used for instructional purposes in the classroom. One would be hard pressed to think of how many teachers and researchers used Thorndike's list to devise teacher-made or commercial tests of spelling and vocabulary, but it is easy to acknowledge that his work contributed greatly to teachers' ability to assess their students' writing abilities in a number of ways.

A significant development in assessment occurred shortly thereafter, when Truman L. Kelley, Giles M. Ruch, and Lewis L. Terman (1923) devised the Stanford Achievement Test. This standardized test gave educators and psychologists the opportunity to test groups of students in a variety of subjects, including language arts. The new test was easy to score and was technically sound—two properties that established assessment as an efficient and popular answer to the call from the Massachusetts Board of Education almost 75 years earlier.

By the late 1920s, assessment had clearly come of age. In fact, Oscar Buros (1978) cited 1927 as "a banner year in testing" (p. 1972). According to Buros, the unreasonably high expectations concerning test use prior to 1927 were being replaced with more modest prospects of tests' usefulness. In addition, textbooks concerning measurement were becoming readily available to prospective test writers, who were using such statistical procedures as correlations and factor analysis to explore their tests' technical characteristics. Buros's comment on the state of assessment in 1927, and its apparent arrested development in intervening years, still speaks volumes: "If you examine these books and the best of the achievement and intelligence tests then available, you might be surprised that so little progress has been made in the past fifty years" (p. 1973).

As the 1930s approached, there was no shortage of methods to assess students' writing abilities. Smith and Wright (1928) listed five tests that assessed "English Composite" (presumably a measure of general English competence), eight tests of "English Usage," eight tests of "Composition," five tests of "Spelling," and three tests assessing "Handwriting."

It was during the Proliferation Period that the practice of making aptitude–achievement comparisons first became popular. In addition to achievement tests, numerous intelligence tests (i.e., tests of academic aptitude) were devised, and it became common practice to set aptitude as the standard to which achievement tests were compared. An example of this line of thinking was offered by Thorndike (1929), which provides interesting information to those involved in the assessment of learning disabilities (LDs) today:

> When tests of achievement are used in connection with measures of capacity, the treatment of each pupil may be made even more fair and fruitful. The pupil gifted with a high degree of native capacity is then expected to do more and better work than the average. He is thus protected against habits of idleness and conceit which might result were he constantly praised for merely exceeding pupils of inferior endowment. Pupils of meager native talents are similarly protected against rebukes, scorn, and discouragement for inferiority in gross attainments. Each pupil's work becomes healthier and more fruitful when appraised in terms of his own capacities. Objective measurement, then, increases the effectiveness of education by setting up standards of achievement in varying capacities. (p. 294)

Several other events occurred during this period that advanced the abilities of test writers to create better products. Bryant and Rivera (1997) identified four contributions as of particular interest:

1. An increased availability of textbooks on psychological and educational measurement.
2. The publication of *Educational, Psychological, and Personality Tests of 1933, 1934, and 1935* (the precursor to the *Mental Measurements Yearbook* series) by Buros (1936), which provided test users with access to critical reviews of published tests.
3. The application of statistical techniques (e.g., factor analysis, coefficient alpha) to aid in the development and validation of tests.
4. The development of aptitude and achievement tests by psychologists who were specially trained in the art of test development.

It is clear that all current authors of writing scales should tip their hats to their early predecessors. There is also little doubt that the work of the early authors made a profound impact on assessment as we know it today and to the advances that were made during the Refinement Period.

Refinement Period

As the Refinement Period emerged, assessment of student abilities via standardized tests had become commonplace for most educators and psychologists. Most professionals had confidence in their abilities and those of test authors. However, the growing number of tests caused some to question the manner in which test results were being used. As a result of these concerns, a period of scrutiny emerged in which measures of ability were closely examined for their technical adequacy.

The American Psychological Association (APA) responded to the concerns of its members by publishing its *Technical Recommendations for Psychological Tests and Diagnostic Techniques* in 1954. This classic contribution to assessment was endorsed by the American Educational Research Association (AERA) and the National Council on Measurement in Education (NCME), thus generalizing the APA's standards to professional educators. Within a year, the AERA and NCME (1954) devised their own document, *Technical Recommendations for Achievement Tests*, which added to the APA publication. The two documents were merged in 1966 under the auspices of the APA, and the new publication was titled *Standards for Educational and Psychological Tests and Manuals* (APA, 1966). The manual and its later revisions have given test authors and critics a blueprint for constructing and evaluating assessment devices.

It was also in the 1960s when specific LDs began to be identified and thus created a new market for tests. Sam Kirk (1962) used the term in his classic text to describe children who were experiencing difficulty in school, yet were doing so without having mental retardation or emotional disturbance. The term had been first used by Emmett Betts in the 1930s (Betts, 1936), but Kirk's use popularized LDs and opened the door for a myriad of aptitude and achievement tests that could be used to help diagnose children as having LDs.

Helmer Myklebust also made an important contribution in the 1960s when he wrote the Picture Story Language Test (PSLT) in 1965. The PSLT was Myklebust's attempt to elicit children's writing samples that could be used to evaluate differences in students with LDs, mental retardation, emotional disturbance, and speech handicaps (Sweetland & Keyser, 1986). The scale examined a student's writing sample for the number of words written, the number of sentences written, the number of words per sentence, grammatical usage, and expression of ideas. Myklebust's work was a model for all later authors of writing tests, and remains a venerable contribution from one of the leaders in special education.

We have noted that earlier during the end of the Pioneering Period and at the beginning of the Proliferation Period, there were those who criticized the use of tests to gauge the abilities of students. Such criticisms were (and still are) also present in the Refinement Period, and they have helped focus attention on the use and misuse of standardized testing. Frank Smith (1982) represented the views of many concerning language arts assessment when he wrote:

> Tests are almost inevitably based on very poor theories of what writing and reading involve; they are constructed by people whose expertise Is in test construction, not in writing and reading. Sometimes it is claimed that tests are atheoretical, which means that no one even gave a thought to what writing and reading involve. When people who have thought about writing and reading are asked to construct tests (of comprehension, for example), they will often say that such tests are impossible and unnecessary. (p. 208)

Along those lines, many professionals have contrasted standardized tests with what are termed "authentic" assessment procedures, vilifying standardized tests while glorifying nonstandardized procedures. In a response to such comparisons, Bryant (1999) wrote:

> Many of the observations are true enough to lead the gullible reader to believe that standardized testing is the work of malevolent trolls, whereas authentic assessment is used by benevolent fairy godfathers and godmothers. In truth, both assessment approaches are valuable tools that, when used by competent pro-

fessionals, provide considerable information about the examinee. (p. 403)

As a result of criticisms aimed at standardized tests, portfolio assessment became a popular alternative to standardized testing, particularly in writing. It has been argued that "portfolios," or collections of student writing samples for assessment and instructional purposes, allow evaluators to monitor student learning and evaluate the effectiveness of instructional programs (McMillan, 1997; Paulson, Paulson, & Meyer, 1991; Rivera & Smith, 1996; Swicegood, 1994; Taylor, 2003; Valencia, 1990; Wolf, 1991). Paulson and colleagues (1991) defined "portfolio assessment" as assessment of

> a purposeful collection of student work that exhibits the student's efforts, progress, and achievements in one or more areas. The collection should include student participation in selecting content, criteria for selection, the criteria for judging merit, and evidence of student self-reflection. (p. 60)

It is interesting to note that for years, portfolio advocates disdained measurement professionals' concerns for technical adequacy. It is hoped that advocates of portfolio assessment will heed White's (1994) cogent recommendation that portfolio assessment adherents "should not repeat the naiveté of an earlier generation of English faculty by ignoring reliability while [portfolio assessment] claims validity, a claim that nobody in measurement can take seriously" (p. 292).

In the 1970s and 1980s, numerous writing tests and assessment procedures were devised to identify student strengths and weaknesses (Maddox, 2003). Many of these tests have been evaluated by Hammill, Brown, and Bryant (1992), who used APA standards for test construction to identify an objective method for evaluating tests' technical adequacy. Their work, titled *A Consumer's Guide to Tests in Print,* lists ratings of popular norm-referenced tests.

A review of Hammill and colleagues' (1992) ratings for writing tests and individually administered general achievement tests with writing components demonstrates that writing measures have indeed improved technically. In fact, the vast majority of the tests reviewed by Hammill and colleagues and of tests published subsequently have garnered acceptable ratings with regard to reliability, validity, and normative statistics. These tests (and their applicable subtests and composites) include the Test of Written Language (3rd edition) (TOWL-3; Hammill & Larsen, 1988)—the Writing composite and the Vocabulary, Style and Spelling, Logical Sentences, Sentence Combining, Thematic Maturity, Contextual Vocabulary, Syntactic Maturity, Contextual Style, and Contextual Spelling subtests; the Basic Achievement Skills Individual Screener (BASIS; Psychological Corporation, 1983)—the Spelling and Writing subtests; the Diagnostic Achievement Battery (3rd edition) (DAB-3; Newcomer, 2001)—the Writing composite and the Spelling, Capitalization and Punctuation, and Written Vocabulary subtests; the Diagnostic Achievement Test for Adolescents (2nd edition) (DATA-2; Newcomer & Bryant, 1992)—the Writing composite and the Spelling and Writing Composition subtests; the Diagnostic Spelling Potential Test (DSPT; Arena, 1982)—the Spelling, Word Recognition, Visual Recognition, and Auditory–Visual Recognition subtests; Scholastic Abilities Test for Adults (SATA; Bryant, Patton, & Dunn, 1991)—the Writing composite and the Spelling and Writing Composition subtests; the Kaufman Test of Educational Achievement (K-TEA; Kaufman & Kaufman, 1985)—the Spelling subtest; the Test of Written Expression (TOWE; McGhee, Bryant, Larsen, & Bryant, 1995)—the Writing composite and the Writing Mechanics and Essay subtests; the Peabody Individual Achievement Test—Revised (PIAT-R; Markwardt, 1989)—the Spelling and Writing subtests; the Test of Adolescent Language (3rd edition) (TOAL-3; Hammill, Brown, Larsen, & Wiederholt, 1994)—the Writing composite and the Writing Vocabulary and Writing Grammar subtests; the Hammill Multiability Achievement Test (HAMAT; Hammill, Hresko, Ammer, Cronin, & Quinby, 1998)—the Writing subtest; the Test of Early Written Language (2nd edition) (TEWL-2; Hresko, Herron, & Peak, 1996)—the Writing Quotient; Wechsler Individual Achievement Test (WIAT; Psychological Corporation, 1992)—the Writing subtest; the Wide

Range Achievement Test (3rd edition) (WRAT-3; Wilkinson, 1993)—the Spelling subtest; the Test of Written Spelling (4th edition) (TWS-4; Larsen, Hammill, & Moats, 2000), Total Spelling; and the Woodcock–Johnson Psycho-Educational Battery—Revised (WJ-R; Woodcock & Johnson, 1989)—the Writing composite and the Dictation and Proofing subtests.

Finally, the Refinement Period has provided educators and psychologists with caveats as to how tests should be used. Simply put, norm-referenced tests generally should not be used to plan instruction, because they simply possess too few items to enable educators to assess individual skills accurately (e.g., spelling words with consonant–vowel–consonant–silent-e configurations). Numerous assessment text authors (e.g., McLoughlin & Lewis, 1990; Salvia & Ysseldyke, 1998) have noted the limitations of norm-referenced tests. Yet these limitations should not be considered evidence that norm-referenced tests have no role in a comprehensive assessment of student performance. Rather, these tests are a valuable contribution that cannot be replicated using criterion-referenced and nonreferenced procedures (Hammill & Bryant, 1991).

To conclude this section, the past century and a half have provided educators and psychologists with a valuable foundation upon which to build. Assessment professionals owe a great deal of thanks to those who dedicated their professional lives to the examination of pupil performance in writing. Such contributions should never be forgotten.

WRITING ASSESSMENT STRATEGIES

In this section, we discuss how standardized tests assess the constructs we have outlined at the beginning of this chapter. We then provide a number of nonstandardized procedures that are currently available to evaluators of writing abilities.

Assessment of Established Constructs Using Standardized Tests

Earlier in this chapter, we have discussed various elements of writing and their importance to the writing process and product. In this section, we discuss how some of the more popular tests assess those elements.

General Writing

Several tests provide overall writing scores or have items that yield an overall writing score. Tests like the TOWL-3 and the DATA-2 use the composite method to yield an overall writing score. In the case of the DATA-2, the results of Spelling and Writing Composition combine to form a Writing Quotient.

The Learning Disabilities Diagnostic Inventory (LDDI; Hammill & Bryant, 1998) is somewhat unique in this regard. This scale's authors did a literature review to identify writing behaviors indicative of specific writing disabilities (i.e., dysgraphia). Raters identify the frequency with which 15 writing behaviors occur (e.g., "Omits endings in words" or Writes sentence fragments"). The norms for the LDDI are based only on students with identified LDs who had writing weaknesses.

Spelling

Spelling is assessed in a variety of ways. By far the most popular form of spelling test involves the use of the word dictation method, wherein the examiner says a word, uses the word in a sentence, and repeats the word (e.g., "Tall. Tom is a very tall man. Tall."). The examinee spells the word on an answer sheet, and the examiner scores the response as correct or incorrect. This approach is used on the DAB-2, DATA-2, TWS-4, DSPT, BASIS, K-TEA, WRAT-3, WJ-R, and WIAT.

Several alternate approaches have also been used with considerable success. For example, the PIAT-R uses a multiple-choice format, in which the examiner says the name of the stimulus word, and the student selects the correct spelling from among four response choices.

The TOWL-3 provides yet another method of gauging students' spelling abilities. Here the examinee says a sentence, which the student writes verbatim. The sentence can be repeated several times, thus reducing the memory load as a factor in assessment. A target word is identified in the sentence (e.g., "red" in "The boy pulled the little red wagon"), which is scored for spelling accuracy. Similar approaches are used in the TOWE and the HAMAT.

The TOWL-3 is the only test we have encountered that generates a norm-referenced score using spelling in context. The test has a student write a story using a stimulus picture (see Figure 18.1), and the examiner counts the number of correctly spelled words written by the examinee. This total constitutes a Contextual Spelling subtest score.

Capitalization and Punctuation

Knowledge of capitalization and punctuation rules is assessed in a number of ways. A common assessment involves proofreading, in which the examinee looks at a sentence that has no capital letters or punctuation marks (e.g., "soon after president lincoln was elected several states led by south carolina seceded from the union"). The sentence is rewritten, with the product examined for correct application of capitalization and punctuation rules (e.g., "Soon after President Lincoln was elected; several states, led by South Carolina, seceded from the union"). This approach is used in the DAB-2. A variant of this method is the dictated-sentence technique, in which a sentence is spoken by the examiner and transcribed by the examinee. This approach uses the same scoring technique as does proofreading and is used with the HAMAT, TOWE, and TOWL-3.

The TOWL-3 assesses application of capitalization and punctuation rules by examining the student's written product. Each rule is given a point value, and these points are summed to achieve what is called the Contextual Style score.

Vocabulary

Several tests examine a student's ability to demonstrate an understanding of word meanings and their application. Two approaches are typically used to assess writing vocabulary. The first approach has the student write a story based on a stimulus set of pictures (see Figure 18.2), and the examiner counts the number of words that have seven or more letters (e.g., "because," "catching"). This approach is used with the DAB-

STORY

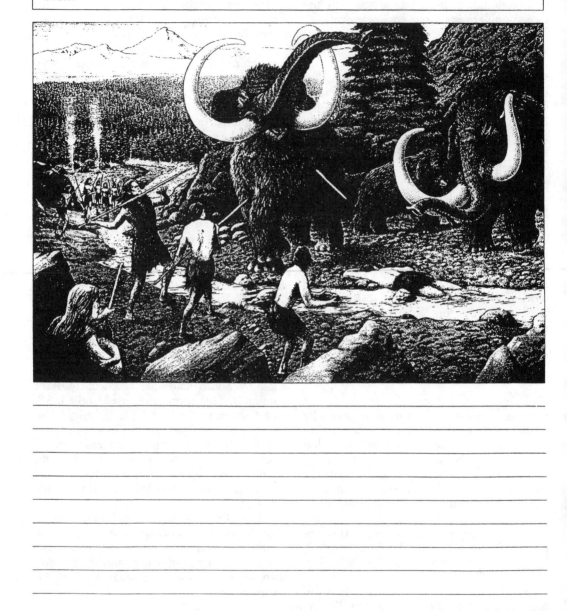

2

FIGURE 18.1. Stimulus picture from Hammill and Larsen's (1988) Test of Written Language (3rd ed.) (TOWL-3). Copyright 1988 by Pro-Ed. Reprinted by permission.

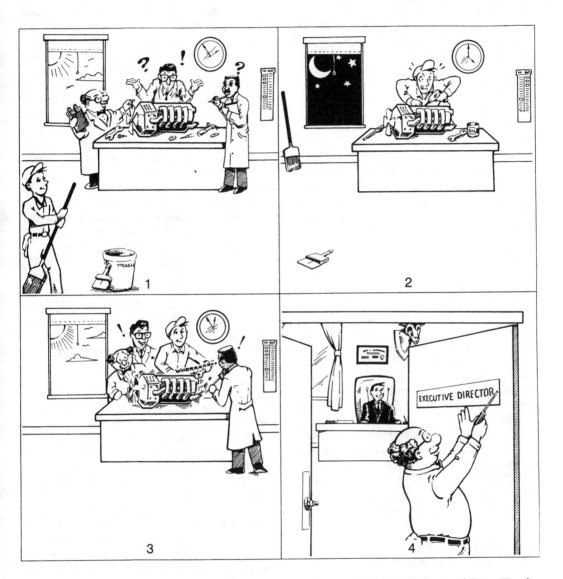

FIGURE 18.2. Stimulus picture from Bryant, Patton, and Dunn's (1991) *Scholastic Abilities Test for Adults (SATA)*. Copyright 1991 by Pro-Ed. Reprinted by permission.

2, DATA-2, TOWE (also as one factor in composition), SATA, and TOWL-3.

The second way to assess vocabulary is used with the TOAL-3 and the TOWL-3. Here, the examinee is shown a word (e.g., "sky"), and then writes a sentence that demonstrates that he or she knows the meaning of the word (e.g., "The sky has a reddish hue as the sun sets over the lake").

Grammar

Knowledge of grammatical structures is assessed via numerous methods. The TOWL-

3 and the TOAL-3 use a sentence-combining technique. With this approach, a student examines sentences (e.g., "I yelled. I cried") and then writes a single sentence that combines the ideas represented in the stimulus sentences (e.g., "I yelled and cried").

The TOWL-3 assesses syntactic maturity by examining the student's writing sample and counting the number of sentences that are written correct syntactically. The total constitutes the Syntactic Maturity raw score.

Ideation

Idea generation is assessed by the TOWL-3 and the TOWE. These techniques examine a student's written product for inclusion of specific elements (e.g., title, use of proper names).

Miscellaneous

Other skills, which are not identified above, are examined by writing tests. For instance, the DSPT examines spelling-related skills of visual recognition and auditory/visual recognition. The TOWL-3 examines an element of semantics by having the student read a sentence that is illogical (e.g., "She was as cold as fire"). The sentence is rewritten by the examinee, and the revised sentence is examined for its correction of the illogicality (e.g., "She was as cold as ice" or "She was as hot as fire"). Finally, the BASIS and the PIAT-R examine written products holistically. Examiners read each passage and classify it on a general scale of competence when compared to samples or criteria provided by the test authors.

Assessment of Writing Skills Using Nonstandardized Procedures

For decades, researchers have provided a variety of nonstandardized methods to assess writing skills (for a discussion of what constitute nonstandardized procedures, see Hammill & Bryant, 1991). Our discussion here focuses on conducting student interviews, creating criterion-referenced inventories, and analyzing written passages. Information obtained with these techniques can be important to members of an assessment team who need to validate the results of

standardized procedures by examining student writing samples.

Conducting Student Interviews

Considerable information can be obtained about a student's writing experiences simply by engaging in an informal discussion. Many students who write poorly don't like to write, because it places them in a position of accentuating their weaknesses or demonstrating thier lack of competence. Frankly, students are taught early to avoid activities that are self-injurious, so it should come as no surprise that this advice generalizes to avoiding tasks that are emotionally debilitating. Such attitudes are easily gleaned though conversation.

Some may choose to use a more formal approach to gaining information about a student's attitudes about writing. In this case, the writing survey depicted in Figure 18.3 may be of interest. As can be seen, Deshler, Ellis, and Lenz (1996) have devised a useful questionnaire that can be completed by the student if he or she is able to read it. If this is not the case, the information can be obtained during an interview, and the interviewer can transcribe the student's responses.

Creating Criterion-Referenced Measures

Criterion-referenced measures can be useful if the purpose of assessment is to identify mastery of specific skills. By far the most popular criterion-referenced tools are those authored by Alfred Brigance. His Comprehensive Inventory of Basic Skills (Brigance, 1999) is an excellent resource for conducting such an assessment. Many people choose to devise their own instruments that are aligned with the particular basal language arts texts used in the school. Or perhaps the publisher of a basal text in use provides its own criterion-referenced measure. Either way, the notion is the same. The writer of the test first identifies the skills being taught (e.g., capitalization rules; see Figure 18.4) and then selects items to represent the skills. Figure 18.5 provides a rudimentary demonstration of the principle by showing four items that assess the skill "Capitalize the pronoun I." Some criterion for mastery is set (usually 90%; in our example, 75%), and the examiner administers the test

Instructions: The questions below ask you to indicate how you feel about different aspects of writing. For each question, circle the number that best shows what you really feel.

| 1 = Strongly agree | 2 = Mostly agree | 3 = Unsure | 4 = Mostly Disagree | 5 = Strongly Disagree |

1 2 3 4 5   1. I think writing about a topic helps you learn about it.

1 2 3 4 5   2. It really does not matter how you go about writing as long as you finish the job.

1 2 3 4 5   3. Writing is a waste of time.

1 2 3 4 5   4. Setting goals before you start writing is important.

1 2 3 4 5   5. Thinking about who will be reading your writing and what the reader already knows about your topic is an important thing to consider when writing.

1 2 3 4 5   6. I like to write.

1 2 3 4 5   7. The approach I'm using for writing now is a lot better than the approach I was using last year.

1 2 3 4 5   8. I am a good writer.

---

1 2 3 4 5   9. Before you actually start writing, creating an outline that shows the organization of the main points you will write about is important.

☐ I *almost never* make an outline before writing because: ☐ I *usually don't* make an outline before writing because: ☐ I *usually do* make an outline before writing, but when I don't, it's because:

(check all that apply to you)

__ I know the writing will be so short that an outline is not needed.
__ I'm not sure how to create outlines.
__ Outlining is too much trouble.
__ I usually forget to outline.
__ Outlining won't make a difference on my grade.

__ I can never think of ideas to note on the outline.
__ I'm not very good at outlining ideas before writing.
__ I usually don't have time to outline.
__ Nobody important will read what I have written.
__ I never end up following the outline anyway.

Other reason? _____

---

1 2 3 4 5   10. I think that editing and revising writing assignments are important.

☐ I *almost never* edit and revise my writing because: ☐ I *usually don't* edit and revise my writing because: ☐ I *usually do* edit and revise my writing, but when I don't, it's because:

(check all that apply to you)

__ I rarely need to edit and revise anything I write.
__ I'm not very good at editing or revising.
__ I usually don't have time to edit and revise.
__ I usually forget to edit and revise.
__ Editing and revising won't make a difference on my grade.

__ I'm not sure how to edit and revise.
__ Editing and revising are too much trouble.
__ Small writing mistakes don't matter.
__ Nobody important will read what I have written.
__ I usually catch mistakes and correct them as I write.

Other reason? _____

FIGURE 18.3. Deshler, Ellis, and Lenz's (1996) Writing Attitudes Survey. Copyright 1996 by Love Publishing Company. Reprinted by permission.

Capitalization Rules
Capitalize the pronoun I.
Capitalize the first word in a sentence.
Capitalize proper adjectives (e.g., Spanish, French).
Capitalize names of cities, states, and countries (e.g., Baltimore, Minnesota, England).
Capitalize titles when used with names (e.g., President Lincoln, General Eisenhower).
Capitalize street names (e.g., Elm Street, Mai Street).
Capitalize names of organizations (e.g., Peace Corps, Cub Scouts).
Capitalize people's first and last names (e.g., Paul Smith, Omar Bradley).
Capitalize first and important words in book and story titles (e.g., *Alice in Wonderland, Paradise Lost*).
Capitalize family titles when used as names (e.g., Father, Mother).

FIGURE 18.4. Sample content for a criterion-referenced measure of capitalization rules.

to determine whether the skill has or has not been mastered.

Assessing Student Writing Samples

In most instances, teachers have collected numerous samples of written work by their

---

Rewrite the following sentences, applying capital letters correctly.

1. Mark and i went to the Store.

_____

2. have you seen the jacket i left on the couch?

_____

3. check to see if tim will go to the store i went to yesterday.

_____

4. when i last saw you, you were only 3 years old.

_____

FIGURE 18.5. Sample items for a criterion-referenced measure of capitalization rules.

---

students. These samples can be examined to identify the extent to which students apply the writing skills they have been taught. Two approaches for examining writing samples are discussed here: "atomistic" and "holistic."

Atomistic scoring procedures focus on specific skills that are displayed by writers. In these assessments, evaluators focus on students' abilities to spell correctly, apply capitalization and punctuation rules appropriately, use proper syntax, and so forth. One such sample scoring template is found in Figure 18.6. Here several questions are asked about a student's ability in capitalization. The examiner peruses the written passage and then responds to the items on the scale. Note that the capitalization scale corresponds to the information used to help create the criterion-referenced measure depicted earlier in this section (see Figure 18.4). Additional scales can be created for selected writing areas and are demonstrated in Figures 18.7 through 18.9. These samples provide means of evaluating punctuation, ideation, and grammar/usage.

An example of a tool that can be used to assess handwriting is provided in Figure 18.10. Note that Bradley-Johnson and Lesiak (1989) examine not only the student's written product, but also the student's posture, writing position, and so forth. This is in line with Frank Smith's (1982) observation that writing is hard work, and that it is important to observe the amount of physical effort expended by the student. Bradley-Johnson's and Lesiak's scale provides for such an assessment.

Holistic scoring is accomplished by reading the passage and giving an overall rating as to the sophistication of the writing sample. In reality, one never evaluates a scale as a whole without considering skills, because the presence or absence of skills is what affects a rater's judgment. For example, two passages may contain exactly the same words, but the passage with numerous spelling errors or written illegibly is likely to receive a lesser rating because of certain skill deficiencies. An example of a holistic scale for evaluating a writing sample is provided in Figure 18.11. The evaluator reads the passage and compares its features to the criteria associated within a specific point value. Thus, if the passage addresses the

Rating Scale for Assessing Application of Capitalization Rules

Examinee: _____ Passage title/topic: _____

The student capitalizes . . .	Yes	No	No example
. . . the pronoun I.			
. . . the first word in a sentence.			
. . . proper adjectives (e.g., Spanish, French).			
. . . names of cities, states, and countries (e.g., Baltimore, Minnesota, England).			
. . . titles when used with names (e.g., President Lincoln, General Eisenhower).			
. . . street names (e.g., Elm Street, Mai Street).			
. . . names of organizations (e.g., Peace Corps, Cub Scouts).			
. . . people's first and last names (e.g., Paul Smith, Omar Bradley).			
. . . first and important words in book and story titles (e.g., *Alice in Wonderland, Paradise Lost*).			
. . . family titles when used as names (e.g., Father, Mother).			

FIGURE 18.6. Sample dichotomous rating scale for atomistic assessment of capitalization skills.

Rating Scale for Assessing Application of Punctuation Rules

Examinee: _____ Passage title/topic: _____

The student uses . . .	Always	Sometimes	Never	Not observed
. . . a period at the end of a sentence.				
. . . a period after abbreviations (e.g., Mrs., Dr.).				
. . . a period after initals in a name (e.g., Paul P. Leech, E. J. Bryant).				
. . . a question mark at the end of an interrogative sentence.				
. . . an exclamation mark to conclude a sentence showing strong emotions.				
. . . an apostrophe in contractions (e.g., don't, can't).				
. . . a comma between the day of the month and the year (e.g., June 8, 2000).				
. . . a comma to separate a city from a state (e.g., Auburn, Maine).				
. . . a comma to separate words in a series (e.g., Tom, Frank, and I).				
. . . a comma to separate a noun in a direct address (e.g., Paul, I like you).				
. . . a comma to set off a quotation in a sentence (e.g., I said, "Thank you").				
. . . a colon between numbers in expressions of time (e.g., 9:15).				
. . . a colon after the greeting in a business letter (e.g., Dear Sir:).				
. . . a hyphen in a fraction (e.g., one-half).				
. . . a hyphen in a telephone number (e.g., 555-8760).				

FIGURE 18.7. Sample rating scale for atomistic assessment of punctuation skills.

Rating Scale for Assessing Ideation

Examinee: _____ Passage title/topic: _____

Ideation skill	Not at all so	Somewhat so	Very much so
There is a theme or topic that runs throughout the passage.			
Ideas are well developed and easily understood.			
Topics are supported by details.			
Paragraphs reflect an organizational structure that provides for a natural flow of ideas.			
The form of the passage is appropriate for its purpose.			
The language and tone are appropriate for the intended audience.			
Characters, if present, are well defined according to their traits.			
Locations, if present, are well described.			

FIGURE 18.8. Sample rating scale for atomistic assessment of ideation.

topic clearly and appropriately explores ideas, shows some depth and complexity of thought, is effectively organized, is well developed with supporting details, and so forth, the evaluator awards a score of 5, signifying a strong written product.

A hybrid holistic–atomistic scoring procedure is demonstrated in Figure 18.12, which depicts a scoring template that examines a variety of skill areas, yet does so in a holistic fashion. Examiners use their experience with children the writer's age to rate skills along a 5-point continuum. In Figure 18.12, skill areas have been clustered according to

Rating Scale for Grammar and Usage

Examinee: _____ Passage title/topic: _____

In the writing passage, the student. . .	Rating (1 is lowest, 5 is highest)				
• . . . used incorrect tense. • . . . shifted tense within the composition. • . . . made frequent word omissions.	1				
• . . . evidenced some, yet inconsistent, use of subject–verb agreement.		2			
• . . . evidenced consistent use of subject–verb agreement. • . . . demonstrated inconsistencies in use of tense.			3		
• . . . evidenced consistent use of subject–verb agreement. • . . . demonstrated consistent competence in use of tense. • . . . used possessives correctly.				4	
• . . . made few or no grammatical errors.					5

FIGURE 18.9. Sample rating scale for atomistic assessment of grammar and usage skills. From Deshler, Ellis, & Lenz (1996). Copyright 1996 by Love Publishing Company. Adapted by permission.

Obtain samples of the student's handwriting from three different days. For each sample ask the student to copy one of the sentences that follow and write the alphabet in capital letters once each day. Use a different sentence each day. These three samples are used to evaluate the student's handwriting with the checklist.

Sentences to Copy

The quick fox jumps over the lazy brown dog.
The strong zebra quickly jumped over five white boxes.
Just now a breeze made the six pine twigs fall very quickly.

If both manuscript and cursive handwriting are to be evaluated, then six samples will be needed (i.e., three samples of manuscript and three of cursive). These six samples should be taken on at least three separate days.

Student's Name: _____

Dates: Sample 1 _____   Sample 2 _____   Sample 3 _____

Manuscript _____   Cursive _____

Writing Behaviors

Paper position appropriate? yes no
    (Parallel with desk for manuscript, 60° from vertical for cursive)

Pencil grip appropriate? yes no
    (An easy three-finger grasp about one inch from the tip of the pencil)

Posture appropriate? yes no
    (Comfortable and functional writing posture e.g., not stooped over or with head on desk)

If left handed, evidence of "hooking?" yes no
    (If yes, target as a goal to eliminate this problem during instruction)

Formation of Lower Case Letters
(For problem letters, include an example, or examples if more than one, of formation problems next to the corresponding letter.)

a ___   b ___   c ___   d ___   e ___   f ___   g ___   h ___   i ___   j ___
k ___   l ___   m ___   n ___   o ___   p ___   q ___   r ___   s ___   t ___
u ___   v ___   w ___   x ___   y ___   z ___

Scoring Formation Errors:
If a formation problem occurs 2 or 3 times for a letter, instruction on this letter is needed. If a formation problem occurs only once for a letter, additional practice with feedback is needed. If no formation problems are noted for a letter, consider this letter mastered.

Formation of Capital Letters

A ___   B ___   C ___   D ___   E ___   F ___   G ___   H ___   I ___   J ___
K ___   L ___   M ___   N ___   O ___   P ___   Q ___   R ___   S ___   T ___
U ___   V ___   W ___   X ___   Y ___   Z ___

FIGURE 18.10. Sample scale for assessing handwriting skills. From Bradley-Johnson and Lesiak (1989). Copyright 1989 by The Guilford Press. Reprinted by permission.

See Scoring Formation Errors for lower case letters for teaching implications for capital letters.

List any letters which are reversed (e.g., b, d,) or inverted (e.g., n, u):

Size of Writing
(If size is a problem for only some letters, indicate this under the Formation of Letters sections.)

Overall handwriting is:
____ too small
____ too large
____ adequate

Spacing
Between letters there is:
____ too much space
____ not enough space (i.e., crowded)
____ adequate space

Between words there is:
____ too much space
____ not enough space
____ adequate space

Words ending at margins are:
____ crowded
____ adequately spaced

Slant
Overall handwriting slant is:
____ inconsistent
____ reasonably consistent

Rate
Handwriting is done:
____ too quickly
____ too slowly
____ at an adequate pace

Alignment
Writing is:
____ sometimes above the lines
____ sometimes below the lines
____ on the lines

Other
There are:
____ writeovers
____ frequent erasures
____ problems with copying near-point material
____ problems with copying far-point material

FIGURE 18.10. *Continued*

conceptual writing and writing conventions, allowing comparisons to be made across the seven skill areas and across the two clusters.

SUMMARY

In this chapter, we have examined the nature of writing and described how it has been assessed and is currently being evaluated. We have discussed the various elements of writing and their importance to the writing process and subsequent products. We have also provided an overview of writing assessment history, in hopes that knowledge of the contributions of assessment experts will provide us with a broader perspective on our assessment efforts to-

Holistic Rating Scale

Examinee: _____ Passage title/topic: _____

Circle the appropriate rating below.

Score of 6: Superior

- Addresses the topic fully and explores ideas thoughtfully.
- Shows substantial depth, fullness, and complexity of thought.
- Demonstrates clear, focused, unified, and coherent organization.
- Is fully developed and detailed.
- Evidences superior use of vocabulary, syntactic variety, and transition; may have a few minor flaws.
- Void of spelling, capitalization, and spelling errors.
- Written neatly (if handwritten).

Score of 5: Strong

- Addresses the topic clearly and explores ideas.
- Shows some depth and complexity of thought.
- Is effectively organized.
- Is well developed with supporting details.
- Evidences control of vocabulary, syntactic variety, and transition; may have some flaws.
- Almost no spelling, capitalization, and spelling errors.
- Written with adequate legibility (if handwritten).

Score of 4: Competent

- Adequately addresses the topic and explores ideas.
- Shows clarity of thought, but may lack complexity.
- Is organized.
- Is adequately developed, with some detail.
- Demonstrates competency in vocabulary and syntax; may have some flaws.
- Some spelling, capitalization, and spelling errors.
- Written legibly (if handwritten).

Score of 3: Weak

- Some distortion of ideas.
- Shows simplistic thought and lacks complexity.
- Has problems with organization.
- Provides few supportive details; may be underdeveloped.
- Demonstrates considerable flaws in vocabulary and syntax.
- Many spelling, capitalization, and spelling errors.
- Sections of the passage have poor legibility (if handwritten).

Score of 2: Weak

- Demonstrates serious inadequacies in one or more of the areas listed in 3 above.

Score of 1: Incompetent

- Fails in the attempt to discuss the topic.
- Is off topic.
- Is so incompletely developed as to suggest or demonstrate incompetence.
- Is wholly incompetent with regard to spelling, capitalization, and punctuation.
- Is nearly or completely illegible.

FIGURE 18.11. Sample holistic scoring guide. From White (1994). Copyright 1994 by Jossey-Bass. Adapted by permission.

Rating Scale for Assessing Overall Writing Competence

Examinee: _____ Passage title/topic: _____

Conceptual writing	Weak				Strong
Ideation	1	2	3	4	5
Vocabulary	1	2	3	4	5
Syntax	1	2	3	4	5
Subtotal					
Writing conventions	Weak				Strong
Spelling	1	2	3	4	5
Capitalization	1	2	3	4	5
Punctuation	1	2	3	4	5
Legibility	1	2	3	4	5
Subtotal					
Total					

FIGURE 18.12. Sample atomistic–holistic rating scale for assessing student writing skills.

day. Finally, we discussed various methods for examining writing competence. For the most part, this discussion has focused on standardized procedures, although we have included a brief discussion of nonstandardized procedures that can be used with writing samples to validate the results of standardized tests.

REFERENCES

American Educational Research Association (AERA) & National Council on Measurement in Education (NCME). (1954). *Technical recommendations for achievement tests.* Washington, DC: National Education Association.

American Psychological Association (APA). (1954). *Technical recommendations for psychological tests and diagnostic techniques.* Washington, DC: Author.

American Psychological Association (APA). (1966). *Standards for educational and psychological tests and manuals.* Washington, DC: Author.

Arena, J. (1982). *Diagnostic Spelling Potential Test.* Novato, CA: Academic Therapy.

Betts, A. B. (1936). *The prevention and correction of reading difficulties.* Evanston, IL: Row, Peterson.

Bradley-Johnson, S., & Lesiak, J. L. (1989). *Problems in written expression: Assessment and remediation.* New York: Guilford Press.

Brigance, A. H. (1999). *Comprehensive Inventory of Basic Skills.* North Bellerica, MA: Curriculum Associates.

Bryant, B. R. (1999). The dynamics of assessment. In W. M. Bender (Ed.), *Professional issues in learning disabilities* (pp. 395–413). Austin, TX: Pro-Ed.

Bryant, B. R., Patton, J., & Dunn, C. (1991). *Scholastic Abilities Test for Adults.* Austin, TX: Pro-Ed.

Bryant, B. R., & Rivera, D. P. (1997). Educational assessment of mathematics skills and abilities. *Journal of Learning Disabilities, 30*(1), 57–68.

Buros, O. K. (1936). *Educational, psychological, and personality tests of 1933, 1934, and 1935* (Rutgers University Bulletin, Vol. 13, No. 1; Studies in Education, No. 9). New Brunswick, NJ: School of Education, Rutgers University.

Buros, O. K. (1978). Fifty years in testing. In O. K. Buros (Ed.), *The eighth mental measurements yearbook* (pp. 1972–1979). Highland Park, NJ: Gryphon Press.

Deshler, D. D., Ellis, E. S., & Lenz, B. K. (1996). *Teaching adolescents with learning disabilities: Strategies and methods.* Denver: Love.

Freeman, F. N. (1914). *Freeman chart for diagnosing faults in handwriting for grades 2 to 8.* New York: Houghton Mifflin.

Gilliland, A. R., & Jordan, R. H. (1924). *Educational measurements and the classroom teacher.* New York: Century.

Greene, H. A., Jorgensen, A. L., & Gerberich, J. R. (1953). *Measurement and evaluation in the elementary school.* New York: Longmans, Green.

Hammill, D. D., Brown, V. L., & Bryant, B. R. (1992). *A consumer's guide to tests in print* (2nd ed.). Austin, TX: Pro-Ed.

Hammill, D. D., Brown, V. L., Larsen, S. C., & Wiederholt, J. L. (1994). *Test of Adolescent Language* (3rd ed.). Austin, TX: Pro-Ed.

Hammill, D. D., & Bryant, B. R. (1991). Standardized assessment and academic intervention. In H. L. Swanson (Ed.), *Handbook on the assessment of learning disabilities: Theory, research, and practice* (pp. 373–406). Austin, TX: Pro-Ed.

Hammill. D. D., & Bryant, B. R. (1998). *Learning Disabilities Diagnostic Inventory.* Austin, TX: Pro-Ed.

Hammill, D. D., Hresko, W. P., Ammer, G., Cronin, M., & Quinby, S. (1998). *Hammill Multiability Achievement Test.* Austin, TX: Pro-Ed.

Hammill, D. D., & Larsen, S. C. (1988). *Test of Written Language* (3rd ed.). Austin, TX: Pro-Ed.

Hillegas, M. B. (1912). *Hillegas Scale for Measurement of English Composition.* New York: Teachers College Record.

Hresko, W. P., Herron, S. R., & Peak, P. (1996). *Test of Early Written Language* (2nd ed.). Austin, TX: Pro-Ed.

Jordan, A. M. (1953). *Measurement in education.* New York: McGraw-Hill.

Kaufman, A. S., & Kaufman, N. L. (1985). *Kaufman Test of Educational Achievement.* Circle Pines, MN: American Guidance Service.

Kelley, T. L., Ruch, G. H., & Terman, L. L. (1923). *Stanford Achievement Test.* Yonkers, NY: World.

Kirk, S. A. (1962). *Educating exceptional children.* Boston: Houghton Mifflin.

Larsen, S. C., Hammill, D. D., & Moats, L. (2000). *Test of Written Spelling* (4th ed.). Austin, TX: Pro-Ed.

Maddox, T. (2003). *Tests* (5th ed). Austin, TX: Pro-Ed.

Markwardt, F. C. (1989). *Peabody Individual Achievement Test—Revised.* Circle Pines, MN: American Guidance Service.

McGhee, R., Bryant, B. R., Larsen, S. C., & Rivera, D. M. (1995). *Test of Written Expression.* Austin, TX: Pro-Ed.

McLoughlin, J., & Lewis, R. B. (1990). *Assessing special students.* Columbus, OH: Merrill.

McMillan, J. (1997). *Classroom assessment.* Boston: Allyn & Bacon.

Myklebust, H. (1965). *Picture Story Language Test.* New York: Grune & Stratton.

Newcomer, P. (2001). *Diagnostic Achievement Battery* (3rd ed.). Austin, TX: Pro-Ed.

Newcomer, P., & Bryant, B. R. (1992). *Diagnostic Achievement Test for Adolescents* (2nd ed.). Austin, TX: Pro-Ed.

Paulson, F. L., Paulson, P. R., & Meyer, C. A. (1991). What makes a portfolio and portfolio? *Educational Leadership, 48*(5), 60–63.

Psychological Corporation. (1983). *Basic Achievement Skills Individual Ccreener.* San Antonio, TX: Author.

Psychological Corporation. (1992). *Wechsler Individual Achievement Test.* San Antonio, TX: Author.

Rivera, D. P., & Smith, D. D. (1996). *Teaching students with learning and behavior problems.* Boston: Allyn & Bacon.

Ruch, G. M., & Stoddard, G. D. (1927). *Tests and measurements in high school instruction.* Chicago: World.

Salvia, J., & Ysseldyke, J. E. (1998). *Assessment* (7th ed.). Boston: Houghton Mifflin.

Smith, F. (1982). *Writing and the writer.* New York: Holt, Rinehart, & Winston.

Smith, H. L., & Wright, W. W. (1928). *Tests and measurements.* New York: Silver, Burdett.

Sweetland, R. C., & Keyser, D. J. (1986). *Tests* (2nd ed.). Austin, TX: Pro-Ed.

Swicegood, P. (1994). Portfolio-based assessment practices. *Intervention in School and Clinic, 30*(1), 6–15.

Taylor, R. L. (2003). *Assessment of exceptional student.* Boston: Allyn & Bacon.

Thorndike, E. L. (1904). *An introduction to the theory of mental and social measurements.* New York: Teachers College, Columbia University.

Thorndike, E. L. (1910). *Thorndike Scale for Handwriting of Children.* New York: Teachers College, Columbia University.

Thorndike, E. L. (1921). *The teacher's word book.* New York: Teachers College, Columbia University.

Thorndike, E. L. (1929). *Elementary principles of education.* New York: Macmillan.

Thorndike, R. L., & Hagen, E. (1955). *Measurement and evaluation in psychology and education.* New York: Wiley.

Tiegs, E. W. (1931). *Tests and measurement for teachers.* Cambridge, MA: Riverside Press.

Valencia, S. (1990). A portfolio approach to classroom reading assessment: The whys, whats, and hows. *The Reading Teacher, 43,* 338–340.

White, E. M. (1994). *Teaching and assessing writing* (2nd ed.). San Francisco: Jossey-Bass.

Wilkinson, G. (1993). *Wide Range Achievement Test* (3rd ed.). Wilmington, DE: Wide Range.

Wolf, K. (1991). The school teacher's portfolio: Issues I design, implementation, and evaluation. *Phi Delta Kappan, 73*(2), 130–136.

Woodcock, R. W., & Johnson, M. (1989). *Woodcock–Johnson Psycho-Educational Battery—Revised.* Chicago: Riverside.

19

Clinical Assessment of Children's Academic Achievement

This chapter focuses primarily on individually administered, norm-referenced measures known as "screeners" or "broad-band measures" of academic achievement. Screeners of academic achievement that assess multiple domains are useful for a myriad of purposes. Since the enactment of Public Law (PL) 94-142, the usage of such instruments has steadily increased. More specifically, the usage of broad-band achievement measures has been central in the diagnosis of learning disabilities (Kamphaus, Slotkin, & DeVincentis, 1990).

This chapter covers academic achievement screeners; specific instruments and their purposes are described. Not all tests of this nature are covered in this text, and exclusion of a test is not a comment on its quality. Instruments have been selected for discussion primarily according to both their frequency of use and their technical adequacy.

A NOTE ON THE DIFFERENCE BETWEEN ACADEMIC ACHIEVEMENT SCREENERS AND DIAGNOSTIC TESTS

It is sometimes difficult to classify the many academic achievement testing selections that are available. Generally speaking, there are two classes of achievement tests: They exist along a continuum from screeners or broad-band measures of achievement to diagnostic tests. Screeners survey a broad range of content areas such as mathematics, reading, and writing, at a wide range of skill levels. Ordinarily, no one content area is probed in depth. However, achievement screeners can be useful in identifying general weak areas for individuals. Once a weak area is identified, skilled psychologists will follow up with diagnostic testing to address that weak area. For example, if a child scores poorly on the Reading Recognition subtest of the Peabody Individual Achievement Test—Revised (PIAT-R), a diagnostic achievement test such as the Woodcock Reading Mastery Test—Revised (WRMT-R) would be administered for the purpose of identifying more specifically which discrete skill or skills are deficient. A caveat is in order here: It is emphasized that screening measures alone are not sufficient to form definitive diagnoses, but that they are considered to be useful preliminary and/or ancillary measures in the assessment process. The following sections cover achievement tests that are considered screeners or broad-band measures.

WIDE RANGE ACHIEVEMENT TEST—3

The Wide Range Achievement Test—3 (WRAT-3; Wilkinson, 1993) is the latest revision of the original WRAT, which was published in 1936 as an adjunct to the Wechsler–Bellevue scales. The WRAT-3 was developed to assess the "codes which are needed to learn the basic skills of reading, spelling, and arithmetic" (Wilkinson, 1993, p. 10). According to Cohen and Spenciner (1998), the precise definition of the word "codes" is unclear, although it is generally assumed that it refers to basic academic skills that are essential in reading, spelling, and arithmetic. This basic tenet of the WRAT-3 has not been changed since its original publication over 60 years ago. Also, many of the items found on the WRAT-3 were first constructed for previous editions of the test. For these reasons, this test has been criticized as being outdated. There is also substantial confusion regarding the name of the test and the skills that it purports to measure. At first glance, a test consumer may assume that the name "Wide Range" implies that a wide range of skills is assessed. However, the name refers to the fact that a wide range of ages is covered (5 years, 0 months to 74 years, 11 months). Furthermore, the names of the subtests, Reading, Spelling, and Arithmetic, may imply that a broad range of skills is assessed within each of these areas. A closer examination of the rationale and descriptions in the test manual, however, indicates that this is not the case.

Administration and Scoring

The WRAT-3 is an individually administered test of academic skills. It consists of two forms, Blue and Tan, with the same number of items for each subtest per form. In addition, both the Blue and Tan forms can be administered (i.e., Combined form). The test consists of three subtests:

1. *Reading.* This subtest is essentially a test of word recognition alone, as opposed to a test that measures more than one reading skill. The individual is required to recognize and name 15 letters and 42 words as presented on a card. Ten seconds are allowed for the individual to respond to each item.

2. *Spelling.* This subtest is a test of written encoding that requires an individual to write his or her name and to write letters (15 items) and words (40 items) from dictation. Fifteen seconds are allowed per item.

3. *Arithmetic.* The Arithmetic subtest is basically a test of computation. The subtest consists of an untimed Oral Arithmetic section in which the examinee is required to read numbers and solve problems that are dictated (15 items), and a timed Written Arithmetic section in which the examinee is required to perform arithmetic computations (40 items) within a 15-minute time limit.

Items are scored as correct or incorrect, and set basal and ceiling rules are used to determine the appropriate number of items to administer. Computerized scoring is available. The total test administration time ranges from 15 to 30 minutes, and the test is relatively quick and simple to score. Raw scores can be converted to standard scores having a mean of 100 and a standard deviation of 15. Scores for each subtest can be computed for the Blue, Tan, and Combined forms. Profile/Analysis forms may be used to display scores graphically. In addition, a score classification scheme is presented in the manual: Very Superior (130 and up), Superior (120–129), High Average (110–119), Average (90–109), Low Average (80–89), Borderline (70–79), and Deficient (69 and below).

Standardization

The standardization sample of the WRAT-3 consisted of 4,433 individuals between the ages of 5 years, 0 months and 74 years, 11 months. The norming process took place during 1992 and 1993, and the sample was selected to approximate 1990 U.S. Census data. The sample was stratified according to variables of age, gender, geographic region, ethnicity, and socioeconomic level (as defined by occupational category). It is unclear how many individuals with disabilities, if any, were included in the sample. Overall, it appears that the obtained normative sample resembles the U.S. population as a whole.

Reliability

Internal-consistency estimates for the WRAT-3 were determined by using coefficient alpha for each test across the standardization sample and for each form (Blue, Tan, and Combined). For the Combined form of the Reading subtest, coefficients ranged from .91 to .97, with a median of .95. On the Blue form, the values ranged from .88 to .95, with a median of .91. On the Tan form, the coefficients ranged from .88 to .94, with a median of .90. For the Combined form of the Spelling subtest, the coefficients ranged from .89 to .97, with a median of .95. On the Blue form, the values ranged from .83 to .95, with a median of .91. On the Tan form, the coefficients ranged from .83 to .94, with a median of .89. On the Combined form of the Arithmetic subtest, the coefficients ranged from .72 to .96, with a median of .92. On the Blue form, the values ranged from .69 to .82, with a median of .86. On the Tan form, the coefficients ranged from .70 to .92, with a median of .85. Alternate-form correlations were also computed to compare the Blue and Tan forms of the WRAT-3. On Reading, correlations ranged from .87 to .99, with a median of .92. Spelling correlations ranged from .86 to .99, with a median of .93; Arithmetic correlations ranged from .82 to .99, with a median of .89. Furthermore, the stability of the WRAT-3 was assessed via test–retest reliability, with an average of 37.4 days in between test administrations, for a sample of 142 individuals between the ages of 6 and 16 years for each form. These coefficients ranged from .91 to .98 overall, with a range of .96 to .98 for Reading, .93 to .96 for Spelling, and .91 to .94 for Arithmetic. Altogether, the presented reliability estimates for the WRAT-3 appear to be adequate.

Validity

Content and construct validity are addressed in the WRAT-3 manual. In terms of content validity, it is reemphasized that the test is intended to measure basic academic skills—specifically, word recognition, spelling from dictation, and arithmetic computation. However, evidence of adequate content validity is not well delineated. Wilkinson (1993) claims that the subtests of the WRAT-3 measure the domains of "all the words in the English language for reading and spelling and the arithmetic compu-

tation problems taught in grades Kindergarten through high school for arithmetic" (p. 176). The Rasch statistic of item separation was used to indicate whether or not adequate numbers of items at varying levels of difficulty were chosen for the test. However, item separation does not directly measure the content validity of a domain. Therefore, it appears that more evidence of content validity is in order.

Construct validity is presented in terms of developmental skills, intercorrelations of the WRAT-3 tests, and relationships with measures of intelligence and achievement. Intercorrelations suggest that the subtests of the WRAT-3 are moderately to highly related to one another. Median intercorrelations were .87, .66, and .70, respectively, for Reading and Spelling, Reading and Arithmetic, and Spelling and Arithmetic. WRAT-3 Combined form scores were correlated with results on the Weschler Intelligence Scale for Children—Third Edition (WISC-III) for a sample of 100 children ages 6–16 years. The WISC-III Verbal IQ scores correlated .70, .69, and .71, respectively, with the WRAT-3 Combined scores on Reading, Spelling, and Arithmetic. WISC-III Performance IQ scores correlated .52, .53, and .67, respectively, with the WRAT-3 Combined scores on Reading, Spelling, and Arithmetic. The Full Scale IQ scores correlated .66, .66, and .73, respectively, with the WRAT-3 Combined scores on Reading, Spelling, and Arithmetic. Correlations for the WRAT-3 Combined scores and WISC-III subtests are also presented: Picture Completion (Reading $r = .47$, Spelling $r = .46$, Arithmetic $r = .49$); Information (Reading $r = .71$, Spelling $r = .63$, Arithmetic $r = .66$); Coding (Reading $r = .44$, Spelling $r = .55$, Arithmetic $r = .54$); Similarities (Reading $r = .68$, Spelling $r = .60$, Arithmetic $r = .66$); Picture Arrangement (Reading $r = .33$, Spelling $r = .31$, Arithmetic $r = .48$); Arithmetic (Reading $r = .54$, Spelling $r = .59$, Arithmetic $r = .66$); Block Design (Reading $r = .41$, Spelling $r = .42$, Arithmetic $r = .64$); Vocabulary (Reading $r = .64$, Spelling $r = .64$, Arithmetic $r = .58$); Object Assembly (Reading $r = .37$, Spelling $r = .30$, Arithmetic $r = .45$); Comprehension (Reading $r = .53$, Spelling $r = .60$, Arithmetic $r = .59$); and Digit Span (Reading $r = .58$, Spelling $r = .64$, Arithmetic $r = .52$).

In a separate study, Wechsler Adult Intelligence Scale—Revised (WAIS-R) scores were correlated with WRAT-3 scores for a sample of 40 adolescents and adults ages 16–63 years. The WAIS-R Verbal IQ scores correlated .63, .59, and .53, respectively, with the WRAT-3 Combined scores on Reading, Spelling, and Arithmetic. WAIS-R Performance IQ scores correlated .31, .28, and .54, respectively, with the WRAT-3 Combined scores on Reading, Spelling, and Arithmetic. WAIS-R Full Scale IQ scores correlated .53, .49, and .60, respectively, with the WRAT-3 Combined scores on Reading, Spelling, and Arithmetic. Correlations for the WRAT-3 Combined scores and WAIS-R subtests are also presented: Picture Completion (Reading $r = .35$, Spelling $r = .19$, Arithmetic $r = .26$); Information (Reading $r = .52$, Spelling $r = .44$, Arithmetic $r = .34$); Similarities (Reading $r = .47$, Spelling $r = .52$, Arithmetic $r = .46$); Picture Arrangement (Reading $r = .39$, Spelling $r = .42$, Arithmetic $r = .43$); Arithmetic (Reading $r = .36$, Spelling $r = .36$, Arithmetic $r = .46$); Block Design (Reading $r = .32$, Spelling $r = .32$, Arithmetic $r = .49$); Vocabulary (Reading $r = .62$, Spelling $r = .58$, Arithmetic $r = .46$); Object Assembly (Reading $r = .05$, Spelling $r = .05$, Arithmetic $r = .25$); Comprehension (Reading $r = .48$, Spelling $r = .43$, Arithmetic $r = .46$); Digit Symbol (Reading $r = .09$, Spelling $r = .24$, Arithmetic $r = .48$); and Digit Span (Reading $r = .45$, Spelling $r = .41$, Arithmetic $r = .35$).

Relationships between the WRAT-3 and the WRAT-R are also presented for a sample of 77 children. Each form of the WRAT-3 was administered on average 82 days after the WRAT-R was given. As a result, correlations between Reading on the WRAT-3 and the WRAT-R ranged from .90 to .95; correlations between Spelling on the WRAT-3 and the WRAT-R ranged from .96 to .99; and correlations between Arithmetic on the WRAT-3 and the WRAT-R ranged from .79 to .85. Correlations of the WRAT-3 Combined form with standardized group achievement tests—for example, the California Test of Basic Skills, 4th edition (CTBS-4), the California Achievement Test Form E (CAT), and the Stanford Achievement Test (SAT)—are also presented. First, WRAT-3 and CTBS-4 scores were correlated for a sample of 46 children ages 8–16 years. The WRAT-3

Reading subtest correlated .69 with Total Reading on the CTBS-4; WRAT-3 Spelling correlated .84 with CTBS-4 Spelling; and WRAT-3 Arithmetic correlated .79 with Total Math on the CTBS-4. Next, scores on the WRAT-3 and the CAT were correlated for a sample of 49 children ages 8–16 years. Results yielded correlations of .72 between WRAT-3 Reading and CAT Total Reading, .77 between WRAT-3 Spelling and CAT Total Spelling, and .41 between WRAT-3 Arithmetic and CAT Total Math. Finally, scores on the WRAT-3 and the SAT were correlated for a sample of 31 children ranging in age from 9 to 15 years. WRAT-3 Reading correlated .87 with SAT Total Reading; WRAT-3 Spelling correlated .76 with SAT Spelling; and WRAT-3 Arithmetic correlated .81 with SAT Total Math. Discriminant analysis was used to determine the utility of the WRAT-3 in special education placement. Of a sample of 222 persons, the WRAT-3 grouped gifted children at 85% accuracy, children with learning disabilities at 72% accuracy, children described as "educable mentally handicapped" (i.e., children with mild mental retardation) at 83% accuracy, and "normal" children at 56% accuracy. As a result, the test developer purports that the WRAT-3 can be a useful tool in making special education placement decisions, although it should not be the only criterion utilized.

Independent validity investigations have been done with the WRAT-3. Vance and Fuller (1995) examined the validity of the WRAT-3 in relationship to the WISC-III for a sample of 60 children ages 6 years, 0 months to 15 years, 8 months who were referred for special education. WRAT-3 Reading correlated with WISC-III Verbal IQ, Performance IQ, and Full Scale IQ .71, .62, and .72, respectively. WRAT-3 Spelling correlated with WISC-III Verbal, Performance, and Full Scale IQ .66, .59, and .68, respectively. Finally, WRAT-3 Arithmetic correlated with Verbal, Performance, and Full Scale IQ .79, .73, and .82, respectively. Smith, Smith, and Smithson (1995) examined the relationship between the WRAT-3 and the WISC-III for a sample of 37 rural children ages 6–16 years who were referred for psychoeducational evaluation. Combined Reading scores on the WRAT-3 correlated with WISC-III Verbal, Performance, and Full Scale IQ .59, .45, and .59, respectively. Combined Spelling scores on the WRAT-3 correlated with WISC-III Verbal, Performance, and Full Scale IQ .51, .51, and .58, respectively. Combined Arithmetic scores on the WRAT-3 correlated with WISC-III Verbal, Performance, and Full Scale IQ .66, .48, and .66, respectively. Although most of the data pertaining to construct validity of the WRAT-3 appear adequate, there are problems pertaining to the definition of the construct itself, as well as with the limited variety of instruments and the limited sample sizes upon which the validity evidence is based.

Summary

The WRAT-3 has a long history, as well as an ample number of users. Its brevity and ease of use make it a popular instrument. However, it does appear to be riddled with numerous problems. First, the terminology used throughout the test (i.e., Reading, Spelling, Arithmetic, and Wide Range) can be problematic. Such terms may imply to some test consumers that the WRAT-3 covers a wide array of skills, which it clearly does not. Instead, it assesses three discrete skills: word recognition, spelling from dictation, and arithmetic computation. Although these skills are outlined in the manual, the test would benefit from revised terminology that better reflects the test content. Also, it should be noted that the WRAT-3 differs from many other screeners of academic achievement in that it assesses considerably fewer skills. In a sense, the WRAT-3 could be considered a "screener of a screener." Clinicians should take care to see that the WRAT-3 is used for screening purposes only. Mabry (1995) criticizes the WRAT-3 for its obsolescence, test content, lack of underlying rationale and philosophy, and insufficient evidence of validity, among other concerns. Cohen and Spenciner (1998) suggest that although the WRAT-3 possesses adequate norms and reliability, that this test should be used solely as a "screening instrument, if at all" (p. 148).

WOODCOCK–McGREW–WERDER MINI-BATTERY OF ACHIEVEMENT

The Woodcock–McGrew–Werder Mini-Battery of Achievement (MBA; Woodcock, McGrew, & Werder, 1994) is a brief academic achievement screening measure that may be used with children and adults from 4 to 95 years of age. This test is designed to expand upon content that is generally found in brief achievement screening measures such as the WRAT-3. Specifically, the MBA contains tests of reading, mathematics, writing, and general knowledge. These tests are highly similar in format and content to those of the Woodcock–Johnson Psycho-Educational Battery—Revised Tests of Achievement (WJ-R ACH), discussed later in this chapter. In fact, WJ-R ACH counterparts for the MBA are presented in the manual, and MBA items were drawn from WJ-R ACH item banks. Each of the MBA tests covers more than one skill, thus providing "more extensive coverage of basic and applied skills than any other brief achievement battery" (p. 219). The authors of the MBA suggest several applications of this instrument: screening for special education referrals; intake screenings in pediatric, geriatric, psychological, medical, and other clinical settings; hiring and job placement decisions; initial screenings of new students in educational settings; and research uses. However, the authors of this instrument also point out that the MBA should be not used without corroborating information to make placement or treatment decisions. Instead, it is recommended that MBA results be utilized to identify potential need for more in-depth evaluations, using instruments such as the WJ-R (Woodcock & Johnson, 1989).

Administration and Scoring

The MBA is an individually administered test of basic academic skills and knowledge designed for use with children and adults ages 4 through 95 years. It consists of a single form and four tests that can be given separately or in any combination. The MBA consists of four subtests presented in an easel format:

1. *Reading.* This test contains three parts. Part A, Identification, has 28 items that assess reading recognition skills. The individual is required to recognize and name letters and words as presented by the examiner. Part B, Vocabulary, has 22 items that assess skills in reading words and supplying

correct meanings. The individual is required to read a stimulus word and supply a word that is opposite in meaning. Part C, Comprehension, consists of 23 items. The individual is required to point to a picture that describes a written phrase, and/or to read passages and identify a missing word. All items on the Reading test are presented in order of difficulty and are not timed. The counterpart for the MBA Reading test is the Broad Reading Cluster of the WJ-R ACH.

2. *Writing*. This test consists of two parts. Part A, Dictation, measures skills in writing responses to questions that involve knowledge of letters, spelling, capitalization, punctuation, and usage. This part contains 32 items and is administered in a traditional spelling test format with the provided MBA Worksheet. Part B, Proofreading, contains 26 items. This task is designed to assess skills in identifying errors in writing, requiring the individual both to identify errors and to specify how errors should be corrected in printed passages as presented by the examiner. Items on the Writing test are organized according to level of difficulty and are not timed. The counterpart for the MBA Writing test is the Basic Writing Skills Cluster on the WJ-R ACH.

3. *Mathematics*. The Mathematics test also consists of two sections. Part A, Calculation, has 29 items intended to measure basic mathematical computations such as addition, subtraction, multiplication, and division. Geometry, trigonometry, and calculus problems are also included. The items are completed on the MBA Worksheet. Part B, Reasoning and Concepts, has 50 items that measure skills in analyzing and solving problems, as well as knowledge of mathematical concepts and terminology. Unlike Calculation, this section requires that the individual decide which mathematical operations to use and which information to include in solving the problems. Examinees may use scratch paper if needed. Items on the Mathematics test are arranged in order of difficulty and are not timed. The counterpart of the MBA Mathematics test is the WJ-R ACH Broad Mathematics Cluster.

4. *Factual Knowledge*. This test assesses knowledge of social studies, science, and the humanities (literature, music, and art). Factual Knowledge contains 59 items that are arranged according to difficulty level, and

the test is not timed. The counterpart of the MBA Factual Knowledge test is the WJ-R ACH Broad Knowledge Cluster.

The four MBA subtests can be given separately or in any combination. The scores from the Reading, Writing, and Mathematics subtests are combined into a Basic Skills Cluster score as an indicator of general overall achievement. The counterpart of the MBA Basic Skills Cluster is the Skills Cluster on the WJ-R ACH. Items are scored as correct or incorrect, and scores should be written on the test record. Set basal and ceiling rules are used to determine the appropriate number of items to administer. The total test administration time is approximately 30 minutes. The MBA includes a computerized program that calculates and reports standard scores having a mean of 100 and a standard deviation of 15, as well as other scores based on entered raw scores. This program also generates a brief narrative report. Hand scoring of the MBA is not an option for anything other than raw scores.

Standardization

The standardization sample of the MBA consisted of 6,026 individuals between the ages of 4 and 95 years. The norming data were collected from 1986 to 1988 and are based on data from a common norming sample with the WJ-R. The sample was stratified according to variables of age, gender, geographic region, race, community size, origin (Hispanic vs. non-Hispanic), funding of college/university (public vs. private), type of college/university (university or 4-year college vs. 2-year college), distribution of adult occupation in the community, distribution of adult occupational status in the community (e.g., employed vs. unemployed), and distribution of adult education in the community. It is unclear whether or not individuals with disabilities were included in the sample. The norming sample was selected to approximate 1980 U.S. Census data. Descriptive standardization data are adequately presented in the MBA manual, and the authors refer the test consumer to the normative information presented in the WJ-R. A more detailed description of norms is provided in the section of this chapter on the WJ-R ACH. Overall, it appears that the obtained normative sample for the MBA closely resembles the U.S. population of 1980. However, these norms are relatively old, especially for a test published in 1994. Kamphaus (1993) suggests a rule of thumb that if the standardization sample is 10 or more years old, the examiner should be cautious about the accuracy of the norms for current use.

Reliability

Internal-consistency reliability coefficients for the MBA were calculated for the four tests as well as the Basic Skills Cluster for individuals ages 5 through 79 years, using the split-half method. It is unclear why data are presented only for individuals in this age range from the standardization sample. Across a sample of 2,675 individuals ages 5–79, reliability coefficients for the Reading test ranged from .88 to .98, with a median of .94. For a sample of 2,666 individuals ages 5–79, the Writing test reliability coefficients ranged from .79 to .97, with a median of .92. For a sample of 2,673 individuals ages 5–79, the Mathematics test reliability coefficients ranged from .70 to .98, with a median of .93. Reliability coefficients for the Factual Knowledge test ranged from .80 to .96, with a median of .87, for a sample of 2,854 individuals ages 5–79. Lastly, the Basic Skills Cluster had reliability coefficients ranging from .90 to .98, with a median of .93, for a sample of 2,838 individuals ages 5–79. Furthermore, the stability of the MBA was assessed via test–retest reliability, with an interval of 1 week separating the two administrations for three samples. For a sample of 52 sixth-grade students, test–retest reliability coefficients were .89 for Reading, .85 for Writing, .86 for Mathematics, .88 for Factual Knowledge, and .96 for the Basic Skills Cluster. In a sample of 53 college students, test–retest reliability coefficients were .86 for Reading, .93 for Writing, .90 for Mathematics, .88 for Factual Knowledge, and .94 for the Basic Skills Cluster. In a sample of 56 adults, test–retest reliability coefficients were .90 for Reading, .94 for Writing, .89 for Mathematics, .89 for Factual Knowledge, and .97 for the Basic Skills Cluster. Overall, the presented reliability estimates for the MBA appear to be ade-

quate. However, internal-consistency estimates would have been more informative if the entire standardization sample had been used, and additional studies of stability with larger samples and longer administration intervals would be useful.

Validity

Content, concurrent, and construct validity are addressed in the MBA manual (Woodcock et al., 1994). In terms of content validity, it is emphasized that the items included in the MBA were chosen for the purpose of offering a brief but extensive sampling of knowledge and basic academic skills. Items were also selected to cover a wide range of ability levels. Though this explanation makes sense, more information pertaining to content validity would be helpful.

Concurrent validity studies were conducted with other popular tests of achievement, using three different samples. Selected correlations are presented here. For a sample of 55 sixth-grade students, MBA Reading test scores correlated .79 with WJ-R ACH Broad Reading, .75 with Kaufman Test of Educational Achievement (K-TEA) Brief Form Reading, .82 with PIAT-R Total Reading, and .64 with WRAT-R Reading. MBA Writing test scores correlated .53 with WJ-R ACH Broad Written Language, .62 with K-TEA Brief Form Spelling, .64 with PIAT-R Written Language Composite, and .57 with WRAT-R Spelling. MBA Mathematics test scores correlated .72 with WJ-R ACH Broad Mathematics, .67 with K-TEA Brief Form Mathematics, .62 with PIAT-R Mathematics, and .66 with WRAT-R Arithmetic. MBA Factual Knowledge test scores correlated .74 with WJ-R ACH Broad Knowledge and .64 with PIAT-R General Information. The MBA Basic Skills Cluster correlated .82 with the WJ-R ACH Skills Cluster. For a sample of 58 college students, MBA Reading test scores correlated .70 with WJ-R ACH Broad Reading, .60 with K-TEA Brief Form Reading, .68 with PIAT-R Total Reading, and .66 with WRAT-R Reading. MBA Writing test scores correlated .74 with WJ-R ACH Broad Written Language, .80 with K-TEA Brief Form Spelling, .70 with PIAT-R Written Language Composite, and .67 with WRAT-R Spelling. MBA Mathematics test scores correlated

.84 with WJ-R ACH Broad Mathematics, .75 with K-TEA Brief Form Mathematics, .82 with PIAT-R Mathematics, and .72 with WRAT-R Arithmetic. MBA Factual Knowledge test scores correlated .77 with WJ-R ACH Broad Knowledge and .53 with PIAT-R General Information. The MBA Basic Skills Cluster correlated .85 with the WJ-R ACH Skills Cluster. In a sample of 59 adults, MBA Reading test scores correlated .75 with WJ-R ACH Broad Reading, .70 with K-TEA Brief Form Reading, .73 with PIAT-R Total Reading, and .70 with WRAT-R Reading. MBA Writing test scores correlated .78 with WJ-R ACH Broad Written Language, .76 with K-TEA Brief Form Spelling, .59 with PIAT-R Written Language Composite, and .78 with WRAT-R Spelling. MBA Mathematics test scores correlated .88 with WJ-R ACH Broad Mathematics, .76 with K-TEA Brief Form Mathematics, .83 with PIAT-R Mathematics, and .75 with WRAT-R Arithmetic. MBA Factual Knowledge test scores correlated .77 with WJ-R ACH Broad Knowledge and .69 with PIAT-R General Information. The MBA Basic Skills Cluster correlated .88 with the WJ-R ACH Skills Cluster.

Furthermore, MBA subtest and Basic Skills Cluster intercorrelation patterns for individuals between the ages of 5 and 79 are reported for the purpose of contributing evidence for construct validity. The median correlations were as follows: Reading with Writing ($r = .80$), Reading with Mathematics ($r = .66$), Reading with Factual Knowledge ($r = .74$), Writing with Mathematics ($r = .65$), Mathematics with Factual Knowledge ($r = .68$), Writing with Factual Knowledge ($r = .68$), Basic Skills Cluster with Reading ($r = .90$), Basic Skills Cluster with Writing ($r = .93$), Basic Skills Cluster with Mathematics ($r = .82$), and Basic Skills Cluster with Factual Knowledge ($r = .76$). The data show that the four MBA subtests measure different but related academic skills. No studies relating the MBA to measures of intelligence are presented. Altogether, there needs to be more clarification pertaining to content and construct validity. Moreover, despite the fact that the data pertaining to concurrent validity appear adequate, studies having a wider variety of instruments and increased sample sizes would enhance claims of validation.

Summary

The MBA is a brief screening measure of academic achievement. It appears to be technically adequate in some respects. However, more recent norms, as well as enhanced reliability and validity studies, would certainly be beneficial. Unfortunately, little independent research has been conducted on the MBA. The content of the MBA covers a broader range of skills than do other brief screeners of achievement (such as the WRAT-3), but it still might be considered a "screener of a screener," as there are yet more comprehensive screening measures of academic achievement. The instrument appears to be quick and easy to use, has close ties with the WJ-R, and comes with a computerized scoring program. Michael (1998) concluded in a review of the MBA that "this reviewer would consider the MBA to be a practical measure requiring a relatively short time (about 30 minutes) to administer and in light of the supporting reliability and validity data would recommend its use" (p. 1142). As always, clinicians should take care to use the MBA for the purposes for which it was intended.

DIFFERENTIAL ABILITY SCALES SCHOOL ACHIEVEMENT TESTS

The Differential Ability Scales School Achievement Tests (DAS ACH; Elliott, 1990a, 1990b) is a portion of the DAS, a comprehensive instrument designed to assess cognitive ability and achievement. Although the DAS covers an age range of 2 years, 6 months to 17 years, 11 months overall, the DAS ACH tests are designed to cover an age range of 6 years, 0 months to 17 years, 11 months. The DAS ACH consists of three tests that measure the basic skills of word reading, spelling, and arithmetic, similar to the WRAT-3. An advantage of the DAS ACH battery is that it shares a common normative sample with the DAS Cognitive battery, thus enhancing ability–achievement comparisons. The test author cautions against misuse of the DAS ACH, stating that these tests should not be considered as measures of general achievement in their respective areas.

Administration and Scoring

The DAS ACH is an untimed, individually administered test of basic academic skills. It consists of three subtests:

1. *Basic Number Skills*. This test consists of a total of 48 items and is generally administered to children ages 6 years, 0 months to 17 years, 11 months. Skills assessed include the recognition and naming of numbers, as well as computation using the four basic arithmetic operations with whole numbers, fractions, decimals, and percentages. Items are presented on the Basic Number Skills worksheet. Low scores on this test may indicate that a child has poor understanding of mathematical operations or numeration, and/or poor attention or motivation.

2. *Spelling*. Like Basic Number Skills, Spelling is administered to children ages 6 years, 0 months to 17 years, 11 months. This 70-item test assesses knowledge and recall of spellings by requiring a child to write words that are dictated to him or her onto the Spelling worksheet. Low scores on the Spelling test may indicate poor knowledge of phonological skills, poor auditory and/or visual memory, or poor auditory discrimination.

3. *Word Reading*. The usual age range for administering Word Reading is 6 years, 0 months to 17 years, 11 months, but on occasion, this test is administered to children as young as 5 years, 0 months. On this 90-item test, word recognition is assessed by having the individual read aloud printed words as presented on the Word Reading card. Low scores on this test may reflect difficulties similar to those described for Spelling.

The DAS ACH tests may be given separately or in any combination desired. Items on each of these tests are scored as correct or incorrect, and set basal and ceiling rules are used to determine the appropriate number of items to administer. The total test administration time is about 15–25 minutes, and the test is relatively simple to score. Raw scores for each test are first converted to "Ability scores," and these can be further converted to standard scores having a mean of 100 and a standard deviation of 15.

Computerized scoring is also available. Furthermore, each of these tests can be subjected to a performance analysis. Performance analysis calls for the clinician to examine the child's responses for the purpose of identifying strengths and weaknesses in terms of more discrete skills. For example, discrete academic skills presented in the Basic Number Skills subtest include multiplying simple fractions and naming a two-digit number. Performance analysis guidelines are presented on the test record forms as well as in the manual. The DAS ACH includes guidelines for testing children with disabilities and children who are not proficient in English. Instructions and suggestions for computing ability–achievement discrepancies are presented as well.

Standardization

The standardization sample for the DAS (and hence for the DAS ACH) consisted of 3,475 children, including 175 children for each 6-month interval for ages 2 years, 6 months to 4 years, 11 months, and 200 children for each 1-year interval for ages 5 years, 0 months to 17 years, 11 months. The standardization process took place from 1987 to 1989, and the sample was selected to approximate U.S. census data as presented in the March 1988 *Current Population Survey*. The sample was stratified according to variables of age, gender, geographic region, race/ethnicity, socioeconomic status (as defined by educational level of parents or guardians), and educational preschool enrollment. Students enrolled in special education classes, with the exclusion of children with severe disabilities, were also included in the normative sample. Overall, it appears that the obtained normative sample for the DAS is representative of the U.S. population.

Reliability

Internal-consistency reliabilities based on item response theory were computed for the DAS ACH, using individuals ages 6 years, 0 months to 17 years, 11 months from the standardization sample. Groups of 200 cases at each 1-year age level were used in the calculations ($n = 2,400$). These coefficients ranged from .82 to .90, with a mean of .87, for Basic Number Skills; .91 to .94, with a mean of .92, for Spelling; and .88 to .95, with a mean of .92, for Word Reading. In addition, the coefficient was computed as .68 for children ages 5 years, 0 months to 5 years, 11 months ($n = 200$) for Word Reading. Indicators of test–retest reliability were also computed. The interval separating the test administrations spanned 2–6 weeks. For children ages 5 years, 9 months to 6 years, 11 months ($n = 67$), test–retest reliability was .79 for Basic Number Skills. On this same test, the reliability was .85 for children ages 12 years, 0 months to 13 years, 11 months ($n = 121$). Test–retest reliability for Spelling was .89 for children ages 5 years, 9 months to 6 years, 11 months ($n = 62$), and .94 for children ages 12 years, 0 months to 13 years, 11 months ($n = 118$). For children ages 5 years, 9 months to 6 years, 11 months ($n = 79$), test–retest reliability was .97 for Word Reading. On this same test, the reliability was .94 for children ages 12 years, 0 months to 13 years, 11 months ($n = 121$). These figures suggest a high degree of item consistency and score stability.

Validity

Internal validity of the DAS as a whole is described in terms of intercorrelations of tests and composites. Correlations between the DAS ACH and the Cognitive battery's General Conceptual Ability (GCA) composite are moderate. Intercorrelations are reported for 2,400 individuals ages 6 years, 0 months to 17 years, 11 months, with 200 cases per 1-year age level. Basic Number Skills, Spelling, and Word Reading correlated with the GCA .60, .52, and .60, respectively. For Verbal Ability on the DAS, correlations were .48, .49, and .59 for Basic Number Skills, Spelling, and Word Reading, respectively. For Nonverbal Reasoning Ability, correlations were .59, .49, and .52 for Basic Number Skills, Spelling, and Word Reading, respectively. For Spatial Ability, correlations were .45, .34, and .40 for Basic Number Skills, Spelling, and Word Reading, respectively. Furthermore, the correlation for Basic Number Skills with Spelling was .56, for Basic Number Skills with Word Reading was .53, and for Word Reading with Spelling was .81.

Several concurrent validity studies are also reported. Correlations of the DAS

ACH and the WISC-R were calculated for a sample of 66 children 8–10 years of age. Basic Number Skills was found to correlate with the WISC-R Verbal IQ, Performance IQ, Full Scale IQ, and Freedom from Distractibility .62, .53, .68, and .69, respectively. Spelling correlated with Verbal IQ, Performance IQ, Full Scale IQ, and Freedom from Distractibility .57, .34, .50, and .47, respectively. Word Reading correlated with the Verbal IQ, Performance IQ, Full Scale IQ, and Freedom from Distractibility .68, .50, .66, and .50, respectively. Moreover, Basic Number Skills correlated .66 with Arithmetic on the WISC-R. For a sample of 60 children 14–15 years of age, Basic Number Skills correlated with the WISC-R Verbal IQ, Performance IQ, Full Scale IQ, and Freedom from Distractibility .66, .40, .68, and .63, respectively. Spelling correlated with Verbal IQ, Performance IQ, Full Scale IQ, and Freedom from Distractibility .57, .34, .55, and .47, respectively. Word Reading correlated with Verbal IQ, Performance IQ, Full Scale IQ, and Freedom from Distractibility .74, .38, .72, and .63, respectively. In addition, it was found that Basic Number Skills correlated .67 with Arithmetic on the WISC-R.

Correlations of the DAS ACH and the Stanford–Binet Intelligence Scale: Fourth Edition (SB4) were calculated for a sample of 55 children 9–10 years of age. DAS ACH Basic Number Skills correlated .55 with SB4 Verbal Reasoning, .56 with Abstract/Visual Reasoning, .69 with Quantitative Reasoning, .28 with Short-Term Memory, and .66 with the Test Composite. DAS ACH Spelling correlated .34 with Verbal SB4 Reasoning, .44 with Abstract/Visual Reasoning, .50 with Quantitative Reasoning, .39 with Short-Term Memory, and .49 with the Test Composite. DAS ACH Word Reading correlated .58 with SB4 Verbal Reasoning, .48 with Abstract/Visual Reasoning, .63 with Quantitative Reasoning, .45 with Short-Term Memory, and .66 with the Test Composite. For a sample of 29 children 7 to 11 years of age with gifted referrals, DAS ACH Basic Number Skills correlated .28 with SB4 Verbal Reasoning, .52 with Abstract/Visual Reasoning, .64 with Quantitative Reasoning, .37 with Short-Term Memory, and .57 with the Test Composite. Spelling correlated .24 with Verbal Reasoning, .36 with Abstract/Visual Reasoning, .43 with Quantitative Reasoning, .35 with Short-Term Memory, and .46 with the Test Composite. DAS ACH Word Reading correlated .50 with SB4 Verbal Reasoning, .51 with Abstract/Visual Reasoning, .52 with Quantitative Reasoning, .43 with Short-Term Memory, and .61 with the Test Composite.

Correlations of the DAS ACH and the Kaufman Assessment Battery for Children (K-ABC) were calculated for a sample of 18–27 children ages 5–7. Correlations of K-ABC Sequential Processing and the DAS ACH yielded values of .58, .49, and .34 for Basic Number Skills, Spelling, and Word Reading, respectively. Correlations with K-ABC Simultaneous Processing yielded values of .38, .38, and .38 for Basic Number Skills, Spelling, and Word Reading, respectively. Correlations with the K-ABC Mental Processing Composite were .66, .51, and .38 for Basic Number Skills, Spelling, and Word Reading, respectively. For K-ABC Achievement, correlations were .64, .60, and .83 for Basic Number Skills, Spelling, and Word Reading, respectively. Correlations between scores on the DAS ACH and the Peabody Picture Vocabulary Test—Revised (PPVT-R) were also reported for a sample of 64 children ages 6 years, 0 months to 10 years, 9 months. The PPVT-R and Basic Numbers Skills correlated .31; Spelling and the PPVT-R correlated .42; and Word Reading and the PPVT-R correlated .48.

In addition, correlations of the DAS ACH with both individually administered and group-administered achievement tests are reported. Correlations were calculated for a sample of 198 children age 7 years and 157 children age 11 years, using the Basic Achievement Skills Individual Screener (BASIS). Basic Number Skills correlated .75 to .79 with the BASIS Mathematics subtest; Spelling correlated .87 to .88 with the BASIS Spelling subtest; and Word Reading correlated .64 to .79 with the BASIS Reading subtest. In a sample of 100 children ages 8–11 years, a correlation of .83 was found between Word Reading and the Total Reading score on the WRMT-R. Correlations with the K-TEA were calculated for a sample of 29 children ages 7–11 years with gifted referrals. Basic Number Skills correlated .84 with the K-TEA Mathematics Compos-

ite; Spelling correlated .85 with the K-TEA Spelling; and Word Reading correlated .85 with the K-TEA Reading Composite. Correlations were also calculated to compare the scores on the DAS ACH with group achievement test results collected from the standardization sample. The group tests included such measures as the CAT, the CTBS, the SAT, and the Iowa Test of Basic Skills. Basic Number Skills correlated .62 with total mathematics scores on the group tests; Word Reading correlated .67 with total reading scores; and Spelling correlated .77 with spelling scores. Furthermore, DAS ACH scores and school grades were correlated for the standardization sample. Basic Number Skills and mathematics grades correlated at .43; Spelling and spelling grades correlated at .60; and Word Reading and reading grades correlated at .48. Overall, these data provide lend adequate support for the validity of the DAS ACH. However, additional studies with larger sample sizes would be more informative.

Summary

The DAS ACH appears to be a useful tool for measuring basic academic achievement skills. Because the DAS ACH examines a limited range of skills, not unlike the WRAT-3, it may be best considered a "screener of a screener." However, the DAS ACH possesses several characteristics that make it worthy of use, including an adequate standardization sample, the ability to make direct comparisons with the DAS Cognitive battery, adequate reliability and validity data, and the availability of performance analysis procedures. Aylward (1992) indicates that the DAS as a whole is a psychometrically sound, well-constructed test.

PEABODY INDIVIDUAL ACHIEVEMENT TEST—REVISED

The PIAT-R (Markwardt, 1989) is the revision of the original PIAT (Dunn & Markwardt, 1970). A normative update has also been released for the PIAT-R (Markwardt, 1997). The only difference between the 1989 and 1997 versions of the PIAT-R is that the 1997 update contains a more current standardization sample. The PIAT-R includes a greater number of items and more contemporary items than its predecessor, and a new subtest, Written Expression, was also added. The PIAT-R is an individually administered achievement test designed to provide a wide range of assessment in six content areas: General Information, Reading Recognition, Reading Comprehension, Mathematics, Spelling, and Written Expression. According to the test author, the PIAT-R is useful in providing a survey of an individual's academic achievement. As such, results of the PIAT-R may be used to determine the need for diagnostic testing. Other purposes include individual evaluation, program planning, school admissions and placement, ability grouping, guidance and counseling, personnel selection, and follow-up evaluation, as well as research uses. Several caveats are presented in the manual, cautioning the test consumer against the limitations of the PIAT-R (e.g., the PIAT-R is not designed to be a diagnostic test of achievement or to provide highly precise measurements of achievement; it is not based on any one curriculum used in schools; and the qualifications of the test consumer may influence the interpretation of the test).

Administration and Scoring

The PIAT-R is an individually administered test of academic achievement for use with individuals ages 5 years, 0 months to 18 years, 11 months. The PIAT-R consists of one form having six subtests presented in an easel format:

1. *General Information.* This subtest contains 100 items. The examinee answers open-ended questions as read aloud by the examiner. Items cover general encyclopedic knowledge in the areas of science, social studies, the humanities, and recreation.

2. *Reading Recognition.* This subtest contains 100 items of two distinct types. Items 1–16 are multiple-choice in format (four alternatives per item) and assess readiness skills. The student is to choose the correct word or picture to demonstrate knowledge of phonics skills. Items 17–100 require the examinee to read aloud words as presented by the examiner.

3. *Reading Comprehension.* The Reading Comprehension subtest contains 82 items designed to measure the individual's understanding of what is read. Each item covers two pages in the Book of Plates. On the first page, the examinee reads a sentence silently; on the second page, he or she chooses one of four pictures that best illustrates the sentence.

4. *Mathematics.* This subtest consists of 100 items in which the examiner reads aloud each item while displaying the four choices to the subject. The content of this test focuses on application of mathematical concepts rather than computation, and the level of difficulty ranges from recognizing numbers to solving trigonometry problems.

5. *Spelling.* Unlike other tests of this nature, the Spelling subtest of the PIAT-R is presented in a multiple-choice format. This subtest consists of 100 items requiring the examinee to accurately recognize letters and correct spellings of words from four given choices.

6. *Written Expression.* This subtest consists of two levels. Level I (19 items) is designed for use with kindergarten and first-grade students and measures readiness skills, including writing one's name, copying letters and words, and writing letters, words, or sentences as dictated by the examiner. Level II is designed for use with students in grades 2–12. Here, the student is asked to write a story in response to one of two picture prompts (A or B) with a time limit of 20 minutes. Stories are scored on 24 criteria relating to content, organization, and mechanics.

Items on the first five subtests are scored as correct or incorrect, and set basal and ceiling rules are used to determine the appropriate number of items to administer. Training exercises or teaching items are provided. The Written Expression subtest is scored differently, and the manual presents a detailed scoring guide for examiner use. A computerized scoring program is also available. The total test administration time is about 60 minutes. Raw scores can be converted to standard scores having a mean of 100 and a standard deviation of 15, among other scores. These scores can be calculated for each subtest. Written Expression is an exception to this; it yields a "developmental scaled score" ranging from 1 to 15, as well as grade-based stanines. In addition, a Total Test Composite score comprising General Information, Reading Recognition, Reading

Comprehension, Mathematics, and Spelling; a Total Reading Composite comprising Reading Recognition and Reading Comprehension; and an optional Written Language Composite comprising Spelling and Written Expression can also be computed. Instructions for determining significant differences between scores are given in the manual. Guidelines for testing individuals with disabilities are also provided for reference. Finally, a Report to Parents form is included in the manual and can be used as an aid in communicating scores.

Standardization

The PIAT-R was renormed between October 1995 and November 1996 to match U.S. census data as depicted in the March 1994 *Current Population Survey.* These updated norms were published in 1997. The standardization sample is linked to those of the K-TEA, the WRMT-R, and the Key-Math—Revised. The sample consisted of 3,429 individuals, including 3,184 students in kindergarten through grade 12 and 245 young adults ages 18–22 years. The sample was stratified according to variables of age, gender, socioeconomic status (i.e., parental education level), race/ethnicity, and geographic region. Gifted and special education status was also considered when constructing the sample. Overall, the sample appears to match census statistics adequately. However, whites are slightly overrepresented, as are individuals from the Southern and North Central regions of the country.

Reliability

In regard to reliability, it should be noted that the original PIAT-R norms from 1989 were used, not those from 1997. Split-half reliability coefficients were calculated for a sample of 1,563 students ages 5–18 years from the original PIAT-R normative sample. Reliability information is also presented according to grade level in the manual, but is not presented here. For the General Information subtest, split-half coefficients ranged from .92 to .96, with a median of .94. Coefficients for Reading Recognition ranged from .94 to .98, with a median of .97. For Reading Comprehension, coefficients ranged from .90 to .96, with a median of

.93. The Total Reading Composite coefficients ranged from .95 to .98, with a median of .97. The Mathematics subtest coefficients ranged from .83 to .98, with a median of .94. Coefficients for Spelling ranged from .91 to .97, with a median of .95. Coefficients for the Total Test Composite ranged from .98 to .99, with a median of .99. Kuder–Richardson reliability coefficients were also calculated for that same sample. For the General Information subtest, coefficients ranged from .93 to .97, with a median of .96. Coefficients for Reading Recognition ranged from .93 to .97, with a median of .96. For Reading Comprehension, coefficients ranged from .92 to .98, with a median of .95. The Total Reading Composite coefficients ranged from .96 to .99, with a median of .97. The Mathematics subtest coefficients ranged from .87 to .98, with a median of .95. Coefficients for Spelling ranged from .90 to .97, with a median of .95. Coefficients for the Total Test Composite ranged from .98 to .99, with a median of .99.

Test–retest reliability was calculated for a sample of 225 individuals ages 6–16 years, with the testing interval being 2–4 weeks. For the General Information subtest, coefficients ranged from .83 to .97, with a median of .90. Coefficients for Reading Recognition ranged from .94 to .98, with a median of .96. For Reading Comprehension, coefficients ranged from .65 to .97, with a median of .90. The Total Reading Composite coefficients ranged from .87 to .98, with a median of .96. The Mathematics subtest coefficients ranged from .67 to .94, with a median of .90. Coefficients for Spelling ranged from .78 to .97, with a median of .90. Coefficients for the Total Test Composite ranged from .88 to .99, with a median of .96. Item response theory reliability coefficients are presented for a sample of 1,560 children ages 5–18 as well. For the General Information subtest, coefficients ranged from .95 to .98, with a median of .97. Coefficients for Reading Recognition ranged from .96 to .99, with a median of .98. For Reading Comprehension, coefficients ranged from .94 to .98, with a median of .96. The Total Reading Composite coefficients ranged from .97 to .99, with a median of .98. The Mathematics subtest coefficients ranged from .91 to .99, with a median of .96. Coefficients for Spelling ranged from .93 to .98, with a median of .97. Coefficients for the Total Test Composite were all .99.

Reliability information pertaining to Written Expression is also presented. Coefficient alpha reliabilities for Level I of Written Expression were calculated for a sample of 437 children in kindergarten and first grade. These values ranged from .60 to .69. For a sample of 45 first graders, test–retest reliability coefficients were calculated for Level I Written Expression with a testing interval of 2–4 weeks. The overall coefficient was .56. Furthermore, interrater reliability was calculated. For a sample of 299 kindergarten children, the interrater reliability was .90, and for a sample of 138 first graders, the interrater reliability was .95. Coefficient alpha reliabilities were also calculated for Level II of Written Expression for samples of children in grades 2–12. For prompt A (n = 530), these values ranged from .69 to .89 with a median of .86; for prompt B (n = 541), these values ranged from .76 to .91, with a median of .88. Interrater reliability for prompt A (n = 537) ranged from .30 to .81, with a median of .58; for prompt B (n = 550), it ranged from .53 to .77, with a median of .67. Alternate-forms reliability coefficients were also presented for a sample of 168 children in grades 3, 5, 7, 9, and 11. The coefficients ranged from .44 to .61 for these grades, and for the total sample it was .63. Overall, the reliability estimates for the PIAT-R are adequate, but this information would be improved if it had been based on the more recent standardization sample. As expected, coefficients are not as impressive for Written Expression, as this subtest requires more subjective scoring.

Validity

Like the reliability information, the validity information for the PIAT-R is based on the 1989 norms. Content validity of the PIAT-R is addressed in terms of the development process for each subtest. Also, according to the test author, that the internal-consistency coefficients indicate that each subtest measures a clear content domain. Furthermore, intercorrelation data support the content validity of each subtest. For a total sample of 715 children ages 5, 7, 9, 11, 13, 15, and 17 years, intercorrelations between subtests

and composites with the Total Test Composite are presented: General Information (r = .78 to .86), Reading Recognition (r = .78 to .95), Reading Comprehension (r = .85 to .93), Total Reading Composite (r = .90 to .96), Mathematics (r = .66 to .87), and Spelling (r = .66 to .92). Construct validity is evidenced through age differentiation of scores, correlations with other tests, and factor analysis. Correlations between scores on the original PIAT and the PIAT-R were calculated for a sample of 273 children ages 6–17. Correlations for Mathematics ranged from .54 to .93, with a median of .78; correlations for Reading Recognition ranged from .68 to .95, with a median of .88; correlations for Reading Comprehension ranged from .63 to .90, with a median of .79; correlations for Spelling ranged from .59 to .92, with a median of .76; correlations for General Information ranged from .46 to .86, with a median of .78; and correlations for the Total Test Composite ranged from .82 to .97, with a median of .91. As further evidence of construct validity, scores on the PIAT-R were correlated with PPVT-R scores for a sample of 1,522 children ages 5–18. For General Information, correlations ranged from .61 to .81, with a median of .72. For Reading Recognition, correlations ranged from .51 to .70, with a median of .62. Correlation coefficients ranged from .54 to .75, with a median of .66, for Reading Comprehension. For the Total Reading Composite, correlations ranged from .52 to .78, with a median of .69. For Mathematics, correlations ranged from .50 to .69, with a median of .56. Correlation coefficients ranged from .28 to .58, with a median of .50, for Spelling. For the Total Test Composite, correlations ranged from .62 to .81, with a median of .72.

The underlying constructs of the PIAT-R were also examined via a factor analysis of subtest intercorrelations for those in grades 2–12 in the standardization sample. Six factors were identified, but three of these factors were found to account for 64.3% of the total variance. Factor I had high loadings for General Information (.71), Reading Comprehension (.52), and Mathematics (.70), appearing to represent a general verbal–educational ability factor. Factor II was characterized by high loadings for Reading Recognition (.73) and Spelling (.75), appearing to represent a more specific verbal factor involving knowledge of letters and phonics. Factor III was marked by modest loadings for Reading Comprehension (.39) and Written Expression, Level II (.39). This factor appears to represent a more complex verbal factor involving knowledge of grammar and syntax. Although the inclusion of factor analyses lends unique evidence of construct validity for the PIAT-R, other forms of validity are certainly missing. For example, no correlations with other measures of achievement or intelligence are provided in the manual. Instead, numerous validity studies on the original PIAT are provided. The utility of this information is questionable, as only about 35% of the items on the PIAT-R are found on the PIAT.

In an independent investigation, Prewett and Giannuli (1991) investigated the relationships among the reading subtests of the PIAT-R, WJ-R ACH, K-TEA, and WRAT-R for a sample of 118 students ages 6 years, 5 months to 11 years, 11 months, referred for psychoeducational evaluation. The correlations among these subtests ranged from .78 to .98. Specifically, the Total Reading Composite of the PIAT-R correlated .88 with Broad Reading on the WJ-R ACH, .93 with the Reading Composite of the K-TEA Comprehensive Form, and .92 with Reading on the WRAT-R. Daub and Colarusso (1996) examined the validity of the reading subtests of the PIAT-R, the WJ-R ACH, and the Diagnostic Achievement Battery—2 (DAB-2) for a sample of 35 children ages 9 years, 3 months to 10 years, 11 months identified as having reading disabilities. The Total Reading Composite of the PIAT-R correlated .82 with Broad Reading on the WJ-R ACH, and .88 with the reading composite on the DAB-2. Although the evidence presented in the PIAT-R manual for validity is supportive, more studies using a wider variety of tests and populations would be worthwhile.

Summary

The PIAT-R is a widely used test of academic achievement. Some clinicians find that the multiple-choice formats of many of the subtests are relatively nonthreatening for special populations of students. Others may criticize this type of response format, in that students are often asked to supply or pro-

duce their own answers for most tasks encountered in school. Costenbader and Adams (1991) indicate that more extensive research with the PIAT-R needs to be conducted with other major instruments. Likewise, Rogers (1992) suggests that more evidence to support concurrent validity is needed, but adds that "the PIAT-R appears to be a useful instrument both to practitioners in the schools and to researchers" (p. 654).

KAUFMAN TEST OF EDUCATIONAL ACHIEVEMENT

The K-TEA (Kaufman & Kaufman, 1985a, 1985b) is an individually administered test of academic achievement that consists of two forms: Brief and Comprehensive. A normative update has also been released for the K-TEA (Kaufman & Kaufman, 1997a, 1997b). The sole difference between the 1989 and 1997 versions of the K-TEA is that the 1997 update contains a more current standardization sample. The Brief Form consists of three subtests: Mathematics, Reading, and Spelling. The Comprehensive Form consists of five subtests: Mathematics Applications, Reading Decoding, Spelling, Reading Comprehension, and Mathematics Computation. Some items have been taken from or are highly similar to ones on the K-ABC. The authors propose several uses appropriate for both forms of the K-TEA, including contributing to a psychoeducational battery; program planning; research; pretesting and posttesting; making placement decisions; student self-appraisal; use by government agencies, such as social services; personnel selection; and measuring adaptive functioning. In addition, the Comprehensive Form is useful for analyses of strengths and weaknesses and for error analysis. Generally, it is recommended that the Brief Form be used for screening and prereferral, and that the Comprehensive Form be used when more detailed information is warranted.

Administration and Scoring

The K-TEA Brief Form is an individually administered test of academic achievement designed for use with children ages 6 years,

0 months to 18 years, 11 months. This test consists of a single form and easel format, and contains items that are completely different from the ones on the K-TEA Comprehensive Form. The K-TEA Brief Form consists of the following subtests:

1. *Mathematics.* This subtest contains 52 items that assess basic arithmetic concepts, applications, numerical reasoning, and computational skills. Items 1–25 consist of computational problems that are completed on the Mathematics Worksheet. Items 26–52 consist of concepts and applications problems; each problem is presented orally, along with an accompanying picture. The examinee may use paper and pencil to complete necessary calculations, but must respond orally.

2. *Reading.* This subtest consists of 52 items that assess reading decoding and comprehension. Items 1–23 assess decoding skills, requiring the examinee to identify printed letters and words as presented. Items 24–52 assess comprehension and require the examinee to respond orally or in gestures to printed instructions as presented by the examiner.

3. *Spelling.* The Spelling subtest consists of 40 items. The examiner reads aloud a word both in isolation and as used in a sentence, and the examinee writes each word on the Spelling Sheet. Alternatively, the examinee may spell the word aloud.

The K-TEA Brief Form generally takes 30 minutes to administer. Items are grouped into units and are scored as correct or incorrect. Verbal responses may be made in languages other than English, provided that the correctness of such responses is easily determined. Set basal and ceiling rules are used to determine the appropriate number of items to administer. Extensive psychometric training is not a prerequisite for administering and scoring the K-TEA Brief Form, although practice is recommended. Separate subtest scores as well as a Battery Composite may be calculated. Among other scores, the K-TEA Brief Form yields standard scores having a mean of 100 and a standard deviation of 15. Computerized scoring is available. The K-TEA Brief Form also permits subtest comparisons for the purpose of identifying general strengths and weaknesses. A graphic

display of descriptive categories is presented in the manual for the purpose of interpreting standard scores: Upper Extreme (130 and above), Well Above Average (120–129), Above Average (110–119), Average (90–109), Below Average (80–89), Well Below Average (70–79), and Lower Extreme (69 and below). A K-TEA Brief Form Report to Parents is also available.

The K-TEA Comprehensive Form is an individually administered test of academic achievement designed for use with children ages 6 years, 0 months to 18 years, 11 months. This test also consists of a single form, but (as noted earlier) contains items that are completely different from the ones on the K-TEA Brief Form. The K-TEA Comprehensive Form consists of the following subtests presented in an easel format:

1. *Mathematics Applications.* This subtest contains 60 items that assess arithmetic concepts and problem-solving applications. Each problem is presented orally, along with an accompanying picture, graph, or the like. The examinee may use paper and pencil to complete necessary calculations, but must respond orally.

2. *Reading Decoding.* This subtest consists of 60 items that assess decoding skills, requiring the examinee to identify and read aloud printed letters and words as presented to him or her.

3. *Spelling.* The Spelling subtest consists of 50 items. The examiner reads aloud a word both in isolation and as used in a sentence, and the examinee writes each word on the Spelling Sheet. Alternatively, the examinee may spell the word aloud.

4. *Reading Comprehension.* This subtest consists of 50 items. For some items, the student is to read passages and answer questions about them. Other items require the student to read printed instructions and to respond orally or in gestures, accordingly.

5. *Mathematics Computation.* This subtest consists of 60 items that measure computational skills involving the four basic arithmetic operations to more complex (e.g., algebraic) operations. The examinee completes the problems on the Mathematics Computation Worksheet.

The K-TEA Comprehensive Form generally takes 60–75 minutes to administer.

Items are grouped into units and are scored as correct or incorrect. Verbal responses may be made in languages other than English, provided that the correctness of such responses is easily determined. Set basal and ceiling rules are used to determine the appropriate number of items to administer. Extensive psychometric training is not a prerequisite for administering and scoring the K-TEA Comprehensive Form, although practice is recommended. Separate subtest scores, as well as a Reading Composite, Mathematics Composite, and Battery Composite, may be calculated. Among other scores, the K-TEA Comprehensive Form yields standard scores having a mean of 100 and a standard deviation of 15. Computerized scoring is available. The K-TEA Comprehensive Form also allows for subtest comparisons for the purpose of identifying general strengths and weaknesses. Furthermore, detailed error analysis procedures are available to provide more refined information pertaining to specific skills. The same graphic display of descriptive categories is presented in the K-TEA Comprehensive Form manual as in the K-TEA Brief Form Manual for the purpose of interpreting standard scores. Finally, a K-TEA Comprehensive Form Report to Parents is also available for use.

Standardization

The K-TEA was renormed between October 1995 and November 1996 to match U.S. census data as depicted in the March 1994 *Current Population Survey*. These updated norms were published in 1997. The standardization sample is the same for the K-TEA Brief Form and Comprehensive Form, and is linked to those of the PIAT-R, the WRMT-R, and the KeyMath—Revised. The sample consisted of 3,429 individuals, including 3,184 students in kindergarten through grade 12 and 245 young adults ages 18–22 years. The sample was stratified according to variables of age, gender, socioeconomic status (i.e., parental education level), race/ethnicity, and geographic region. Gifted and special education status was also considered in constructing the sample. Overall, the sample appears to match census statistics adequately. However, whites are slightly overrepresented, as are individuals from the Southern and North Central regions of the country.

Reliability

Reliability data are based on the original K-TEA norms from 1985. Internal-consistency reliability coefficients for the K-TEA Brief Form were calculated for each subtest as well as the Battery Composite across 589 individuals ages 6–18 years from the standardization sample. Coefficients were also presented in the manual according to grade level, but are not presented here. Reliability coefficients for the Mathematics subtest ranged from .81 to .92, with a mean of .87. For the Reading subtest, the coefficients ranged from .83 to .97, with a mean of .91. For the Spelling subtest, reliability coefficients ranged from .79 to .96, with a mean of .89. Reliability coefficients for the Battery Composite ranged from .91 to .98, with a mean of .95. Test–retest reliability was also assessed for a sample of 153 students in grades 1–12, with an average testing interval of 1 week. In a sample of 79 students in grades 1–6, test–retest coefficients were .88 for Mathematics, .84 for Reading, .90 for Spelling, and .94 for the Battery Composite. In a sample of 74 students in grades 7–12, test–retest coefficients were .85 for Mathematics, .85 for Reading, .84 for Spelling, and .92 for the Battery Composite. A sort of "alternate-forms" reliability is also presented, using the Brief Form (Mathematics, Reading, Spelling, and Battery Composite) and the Comprehensive Form (Mathematics Composite, Reading Composite, Spelling, and Battery Composite) for a sample of 576 children ages 6–18 years. For Mathematics, correlations ranged from .79 to .90, with a mean of .85. For Reading, correlations ranged from .68 to .95, with a mean of .83. Correlations on Spelling ranged from .86 to .94, with a mean of .90. Finally, correlations for the Battery Composite ranged from .90 to .97, with a mean of .93.

As with the K-TEA Brief Form, reliability data pertaining to the K-TEA Comprehensive Form are based on the 1985 norms. Internal-consistency reliability coefficients for the K-TEA Comprehensive Form were calculated for each subtest and composite for 2,476 individuals ages 6 to 18 years from the normative sample. Coefficients were also presented in the manual according to grade level, but are not presented here. Reliability coefficients for the Mathematics Applications subtest ranged from .86 to .94, with a mean of .92. For the Mathematics Computation subtest, the coefficients ranged from .83 to .97, with a mean of .92. These two tests combine to form the Mathematics Composite, for which reliability coefficients ranged from .93 to .98, with a mean of .95. For the Reading Decoding subtest, the coefficients ranged from .91 to .97, with a mean of .95. Coefficients for the Reading Comprehension subtest ranged from .89 to .96, with a mean of .93. These two subtests combine to form the Reading Composite, for which reliability coefficients ranged from .94 to .98, with a mean of .97. For the Spelling subtest, reliability coefficients ranged from .88 to .96, with a mean of .94. Finally, reliability coefficients for the Battery Composite ranged from .97 to .99, with a mean of .98. As a measure of stability, test–retest coefficients are presented for a sample of 172 individuals in grades 1–12, with an average testing interval of about 1 week. In a sample of 85 students in grades 1–6, test–retest coefficients were .90 for Mathematics Applications, .83 for Mathematics Computation, .93 for Mathematics Composite, .95 for Reading Decoding, .92 for Reading Comprehension, .96 for the Reading Composite, .95 for Spelling, and .97 for the Battery Composite. In a sample of 87 students in grades 7–12, test–retest coefficients were .94 for Mathematics Applications, .92 for Mathematics Computation, .96 for Mathematics Composite, .91 for Reading Decoding, .90 for Reading Comprehension, .94 for the Reading Composite, .96 for Spelling, and .97 for the Battery Composite. The information pertaining to a variety of "alternate-forms" reliability is the same as that presented for the Brief Form (see above). Altogether, the estimates of reliability for the K-TEA appear to be strong. However, such information needs to be calculated with the normative update to make it more current.

Validity

Content validity for the K-TEA Brief Form was described in terms of the item selection process. The test authors indicated that content validity was in part established through consultation with curriculum experts in each subject area. In addition, item analysis procedures such as the Rasch–Wright and Angoff methods were utilized. Mean intercorrelations are presented for the K-TEA Brief Form for a sample of 589 individuals ages 6–18 years from the normative data. Mathematics correlated with Reading and Spelling .63 and .55, respectively, and Spelling correlated .65 with Reading.

Evidence of construct validity is presented in terms of age differentiation in the K-TEA Brief Form. Also, correlations were computed between the subtests and the Battery Composite for a sample of 589 children ages 6–18 years. Correlation coefficients for Reading and the Battery Composite ranged from .62 to .86, with a mean of .79. Correlations for Mathematics ranged from .75 to .93, with a mean of .84. For Spelling, correlations ranged from .68 to .90, with a mean of .81. Evidence of concurrent validity is also presented. For a sample of 198 students in grades 1–12, correlations between Reading on the K-TEA Brief Form and Reading on the WRAT ranged from .61 to .74. For Mathematics on the K-TEA Brief Form and Arithmetic on the WRAT, correlations ranged from .42 to .84 in a sample of 200 students in grades 1–12. For K-TEA Brief Form Spelling and WRAT Spelling, correlations ranged from .43 to .87 in a sample of 200 students in grades 1–12. For a sample of 52 students in grades 1–12, correlations were calculated between the K-TEA Brief Form and the PIAT. The correlation between the K-TEA Brief Form Mathematics subtest and Mathematics on the PIAT was .59. Reading on the K-TEA Brief Form correlated .78 with Reading Recognition and .80 with Reading Comprehension on the PIAT. Spelling on the K-TEA Brief Form correlated .68 with Spelling on the PIAT. Finally, the K-TEA Brief Form Battery Composite correlated .84 with the Total Test score on the PIAT.

Correlations between the K-TEA Brief Form and the K-ABC are also presented for a sample of 105 children ages 6–12 years. For this total sample, Mathematics on the K-TEA Brief Form correlated .39 to .45 with K-ABC Sequential Processing, .36 to

.58 with Simultaneous Processing, .52 to .60 with the Mental Processing Composite, .19 to .66 with Nonverbal, .60 to .71 with Achievement, .26 to .37 with Faces and Places, .71 to .78 with Arithmetic, .32 to .42 with Riddles, .26 to .55 with Reading/Decoding, and .57 to .66 with Reading/Understanding. Reading on the K-TEA Brief Form correlated .27 to .38 with K-ABC Sequential Processing, .36 to .46 with Simultaneous Processing, .46 to .48 with the Mental Processing Composite, .22 to .59 with Nonverbal, .73 to .82 with Achievement, .28 to .43 with Faces and Places, .55 to .63 with Arithmetic, .30 to .54 with Riddles, .45 to .90 with Reading/Decoding, and .78 to .95 with Reading/Understanding. Spelling on the K-TEA Brief Form correlated .37 to .41 with K-ABC Sequential Processing, .11 to .21 with Simultaneous Processing, .23 to .39 with the Mental Processing Composite, .21 to .23 with Nonverbal, .52 to .75 with Achievement, .32 to .33 with Faces and Places, .42 to .50 with Arithmetic, .18 with Riddles, .63 to .86 with Reading/Decoding, and .46 to .79 with Reading/Understanding. The Battery Composite on the K-TEA Brief Form correlated .44 to .48 with K-ABC Sequential Processing, .33 to .47 with Simultaneous Processing, .51 to .54 with the Mental Processing Composite, .22 to .60 with Nonverbal, .77 to .84 with Achievement, .34 to .39 with Faces and Places, .63 to .76 with Arithmetic, .26 to .45 with Riddles, .58 to .90 with Reading/Decoding, and .78 to .92 with Reading/Understanding.

Lastly, for a total sample of 580 children in grades 1–12, scores on the K-TEA Brief Form and the PPVT-R were correlated. For Mathematics, correlations with PPVT-R scores ranged from .25 to .46. For Reading, correlations with PPVT-R scores ranged from .42 to .66. For Spelling, correlations with PPVT-R scores ranged from .25 to .42. Correlations between the Battery Composite and PPVT-R scores ranged from .35 to .59.

Content validity for the K-TEA Comprehensive Form was also described in terms of the item selection process. The test authors indicated that content validity was in part established through consultation with curriculum experts in each subject area. In addition, item analysis procedures such as the Rasch–Wright and Angoff methods were utilized. Mean intercorrelations are presented for the K-TEA Comprehensive Form for 2,476 individuals ages 6–18 years from the standardization sample. The Mathematics Composite correlated with the Reading Composite and Spelling .74 and .64, respectively. Spelling correlated .81 with the Reading Composite. Evidence of construct validity is presented in terms of age differentiation in the K-TEA Comprehensive Form. Also, correlations were computed between the subtests and the Battery Composite for a sample of 2,476 children ages 6–18 years. Correlation coefficients for Reading Decoding and the Battery Composite ranged from .83 to .93, with a mean of .87. For Reading Comprehension, correlations ranged from .84 to .92, with a mean of .88. Correlations for Mathematics Applications ranged from .72 to .91, with a mean of .84. Correlations for Mathematics Computation ranged from .73 to .90, with a mean of .82. For Spelling, correlations ranged from .76 to .91, with a mean of .85.

Evidence of concurrent validity is also presented for the K-TEA Comprehensive Form. For a sample of 199 students in grades 1–12, correlations were computed between Reading on the WRAT and reading scores on the K-TEA Comprehensive Form. For Reading Decoding, correlations ranged from .67 to .90; for Reading Comprehension, they ranged from .51 to .78; and for the Reading Composite, they ranged from .65 to .89. For a sample of 201 students in grades 1–12, correlations between Arithmetic on the WRAT and Mathematics Applications, Mathematics Computation, and Mathematics Composite were .35 to .66, .34 to .52, and .37 to .66, respectively. For a sample of 201 students in grades 1–12, correlations ranged from .43 to .84 for the K-TEA Comprehensive Form Spelling and WRAT Spelling. For a sample of 52 students in grades 1–12, correlations were calculated between the K-TEA Comprehensive Form and the PIAT. The correlation between Mathematics on the PIAT and Mathematics Applications, Mathematics Computation, and the Mathematics Composite were .72, .63, and .75, respectively. Correlations between Reading Recognition on the PIAT and Reading Decoding, Reading Comprehension, and the Reading Composite were .84, .73, and .82, respectively. For

Reading Comprehension on the PIAT, correlations were .81, .74, and .82 with Reading Decoding, Reading Comprehension, and the Reading Composite, respectively. Spelling on the PIAT correlated .78 with Spelling on the K-TEA Comprehensive Form. Finally, the K-TEA Comprehensive Form Battery Composite correlated .86 with the Total Test score on the PIAT.

Correlations between the K-TEA Comprehensive Form and the K-ABC are also presented for a sample of 106 children ages 6 years, 0 months to 12 years, 6 months. For this total sample, the Mathematics Composite on the K-TEA Comprehensive Form correlated .39 to .55 with K-ABC Sequential Processing, .43 to .66 with Simultaneous Processing, .63 to .67 with the Mental Processing Composite, .29 to .68 with Nonverbal, .69 to .76 with Achievement, .25 to .32 with Faces and Places, .79 to .85 with Arithmetic, .38 to .54 with Riddles, .34 to .59 with Reading/Decoding, and .63 to .66 with Reading/Understanding. The Reading Composite on the K-TEA Comprehensive Form correlated .45 to .54 with K-ABC Sequential Processing, .34 to .54 with Simultaneous Processing, .50 to .64 with the Mental Processing Composite, .19 to .56 with Nonverbal, .80 to .84 with Achievement, .27 to .48 with Faces and Places, .59 to .69 with Arithmetic, .24 to .61 with Riddles, .75 to .89 with Reading/Decoding, and .74 to .92 with Reading/Understanding. Spelling on the K-TEA Comprehensive Form correlated .45 with K-ABC Sequential Processing, .14 to .30 with Simultaneous Processing, .30 to .47 with the Mental Processing Composite, .19 to .23 with Nonverbal, .51 to .77 with Achievement, .28 to .30 with Faces and Places, .45 to .56 with Arithmetic, .17 to .19 with Riddles, .60 to .88 with Reading/Decoding, and .43 to .83 with Reading/Understanding. The Battery Composite on the K-TEA Comprehensive Form correlated .51 to .55 with K-ABC Sequential Processing, .38 to .58 with Simultaneous Processing, .56 to .67 with the Mental Processing Composite, .25 to .61 with Nonverbal, .83 to .84 with Achievement, .27 to .43 with Faces and Places, .73 to .80 with Arithmetic, .28 to .55 with Riddles, .65 to .85 with Reading/Decoding, and .76 to .86 with Reading/Understanding.

Next, for a total sample of 1,054 children in grades 1–12, scores on the K-TEA Comprehensive Form and the PPVT-R were correlated. For the Reading Composite, correlations with PPVT-R scores ranged from .45 to .67. For the Mathematics Composite, correlations ranged from .41 to .54. For Spelling, correlations with PPVT-R scores ranged from .29 to .46. Correlations between the Battery Composite and PPVT-R scores ranged from .47 to .63. For a second sample of 1,402 children in grades 1–12, scores on the K-TEA Comprehensive Form and the PPVT-R were correlated. For the Reading Composite, correlations with PPVT-R scores ranged from .57 to .68. For the Mathematics Composite, correlations ranged from .49 to .64. For Spelling, correlations with PPVT-R scores ranged from .40 to .51. Correlations between the Battery Composite and PPVT-R scores ranged from .57 to .70.

Lastly, concurrent validity studies involving group achievement tests are presented. The correlations between Reading on the SAT (n = 53), the Metropolitan Achievement Tests (n = 41), and the Comprehensive Test of Basic Skills (n = 43) and the K-TEA Comprehensive Form Reading Composite were .79, .75, and .73, respectively. The correlations between Mathematics on the SAT (n = 54), the Metropolitan Achievement Tests (n = 41), and the Comprehensive Test of Basic Skills (n = 43) and the K-TEA Comprehensive Form Mathematics Composite were .78, .74, and .87, respectively. The correlations between Composite scores on the SAT (n = 42), the Metropolitan Achievement Tests (n = 30), and the Comprehensive Test of Basic Skills (n = 35) and the K-TEA Comprehensive Form Battery Composite were .85, .80, and .90, respectively.

In an independent investigation, Lavin (1996a) examined the relationship between the WISC-III and the K-TEA Comprehensive Form for a sample of 72 children ages 7–16 years with emotional disabilities. WISC-III Full Scale IQ correlated .66 with Mathematics Applications, .54 with Mathematics Computation, .38 with Spelling, .51 with Reading Decoding, .53 with Reading Comprehension, .53 with the Reading Composite, and .65 with the Mathematics Composite. WISC-III Verbal IQ correlated .64 with Mathematics Applications, .52 with Mathematics Computation, .55 with

Spelling, .63 with Reading Decoding, .67 with Reading Comprehension, .60 with the Reading Composite, and .57 with the Mathematics Composite. WISC-III Performance IQ correlated .37 with Mathematics Applications, .27 with Mathematics Computation, .05 with Spelling, .13 with Reading Decoding, .10 with Reading Comprehension, .19 with the Reading Composite, and .42 with the Mathematics Composite.

Overall, the presented indices of validity appear to be adequate, although more studies using a wider variety of tests and including the updated norms would be desirable. Specifically, some studies should be conducted using special populations, as these are included in the normative sample.

Summary

The K-TEA is a measure of academic achievement that is still in its first edition, although a normative update has been released. Worthington (1987) describes the K-TEA as a technically strong instrument with more than adequate reliability and validity. As such, the K-TEA must be considered a prominent competitor in the field of achievement assessment.

WOODCOCK–JOHNSON PSYCHO–EDUCATIONAL BATTERY–REVISED, TESTS OF ACHIEVEMENT

The WJ-R ACH (Woodcock & Johnson, 1989; Woodcock & Mather, 1989) is one of two components of the WJ-R (Woodcock & Johnson, 1989). The original WJ was published in the 1970s (Woodcock & Johnson, 1977). The other component of the battery is the Woodcock–Johnson Tests of Cognitive Ability (WJ-R COG). The WJ-R COG was developed according to the Horn–Cattell theory of Gf and Gc (fluid and crystallized abilities), as noted elsewhere. Certain portions of the WJ-R ACH are also supportive of this framework. The WJ-R COG and WJ-R ACH were conormed, allowing the examiner to make meaningful ability–achievement comparisons. In comparison to the original WJ ACH, the WJ-R ACH has been improved in a number of ways; it includes two parallel achievement batteries, as well as four new subtests. The

WJ-R ACH is an individually administered test of achievement designed to provide a complete assessment of reading, mathematics, written language, and general knowledge. Specific tests may be selected to suit a variety of testing purposes. The test authors suggest several uses of the WJ-R ACH in the manual, including diagnosis, determination of psychoeducational discrepancies, individual program planning, program placement, guidance, assessing growth, program evaluation, and research. A Spanish-language version of the entire battery, called the Batería Woodcock–Muñoz—Revisada (Woodcock & Muñoz-Sandoval, 1996), is also available.

Administration and Scoring

The WJ-R ACH is an individually administered test of academic achievement designed for use with individuals ages 2–95 years. The WJ-R ACH consists of two parallel forms, A and B, in an easel format. Each form, in turn, consists of a Standard Battery and a Supplemental Battery. Clinicians may select various combinations of tests to administer for any given situation, and a Selective Testing Table is provided in the manual for reference. The Standard Battery contains nine subtests as follows:

1. *Letter–Word Identification* (Test 22). This test consists of 57 items. The first 5 items require the individual to match a rebus with an actual picture of an object. The remaining items require the individual to orally identify letters and words presented in isolation.

2. *Passage Comprehension* (Test 23). This test consists of 43 items. The first 4 items require the individual to point to a picture represented by a phrase. The remaining items require the individual to read a short passage and identify a missing word.

3. *Calculation* (Test 24). The Calculation test consists of 58 items. The individual solves problems in a paper-and-pencil format as presented in the Subject Response Booklet. Problems involve basic arithmetic operations up to trigonometric and calculus operations.

4. *Applied Problems* (Test 25). This test consists of 60 items requiring the individual to solve practical mathematical problems. If

needed, the examinee may make calculations on the provided Applied Problems Worksheet portion of the Subject Response Booklet, but the response must be given orally.

5. *Dictation* (Test 26). The Dictation test consists of 56 items, and responses are written in the designated portion of the Subject Response Booklet. Items 1–6 assess prewriting skills such as drawing and copying. The remaining items assess the subject's skill in providing written responses to questions pertaining to knowledge of letters, spelling, punctuation, capitalization, and word usage.

6. *Writing Samples* (Test 27). This test consists of 30 items that require the individual to write responses to a variety of instructions. Responses are recorded in the designated section of the Subject Response Booklet.

7. *Science* (Test 28). The Science test consists of 49 items covering content in the biological and physical sciences. The first eight items require pointing responses from the examinee, whereas for the remainder of the items, the examinee must respond orally to questions posed by the examiner.

8. *Social Studies* (Test 29). Like the Science test, Social Studies consists of 49 items. The items cover content from history, government, geography, economics, and the like. The first six items require pointing responses, whereas the remainder of the items require oral responses to questions read aloud by the examiner.

9. *Humanities* (Test 30). The Humanities test consists of 45 items that assess an individual's knowledge in art, music, and literature. The first five items require pointing responses, whereas the remainder of the items require oral responses to questions read aloud by the examiner.

The Supplemental Battery contains the following five subtests:

1. *Word Attack* (Test 31). This test consists of 30 items that assess the individual's ability to apply rules of phonics and structural analysis in reading aloud unfamiliar or nonsense words.

2. *Reading Vocabulary* (Test 32). Part A, Synonyms, consists of 34 items in which the examinee must state a word similar in meaning to the one presented. Part B, Antonyms, consists of 35 items in which the examinee must state a word opposite in meaning to the one presented.

3. *Quantitative Concepts* (Test 33). This test consists of 48 items that require the examinee to respond to questions involving mathematical concepts and terminology.

4. *Proofing* (Test 34). Proofing consists of 36 items in which the examinee must identify and explain how to correct a mistake (e.g., punctuation, spelling, etc.) in a printed passage.

5. *Writing Fluency* (Test 35). This test consists of 40 items in which the examinee must write a sentence that relates to a given stimulus picture and includes three given words. Answers are recorded in the designated portion of the Subject Response Booklet, and there is a 7-minute time limit.

Additional test scores may be obtained for Punctuation and Capitalization, Spelling, and Usage. Responses from the Dictation and Proofing tests are used to obtain these scores. Furthermore, a Handwriting test score may be obtained from the Writing Samples test.

Various combinations of tests from the WJ-R ACH Standard Battery yield five cluster scores: Broad Reading (Letter–Word Identification and Passage Comprehension); Broad Mathematics (Calculation and Applied Problems); Broad Written Language (Dictation and Writing Samples); Broad Knowledge (Science, Social Studies, and Humanities); and Skills (Letter–Word Identification, Applied Problems, and Dictation). Supplemental Battery cluster scores may also be computed: Basic Reading Skills (Letter–Word Identification and Word Attack); Reading Comprehension (Passage Comprehension and Reading Vocabulary); Basic Mathematics Skills (Calculation and Quantitative Concepts); Mathematics Reasoning (Applied Problems); Basic Writing Skills (Dictation and Proofing); and Written Expression (Writing Samples and Writing Fluency). Of further note, the following tests and clusters can be used as a measure of quantitative ability (Gq) when one is analyzing cognitive factors of the WJ-R COG: Calculation, Applied Problems, Quantitative Concepts, and Broad Mathematics. Writing Fluency may be used as a measure of processing speed (Gs), and Word Attack may be used as a measure of auditory processing (Ga). Science, Social Studies, and Humanities may be used as measures of comprehension–knowledge (Gc). Moreover, Letter–Word Identification, Applied Problems, Dictation, Science, Social Studies, and Humanities, as well as the Broad Knowledge and Skills Clusters may be used as Early Development (EDev) measures.

Items on most of the tests are scored as correct or incorrect, with the exception of Writing Samples, which is scored 2, 1, or 0. Writing Fluency, Punctuation and Capitalization, Spelling, Usage, and Handwriting also have differing scoring criteria. Set basal and ceiling rules are used to determine the appropriate number of items to administer. Teaching items are provided. The total test administration time varies according to how many tests are administered, but generally ranges from 20 minutes to over an hour. As the WJ-R ACH is lengthier and somewhat more complex than other measures of achievement, the authors recommend that the training steps outlined in the manual be followed before attempts are made to administer the test. Raw scores can be converted to standard scores having a mean of 100 and a standard deviation of 15, among other scores. These scores can be calculated for each individual test and for each cluster, provided that the appropriate tests are given. Furthermore, instructions for determining significant intra-achievement and ability–achievement discrepancies are outlined in the manual. A classification guide for standard scores and percentile ranks is provided in the manual: Very Superior (standard scores of 131 and above), Superior (121–130), High Average (111–120), Average (90–110), Low Average (80–89), Low (70–79), and Very Low (69 and below). Alternate descriptive labels are also provided—for example, Mentally Deficient (69 and below)—but these are excessively evaluative in nature. Guidelines for testing preschoolers, individuals with disabilities, and those with language differences are also provided for reference. However, it should be noted that if English is not the primary language of the examinee, attempts to translate the WJ-R ACH should not be made. As mentioned previously, a Spanish-language version has been published for use with persons whose primary language is Spanish. Many clinicians find the WJ-R ACH somewhat cumbersome to score; however, computerized scoring and reporting are available to ease the scoring process.

Standardization

The WJ-R ACH was conormed with the WJ-R COG. As mentioned previously in this chapter, the normative sample for the MBA was also derived from this sample. The WJ-R ACH was normed between September 1986 and August 1988. The standardization sample was selected to match 1980 U.S. Census statistics. The sample consisted of 6,359 individuals in over 100 of the U.S. communities. The preschool sample consisted of 705 subjects ages 2–5; the school–age sample consisted of 3,245 individuals in kindergarten through 12th grade, the college/university sample was composed of 916 subjects; and the non-school adult sample consisted of 1,493 subjects ages 14–95 years. The sample was stratified according to variables of age, gender, geographic region, race, community size, origin (Hispanic vs. non-Hispanic), funding of college/university (public vs. private), type of college/university (university or 4-year college vs. 2-year college), distribution of adult occupation in the community, distribution of adult occupational status in the community (e.g., employed vs. unemployed), and distribution of adult education in the community. It is unclear whether individuals with disabilities were accounted for in the sample. Overall, it appears that the obtained normative sample for the WJ-R ACH closely resembles the U.S. population of 1980. However, these norms are relatively old. As with the MBA, Kamphaus (1993) suggests that if the standardization sample is 10 or more years old, the examiner should be cautious about the accuracy of the norms for current use.

Reliability

The split-half method corrected by the Spearman–Brown formula was used to estimate internal consistency for the WJ-R ACH. Figures are presented for each age level, based on the data for all subjects at that level in the norming sample who took each test. Average reliabilities for forms A and B are presented. It should be noted that although the norming sample is based on persons ages 2–95 years, reliability information is presented only for those ages 2–79 years. First, reliabilities are presented for the Standard Battery. For Letter–Word Identification, reliability coefficients ranged from .88 to .98, with a median of .92. For Passage Comprehension, the coefficients ranged from .78 to .96, with a median of .90. Coefficients for Calculation ranged from .89 to .98, with a median of .93. For Applied Problems, the coefficients ranged from .84 to .97, with a median of .91. For Dictation, the values ranged from .83 to .96, with a median of .92. Coefficients for Writing Samples ranged from .85 to .98, with a median of .93. For Science, values ranged from .79 to .94, with a median of .87. For Social Studies, the coefficients ranged from .75 to .96, with a median of .87. Coefficients for Humanities ranged from .83 to .95, with a median of .87.

Next, reliability information is presented for the Supplemental Battery. For Word Attack, the split-half reliability coefficients ranged from .87 to .95, with a median of .91. Reading Vocabulary coefficients ranged from .88 to .97, with a median of .93. For Quantitative Concepts, the values ranged from .76 to .91, with a median of .86. For Proofing, the coefficients ranged from .85 to .96, with a median of .91. The coefficients for Writing Fluency ranged from .59 to .87, with a median of .76. For Punctuation and Capitalization, the values ranged from .78 to .95, with a median of .86. For Spelling, the coefficients ranged from .85 to .96, with a median of .89. The coefficients for Usage ranged from .81 to .94, with a mean of .84.

Reliability coefficients are also presented for cluster scores. For Broad Reading, the coefficients ranged from .90 to .98, with a median of .95. The coefficients for Broad Mathematics ranged from .93 to .99, with a median of .95. The coefficients for Broad Written Language ranged from .85 to .98, with a median of .94. For Broad Knowledge, the values ranged from .91 to .98, with a median of .94. For Skills, the coefficients ranged from .94 to .99, with a median of .96. For Basic Reading Skills, the values ranged from .93 to .98, with a median of .96. Coefficients for Reading Compre-

hension ranged from .90 to .97, with a median of .95. For Basic Mathematics Skills, the values ranged from .89 to .97, with a median of .94. For Mathematics Reasoning, the coefficients ranged from .84 to .97, with a median of .91. Coefficients for Basic Writing Skills ranged from .91 to .98, with a median of .94. Lastly, coefficients for Written Expression ranged from .87 to .97, with a median of .93. These indices of internal consistency are quite adequate. Test–retest reliability information is not presented in the manual; however, more detailed information pertaining to reliability can be found in the WJ-R technical manual (McGrew, Werder, & Woodcock, 1991).

Validity

Content, concurrent, and construct validity are addressed for the WJ-R ACH. Content validity is described in terms of the item selection process. The authors indicated that expert opinion was used in developing the test content, and that the tests were designed to provide a sampling of skills in a number of areas. This area of validity could profit from more explanation.

Concurrent validity investigations are presented in the test manual. For a sample of 62 children ages 2 years, 6 months to 3 years, 7 months, correlations with the Boehm Test of Basic Concepts—Preschool Version of .61 and .53 were found for the WJ-R ACH Broad Knowledge Cluster and Skills Cluster, respectively. For this same sample, the Broad Knowledge Cluster and Skills Cluster correlated .61 and .49, respectively, with the Bracken Basic Concepts Scale. Also for this same sample, the Broad Knowledge Cluster and Skills Cluster correlated .63 and .52, respectively, with the PPVT-R. Broad Knowledge and Skills correlated .32 and .29, respectively, with Expressive Vocabulary on the K-ABC for this same sample. Broad Knowledge and Skills correlated .29 and .10, respectively, with Faces and Places on the K-ABC. For a sample of 30 children ages 2 years, 6 months to 3 years, 7 months, Broad Knowledge and Skills correlated .72 and .63, respectively, with Arithmetic on the K-ABC. For this same sample, correlations of .47 and .24 were found between the Broad Knowledge and Skills, respectively, and Riddles on the K-ABC. Lastly, for the sample of 62 children of this same age group, Broad Knowledge and Skills correlated .61 and .52, respectively, with the Total Achievement score on the K-ABC.

Next, concurrent validity studies are presented for a sample of 70 children age 9. Selected correlations are presented here. Broad Reading correlated as follows with these measures: BASIS Reading (r = .63), K-ABC Reading Composite (r = .80), K-TEA Reading Composite (r = .85), PIAT Reading Composite (r = .86), and WRAT-R Reading (r = .83). Broad Mathematics correlated as follows with these measures: BASIS Math (r = .71), K-ABC Arithmetic (r = .71), K-TEA Mathematics Composite (r = .83), PIAT Mathematics (r = .41), and WRAT-R Mathematics (r = .63). Broad Written Language correlated as follows with these measures: BASIS Spelling (r = .63), K-TEA Spelling (r = .68), PIAT Spelling (r = .53), and WRAT-R Spelling (r = .69). Finally, Broad Knowledge correlated .64 with General Information on the PIAT. Concurrent validity studies are also presented for a sample of 51 adolescents age 17. Broad Reading correlated as follows with these measures: BASIS Reading (r = .36), K-TEA Reading Composite (r = .49), PIAT Reading Composite (r = .68), and WRAT-R Reading (r = .57). Broad Mathematics correlated as follows with these measures: BASIS Mathematics (r = .65), K-TEA Mathematics Composite (r = .73), PIAT Mathematics (r = .74), and WRAT-R Mathematics (r = .72). Broad Written Language correlated with these measures as follows: BASIS Spelling (r = .48), K-TEA Spelling (r = .53), PIAT Spelling (r = .62), and WRAT-R Spelling (r = .69). Finally, Broad Knowledge correlated .66 with General Information on the PIAT.

Construct validity is presented in terms of intercorrelation patterns. Although other indices of construct validity would be useful, these intercorrelations are supportive of the domains represented on the WJ-R ACH. Intercorrelations are presented for the individual tests and the cluster scores. Selected figures are presented here. For children age 6 in the standardization sample, Broad Reading correlated .94 and .96 with Basic Reading Skills and Reading Comprehension, respectively. At this same age, Broad Mathematics correlated .93 and .82 with Basic Mathematics Skills and Mathematics Reasoning, respectively. Furthermore, Broad Written Language correlated .87 and .96 with Basic Writing Skills and Written Expression, respectively. Further evidence of construct validity would be desirable with other measures using a variety of populations.

In an independent study, Lavin (1996b) examined the relationship between the WJ-R ACH and the WISC-III for a sample of 85 children ages 6 to 16 years with emotional disabilities. WISC-III Full Scale IQ scores correlated with WJ-R ACH measures as follows: Letter–Word Identification (r = .34), Passage Comprehension (r = .39), Calculation (r = .46), Applied Problems (r = .58), Broad Reading (r = .36), and Broad Mathematics (r = .52). WISC-III Verbal IQ scores correlated with WJ-R ACH measures as follows: Letter–Word Identification (r = .41), Passage Comprehension (r = .51), Calculation (r = .47), Applied Problems (r = .60), Broad Reading (r = .47), and Broad Mathematics (r = .54). WISC-III Performance IQ scores correlated with WJ-R ACH measures as follows: Letter–Word Identification (r = .16), Passage Comprehension (r = .14), Calculation (r = .32), Applied Problems (r = .38), Broad Reading (r = .13), and Broad Mathematics (r = .36). As expected, higher correlations were found with Verbal IQ. Although more information pertaining to validity is presented in the WJ-R technical manual (McGrew et al., 1991), additional studies of concurrent validity and construct validity would be informative.

Summary

The WJ-R ACH is a popular broad-band achievement test. It is a flexible instrument, in that the clinician may choose different combinations of tests to administer for varying purposes. Although much of the reliability and validity information presented for the WJ-R ACH is strong, additional information would be beneficial for the test consumer. It also appears that the WJ-R ACH could benefit from a normative update, since current norms are based on a sampling using 1980 U.S. Census data. In fairness, however, the third edition of the WJ is in the final stages of completion at press time. Until then, despite these problems, Lee (1995) suggests that the WJ-R "represents a significant advancement in the field of cognitive and achievement testing" (p. 1117).

WOODCOCK–JOHNSON III TESTS OF ACHIEVEMENT

The third edition of the Woodcock–Johnson III Tests of Achievement (WJ-III ACH) was published after this book was in press. Like its predecessor, the WJ-III ACH (Woodcock, McGrew, & Mather, 2001b) is one of two components of the Woodcock–Johnson III (Woodcock, McGrew, & Mather, 2001a). I will briefly highlight major changes and features here. The reader is referred to the test manuals for further details. The Woodcock–Johnson III was developed according to the Cattell-Horn-Carroll theory of cognitive abilities, encompassing several broad ability factors: Comprehension-Knowledge (Gc), Fluid Reasoning (Gf), Visual-Spatial Thinking (Gv), Auditory Processing (Ga), Processing Speed (Gs), Long-Term Retrieval (Glr), Short-Term Memory (Gsm), Reading-Writing (Grw), and Mathematics (Gq). In comparison to its two predecessors, the WJ-III ACH has been improved in a number of ways. It includes two parallel achievement batteries as well as seven new subtests. The 22 tests are organized into a standard battery and extended battery. Clinicians may select a variety of combinations of tests to administer for any given situation, and a Selective Testing Table is provided in the manual for reference (Mather & Woodcock, 2001). New subtests include:

1. *Reading Fluency (Grw)*. This test consists of 98 items. The individual is required to read simple sentences, decide if the statement is true, and circle an answer of "Yes" or "No." Three minutes are allotted for this task.
2. *Story Recall (Gc)*. The Story Recall test consists of 10 stories of increasing length. The individual is required to listen to selected stories and recall them from memory. A Delayed Story Recall subtest is also included in the battery.
3. *Understanding Directions (Gc)*. This task requires the test taker to listen to orally presented instructions and then follow the directions by pointing to specified objects in a given picture. Six pictures or scenes are included.
4. *Math Fluency (Gq)*. The Math Fluency task includes 160 simple arithmetic facts. The individual is required to solve as many problems as possible within 3 minutes.
5. *Writing Fluency (Grw)*. This test consists of 40 items in which the examinee must write a sentence that relates to a given stimulus picture and includes three given words. Answers are recorded in the designated portion of the Subject Response Booklet, and there is a 7-minute time allotment.
6. *Spelling of Sounds (Ga)*. The 28 items on this subtest require the individual to write single letters of sounds. As such, the task measures phonological and orthographic coding ability.
7. *Sound Awareness (Ga)*. This test assesses phonological ability, requiring the individual to identify rhyming words, as well as delete, substitute, and reverse sounds in words.

Notably, the Science, Social Studies, and Humanities subtests from the WJ-R ACH are now represented by one test of Academic Knowledge (Gc).

Eight new interpretive clusters have been added to this edition. In all, there are 19 overlapping clusters, including Broad Reading, Oral Language, Listening Comprehension, Academic Knowledge, and Phonemic Awareness. The WJ-III ACH manual (Mather & Woodcock, 2001) provides detailed information regarding testing accommodations, item scoring procedures, and interpretation. Practice exercises are included in the manual, and a training workbook (Wendling & Mather, 2001) is also available. The WJ-III Compuscore and Profiles Program (Schrank & Woodcock, 2001) has completely replaced the hand-scoring option. As such, no normative tables have been published, making it impossible for examiners to check scoring. The standardization sample, based on U.S. Census projections for the year 2000, is impressive in size and stratification ($N = 8,818$). Like the WJ-R ACH, this test is designed for use with individuals 2 to 90+ years of age.

Information on reliability and validity is provided in the technical manual (McGrew & Woodcock, 2001). The split-half method was used to estimate internal consistency for the WJ-III ACH. Median internal consistency reliability coefficients for the 22 subtests range from .76 to .97, and for the clusters, .85 to .96. Interrater reliability studies were conducted for subtests involving a degree of subjectivity (i.e., Writing Samples), ranging from .93 to .99. Stability was measured via two test–retest studies. Median coefficients ranged from .69 to .96. Although information regarding standard error, item difficulty, and response is provided to support alternate-form equivalence, an alternate-form reliability study was only conducted for the Passage Comprehension subtest. Evidence for content, construct, and concurrent validity is presented in the manual as well. Confirmatory factor analyses and correlations between cluster scores presented are support for content validity. Correlations for achievement clusters generally ranged from .50 to .70. Concurrent validity studies were conducted with the KTEA and WIAT for a sample of children in grades 1 through 8 ($N \cong 50$). For example, the Reading Composite of the KTEA and the Broad Reading Cluster of the WJ-III ACH correlated at .76. The Math Composite of the WIAT and the Broad Math Cluster of the WJ-III ACH correlated at .70. Overall, the technical qualities of the WJ-III ACH appear to be fairly solid.

In my experience and that of my colleagues, the WJ-III ACH is an appealing broadband test of academic achievement. However, some debate has arisen as to whether the Story Recall and Understanding Directions subtests are adequate measures of oral language, in that each task relies heavily upon auditory memory. The utility of the fluency subtests remains to be seen. Also of concern is the absence of normative tables and hand scoring procedures. Additionally, Sattler (2001) indicates that "more information is needed about its psychometric properties" (p. 607). Due to the recency of the WJ-III ACH, independent reviews of the test, as well as research studies, are scant. However, this author expects that the WJ-III ACH will receive much attention in forthcoming years.

WECHSLER INDIVIDUAL ACHIEVEMENT TEST

The Wechsler Individual Achievement Test (WIAT; Psychological Corporation, 1992) is an individually administered test of academic achievement that was designed to cover all of the achievement areas of learning disability as defined in the Individuals with Disabilities Education Act: oral expression, listening comprehension, written expression, basic reading skill, reading comprehension, mathematics calculation, and mathematics reasoning. The WIAT Comprehensive Battery contains eight subtests overall, and a WIAT Screener consisting of three of the eight subtests is also published. It is stated in the manual that the WIAT is to be considered as a single piece in the assessment context, and that the clinician should take care to gather client information from multiple sources. In this context, the WIAT can be used to assist in diagnosis, placement, program planning, and intervention. Of further note, the WIAT is the only achievement test that is directly linked to the WISC-III, Wechsler Preschool and Primary Scale of Intelligence—Revised (WPPSI-R), and WAIS-R. This advantage allows for more precise ability–achievement comparisons.

Administration and Scoring

The WIAT, an individually administered test having an easel format, is designed for use with children and adolescents ages 5 years, 0 months to 19 years, 11 months. This test consists of a single form with the following subtests:

1. *Basic Reading.* This subtest contains 55 items that assess decoding and word-reading ability. Items 1–7 contain picture cues and require pointing responses only. Items 8–55 require the examinee to read aloud printed words as presented by the examiner. Items are scored as correct or incorrect.

2. *Mathematics Reasoning.* This subtest contains 50 items that assess the ability to reason mathematically. The examinee is to respond orally, point, or write answers to questions posed by the examiner. For some problems, visual stimuli are provided. The examinee may use pencil and paper if needed. Items are scored as correct or incorrect.

3. *Spelling.* This subtest consists of 50 items. Items 1–6 require the examinee to write single letters, and items 7–50 require the examinee to write words as dictated by the examiner. Responses are written in the designated section of the Response Booklet. Items are scored as correct or incorrect.

4. *Reading Comprehension.* The items on this 38-item subtest are designed to measure an individual's ability to comprehend printed passages. Items 1–8 contain a one-sentence passage accompanied by a picture. The remaining items contain longer passages without picture cues. For all items, the examinee is to read the passage and respond orally to a question asked by the examiner. Items are scored as correct or incorrect.

5. *Numerical Operations.* This subtest contains 40 problems that the examinee is to answer in the provided Response Booklet. The first four items require the examinee to write numeral dictated by the examiner. The remaining items require the examinee to solve problems covering basic arithmetic operations to algebraic equations. Items are scored as correct or incorrect.

6. *Listening Comprehension.* This subtest consists of 36 items that assess the ability to comprehend orally presented information. Items 1–9 require the individual to point to one of four pictures correctly describing a word spoken by the examiner. The remaining items require the examinee to listen to a passage read aloud by the examiner and to answer one or more questions about it. A corresponding stimulus picture is presented for each of these items. Items are scored as correct or incorrect.

7. *Oral Expression.* This subtest contains 16 items intended to assess the ability to express words, give directions, and describe scenes. For items 1–10, the examiner presents a picture depicting a word and defines the word. In turn, the examinee is to respond orally to these clues with the correct word. Items 11–12 require the individual to describe orally a scene depicted in a stimulus picture; items 13–14 require the individual to look at a map and describe how to get to one location from another; and items 15–16 require the examinee to describe the steps needed in order to complete an action. Items are scored according to given sets of criteria, for a total possible raw score of 40 points.

8. *Written Expression.* This subtest is administered only to students in grades 3–12. The examinee is given 15 minutes to write in response to one of two prompts. Responses are written in the designated section of the Response Booklet. The Written Expression subtest is scored analytically and holistically

according to a given set of criteria, for a total possible raw score of 24 points.

The WIAT Comprehensive Battery takes 30–60 minutes to administer in general, depending on the age of the individual. Written Expression is the only timed subtest, although suggested time limits are given for the other subtests. Items on Basic Reading, Mathematics Reasoning, Spelling, Numerical Operations, Reading Comprehension, and Listening Comprehension are scored as correct or incorrect. However, Reading Comprehension and Listening Comprehension, as well as Oral Expression and Written Expression, are scored somewhat subjectively in nature. Scoring guidelines and examples are provided in the manual. Teaching is allowed for certain items. Set basal and ceiling rules are used to determine the appropriate number of items to administer. Guidelines for testing special populations are provided. Extensive psychometric training is not a prerequisite for administering and scoring the WIAT, although practice is recommended. The WIAT also includes skills analysis procedures, allowing for more in-depth examination of the individual's performance. Furthermore, detailed procedures for determining ability–achievement discrepancies are provided. Among other types of scores, the WIAT yields standard scores having a mean of 100 and a standard deviation of 15. These scores can be calculated for each of the eight subtests, in addition to a Reading Composite, Mathematics Composite, Language Composite, Writing Composite, and Total Composite for the Comprehensive Battery. The WIAT Screener consists of the same Basic Reading, Mathematics Reasoning, and Spelling subtests as found on the WIAT Comprehensive Battery. The Screener takes about 10–15 minutes to administer. Although not really necessary, separate WIAT Screener test protocols are marketed. Computerized scoring and reporting programs are available.

Standardization

The standardization sample of the WIAT was selected to match March 1988 U.S. Census data. The sample was composed of 4,252 individuals ages 5 years, 0 months to 19 years, 11 months, in grades K–12. The sample was stratified according to variables of age, grade, sex, race/ethnicity, geographic region, and parent education. In addition, it is noted that 6% of the normative sample consisted of children classified as having learning disabilities, speech/language impairments, emotional disturbances, or physical impairments. Another 4.3% of the sample consisted of children served in gifted programs, and 1.4% of the sample was classified as having borderline or mild mental retardation; however, separate norms are not presented for these groups. Finally, a linking sample is described. This sample consisted of 1,284 children who were administered either the WPPSI-R, WISC-III, or WAIS-R. The sample slightly overrepresented those with parents having higher education levels and those living in the Southern region of the United States. Weighting procedures were used to adjust race/ethnicity proportions to U.S. census data. Overall, the WIAT standardization sample closely matches the U.S. population as described in the 1988 census.

Reliability

Split-half reliability coefficients were used to estimate internal consistency across the standardization sample for the WIAT. These are presented according to both age and grade; age-based coefficients are presented here. For Basic Reading, reliability coefficients ranged from .87 to .95, with a mean of .92. Coefficients for Mathematics Reasoning ranged from .74 to .92, with a mean of .89. Spelling coefficients ranged from .80 to .93, with a mean of .90. Reading Comprehension coefficients ranged from .81 to .93, with a mean of .88. Numerical Operations had coefficients ranging from .69 to .91, with a mean of .85. For Listening Comprehension, values ranged from .80 to .88, with a mean of .83. Oral Expression coefficients ranged from .88 to .92, with a mean of .91. Written Expression coefficients ranged from .76 to .84. Coefficients for the Reading Composite ranged from .90 to .97, with a mean of .95. For the Mathematics Composite, coefficients ranged from .83 to .95, with a mean of .92. Coefficients for the Language Composite ranged from .88 to .93, with a mean of .90. For the Writing Composite, the values

ranged from .89 to .92, with a mean of .90. The Total Composite coefficients ranged from .94 to .98, with a mean of .97. For the Screener, coefficients ranged from .91 to .97, with a mean of .96.

In addition, test–retest reliability was assessed for a sample of 367 children in grades 1, 3, 5, 8, and 10. The median interval between testing was 17 days, ranging from 12 to 52 days. The average test–retest reliability coefficients across this sample were as follows: Basic Reading ($r = .94$), Mathematics Reasoning ($r = .89$), Spelling ($r = .94$), Reading Comprehension ($r = .85$), Numerical Operations ($r = .86$), Listening Comprehension ($r = .76$), Oral Expression ($r = .68$), Written Expression ($r = .77$), Reading Composite ($r = .93$), Mathematics Composite ($r = .91$), Language Composite ($r = .78$), Writing Composite ($r = .94$), Total Composite ($r = .96$), and Screener ($r = .95$). Because the Reading Comprehension, Listening Comprehension, Oral Expression, and Written Expression subtests require more judgment in scoring, studies of interscorer agreement were conducted. Fifty protocols were randomly selected from the standardization sample, including protocols from each grade level. Four raters independently scored responses on all 50 protocols for these four subtests. For Reading Comprehension and Listening Comprehension, the mean interscorer agreement was .98. The mean for Oral Expression was .93. Average correlations for Written Expression were .89 for prompt 1 and .79 for prompt 2. Overall, indices for reliability on the WIAT appear quite adequate.

Validity

Information pertaining to content, construct, and criterion-related validity is presented in the WIAT manual. Several goals guided the development of the WIAT. One of the aims was to develop an achievement test that reflected current curricular trends. A second goal was to link the WIAT to the Wechsler intelligence scales to promote meaningful ability–achievement comparisons. Third, the WIAT was designed to reflect the seven areas of achievement specified in the Individuals with Disabilities Education Act that may be used to identify children with learning disabilities. Subtest and item specifications, field testing, and item analysis procedures are described at length in the manual, and a clear scope and sequence chart of curricular objectives addressed is included. Overall, the information pertaining to content validity appears to be adequate.

Construct validity is evidenced by intercorrelations among the subtests, correlations with the Wechsler intelligence scales, and studies of group differences. As a whole, the intercorrelation patterns confirm expected relationships among the subtests and composites. For example, at age 7 years, the Reading Composite correlated .98 with Basic Reading and .95 with Reading Comprehension. At this same age, the Mathematics Composite correlated .96 with Mathematics Reasoning and .91 with Numerical Operations. The Language Composite correlated .82 with Listening Comprehension and .90 with Written Expression. As an additional measure of construct validity, correlations with the Wechsler intelligence scales are presented. For children in the linked sample at age 5 years, 0 months to 5 years, 11 months, scores on the WPPSI-R and the WIAT were correlated. Verbal IQ correlated as follows: Mathematics Composite ($r = .65$), Language Composite ($r = .65$), Screener ($r = .62$), and Total Composite ($r = .70$). Performance IQ correlated as follows: Mathematics Composite ($r = .61$), Language Composite ($r = .54$), Screener ($r = .53$), and Total Composite ($r = .59$). Full Scale IQ correlated as follows: Mathematics Composite ($r = .70$), Language Composite ($r = .67$), Screener ($r = .63$), and Total Composite ($r = .71$). For children ages 6–16 years, scores on the WIAT were correlated with scores on the WISC-III. Verbal IQ correlated as follows: Reading Composite ($r = .50–.81$), Mathematics Composite ($r = .62–.78$), Language Composite ($r = .40–.71$), Writing Composite ($r = .49–.67$), Screener ($r = .59–.84$), and Total Composite ($r = .69–.84$). Performance IQ correlated as follows: Reading Composite ($r = .31–.55$), Mathematics Composite ($r = .44–.63$), Language Composite ($r = .30–.55$), Writing Composite ($r = .32–.45$), Screener ($r = .41–.61$), and Total Composite ($r = .46–.61$). Full Scale IQ correlated as follows: Reading Composite ($r = .48–.75$), Mathematics Composite ($r = .65–.79$), Lan-

guage Composite ($r = .49–.68$), Writing Composite ($r = .51–.60$), Screener ($r = .55–.81$), and Total Composite ($r = .53–.80$). Lastly, correlations were calculated between the WIAT and WAIS-R for the sample of adolescents ages 17 years, 0 months to 19 years, 11 months. Verbal IQ correlated as follows: Reading Composite ($r = .77$), Mathematics Composite ($r = .73$), Language Composite ($r = .57$), Writing Composite ($r = .63$), Screener ($r = .76$), and Total Composite ($r = .83$). Performance IQ correlated as follows: Reading Composite ($r = .54$), Mathematics Composite ($r = .66$), Language Composite ($r = .27$), Writing Composite ($r = .52$), Screener ($r = .64$), and Total Composite ($r = .62$). Full Scale IQ correlated as follows: Reading Composite ($r = .74$), Mathematics Composite ($r = .77$), Language Composite ($r = .49$), Writing Composite ($r = .64$), Screener ($r = .78$), and Total Composite ($r = .81$). Finally, several studies were conducted with various clinical groups (e.g., children with mental retardation). Scores for such groups were compared with those of the standardization sample. Expected differences were found, verifying the construct validity of WIAT interpretations. Overall, these indices of construct validity appear adequate. Studies using other major measures of intelligence would also be of interest, however.

Criterion-related validity evidence is demonstrated through comparisons with other achievement tests, grades, and special education classification. The BASIS was administered to a sample of 80 children in grades 3 and 8. Across this group, BASIS Reading correlated .80 with WIAT Basic Reading and .81 with Reading Comprehension. Correlations with BASIS Mathematics were .82 with WIAT Mathematics Reasoning and .79 with Numerical Operations. BASIS Spelling correlated .88 with Spelling on the WIAT. Scores on the WIAT and the K-TEA were correlated for a sample of 28 children ages 6–16 years. K-TEA Reading Decoding and WIAT Basic Reading correlated .86; K-TEA Reading Comprehension and WIAT Reading Comprehension correlated .78; K-TEA Mathematics Applications and WIAT Mathematics Reasoning correlated .87; K-TEA Mathematics Computation and WIAT Numerical Operations correlated .81; and K-TEA Spelling and WIAT

Spelling correlated .73. Scores on the WRAT-R and the WIAT were correlated for a sample of 251 children ages 7–19 years. WRAT-R Reading correlated .84 with WIAT Basic Reading; WRAT-R Arithmetic correlated .77 with WIAT Numerical Operations; and WRAT-R Spelling correlated .84 with WIAT Spelling. Furthermore, scores on the WJ-R ACH and the WIAT were correlated for a sample of 43 children ages 7–14 years. WJ-R ACH Letter–Word Identification correlated .79 with WIAT Basic Reading; WJ-R ACH Passage Comprehension correlated .74 with WIAT Reading Comprehension; WJ-R ACH Calculations correlated .68 with WIAT Numerical Operations; WJ-R ACH Applied Problems correlated .67 with WIAT Mathematics Reasoning; and WJ-R ACH Dictation correlated .72 with WIAT Written Expression and .88 with Spelling. Scores on the DAS ACH and the WIAT were correlated for a sample of 29 children ages 8 to 13. DAS ACH Word Reading correlated .82 with WIAT Basic Reading and .42 with Reading Comprehension; DAS ACH Basic Number Skills correlated .75 with WIAT Mathematics Reasoning and .70 with Numerical Operations; and DAS ACH Spelling correlated .86 with WIAT Spelling. For a sample of 51 children ages 6–16 years, scores on the WIAT and the PPVT-R were correlated as well. WIAT Basic Reading, Reading Comprehension, and Listening Comprehension correlated .68, .68, and .75, respectively, with the total score on the PPVT-R. Correlations between the composite scores of the WIAT and composite scores of group-administered achievement are also presented. 944 children ages 6–19 years were administered the SAT, the Iowa Test of Basic Skills, or the CAT in addition to the WIAT. Average correlations between the WIAT Reading Composite and the Total Reading scores on these group measures ranged from .72 to .78; average correlations between the WIAT Mathematics Composite and the Total Mathematics scores on the group measures ranged from .64 to .77; and correlations between WIAT Spelling and the Spelling scores on the group measures ranged from .70 to .77. In addition, teacher-assigned grades were obtained for a sample of 897 children 6–19 years of age. Reading grades correlated .42 with scores on the WIAT Reading Compos-ite, and mathematics grades correlated .43 with scores on the WIAT Mathematics Composite.

Independent validity studies of the WIAT have also been conducted. Gentry, Sapp, and Daw (1995) compared scores on the WIAT and the K-TEA Comprehensive Form for a sample of 27 children with emotional disturbances, whose ages ranged from 12 years, 9 months to 18 years, 1 month. K-TEA Reading Decoding correlated .88 with WIAT Basic Reading; K-TEA Reading Comprehension correlated .79 with WIAT Reading Comprehension; K-TEA Mathematics Applications correlated .89 with WIAT Mathematics Reasoning; K-TEA Mathematics Computation correlated .91 with WIAT Numerical Operations; and K-TEA Spelling correlated .85 with WIAT Spelling. Slate (1994) compared WISC-III and WIAT scores for a sample of 202 students with specific learning disabilities (mean age 11 years, 4 months), 115 students with mental retardation (mean age 11 years, 5 months), and 159 students who did not qualify for special education (mean age 9 years, 8 months). The following correlations were found across these groups (N = 476) between the following WIAT measures and WISC-III Full Scale IQ: Basic Reading (r = .52), Reading Comprehension (r = .71), Mathematics Reasoning (r = .81), Numerical Operations (r = .70), Spelling (r = .57), Listening Comprehension (r = .70), Oral Expression (r = .45), and Written Expression (r = .36). For WISC-III Verbal IQ, the correlations with WIAT measures were as follows: Basic Reading (r = .62), Reading Comprehension (r = .73), Mathematics Reasoning (r = .81), Numerical Operations (r = .66), Spelling (r = .63), Listening Comprehension (r = .69), Oral Expression (r = .52), and Written Expression (r = .42). For WISC-III Performance IQ, the correlations with WIAT measures were as follows: Basic Reading (r = .30), Reading Comprehension (r = .49), Mathematics Reasoning (r = .65), Numerical Operations (r = .59), Spelling (r = .38), Listening Comprehension (r = .55), Oral Expression (r = .28), and Written Expression (r = .20). For the WISC-III Verbal Comprehension Index, WIAT correlations were the following: Basic Reading (r = .62), Reading Comprehension (r = .72), Mathematics Reasoning ($r = .73$), Numerical Operations ($r = .61$), Spelling ($r = .59$), Listening Comprehension ($r = .66$), Oral Expression ($r = .47$), and Written Expression ($r = .39$). For the WISC-III Perceptual Organization Index, WIAT correlations were these: Basic Reading ($r = .25$), Reading Comprehension ($r = .46$), Mathematics Reasoning ($r = .53$), Numerical Operations ($r = .39$), Spelling ($r = .25$), Listening Comprehension ($r = .44$), Oral Expression ($r = .14$), and Written Expression ($r = .08$). For the WISC-III Freedom from Distractibility Index, WIAT correlations were as follows: Basic Reading ($r = .64$), Reading Comprehension ($r = .73$), Mathematics Reasoning ($r = .75$), Numerical Operations ($r = .50$), Spelling ($r = .66$), Listening Comprehension ($r = .43$), Oral Expression ($r = .51$), and Written Expression ($r = .43$). Although the WIAT manual includes numerous informative validity studies, additional investigations using a wider variety of populations and instruments would be helpful.

Summary

The WIAT is a screener or broad-band measure of academic achievement that appears to have a representative standardization sample, adequate to strong psychometric characteristics, and a sensible rationale. Furthermore, its connection to the Wechsler intelligence scales makes the WIAT an appealing choice for use with children referred for learning problems. In a review of this test, Ackerman (1998) indicates that the WIAT seems to be an instrument worthy of use, but that additional "empirical evidence supporting its effectiveness needs to be gathered" (p. 1128). It is highly likely that the WIAT will become a mainstay in the arena of academic achievement.

WECHSLER INDIVIDUAL ACHIEVEMENT TEST—SECOND EDITION

Just recently, the Psychological Corporation released the second edition of the Wechsler Individual Achievement Test—Second Edition (WIAT; 2002a, 2002b, 2002c). Major changes and features are highlighted in this section. The reader is referred to the test manuals for further details. The WIAT-II

was developed as an expansion of its predecessor. As such, the WIAT-II reflects several improvements, including updated and modified subtests, the addition of a phonological decoding subtest, and an extended age range. Clinicians may choose to administer any combination of tests desired.

The reading tasks of the WIAT-II are more comprehensive than those found on the original WIAT. The Pseudoword Decoding subtest was added as a measure of phonetic decoding skills. Furthermore, the Word Reading (formerly Basic Reading) and Reading Comprehension subtests contain a wider range and variety of skills. Reading rate and fluency can be measured as part of the Reading Comprehension task. The Mathematics subtests were updated to include a wider range of items and to facilitate error analysis. The Spelling and Written Expression subtests of the WIAT-II assess lower-level skills, as well as advanced composition. Scoring criteria for the writing tasks are more detailed and provide more diagnostics information. The Listening Comprehension and Oral Expression subtests of the WIAT-II have been significantly modified and expanded to measure more discrete skills.

Five composite scores may be calculated, including Reading, Mathematics, Written Language, Oral Language, and a Total Composite. The examiner's manual and the scoring supplements (Psychological Corporation, 2002a, 2002b, 2002c) provide detailed information regarding testing accommodations, item scoring procedures, and interpretation. Examples are included. Computerized scoring for the WIAT-II is available, but it may be hand scored if preferred. The standardization sample included 5,586 individuals, ages 4 to 85. The sample characteristics were based on U.S. Census data from 1998.

Information on reliability and validity is provided in the examiner's manual (Psychological Corporation, 2002a). The split-half method was used to estimate internal consistency for the WIAT-II. Average age-based internal consistency reliability coefficients for the nine subtests ranged from .80 to .97, and for the composites, .89 to .98. Grade-based coefficients are also presented. Interrater reliability studies were conducted for subtests requiring more judgment in scoring (i.e., Written Expression), ranging from .71 to .99. Stability was measured via test–retest studies. Average coefficients ranged from .85 to .98. Evidence for content, construct, and concurrent or criterion-related validity is presented in the manual as well. Intercorrelations were supportive of the WIAT-II structure. Concurrent validity studies were conducted with the WRAT-3, DAS ACH, and WIAT for relatively small samples of children ($N \leq 100$). For example, the Reading Composite of the WIAT and WIAT-II correlated at .91. However, the Oral Language composite of each test correlated at only .50, perhaps due to the substantive changes in the WIAT-II subtests. WIAT-II subtests (Word Reading, Numerical Operations, and Spelling) correlated in the .70s with their WRAT-3 counterparts. The Word Reading subtest of the DAS ACH correlated only .37 with its WIAT-II counterpart, whereas coefficients for Spelling and Basic Number Skills were in the .70s with the like WIAT-II tasks. Overall, the technical qualities of the WIAT-II appear to be fairly sound, although further information would be desirable.

In my experience and that of my colleagues, the WIAT-II is less attractive than its previous edition. Problems with the floor of the Reading Comprehension subtest have been observed. Generally speaking, the scoring procedures and the actual test protocol are considered to be unduly complicated. Furthermore, starting and stopping rules often seem flawed in that scores may be based on a limited number of responses, depending on the range of items the examiner is allowed to administer. The addition of the Pseudoword Decoding subtest and the improvements made to the Written and Oral Language subtests appear favorable. As the WIAT-II becomes more widely used, it will likely undergo considerable review and be included in research studies.

CONCLUSIONS

This chapter has taken the reader on a tour of numerous screening measures of academic achievement. Again, even more testing options than the ones presented here are available. Screening instruments, when used appropriately, can be useful assessment tools for a variety of purposes. Time constraints imposed by school systems and managed health care have certainly contributed to the increasing popularity and use of screening instruments. It is highly likely that screening measures will continue to improve, and that new ones will be developed and researched.

CHAPTER SUMMARY

- Screeners of academic achievement are useful for numerous purposes when the administration of comprehensive instruments is not feasible.
- Academic achievement screeners survey a broad range of content areas such as reading, mathematics, and writing at a wide range of skill levels; diagnostic achievement tests are given to probe an academic area in depth.
- The WRAT-3 is a brief screener of achievement designed for use with individuals ages 5 years, 0 months to 74 years, 11 months.
- The MBA is a brief screener of achievement intended for use with children and adults ages 4 through 95 years.
- The DAS ACH consists of three school achievement tests as a part of the DAS. These tests are to be used with children ages 6 years, 0 months to 17 years, 11 months.
- The PIAT-R is an individually administered achievement test designed to cover six content areas for children ages 5 years, 0 months to 18 years, 11 months.
- The K-TEA is an achievement test that consists of Brief and Comprehensive Forms, and is designed for use with children ages 6 years, 0 months to 18 years, 11 months.
- As a part of the WJ-R, the WJ-R ACH is an individually administered test of academic achievement designed for use with individuals ages 4 to 95. The newly published third edition (WJ-III ACH) retains many features from the previous version and has been enhanced.
- The WIAT is a broad-band measure of academic achievement intended for use with individuals ages 5 years, 0 months to 19 years, 11 months. Recently, the

WIAT-II was released. It covers a wider range than its predecessors.

REFERENCES

Ackerman, T. (1998). Review of the Wechsler Individual Achievement Test. In J. C. Impara & B. S. Plake (Eds.), *The thirteenth mental measurements yearbook* (pp. 1125–1128). Lincoln: University of Nebraska Press.

Aylward, G. P. (1992). Review of the Differential Ability Scales. In J. J. Kramer & J. C. Impara (Eds.), *The eleventh mental measurements yearbook* (pp. 281–282). Lincoln: University of Nebraska Press.

Cohen, L. G., & Spenciner, L. J. (1998). *Assessment of children and youth.* New York: Addison Wesley Longman.

Costenbader, V. K., & Adams, J. W. (1991). A review of the psychometric and administrative features of the PIAT-R: Implications for the practitioner. *Journal of School Psychology, 29,* 219–228.

Daub, D., & Colarusso, R. P. (1996). The validity of the WJ-R, PIAT-R, and DAB-2 reading subtests with students with learning disabilities. *Learning Disabilities Research and Practice, 11*(2), 90–95.

Dunn, L. M., & Markwardt, F. C. (1970). *Peabody Individual Achievement Test.* Circle Pines, MN: American Guidance Service.

Elliott, C. D. (1990a). *Administration and scoring manual for the Differential Ability Scales.* New York: Psychological Corporation.

Elliott, C. D. (1990b). *Introductory and technical handbook for the Differential Ability Scales.* New York: Psychological Corporation.

Gentry, N., Sapp, G. L., & Daw, J. L. (1995). Scores on the Wechsler Individual Achievement Test and the Kaufman Test of Educational Achievement—Comprehensive Form for emotionally conflicted adolescents. *Psychological Reports, 76,* 607–610.

Kamphaus, R. W. (1993). *Clinical assessment of children's intelligence.* Boston: Allyn & Bacon.

Kamphaus, R. W., Slotkin, J., & DeVincentis, C. (1990). Clinical assessment of children's academic achievement. In C. R. Reynolds & R. W. Kamphaus (Eds.), *handbook of psychological and educational assessment of children: intelligence and achievement* (pp. 552–568). New York: The Guilford Press.

Kaufman, A. S., & Kaufman, N. L. (1985a). *Brief Form manual for the Kaufman Test of Educational Achievement.* Circle Pines, MN: American Guidance Service.

Kaufman, A. S., & Kaufman, N. L. (1985b). *Comprehensive Form manual for the Kaufman Test of Educational Achievement.* Circle Pines, MN: American Guidance Service.

Kaufman, A. S., & Kaufman, N. L. (1997a). *Brief Form manual for the Kaufman Test of Educational Achievement: Normative update.* Circle Pines, MN: American Guidance Service.

Kaufman, A. S., & Kaufman, N. L. (1997b). *Comprehensive Form manual for the Kaufman Test of Edu-cational Achievement: Normative update.* Circle Pines, MN: American Guidance Service.

Lavin, C. (1996a). The relationship between the Wechsler Intelligence Scales for Children-Third Edition and the Kaufman Test of Educational Achievement. *Psychology in the Schools, 33,* 119–123.

Lavin, C. (1996b). Scores on the Wechsler Intelligence Scale for Children—Third Edition and Woodcock-Johnson Test of Achievement—Revised for a sample of children with emotional handicaps. *Psychological Reports, 79,* 1291–1295.

Lee, S. W. (1995). Review of the Woodcock–Johnson Psycho-Educational Battery—Revised. In J. C. Conoley & J. C. Impara (Eds.), *The twelfth mental measurements yearbook* (pp. 1116–1117). Lincoln: University of Nebraska Press.

Mabry, L. (1995). Review of the Wide Range Achievement Test—3. In J. C. Conoley & J. C. Impara (Eds.), *The twelfth mental measurements yearbook* (pp. 1108–1110). Lincoln: University of Nebraska Press.

Markwardt, F. C., Jr. (1989). *Manual for the Peabody Individual Achievement Test—Revised.* Circle Pines, MN: American Guidance Service.

Markwardt, F. C., Jr. (1997). *Manual for the Peabody Individual Achievement Test—Revised: Normative update.* Circle Pines, MN: American Guidance Service.

Mather, N., & Woodcock, R. W. (2001). *Examiner's Manual: Woodcock–Johnson III Tests of Achievement.* Itasca, IL: Riverside.

McGrew, K. S., Werder, J. K., & Woodcock, R. W. (1991). *WJ-R technical manual.* Allen, TX: DLM Teaching Resources.

McGrew, K. S., & Woodcock, R. W. (2001). *Technical Manual: Woodcock–Johnson III.* Itasca, IL: Riverside.

Michael, W. B. (1998). Review of the Woodcock–Mc-Grew–Werder Mini-Battery of Achievement. In J. C. Impara & B. S. Plake (Eds.), *The thirteenth mental measurements yearbook* (pp. 1140–1142). Lincoln: University of Nebraska Press.

Prewett, P. N., & Giannuli, M. M. (1991). The relationship among the reading subtests of the WJ-R, PIAT-R, K-TEA, and WRAT-R. *Journal of Psychoeducational Assessment, 9,* 166–174.

Psychological Corporation. (1992). *Manual for the Wechsler Individual Achievement Test.* San Antonio, TX: Author.

Psychological Corporation. (2002a). *Wechsler Individual Achievement Test—Second Edition: Examiner's manual.* San Antonio, TX: Author.

Psychological Corporation. (2002b). *Wechsler Individual Achievement Test—Second Edition: Scoring and normative supplement for grades preK-12.* San Antonio, TX: Author.

Psychological Corporation. (2002c). *Wechsler Individual Achievement Test—Second Edition: Supplement for college students and adults.* San Antonio, TX: Author.

Rogers, B. G. (1992). Review of the Peabody Individual Achievement Test—Revised. In J. J. Kramer & J. C. Impara (Eds.), *The eleventh mental measurements yearbook* (pp. 652–654). Lincoln: University of Nebraska Press.

Sattler, J. M. (2001). *Assessment of children: Cognitive applications* (4th ed.). San Diego, CA: Author.

Schrank, F. A., & Woodcock, R. W. (2001). *WJ III Compuscore and Profiles Program: Woodcock–Johnson III* [Computer software]. Itasca, IL: Riverside.

Slate, J. R. (1994). WISC-III correlations with the WIAT. *Psychology in the Schools, 31,* 278–285.

Smith, T. D., Smith, B. L., & Smithson, M. M. (1995). The relationship between the WISC-III and the WRAT-3 in a sample of rural referred children. *Psychology in the Schools, 32,* 291–295.

Vance, B., & Fuller, G. B. (1995). Relation of scores on the WISC-III and the WRAT-3 for a sample of referred children and youth. *Psychological Reports, 76,* 371–374.

Wendling, B. J., & Mather, N. (2001). *Woodcock–Johnson III Tests of Achievement: Examiner's training workbook.* Itasca, IL: Riverside.

Wilkinson, G. S. (1993). *Administration and scoring manual for the Wide Range Achievement Test—3.* Wilmington, DE: Jastak Associates.

Woodcock, R. W., & Johnson, M. B. (1977). *Woodcock–Johnson Psycho-Educational Battery.* Allen, TX: DLM Teaching Resources.

Woodcock, R. W., & Johnson, M. B. (1989). *Woodcock–Johnson Psycho-Educational Battery—Revised.* Allen, TX: DLM Teaching Resources.

Woodcock, R. W., & Mather, N. (1989). *WJ-R Tests of Achievement: Examiner's manual.* Allen, TX: DLM Teaching Resources.

Woodcock, R. W., McGrew, K. S., & Werder, J. K. (1994). *Woodcock–McGrew–Werder Mini-Battery of Achievement.* Chicago: Riverside.

Woodcock, R. W., McGrew, K. S., & Mather, N. (2001a). *Woodcock–Johnson III.* Itasca, IL: Riverside.

Woodcock, R. W., McGrew, K. S., & Mather, N. (2001b). *Woodcock–Johnson III Tests of Achievement.* Itasca, IL: Riverside.

Woodcock, R. W., McGrew, K. S., & Mather, N. (2001c). *Woodcock–Johnson III Tests of Cognitive Abilities.* Itasca, IL: Riverside.

Woodcock, R. W., & Muñoz-Sandoval, A. F. (1996). *Batería Woodcock–Muñoz—Revisada.* Chicago: Riverside.

Worthington, C. F. (1987). Testing the test: Kaufman Test of Educational Achievement, Comprehensive Form and Brief Form. *Journal of Counseling and Development, 65,* 325–327.

PART IV

SPECIAL TOPICS IN MENTAL TESTING

20

Conceptual and Technical Problems in Learning Disability Diagnosis

CECIL R. REYNOLDS

For many years, the diagnosis and evaluation of learning disability (LD) have been the subjects of almost constant debate in the professional, scholarly, and lay literature, but this has been especially true since the passage of Public Law (PL) 94-142. The lack of consensus regarding the definition of LD is reflected in the day-to-day implementation of PL 94-142 and its successor legislation, known as the Individuals with Disabilities Education Act (IDEA); in the absence of a readily operationalized definition, many clinicians and administrative agencies, particularly school districts, experience difficulty in deciding who is eligible for services. Both under- and overidentification of children with LD create significant problems. Undercounting deprives such children of special services to which they are entitled; overcounting results in the inappropriate placement of students who do not have disabilities, loss of valuable staff time, and increased expense of operating programs (Chalfant, 1984). Overcounting thus drains resources from other programs and students; if it continues to be rampant, it could result in the demise of LD programs altogether. Errors in LD diagnosis will never be completely eliminated, but the amount of error must be reduced as much as possible, while still insuring that as many children with LD as possible receive the special services to which they are entitled.

FEDERAL AND STATE CRITERIA: THE "SEVERE DISCREPANCY" COMPONENT

Two broad factors seem to determine who has an LD: (1) the prevailing definition of LD, and (2) how that definition is applied on a day-to-day basis in practice. The rules and regulations implementing PL 94-142 provide a definition of LD for use by all states receiving federal funds for special education program that remains essentially unchanged in revisions under IDEA through 2002. According to this definition, the diagnosis

is made based on (1) whether a child does not achieve commensurate with his or her age and ability when provided with appropriate educational experience and (2) whether the child has a severe discrepancy between achievement and intellectual ability in one or more of seven areas relating to communication skills and mathematical abilities.

These concepts are to be interpreted in a case by case basis by the qualified evaluation team members. The team must decide that the discrepancy is not primarily the result of (1) visual, hearing, or motor handicaps; (2) mental retardation; (3) emotional disturbance; or (4) environmental, cultural, or economic disadvantage. (Rules and Regulations Implementing Education for All Handicapped Children Act of 1975, 1977, p. 655082)

Although this definition gives some guidance, the field has generally regarded it as vague, subjective, and resulting in diagnosis by exclusion in many cases. Operationalization of the federal definition has varied tremendously across states, resulting in great confusion and disagreement over who should be served as having LD. In fact, the probability of LD diagnosis in the schools varies by a factor of nearly 5, purely as a function of a child's state of residence.

This definition is mandated by federal law only for use by public schools and related agencies that accept federal funding for children with disabilities, including LD. Apparently because schools are where children are served in the vast majority of cases, because schools often pay for outside evaluations, and because other agencies tend to look toward federal directives as a safe haven in the current litigious era, this definition or a close variant is the most often encountered in practice as well as in clinical texts (e.g., Hynd & Willis, 1988). Interpretations of the definition abound in private and clinic practices, just as in the schools, with greater disparities even than in educational settings.

A review by Chalfant (1984) of state education agency (SEA) definitions across the United States identifies five major components that appear to be reasonably consistent across states. Such a review of private clinical settings and mental health agencies is improbable and would seem to offer little in the way of clarification. In addressing problems of LD diagnosis, Chalfant's major components offer a sound beginning.

1. "Failure to achieve," or perhaps more aptly, "school failure," represents a lack of academic attainment in one of the principal areas of school learning; this lack is sometimes seen as relative to grade placement and sometimes as compared to intellectual potential for achievement.

2. "Psychological process disorders" are disorders in one or more of the basic psychological processes that are believed to underlie school learning. Though never listed or defined in their entirety, such processes include attention and concentration, understanding and using written and spoken language, conceptualization, and information processing of all types.

3. "Exclusionary criteria" require that the observed symptoms not be due to other factors, such as sensory incapacity; mental retardation; emotional disturbances; or educational, economic, or related disadvantages.

4. "Etiology," probably the most ill defined of all factors, typically reflects a student's medical and developmental histories, which must be evaluated in order to locate factors believed to be causative in LD. These include a history of brain injury or substantive neurological problems, motor coordination, hyperactivity, delayed speech and language development, and pre- or perinatal difficulties.

5. The federal regulations specify that a child's failure to achieve commensurate with age and ability must result in a "severe discrepancy between achievement and intellectual ability" in one or more of the seven areas listed in the federal regulations. It is important to note that many states seem to ignore the "and intellectual ability" component of this definition, focusing only on the mean achievement level of all children of the same age, regardless of ability.

All five components are important, and each should be addressed in the diagnosis of LD, case by case. Each is hindered by problems of operational and technical clarity. Often no etiological factors are present. Rigid use of exclusionary criteria prohibits a finding of "multiple disabilities." Just what is to be considered a "psychological process," and are there any other "processes"? How is a severe discrepancy" to be determined? Endless questions remain before objective diagnosis of LD will occur, yet much can be done at present.

As Chalfant (1984) has argued, I agree that the "psychological process" and "severe discrepancy" components of the definition are the most salient and the most promising areas to pursue. This chapter focuses on the problems of the "severe discrepancy" criterion, examining conceptual and technical problems of the past and present, as well as reviewing a proposed solution (Reynolds, 1984).

The "severe discrepancy" component is featured here not only because it is the most pervasive of Chalfant's (1984) components, but for the same reason it was included in the federal definition initially. When the rules and regulations for PL 94-142 were being developed, many experts in the field testified before Office of Education hearings, submitted numerous papers and related documentation, and were brought together for discussion and debate at open meetings. When the results of these hearings and debates are examined, the reason for the particular emphasis of the PL 94-142 definition becomes clear. The only consensus regarding definition or characteristics of this thing called LD was that it resulted in a major discrepancy between what one would expect academically of children with LD and the level at which they were actually achieving.

The importance of the "severe discrepancy" statement in the federal definition quoted above was immediately obvious, just as was the potentially subjective nature of the term, especially as it may be applied to individual cases. In an effort to provide guidance in determining a severe discrepancy" between expected and obtained academic levels, several formulas were proposed by the Bureau of Education for the Handicapped (now the Office of Special Education and Rehabilitation). Some of the formulas defined an expected grade equivalent (EGE), and others went further to provide cutoffs for a severe discrepancy. Some of the formulas considered included the following (CA stands for chronological age, MA for mental age):

Formula 5 is the formula for determining a severe discrepancy that was proposed by the bureau in 1976 in the process of setting up rules and regulations for implementation of PL 94-142. This formula was published in the *Federal Register,* and considerable commentary was gathered.

Much of the commentary has been reviewed (Danielson & Bauer, 1978). All of these various formulas were ultimately rejected for a host of interrelated reasons, though most centered around their mathematical inadequacy (see Berk, 1984, Ch. 4). Though more is said on this subject later, these formulas attempted mathematical operations that are not considered appropriate to the level of measurement being employed. The various formulas proffered used age and grade equivalents (which as scaling metrics are only ordinal-level data), and treated them as interval-scale and sometimes even ratio-scale data in some formulas (e.g., Formula 5). Thus the various additions, subtractions, divisions, and ratios proposed in these formulas were essentially meaningless and in all cases misleading. In the final rules and regulations, no criteria for "severe discrepancy" were offered, and agencies were left to develop their own individual criteria for implementing the federal definition.

The present chapter continues addressing the need for objective diagnosis in more detail, and then looks at the reasons why there are such tremendous disparities in the numbers of children identified as having LD from one locale to another; examines the forms of bias (including over- and underidentification) taken by different models of severe discrepancy; and proposes a specific

$$EGE = \text{no. years in school} \times \frac{IQ}{100} + 1.0 \qquad \text{(Formula 1)}$$

$$EGE = \frac{IQ \times CA}{100} - 5 \qquad \text{(Formula 2)}$$

$$EGE = (MA + CA + \text{grade age})/3 - 5 \qquad \text{(Formula 3)}$$

$$EGE = (2MA + CA)/3 - 5 \qquad \text{(Formula 4)}$$

$$\text{Severe discrepancy} = CA \frac{IQ}{300} + 0.17 = 2.5 \qquad \text{(Formula 5)}$$

approach that seems to solve most problems occurring in other models of determining a severe discrepancy. Finally, setting cutoff scores and choosing appropriate tests are addressed along with the issue of who should be diagnosing LD.

OBJECTIVE DETERMINATION OF A SEVERE DISCREPANCY

Clinical judgment has a revered and appropriate place in all diagnostic decision making. Even though it has been amply demonstrated that statistical or actuarial approaches are always as good as—and often better than—clinical judgment (Meehl, 1954; Wiggins, 1981), people should play the central role in making decisions about people. Clinical judgment, however, must be guided by statistical criteria whenever possible. A uniform approach to determining severe discrepancy seems an opportune point of departure for giving empirical guidance in LD diagnosis, particularly because the profession generally accepts the salience of the criterion (Reynolds, 1984) and because of its reason for inclusion in LD definition in the first place. Most states, in fact, require the demonstration of a severe discrepancy for diagnosis of LD. It is important to note, however, that determining a severe discrepancy does not constitute the diagnosis of LD; it only establishes that the primary symptom of LD exists. A severe discrepancy is a necessary but insufficient condition for a diagnosis of LD; the remaining four factors discussed by Chalfant (1984) demand serious consideration. Determining a severe discrepancy requires considerable statistical sophistication, but computers and easily used programs for calculating severe discrepancies are now so widely available (e.g., Reynolds & Stanton, 1988) that previously cumbersome and lengthy computational demands are no longer a problem.

DIFFERENCES IN PREVALENCE RATES ACROSS AND WITHIN STATES

The various models for determining a severe discrepancy in use among SEAs, private agencies, and individual clinicians are count-

less. They range from application of previously rejected federal formulas to the use of constant grade equivalent discrepancies (e.g., performance 2 years below grade level for age) to regulations requiring an achievement deficit and a processing strength (i.e., a processing skill that exceeds general intellectual functioning) to attempts at application of several different regression models of aptitude–achievement differences. Many variations of these "models" are evident in written guidelines, though some agencies provide no guidelines beyond those given in the federal definition. Each of these procedures, whether intentional or not, sets a mathematical limit on the number of children who can be identified as having LD. Although other factors such as referral rates will affect the actual number of children identified, the range of incidence of figures easily can vary from less than 2% to more than 35% of a random sample of the population, depending upon which agency's criteria are being applied. These percentages assume a 100% referral rate and the use of a single aptitude or intelligence measure and a single achievement measure. As more tests (or multiple scores from only two tests) are employed, these percentages increase dramatically.

In the context of a 2-hour psychoeducational evaluation, it is not uncommon for various models to allow an astute diagnostician to diagnose (conservatively estimated) between 50% and 80% of a random sample of the population as having LD. Much of this problem is due to a psychometric naivete that permeates much of the rule making for diagnosis at the SEA level, as well as in other federal and state agencies; it is also due in part to certain myths harbored by many clinicians about how test scores behave.

As an example, consider that some states have adopted a model of the "severe discrepancy criterion whereby children who exhibit a difference of one standard deviation (1 SD) between aptitude and achievement (when both tests' scores are expressed on a common scale) are eligible for a diagnosis of LD by a multidisciplinary team. Since 1 SD below the mean of a normal distribution (assuming that we are only interested in cases where achievement is below aptitude) falls at about the 16th percentile, many believe this to create a pool of eligibility of 16% of the population, Other states use 1.5 *SD*s as a criterion, hoping to generate a pool of about 6% eligibility in the population (obviously, setting different cutting scores will create disparities in the number of children identified). Such inferences are faulty for several reasons.

The concept of *SD* refers to a distribution of scores. If two scores are positively correlated, the distribution of scores created by subtracting the scores of a set of students on both tests from one another will not be the same as the two univariate distributions; the *SD* of this newly created distribution will be significantly smaller than that of the two original distributions. The Wechsler Intelligence Scale for Children—Third Edition (WISC-III, Wechsler, 1991) Verbal and Performance IQs (VIQ and PIQ) are normed on the same sample of children, are scaled to the same mean (100) and *SD* (15), and are correlated about .60 to .65. A difference of"1 *SD*" between these two scores (15 points) occurs in 25% of the population, independent of the direction of the difference. In a truly random sample of the population (allowing IQ to range from about 45 to 155), the 1-*SD* criterion, with the direction of the difference specified, would declare only 12.5% of the population eligible. Most criteria, however, have an exclusionary clause and do not allow children with IQs in the lower ranges to be considered (e.g., IQ < 85). This will further reduce the number of children eligible, usually quite unbeknownst to the individual writing such a rule. Such criteria also fail to consider the regression of IQ on achievement or the joint distributions of multiple-difference score distributions when more than one aptitude or achievement score is being considered. Such factors will also wreak havoc with the anticipated results of the measurement models promulgated under various state guidelines.

This discussion could be carried further, but need not be here. The tremendous disparities in measurement models adopted by various agencies within their written LD guidelines; the varying levels of expertise with which the models have been implemented; and the variance of individual clinicians in their daily practice are obvious, major contributing factors to the differences in the relative proportions of children diagnosed as having LD from agency to agency and among the states. Lack of specific definition; improper application or lack of application of the "severe discrepancy" criterion; and the failure to develop appropriate mathematical models with references to the criterion are the primary, and certainly interrelated, difficulties in this regard.

FALSE POSITIVES AND FALSE NEGATIVES IN CURRENT PRACTICE

Given current practices, what types of children are being served as having LD who may not actually have LD? Who is being missed? The response to these two questions is a direct function of the measurement model being addressed; in other words, the answer is a resounding "It depends." Given the diversity of models of "severe discrepancy," no specific reply may be given, but it is possible to evaluate the types of systematic errors likely to be made under various models that may be applied. A general comparison of some of the various models to be considered may be found in Table 20.1. Ultimately, each of these models is evaluated in detail, particularly as it deals with the IQ–achievement relationship.

Grade-Level Discrepancy Models

"Grade-level discrepancy models" are models such as "2 years below grade level for age" or even models prescribing performance levels that may change over grades. An example of the latter might be 1 year below grade level for age in first through sixth grades; 1~ years for seventh through ninth grades; and 2 years for 10th through 12th grades. Note that the specific discrepancy required here is not under examination, but rather the general model expressed in such a position. These models frequently may have attached to them additional exclusionary criteria, such as no IQs below 85 or perhaps below 70. These models, which are still prevalent (though not to the extent they were some years ago), overidentify children who fall into the "slow-learning" range of intellectual skill (i.e., 70 < IQ < 90) as having LD. Although these children certainly have problems with academic attainment, and some certainly have LD, most of these children are functioning academically at a level quite con-

TABLE 20.1. Responsiveness of Certain General Models of Severe Discrepancy to Critical Variables

	Deviation from grade level	Expectancy formulas	Simple-difference, standard-score comparisons	Regression discrepancy analysis
Ease of implementation	Yes	Questionable	Yes, if values are tabled	Yes, if values are tabled
Years in school	No	Some	No	No
Increasing range and variability of scores at upper grades	Yes, if a graduated procedure	Questionable	Yes	Yes
Systematic and consistent treatment of IQ–achievement interrelationship	No	Questionable	No	Yes
Error of measurement	No	No	Yes	Yes
Regression toward mean	No	No	No	Yes
A priori approximation of incidence[a]	No	No	No	No
Comparability of norms[b]	N/A	No	Yes, certain group tests; possibly certain individual tests	Yes, certain group tests; possibly certain individual tests

Note. N/A, not applicable. From Cone and Wilson (1981). Copyright 1981 by the Council on Learning Disabilities. Adapted by permission.
[a]All discrepancy criteria ultimately set an incidence figure, though this figure will be particularly difficult to estimate under some models. Criteria usually are not adopted on this basis, however.
[b]This variable is treated in greater detail in a later section of this chapter.

sistent with their age and overall level of intellectual ability. As such, no severe discrepancy between expected and obtained achievement levels is present. These children do exhibit mild intellectual disabilities and present problems for teachers in regular classrooms; thus there exists much pressure to place these children in special education programs. Nevertheless, the intent of PL 94-142 was not to provide services in special education for these children. Rather, they should be served in the regular education program, with appropriate assistance made available to their classroom teachers.

On the other hand, the use of grade-level discrepancy criteria will deny LD services to children with above-average IQs who should be served in special education. Whereas a sixth grader with an IQ of 85 who is reading 2 years below grade level for age (equivalent to an achievement score of about 80–85 on an IQ scale) is eligible for services under these models (though the student's achievement is commensurate with his or her IQ level), a sixth grader with an IQ of 160 who is reading at or just below grade level (say, with a reading score of 90–100 on an IQ scale) is not eligible. Although the multidisciplinary team will certainly want to consider other information prior to making a determination, it seems inconsistent with the concept of LD that the former child should be eligible and the latter not eligible for services. The use of grade-level discrepancy models will result in systematic overidentification of children with IQs below 100 as LD, and systematic underidentification of children with IQs of more than 100. Only for children with IQs of precisely 100 is there no bias in diagnosis with these models.

Standard-Score Comparison Models

Standard-score comparison models are generally more appropriate than models employing grade-level discrepancy, but can also result in bias in eligibility. Many standard-score models currently in effect do not take into account the regression of IQ on achievement. Such models will systematically include as having LD more children with IQs over 100 than should be otherwise justifiable. Conversely, children with IQs below 100 will be excluded in unacceptable numbers. This is exactly the opposite of what happens with grade-level discrepancy models; as noted, it occurs because of the well-known regression between IQ and achievement. Common clinical methodology leads one to believe that children with a mean IQ of 130 will have a mean equivalent achievement score of 130. However, given the magnitude of most concurrent validity coefficients (assuming values in the low .70s), the mean achievement level of children with obtained IQ of 130 will be in the range of 121–123. Thus the "expected" achievement level of a child with an IQ of 130 is not 130 at all, but 121–123. For the child with a low IQ, the reverse happens: The expected achievement level of a child with an IQ of 85 will be about 88–89. This produces the over- and underidentification phenomenon as a function of IQ, noted above.

In addition, standard-score models that attempt to define a "severe discrepancy" on the basis of the frequency of occurrence of a discrepancy between an obtained aptitude and an obtained achievement score, on the basis of the *SD* of the two univariate distributions (i.e., the intelligence and the achievement score distributions taken independently), will miss the desired frequency significantly. This problem has been discussed earlier. It will also bias diagnosis systematically as a function of IQ, in addition to identifying far fewer children than its progenitors believe. This problem may be amplified when the reliabilities of the two scales are dissimilar.

Grade-Level Exclusionary Models

Some school districts and clinicians exclude children who do not score below grade level, regardless of any discrepancy among IQ, expected achievement level, and obtained achievement level, and regardless of the type of mathematical model applied. Any such exclusionary model will result in the systematic denial of services to children with IQs above 100; the higher the IQ, the more likely the denial of services. Yet these are likely to be just the children who stand to benefit most from services for LD.

Failure to Consider Multiple Comparisons

Typically, the determination of a "severe discrepancy" under any of the models presented above is based on a comparison between two scores, one a measure of aptitude and the other a measure of achievement. Rarely are only two scores compared, however. More typical is the case where, for example, all three WISC-III IQs are compared to a series of achievement scores, resulting in from 9 to 15 actual comparisons. Unless the multivariate or joint distributions are considered, the number of children found to have a severe discrepancy" will be substantially greater than anticipated, resulting in significant overidentification in each segment of the population. In the case of multiple comparisons, the likelihood of chance occurrences of severe discrepancies is large.

Summary

The question of who is served as having LD who does not actually have LD is a complex one; the answer depends upon the particular model of severe discrepancy being employed and its precise method of implementation. Given the most prevalent LD criteria, the prominence of grade-level exclusionary criteria, and biases in the referral process favoring children with low IQ and low achievement, it appears that the largest group of children being served as having LD who may not in fact have LD consists of children in the borderline and low-average range. These children are difficult to instruct in regular education classrooms, but may not be severely impaired educationally. Such children indeed have mild disabilities; however, they should be served, under current legislation, in the regular education program with support services (e.g., consultation from professional school psychologists) available to their classroom teachers.

DETERMINING A SEVERE DISCREPANCY: STANDARD-SCORE APPROACHES

At best, determining a severe discrepancy is at once crucial, complex, controversial, and hotly debated. In order to avoid biasing diagnosis as a function of IQ, a regression model of some type must be adopted. To avoid measurement error, the simple-difference score must be reliable; the difference must be relatively infrequent in the normal population if it is to indicate an abnormal state (LD decidedly is not normal, but is a pathological state).

Formulas such as the five given earlier, and variations of these formulas that in any way involve the use of grade equivalents or age equivalents, are rejected as grossly inadequate and misleading. Although the reasons for this are many, age and grade equivalents do not possess the necessary mathematical properties for use in any kind of discrepancy analysis. (These problems are discussed at length in a variety of sources. The interested reader will find most relevant information in Angoff, 1971; Birk, 1984; Reynolds, 1981a; and Thorndike & Hagen, 1977.) In addition to these problems, grade equivalents have other features that make them undesirable, including their ease of misinterpretation, their lack of relation to curriculum markers (though they appear directly related), and their more general imprecision.

Only standard-score models have any real potential for solution to the question of severe discrepancy. The following presentations thus employ only standard or scaled scores, typically of the age-corrected deviation score genre, such as those employed by the current Wechsler scales, the Kaufman Assessment Battery for Children (K-ABC), and related scales. Other means of determining a severe discrepancy will probably result in a biasing of the diagnostic process, producing misclassification of an inordinate number of children.

Reliability of a Discrepancy

As noted above, the difference between a child's scores on the aptitude and achievement measures should be large enough to indicate, with a high degree of confidence (i.e., $p < .05$), that it is not due to chance or to errors of measurement (see also Reynolds, 1981a). This requires an inferential statistical test of the hypothesis that the aptitude and achievement scores for the child in question are the same. Payne and Jones (1957) first introduced such a test to interpret individual variation in scores within tests of intelligence. More complex calculations involving the reliabilities of the re-

spective scales and the correlation between the two measures have been proffered (e.g., Salvia & Ysseldyke, 1981), but the simpler computational formula shown below is the algebraic equivalent of the more complex formulas (Reynolds & Willson, 1984; Willson & Reynolds, 1984; Zimmerman & Williams, 1982). The test for significance of the difference of two obtained scores ($X_i - Y_i$) when the scores are expressed as z-scores is as follows:

$$z = \frac{X_i - Y_i}{\sqrt{2 - r_{xx} - r_{yy}}} \qquad \text{(Formula 6)}$$

In Formula 6, X_i and Y_i represent the individual child's score on an aptitude measure X and an achievement measure Y, and r_{xx} and r_{yy} represent the respective internal-consistency reliability estimates for the two scales. These reliability estimates should be based on the responses of the standardization sample of each test and should be age-appropriate for the child being evaluated; they are most often reported in test manuals. Several factors can spuriously inflate reliability estimates. For example, reliability estimates based on item scores across an age range of more than 1 year will be spuriously inflated (see Stanley, 1971). The test statistic is a z-score that is referred to as the normal curve. For a one-tailed test with $p = .05$, the critical value of $z = 1.65$. If $z > 1.65$, one can be sufficiently confident that the difference is not due to errors inherent in the two tests. Although a one-tailed test at the .05 level is probably justifiable for evaluating children referred for the possibility of LD, a two-tailed test or a higher level of confidence (e.g., $p = .01$) would provide a more conservative measure of observed differences. For a two-tailed test, the critical value of z at $p = .05$ is 1.96. All other critical values can be determined from any table of values of the normal curve.

After reliability has been established, the frequency of occurrence of a difference score must be evaluated.

Frequency of a Discrepancy

In evaluating the frequency of a discrepancy score, one must first decide what type of discrepancy score to assess (e.g., a residualized difference between predicted and obtained achievement scores, differences between estimated true scores and residualized true scores, true-difference scores, etc.). In part, this decision depends upon how one interprets the PL 94-142 definition of LD.

To establish that a discrepancy is severe, one must decide which of the following two questions to address:

1. Is there a severe discrepancy between this child's score on the achievement measure and the average achievement score of all other children with the same IQ as this child?
2. Is there a severe discrepancy between 2. Is there a severe discrepancy between this child's measured achievement level and this child's measured level of intellectual functioning?

Both of these questions involve intraindividual variations in test performance (as opposed to purely interindividual norm-referenced comparisons). Although this is obvious in the case of the second question, it may not be so evident for the first, which involves an intraindividual comparison because the determination of the "average achievement score of all other children with the same IQ" is based upon the IQ obtained by the individual child in question. Though both of these are clearly intraindividual-difference models, the mathematical models for answering these two questions differ considerably.

The former appears to be the more pressing question for evaluating children with learning problems and is the more consistent with the intent of PL 94-142, because the aptitude or ability one wants to define is the aptitude or ability to achieve in academic areas (Reynolds, 1984, 1985b). Evaluating the second question is easier in terms of calculation; one can follow Kaufman's (1979) or our (Reynolds & Gutkin, 1981) recommended methodology for assessing VIQ–PIQ differences on the Wechsler scales. Several approaches to the first question have been proffered.

The Simple-Difference-Score Model

The simple-difference-score distribution approach defines as the appropriate discrepancy score the simple differences between the

obtained aptitude score and the obtained achievement score when both measures are expressed on a common scale $(X_i - Y_i)$, where X_i is the individual child's score on an aptitude measure and Y_i is the same child's score on an achievement measure. This model was one of the first attempts to use standard scores to assess the frequency of a discrepancy, and is appealing in its ease of use and its superficial elegance. It has an intuitive appeal, much as does the use of grade equivalents. In this model, the frequency of occurrence of a discrepancy $(X_i - Y_i)$ of a given magnitude is calculated, and the precise percentage of children showing such a discrepancy is readily apparent. In the absence of detailed information on the joint distribution of the two measures, the frequency of occurrence of any given discrepancy can be determined by the following formula, which also estimates a "severe discrepancy":

$$\text{Severe discrepancy} = SD\, z_a\sqrt{2 - 2\, r_{xy}}$$

(Formula 7)

In Formula 7, SD represents the standard deviation of the two scales (scaled to a common metric), and z_a is the z-score corresponding to the point on the normal curve that designates the frequency of occurrence of a "severe discrepancy. The r_{xy} term is simply the correlation between the two measures. The formula estimates, assuming that the distribution of difference scores is perfectly normal, the percentage of the population showing a simple difference of the specific magnitude of interest (independent of the direction of the difference), since the SD of the difference-score distribution will be equal to $SD\sqrt{2 - 2r_{xy}}$. A guideline for determining a value of z_a to indicate that a discrepancy is severe is described in a later section.

The use of this model is common in certain aspects of clinical assessment and diagnosis, most prominently in the evaluation of the meaning of VIQs and PIQs on the Wechsler scales (Kaufman, 1979; Reynolds & Gutkin, 1981). In this context, the simple-difference-score distribution is of considerable value, and discussions of its application can be found in the references above. In the evaluation of aptitude versus achievement or expected versus obtained levels of academic function, however, the simple-difference-score model is inadequate, primarily because it fails to account for regression effects in the relation between IQ and achievement. And, in diagnosing and evaluating LD, we are always interested in the regression of IQ on achievement. The results of failure to account for regression effects have been discussed previously and need not be reiterated here. However, the simple- difference-score model fails on this criterion. It will systematically overestimate the frequency of LD among those with above-average ability and systematically underestimate the frequency of LD among those with below-average ability (when both are expressed in z-score form). This is not theory; it is an unavoidable factual consequence of the positive correlation between aptitude and achievement. Thus with the simple-difference-score model, the number of children identified as having LD will be much greater among those of above-average ability. There is no theoretical or logical reason to believe that this reflects the state of nature. Though recommended by Hanna, Dyck, and Holen (1979), this model, despite its simplicity and ease of application, must be rejected on mathematical as well as theoretical grounds. Its use in the assessment of aptitude–achievement differences seems unsound.

Several similar models have been proposed, including one by McLeod (1979) that attempts to account for regression and for measurement error in the process of diagnosis. Elsewhere (Reynolds, 1984), I have critiqued these various models; all fall far short of their promise, typically on technical grounds, but some on conceptual grounds as well.

Regression Modeling of Severe Discrepancy

To assess the first question above, a regression model (i.e., a mathematical model that accounts for the imperfect relationship between IQ and achievement) is required. Once regression effects have been assessed, the frequency of occurrence of the difference between the academic performance of the child in question and all other children having the same IQ can be determined. The correct model specifies that a severe discrepancy between aptitude (X) and achievement (Y) exists when, assuming the two tests are scaled to a common metric,

$$\hat{Y} - Y_i > SD_y z_a \sqrt{1 - r_{xy}^2} \qquad \text{(Formula 8)}$$

where

Y_i is the child's achievement score
X_i is the child's aptitude score
$\hat{Y}$ is the mean achievement score for all children with IQ = X_i
SD_y is the standard deviation of Y
z_a is the point on the normal curve corresponding to the relative frequency needed to denote "severity"
r_{xy}^2 is the square of the correlation between the aptitude and achievement measures

It is necessary to use $\hat{Y} - Y_i$ as the discrepancy score, because IQ and achievement are not perfectly correlated. For example, if the IQ and achievement tests have the same mean and standard deviation (mean = 100, $SD = 15$) and if they correlate at .60, then the average achievement score for all children with IQs of 80 is 88 and for all children with IQs of 120 is 112. Therein lies the need to compare the achievement level of all other children with the same IQ. The term $\hat{Y}$ is calculated through use of a standard regression equation. When all scores are expressed in z-score form (mean = 0, $SD = 1$), the simplest form to use for all mathematical calculations, Y is easily determined to be

$$Y_z = r_{xy} X_z \qquad \text{(Formula 9)}$$

where

Y_z is the mean score on Y, in z-score form, of all children with IQ = X
r_{xy} is the correlation between X and Y
X_z is the child's score on X (the IQ or aptitude measure) in z-score form

Since few test manuals provide z-scores and most do not like to make the conversion for this purpose, a formula for use on a calculator is given below:

$$\hat{Y} = \left[r_{xy} \left(\frac{X - \overline{X}}{SD_x} \right) \right] SD_x + \overline{X} \qquad \text{(Formula 10)}$$

These terms should all be familiar; the previously undefined values are $\overline{X}$ (the mean of X; e.g., on the WISC-III, 100) and SD_x (the standard deviation of X; e.g., on the WISC-R, 15). The only piece of information required to calculate Formula 8 that is not given in all test manuals, besides the child's own score on the tests, is the correlation between the aptitude and the achievement measure. This must usually be obtained from a literature review or estimated, although for some tests (most notably the K-ABC), many aptitude–achievement correlations are given in test manuals (see, e.g., Kamphaus & Reynolds, 1987).

The correlation r_{xy} can also be estimated. Using data from national standardizations of several major intelligence and achievement tests, we (Reynolds & Stanton, 1988) have developed Formula 11 to estimate r_{xy} when it is unknown, although the equation's accuracy is far from the degree desired.

$$r_{xy} = \sqrt{0.5} \sqrt{r_{xx}r_{yy}} \qquad \text{(Formula 11)}$$

The values r_{xx} and r_{yy} are the internal-consistency reliability coefficients for the aptitude and the achievement measures in question.

Now that $\hat{Y}$ can always be calculated exactly or estimated reasonably when r_{xy} is unknown, we can return to Formula 8. In this equation, the term $SD_y \sqrt{1 - r_{xy}}$ is the standard deviation for the distribution $\hat{Y} - Y_i$. Since this distribution is normal, we can estimate the frequency of occurrence of any given difference $(\hat{Y} - Y_i)$ with great accuracy. Thus z_a is the number of standard deviations between the two scores $(\hat{Y} - Y_i)$ that corresponds to the point of "severity" on the normal curve. Next, we must establish a value of z_a, a controversial matter in itself.

Establishing a Value for z_a in Discrepancy Models

There are no strictly empirical criteria or research methods for establishing a value for z_a for any of the models above. This is true because there is no consensus regarding the definition of LD generally, and specifically none that would allow the generation of a *true and globally accepted* estimate of the prevalence of the group of disorders subsumed under the term "LD." To complicate this issue further, there is no professional consensus in the LD community regarding whether it is better to risk identifying some children as having LD who do not in fact have LD, in hopes that nearly all children with true LD will receive services, or to risk identifying as not having LD a significant number of children who do in fact have LD, in order to identify as few children without LD as having LD as possible. However, under the latter scenario, as well as with the assumption of an equal-risk model (associated equal risks with both types of diagnostic errors, false positives and false negatives), the proper procedure would be not to identify *any* children as having LD, since the proportion of the population who exhibit this disorder is so small (e.g., see Schmidt's [1974~ discussion of probability and utility assumptions). Such a consensus, coupled with valid estimates of prevalence, would provide considerable guidance in establishing a recommended value of z_a. In the absence of such guidance, one may relay only upon rational, statistical, and traditional criteria for guidance.

It has been argued previously that for a discrepancy to be considered severe, it should occur relatively infrequently in the normal population of individuals under consideration (see also Kamphaus & Reynolds, 1987; Reynolds, 1984). Of course, "relatively infrequently" is open to the same problems of interpretation as is "severe discrepancy." Strong tradition and rational arguments exist in psychology, particularly in the field of mental retardation, that "severity" should be defined as 2 SDs from the mean of the distribution under consideration. With regard to a diagnosis of mental retardation, we define a score 2 SDs below the mean of an intelligence scale as a severe intellectual problem, making an individual eligible (provided that other criteria are met) for a diagnosis of mental retardation. Qualitative descriptions such as "mental or cognitive deficiency" or "lower extreme" are common designations below this point in the distribution. At the opposite end of the curve, most definitions of intellectual giftedness refer to IQs falling 2 SDs or more above the mean, with descriptions such as "very superior ability" and "upper extreme" being common. These practices are widely accepted.

In the field of inferential statistics, confidence levels of .05 in an inference or judgment that a hypothesis is to be rejected are the accepted standard in the field. The .05 figure corresponds, roughly, to two standard errors (2 SEs; for a two-tailed test) of the difference being evaluated or to 2 SDs from the mean of the distribution of the test statistic employed (e.g., z, t, F, etc.). There is thus considerable precedent in the social as well as physical sciences for implementation of 2 SDs as the criterion for characterizing a discrepancy as "severe." (For a .05 level of confidence, the actual value of z is 1.96 rather than 2.00, but is certainly close enough to the 2.00 value to support its use.) Thus a value of $z_a = 2.00$ is recommended for determining whether a difference score is severe. This value needs further qualification, however.

Since a difference score, whether defined as $\hat{Y} - Y_i$ or some other value, will be less than perfectly reliable, we must somehow consider this unreliability in defining a severe discrepancy. If we consider it a greater risk to fail to identify as having LD a child who has LD than to identify by mistake a child as having LD who may not have LD, then we can propose a reasonable solution. Note that without this assumption, we would minimize total errors by not identifying *any* children as having LD. Although several methods of accounting for potential unreliability in a discrepancy score are possible, the concept of the confidence interval is both popular and applicable. Adopting the traditional .05 confidence level for a one-tailed test, we can define the value of z_a corrected for unreliability as 2 and reduce the final cutoff score by 1.65 $SE_{\hat{Y}-Y_i}$ thus giving protection corresponding to the one-tailed .05 confidence level times the standard error of the relevant difference score. (A one-tailed value is clearly appropriate here, since we must decide in advance which side to protect; both sides cannot be protected.)

The final model, then, specifies that a severe discrepancy exists between a child's current level of achievement (Y_i) and the mean level of achievement of all other children with the same IQ ($\hat{Y}$; see Formula 10) equals or exceeds the value given in Formula 12 below.

$$\hat{Y} - Y_i \geq 2\,SD_y\,\sqrt{1 - r_{xy}^2} - 1.65\,SE_{\hat{Y}-Y_i}$$
$$\text{(Formula 12)}$$

The calculation of the standard error of $\hat{Y} - Y_i$ ($SE_{\hat{Y}-Y_i}$) is explained in detail elsewhere (Reynolds, 1984) and need not be repeated. Its use is clearly optional, although it does seem advisable to account for error in the process. It is important to note here that this is not the type of measurement error assessed by Formula 6.

The number of children eligible for a diagnosis of LD under these two formulas will vary as a function of the standard error of the difference scores. If $r_{xy} = .60$ and $r_{xx} = r_{yy} = .90$ (a quite realistic set of assumptions), the new cutoff for $z = 1.393$ instead of 2.00. This new value corresponds to 8.2% of the total population for consideration as having LD. A one-tailed confidence interval is appropriate here, because we are only interested in preventing false negatives in diagnosis of children with LD, so only one side needs protection. As noted previously, to guard against over-identification (false positives), the best procedure would be not to identify any children as having LD, since the prevalence is so low. Once can make an argument for serving only the most severely disabled children with LD as a compromise in reducing false positives, but still providing services to some children and consequently increasing the number of false negatives (see Figure 20.1). Under these circumstances, the expressions in Formula 12 would be changed to "+ 1.65 $SE_{\hat{Y}-Y_i}$." This protects the opposite side of the region of severity. The region of "severe discrepancy" under each consideration is depicted in Figure 20.2. One should be cautioned that such

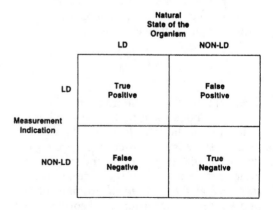

FIGURE 20.1. Possible outcomes when considering a diagnosis of LD.

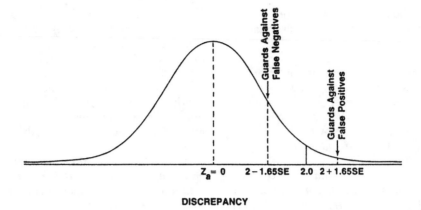

FIGURE 20.2. Illustration of confidence intervals designed to guard against the false-positive or false-negative diagnoses depicted in Figure 20.1.

a restrictive application of a criterion of severity would result in significantly less than 1% of the population of school-age children being eligible for an LD diagnosis.

This calculation (Formula 12) allows us to identify more children than are likely to have true LD; on the other hand, it accounts for many possible inaccuracies in the process that might inhibit identification of a child with true LD, with the exception of the problem of multiple comparisons (i.e., when one compares multiple IQs with many achievement scores; see Reynolds, 1984, for discussion). The other four components of the most prevalent LD definitions, as previously presented, may then be evaluated to make the final judgment regarding whether or not a child is entitled to and in need of services for the LD.

The procedures outlined above can certainly objectify determination of severe discrepancy in LD diagnosis. However, it bears repeating here that not all children who have a severe discrepancy between aptitude and achievement in fact have LD. Even a quick reading of the statutory definition shows that many other factors may cause such a discrepancy, and the reasoned use of clinical judgment is clearly appropriate. However, clinical judgment is wrong at least as often and typically more often than empirical, actuarial judgments. We may think that with regard to LD diagnosis we "know one when we see one," but if there is no "severe discrepancy," chances are we are wrong.

The procedure outlined above provided guidance for the objective determination of a severe discrepancy. It is crucial to bear in mind, however, that mathematical manipulations cannot transform the quality of the initial data, The next section reviews the requisite characteristics of the test and assessment data to be included in evaluating a severe discrepancy.

QUALITY OF INPUT DATA

The quality of the input or test data used is crucial in assessing a discrepancy. Tests with poor psychometric characteristics (especially with low internal-consistency reliability estimates) can be misleading or can fail to detect a severe discrepancy (see also Reynolds, 1986). This section provides standards for tests to be used in the assessment of a potentially severe discrepancy. Though one will not always be able to choose tests that meet all of these standards, the more that can be met, the better. Of course, the characteristics of the examiner(s)—that is, the person(s) gathering the data—are of equal or possibly even greater importance. More is said on this topic in the next section.

1. *A test should meet all requirements stated for assessment devices in the rules and regulations for implementing IDEA.* This not only is a requirement of law, but is consistent with good professional practice. For example, administering a test in accor-

dance with the instructions provided by the test maker is prerequisite to interpretation of a test's scores. If a standardized test is not given precisely according to the instructions provided, inestimable amounts of error are introduced, and norm-referenced scores are no longer interpretable. Thus all personnel evaluating children with educational problems must be conversant with the requirements of PL 94-142 and adhere closely to these standards.

2. *Normative data should meet contemporary standards of practice and should be provided for a sufficiently large, nationally stratified random sample of children.* In practice, this standard is nearly impossible to meet in all respects. Yet it is important to approximate it as closely as possible, because standardization samples are crucial to establishing levels of performance for comparison purposes. To know that an individual answered 60 out of 100 questions correctly on an achievement test and 75 out of 100 questions correctly on an intelligence test conveys very little information. On which test did this individual earn the better score? Without knowledge of how a specified reference group has performed on these tests, one cannot answer this question.

Raw scores on a test, such as the number or percentage of correct responses, take on meaning only when they are evaluated against the performance of a normative or reference group. For convenience, raw scores are typically converted to standard or scaled scores of some type. The reference group from which the norms are derived is defined prior to the standardization of the test. Once the appropriate reference population has been defined, a random sample of this group is tested under procedures as nearly identical as possible, with the same administration, scoring, timing rules, and the like for all. This group is known as the "standardization sample."

Ebel (1972) and Angoff (1971) have discussed a number of conditions necessary for the appropriate development and use of normative reference group data. The following are taken, with some elaboration, principally from these two sources. Some of these conditions place requirements on the test being normed, some on the psychological trait being measured, and others on the test user. All affect test score interpretation.

a. *The psychological trait being assessed must be amenable to at least ordinal scaling.* If a nominal scale were employed, only the presence or absence of the trait would be of interest, and relative amounts of the trait could not be determined; under this unusual condition, norms would be superfluous if not distracting or misleading. Intelligence and achievement tests typically meet this criterion.

b. *The test must provide an adequate operational definition of the trait under consideration.* With a proper operational definition, other tests can be constructed to measure the same trait and should yield comparable scores for individuals taking both tests.

c. *The test should assess the same psychological construct throughout the entire range of performance.* Some achievement tests obviously fail this criterion. Various versions of the Wide Range Achievement Test, for example, measure only what can generously be construed as prereading and prespelling skills at lower ranges of performance on these subtests. Continuous norms and scaling across different variables is confusing at best.

d. *The normative reference group should consist of a large random sample that is representative of the population to whom the test will be administered or performance compared.* Of course, truly random samples for test standardization are not even remotely possible, since individuals must agree to participate. As soon as one parent refuses to allow a child to be tested, the sample is no longer random. To help with this problem, most test-publishing companies stratify their samples according to demographic characteristics of the population, and then compare the outcome to actual population characteristics to see how closely the elusive perfect sample has been approximated. Despite some quite unrealistic opinions to the contrary (e.g., Hopkins & Hodge, 1984), this is an excellent strategy for developing standardization samples, as is exemplified in such standardization projects as those for the WISC-III and the K-ABC.

e. *The sample of examinees from the population should* "have been tested under standard conditions, and . . . take the tests as seriously, but no more so, than other students to be tested later for whom the norms are needed" (Ebel, 1972, p. 488).

f. *The population sampled must be relevant to the test and to the purpose for which the test is to be employed.* Because the point about purpose is so often misinterpreted (especially with regard to the evaluation of exceptional children—the children we most often assess), many adequately normed psychological tests are maligned for failure to include enough children with disabilities in their normative samples. The major intelligence scales designed for use with children (i.e., the various Wechsler scales, the K-ABC, and the McCarthy Scales of Children's Abilities) have been normed on stratified random samples of children representative of children in the United States at large. With these as the reference groups, scores from these scales may be correctly interpreted as providing an indication of a child's current intellectual standing with regard to other children in the United States. Some authors (e.g., Salvia & Ysseldyke, 1981) criticize tests such as the McCarthy Scales as inappropriate for measuring the intellectual levels of various categories of exceptional children, because large numbers of these children were not included in the test's standardization sample. Whether this is a valid criticism depends upon the purpose to which the test is applied. If knowledge about the intellectual functioning of a child with LD relative to age-mates in the United States is desired, comparing the child's performance on an IQ test to that of other children with LD is inappropriate. However, if we are interested in learning how the child compares intellectually to other children with LD, then a reference group of such children is appropriate (although the latter information is not frequently sought, and it has not been shown to be more useful in developing appropriate intervention strategies).

Salvia and Ysseldyke (1981) contend that it is inappropriate to base predictions of future intellectual or academic performance on test scores for an exceptional child that have been derived through comparison with the performance of the larger, normal population. To make predictions, they would require that the reference group have similar sociocultural background, experience, and disabling conditions. Although this may be

an appropriate—indeed, a noble—hypothesis for research study, implementation must await empirical verification, especially since the idea runs counter to traditional practice and considerable evidence. All interpretations of test scores should be guided principally by empirical evidence. Once norms have been established for a specific reference group, the generalizability of the norms becomes a matter of actuarial research. Just as norms based on one group may be inappropriate, a priori acceptance of either hypothesis would be incorrect (Reynolds & Brown, 1984). Current evidence demonstrates rather clearly that test scores predict most accurately (and equally well for a variety of subgroups) when based on a large, representative random sample of the population (e.g., Hunter, Schmidt, & Rauschenberger, 1984; Jensen, 1980; Reynolds, 1982). Exceptions will be found, however. The System of Multicultural Pluralistic Assessment (SOMPA; Mercer & Lewis, 1979), for example, was normed on a large sample of children from California. However, despite the size and representative nature of this sample of children in California, these norms have not withstood empirical evaluation for children in other states, such as Arizona, Texas, and Florida.

g. *Normative data should be provided for as many different groups as may be useful for comparisons of an individual.* Although this may at first glance seem contradictory to the foregoing conclusions, there are instances when it is useful to know how a child compares to members of other specific subgroups; whenever possible, such data should be made available. The more good reference groups available for evaluating a child's performance on a test, the more useful the test may become.

Once the reference group has been obtained and tested, tables of standardization or scaled scores are developed. These tables are based on the responses of the standardization sample and are called "norms tables."

3. *Standardization samples for tests whose scores are being compared must be the same or highly comparable.* Under the best of all conditions, the aptitude, achievement, or other tests on which children are being compared to themselves or to others

should be conormed; that is, their standard-ization samples should consist of precisely the same children. When this is not possible, the norms for each test should be based on comparable samplings of the same population that meet all of the requirements stated under point 2 above. Standardization of the scales should have been undertaken in the same general time period, or else equating studies should be done. Scales normed on different samples and at different times are not likely to have the same means and SDs across samples, even though they may be scaled to a common metric within their respective samples. This gives the two tests the appearance of actually having the same mean and the same SD, even though this may not at all be true. Ample evidence demonstrates that general levels of performance on aptitude and achievement measures vary in the population across time. As just one example, the population mean level of performance on the 1949 WISC is now very close to 110, and the 1974 revision (the WISC-III) now has a mean of nearly 110, though both are scaled within their respective normative samples to a mean of 100. Use of an achievement test normed in 1984 and an intelligence test normed in 1970 would add approximately 3 points to the size of the intelligence–achievement score difference for children with achievement levels below their IQ, purely as an artifact of the times when the two tests were standardized. In the face of the paucity of conormed scales, using highly similar samples tested at a similar time (or with equating studies completed) is acceptable, but conorming will always be superior, provided that the sample meets the conditions of point 2.

4. *For diagnostic purposes, individually administered tests should be used.* For purely screening purposes (e.g., referral for comprehensive evaluation), group-administered tests may be appropriate, though for young children individual screening is preferable (Reynolds & Clark, 1983). For all children, but especially for children with disabilities, too many uncontrolled and unnoticed factors can affect test performance in an adverse manner. The test administrator is more likely to detect these factors under the conditions of individual assessment, where close observation of the child is possible.

Furthermore, individual assessment is more conducive to the use of special adaptations and testing procedures that may be required. Finally, individual assessment allows for careful clinical observation of the child during performance of a variety of academic and intellectual tasks, which is central to the proper assessment of learning problems for children of all ages (Kaufman, 1979; Reynolds & Clark, 1983). Generally, individual assessment affords a better opportunity to maximize the child's performance and provides higher-quality data from which to devise interventions.

5. *In the measurement of aptitude, an individually administered test of general intellectual ability should be used.* Such a test should sample a variety of intellectual skills; basically, it should be a good measure of what psychologists refer to as "g," the general intellectual ability that permeates performance on all cognitive tasks. If ability tests are too specific, a single strength or weakness in the child's ability spectrum may inordinately influence the overall estimation of aptitude. It is also important to assess multiple abilities in deriving a remedial or instructional plan for a handicapped student and in preventing ethnic bias (Reynolds, 1982). Highly specific ability measures (e.g., the Bender–Gestalt, the Columbia Mental Maturity Scale, the Peabody Picture Vocabulary Test—Revised) are necessary complements to a good assessment, but are inadequate for estimating the general ability level of handicapped children. In the assessment of LD, it is important that the chosen measure of aptitude not be influenced adversely by the child's area of specific disability. For example, a measure of intelligence that relies heavily upon expressive vocabulary and assessment of general funds of information for a child with a reading disability may be inappropriate. Since acquisition of general information and vocabulary development occur largely as a function of reading, such an intelligence measure is likely to underestimate the ability level of such a child.

6. *Age-based standard scores should be used for all measures, and all should be scaled to a common metric.* The formulas presented earlier for deriving severe discrepancies require the use of at least interval data. Scoring systems such as age or grade equivalents, which are essentially ordinal

scales, should be avoided whenever score comparisons are to be made. Such scores may be helpful for purely descriptive purposes, but they are unacceptable for comparing scores of individuals or groups except under special, infrequent circumstances. Scores that are ratios of age and/or grade equivalents, such as IQs derived from the traditional formula of (MA/CA) × 100, are also inappropriate. Grade-based standard scores are inappropriate as well. In setting forth the "severe discrepancy" criterion, PL 94-142 specifically notes that a child's achievement should not be commensurate with his or her age and ability; thus, age is properly considered in age-based standard scores. The scores should be corrected at appropriate intervals. Age groupings for the derivation of standard scores may cover from 2 to 6 months, but in no case should groups extend more than 6 months for children below age 6 years or more than 12 months for children above 6 years.

Age and grade equivalents remain immensely popular, despite their serious psychometric deficiencies and misleading nature. In most instances relevant to diagnosis, grade equivalents are abused because they are assumed to have scaled-score properties when they in fact represent only an ordinal scale of measurement. Grade equivalents ignore the dispersion of scores about the mean when the dispersion is constantly changing from grade to grade. Under no circumstances do grade equivalents qualify as standard scores. The calculation of a grade equivalent is quite simple. When a test is administered to a group of children, the mean raw score is calculated at each grade level, and this mean raw score then is called the "grade equivalent" for a raw score of that magnitude. If the mean raw score for beginning fourth grade (grade 4.0) on a reading test is 37, then any person earning a score of 37 on the test is assigned a grade equivalent of 4.0. If the mean raw score for beginning fifth grade (5.0) is 38, then a score of 38 would receive a grade equivalent of 5.0. However, a raw score of 37 could represent a grade equivalent of 3.8; 38 could be 4.0; and 39 could be 5.0. Thus differences of 1 raw-score point can cause dramatic differences in the grade equivalents received, and the differences will be inconsistent in magnitude across grades.

Table 20.2 illustrates the problems associated with the use of grade equivalents in

TABLE 20.2. Standard Scores and Percentile Ranks Corresponding to Performance "Two Years Below Grade Level for Age" on Four Major Reading Tests

Grade placement	Two years below placement	Wide Range Achievement Test		Peabody Individual Achievement Test[a]		Woodcock Reading Mastery Test[b]		Stanford Diagnostic Reading Test[b]	
		SS[c]	%R[d]	SS	%R	SS	%R	SS	%R
1.5	Pk.5	65	1	—		—		—	
2.5	K.5	72	3	—		—		—	
3.5	1.5	69	2	—		64	1	64	1
4.5	2.5	73	4	75	5	77	6	64	1
5.5	3.5	84	14	85	16	85	16	77	6
6.5	4.5	88	21	88	21	91	27	91	27
7.5	5.5	86	18	89	23	94	34	92	30
8.5	6.5	87	19	91	27	94	34	93	32
9.5	7.5	90	25	93	32	96	39	95	37
10.5	8.5	85	16	93	32	95	37	95	37
11.5	9.5	85	16	93	32	95	37	92	30
12.5	10.5	85	16	95	37	95	37	92	30

[a]Reading Comprehension subtest only.
[b]Total test.
[c]All standard scores in this table have been converted for ease of comparison to a common scale having a mean of 100 and a standard deviation of 15.
[d]Percentile rank.

evaluating a child's academic standing relative to his or her peers. Frequently in research, as well as in clinical practice, children of normal intellectual capacity are diagnosed as having LD through the use of grade equivalents when they perform "2 years below grade level for age" (or some variant of this, such as $1\frac{1}{2}$ years below) on a test of academic attainment. The use of this criterion for the diagnosis of LD or other academic disorders is clearly inappropriate (Reynolds, 198 la). As shown in Table 20.2, a child with a grade equivalent reading score 2 years below the appropriate grade placement for his or her age may or may not have a reading problem. At some ages, this score would be well within the average range; at others, it may indicate a severe reading problem. If math, spelling, or science were to be added to this table, the percentile ranks in each column would be quite different, adding to the difficulties of interpretation.

Grade equivalents are also used as standards of performance, which they clearly are not. Contrary to popular belief, grade equivalents do not indicate what level of reading text a child should be using. Grade equivalent scores on tests simply do not have a one-to-one correspondence with reading series placement or the various formulas for determining readability levels.

Grade equivalents are also inappropriate for use in any sort of discrepancy analysis of an individual's test performance or for use in many statistical procedures (Reynolds, 1981a). First, the growth curve between age and achievement in basic academic subjects flattens out at upper grade levels. In Table 20.2, for instance, there is very little change in standard-score values corresponding to 2 years below grade level for age after about seventh or eighth grade. In fact, grade equivalents have almost no meaning in reading at this level, since reading instruction typically stops by high school. Thus grade equivalents really only represent extrapolations from earlier grades. Since the average reading level in the population changes very little after junior high school, grade equivalents at these ages become virtually nonsensical, with large fluctuations resulting from a raw-score difference of 2 or 3 points on a 100-item test. In math and other areas where instruction specifically

continues, this is not the case, but it only adds to our overall problem.

Second, grade equivalents assume that the rate of learning is constant throughout the school year and that there is no gain or loss during summer vacation. Third, grade equivalents involve an excess of extrapolation. Since tests are not administered during every month of the school year, scores between the testing intervals (often a full year) must be extrapolated on the assumption of constant growth rates. Interpretation of frequently extrapolated values based on an assumption of constant growth rates is fundamentally just silly. Fourth, different academic subjects are acquired at different rates, and performance varies across content areas. Thus "2 years below grade level for age" may indicate much more serious deficiency in math, for example, than in reading comprehension.

Finally, grade equivalents exaggerate small differences in performance between individuals and for a single individual across tests. Some test authors even caution users on test record forms that standard scores only, and not grade equivalents, should be used for comparison purposes. The Wide Range Achievement Test (WRAT; Jastak & Jastak, 1978) includes a caution at the bottom of the child's test record form stating that standard scores only and not grade equivalents should be used for interpretive purposes. Despite this caution, many school psychologists and educational diagnosticians persist in reporting grade equivalents for the WRAT as well as for other achievement tests. The popularity of these scores is based primarily on misconceptions regarding their psychometric properties.

The principal advantage of using standardized or scaled scores with children lies in the comparability of score interpretation across age. By "standard scores," of course, are meant scores that are scaled to a constant mean and SD, such as the Wechsler deviation IQ, rather than the ratio IQ scores employed by the early Binet and the Slosson Intelligence Test, which give the false appearance of being scaled scores. Ratio IQs or other types of quotients have many of the same problems as grade equivalents and should be avoided for many of these same reasons. The SD of the Slosson Intelligence Test varies from approximately 11 to as much as 32, depending upon the age group under consideration; this causes major problems in interpretation and explanation of performance to teachers and parents. Standard scores of the deviation IQ type have the same percentile rank across age, since they are based not only on the mean but on the variability in scores about the mean at each age level. Grade and age equivalents do not consider the dispersion of scores about the mean.

Standard scores are more accurate and precise. Extrapolation of scores to arrive at an exact score point is typically not necessary, whereas the opposite is true of grade equivalents. Extrapolation is also typically not necessary for scores within 3 SDs of the mean, which accounts for more than 99% of all scores encountered.

Scaled scores can be set to any desired mean and SD (the fancy of the test author is not infrequently the principal determinant).

Fortunately, a few scales can account for the vast majority of standardized tests. Table 20.3 depicts the relationship among various scaled-score systems. If the standardization samples of the two tests are the same or are highly comparable, and the reliability coefficients for the two scales are reasonably similar, then Table 20.3 can also be used to equate scales to a common metric for ease of comparison. To use Table 20.3 for this purpose, one should enter the column corresponding to the mean and SD for the test in question and locate the child's score; read to the far left column (headed $\overline{X} = 0$, $SD = 1$); and repeat this procedure for other tests one wishes to place on the same scale.

7. *The measures employed should demonstrate a high level of reliability, which should be documented in the technical manual accompanying the test.* The specific scores employed in the various discrepancy formulas should have associated internal-

TABLE 20.3. Conversion of Standard Scores Based on Several Scales to a Commonly Expressed Metric

$\overline{X} = 0$ $SD = 1$	$\overline{X} = 0$ $SD = 3$	$\overline{X} = 36$ $SD = 6$	$\overline{X} = 50$ $SD = 10$	$\overline{X} = 50$ $SD = 15$	$\overline{X} = 100$ $SD = 15$	$\overline{X} = 100$ $SD = 16$	$\overline{X} = 100$ $SD = 20$	$\overline{X} = 500$ $SD = 100$	Percentile rank
2.6	.8	52	76	89	139	142	152	760	99
2.4	17	51	74	86	136	138	148	740	99
2.2	17	49	72	83	133	135	144	720	99
2.0	16	48	70	80	130	132	140	700	98
1.8	15	47	68	77	127	129	136	680	96
1.6	15	46	66	74	124	126	132	660	95
1.4	14	44	64	71	121	122	128	640	92
1.2	14	43	62	68	118	119	124	620	88
1.0	13	42	60	65	115	116	120	600	84
0.8	12	41	58	62	112	113	116	580	79
0.6	12	40	56	59	109	110	112	560	73
0.4	11	38	54	56	106	106	108	540	66
0.2	11	37	52	53	103	103	104	520	56
0.0	10	36	50	50	100	100	100	500	50
−0.2	9	35	48	47	97	97	96	480	42
−0.4	9	34	46	44	94	94	92	460	34
−0.6	8	33	44	41	91	90	88	440	27
−0.8	8	31	42	38	88	87	84	420	21
−1.0	7	30	40	35	85	84	80	400	16
−1.2	6	29	38	32	82	81	76	380	12
−1.4	6	28	36	29	79	78	72	360	8
−1.6	5	26	34	26	76	74	68	340	5
−1.8	5	25	32	23	73	71	64	320	4
−2.0	4	24	30	20	70	68	60	300	2
−2.2	3	23	28	17	67	65	56	280	1
−2.4	3	21	26	14	64	62	52	260	1
−2.6	2	20	24	11	61	58	48	240	1

consistency reliability estimates (where possible) of no less than .80 and preferably of .90 or higher. Coefficient alpha is the recommended procedure for estimating reliability, and should be reported routinely for each age level in the standardization sample of the test at not more than 1-year intervals. It is recognized that alpha will not be appropriate for all measures. Test authors and publishers should routinely use alpha where appropriate and should provide other reliability estimates as may be appropriate to the nature of the test. When alpha is not reported, an explanation should be given. Authors and publishers should he careful not to inflate reliability estimates spuriously through inappropriate sampling or other computational methods (Stanley, 1971). Internal-consistency reliability (e.g., alpha) will almost always be the most appropriate reliability estimate for intelligence and achievement tests. Internal-consistency estimates are the most appropriate of all reliability estimates for these tests because they best determine the accuracy of test scores.

8. *The validity coefficient* r_{xy}, *which represents the relationship between the measures of aptitude and achievement, should be based on an appropriate sample.* This sample should consist of a large, stratified random sample of normally functioning children. A large sample is necessary to reduce the sampling error in r_{xy} to an absolute minimum, since variations in r_{xy} will affect the calculation of a severe discrepancy and affect the distribution of difference scores, which is the area of greater concern. Normally functioning children are preferred for the samples, because the definition of "severe discrepancy" is based in part on the frequency of occurrence of the discrepancy in the normal population. When conorming of aptitude and achievement measures is conducted, this problem is simplified greatly, since r_{xy} can be based on the standardization sample of the two measures (which should meet the standards in point 2 above) without any children with disabilities included. Some states (notably California) use validity coefficients based in estimates derived from research using children with disabilities. This practice is not recommended, because the IQ and achievement score distributions of such children are not normal; thus they restrict the range of scores and

lower the correlation between IQ and achievement, making it appear artificially smaller than it is in reality.

9. *The validity of test score interpretations should be clearly established.* Though clearly stated in the rules and regulations for IDEA, this requirement should receive special emphasis, particularly with regard to Cronbach's (1971) discussion of test validation. Validation with normal samples is insufficient for application to diagnosis of disabling conditions; validity should be demonstrated for exceptional populations. This requirement is an urgent one, especially in certain areas of achievement where few adequate scales exist. To determine deviations from normality, validation with normal samples should typically be regarded as sufficient. This requirement does not require separate normative data for each handicapping condition. The generalizability of norms and of validity data is in part a function of the question one seeks to answer with the test data and is ultimately an empirical question (Reynolds, Gutkin, Elliot, & Witt, 1984).

10. *Special technical considerations should be addressed when one uses performance-based measures of achievement (e.g., writing skill).* Some measures, such as written expression, involve special problems of reliability and validity. This is also true of such tasks as the Wechsler Vocabulary and Comprehension measures, in which examiners are frequently called upon to make fine distinctions regarding the quality of a response. Interrater reliability of scoring on any measure calling for judgments by the examiner should be reported and should be .85 to .90 or higher. Highly speeded and primarily memory-based tasks will also pose special technical problems that must be addressed.

11. *Bias studies on the instruments in use should be reported.* Criterion-related validity should receive emphasis in this regard, but not to the exclusion of other studies of bias. Bias should be addressed with respect to appropriate demographic variables that may moderate the test's validity. At a minimum, these should include race, sex, and socioeconomic status (though not necessarily simultaneously). In the assessment and diagnosis of LD in particular, sex bias needs to he investigated, since boys outnumber

girls in classes for those with LD by about 3.5 to 1. The procedures for evaluating bias in all aspects of a test are presented in a comprehensive form in Berk (1982) and in Jensen (1980). Although measures that exhibit little or no statistical bias are the measures of choice, other measures can be used with appropriate correction.

All of the points made above should be considered in the evaluation of test data used for determining a severe discrepancy. It bears repeating that the discrepancy formulas presented here yield results that are only as reliable as the test data used in them. Integrally related to the quality of test data are the characteristics of the examiner; the next section explores this issue.

WHO SHOULD BE DIAGNOSING LD?

In the public schools, in one sense, the question of who should be diagnosing LD has been resolved by IDEA. According to the rules and regulations implementing this law, only a multidisciplinary team is empowered to diagnose disabling conditions of any type in the schools. It remains legitimate to ask, however, who should be doing the primary assessment of the discrepancy criterion (as well as the psychological process criterion) and interpreting these results to the team. It would be convenient to proffer a job title and move on; however, the educational and certification requirements for any given job in the schools vary greatly from state to state. This variation is troublesome, because the quality of the personnel conducting the diagnosis or interpreting it to the team and to the parents is as important to the diagnosis of LD as the quality of the data and the objectivity of the definition.

The task of LD diagnosis is the most difficult of all psychoeducational diagnostic tasks; thus the most highly trained personnel available should be reserved for assignment to evaluating children with potential LD. This is clearly not what has been happening in practice. Although accurate diagnosis of LD in school-age children is considered the most difficult type of diagnosis mandated by IDEA, it is precisely the area of evaluation and diagnosis most often relegated to the least qualified, most poorly

trained diagnostic personnel in the schools. Arguments and data (Bennett, 1981; Bennett & Shepherd, 1982) clearly show that the specialists and diagnosticians commonly assigned the task of LD diagnosis do not possess the requisite knowledge of tests and measurements to allow them to interpret test scores adequately. On a test of beginning-level measurement concepts, Bennett and Shepherd's (1982) LD specialists answered barely 50% of the questions correctly. A group of first-year graduate students in an introductory measurement class answered more than 70% of the same questions correctly. Using the best-trained staff will not solve the problems involved in diagnosis and evaluation of children with LD, but it would be a step in the right direction. Who precisely are the best-trained staff members will vary from state to state; the point is that this subject desperately needs attention.

Personnel such as psychiatrists and social workers are often legally acceptable diagnosticians for LD, but have no training in psychological or educational assessment. Without the assistance of a qualified psychologist, it is doubtful that accurate diagnoses will occur. Psychologists who diagnose LD need specialized training as well—not only in psychopathology, hut in psychometrics and special education (areas poorly treated in many clinical programs).

CONCLUSION

This chapter reviews the state of the art in determining a "severe discrepancy" between a child's achievement and his or her age and ability. Other factors to be considered in this determination are found in IDEA and in Chalfant (1984), but are also dictated by the theoretical approach adopted. The state of the art in determining a severe discrepancy is known, but now needs to be implemented. As implementation moves forward, we need to turn our attention toward objectification of the remaining four key aspects of LD diagnosis reviewed in Chalfant (1984). Next, given the relative importance of these five factors, we should tackle the "psychological process" criterion. This criterion is absolutely crucial, but must of necessity be theory-driven. However controversial and complex the issues may be, we must move forward on all fronts.

It is inappropriate at this stage to recommend a single, specific theoretical model from which to assess LD. What is imperative, however, is that *a clear theoretical rationale is necessary for a coherent diagnosis and evaluation of children with LD.* Consequently, at least at the local education agency level if not at the SEA level, the theoretical and conceptual basis for any given criteria for designating a child as having LD should be clearly stated and understood by district diagnostic personnel, and its supporting body of literature should be cited (Reynolds, 1985a). Clinicians need to adopt a theoretical model and to strive earnestly for internal consistency in their own case-by-case work. It is less important at this stage of inquiry in the discipline just which theoretical or conceptual model is adopted than it is that a theoretical model be clearly stated and implemented at a state-of-the-art level. To do less is to cheat the children we seek to serve.

REFERENCES

Angoff, W. H. (1971). Scales, norms, and equivalent scores. In H. L. Thorndike (Ed.), *Educational measurement* (2nd ed.). Washington, DC: American Council on Education.

Bennett, H. E. (1981). Professional competence and the assessment of exceptional children. *Journal of Special Education, 15,* 437–446.

Bennett, H. E., & Shepherd, M. J. (1982). Basic measurement proficiency of learning disability specialists. *Learning Disability Quarterly, 5,* 177–184.

Berk, H. A. (Ed.). (1982). *Handbook of methods for detecting test bias.* Baltimore: Johns Hopkins University Press.

Berk, B. A. (1984). *Screening and diagnosis of children with learning disabilities.* Springfield, IL: Charles C Thomas.

Chalfant, J. C. (1984). *Identifying learning disabled students: Guidelines for decision making.* Burlington, VT: Northeast Regional Resource Center.

Cone, T., & Wilson, L. (1981). Quantifying a severe discrepancy: A critical analysis. *Learning Disability Quarterly, 4,* 359–371.

Cronbach, L. J. (1971). Test validation. In B. L. Thorndike (Ed.), *Educational measurement* (2nd ed.). Washington, DC: American Council on Education.

Danielson, L. C., & Bauer, J. W. (1978). A formula-based classification of learning disabled children: An examination of the issues. *Journal of Learning Disabilities, 11,* 163–176.

Ebel, B. (1972). *Essentials of educational measurement* Englewood Cliffs, NJ: Prentice-Hall.

Hanna, C., Dyck, N., & Holen, M. (1979). Objective analysis of aptitude-achievement discrepancies in LD classification. *Learning Disability Quarterly, 2,* 32–38.

Hopkins, H., & Hodge, S. (1984). Review of the Kaufman Assessment Battery (K-ABC) for Children. *Journal of Counseling and Human Development, 63,* 105–107.

Hunter. J. E., Schmidt, F. L., & Rauschenberger, J. (1984). Methodological, statistical, and ethical issues in the study of bias in psychological tests. In C. R. Reynolds & B. T. Brown (Eds.), *Perspectives on bias in mental testing.* New York: Plenum Press.

Hynd, C., & Willis, W. (1988). *Pediatric neuropsychology.* New York: Grune & Stratton.

Jastak, J. E., & Jastak, S. (1978). *Wide Range Achievement Test.* Wilmington, DE: Jastak Associates.

Jensen, A. R. (1980). *Bias in mental testing.* New York: Free Press.

Kamphaus, R. W., & Reynolds, C. B. (1987). *Clinical and research applications of the K-ABC.* Circle Pines, MN: American Guidance Service.

Kaufman, A. S. (1979). *Intelligent testing with the WISC-R.* New York: Wiley-Interscience.

McLeod, J. (1979). Educational underachievement: Toward a defensible psychometric definition. *Journal of Learning Disabilities, 12,* 42–50.

Meehl, P. E. (1954). *Clinical versus statistical prediction.* Minneapolis: University of Minnesota Press.

Mercer, J., & Lewis, J. (1979). *System of Multicultural Pluralistic Assessment: Technical manual.* New York: Psychological Corporation.

Payne, R. W., & Jones, H. G. (1957). Statistics for the investigation of individual cases. *Journal of Clinical Psychology, 13,* 115–121.

Reynolds, C. R. (1981a). The fallacy of "two years below grade level for age" as a diagnostic criterion for reading disorders. *Journal of School Psychology, 19,* 350–358.

Reynolds, C. R. (1982). The problem of bias in psychological assessment. In C. R. Reynolds & T. B. Gutkin (Eds.), *The handbook of school psychology.* New York: Wiley.

Reynolds, C. R. (1984). Critical measurement issues in learning disabilities. *Journal of Special Education, 18,* 451–476.

Reynolds, C. B. (1985a). Measuring the aptitude–achievement discrepancy in learning disability diagnosis. *Remedial and Special Education, 6,* 37–55.

Reynolds, C. R. (1985b). Toward objective diagnosis of learning disabilities. *Special Services in the Schools, 1,* 161–176.

Reynolds, C. R. (1986). Assessment of exceptional children. In B. T. Brown & C. B. Reynolds (Eds.), *Psychological perspectives on childhood exceptionality.* New York: Wiley-Interscience.

Reynolds, C. R., & Brown, B. T. (1984). An introduction to the issues. In. R. Reynolds & B. T. Brown (Eds.), *Perspectives on bias in mental testing.* New York: Plenum Press.

Reynolds, C. R., & Clark, J. A. (1983). Cognitive assessment of the preschool child. In B. Bracken & K. Paget (Eds.), *Psychoeducational assessment of the preschool child.* New York: Grune & Stratton.

Reynolds, C. R., & Gutkin, T. B. (1981). Test scatter on the WPPSI: Normative analyses of the standardization sample. *Journal of Learning Disabilities, 14,* 460–464.

Reynolds, C. R., Gutkin, T. B., Elliot, S. N., & Witt, J. C. (1984). *School psychology: Essentials of theory and practice.* New York: Wiley.

Reynolds, C. R., & Stanton, H. C. (1988). *Discrepancy determinator 1.* Bensalem, PA: TRAIN.

Reynolds, C. R., & Willson, V. L. (1984, April). *Another look at aptitude–achievement discrepancies in the evaluation of learning disabilities.* Paper presented at the annual meeting of the National Council on Measurement in Education, New Orleans, LA.

Rules and Regulations Implementing Education for All Handicapped Children Act of 1975, PL 94-142, 42 Fed. Reg. 42474 (1977).

Salvia, J., & Ysseldyke, J. (1981). *Assessment in special and remedial education* (2nd ed.). Boston: Houghton Mifflin.

Schmidt, F. L. (1974). Probability and utility assumptions underlying use of the Strong Vocational Interest Blank. *Journal of Applied Psychology, 4,* 456–464.

Silverstein, A. B. (1981). Pattern analysis as simultaneous statistical inference. *Journal of Consulting and Clinical Psychology, 50,* 234–240.

Stanley, J. C. (1971). Reliability. In R. L. Thorndike (Ed.), *Educational measurement* (2nd ed.). Washington, DC: American Council on Education.

Thorndike, R. L., & Hagen, E. (1977). *Measurement and evaluation in education and psychology.* New York: Wiley.

Wechsler, D. (1991). *The Wechsler Intelligence Scale for Children—Third Edition.* San Antonio, TX: Psychological Corporation.

Wiggins, J. S. (1981). Clinical and statistical prediction: Where are we and where do we go from here? *Clinical Psychology Review, 1,* 3–18.

Willson, V. L., & Reynolds, C. R. (1984). Another look at evaluating aptitude–achievement discrepancies in the diagnosis of learning disabilities. *Journal of Special Education, 18,* 477–487.

Zimmerman, D. W., & Williams, R. H. (1982). The relative error magnitude in three measures of change. *Psychometrika, 47,* 141–147.

21

Visual–Motor Assessment of Children

JACK A. CUMMINGS
JESSICA A. HOIDA
GREGORY R. MACHEK
JASON M. NELSON

The primary rationale for psychological assessment is to promote a child's successful adaptation to the environment (Yeates & Taylor, 1998). Whether the environment is the school setting, community, or home, assessment data should inform intervention decisions that facilitate academic achievement, improve peer relations, enhance family interactions, and/or increase the likelihood of the child's success at negotiating the complex systems in the broader context of the community. When assessment is conceptualized to promote adaptation, it is essential that the psychologist understand the context within which the child is expected to perform. Assessment is bounded by the ecological setting. This contrasts sharply with assessment that takes as its focus a within-child perspective.

Too often, psychologists have been content to offer a nomothetic approach to assessment. The performance of the individual is compared to the norm group, and the individual becomes a composite of standard scores. Reporting these scores overshadows insights into the individual's motivation, problem solving, persistence, self-monitoring, reflectivity, and sense of self-efficacy.

Kaufman (1979; Kaufman & Lichtenberger, 2000) endorses a hypothesis-testing approach to the interpretation of a child's performance. Within this approach, the role of the psychologist is to develop hypotheses about the child from various sources (behavioral observations, background information, developmental history, test results, etc.). Hypothesis generation and testing are processes occurring continually during an assessment. As noted by Cummings (1986), it is critical that the examiner not adopt an attitude of attempting to verify or confirm hypotheses. Rather, evidence that would either support or negate a given hypothesis must be considered sequentially. Confirmatory assessment is a dangerous practice that may lead to a search for pathology, rather than an appropriate and fair assessment of an individual. This is not a minor semantic difference; it is an important aspect of a psychologist's philosophy of assessment.

The assessment of visual–motor functioning is complex. Benton and Tranel (1993) categorize visually related disorders as visual-perceptive, visual–spatial, and visual–constructive. Visual-perceptive problems may include visual object agnosia or an inability to visually analyze or synthesize. Visual–spatial difficulties may be observed when an individual is unable to localize points in space, has defective judgment of direction and distance, or lacks topographical orientation. Visual–constructive disorders may be reflected by difficulty in assembling parts of a whole or in the graphomotor aspect of performance. To complete a visual–motor task successfully, an individual must have not only adequate visual acuity, but the abilities to attend to a stimulus, analyze the stimulus through a process of deconstruction, plan the sequential execution of the drawing, continually monitor the outcome of the act of drawing, and make appropriate adjustments while drawing. An adequate pencil grip, persistence, recognition of errors, and careful monitoring all contribute to a successful performance.

We recommend a data-based, eclectic approach to psychological assessment. It is imperative that professionals use assessment tools that have been demonstrated to exhibit adequate technical qualities in the form of validity and reliability. Results of visual–motor tests should be weighed in a manner consistent with hypothesis testing, where evidence is considered from behavioral observations, interview data, other psychological or neuropsychological test data, and other data relative to improving the child's adaptation in the environments central to the referral question. It should be emphasized that the hallmark of a high-quality assessment is that it is responsive to the referral question.

The remainder of this chapter is divided into three sections. The first section includes reviews of common measures of visual–motor functioning. Among the measures covered are the Bender–Gestalt Test and several of its scoring systems; the Developmental Test of Visual–Motor Integration (VMI); the Wide Range Assessment of Visual–Motor Abilities (WRAVMA); the Rey–Osterrieth Complex Figure (ROCF) and its Developmental Scoring System (DSS); and the Motor-Free Visual Perception Test—Revised (MVPT-R). The second section of the chapter focuses on the distinction between a product-oriented and a process-oriented approach to assessment. In this section, the role of keen observation is stressed. The third section of the chapter ex-

amines the relationship between visual–motor functioning and academic achievement. The chapter concludes with commentary on past reservations expressed about visual–motor assessment of children, as well as a case study.

COMMON MEASURES OF VISUAL–MOTOR FUNCTIONING

Despite predictions of the demise of visual–motor assessment, these measures continue to enjoy frequent use by psychologists. Watkins, Campbell, Nieberding, and Hallmark (1995) surveyed 1,000 randomly selected American Psychological Association (APA) members "who identified their psychology specialty as clinical" (p. 54). They received 421 usable returns. The clinical psychologists were distributed across seven types of work settings: private practice, mental hospital, general hospital, community mental health center/outpatient clinic, university department, medical school, and others. The Bender–Gestalt (along with the Wechsler scales, the Minnesota Multiphasic Personality Inventory—2, the Thematic Apperception Test, and sentence completion) was consistently among the top-ranked procedures, based on frequency of use across the settings. For all but medical school settings, the Bender–Gestalt was ranked in the top 10 most frequently used procedures. Watkins and colleagues concluded that there has been little change in the frequency of use of various measures since the 1960s. Based on the introduction of behavioral assessment techniques, Hunsley (1996) questioned this conclusion. Hunsley suggested that Watkins and colleagues failed to consider the impact of behavioral approaches on current practices of clinical psychologists. However, Watkins, Campbell, Nieberding, and Hallmark (1996) responded with a table providing a breakdown of psychologists by theoretical orientation. Self-identified behavioral psychologists reported that the Bender–Gestalt was the 10th most frequently used measure, while self-identified cognitive psychologists ranked it 5th. Piotrowski and Zalewski (1993) surveyed APA-accredited training programs and likewise found that visual–motor measures continue to have a place in the preparation of psychologists.

Most of the measures reviewed in this section of the chapter are administered via paper and pencil (e.g. the Bender–Gestalt Test, the VMI). These tests typically require examinees to draw or copy various geometric shapes onto a sheet of paper. Their productions are scored for errors or various types of deviations (e.g., failure to integrate parts, rotations, expansion, etc.). Similarly, the WRAVMA uses a paper-and-pencil format to assess visual–motor skills, but also measures visual–spatial skills via a matching task and fine motor skills via a pegboard task. The ROCF uses a single complex figure as a stimulus for examinees to copy. The following sections address issues surrounding the administration, scoring, and psychometric properties of the aforementioned visual–motor instruments.

The Bender Visual–Motor Gestalt (Bender–Gestalt) Test

In the past six decades, the Bender Visual–Motor Gestalt Test, more commonly referred to as the Bender–Gestalt, has been the best-known and most widely used measure of visual–motor functioning. The Bender–Gestalt Test was developed in 1938 by Lauretta Bender. Bender was working at Bellevue Hospital when she became interested in Gestalt psychologists' study of visual perception in humans. One such psychologist, Wertheimer (1923), had developed approximately 30 Gestalt designs; Bender adapted nine of these figures and began using them with her patients. The Bender–Gestalt Test evolved from her work with these nine designs. Although Bender never proposed a standardized scoring system, she did provide, in the original monograph, guidelines for identifying patterns of errors that could be used to assist the diagnosis of schizophrenia and other neuroses (Bender, 1938). Later, Bender (1946) published a second manual of instructions for the Bender–Gestalt Test.

Description of Stimuli and Administration

The Bender–Gestalt Test is composed of nine designs. The examiner presents each card, starting with A and then proceeding in numerical order from 1 through 8. The examinee is asked to copy the designs onto an unlined sheet of $8\frac{1}{2}'' \times 11''$ paper. Koppitz (1964, p. 15) suggests the following instructions: "I have nine cards here with designs on them for you to copy. Here is the first one. Now, go ahead and make one just like it." The designs are presented one at a time. There is no time limit, and the test usually requires about 6 minutes to administer.

Early Scoring Systems

Billingslea (1948) was the first to attempt to provide an objective scoring system for the Bender–Gestalt Test. His system initially consisted of 38 "factors" and 137 "indices," many of which required precise measurement. His procedure proved extremely time-consuming; in fact, Billingslea (1948) reported a scoring time of 15 hours per protocol. Subsequently, he reduced the number of factors to 25 and the number of indices to 63. However, the Billingslea scoring system failed to achieve widespread use.

The Pascal–Suttell (1951) and the Hain (1964) scoring systems are frequently mentioned in the research literature. Pascal and Suttell attempted to provide a system capable of distinguishing persons with psychogenic disorders from those without such disorders. The system was standardized on a sample of psychiatric patients and a matched group of individuals without mental illness. The sample included 474 persons ages 15–50, and was stratified by age and education. The scoring system involves the identification of 105 possible errors in the reproduction of the designs. Each error is weighted from 2 to 8; these weighted scores are summed and converted to a standard score, based on education. The authors reported an interrater reliability of .90. The test–retest stability coefficient, for a time interval of 24 hours, was reported as .71. Summarizing two studies, Pascal and Suttell cited diagnostic accuracy figures ranging from .76 to .83. The popularity of the Pascal–Suttell system has waned in the past few decades; some have pointed to the complexity and time-consuming nature of the scoring system as factors that have limited its use (Lacks, 1984). However, Marsico and Wagner (1991), using the Pascal–Suttell scoring system, found that one item (item 7) was almost (73%) as accurate in discriminating patients with organic mental disorders from those without as the total score (74%). If these findings hold true with further research, using only item 7 and the Pascal–Suttell system could significantly reduce time spent on scoring, at least in screening for organicity. Research by Marsico and Wagner (1990) has also shown that the Pascal–Suttell system is as good as or better than other scoring systems in detecting organic problems. However, we believe that other systems may be more attractive to clinicians, due to the time-consuming scoring process of the Pascal–Suttell system.

The Koppitz Developmental Bender–Gestalt Test Scoring System

The Koppitz Developmental Bender–Gestalt Test Scoring System (Koppitz, 1964) has emerged as one of the most commonly used systems with children in both school and clinical settings (Neale & McKay, 1985). As suggested in the title of her scoring system, Koppitz emphasized that the Bender–Gestalt Test, when used with children, must be seen as a developmental test. Her scoring system, also known as the Developmental Scoring System or simply as the "Koppitz system," entails the identification of 30 mutually exclusive errors that are scored as either present or absent. Four major types of errors are scored: rotations, distortions, errors of integration, and errors of perseveration. Koppitz (1975) provided numerous clear examples of these errors and when they should be scored. The errors are summed to produce a Total Bender Developmental Score, which is a raw score. The highest possible score attainable on the test is 30, though, according to Koppitz, scores above 20 are rare. Koppitz provided information that enabled the transformation of the Total Developmental Score to age equivalents and to percentile ranks, based on the 1974 restandardization data (see below). In addition, Furr (1970) has published a table of standard scores ($M = 100$, $SD = 15$) for the Bender–Gestalt, based on Koppitz's (1964) original normative information.

The Koppitz system was restandardized in 1974 (Koppitz, 1975). This restandardization included a sample of 975 elementary school pupils ranging in age from 5 years, 0 months to 10 years, 11 months. Children from the following geographic regions were included: 15% from the West, 2% from the South, and 83% from the Northeast. In terms of racial/ethnic composition, 86% of the sample was white, 8.5% black, 4.5% Mexican American or Puerto Rican, and 1% Asian American. Seven percent of the students were from rural areas, 31% from small towns, 36% from the suburbs, and 26% from large metropolitan areas. Koppitz did not provide information regarding the gender or socioeconomic status of the sample. In addition, there are obvious problems with the geographical representativeness of the sample: the Northeast was highly overrepresented, whereas the South, Midwest, and West were underrepresented.

Koppitz (1975) presented the results from 31 studies, which produced a range of interjudge reliabilities from .79 to .99. Further research on the interjudge reliability of the Koppitz system reveals figures clustering around .90. Neale and McKay (1985) reported an interjudge reliability of .92. Aylward and Schmidt (1986) found interjudge reliabilities of .93, .86, and .87; these results were derived from comparisons of total Koppitz scores. Aylward and Schmidt's study, however, revealed lower interjudge reliabilities (ranging from .71 to .94) when individual error items were analyzed.

An important dimension of any test score is its stability. Nine studies of the test–retest stability of Koppitz system scores were presented by Koppitz; these studies examined scores obtained from children of varying grade levels and at various testing intervals. Test–retest stability coefficients ranging from .50 to .90 were reported. Although there appears to be no identifiable pattern of stability variation based on grade level, the length of the interval between initial testing and retesting is critical to the stability of the scores. The pattern indicates that the scores decrease as the length of the interval between the initial testing and the retesting increases. This pattern is not surprising, given the developmental nature of the test. Normally, a child's visual–motor integration skills will improve as the child develops; therefore, the greater the interval between the initial testing and retesting, the greater the opportunity for the child's visual–motor skills to have improved. This improvement will influence the child's performance on the test. The emergence of the Koppitz system as one of the most commonly used scoring systems coincided with the increased usage of the Bender–Gestalt Test with children (Lacks, 1984).

Although the Koppitz system was standardized on children, others have sought to determine its applicability with preadolescent and adolescent populations. For example, Bolen, Hewett, Hall, and Mitchell (1992) examined the claim by Koppitz that the normal child's visual–motor functioning is developed enough by 11 years to preclude the Bender–Gestalt Test's usefulness with older children. Their results showed that the use of the Koppitz system revealed errors among all age groups between 11 years, 6 months and 15 years, 11 months of age. Bolen and colleagues concluded that visual–motor integration functioning may be measurable for an adolescent population; they called for further research on increasing the standardization sample to include children from 11 years, 6 months to 15 years, 11 months of age, or to create a scoring system specifically for the adolescent population. Shapiro and Simpson (1995) provided further support for the use of the Koppitz system with older children. Using a sample of adolescents with behavioral and emotional disturbances, these researchers found that perceptual skills, as measured by specific Wechsler Intelligence Scale for Children—Revised (WISC-R) subtests, correlated with Koppitz Total Developmental Scores. They concluded that the Bender–Gestalt Test seemed to have some ability to assess ongoing visual–motor development through adolescence. This ability corresponds with the severity of the impairment: The utility of the instrument increases with the severity of the impairment. Shapiro and Simpson (1995) also suggested that further research could lead to a more discernible scoring system for adolescents. They cautioned that it is inappropriate to use the Bender–Gestalt on such populations before applicable normative data are established. Similarly, the Koppitz system has been used by some researchers on adult populations. This is not advisable, because the norms provided by Koppitz were established with a sample of children. The Lacks scoring system, described next, is more appropriate for use with adults.

The Lacks Adaptation of the Hutt–Briskin Scoring System

Patricia Lacks published a second edition of her 1984 book, *Bender Gestalt Screening for Brain Dysfunction*, in 1999. Using Hutt and Briskin's (1960) list of 12 essential discriminators for the Bender–Gestalt Test as the basis for her scoring method, Lacks (1999) has provided a rich set of drawings to guide scoring. Examples of various errors are illustrated, as are correct exemplars that should not be scored as errors. Although the Lacks system of scoring is intended for adults, the criteria have merit as a framework from which the psychologist may develop internal norms to interpret children's production of Bender–Gestalt designs. The 12 criteria include rotation (orientation of the major axis by 80–180 degrees); overlapping (difficulty drawing the parts of the designs that overlap); simplification (simplifying all or part of the design); fragmentation (failing to capture the Gestalt of the design); retrogression (the individual is capable of rendering an accurate design, but instead draws a more primitive figure); perseveration (continuing elements of a previous design or drawing more than what the stimulus calls for); collision (drawing separate figures as overlapping); impotence (the individual recognizes that the production is incorrect, but is incapable of fixing it); closure (failure to complete figures); motor incoordination (irregular, not smooth lines); angulation (inability to render angles); and cohesion (irregularities in size).

The Modified Version of the Bender–Gestalt Test, and the Qualitative Scoring System

The Qualitative Scoring System (QSS) was developed for use with the Modified Version of the Bender–Gestalt Test for Preschool and Primary School Children (Brannigan & Brunner, 1989, 1996, 2002). The Modified Version eliminated three of the designs from the original Bender–Gestalt Test and retained designs A, 1, 2, 4, 6, and 8. The test was modified to make it more appropriate for younger children by eliminating some of the more difficult designs. A sample of 1,160 children, ranging in age from 4 years, 6 months to 8 years, 5 months, was used to standardize the Modified Version. The children were drawn from New York, Pennsylvania, West Virginia, Wisconsin, Minnesota, Wyoming, and Texas. Brannigan and Brunner (1996) did not specify the proportion of the sample that came from each state. There was adequate representation across the age levels for the standardization.

The QSS uses a 6-point rating scale that allows for an individual score for each design, as well as a total score for all designs. Individual design scores can range from 0 to 5 points, whereas the highest possible overall score is 30 points. Research by Moose and Brannigan (1997) on the concurrent validity of the Modified Version of the Bender–Gestalt Test has shown significant correlation ($r = .54$) with the VMI (Beery, 1989). Research has also been conducted comparing the QSS with the Koppitz system and assessing their concurrent validity with other visual–motor measures. Schachter, Brannigan, and Tooke (1991) found that the QSS accounted for nearly twice as much variance in VMI scores as the Koppitz system did.

In addition to strong concurrent validity, research has supported the interscorer reliability of the Modified Version of the Bender–Gestalt Test. Fuller and Vance (1995) found correlation coefficients ranging from .74 to .80 between two previously untrained licensed psychologists scoring the six individual designs. Some caution should be exercised when considering these results due to the sample size ($n = 48$). Furthermore, the representativeness of the sample prevents generalizability, because participants were predominantly white and were drawn from a limited geographic region.

Finally, the utility of the Modified Version of the Bender–Gestalt Test and the QSS in predicting academic achievement has been investigated. Brannigan and Brunner (1993) compared the validity of the QSS and the Koppitz system in predicting academic achievement scores of first- and second-grade students. They found that the QSS showed significantly higher correlation coefficients than the Koppitz system with the Otis–Lennon School Ability Test among second graders. However, differences did not reach significance for the first-grade sample.

Further evidence for the predictive validity of the Modified Version and the QSS has been found by Brannigan, Aabye, Baker, and Ryan (1995). Their study used 409 first- through fourth-grade students in a predominantly white, rural setting. Results showed that the QSS and the Koppitz system both significantly correlated with the Metropolitan Achievement Test. The QSS, however, correlated higher than the Koppitz system on all achievement subtests, and correlation differences were found to be significantly higher in five areas (second-grade math, third-grade reading and language, and fourth-grade reading and language). Again, however, caution should be used in generalizing such findings to populations that do not share similar demographic characteristics.

The Developmental Test of Visual–Motor Integration

The VMI is now in its fourth edition (Beery, 1997a, 1997b). The original version of the VMI was published in 1967, with subsequent versions published in 1982 and 1989. The VMI was designed to correspond with the child's acquisition of sequential developmental abilities. According to Beery (1997b), the purposes of the VMI are "to help identify, through early screening, children who may need special assistance, to obtain needed services, to test the effectiveness of educational and other interventions, and to advance research" (p. 5).

The fourth edition of the VMI makes use of three additional items, bringing the total number of items to 27. The 27 figures of the VMI are arranged from simple to complex; two of these figures are from the Bender–Gestalt Test. Unlike the Bender–Gestalt Test, the VMI presents the designs in a protocol. Each page is divided into six blocks. The three blocks on the upper portion of the page contain designs; the child is instructed to copy each stimulus design into the corresponding empty block below. In comparison to the Bender–Gestalt Test, the VMI is more structured, in that the stimuli are printed on the page and there are boundaries within which each design is to be copied.

The child's reproductions are scored as either "pass" or "fail." The manual (Beery,

1997b) provides numerous scoring examples; in addition to these examples, developmental comments are included to assist in the interpretation of a child's performance. A total raw score is computed by adding the number of figures passed. The manual provides a table that allows for the conversion of raw scores to developmental age equivalents. Additional tables are provided that allow the raw scores to be converted into either percentile ranks or standard scores. The standard scores are based on a mean of 10 and a standard deviation of 3 points. The scoring of the VMI takes into account the fact that older children will occasionally rush through simple designs and consequently fail them. In a case where it is obvious that a child or adolescent failed to give adequate attention to one of the simpler designs and later demonstrated ample visual–motor skill with more complex designs, the examiner is encouraged not to score the earlier designs as errors. It should be noted that this does not mean when a complex, difficult item is passed that all preceding errors are forgiven. Rather, the examiner is encouraged to use clinical judgment.

The 1997 edition of the VMI was normed on 2,734 children. The standardization sample closely reflected the 1990 U.S. Census data by gender, ethnicity, geographic region, and socioeconomic level. Standardization data are provided for ages 3 through 17. Beery (1997b) suggested that the VMI is appropriate for individuals "ages 3 to adult" (p. 26). Although standardarization data are not provided for adults, Hall, Pinkston, Szalda-Petree, and Coronis (1996) found evidence to support the VMI's ability to assess graphomotor ability in adults from 60 to 92 years of age. Their investigation found that the VMI was sensitive to differences according to age.

Beery (1997b) reported various reliability coefficients. With respect to interscorer reliability, two independent scorers rated 100 random protocols from the standardization sample. The reliability coefficients from this effort were reported to be .94 for Visual–Motor Integration, .98 for the Visual subtest, and .95 for the Motor subtest. The manual also reported similarly high interrater reliability coefficients for previous versions of the instrument. However, Beery acknowledged that high interrater reliabili-

ties may be particularly dependent on thorough training of those scoring the test. The manual (Beery, 1997b) reports that split-half internal-consistency correlations (.88) were slightly higher than the average correlations from the 1988 norming studies (.85). Test–retest coefficients were derived using 122 children from 6 to 10 years of age. The interval between test administrations was 3 weeks. The coefficients were .87 for Visual–Motor Integration, .84 for the Visual subtest, and .83 for the Motor subtest.

Beery (1997b) also provided information on the validity of the VMI. In a study of concurrent validity, 122 kindergarten through fifth-grade students in regular education were administered the VMI, the Copying subtest of the Developmental Test of Visual Perception, and the Drawing subtest of the WRAVMA. Correlation coefficients of .52 with the WRAVMA Drawing subtest and .75 with the Developmental Test of Visual Perception Copying subtest were found. Studies using previous versions of the VMI have found correlations with the Bender–Gestalt Test ranging from .29 to .93, with a median of .56. Beery suggested that the VMI has good predictive validity when used in combination with other measures. Examples given by Beery include prediction of achievement at the kindergarten and first-grade level when used in conjunction with a test for auditory–vocal association; prediction of Science Research Associates Reading, Language Arts, and Mathematics between entering kindergarten and the end of first grade; correspondence of kindergarten scores with sixth-grade reading classification, when used with three other measures as part of the Florida Kindergarten Screening Test; and predictions of school grade failures or retentions, especially when the VMI is used in conjunction with pediatricians' ratings.

Other research points to limitations in the VMI's predictive validity, especially when it is used on children above the first grade. For example, Hagborg and Aiello-Coultier (1994) compared the relationship between scores on the third revision of the VMI and teacher ratings of written language for 73 second- through seventh-grade students with learning disabilities. After controlling for socioeconomic status, achievement, and intelligence, Hagborg and Aiello-Coultier found that the VMI correlated only with handwriting (a finding that has been previously established) and not with other areas of writing skills.

The Wide Range Assessment of Visual–Motor Abilities

The WRAVMA (Adams & Sheslow, 1995) is similar to the VMI, in that it is made up of tasks to measure three abilities: visual–motor integration, visual–spatial skills, and fine motor skills. Like the VMI, the WRAVMA uses a paper-and-pencil task in which the child draws geometric forms and a matching task that does not require motor skills. A difference between the WRAVMA and the VMI is its use of a pegboard rather than a tracing task to assess fine motor skills. The manual states that the WRAVMA measures visual–motor, visual–spatial, and fine motor skills because of their relevance to children's school activities. Adams and Sheslow (1995) stated that all of these abilities are necessary for the child to be able to engage in the most fundamental school activities, such as copying from the chalkboard or writing. Because of the WRAVMA's use of tasks other than simply copying geometric shapes, the test developers stated that it is "uniquely suited to evaluate visual–motor ability because of its capability of making meaningful psychometric distinctions between important contributing sub-areas" (p. 3).

The manual reported that the three tests making up the WRAVMA may be administered alone or together. The Drawing test is the same type of task as the Bender–Gestalt Test and the VMI, requiring the child to copy designs that become increasingly difficult. The Matching test eliminates the use of motor skills by requiring the child to pick from a series of items the one that "goes best" with the stimulus item. Finally, the Pegboard test requires examinees to place small pegs into a pegboard as fast as they can in 90 seconds. This is done separately for each hand.

The scoring system of the WRAVMA is convenient. On the Drawing test, each item is worth 1 point, but often several criteria need to be met in order to receive credit. These criteria are printed on the test protocol and simply need to be checked off when the examiner is analyzing the child's drawings. One point is also given for each correct item on the Matching test and for each peg placed in the pegboard within the time limit of the Pegboard test. Tables are provided to convert these scores to standard scores. Other tables are provided to determine age equivalents, percentile scores, and significant differences between tests.

The test developers standardized all three tests on the same sample of children. The standardization sample was made up of 2,282 children ranging in age from 3 to 17 years. Adams and Sheslow (1995) reported that the sample's selection was based on demographic data from the 1990 U.S. Census. Twenty-five age groups were used, with 6-month intervals up to 12 years, and then 1-year intervals from 13 to 17 years. Gender breakdown was comparable to that of the nation at large, with 49.78% females and 50.22% males. Ethnicity was broken down into four groups: white, black, Hispanic, and other. The ethnic breakdown was as follows: 76.6% white, 12.3% black, 7.2% Hispanic, and 3.8% other. Hispanics were somewhat underrepresented compared to their presence in the 1990 U.S. Census (9%). Standardization was also completed in four regions of the country: 23.1% from the East, 22% from the North Central, 35.4% from the South, and 19.5% from the West. These percentages were similar to the census data. Lastly, the test developers attempted to represent socioeconomic levels in their sample according to those in the nation at large. They did this by breaking the sample down according to the highest occupational level of the custodial parents. These occupational groups, such as "managerial and professional" and "service, farming, and fishing occupations," were also roughly equivalent to those in the U.S. census report. Overall, the WRAVMA's standardization sample was representative of the U.S. population as a whole.

With respect to the reliability of the instrument, the manual reported on internal-consistency, test–retest, and interrater reliability. Reliability coefficients for the total sample were .93 on the Drawing test and .95 on the Matching test. Internal consistency was measured by coefficient alphas and corrected split-half correlations. For the Drawing test, coefficient alphas ranged from .63 to .82, with a mean of .75; split-half coefficients ranged from .69 to .89, with a mean of .81. On the Matching test, coefficient alphas ranged from .65 to .89, with a mean of .81; split-half coefficients ranged from .68 to .92, with a mean of .84. The manual also reported that test–retest stability of the WRAVMA, based on its Composite Score, was .86. Finally, the test developers assessed the interrater reliability of the measure. Adams and Sheslow (1995) reported that only one test on the WRAV-MA, the Drawing test, may result in errors in scoring; thus only this test was examined for interrater reliability. The manual report-ed that a study examined 39 Drawing test protocols and found correlations of .96 and .97 between three examiners. Overall, ade-quate evidence is provided to document the reliability of the WRAVMA.

Adams and Sheslow (1995) also reported evidence for the WRAVMA's content validi-ty, using an item separation reliability index from a Rasch analysis. Item separation in-dices ranged from .92 to .99 across age groups. The test developers stated, "Such high indices demonstrate that the items se-lected for the respective tests work together to define and measure a variable accurate-ly" (p. 131). The manual reported on the construct validity of the test by showing its relationship with other types of measures, such as intelligence tests and academic achievement tests. A correlation of .44 was found between the Drawing test and the WISC-III Full Scale IQ. The Matching test and the Pegboard test had correlations with the Full Scale IQ of .47 and .39, respective-ly. These correlations are moderate. When compared to the Reading, Spelling, and Arithmetic scores of the Wide Range Achievement Test—3 (WRAT-3), correla-tions ranged from .31 to .46 on the three WRAVMA tests. The test developers stated that these results supported their hypothesis that there would be a moderately high rela-tionship between the WRAT-3 and the WRAVMA. As reported by the manual, studies were also conducted to assess the concurrent validity of the instrument. A cor-relation of .76 was found between the Drawing test of the WRAVMA and the VMI. To test the concurrent validity of the Matching test, the test developers compared it to the MVPT-R and found a .54 correla-tion. Lastly, the Pegboard test of the

WRAVMA and the Grooved Pegboard Test were compared. A correlation of .35 was found between the dominant-hand Peg-board test score of the Grooved Pegboard Test and the dominant-hand Pegboard Test score of the WRAVMA. Adams and Shes-low (1995) concluded that these results may be related to the inadequate norming of the Grooved Pegboard Test.

Apart from the reliability and validity studies reported in the manual for the in-strument, no other studies of the WRAVMA were located after a thorough computer search of both ERIC and PSYCHinfo data-bases. Further independent research would aid in determining the usefulness of the WRAVMA in accurately assessing the visu-al–motor ability of children.

The Rey–Osterrieth Complex Figure and the Developmental Scoring System

The ROCF (Bernstein & Waber, 1996; Rey, 1941) differs from other perceptual mea-sures, in that it consists of only one rather complex figure. The manual for the ROCF's DSS (Bernstein & Waber, 1996) explained that the figure was originally developed by André Rey to examine the cognitive abilities of people suffering from brain damage. By obtaining normative data from children and adults, Paul Osterrieth subsequently stan-dardized the production of Rey's figure in 1941. This early scoring system was mostly quantitative and did not address more qual-itative factors, such as developmental con-gruency. Whereas the ROCF was originally used primarily for adults with brain dam-age, the focus has shifted more recently to use with children. This is largely due to ob-served comparabilities as well as fundamen-tal differences between reproductions of the ROCF by adults and children with brain damage who were referred for learning problems (Bernstein & Waber, 1996). Bern-stein and Waber (1996) note that their DSS (Waber & Holmes, 1985) was created large-ly to address the question of how much of the distortion in a child's production of the ROCF was a factor of underlying neurolog-ical pathology, and how much might be ex-plained by normal developmental progres-sion.

The manual for the DSS (Bernstein & Waber, 1996) referred to studies done by

Waber and Holmes (1985, 1986) that provide the normative data for the scoring system. These studies included 454 children from kindergarten through grade 8, who came from middle- to lower-middle-class schools in one school district in the northeastern United States. Their ages ranged from 5 to 14 years, and there was equal representation by gender. Bernstein and Waber (1996) stated that about 90% of the children were right-handed and that none of the children were screened for learning difficulties. Analysis of the scored protocols showed that there was an improvement in copying the figure with age. This analysis demonstrated certain developmental progressions (e.g., younger children typically depicted the left side of the figure more accurately than the right). Thus normative scores, given at 1-year intervals, are available.

There are limitations to the normative sample used for the DSS. One is the small number of participants, leading to relatively low representative numbers after division into age groups. The largest single age group (13-year-olds) included 60 children, whereas the 5-year-old group had only 24 children in it. Another limitation is the lack of geographical representation, because all the children came from one school district. In addition, it is not possible to assess the racial representativeness of the normative sample, because the authors did not include such information in the manual. One other possible limitation has to do with the way in which the tests for the sample group were administered: All children except the kindergartners were administered the ROCF in a group classroom setting. There is no other evidence in the manual to suggest that the ROCF should be used as a group-administered test.

Materials needed for the test include the DSS manual, a DSS scoring booklet, three DSS response sheets, an ROCF stimulus card, and five colored felt-tipped pens. The manual states that using different-colored pens during a single administration both allows the examiner to track the child's progress and enables comparisons across children. The amount of time that the examinee uses each color is dependent on the child's age, with younger children using each pen for a longer time. The administration of the test includes three separate draw-

ing conditions: Copy, Immediate Recall, and Delayed Recall. For the Copy condition, the stimulus card and the response sheet are placed in front of the child, and he or she is asked to make a copy of the ROCF design. Verbal encouragement is allowed if the child is hesitant, and the examiner must cue the child when it is time to switch pens. When the child is finished, the response sheet and the stimulus card are taken away, and a blank response sheet is presented. The child is then asked to draw as much as he or she remembers of the design. During this Immediate Recall phase, the child does not need to switch pen colors. Encouragement can be given if necessary, but verbal cuing for producing elements of the ROCF should be used as a last resort, and should not include reference to specific forms of the figure. After the child cannot remember any more, the materials are again removed, and the examiner engages the child in a series of mostly verbal tasks for about 15–20 minutes. After this period, the child is again given a blank response sheet and pen, and is asked to produce as much of the original figure as he or she can from memory. For this Delayed Recall phase, verbal encouragement may be needed, and the examiner can ask the child whether he or she remembers a particular element of the original figure from which to begin drawing. At no point during the entire testing period is the child told that he or she will be drawing the figure again from memory.

The DSS gives scores for Organization, Accuracy, and Errors, and also gives a Style rating. These three scores and the Style rating are calculated for the Copy, Immediate Recall, and Delayed Recall efforts. The Organization score ranges from 1 to 13 and is based on 24 criterial features for the Copy condition, and 16 criterial features for the Immediate Recall and Delayed Recall conditions. Examples of criterial features include alignments and intersections. The Style rating distinguishes ROCF reproductions into three main categories: Part-Oriented, Intermediate, and Configurational. The Style rating also uses criterial features, and cannot be determined until Organization has been scored. Specifically, the Style rating looks for elements such as continuity in the lines drawn. The Accuracy score is derived independently of any of the other scores, including the Style rating. Accuracy is simply the sum of all the lines represented in the child's reproduction of the ROCF. The manual suggests that the Accuracy score may be particularly useful to the two Recall conditions, where the amount of information remembered from the initial drawing may be relevant. The Error score is derived by counting four different types of distortions: Rotations, Perseverations, Misplacements, and Conflations.

Although the ROCF consists of only one figure, its complexity, as well as the administration procedure of the DSS, sets it apart from other tests of visual–motor integration. It may appear that the Error score from the Copy condition would correlate most accurately with other visual–motor integration measures; however, no empirical data support this claim, and the manual (Bernstein & Waber, 1996) specifically stated that "diagnostic inferences cannot be based on the Copy condition alone" (p. 43). Bernstein and Waber (1996) also suggested that the analysis of the ROCF testing using the DSS should be equally reliant on qualitative and quantitative data. Such an approach should look at the processes and behaviors that come about as a result of the administration, as well as the quantified scores. That the scores should not stand alone is made more apparent by the manual's admission of the relatively wide range of variability among the distribution of scores for the DSS normative sample.

Bernstein and Waber (1996) reported interrater reliability coefficients for the Copy productions at .95. Interrater reliability for the Recall productions were given as .94. Reliabilities for Style ratings were .88 and .87 for Copy and Recall productions, respectively. The manual explained that test–retest reliabilities were intentionally not calculated, because the clinical utility of the figure lies partly in its novelty. Therefore, any administrations subsequent to the initial one would be confounded by the examinee's lack of naiveté about the figure.

Bernstein and Waber (1996) also noted adequate validity for the DSS from studies where correlations were computed between clinical ratings and DSS ratings ($r = .82$) of the Copy productions. Correlations computed between objective DSS ratings and clinical ratings on Style were .78 for Copy

productions. In addition, an agreement of .87 was noted for the Recall productions. As further evidence of validity, the manual referenced a variety of studies that demonstrated the adequacy of the ROCF and DSS in discriminating nonpathological from pathological populations. Specifically, the authors cited studies that used the ROCF to distinguish children with learning disabilities, attention-deficit/hyperactivity disorder (ADHD), sensory deficits, treatment-related central nervous system effects, neurodevelopmental disorders, and acquired head injuries, as well as high-risk infants, from children without these conditions.

In the DSS manual, Bernstein and Waber (1996) also included a section on interpretation of the production results within a neuropsychological brain–behavior framework. This section elucidated how results may be analyzed in reference to possible neuroanatomical axes (specifically, the lateral, anterior–posterior, and cortical–subcortical). Since the ROCF, as scored by the DSS, includes both Immediate Recall and Delayed Recall phases, visual–spatial memory may be assessed. For obtaining clinically useful information, Bernstein and Waber advocated the use of both the Copy and the two Recall conditions. Differences among these conditions can reveal how the child encoded the stimulus. For instance, in the Copy condition alone, the child may provide a line by line reproduction. Once the stimulus is removed, the child's rendering gives cues to the manner in which the child encoded the whole.

Among the measures reviewed in this chapter, the ROCF is receiving the most attention in the neuropsychological literature. Ruffolo, Javorsky, Tremont, Westervelt, and Stern (2001) describe the ROCF as a commonly used measure of "visuospatial skills, visuoconstruction, visual memory, and executive functioning" (p. 299). Recent investigations provide documentation of the diverse uses for the ROCF, Hinshaw, Carte, Sami, Treuting, and Zupan (2002) reported significant differences in ROCF. Organization and Error Proportion for preadolescent girls with ADHD as contrasted with matched controls. Henry (2001) examined the organizational strategies and visual–motor skills of children living in rural Amazonia. Hubley and Tremblay (2002) reported that children with unilateral right-hemisphere injury at an early age experienced more difficulty reproducing from memory a figure organized around the central rectangle, as contrasted with children with early left-hemisphere brain injuries. Smith, Elliott, and Lach (2002) used the ROCF to investigate children with epilepsy by comparing the compatability of candidates for surgical intervention with those not deemed appropriate surgical candidates.

The Motor-Free Visual Perception Test—Revised

The MVPT-R (Colarusso & Hammill, 1995) was developed to assess visual perception without the confounding motor components that typify such measures as the Bender–Gestalt Test. The child is only required to point to correct responses, rather than to draw various shapes and figures. If the child is unable to point, the examiner is allowed to point to each choice and ask him or her which one is correct. Colarusso and Hammill (1995) suggested that a comprehensive assessment of visual–motor abilities should include a motor-free test along with a test of visual–motor integration, so as to determine whether a problem is due to poor visual-perceptual skills or to deficits in motor abilities.

The test consists of 40 items that require the child to match a stimulus figure with one of four choices. These items are presented in the following ways: presenting the stimulus figure and asking the child to choose an alternative that is exactly the same; presenting the stimulus and requiring the child to choose one that is similar to it, but that "might be smaller, bigger, darker, or turned on its side"; presenting the stimulus figure separately for 5 seconds, taking the figure away, and then giving the alternative choices; presenting a partially drawn stimulus figure and asking the child to choose which one of the alternative figures it would be like if completely drawn; and presenting the stimulus and asking the child which of the alternatives is different. Colarusso and Hammill reported that these items were selected to represent five facets of visual perception: spatial relations, visual discrimination, figure–ground perception, visual closure, and visual memory. However-

er, Colarusso and Hammill cautioned that the test was developed only to give a general estimate of visual-perceptual ability and not to "identify specific deficits or strengths in the sub-areas of visual perception" (p. 8).

A group of 912 children ages 4–11 years constituted the standardization sample. The revision of the MVPT increased the upper age range of the norms of the original test by 3 years. Colarruso and Hammill (1995) reported that these children were "not identified as having motor, sensory, and learning disabilities" (p.13). The sample has several limitations, however. First, subjects were selected from only two geographic areas of the country, Georgia and California, and therefore do not accurately represent the general U.S. population in this regard. In addition, no information was reported on socioeconomic backgrounds of the children in the sample. Finally, although the manual did report the ethnic breakdown of the sample, African Americans were underrepresented, making up only 10% of the sample when their representation in the general population was 15%. Due to these limitations, one should exercise caution when attempting to interpret normative scores from the MVPT-R.

Despite the addition of four new items, Colarusso and Hammill (1995) chose not to report on updated reliability and validity studies of the MVPT-R. The test developers stated that due to the high correlation between the MVPT-R and the MVPT ($r = .85$), the psychometric properties of the original should also hold for the revised version. Therefore, the following report of reliability and validity is based on studies of the original MVPT. The reliability estimates were generally in the borderline–adequate range. With the exception of a Kuder–Richardson 20 coefficient of .71 for 4-year-olds, the coefficients ranged from .78 to .82 for the other age levels. The test–retest stability was also borderline–adequate; the stability coefficients ranged from .77 to .83.

Validation efforts included a content analysis and "three types of construct validity . . . age differentiations, correlations with similar tests, and internal consistency" (Colarusso & Hammill, 1995, p. 22). The discussion of details regarding the content analysis is inadequate. It is merely stated that the items were developed and retained relative to the five facets of visual perception listed above. However, supporting evidence is presented for age differentiation. The concurrent validation efforts revealed significant overlap with the Frostig Developmental Test of Visual Perception (Frostig, Maslow, Lefever, & Whittlesey, 1964). Modest correlations of the MVPT (.32 and .31, respectively) were reported with the Pinter–Cunningham Primary Test (Pinter & Cunningham, 1965) and with the Slosson Intelligence Test (Slosson, 1963).

The correlations of the MVPT with measures of academic achievement were also modest. The median correlation was .38. Colarusso and Hammill (1995) acknowledged the limited degree of overlap, stating that "no claims are made regarding the relationship of the ability tapped to reading or to any other school skills; actually, our validity findings suggest that little commonality exists between the constructs assessed by the original MVPT and measures of school achievement or intelligence" (p. 8).

In a review, Rosen (1985) raised a significant question about the use of the test. "If the MVPT is a measure of 'motor-free' visual perception, we need to know how important it is to measure such an ability and what useful or critical outcomes do motor-free visual perception contribute to" (p. 1418).

PRODUCT VERSUS BEHAVIOR

Regardless of whether the clinician uses the Bender–Gestalt, the VMI, the WRAVMA, or the MVPT-R, an important point that is often overlooked by less experienced clinicians is the difference between product and behavior. The scoring systems for the common paper-and-pencil visual–motor measures addressed above focus on product; that is, what a child draws is scored in a quantitative fashion. In contrast, the more experienced practitioner attends to the process, observing the child's behavior while the child is producing the drawing. It is the observation of the act that leads to greater insight and understanding of the child's strengths and difficulties. Graf and Hinton (1997) supported the use of process observation with the VMI, stating that clinical observation of student behaviors (e.g., pace, distractibility, fine motor skill, moti-

vation, reflectiveness, compulsiveness) in interpreting test scores is needed. Sattler (1992, p. 360) also emphasized the importance of observation in the assessment process, and provided a comprehensive list of observation questions specifically related to visual–motor tests. Sattler's questions have provided us with the foundation for creating Table 21.1. Drawing attention to the process is not intended to diminish the importance of a careful analysis of the product, but rather to highlight the stream of behavior that results in the scored designs. This point is critical in the context of Kirkwood, Weiler, Holms Bernstein, Forbes, and Waber's (2001) observation that most children referred for learning difficulties were able to improve their performance with structured feedback.

Developing a sense of "internal norms" for process behaviors requires keen observation of both typical and atypical children. The former are an important group to watch; too often clinicians assume age-appropriate behavior patterns to be atypical, because they are rarely confronted with the task of carefully observing typical children. A good illustration of this point is provided in the literature on the WISC-R. Kaufman (1976) asked experienced clinicians to estimate the Verbal–Performance discrepancies of "normal" children. The clinicians grossly underestimated the magnitude of these discrepancies. They assumed that since so many of the children referred for learning problems were exhibiting discrepancies of 10–15 points or more, normal children would exhibit 3- or 4-point discrepancies. Analysis of the standardization data collected on normal children proved that discrepancies of 12 points or more occurred in large numbers of children who had not been referred for special education services. The important implication is that without a good foundation in typical behavior patterns, a clinician will arrive at erroneous conclusions. Because clinicians have the most contact with children who have been referred because they are experiencing difficulties in a setting, it is incumbent on the practitioners to observe nonexceptional children. The problem of developing internal norms based on an atypical sample may be avoided by vigilant observation of typical children.

Haywood (1986) made an excellent point when she suggested that the most efficient

TABLE 21.1. Questions to Consider during Observation of a Child Working on a Visual–Motor Task

Graphomotor behavior

How does the child hold the pencil? Which hand?

Can the tightness of the grip be seen by discoloration of the thumb and/or fingernails?

As reflected by line intensity, how much pencil pressure is placed on the page?

Is pencil pressure evident in wear on the pencil point? Broken pencil points?

How does the child hold the paper in place?

Is the child able to see what is produced in the act of writing?

Does the method of writing block the view?

Child's analysis of the stimuli

Does the child adequately attend to the stimuli?

How does the child analyze the stimuli? Systematically? Impulsively?

Does the analysis take an inordinate amount of time? Or too little time?

Does the child manipulate the stimulus by rotating it? Or by tilting or turning the head?

Production

How meticulous is the child in the production of each figure?

Is there a difference in performance over time? Are early figures drawn with care, while later figures reflect carelessness?

Is fatigue a factor?

Does the child recognize aspects of the drawing that were incorrectly produced?

Are there attempts to erase and redraw portions of designs that were perceived to be in error? Are second and third attempts more carefully executed?

Does the child ignore mistakes and proceed as if they were not recognized?

Is the drawing a struggle for the child?

How does the child tolerate the frustration of not being able to render a design correctly?

Verbal cues

What does the child say about his or her visual–motor abilities, writing skills, or coordination?

Is visual–motor skill recognized as a strength or weakness?

Does the child attribute difficulties to internal or external causes?

What does the child say that gives clues to self-efficacy?

Note. Data from Sattler (1992).

way to refine one's observational skills is to focus on specific body movements. She used "walking" to illustrate the way to break down a behavior. One can scrutinize the heel strike pattern, trunk rotation, synchronous–asynchronous arm swing, elbow flexion, or knee flexion. Likewise, one may watch children engaged in writing. Again, the initial focus is on specific body parts and their contributions to the act. After the parts are scrutinized, the entire Gestalt of the act should be sought. Again, Table 21.1 provides a set of questions to consider while observing a child's visual–motor behavior. It is suggested that the examiner observe the child's approach to holding and using the pencil, the way the child analyzes the stimuli, the modifications the child makes in the production process, and the verbal statements that the child makes. By careful observation and listening, the examiner will have a more complete understanding of the child's visual–motor skills.

Familiarity with symptoms associated with various eye difficulties is another way for clinicians to enhance their observation skills. Knowledge of children's behaviors when they are experiencing eye problems will reduce the possibility of overlooking a potential visual acuity problem. Most of the symptoms may be observed in the context of the individual psychological evaluation or the classroom. In some cases, the child's teacher will report the presence of a symptom; the psychologist should follow up such a report with questions on the presence of other visual acuity symptoms. When a visual problem is suspected, a referral should be made for a comprehensive eye examination. It should not be assumed that because a child has passed eye screening, there is no possibility of a visual acuity problem. Extensive information on vision and eye disorders may be found at the Web site of the National Eye Institute of the U.S. National Institutes of Health (see http://www.nei.nih.gov/publications/US-sources.htm).

A CAUTIONARY NOTE ABOUT THE RELATIONSHIP BETWEEN ACADEMIC ACHIEVEMENT AND VISUAL–MOTOR SKILLS

Visual–motor assessment results have often been used to support assessment results for students referred with learning difficulties, and numerous researchers have reported statistically significant correlations between visual–motor test performance and performance on measures of academic achievement (Graf & Hinton, 1997). Koppitz and her colleagues (Koppitz, 1975; Koppitz, Mardis, & Stephens, 1961; Koppitz, Sullivan, Blyth, & Shelton, 1959) did a series of investigations examining the relationship of her scoring system for the Bender–Gestalt to first- and second-grade achievement. Likewise, other researchers have examined the magnitude of variance shared by the Bender–Gestalt and various measures of academic achievement (Carter, Spero, & Walsh, 1978; Henderson, Butler, & Goffeney, 1969; Keogh, 1965; Norfleet, 1973; Obrzut, Taylor, & Thweatt, 1972). Generally, the findings of these investigations indicate that children who reproduce the Bender–Gestalt designs with numerous errors are also those who have difficulty in attaining basic academic skills. Tolor and Brannigan (1980) pointed out that although these correlations are statistically significant (usually ranging from .30 to .50), the Bender–Gestalt provides little additional predictive power after one controls for the effect of intelligence. When the Bender–Gestalt has been observed to increase the power of prediction in regression studies, it has usually been in studies focusing on reading achievement in the early elementary grades (Tolor & Brannigan, 1980).

Lesiak (1984) reviewed 32 empirical investigations pertaining to the use of the Bender–Gestalt as a predictor of reading achievement. These investigations were divided into two categories: studies in which the Bender–Gestalt was administered concurrently with measures of reading achievement, and studies in which the Bender–Gestalt was used to differentiate children who read well from those who read poorly. Lesiak (1984) drew two conclusions from her review. The first was that the Bender–Gestalt is inferior to broad-based reading readiness tests as a predictor of reading skills. She stated that the Bender–Gestalt "adds little or nothing to the predictive validity of most standardized reading readiness tests" (Lesiak, 1984, p. 402). Lesiak's second conclusion was that the Bender–Gestalt is not *consistent* in dif-

ferentiating between children who read well and those who read poorly. Lesiak ended her article by questioning the utility of the Bender–Gestalt as a measure to be included in a diagnostic reading battery.

In a comprehensive meta-analysis, Kavale (1982) reported findings that both supported and challenged Lesiak's (1984) and Tolor and Brannigan's (1980) conclusions. Kavale (1982) integrated the findings of 161 studies and 1,571 correlations in an attempt to clarify the relationship between visual perception skills and reading achievement. The analysis represented an aggregation of results from 32,500 subjects whose mean age was 7.88 years. Kavale reported that the mean correlation between visual perception and reading ability was .375, which is consistent with Lesiak's conclusion. Likewise, when he used traditional factor-analytic procedures with the composite correlation matrix (principal components with varimax rotation), he found that visual perception did not break out as a unitary skill, but rather loaded across reading, cognitive, and visual differentiation factors. In order to clarify the relationship further, he used a canonical correlation analysis (a procedure that is sensitive to the contributions of respective variables). From his review of the canonical correlation and additional multiple-regression analyses, Kavale concluded that visual perception accounted for "moderate proportions of the total shared variance in reading ability" (1982, p. 51).

More recently, Kilpatrick and Lewandowski (1996) assessed the ability of the Bender–Gestalt to differentiate between students with and without learning disabilities. Their findings—that classification accuracies were at the chance level (50%), and that the two groups had equal percentages of poor and age-appropriate scores—led them to conclude that the validity of the Bender–Gestalt as a component of an assessment for learning disabilities is suspect. Other 1990s research on the relationship between visual–motor and academic achievement has attempted to address methodological flaws of earlier studies by controlling for mediating variables such as intelligence and by using more than one test of visual–motor skill (Goldstein & Britt, 1994). Goldstein and Britt (1994) administered the Test of Visual–Motor Skills (Gardner, 1986), the VMI (Beery, 1989), the Bender–Gestalt (Koppitz, 1975), the WISC-R (Wechsler, 1974), and the Woodcock–Johnson Tests of Achievement (Woodcock & Johnson, 1977) to a group of elementary-age students who were referred for suspected learning disabilities. Results supported those found by Lesiak (1984) and Wright and DeMers (1982), demonstrating that although visual–motor test scores had significant correlations with academic achievement scores, the majority of visual–motor measures did not account for unique variance in achievement scores unrelated to intelligence (Goldstein & Britt, 1994). The exception to these findings was the Test of Visual–Motor Skills, which accounted for a small amount (7.5%) of variance in mathematics achievement beyond that accounted for by intelligence scores.

Although most studies have not considered the relationship between visual–motor skills and written language achievement, this is one relationship in which there appears at least to be some face validity. That is, similar skills may be required for portions of the tasks of both copying shapes and writing. Hagborg and Aiello-Coultier (1994) investigated the relationship between visual–motor skills (measured by the VMI) and written language achievement (measured by teacher ratings) and found that after intelligence, achievement, and socioeconomic status of students were accounted for, the VMI was not a good predictor of written language achievement. In fact, the researchers recommended that clinicians rely on work samples before using the VMI for this purpose (Hagborg & Aiello-Coultier, 1994). Graf and Hinton (1997) also offered support for this recommendation, by pointing out that teacher observations (e.g., of letter reversals, writing problems, copying difficulties) may be as useful as the VMI, even when used in conjunction with the WISC-III (Wechsler, 1991).

A concern linked to the ability of visual–motor assessment to predict achievement of school-age children is the relationship of visual–motor skills to the attainment of basic academic skills (learning to read or solve arithmetic problems). Kephart (1967), Delacato (1966), and Ayres (1980) are representative of those who consider basic visual–motor learning to be a prerequisite to

the attainment of academic skills. Along a similar vein, the Getman (1965) and Frostig and colleagues (1964) approaches emphasize the role of visual–motor processes. Lerner (1986) pointed out that early Western philosophers acknowledged a relationship between motor development and learning. She stated that Plato's first level of education was gymnastics, and that Spinoza recommended teaching the body so the mind could reach an intellectual level of thought.

Kephart, Delacato, Ayres, Getman, and Frostig and colleagues agree that if an individual is evaluated and subsequently judged to be deficient in a motor, perceptual–motor, or perceptual skill, a training program should be aimed at developing the specific skill or a constellation of abilities. For instance, within Kephart's (1967) perspective, if an individual is judged deficient in ocular control, a five-stage ocular training procedure should provide the basis for developing the skill. First, the child is taught to follow an object with his or her eyes. In essence, the eyes are taught to move in different directions—laterally, vertically, diagonally, and in circles. In the second stage, the target to be followed is switched to a small flashlight. The third stage increases the demands on the child's motor skill by having the child follow the light source with eyes and with a finger. The child must move eyes and finger in concert to follow the movements of the light. In the fourth stage, a tactile/kinesthetic element is added by having the child touch the light while it is moved in various directions. In the final stage of ocular training, the child is given a ball to hold, and the teacher moves the ball in different directions. The child holds the ball with both hands and is instructed to watch the movements of the ball.

A conceptualization emphasizing the role of visual–motor functioning is Ayres's (1980) sensory–motor integration approach. The emphasis within this approach is not on teaching specific and discrete skills, but rather on enhancing the brain's ability to learn. It is assumed that normal neural development proceeds along an orderly sequence; thus therapy is designed to enhance and facilitate this neural sequence of development. Among the training activities are various balancing acts, tactile stimulation, and swinging a child who is either sitting or lying in a hammock (vestibular stimulation).

Lerner (1986) concluded that research investigations have failed to yield conclusive evidence that motor training exercises improve academic learning skills. She based this conclusion on reviews by Goodman and Hammill (1973) and Hammill, Goodman, and Wiederholt (1974). Hoehn and Baumeister (1994) have extended Lerner's conclusions, based on an evaluation and critique of empirical studies on sensory integration training, by concluding not only that this treatment is unproven, but that it is "a demonstrably ineffective, primary or adjunctive treatment for learning disabilities and other disorders" (p. 348). Others, such as Reynolds (1981), have come to a similar conclusion. Reynolds noted that the problem rests within a deficit-based model of remediation. The focus of the assessment is on the weakness that the child exhibits, and the training is aimed at the weakness. Taking a neurological perspective, Reynolds stated that when "viewed from contemporary neuropsychological models, the deficit approach to remediation is doomed to failure since it takes damaged or dysfunctional areas of the brain and focuses training specially on these areas" (1981, p. 343).

Kamphaus and Reynolds (1987), Kaufman (1979), and Reynolds (1981) have all suggested that remediation should be designed within the context of the child's strengths. Rather than attempting to remediate the child's weaknesses, the clinician should locate strengths and use these to accomplish the same objectives; the notion is that a child's strengths are used to circumvent weaknesses. Reynolds framed this within Luria's neuropsychological model of intelligence. That is, an intact complex functional system is used to take over and accomplish what would have normally been done by the dysfunctional system.

CONCLUDING COMMENTS AND CASE STUDY

Cummings and Laquerre (1990), in the chapter on visual–motor assessment in the first edition of this handbook, concluded that the psychometric properties of the available visual–motor measures were inadequate. That blanket caution is unnecessary in the present chapter. The VMI now has a nationally representative standardization sample with evidence of reliability and validity, as does the WRAVMA.

Salvia and Ysseldyke (1998) expressed serious reservations over the use of current visual–motor measures. They suggested that the assessment of visual–motor skills is "incredibly problematic" (p. 596). They expressed the same concern over the technical adequacy of the measures that Cummings and Laquerre did in 1990, and added concern over the lack of evidence for effective interventions to address deficits in perceptual–motor functioning. If one takes a deficit-focused approach to intervening with children who exhibit problems, then we concur with Salvia and Ysseldyke. It would be inappropriate to establish an intervention to develop a child's visual–motor skills, especially when the real intent is to improve a child's reading skills.

In the introduction to this chapter, we have noted that a child's success with a visual–motor task is a function of multiple systems working together. The individual must have adequate visual acuity, attend to a stimulus, analyze the stimulus through a process of deconstruction, plan the execution of the drawing, continually monitor the outcome of the act of drawing, and make appropriate adjustments during the process. The examiner must therefore have an understanding of the multifaceted aspects of the act of rendering a successful drawing. Table 21.1 should assist the examiner in raising hypotheses about where the child's difficulties reside. By forming hypotheses and then proceeding to the careful collection of evidence to test (not merely to confirm) each hypothesis, the psychologist is able to develop a picture of the child's abilities. The emergence of an accurate description of the child's current functioning represents a good starting point, but will only help the child if the results lead to interventions that have meaning within the context of the environment. To illustrate this point, a case study is used to conclude the chapter.

Jean, age 13, was referred because of concerns about her difficulty with writing, concern over a recent downturn in grades, and a generally poor attitude toward school.

One of the goals of the assessment was to determine the cause(s) for the recent drop in academic performance. Independent interviews with Jean and her parents indicated that she had consistently found school difficult, but with support had managed to obtain A's and B's. In fourth grade, she had been placed on Ritalin because of her reported inattentiveness and hyperactivity in the classroom. The medication was discontinued after a year; it was noted that Jean had had an exceptional teacher during the school year in which the medication was stopped. Jean was given a battery of cognitive, academic achievement, and visual–motor measures. Her Full Scale, Verbal, and Performance scores on the WISC-III placed her in the "very superior" range of intellectual functioning. Her conversation with the examiner was highly sophisticated, making her appear older than her chronological age. Without prompting, she engaged the examiner in discussions of hiking and nature. In the preceding summer, she had gone with adults on a 3-week hike, crossing a segment of the Rockies.

In contrast to her oral language and perceptual organization skills, her Processing Speed Index score on the WISC-III was significantly lower, primarily as a function of a low score on Coding. While copying the symbols on Coding, she labored to draw each one. Even though she had drawn various symbols multiple times, each instance appeared to require the effort of a new task. The copying of each Coding item was slow and laborious, with numerous glances back to the stimulus to make sure she was getting it right. She appeared to have difficulty making the pencil go in the direction she intended. However, the quality of the final product was good. No reversals, rotations, or distortions were observed. Jean's performance on the VMI was similar to what was observed during Coding: She slowly drew the designs, and hesitated multiple times in the process of drawing each figure.

On the academic achievement measures, Jean's performance was consistent with her intellectual skills reflected by the WISC-III. Her reading and math scores were in the "very superior" range, but she struggled with the task of writing. Her cursive writing was slightly quicker and more legible than her printing, but both took her three to four times as long as they took for peers her same age. This was evident both when she attempted to write orally presented spelling words and when she tried to write sentences to correspond to pictures. The most challenging task was to write a story. She hesitated and grew increasingly anxious before being able to write three sentences that had many misspellings. Proper nouns and words that began sentences were inconsistently capitalized. Commas and periods were omitted in more than half of the appropriate locations. Numerous words were misspelled. In two instances, she spelled the same words correctly and incorrectly in the same passage. During the assessment, she spontaneously commented about her frustration with writing and her inability to express her ideas in writing. Analysis of her work samples and feedback from her teachers confirmed that she exhibited the same writing blocks in the classroom. She confided that she feared her problems with ADHD were returning.

Jean was highly articulate and performed well in all areas except visual–motor and writing skills. Because she lacked strategies for writing, she was encouraged to approach writing in stages: generating initial ideas, outlining, writing a rough draft, editing, and completing a final draft. A mnemonic was provided to assist with her editing (CUPS—capitalization, understanding, punctuation, spelling). She was asked to read her work out loud in a word-by-word fashion, to catch words she may have omitted from a rough draft; this was the "understanding" portion of the CUPS procedure. Because she had access to a computer in the home, her parents agreed to obtain voice recognition software so she could verbalize her ideas and get a good start on writing. Jean's teachers were willing to allow her to use a computer for independent written assignments in the classroom. She was able to produce much more when the keyboard was substituted for handwritten input.

Consistent with Kamphaus and Reynolds (1987), Kaufman (1979), and Reynolds (1981), recommendations were developed that would take advantage of Jean's strengths. Rather than attempt to train her psychomotor skills, the examiner and teachers sought alternative strategies to allow her to express her thoughts. These accommodations had to be considered within the context of what was available in the home and how much her teachers were willing to adapt to her needs in the classroom. As noted at the start of the chapter, the goal of any assessment should be to promote an individual's adaptations to the environment. The case of Jean reveals that accomplishing this goal may also require changes in the environment to accommodate strengths or weaknesses of the individual.

REFERENCES

Adams, A., & Sheslow, D. (1995). *Wide Range Assessment of Visual–Motor Abilities*. Wilmington, DE: Wide Range.

Aylward, E. H., & Schmidt, S. (1986). An examination of three tests of visual–motor integration. *Journal of Learning Disabilities, 19,* 328–330.

Ayres, A. J. (1980). *Southern California Sensory Integration Tests—Revised*. Los Angeles, CA: Western Psychological Services.

Beery, K. E. (1989). *The Developmental Test of Visual–Motor Integration: Administration, scoring, and teaching manual* (3rd ed., rev.). Cleveland, OH: Modern Curriculum Press.

Beery, K. E. (1997a). *The Beery–Buktenica Developmental Test of Visual–Motor Integration* (4th ed., rev.). Cleveland, OH: Modern Curriculum Press.

Beery, K. E. (1997b). *The Beery–Buktenica Developmental Test of Visual–Motor Integration: Administration, scoring, and teaching manual* (4th ed., rev.). Cleveland, OH: Modern Curriculum Press.

Bender, L. (1938). *A visual–motor gestalt test and its clinical use* (Research Monograph No. 3). New York: American Orthopsychiatric Association.

Bender, L. (1946). *Instructions for the use of the Visual Motor Gestalt Test*. New York: American Orthopsychiatric Association.

Benton, A., & Tranel, D. (1993). Visuoperceptual, visuospatial, and visuoconstructive disorders. In K. M. Heilman & E. Valenstein (Eds.), *Clinical neuropsychology* (3rd ed., pp. 165–212). New York: Oxford University Press.

Bernstein, J. H., & Waber, D. P. (1996). *Developmental scoring system for the Rey–Osterrieth Complex Figure*. Odessa, FL: Psychological Assessment Resources, Inc.

Billingslea, F. (1948). The Bender–Gestalt: An objective scoring method and validating data. *Journal of Clinical Psychology, 4,* 1–27.

Bolen, L. M., Hewett, B. J., Hall, C. W., & Mitchell, C. C. (1992). Expanded Koppitz scoring system of the Bender Gestalt Visual–Motor Test for Adolescents: A pilot study. *Psychology in the Schools, 29,* 113–115.

Brannigan, G. G., Aabye, S., Baker, L. A., & Ryan, G. T. (1995). Further validation of the qualitative scoring system for the Modified Bender–Gestalt Test. *Psychology in the Schools, 32,* 24–26.

Brannigan, G. G., & Brunner, N. A. (1989). *The Modified Version of the Bender–Gestalt Test for Preschool and Primary School Children*. Brandon, VT: Clinical Psychology.

Brannigan, G. G., & Brunner, N. A. (1993). Comparison of the qualitative and developmental scoring systems for the Modified Version of the Bender–Gestalt Test. *Journal of School Psychology, 31,* 327–330.

Brannigan, G. G., & Brunner, N. A. (1996). *The Modified Version of the Bender–Gestalt Test for Preschool and Primary School Children*. Brandon, VT: Clinical Psychology.

Brannigan, G. G., & Brunner, N. A. (2002). *Guide to the Qualitative Scoring System for the modified version of the Bender–Gestalt Test*. Springfield, IL: Charles C Thomas.

Carter, D., Spero, A., & Walsh, J. (1978). A comparison of the Visual Aural Digit Span and the Bender–Gestalt as discriminators of low achievement in the primary grades. *Psychology in the Schools, 15,* 194–198.

Colarusso, R. P. & Hammill, D. D. (1995). *Manual for the Motor-Free Visual Perception Test—Revised*. Novato, CA: Academic Therapy.

Cummings, J. A. (1986). Projective drawings. In H. M. Knoff (Ed.), *The assessment of child and adolescent personality* (pp. 199–244). New York: Guilford Press.

Cummings, J. A., & Laquerre, M. (1990). Visual–motor assessment. In C. R. Reynolds & R. W. Kamphaus (Eds.), *Handbook of psychological and educational assessment of children: Intelligence and achievement* (pp. 593–610). New York: Guilford Press.

Delacato, C. (1966). *Neurological organization and reading*. Springfield, IL: Charles C Thomas.

Frostig, M., Maslow, P., Lefever, D. W., & Whittlesey, J. R. B. (1964). The Marianne Frostig Developmental Test of Visual Perception. *Perceptual and Motor Skills, 19,* 463–499.

Fuller, G. G., & Vance, B. (1995). Interscorer reliability of the Modified Version of the Bender–Gestalt Test for Preschool and Primary School Children. *Psychology in the Schools, 32,* 264–266.

Furr, K. D. (1970). Standard scores for the Koppitz Developmental Scoring System. *Journal of Clinical Psychology, 16,* 78–79.

Gardner, M. F. (1986). *Test of Visual–Motor Skills: Manual*. San Francisco: Children's Hospital of San Francisco.

Getman, G. (1965). The visual–motor complex in the acquisition of learning skills. In J. Hellmuth (Ed.), *Learning disabilities* (Vol. 1, pp. 47–76). Seattle, WA: Special Child.

Goldstein, D. J., & Britt, T. W., Jr. (1994). Visual–motor coordination and intelligence as predictors of reading, mathematics, and written language ability. *Perceptual and Motor Skills, 78,* 819–823.

Goodman, L., & Hammill, D. (1973). The effectiveness of the Kephart–Getman activities in developing perceptual-motor and cognitive skills. *Focus on Exceptional Children, 9,* 1–9.

Graf, M., & Hinton, R. N. (1997). Correlations for the

Developmental Visual–Motor Integration Test and the Wechsler Intelligence Scale for Children—III. *Perceptual and Motor Skills, 84,* 699–702.

Hagborg, W. J., & Aiello-Coultier, M. (1994). The Developmental Test of Visual–Motor Integration—3R and teachers' ratings of written language. *Perceptual and Motor Skills, 79,* 371–374.

Hain, J. D. (1964). The Bender Gestalt Test: A scoring method of identifying brain damage. *Journal of Clinical Psychology, 25,* 268–271.

Hall, S., Pinkston, S. L., Szalda-Petree, A. C., & Coronis, A. R. (1996). The performance of healthy older adults on the Continuous Visual Memory Test and the Visual–Motor Integration Test: Preliminary findings. *Journal of Clinical Psychology, 52,* 449–454.

Hammill, D., Goodman, L., & Wiederholt, J. (1974). Visual–motor processes: Can we train them? *The Reading Teacher, 28,* 467–478.

Haywood, K. M. (1986). *Life span motor development* Champaign, IL: Human Kinetics.

Henderson, N. B., Butler, B. V., & Goffeney, B. (1969). Effectiveness of the WISC and Bender–Gestalt Test in predicting arithmetic and reading achievement for white and non-white children. *Journal of Clinical Psychology, 25,* 268–271.

Henry, G. K. (2001). The Rey figure in Amazonia: Effects of jungle living on childrens' copy performance. *Developmental Neuropsychology, 19,* 32–39.

Hinshaw, S. P., Carte, E. T., Sami, N., Treuting, J. J., & Zupan, B. A. (2002). Preadolescent girls with attention-deficit/hyperactivity disorder: II. Neuropsychological performance in relation to subtypes and individual classification. *Journal of Consulting and Clinical Psychology, 70,* 1099–1111.

Hoehn, T. P., & Baumeister, A. A. (1994). A critique of the application of sensory integration therapy to children with disabilities. *Journal of Learning Disabilities, 27*(6), 338–350.

Hubley, A. M., & Tremblay, D. (2002). Comparability of total score performance on the Rey–Osterrieth Complex Figure and modified Taylor Complex Figure. *Journal of Clinical and Experimental Neuropsychology, 24,* 370–382.

Hunsley, (1996). Assessment practices of clinical psychologists. *Professional Psychology: Research and Practica, 27,* 315–316.

Hutt, M. L., & Briskin, G. J. (1960). *The clinical use of the revised Bender Gestalt Test.* New York: Grune & Stratton.

Kamphaus, R. E., & Reynolds, C. B. (1987). *Clinical and research applications of the K-ABC.* Circle Pines, MN: American Guidance Service.

Kaufman, A. S. (1976). A new approach to the interpretation of test scatter on the WISC-R. *Journal of Learning Disabilities, 9,* 160–168

Kaufman, A. S. (1979). *Intelligent testing with the WISC-R.* New York: Wiley.

Kaufman, A. S., & Lichtenberger, E. O. (2000). *Essentials of WISC-III and WPPSI-R assessment.* New York: John Wiley.

Kavale, K. A. (1982). Meta-analysis of the relationship between visual perceptual skills and reading

achievement. *Journal of Learning Disabilities, 15,* 42–51.

Keogh, B. K. (1965). The Bender–Gestalt as a predictive and diagnostic test of reading performance. *Journal of Consulting Psychology, 29,* 83–84.

Kephart, N. (1967). Perceptual–motor aspects of learning disabilities. In E. C. Frierson & W. B. Barbe (Eds.), *Educating children with learning disabilities* (pp. 405–413). New York: Appleton-Century-Crofts.

Kilpatrick, D. A., & Lewandowski, L. J. (1996). Validity of screening tests for learning disabilities: A comparison of three measures. *Journal of Psychoeducational Assessment, 14,* 41–53.

Kirkwood, M. W., Weiler, M. D., Holms Berstein, J., Forbes, P. W., & Waber, D. P. (2001). Sources of poor performance on the Rey–Osterrieth Complex Figure Test among children with learning difficulties: A dynamic assessment approach. *Clinical Neuropsychologist, 15,* 345–356.

Koppitz, E. M. (1964). *The Bender Gestalt Test with young children.* New York: Grune & Stratton.

Koppitz, E. M. (1975). *The Bender Gestalt Test with young children: Vol. 2. Research and application, 1963–1973.* New York: Grune & Stratton.

Koppitz, E. M., Sullivan, J., Blyth, D., & Shelton, J. (1959). Prediction of first grade school achievement with the Bender Gestalt Test and Human Figure Drawings. *Journal of Clinical Psychology, 15,* 432–435.

Koppitz, E. M., Mardis, V., & Stephens, T. (1961). A note on screening school beginners with the Bender Gestalt Test. *Journal of Educational Psychology, 52,* 80–81.

Lacks, P. (1984). *Bender Gestalt screening for brain dysfunction.* New York: Wiley.

Lacks, P. (1999). *Bender Gestalt screening for brain dysfunction* (2nd ed.). New York: Wiley.

Lacks, P. (2000). Visuoconstructive abilities. In G. Groth-Marnat (Ed.), *Neuropsychological Assessment in clinical practice: A guide to test interpretation and integration* (pp. 401–436). New York: Wiley.

Lerner, J. (1986). *Learning disabilities.* Boston: Houghton Mifflin.

Lesiak, J. (1984). The Bender Visual–Motor Gestalt Test: Implications for the diagnosis and prediction of reading achievement. *Journal of School Psychology, 22,* 391–405.

Marsico, D. S., & Wagner, E. E. (1990). A comparison of the Lacks and Pascal–Suttell Bender–Gestalt scoring methods for diagnosing brain damage in an outpatient sample. *Journal of Clinical Psychology, 46,* 868–877.

Moose, D., & Brannigan, G. G. (1997). Comparison of preschool children's scores on the modified version of the Bender–Gestalt Test and Developmental Test of Visual–Motor Integration. *Perceptual and Motor Skills, 85,* 766.

Neale, M. D., & McKay, M. F. (1985). Scoring the Bender–Gestalt Test using the Koppitz Developmental System: Interrater reliability, item difficulty and scoring implications. *Perceptual and Motor Skills, 60,* 627–636.

Norfleet, M. (1973). The Bender Gestalt as a group screening instrument for first grade potential. *Journal of Learning Disabilities, 6,* 383–388.

Obrzut, J. E., Taylor, H. D., & Thweatt, R. C. (1972). Re-examination of Koppitz Developmental Scoring System. *Perceptual and Motor Skills, 34,* 279–282.

Pascal, G. R., & Suttell, B. J. (1951). *The Bender Gestalt Test: Quantification and validity for adults.* New York: Grune & Stratton.

Pinter, R., & Cunningham, B. V. (1965). *Pinter–Cunningham Primary Test* (rev. ed.). New York: Harcourt, Brace & World.

Piotrowski, C., & Zalewski, C. (1993). Training in psychodiagnostic testing in APA-approved PsyD and PhD clinical psychology programs. *Journal of Personality Assessment, 61,* 394–405.

Rey, A. (1941). L'examen psychologique dans le cas d'encephalopathie traumatique. *Archives de Psychologie, 28,* 286–340.

Reynolds, C. R. (1981). Neuropsychological assessment and the habilitation of learning: Considerations in the search for the aptitude × treatment interaction. *School Psychology Review, 10,* 343–349.

Rosen, C. L. (1985). Review of the Motor-Free Visual Perception Test. In J. V. Mitchell (Ed.), *The ninth mental measurements yearbook* (Vol. 2, pp. 1398–1399). Lincoln: University of Nebraska Press.

Ruffolo, J. S., Javorsky, D.J., Tremont, G., Westervelt, H. J., & Stern, R. (2001). A comparison of administration procedures for the Rey–Osterrieth Complex Figure: Flowcharts versus pen switching. *Psychological Assessment, 13,* 299–305.

Salvia, J., & Ysseldyke, J. E. (1998). *Assessment* (7th ed.). Boston: Houghton Mifflin.

Sattler, J. M. (1992). *Assessment of children* (rev. 3rd ed.). San Diego, CA: Author.

Schachter, S., Brannigan, G. G., & Tooke, W. (1991). Comparison of the scoring systems for the modified version of the Bender–Gestalt Test. *Journal of School Psychology, 29,* 265–269.

Shapiro, S. K., & Simpson, R. G. (1995). Koppitz scoring system is a measure of Bender–Gestalt performance in behaviorally and emotionally disturbed adolescents. *Journal of Clinical Psychology, 51,* 108–112.

Slosson, R. L. (1963). *Slosson Intelligence Test.* East Aurora, NY: Slosson Educational.

Smith, M. L., Elliott, I. M., & Lach, L. (2002). Cognitive skills in children with intractable epilepsy: Comparison of surgical and nonsurgical candidates. *Epilepsia, 43,* 631–637.

Tolor, A., & Brannigan, G. C. (1980). *Research and clinical applications of the Bender–Gestalt Test.* Springfield, IL: Charles C Thomas.

Waber, D. P., & Holmes, J. M. (1985). Assessing children's copy productions of the Rey–Osterrieth Complex Figure. *Journal of Clinical and Experimental Neuropsychology, 7,* 264–280.

Waber, D. P., & Holmes, J. M. (1986). Assessing children's memory productions of the Rey–Osterrieth Complex Figure. *Journal of Clinical and Experimental Neuropsychology, 8,* 563–580.

Wagner, E. E., & Marsico, D. S. (1991). Redundancy in the Pascal–Suttell Bender–Gestalt scoring system: Discriminating organicity with only one design. *Journal of Clinical Psychology, 47,* 261–263.

Watkins, C. E., Campbell, V. L., Nieberding, R., & Hallmark, R. (1995). Contemporary practice of psychological assessment by clinical psychologists. *Professional Psychology: Research and Practice, 26,* 54–60.

Watkins, C. E., Campbell, V. L., Nieberding, R., & Hallmark, R. (1996). On Hunsley, Warangue, and hoopla. *Program Psychology: Research and Practica, 27,* 316–318.

Wechsler, D. (1974). *Manual for the Wechsler Intelligence Scale for Children—Revised.* New York: Psychological Corporation.

Wechsler, D. (1991). *Manual for the Wechsler Intelligence Scale for Children—Third Edition.* San Antonio, TX: Psychological Corporation.

Wertheimer, M. (1923). Studies in the theory of Gestalt psychology. *Psychologische Forschung, 4,* 301–350.

Woodcock, R. W., & Johnson, M. B. (1977). *Woodcock–Johnson Psycho-Educational Battery.* Boston: Teaching Resources Corporation.

Wright, D., & DeMers, S. T. (1982). Comparison of the relationship between two measures of visual–motor coordination and academic achievement. *Psychology in the Schools, 19,* 473–477.

Yeates, K. O., & Taylor, H. G. (1998). Neuropsychological assessment of older children. In G. Goldstein, P. D. Nussbaum, & S. R. Beers (Eds.), *Neuropsychology* (pp. 35–61). New York: Plenum Press.

22

Bias in Assessment of Aptitude

CECIL R. REYNOLDS
STEVEN M. KAISER

The issue of bias in testing has been a source of intense and recurring social controversy throughout the history of mental measurement. Discussions pertaining to test bias are frequently accompanied by emotionally laden polemics decrying the use of mental tests with any minority group member, since ethnic minorities have not been exposed to the cultural and environmental circumstances and values of the white middle class. Intertwined within the general issue of bias in tests has been the more specific question of whether intelligence tests should be used for educational purposes. Although scientific and societal discussion pertaining to differences among groups on measures of cognitive or intellectual functioning in no way fully encompasses the broader topic of bias in mental measurement, there is little doubt that the so-called "IQ controversy" has received the lion's share of public scrutiny over the years. It has been the subject of numerous publications in the more popular press (see Gould, 1981, or Jensen, 1980, Ch. 1), and court actions and legislation have addressed the use of IQ tests within schools and industry (e.g., *Diana v. State Board of Education*, 1970; *Griggs v. Duke Power Co.*, 1971; *Hobson v. Hansen*, 1967; *Larry P. v. Riles*, 1979).

The controversy has been fueled by actions taken by organizations such as the Association of Black Psychologists (ABP). In 1969, ABP adopted a policy statement supporting parents who refused achievement, aptitude, performance, and intellectual testing of their children for purposes related in any way to "labeling," to placement in "special" classes, to "tracking," and/or to the perpetuation of inferior educational opportunities for blacks. However, as it turned out, ABP defined all applications of psychological tests as falling within these boundaries. Positions taken by groups such as the ABP (and by individuals) have served psychology's purposes well by raising professional and societal awareness regarding the use of testing with minority populations. However, the early denunciations of probable bias in mental measurements with any groups other than the white middle class often lacked sound empirical backing, and political posturing with rather strong language concerning discrimination, racism, and the "genocide" of minorities (e.g., Jackson, 1975; Williams, 1970, 1974) was common.

This chapter focuses on the empirical evaluation of test bias, with particular emphasis placed upon statistical criteria and methods for investigating possible biases in mental measurements. Brief discussions of the major historical developments leading up to the present subspecialty of bias research in testing, as well as of examiner effects, labeling, and litigation pertaining to testing between and among populations, are also presented. Contrary to the state of bias research some 30 years ago, when the concerns described here reached a state of crisis, a considerable body of research and rather sophisticated techniques to detect bias have been generated within the field. There is little doubt that empirical investigations and methods will continue to grow in the decades to come.

GENERAL CONSIDERATIONS IN BIAS RESEARCH

A Brief Historical Review

The issue of bias in mental testing has been important to the study of individual differences and to social policy since Binet first offered a series of graduated intellectual tasks for purposes of placing a child and tracking his or her growth in terms of level of cognitive development. The work of Galton has been noted over the years to be the most important precursor to the modern mental testing movement. He is perhaps best known for establishing the first anthropometric laboratory, where, for a small fee, persons could perform sensory and motor tasks and be provided with their relative standing in regard to group data gathered during the course of Galton's research. Galton's views were a strong contributing factor to the *Zeitgeist* of his era concerning individual differences. He felt that human intelligence was built upon elementary sensations because sensations were the gateway to the mind, and that intelligence could be assessed through the measurement of such simple functions. Galton also believed that level of intellectual functioning was largely genetically determined and that it was a highly heritable trait.

By the beginning of the 20th century, attempts to validate a link between sensation

and intellect had proved discouraging. Independent estimates of intellectual ability (e.g., teachers' ratings, academic standing, occupational achievement, etc.) did not correlate with acuity data (Heidbreder, 1933), and researchers such as Cattell (an American disciple of Galton and the first to coin the term "mental measurement") gradually abandoned attempts to analyze intelligence via the senses in favor of tasks that presumably demanded reasoning, problem solving, the acquisition of knowledge—"thinking," if you will—for successful execution. However, despite the general abandonment of his theory, Galton had a profound impact upon the fields of differential psychology and mental measurement. He developed and implemented twin studies, questionnaire studies, and correlational studies in his investigations of human intellect. As Fancher (1979) has noted, "Among his important contributions was the very idea that tests could be employed to measure psychological differences between people. . . . He thus elevated the scientific study of individual differences to the level of a major psychological specialty with important social implications" (p. 254). Galton's heriditarian views were influential as well and were retained long past the demise of his original theories of intellect.

Binet and Simon tackled the problem of developing a reliable measure of intellectual ability near the start of the 20th century, in response to a social concern and in direct competition with Galtonian wisdom. The French Ministry of Education was interested in formulating a means by which children with intellectual retardation could be selected for special educational attention. This historical note seems an odd juxtaposition, considering that one reason why intelligence testing has been more recently condemned is that the practice is thought to relegate children with low scores to inferior, "dead-end" educational programming as opposed to providing a means of selection for treatment. Binet concluded that the measurement of intellectual functioning necessitated the use of tasks that would tap complex mental processes. He found particularly enticing the notion of systematically evaluating an individual's relative ability in the (then-presumed) intellectual faculty of judgment. Binet rejected the premise that lower-order sensory acuity measures could adequately reflect human thought processes, and argued that individual differences in human intellect were more readily apparent in functions such as memory, verbal comprehension, reasoning, and judgment.

The Binet–Simon scales (Binet & Simon, 1905) were quickly translated and embellished throughout the world. The scales had a strong advocate in the United States in Goddard, who translated the scales into English; in 1909, Goddard recommended to the American Association for the Study of the Feeble-Minded that scores from the scales be used to classify "mentally deficient" persons (Pintner, 1923). The apparent accuracy of the Binet–Simon system served to kindle interest in the application of intelligence testing for a wide variety of social purposes within the United States. Inspection of early psychological texts and journals before and after World War I shows that research, social policy, and theory related to mental measurement were ubiquitous. There is also clear evidence of concern surrounding the differential impact of mental testing across groups.

Pintner and Keller (1922) collected voluminous data on national and racial groups and reported a wide variation in median IQ. Further analyses separated those children whose parents did and did not speak English in the home; results of testing with the Binet placed children from non-English-speaking homes an average of 8 points below children whose families spoke English in the home. Nonverbal intellectual testing, however, served to increase the scores of the non-English home environment group. Pintner and Keller concluded that "those children who hear a foreign language in their homes may suffer a serious handicap when tested only by revisions of the Binet Test" (1922, p. 222). Although many regard the issue of test bias as a product of relatively recent social concerns, the educational and psychological literature from this earlier era (e.g., Kohs, 1923; Pintner, 1923; Pressey & Pressey, 1922) readily attests to the fact that scholars were concerned about factors other than innate intelligence affecting (and presumably biasing) mental measurement test performance. Freeman's (1926) text provides a fairly representative example of what psychologists and educators read then,

and still read to a certain extent today. The position statement also illustrates the long-standing and rocky relationship between the practical uses of mental measurement and the theoretical exploration of environmental and genetic factors on intellectual development. Freeman summarized:

> The detailed examination of the scientific evidence which is at hand indicated the correctness of the moderate view as contrasted with ethnic extreme. . . . [O]ne may regard intelligence tests as an entirely new and perfect instrument for detecting native capacity. At the other extreme [one may discount them and regard them as merely somewhat improved instruments for measuring the results of teaching. The consideration of the historical development of tests, in common with an analysis of their results, shows that neither of these views is correct. Intelligence tests have made a marked advance toward the measurement of native capacity, but these scores are still influenced to a considerable degree by the effects of training, and in their interpretation this influence must always be taken into account. (pp. 474–475)

The Nature–Nurture Issue

Bond (1981) observes that there has been a strong tendency by both professionals and the lay public alike to draw conclusions regarding the relative impact of genetic and environmental factors on test performance if mean performance levels among groups are disparate and those tests in use are shown not to be biased in a statistical sense. Bond goes on to point out that the discussion pertaining to race differences in intelligence is a major reason why bias research and intelligence testing have remained such volatile social issues. He asks the reader to consider this statement: "Test results indicate that white students, on the average, achieve higher levels of competence in most academic subjects than black students, on the average" (p. 56). The statement, viewed objectively, merely addresses a presumed result of past academic achievement and does not provide an etiology for the observed difference. However, consider this statement: "Test results indicate that white students as a group possess greater aptitude for academic work than black students" (p. 56). The seemingly minor change in language quickly elevates the statement into the realm of "genetic" or "innate" superiority of one group over another, and understandably triggers a decidedly emotional response.

The investigation of test bias can proceed unabated without attention to the "nature–nurture" question. This is not to say that the relative impact of endowment and experience on human intellectual development is not a viable issue in the scientific arena. It is, but our methodology is inadequate at present to permit convincing conclusions to be drawn. The "nature–nurture" question has been a part of the human quest for self-comprehension since the time humans were able to formulate the question. Jensen (1980) has clearly stated that research on test bias ought not to be confused with polemic discussion pertaining to genetic and environmental contributions to individual differences. He notes that data obtained from all test scores are measures of phenotypic and not genotypic expression. A "phenotype," in scientific usage, is the detectable expression of the interaction of a genotype with the environment. Consequently, investigation of test bias is, by its very nature, investigation of possible bias in the measurement of phenotypes. If bias is not found in a statistical sense within a test, conclusions drawn concerning genetic differences between/among groups using the "nonbiased" measure are simply another set of assertions requiring further investigation. Such a finding only means that we can research genetic and environmental contributions to individual differences without the contamination of nominally induced score aberrations.

Although Jensen (1980) takes the stand that advancement in psychometric knowledge is a vital component to a better understanding of the reasons underlying individual and group differences, he concludes:

> The answers to questions about test bias surely need not await a scientific consensus on the so-called nature–nurture question. A proper assessment of test bias, on the other hand, is an essential step towards a scientific understanding of the observed differences in all the important educational, occupational, and social correlates of test scores. Test scores themselves are merely correlates, predictors, and indicators of other socially important variables, which would not be altered in the least if tests

did not exist. The problem of individual differences and group differences would not be made to disappear by abolishing tests. One cannot treat a fever by throwing away the thermometer. (p. xi)

Jensen's oft-cited comments in the *Harvard Educational Review* concerning the possible role of genetics as a causative factor for the consistent disparity reported (see Shuey, 1966) in mean IQs between blacks and whites seems an odd twist in comparison to the passage quoted above. And yet the two positions are not discordant if one is able to separate systematic *investigation* of bias in tests and measures from *estimation* of the relative impact of constitution and environment upon test scores. It is interesting to note that both environmental proponents and genetic proponents in the nature–nurture issue have defended their positions using essentially the same data. Loehlin, Lindzey, and Spuhler (1975, Ch. 10) conclude that because data seem to favor both camps, resolution of the issue is in no way imminent. Rosenthal (1975) has analyzed the available evidence concerning heredity and behavior, including three commonly applied research strategies: family studies, twin studies, and adoption studies. Although research using these methodologies has reaffirmed the significance of genetic factors in the formation of a variety of human traits (Cancro, 1971; Loehlin et al., 1975; Minton & Schneider, 1980; Rosenthal, 1975; Tyler, 1965), it is now generally agreed that heredity and environment operate *interactively* in determining traits, with the influence of each depending upon the action of the other (Minton & Schneider, 1980).

Tyler (1965) has suggested that the most important information to be gleaned from this domain of research is not the proportional contribution of nature and nurture (i.e., what "percentage" each is responsible for) in the making of traits or abilities, but the amenability of traits or abilities to change and the ways in which change can be effectively carried out. Minton and Schneider (1980) have endorsed Tyler's position, stressing that "genetic" does not automatically imply a low level of modifiability, nor does "environmental" signal that a trait or ability is easily changeable. The authors point out that certain genetically based disorders such as phenylketonuria can be readily prevented by the environmental adjustment of diet, whereas social workers, psychologists, and other social service providers frequently find it impossible to modify deviant behaviors generally assumed to be a direct function of environmental circumstances. Finally, Steinberg (1985)—in response to Jensen's (1985) summary statements concerning the large role played by the factor of general intelligence (or "*g*") in group differences seen with intelligence tests—provides a perspective clearly intended to engender further thought on testing and the nature–nurture issue. Although Steinberg accepts the *g* data as scientifically viable at present, he adds that research along this line continues to "answer none of the more interesting and timely questions, such as why the score difference holds, what can be done to remedy it, or why the difference matters in the first place" (p. 244).

Mean Score Differences as Test Bias

A popular lay view has been that differences in mean levels of performance on cognitive or ability tasks among groups constitute bias in tests; however, such differences alone clearly are not evidence of test bias. A number of writers in the professional literature have mistakenly taken this position (Alley & Foster, 1978; Chinn, 1979; Hilliard, 1979; Jackson, 1975; Mercer, 1976; Williams, 1974; Wright & Isenstein, 1977). Those who support this definition of test bias correctly state that there is no valid a priori scientific reason to believe that intellectual or other cognitive performance levels should differ across race. It is the inference that tests demonstrating such differences are inherently biased because there can in reality be no differences that is fallacious. Just as there is no a priori basis for deciding that differences exist, there is no a priori basis for deciding that differences do not exist. From the standpoint of the objective methods of science, a priori or premature acceptance of either hypothesis ("differences exist" vs. "differences do not exist") is untenable. As stated by Thorn dike (1971), "The presence (or absence) of differences in mean score between groups, or of differ-

ences in variability, tells us nothing directly about fairness" (p. 64). Likewise, Jensen (1976) notes, "Score differences per se, whether between individuals, social classes, or racial groups, obviously cannot be a criterion of bias" (p. 341). Some adherents to the "mean score differences as bias" viewpoint also require that the distribution of test scores in each population or subgroup be identical before one can assume that the test is fair: "Regardless of the purpose of a test or its validity for that purpose, a test should result in distributions that are statistically equivalent across the groups tested in order for it to be considered nondiscriminatory for those groups" (Alley & Foster, 1978, p. 2). Portraying a test as biased regardless of its purpose or validity is psychometrically naive. Mean score differences and unequivalent distributions have been the most uniformly rejected of all criteria examined by sophisticated psychometricians involved in investigating the problems of bias in assessment. Differences among ethnic groups in mental test scores are among the best-documented phenomena in psychology, and they have persisted over time at relatively constant levels (Reynolds & Gutkin, 1980c).

Jensen (1980) has discussed the "mean score differences as bias" position in terms of the egalitarian fallacy. The egalitarian fallacy contends that all human populations are in fact identical on all mental traits or abilities. Any differences with regard to any aspect of the distribution of mental test scores indicates that something is wrong with the test itself. Such an assumption is totally scientifically unwarranted. There are simply too many examples of specific abilities and even sensory capacities that have been shown to differ unmistakably across human populations. The result of the egalitarian assumption, then, is to remove the investigation of population differences in ability from the realm of scientific inquiry. Logically followed, this fallacy leads to other untenable conclusions as well. Torrance (1980), an adherent of the cultural bias hypothesis, pointed out that disadvantaged black children occasionally earn higher scores on creativity tests—and therefore have more creative ability—than many white children because their environment has forced them to learn to "make do" with less and with simpler objects. The egalitarian assumption would hold that this is not true, but rather that the content of the test is biased against white or high-socioeconomic-status (high-SES) children.

The attachment of minorities to the "mean score differences as bias" definition is probably related to the nature–nurture controversy at some level. Certainly data reflecting racial differences on various aptitude measures have been interpreted to indicate support for a hypothesis of genetic differences in intelligence and to imply that one race is superior to another. However, as discussed previously, the so-called nature–nurture issue is not an inextricable component of bias investigation. Assertions as to the relative impact of genetic factors on group ability levels step into a new arena of scientific inquiry, with differing bodies of knowledge and methods of research. Suffice it to say that in the arena of bias investigation, mean differences on aptitude or achievement measures among selected groups are not evidence per se that the measures are biased.

Culture-Free Tests, Culture Loading, and Culture Bias

A third area of bias investigation that has been confusing in both the professional (e.g., Alley & Foster, 1978; Chinn, 1979) and the lay literature has been the interpretation of culture loading and culture bias. A test can be culture-loaded without being culturally biased. "Culture loading" refers to the degree of cultural specificity present in the test or individual items of the test. Certainly, the greater the cultural specificity of a test item, the greater the likelihood of the item's being biased when it is used with individuals from other cultures. The test item "Who was the first president of the United States?" is a culture-loaded item. However, the item is general enough to be considered useful with children in the United States. The cultural specificity of the item is too great, however, to allow the item to be used on an aptitude measure of 10-year-old children from other countries. Virtually all tests in current use are bound in some way by their cultural specificity. Culture loading must be viewed on a continuum from general (defining the culture in a broad, liberal sense) to specific (defining the culture in narrow, highly distinctive terms).

A variety of attempts have been made to develop a "culture-free" (sometimes referred to as "culture-fair") intelligence test (Cattell, 1979). However, the reliability and validity of these tests are uniformly inadequate from a psychometric perspective (Anastasi, 1986; Ebel, 1979). The difficulty in developing a culture-free measure of intelligence lies in the test's being irrelevant to intellectual behavior within the culture under study. Intelligent behavior is defined within human society in large part on the basis of behavior judged to be of value to the survival and improvement of the culture and the individuals within the culture. A test that is "culture-free," then, cannot be expected to predict intelligent behavior within a variety of cultural settings. Once a test has been developed within a culture (a culture-loaded test), its generalizability to other cultures or subcultures within the dominant societal framework becomes a matter for empirical investigation.

Jensen (1980) admonishes that when one is investigating the psychometric properties of culture-loaded tests across differing societies or cultures, one cannot assume that simple inspection of the content will determine which tests or items are biased against those cultures or societies not represented in the tests or item content. Tests or items that exhibit characteristics of being culturally loaded cannot be determined to be biased with any degree of certainty unless objective statistical inspection is completed. Jensen refers to the mistaken notion that anyone can judge tests and/or items as being "culturally unfair" on superficial inspection as the "culture-bound fallacy."

The Question of Labeling Effects

The relative impact of placing a label on a child's behavior or developmental status has also been a hotly discussed issue within the field of psychometrics in general, and bias investigation in particular. The issue has undoubtedly been a by-product of the practice of using intellectual measures for the determination of mental retardation. Although the question of labeling effects is a viable and important one, it requires consideration in bias research only in much the same way as does the ongoing debate surrounding the nature–nurture question. However, there are some important considerations regarding bias in referral for services, diagnosis, and labeling, which no interested student of the diagnostic process in psychology can afford to ignore.

Rosenthal is the researcher most closely associated with the influence of labeling upon teachers' and parents' perceptions of a child's ability and potential. Even though his early studies had many methodological and statistical difficulties, labeling effects have been shown in some subsequent experimental studies (e.g., Critchley, 1979; Foster & Ysseldyke, 1976; Jacobs, 1978), but not in others (e.g., MacMillan, Jones, & Aloia, 1974; McCoy, 1976). However, these studies have generally been of a short-term nature, and have usually been conducted under quite artificial circumstances. Typically, participants are asked to rate the behavior or degree of pathology of a child seen on videotape. Categorical labels for the child are systematically varied while the observed behaviors remain constant. The demand characteristics of such a design are substantial. Long-term effects of labeling and special education placement in real-life situations have been examined less vigorously. Comparisons of the effects of formal diagnostic labels with the informal, often cursory, personal labeling process that occurs between teachers and children over the course of a school year, and that is subsequently passed on to the next grade via the teachers' lounge (Dworkin & Dworkin, 1979), need to be made. The strict behaviorist position (Ross, 1974, 1976) also contends that formal diagnostic procedures are unnecessary and potentially harmful because of labeling effects. However, whether or not the application of formal labels has detrimental effects on children remains an open question now, much as it did at the conclusion of a monumental effort to address these important questions well over 25 years ago (Hobbs, 1975).

Even without the application of formal, codified labels by psychologists or psychiatrists, the mental labeling, classification, and appraisal of individuals by people with whom they come into contact are common, constant occurrences (Reynolds, 1979c). Auerbach (1971) found that adults often interpret early learning difficulties as primarily emotional disturbances, unrelated to learning problems. According to Bower (1974), children who start the first grade below the mean age of their classmates and are below average in the development of school readiness skills or have behavior problems are more likely to be regarded by school staff as having emotional disturbances and are more likely to be referred to residential placement than their peers. The American Psychological Association (1970) acknowledges that such constant appraisal of individuals occurs at the informal level, and in an official position statement takes the stance that specialized, standardized psychological techniques have been developed to supersede our informal, often casual approach to the appraisal of others. The specialized psychological techniques available to the trained examiner add validity and utility to the results of such appraisals. The quantification of behavior permits systematic comparisons of individuals' characteristics with those of a selected reference or norm group. It is not unreasonable to anticipate that the informal labeling of children so often indulged in by teachers and parents is substantially more harmful than accurate psychoeducational diagnostics intended to accrue beneficial activity toward the child. Should noncategorical funding for services to exceptional children become a reality (Gutkin & Tieger, 1979), or should the use of normative assessment ultimately be banned, the informal labeling process will continue and in all likelihood will exacerbate children's problems.

From the standpoint of *test* bias issues, the question of labeling children or not labeling children is moot. Test bias is concerned with the accuracy of such labels across some nominal grouping system (typically, race, sex, and SES have been the variables of interest). It is a question of whether race, sex, or any other demographic variable of interest influences the diagnostic process or the placement of a child in special programs, independent of the child's cognitive, emotional, and behavioral status. Several well-designed studies have investigated the influences of race and SES on the class placement recommendations of school psychologists (i.e., bias in test interpretation). One of the studies investigated teacher bias as well.

Frame (1979) investigated the accuracy of school psychologists' diagnoses and consistency of treatment plans, with regard to bias effects associated specifically with race and SES. In Frame's study, 24 school psychologists from a number of school districts diagnostically rated and provided treatment plans for hypothetical cases in which all information except race, SES, and the achievement level of the child's school was held constant. No differences in the accuracy of diagnosis (as defined by interrater reliability) occurred as a function of race or SES. Differences did occur with regard to treatment recommendations, however. With all other data held constant, lower-SES black children were less likely to be recommended for special education placement than their white counterparts or higher-SES black children. A more general trend was for higher-SES children to be recommended for special class placement more often than children of lower SES.

In a similar vein, Matuszek and Oakland (1979) asked whether SES and race influenced teacher or psychologist placement recommendations, independent of other characteristics such as adaptive behavior, IQ, and classroom achievement levels. This study included 76 teachers, 53 psychologists, and 106 child studies. Matuszek and Oakland concluded that "The data from this study clearly indicate that they [psychologists] did not make different recommendations on the basis of race" (1979). Consistent with the results of Frame (1979), psychologists were more likely to recommend special class placement for high-SES children than for low-SES children when other variables were held constant. Teachers showed no bias in regard to special education placement recommendations on the basis of race or SES. Upon investigating special education placement recommendations as a function of minority group status (black, Native American, or Asian American), Tomlinson, Acker, Canter, and Lindborg (1977) reported that psychologists recommended special education resource services more frequently for minority than for white children. Placement in a special education class, however, was recommended more frequently for white than for minority children. A rather extensive study of placement in classes for so-called "educable

mentally retarded" ("EMR") children in California also failed to find any racist intent in the placement of minority children in special classes (Meyers, MacMillan, & Yoshida, 1978). In fact, the tendency was not to place black children in special education classes, even though they might be failing in the regular classroom. An even earlier study by Mercer (1971), one of the major critics of IQ testing with minorities, reached the same conclusion.

The general tendency not to label black children also extends to community mental health settings. Lewis, Balla, and Shanok (1979) reported that when black adolescents were seen in mental health settings, behaviors symptomatic of schizophrenia, paranoia, and a variety of psychoneurotic disorders were frequently dismissed as only "cultural aberrations" appropriate to coping with the frustrations created by the antagonistic white culture. Lewis and colleagues further noted that white adolescents exhibiting similar behaviors were given psychiatric diagnoses and referred for therapy and/or residential placement. Lewis and colleagues contended that this failure to diagnose mental illness in the black population acts as bias in the denial of appropriate services. A tendency for psychologists to regard depressed performance on cognitive tasks by blacks and low-SES groups as a "cultural aberration" has also been shown. An early empirical study by Nalven, Hofmann, and Bierbryer (1969) demonstrated that psychologists generally rated the "true intelligence" of black and low-SES children higher than that of white and middle-class children with the same Wechsler Intelligence Scale for Children (WISC) IQ. This tendency to "overrate" the intellectual potential of black and low-SES children probably accounts, at least in part, for psychologists' reluctance to recommend special education placement for these children; it could also be viewed as a discriminatory denial of services, depending on whether the provision of services is considered beneficial or harmful to the individual.

These studies clearly indicate that the demographic variables of race and SES do not, independent of other pupil characteristics, influence or bias psychologists' diagnostic or placement behavior in a manner that would cause blacks or lower-SES children to be labeled inaccurately or placed inappropriately or in disproportionate numbers in special education programs. The empirical evidence, rather, argues in the opposite direction: Black and low-SES children are *less* likely to be recommended for special education class placement than their white or high-SES peers with similar cognitive, behavioral, and emotional characteristics. The data simply do not support Williams's (1970) charge that black children are placed in special education programs on the basis of race or test bias against blacks. When referrals for placement in gifted programs are considered separately from "referrals" generally, the disproportionate representation of minorities in special education programs can be accounted for by the disproportionately higher incidence of referral among minority student populations (Tomlinson et al., 1977; Waits & Richmond, 1978).

Early Bias Research

Jensen (1980) reports that the first attempts to investigate bias in mental tests were restricted to the exploration of certain internal characteristics of items within any given measure. More specifically, emphasis was placed on the relative impact of SES differences on item performance. Earlier thinking in the mental test movement followed the logic that if mental tests did in fact measure some general trait presumed to be "within" the individual, then items ought not to discriminate strongly between or among social classes. Items most discriminating in this regard were considered suspect and, in essence, biased. Jensen further notes that this genre of research (the investigation of group × item interactions, in modern statistical parlance) proved faulty and consequently inconclusive, because the influence of chronological age on the type of task under inspection requires control and because content inspection of items reveals little information about an item's underlying structure. Concerning the latter, there is little or no scientific rationale behind the contention that highly discriminatory items are, by default, biased if it can be demonstrated that those items are tapping different aspects of intellectual ability (e.g., if those items load more highly on *g*) than items presumably less biased as determined by minimal differences across levels of SES. In effect, it can be argued that those high-discrimination items under inspection are adequately measuring a unique aspect of intellectual functioning and not differing levels of SES per se, if the high discrimination items can be shown to exhibit unique psychometric properties.

Two doctoral dissertations completed at midcentury served to propel bias research into a new arena of sophistication. Both dissertations deserve special notice because they attempted to address directly the issue of cultural fairness of commonly used tests of the period; were ambitious in their scope; and served to demonstrate that an awkward, seemingly unruly research topic was amenable to systematic investigation.

Eells (see Eells, Davis, Havighurst, Herrick, & Typer, 1951) tested the hypothesis that the SES of a child's environment was, on the average, related to mean IQ differences, because children were exposed to qualitatively different experiences in such factors as vocabulary spoken at home and discussion of topics that would seem to expand a youngster's general knowledge and reasoning skills. Eells postulated that the intellectual demands of various mental tests were more closely aligned to the environment of high-SES than to that of low-SES groups, and consequently reflected in mean score differences the extent to which any given youngster experienced a more "stimulating" environment. Eells proceeded with an ambitious project, including thousands of children, a lengthy battery of commonly used tests of the time, and demographic data related to family SES. High-, middle-, and low-SES groups were created from family economic/social data; for the low-SES group, further divisions were made along ethnic lines. Children were either 9, 10, 13, or 14 years of age.

Briefly, Eells translated the percentage of children passing each item (there were 658 items in all) with respect to age and economic groupings into a normalized index, and thus transformed item difficulty level into an interval scale. It should be noted here that the percentage of children passing any given item cannot realistically be considered as a product of a flat distribution; consequently, comparisons based on these percentages are misleading. For example, although intervals may appear to be equal (say, .50 and .55, and .90 and .95—both representing a .05 percentage difference), they fail to take into account the distribution of item performance on mental tasks, generally assumed to be normal because of the normal distribution within the population of intellectual ability.

Jensen (1980) notes that Eells's data revealed sizable variation in terms of item difficulties across low- and high-SES groups and across the age ranges tested. Although virtually all items investigated reflected superiority of the high-SES group over the low-SES group, magnitudes fluctuated, as seen by discordant percentages of items that reached statistically significant levels among the differing age groupings. Eells also found that ethnic groupings did not appreciably influence test item performance, as groups (Eells divided subjects into an "ethnic" group and an "old American" group) fared about as well on most items. Furthermore, the largest status differences were found to be greater on easier test items, defined as those items with less verbal and less general informational content. This finding ran contrary to Eells's anticipated results, although he did not find that status differences were, in general, greater with items that demanded stronger verbal skills and information presumably more accessible to high-SES youngsters of the time. Finally, Eells examined patterns in the choice of multiple-choice distractors between high-SES and low-SES groups. He found that high-SES students tended to select with greater frequency more plausible distractors—ones closer to the correct answers—than did low-SES students. Low-SES students appeared to guess more, as their overall patterns across items were random in comparison.

Although Eells conceded that his data were less than consistent, he nonetheless became the first to advocate clearly and strongly the development and use of culture-fair tests. His research effort undoubtedly served to accelerate interest in the empirical aspects of bias investigation, as well as to heighten sensitivity to those aspects of test items that might have a differential impact between/among groups. Yet his main desire—to design culture-fair tests that would eliminate bias—failed in rather short order. A second dissertation from this period yielded more consistent data with regard to the issue of culture fairness and the culture-bound fallacy, and also remains as a hallmark in bias research.

McGurk (1951) addressed the question of whether items from commonly used intelligence tests could be determined, through inspection by qualified persons, to be culturally biased. He enlisted 78 judges with presumed sensitivity (e.g., professors of psychology and sociology, teachers, counselors, etc.) to the cultural content within tasks, and asked each to rate selected items as being low, neutral, or high in cultural content. McGurk's aim was to find those items from intellectual tests that the judges consistently rated as being most and least culturally loaded. Definition was left up to the individual opinion, and ultimately high or low cultural content was decided upon when a significant proportion of the judges made the same classification of individual items. What "fell out" from the first stage of the project were 103 items felt to be highly culturally loaded and 81 items considered generally culture-free by the experts.

McGurk (1951) made comparisons of performances by black and by white high school seniors on the 184 items. He then selected 37 pairs of items from these data, matched on the basis of difficulty levels (determined by percentage passing). Each pair included a least and a most culturally loaded item, as determined by the judges, that black and white students had subsequently passed in similar numbers. The 37 pairs were then administered to a large sample of white students and a smaller sample of blacks in both Pennsylvania and New Jersey. Because McGurk had such a surplus of white students, he was able to create black–white pairs who had similar curriculum exposure and who had attended the same school district, including present placement at the time of testing. Pairings were also made to match social and economic factors.

McGurk's (1951) carefully planned study yielded some interesting results. First, mean differences on items characterized as least and most culturally loaded ran contrary to what one might expect if one assumed that whites would do better on more culturally bound tasks. In fact, black–white mean differences on the items judged least culturally loaded were twice as great as differences on the items judged most culturally loaded. McGurk determined that blacks performed, relatively speaking, better on those items classified as most culturally loaded, even when item difficulty was held constant. Second, correlations between item difficulties showed similar magnitude between the least and most loaded questions, providing strong evidence that blacks and whites showed similar patterns on the relative difficulties of items. Third, further analysis of selected low-SES and high-SES groups revealed that whites showed greater differences between low- and high-SES groups on the most culturally loaded items. However, blacks evidenced a pattern opposite to the white group: Black differences between the low- and high-SES students were found to be greater within the least culturally loaded items and weaker with those items judged high in culture content.

Where Can Research Go?

Harrington (1975, 1984) has taken a quite different, experimentally oriented approach to the issue of test bias. Whereas Eells's and McGurk's work shows where bias investigation has come from, Harrington perhaps shows the myriad of avenues of investigation for the future. In earlier research, Harrington (1968a, 1968b) suggested that the existence of genetic × environmental interactions in intelligence could affect item selection in the construction of intelligence tests, in a manner resulting in bias (mean differences in total test scores) against minorities. Harrington has thus raised the issue of representation in the test development sample, but from a slightly different perspective than that of other researchers. Many have argued that the small numbers of minority children in standardization samples are unable to exert any significant impact on the item analysis data, and that the content of the test subsequently becomes biased against groups with less than majority representation. Harrington's (1975, 1976) approach to researching this question is both innovative and interesting. Harrington first began by creating experimental populations of rats with varying proportions of "minority" composition (group membership was defined on a genetic basis). For his experimental populations, Harrington used six species of rats from ge-

netically homogeneous groups. Harrington then set out to develop six intelligence tests, using standard psychometric procedures. Six test development populations were developed with varying degrees of minority group representation. Items for use in test development for each population were the same and consisted of a large number of performance measures on black and/or white Hebb–Williams-type mazes (Hebb–Williams mazes are accepted standard tasks for the measurement of rat intelligence).

After the administration of all items to each of the six populations, a test was constructed separately for each population. Following traditional psychometric practice, internal-consistency analyses were undertaken, and items showing the greatest item–total correlations within each population were retained for the "IQ test" for that population. A total of 50 items were retained within each of the six populations. Harrington then hypothesized that if minority group representation in the population did not affect item selection, the six measures would be essentially equivalent forms (i.e., group performance would be independent of the test form employed). To test this hypothesis, Harrington randomly sampled each of the six test development populations and administered all six of the newly developed tests to the new grouping of subjects.

There were significant positive correlations between the group mean on any individual test and the degree of group representation in the population used to develop the test. For example, for test A, group A had the greatest representation in the test development sample and the highest mean score on the instrument subsequently developed; for test B, group C had the greatest proportionate representation and the highest score on that instrument. Harrington (1984) concluded that the greater the proportional representation of a homogeneous group in the test base population (the test development sample), the higher the mean score of the group on the test derived on that population.

From some further analyses of this data set, Harrington concluded that it is not possible for tests developed and normed on a white majority to have equivalent predictive validity with blacks or any other minority group. Harrington also contends that the generalization of his results with animals to humans is direct and not analogical, since his experiments are a direct empirical test of common psychometric assumptions and practice. Harrington's comments on predictive validity are particularly crucial, since, as will be seen, most definitions of test bias rely heavily on the differential prediction of some specified criterion (Anastasi, 1986; Bartlett & O'Leary, 1969; Cleary, 1968; Cleary, Humphreys, Kendricks, & Wesman, 1975; Cronbach, 1970; Darlington, 1971; Einhorn & Bass, 1971; Hunter & Schmidt, 1976; Hunter, Schmidt, & Hunter, 1979; Kallingal, 1971; Kennedy, 1978; Linn & Werts, 1971; Potthoff, 1966; Reynolds, 1978, 1980b, 1980c; Reynolds, Bossard, & Gutkin, 1980; Reynolds & Gutkin, 1980a).

Although Harrington's (1975, 1976) results are impressive and seem to call into question certain of the basic psychometric assumptions underlying test construction (particularly as they apply to the development of intelligence tests), his generalizations fail on three major points. First, as will be seen later in this chapter, intelligence and other aptitude tests have repeatedly been shown to have equivalent predictive validity across racial groupings in a variety of circumstances with a fairly diverse set of criterion measures.

Second, well-documented findings that Japanese Americans, Chinese Americans, and Jewish Americans typically score as well as or better than Americans of Christian European descent on traditional intelligence tests and tests of some specific aptitudes (Gross, 1967; Marjoribanks, 1972; Tyler, 1965; Willerman, 1979) are entirely contradictory to Harrington's (1975, 1976) results, given these groups' proportionately small representation in the test development population of such instruments. Neither can Harrington's theory explain why African infants, with zero representation in the standardization samples of such instruments as the Bayley Scales of Infant Development (Bayley, 1969), consistently score at higher levels than do American infants (Gerber & Dean, 1957; Leiderman, Babu, Kagia, Kraemer, & Leiderman, 1973; Warren, 1972). In addition, Harrington's theory cannot explain why Canadian children of French descent and American children earn approximately equivalent scores on the Wechsler Intelligence Scale for Children—Revised (WISC-R) Information subtest (Beauchamp, Samuels, & Griffore, 1979), or why native Eskimos and white Canadian children earn equivalent scores on Raven's Progressive Matrices (MacArthur, 1968). Again, such findings are in direct contradiction to predictions drawn from Harrington's results.

Third, Harrington's theory of minority–majority group score differences cannot account for different *patterns* of cognitive performance between minority groups (Bogen, DeZure, Tenhouten, & Marsh, 1972; Dean, 1979a; Dershowitz & Frankel, 1975; Reynolds, McBride, & Gibson, 1979; Vance, Hankins, & McGee, 1979; Willerman, 1979). Different patterns of performance under Harrington's model imply differential bias in item selection, depending on the type of test involved. The degree of differential bias would also have to remain relatively constant across a number of different test batteries and test development samples with varying degrees of minority representation. This is at present an untenable assumption. Furthermore, there is evidence that SES is most strongly related to *level* of performance and race to *pattern* of performance (Jensen & Reynolds, 1982; Willerman, 1979). How this type of differential effect of test scores by minority category could occur under the Harrington model is not clear.

Hickman and Reynolds (1986) attempted to replicate Harrington's work, using large samples of black and white children taken from a stratified random sampling of children throughout the United States. Using item data collected during the national standardization of the Kaufman Assessment Battery for Children (K-ABC), the investigators selected items for three intelligence scales separately under two conditions: A set of "black" tests was created using only responses of the black children, and a set of "white" tests was created using only the responses of the white children. The item data used to create the "black" IQ tests were taken from a test development sample where the proportionate representation of blacks was 100% and whites was 0%. For the "white" IQ test, the test development sample used to select items was 100% white. This set of circumstances created the most extreme of conditions conducive to finding the Harrington effect. However, the pattern of race differences on the tests so created was contrary to Harrington's predictions: The pattern was totally unaffected by use of the Harrington procedure to select items for each of the tests. Whether items were selected from an analysis of the all-black sample or the all-white sample, the resulting pattern of mean differences was the same as when population proportionate sampling was used—the method Harrington contends is responsible for biasing item selection against minorities.

The Harrington effect has not been demonstrated with human subjects, despite attempts to do so under rather favorable conditions. Why it does not is uncertain; further research seems necessary to clarify this effect so amply demonstrated with Harrington's animal studies, yet failing to materialize with humans.

AREAS OF GENERAL CONCERN

Many potentially legitimate objections to the use of educational and psychological tests with minorities have been raised by black and other minority psychologists. Too frequently, the objections of these groups are viewed as facts without a review of any empirical evidence (e.g., Council for Exceptional Children, 1978; Hilliard, 1979). The problems most often cited in the use of tests with minorities typically fall into the following categories:

1. *Inappropriate content.* Black or other minority children have not been exposed to the material involved in the test questions of other stimulus materials. The tests are felt to be geared primarily toward white middle-class homes and values,

2. *Inappropriate standardization samples.* Ethnic minorities are underrepresented in the collection of normative reference group data. Williams (cited in Wright & Isenstein, 1977) criticized the WISC-R (Wechsler, 1974) standardization sample for including blacks only in proportion to the U.S. total population. Out of 2,200 children in the WISC-R standardization sample, 330 were members of minority groups. Williams contends that such small actual representation has no impact on the test. In earlier

years, it was not unusual for standardization samples to be all white (e.g., the original WISC; Wechsler, 1949).

3. *Examiner and language bias.* Since most psychologists are white and primarily speak only standard English, it is thought that they intimidate black and other ethnic minority children. They are also unable to communicate accurately with minority children. Lower test scores for minorities, then, are said to reflect only this intimidation and difficulty in the communication process, not lower ability levels.

4. *Inequitable social consequences.* It is argued that as a result of bias in educational and psychological tests, minority group members, who are already at a disadvantage in the educational and vocational markets because of past discrimination, are disproportionately relegated to dead-end educational tracks and thought to be unable to learn. Labeling effects also fall under this category.

5. *Measurement of different constructs.* Related to point 1 above, this position asserts that the tests are measuring significantly different attributes when used with minority children than when used with children from the white middle-class culture. Mercer (1979), for example, has contended that when IQ tests are used with minorities, they are measuring only the degree of "Anglocentrism" (adherence to white middle-class values) of the home.

6. *Differential predictive validity.* Although tests may accurately predict a variety of outcomes for white middle-class children, it is argued that they fail to predict any relevant criteria at an acceptable level for minority group members. Corollaries to this objection are a number of competing positions regarding the selection of an appropriate common criterion against which to validate tests across cultural groupings. Many black psychologists consider scholastic or academic attainment levels to be biased as criteria.

THE PROBLEM OF DEFINITION

The definition of test bias has produced considerable, and as yet unresolved, debate among measurement and assessment experts (Angoff, 1976; Bass, 1976; Bernal,

1975; Cleary et al., 1975; Cronbach, 1976; Darlington, 1971, 1976, 1978; Einhorn & Bass, 1971; Flaugher, 1978; Gordon, 1984; Gross & Su, 1975; Humphreys, 1973; Hunter & Schmidt, 1976, 1978; Linn, 1976; McNemar, 1975; Novick & Petersen, 1976; Petersen & Novick, 1976; Reschly, 1980; Reynolds, 1978; Reynolds & Brown, 1984; Sawyer, Cole, & Cole, 1976; Schmidt & Hunter, 1974; Thorndike, 1971). Although the resulting debate has generated a number of selection models with which to examine bias, selection models focus on the decision-making system and not on the test itself. The various selection models are discussed at some length in Hunter and Schmidt (1974), Hunter, Schmidt, and Rauschenberger (1984), Jensen (1980), Petersen and Novick (1976), and Ramsay (1979). The choice of a decision-making system (especially a system for educational decision making) must ultimately be a societal one; as such, it will depend to a large extent on the value system and goals of the society. Thus, before a model for test use in selection can be chosen, it must be decided whether the ultimate goal is equality of opportunity, equality of outcome, or representative equality (these concepts are discussed in more detail in Nichols, 1978).

"Equality of opportunity" is a competitive model wherein selection is based on ability. As more eloquently stated by Lewontin (1970), under equality of opportunity "true merit . . . will be the criterion of men's earthly reward" (p. 92). "Equality of outcome" is a selection model based on ability deficits. Compensatory and remedial education programs are typically constructed on the basis of the equality-of-outcome model. Children of low ability or children believed to be at high risk for academic failure are selected for remedial, compensatory, or other special educational programs. In a strictly predictive sense, tests are used in a similar manner under both of these models. However, under equality or opportunity, selection is based on the prediction of a high level of criterion performance; under equality of outcome, selection is determined by the prediction of "failure" or a preselected low level of criterion performance. Interestingly, it is the failure of compensatory and remedial education programs to bring the disadvantaged learner to "average" levels of performance that has resulted in the charges of test bias now in vogue.

The model of "representative equality" also relies on selection, but selection that is proportionate to numerical representation of subgroups in the population under consideration. Representative equality is typically thought to be independent of the level of ability within each group; however, models can be constructed that select from each subgroup the desired proportion of individuals (1) according to relative ability level of the group, (2) independent of group ability, or (3) according to some decision rule between these two positions. Even under the conditions of representative equality, it is imperative to employ a selection device (test) that will rank-order individuals within groups in a reliable and valid manner. The best way to insure fair selection under any of these models is to employ tests that are equally reliable and equally valid for all groups concerned. The tests employed should also be the most reliable and most valid for all groups under consideration. The question of test bias per se then becomes a question of test validity. Test use (i.e., fairness) may be defined as biased or nonbiased only by the societal value system; at present, this value system is leaning strongly toward some variant of the representative-equality selection model. As noted above, all models are facilitated by the use of a nonbiased test. That is, the use of a test with equivalent cross-group validities makes for the most parsimonious selection model, greatly simplifying the creation and application of the selection model that has been chosen.

This leads to the essential definitional component of test bias. "Test bias" refers in a global sense to *systematic* error in the estimation of some "true" value for a group of individuals. The key word here is "systematic"; all measures contain error, but this error is assumed to be random unless shown to be otherwise. Bias investigation is a statistical inquiry that does not concern itself with culture loading, labeling effects, or test use/test fairness. Concerning the last of these, Jensen (1980) comments,

[U]nbiased tests can be used unfairly and biased tests can be used fairly. Therefore, the concepts of bias and unfairness should be kept distinct. . . . [A] number of different, and often mutually contradictory, criteria for fairness have been proposed, and no amount of statistical or psychometric reasoning per se can possibly settle any arguments as to which is best. (pp. 375–376)

There are three types of validity as traditionally conceived: content, construct, and predictive (or criterion-related). Test bias may exist under any or all of these categories of validity. Though no category of validity is completely independent of any other category, each is discussed separately here for the purpose of clarity and convenience. (All true evidence of validity is as likely as not to be construct validity, and the other, more detailed divisions are for convenience of discussion.) Frequently encountered in bias research are the terms "single-group validity" and "differential validity." "Single-group validity" refers to the phenomenon of a test's being valid for one group but not another. "Differential validity" refers to a condition where a test is valid for all groups concerned, but the degree of validity varies as a function of group membership. Although these terms have been most often applied to predictive or criterion-related validity (validity coefficients are then examined for significance and compared across groups), the concepts of single-group and differential validity are equally applicable to content and construct validity.

RESEARCH STRATEGIES AND RESULTS

The methodologies available for research into bias in mental tests have grown rapidly in number and sophistication over the last three decades. Extensive reviews of the questions to be addressed in such research and their corresponding methodologies are available in Jensen (1980), Reynolds (1982), and Reynolds and Brown (1984). The most popular methods are reviewed below, along with a summary of findings from each area of inquiry. The sections are organized primarily by methodology within each content area of research (i.e., research into content, construct, and predictive validity).

Bias in Content Validity

Bias in the item content of intelligence tests is one of the favorite topics of those who de-

cry the use of standardized tests with minorities (e.g., Hilliard, 1979; Jackson, 1975; Williams, 1972; Wright & Isenstein, 1977). As previously noted, the earliest work in bias centered around content. Typically, critics review the items of a test and single out specific items as being biased because (1) the items ask for information that minority or disadvantaged children have not had equal opportunity to learn; and/or (2) the scoring of the items is improper, since the test author has arbitrarily decided on the only correct answer and minority children are inappropriately penalized for giving answers that would be correct in their own culture but not that of the test maker; and/or (3) the wording of the questions is unfamiliar, and a minority child who may "know" the correct answer may not be able to respond because he or she does not understand the question. Each of these three criticisms, when accurate, has the same basic empirical result: The item becomes relatively more difficult for minority group members than for the majority population. This leads directly to a definition of content bias for aptitude tests that allows empirical assessment of the phenomenon.

> An item or subscale of a test is considered to be biased in content when it is demonstrated to be relatively more difficult for members of one group than for members of another in a situation where the general ability level of the groups being compared is held constant and no reasonable theoretical rationale exists to explain group differences on the item (or subscale) in question.

With regard to achievement tests, the issue of content bias is considerably more complex. Exposure to instruction, general ability level of the group, and the accuracy and specificity of the sampling of the domain of items are all important variables in determining whether the content of an achievement test is biased (see Schmidt, 1983). Research into item (or content) bias with achievement tests has typically, and perhaps mistakenly, relied on methodology appropriate for determining item bias in aptitude tests. Nevertheless, research examining both types of instruments for content bias has yielded quite comparable results.

One method of locating "suspicious" test items requires that item difficulties be determined separately for each group under consideration. If any individual item or series of items appears to be exceptionally difficult for the members of any group, relative to other items on the test, the item is considered potentially biased and removed from the test. A more exacting and widespread approach to identifying biased items involves analysis of variance (ANOVA) and several closely related procedures wherein the group × item interaction term is of interest (e.g., Angoff & Ford, 1973; Cardall & Coffman, 1964; Cleary & Hilton, 1968; Plake & Hoover, 1979; Potthoff, 1966; Stanley, 1969).

The definition of content bias set forth above actually requires that the differences between groups be the same for every item on the test. Thus, in the ANOVA procedure, the group × item interaction should not yield a significant result. Whenever the differences in items are not uniform (a significant group × item interaction does exist), one may contend that biased items exist. Earlier in this area of research, it was hoped that the empirical analysis of tests at the item level would result in the identification of a category of items having similar content as biased, and that such items could then be avoided in future test development (Flaugher, 1978). Very little similarity among items determined to be biased has been found. No one has been able to identify those characteristics of an item that cause the item to be biased. It does seem that poorly written, sloppy, and ambiguous items tend to be identified as biased with greater frequency than those items typically encountered in a well-constructed standardized instrument. The variable at issue then may be the item reliability. Item reliabilities are typically not large, and poorly written or ambiguous test items can easily have reliabilities approaching zero. Decreases in reliability are known to increase the probability of the occurrence of bias (Linn & Werts, 1971). Informal inventories and locally derived tests are much more likely to be biased than professionally written standardized tests that have been scrutinized for bias in the items and whose item characteristics are known.

Once items have been identified as biased under the procedures described above, attempts have been made to eliminate "test bias" by eliminating the offending items and rescoring the tests. As pointed out by Flaugher (1978) and Flaugher and Schrader (1978), however, little is gained by this tactic. Mean differences in performance between groups are affected only slightly, and the test becomes more difficult for everyone involved, since the eliminated items typically have moderate to low difficulty. When race × item interactions have been found, the interaction typically accounts for a very small proportion of variance. For example, in analyzing items on the WISC-R, Jensen (1976), Sandoval (1979), and Mille (1979) found the group × item interaction to account for only 2%–5% of the variance in performance. Using a similar technique with the Wonderlic Personnel Test, Jensen (1977) found the race × item interaction to account for only about 5% of the test score variance. Thus the elimination of the offending items can be expected to have little, if any, significant effect. These analyses have been of a post hoc nature (i.e., after the tests have been standardized), however, and the use of empirical methods for determining item bias during the test development phase (as with the K-ABC) is to be encouraged.

With multiple-choice tests, another level of complexity is added to the examination of content bias. With a multiple-choice question, three or four distractors are typically given in addition to the correct response. Distractors may be examined for their attractiveness (the relative frequency with which they are chosen) across groups. When distractors are found to be disproportionately attractive for members of any particular group, the item may be defined as biased. When items are constructed to have an equal distribution of responses to each distractor for the total test population, then chi-square can be used to examine the distribution of choices for each distractor for each group (Burrill, 1975).

Jensen (1976) investigated the distribution of wrong responses for two multiple-choice intelligence tests, the Peabody Picture Vocabulary Test (PPVT) and Raven's Progressive Matrices (the Raven). Each of these two tests was individually administered to 600 white and 400 black children between the ages of 6 and 12. The analysis of incorrect responses for the PPVT indicated that the errors were distributed in a nonrandom fashion over the distractors for a large number of items. However, no racial bias in response patterns occurred, since the disproportionate choice of distractors followed the same pattern for blacks and whites. On the Raven, blacks made different types of errors than whites, but only on a small number of items. Jensen followed up these items and compared the black response pattern to the response pattern of white children at a variety of age levels. For every item showing differences in black–white response patterns, the black response could be duplicated by the response patterns of whites approximately 2 years younger than blacks.

Veale and Foreman (1983) have advocated inspecting multiple-choice tests for bias in distractor or "foil" response distribution as a means of refining tests *before* they are finalized for the marketplace. They note that there are many instances whereby unbiased external criteria (such as achievement or ability) or culturally valid tests are not readily accessible for detecting bias in the measure under study. Veale and Foreman add that inspection of incorrect responses to distractor items can often lead to greater insight concerning cultural bias in any given question than would inspection of percentage of correct responses across groups. Veale and Foreman provide the statistical analyses for their "overpull probability model" along with the procedures for measuring cultural variation and diagramming the source of bias within any given item. Consider the following example provided by the authors:

Pick out the correct sentence below:
(A) Janie takes her work seriously.
(B) Janie work take too much time.
(C) Working with books are my favorite thing.
(D) Things people like to do is their business.

(Veale & Foreman, 1983)

In this example, blacks are strongly attracted to distractor D, while other groups are more inclined to pick C, as seen by Veale and Foreman's "overpull" computations. The D distractor, at face value, may be having a differential impact on black performance because of the "street" language presumed to be more common in the black culture. There is also the question upon further inspection as to whether the stem of this particular item provides clear direction (i.e., "correct *standard* English") to the testee. Knowledge of the differential response patterns across groups allows for item refinement, and subsequent statistical inspection can insure that distractors are not overly attractive or distracting to one group or another in revised format.

Investigation of item bias during test development is certainly not restricted to multiple-choice items and methods such as those outlined by Veale and Foreman. The possibilities are numerous (see Jensen, 1980, Ch. 9). For example, Scheuneman (1987) has used the results of linear methodology on Graduate Record Examination (GRE) item data to show some interesting influences on black–white performance when item characteristics (e.g., vocabulary content, one true or one false answer to be selected, diagrams to be used or not used, use of antonym items, etc.) are uniformly investigated. Although Scheuneman indicates that future research of this type should reduce the number of variables to address (there are 16 hypotheses), the results nonetheless suggest that bias or content research across groups is a viable way in which to determine whether differential effects can "be demonstrated through the manipulation of relatively stable characteristics of test items" (p. 116). Scheuneman presented pairs of items, with the designated characteristic of a question format under study present in one item and absent or modified in the other. Paired experimental items were administered in the experimental section of the GRE General Test, given in December 1982. Results indicated that certain "item elements"—common in general form to a variety of questions—appeared to have a differential impact on black and white performance. For example, significant group × version interactions were seen for one correct true versus one correct false response and for adding/modifying prefixes/suffixes to the stimulus word in antonym items. The question is thus raised as to whether the items showing differential impact are measuring the content domain (e.g., verbal, quantitative, or analytical thinking) as opposed to an aspect of "element" within the presentation to some degree. Scheuneman concludes that more research is needed to establish ways in which more systematic rules and procedures of test construction can be developed.

Another approach to the identification of biased items has been pursued by Jensen (1976). According to Jensen, if a test contains items that are disproportionately difficult for one group of examinees as compared to another, the correlation of P decrements between adjacent items will be low for the two groups. ("P decrement" refers to the difference in the difficulty index, P. from one item of a test to the next item. Typically, ability test items are arranged in ascending order of difficulty.) Jensen (1974, 1976) also contends that if a test contains biased items, the correlation between the rank order of item difficulties for one race with another will also be low. Jensen (1974, 1976, 1977) calculated cross-racial correlation of item difficulties for large samples of black and white children on five major intelligence tests: the PPVT, the Raven, the Revised Stanford–Binet Intelligence Scale: Form L-M, the WISC-R, and the Wonderlic Personnel Test. Cross-racial correlations of P decrements were reported for several of the scales. Jensen's results are summarized in Table 22.1, along with the results of several other investigators also employing Jensen's methodology.

As is readily apparent in Table 22.1, little evidence to support any consistent content

bias within any of the scales investigated was found. The consistently large magnitude of the cross-racial correlations of P decrements is impressive and indicates a general lack of content bias in the instruments as a whole. As previously noted, however, some individual items were identified as biased; yet they collectively accounted for only 2%–5% of the variance in performance differences and showed no detectable pattern in item content.

Another approach to this question is to use the partial correlation between a demographic or other nominal variable and item score, where the correlation between total test score and the variable of interest has been removed from the relationship. If a significant partial correlation exists, say, between race and an item score after the race–total test score relationship has been partialed out, then the item is performing differentially across race within ability level. Bias has been demonstrated at this point under the definition offered above. The use of the partial correlation (typically a partial point-biserial P) is the simplest and perhaps the most powerful of the item bias detection approaches, but its development is relatively recent, and its use is not yet common. An example of its application may be found in Reynolds, Willson, and Chatman (1984).

A common practice since the 1970s has been a return to including expert judgment by professionals and members of minority

TABLE 22.1. Cross-Racial Analysis of Content Bias for Five Major Intelligence Scales

	Cross-racial correlation of rank order of item difficulties[a]	
Scale	Black–white correlations[b]	White–Mexican American correlations[b]
Peabody Picture Vocabulary Test (Jensen, 1974b)	.99 (.79), .98 (.65)	.98 (.78), .98 (.66)
Raven's Progressive Matrices (Jensen, 1974b)	.99 (.98), .99 (.96)	.99 (.99), .99 (.97)
Stanford–Binet Intelligence Scale (Jensen, 1976)	.96	
Wechsler Intelligence Scale for Children—Revised		
(Jensen, 1976)	.95	
(Sandoval, 1979)[c]	.98 (.87)	.99 (.91)
(Mille, 1979) (1949 WISC)	.96, .95	
Wonderlic Personnel Test (Jensen, 1977)	.94 (.81)	

[a]Correlation of P decrements across race is included in parentheses if reported.
[b]Where two sets of correlations are presented, data were reported separately for males and females and are listed males first. The presence of a single correlation indicates that data were pooled across gender.
[c]Median values for the 10 WISC-R subtests excluding Digit Span and Coding.

groups in the item selection for new psychological and educational tests. This approach was used in development of the K-ABC, the revision of the Wechsler Preschool and Primary Scale of Intelligence (WPPSI-R), the PPVT-R, and a number of other contemporary tests. The practice typically asks for an "armchair" inspection of individual items as a means of locating and expurgating biased components to the measure under development. Since, as previously noted, no detectable pattern or common characteristic of individual items statistically shown to be biased has been observed (given reasonable care in the item-writing stage), it seems reasonable to question the "armchair" approach to determining biased items. The bulk of scientific data since the pioneering work of McGurk (1951) has not supported the position that anyone can—upon surface inspection—detect the degree to which any given item will function differentially across groups (Shepard, 1982). Several researchers since McGurk's time have identified items as being disproportionately more difficult for minority group members than for members of the majority culture and have subsequently compared their results with a panel of expert judges. The data have provided some interesting results.

Although examples of the failure of judges to identify biased items now abound, two studies demonstrate this failure most clearly. After identifying the eight most racially discriminating and eight least racially discriminating items on the Wonderlic Personnel Test, Jensen (1976) asked panels of five black psychologists and five white psychologists to sort out the eight most and eight least discriminating items when only these 16 items were presented to them. The judges sorted the items at a level no better than chance. Sandoval and Mille (1979) conducted a somewhat more extensive analysis, using items from the WISC-R. These two researchers had 38 black, 22 Mexican American, and 40 white university students from Spanish, history, and education classes identify items from the WISC-R that would be more difficult for a minority child than a white child and items that would be equally difficult for each group. A total of 45 WISC-R items were presented to each judge; these items included the 15 most difficult items for blacks as compared to whites, the 15 most difficult items for Mexican Americans as compared to whites, and the 15 items showing the most nearly identical difficulty indices for minority and white children. The judges were asked to read each question and determine whether they thought the item was (1) easier for minority than for white children, (2) easier for white than for minority children, or (3) of equal difficulty for white and minority children. Sandoval and Mille's results indicated that the judges were not able to differentiate accurately between items that were more difficult for minorities and items that were of equal difficulty across groups. The effects of the judges' ethnic background on the accuracy of item bias judgments were also considered. Minority and nonminority judges did not differ in their ability to identify accurately biased items, nor did they differ with regard to the type of incorrect identification they tended to make. Sandoval and Mille's two major conclusions were that "(1) judges are not able to detect items which are more difficult for a minority child than an Anglo child, and (2) the ethnic background of the judge makes no difference in accuracy of item selection for minority children" (p. 6). In each of these studies, the most extreme items were used, which should have given the judges an advantage.

Anecdotal evidence is also available to refute the assumption that "armchair" analyses of test bias in item content are accurate. Far and away, the most widely cited example of a biased intelligence test item is item 6 of the WISC-R Comprehension subtest: "What is the thing to do if a boy (girl) much smaller than yourself starts to fight with you?" This item is generally considered to be biased against black children in particular, because of the scoring criteria. According to the item's critics, the most logical response for a black child is to "fight back," yet this is a 0-point response. The correct (2-point) response is to walk away and avoid fighting with the child—a response that critics claim invites disaster in the black culture, where children are taught to fight back and would not 'know" the "correct white response. Black responses to this item have been empirically investigated in several studies, with the same basic results: The item is relatively easier for black children than for white children. When all items on the WISC-R are ranked separately according to the difficulty level for blacks and whites, this item is the 42nd least difficult item (where 1 represents the easiest item) for black children and the 47th least difficult for white children (Jensen, 1976). Mille (1979), in a large-*n* study of bias, reached a similar conclusion, stating that this item "is relatively easier for blacks than it is for whites" (p. 163). The results of these empirical studies with large samples of black and white children are unequivocal: When matched for overall general intellectual skill, more black than white children will get this item correct—the very item most often singled out as a blatant example of the inherent bias of intelligence tests against blacks (see also Reynolds & Brown, 1984).

Even without empirical support for its accuracy, a number of prestigious writers support the continued use of the "face validity" approach of using a panel of minority judges to identify "biased" test items (Anastasi, 1986; Kaufman, 1979; Sandoval & Mille, 1979). Those who support the continued use of this technique see it as a method of gaining greater rapport with the public. As pointed out by Sandoval and Mille (1979), "Public opinion, whether it is supported by empirical findings, or based on emotion, can serve as an obstacle to the use of a measurement instrument" (p. 7). The elimination of items that are offensive or otherwise objectionable to any substantive segment of the population for whom the test is intended seems an appropriate action that may aid in the public's acceptance of new and better psychological assessment tools. However, the subjective-judgment approach should not be allowed to supplant the use of more sophisticated analyses in the determination of biased items. The subjective approach should serve as a supplemental procedure, and items identified through this method (provided that some interrater agreement can be obtained—an aspect of the subjective method yet to be demonstrated) as objectionable can be eliminated when a psychometrically equivalent (or better) item can be obtained as a replacement and the intent of the item is kept intact (e.g., with a criterion-referenced measure, the new item must be designed to measure the same objective). The reliability, construct validity, and predictive validity of measures

should not suffer any substantial losses for the purposes of increasing face validity.

Researchers such as Tittle (1982) have stressed that the possibility of and need for cooperation between those advocating statistical validity and those advocating face validity in nonbiased test construction are greater than one might think, given the above-cited research. Judgmental analysis allows for the *perception* of fairness in items, tests, and evaluations, and this perception should not be taken lightly. Tittle argues that "judgmental methods arise from a different, nonstatistical ground. In examining fairness or bias primarily on statistical grounds, we may again be witnessing a technical solution to a problem that is broader than the technical issues" (p. 34). Tests under construction should include definitive information concerning the nonbiased nature of the measure from a statistical standpoint, in addition to support by minority groups or other interested parties who have had the opportunity to inspect the test for the perception of fairness. Tittle notes that Cronbach (1980) does not find the issue of fairness as determined by subjective judgment to be outside the realm of test validation. Cronbach states, "The politicalization of testing ought not [to] be surprising. Test data influence the fortunes of individuals and the support given to human service programs" (p. 100). Tittle (1975, 1982) argues that the general field of test development requires greater consensus regarding specific, multidimensional steps taken in formulating "fair" measures, because "fairness" in testing will never be realistically viewed by the public from a unidimensional statistical standpoint. She concludes:

> In the test development setting there needs to be a closer examination [of] and agreement on the test development process, the judgmental and statistical data that are used as the basis to identify the final set of test items. Such agreement would permit both users and developers to reach a conclusion as to whether a test is "fair" for a particular subgroup, e.g., minorities and women. (p. 33)

Berk (1982) has proposed a three-step process for test development that responds to many of the issues outlined by Tittle. Berk's conceptualization includes (1) judgmental review to explore for content that is, for example, stereotypic, culture-specific, or offensive in language; (2) statistical analyses to detect performance discrepancies between/ among groups; and (3) a posteriori analysis of statistical data to determine whether item or test bias is present and, if so, to make appropriate adjustments. He argues that the way in which bias is perceived by society and the empirical methodologies used to detect bias require unification of the statistical and judgmental viewpoints if an equitable and lasting solution to "fair" test development is to be realized.

Thus far, this section has focused on the identification of biased items. Several studies evaluating other hypotheses have provided data that are relevant to the issue of content bias of intelligence tests, specifically the WISC-R.

Jensen and Figueroa (1975) investigated black–white differences in mental test scores as a function of differences in Level I (rote learning and memory) and Level II (complex cognitive processing) abilities. These researchers tested a large number of blacks and whites on the WISC-R Digit Span subtest and then analyzed the data separately for digits forward and digits backward. The content of the digits-forward and digits backward procedures is the same. Thus, if score differences are due only to bias in content validity, score differences across race should remain constant for the two tasks. On the other hand, since the information-processing demands of the two tasks are quite different, the relative level of performance on the two tasks should not be the same if blacks and whites differ in their ability to process information according to the demands of the two tasks. Jensen and Figueroa found the latter to be the case. The black–white score difference on digits backward was more than twice the magnitude of the difference for digits forward. Granted, this methodology can provide only indirect evidence regarding the content validity of an instrument; however, its importance is in providing a different view of the issues and an alternative research strategy. Since the Jensen and Figueroa results do not indicate any content bias in the Digit Span subtest, they add to a growing body of literature that strongly suggests the lack of cultural bias in well-constructed, standardized tests.

Another study (Reynolds & Jensen, 1983) examined each of the 12 WISC-R subtests for cultural bias against blacks, using a variation of the group × item ANOVA methodology discussed earlier. Reynolds and Jensen (1983) matched 270 black children with 270 white children from the WISC-R standardization sample on the basis of gender and WISC-R Full Scale IQ. IQs were required to match within one standard error of measurement (about 3 points). When multiple matching cases were encountered, children were matched on the basis of SES. Matching the two groups of children on the basis of the Full Scale IQ essentially equated the two groups for g. Therefore, examining black–white differences in performance on each subtest of the WISC-R made it possible to determine which, if any, of the subtests were disproportionately difficult for blacks or whites. A significant F ratio in the multivariate analysis of variance (MANOVA) for the 12 WISC-R subtests was followed with univariate F tests between black and white means on each of the 12 WISC-R subtests. A summary of the Reynolds and Jensen results is presented in Table 22.2. Blacks exceeded whites in performance on two subtests: Digit Span and Coding. Whites exceeded blacks in performance on three subtests: Comprehension, Object Assembly, and Mazes. A trend was apparent for blacks to perform at a higher level on the Arithmetic subtest, while whites tended to exceed blacks on the Picture Arrangement subtest. Although these results can be interpreted to indicate bias in several of the WISC-R subtests, the actual differences were very small (typically on the order of 0. 10–0.15 standard deviation), and the amount of variance in performance associated with ethnic group membership was less than 5% in each case. The results are also reasonably consistent with Jensen's theory of mental test score differences and their relationship to Level I and Level II abilities. The Digit Span and Coding subtests are clearly the best measures of Level I abilities on the WISC-R, while Comprehension, Object Assembly, and Mazes are more closely associated with Level II abilities.

From a large number of studies employing a wide range of methodology, a relatively clear picture emerges: Content bias in

TABLE 22.2. Means, Standard Deviations, and Univariate F's for Comparison of Performance on Specific WISC-R Subtests by Groups of Blacks and Whites Matched for WISC-R Full Scale IQ

WISC-R variable	Blacks		Whites		D^a	F^b	p
	$\overline{X}$	SD	$\overline{X}$	SD			
Information	8.40	2.53	8.24	2.62	−.16	0.54	NS
Similarities	8.24	2.78	8.13	2.78	−.11	0.22	NS
Arithmetic	8.98	2.62	8.62	2.58	−.36	2.52	.10
Vocabulary	8.21	2.61	8.27	2.58	+.06	0.06	NS
Comprehension	8.14	2.40	8.58	2.47	+.44	4.27	.05
Digit Span	9.51	3.09	8.89	2.83	+.62	6.03	.01
Picture Completion	8.49	2.88	8.60	2.58	+.11	0.18	NS
Picture Arrangement	8.45	2.92	8.79	2.89	+.34	1.78	.10
Block Design	8.06	2.54	8.33	2.76	+.27	1.36	NS
Object Assembly	8.17	2.90	8.68	2.70	+.51	4.41	.05
Coding	9.14	2.81	8.65	2.80	−.49	4.30	.05
Mazes	8.69	3.14	9.19	2.98	+.50	3.60	.05
Verbal IQ	89.63	12.13	89.61	12.07	−.02	0.04	NS
Performance IQ	89.29	12.22	90.16	11.67	+.87	0.72	NS
Full Scale IQ	88.61	11.48	88.96	11.35	+.35	0.13	NS

Note. NS, not significant.
^{a}White $\overline{X}$–black $\overline{X}$ difference.
^{b}Degrees of freedom = 1, 538.

well-prepared standardized tests is irregular in its occurrence, and no common characteristics of items that are found to be biased can be ascertained by expert judges (minority or nonminority). The variance in group score differences on mental tests associated with ethnic group membership when content bias has been found is relatively small (typically ranging from 2% to 5%). Even this small amount of bias has been seriously questioned, as Hunter (1975) describes such findings basically as methodological artifacts. Although the search for common "biased" item characteristics will continue, and psychologists must pursue the public relations issues of face validity, "armchair" claims of cultural bias in aptitude tests have found no empirical support in a large number of actuarial studies contrasting the performance of a variety of racial groups on items and subscales of the most widely employed intelligence scales in the United States; neither differential nor single-group validity has been demonstrated.

Bias in Construct Validity

There is no single method for the accurate determination of the construct validity of educational and psychological tests. Defin-

ing bias in construct validity thus requires a general statement that can be researched from a variety of viewpoints with a broad range of methodology. The following rather parsimonious definition is preferred:

> Bias exists in regard to construct validity when a test is shown to measure different hypothetical traits (psychological constructs) for one group than for another, or to measure the same trait but with differing degrees of accuracy.

As befits the concept of construct validity, many different methods have been employed to examine existing tests for potential bias in construct validity. One of the most popular and necessary empirical approaches to investigating construct validity is factor analysis (Anastasi, 1986; Cronbach, 1970). Factor analysis, as a procedure, identifies clusters of test items or clusters of subtests of psychological or educational tests that correlate highly with one another, and less so or not at all with other subtests or items. It thus allows one to determine patterns of interrelationships of performance among groups of individuals. For example, if several subtests of an intelligence scale load highly on (are members of) the same factor, then if a group of individuals score high on one of these subtests, they would be expected to score at a high level on other subtests that load highly on that factor. Psychologists attempt to determine, through a review of the test content and correlates of performance on the factor in question, what psychological trait underlies performance; or, in a more hypothesis-testing approach, they will make predictions concerning the pattern of factor loadings. Hilliard (1979), one of the more vocal critics of IQ tests on the basis of cultural bias, has pointed out one of the potential areas of bias in comparisons of the factor-analytic results of tests across races:

> If the IQ test is a valid and reliable test of "innate" ability or abilities, then the factors which emerge on a given test should be the same from one population to another, since intelligence" is asserted to be a set of mental processes. Therefore, while the configuration of scores of a particular group on the factor profile would be expected to differ, logic would dictate that the factors themselves would remain the same. (p. 53)

Although researchers do not necessarily agree that identical factor analyses of an instrument speak to the innateness of the abilities being measured, consistent factor-analytic results across populations do provide strong evidence that whatever is being measured by the instrument is being measured in the same manner and is, in fact, the same construct within each group. The information derived from comparative factor analysis across populations is directly relevant to the use of educational and psychological tests in diagnosis and other decision-making functions. Psychologists, in order to make consistent interpretations of test score data, must be certain that a test measures the same variable across populations.

Two basic approaches, each with a number of variations, have been employed to compare factor-analytic results across populations. The first and more popular approach asks how similar the results are for each group; the second and less popular approach asks whether the results show a statistically significant difference between groups. The most sophisticated approach to the latter question has been the work of Jöreskog (1969, 1971) in simultaneous factor analysis in several populations. Howev-

er, little has been done with the latter approach within the context of test bias research, and Jöreskog's methods can be quite abstruse.

Mille (1979) has demonstrated the use of a simpler method (actually developed by Jensen and presented in detail in Jensen, 1980) for testing the significance of the difference between factors for two populations. In Mille's method, all factor loadings are converted to Fisher's z-scores. The z-scores for corresponding factors are paired by variable and then subtracted. The differences in factor loadings, now expressed as differences in z-scores, are squared. The squared scores are summed and the mean derived. The mean of the squared differences is then divided by the following quantity:

$$\frac{1}{n_1 - 3} + \frac{1}{n_2 - 3}$$

where n_1 is the number of subjects in group 1 and n_2 is the number of subjects in group 2. This division yields a test statistic that is distributed as a chi-square with 1 degree of freedom. Mille's methodology has also received little use in the bias in assessment literature. As one part of a comprehensive internal analysis of test bias on the 1949 WISC, Mille compared the first principal-component factoring across race for blacks and whites at the preschool, first-grade, third-grade, and fifth-grade levels. This factor, often thought of as a measure of g, did not differ significantly across race at any age level. Mille's results with the WISC indicate that factor loadings on g are essentially equivalent and that when score differences occur between groups, the differences reflect whatever is common to all variables that make up the test, rather than some personological or moderator variable that is specific to one group.

A number of techniques have been developed to measure the similarity of factors across groups. Katzenmeyer and Stenner (1977) described a technique based essentially on factor score comparisons. A "factor score" is a composite score derived by summing an individual's weighted scores on all variables that appear on a factor. Weights are derived from factor analysis and are directly related to the factor loadings of the variables. According to Katzen-meyer and Stenner's procedure, factor scores are first derived based on the combined groups of interest (e.g., the scores of blacks and whites as a single, homogeneous group are factor-analyzed). Then the scores of each group are factor-analyzed separately, and factor scores are again determined. The correlation between the factor scores from the total-group analysis and the factor scores from the single-group analysis is then used as an estimate of the factorial similarity of the test battery across groups. The method is actually somewhat more complex, as described by Katzenmeyer and Stenner, and has not been widely employed in the test bias literature; however, it is a practical technique with many utilitarian implications and should receive more attention in future literature.

The two most common methods of determining factorial similarity or factorial invariance involve the direct comparison of factor loadings across groups. The two primary techniques for this comparison are (1) the calculation of a coefficient of congruence (Harman, 1976) between the loadings of corresponding factors for two groups; and (2) the simple calculation of a Pearson product–moment coefficient of correlation between the factor loadings of the corresponding factors. The latter technique, though used with some frequency, is less satisfactory than the use of the coefficient of congruence, since in the comparison of factor loadings certain of the assumptions underlying the Pearson r may be violated. When one is determining the degree of similarity of factors, a value of .90 or greater is typically, though arbitrarily, taken to indicate equivalent factors (factorial invariance). However, the most popular methods of calculating factorial similarity produce quite similar results (Reynolds & Harding, 1983), at least in large-n studies.

In contrast to Hilliard's (1979) strong statement that studies of factorial similarity across race have not been reported in the technical literature, a number of such studies have appeared since 1980, dealing with a number of different tests. The focus here is primarily on studies comparing factor-analytic results across races for aptitude tests.

Because the WISC (Wechsler, 1949) and its successor, the WISC-R (Wechsler, 1974), have been the most widely employed individual intelligence tests with school-age children, it is appropriate that the cross-race structure of these two instruments has received extensive investigation for both nonexceptional and referral populations of children. Using a large, random sample, Reschly (1978) compared the factor structure of the WISC-R across four racially identifiable groups: whites, blacks, Mexican Americans, and Native American Papagos, all from the southwestern United States. Consistent with the findings of previous researchers with the 1949 WISC (Lindsey, 1967; Silverstein, 1973), Reschly reported substantial congruency of factors across races when the two-factor solutions were compared (the two-factor solution typically reiterated Wechsler's a priori grouping of the subtests into a Verbal and a Performance, or nonverbal, scale). The 12 coefficients of congruence for comparisons of the two-factor solution across all combinations of racial groupings ranged only from .97 to .99, denoting factorial equivalence of this solution across groups. Reschly also compared three-factor solutions (three-factor solutions typically include Verbal Comprehension, Perceptual Organization, and Freedom from Distractibility factors), finding congruence only between whites and Mexican Americans. These findings are also consistent with previous research with the WISC (Semler & Iscoe, 1966). The g factor present in the WISC-R was shown to be congruent across race, as was also demonstrated by Mille (1979) for the WISC. Reschly (1978) concluded that the usual interpretation of the WISC-R Full Scale IQ as a measure of overall intellectual ability appears to be equally appropriate for whites, blacks, Mexican Americans, and Native American Papagos. Jensen (1985) has presented compelling data indicating that the black–white discrepancy seen in major tests of aptitude reflects primarily the g factor. Reschly also concluded that the Verbal–Performance scale distinction on the WISC-R is equally appropriate across race, and that there is strong evidence for the integrity of the WISC-R's construct validity for a variety of populations.

Support for Reschly's (1978) conclusions is available from a variety of other studies of the WISC and WISC-R. Applying a hierarchical factor-analytic method developed by Wherry and Wherry (1969), Vance and Wallbrown (1978) factor-analyzed the intercorrelation matrix of the WISC-R subtests for 150 referred blacks from the Appalachian region of the United States. The two-factor hierarchical solution determined for Vance and Wallbrown's blacks was highly similar to hierarchical factor solutions determined for the standardization samples of the Wechsler scales generally (Blaha, Wallbrown, & Wherry, 1975; Wallbrown, Blaha, & Wherry, 1973). Vance and Wallbrown's results with the WISC-R are also consistent with a previous hierarchical factor analysis with the 1949 WISC for a group of disadvantaged blacks and whites (Vance, Huelsman, & Wherry, 1976).

Several more recent studies comparing the WISC-R factor structure across races for nonexceptional and referral populations of children have also provided increased support for the generality of Reschly's (1978) conclusions and the results of the other investigators cited above. Oakland and Feigenbaum (1979) factor-analyzed the 12 WISC-R subtests' intercorrelations separately for stratified (race, age, sex, SES) random samples of nonexceptional white, black, and Mexican American children from an urban school district of the northwestern United States. Pearson r's were calculated between corresponding factors for each group. For the g factor, the black–white correlation between factor loadings was .95, the Mexican American–white correlation was .97, and the black–Mexican American correlation was .96. Similar comparisons across all WISC-R variables produced correlations ranging only from .94 to .99. Oakland and Feigenbaum concluded that the results of their factor analyses "do not reflect bias with respect to construct validity for these three racial–ethnic . . . groups" (1979, p. 973).

Gutkin and Reynolds (1981) determined the factorial similarity of the WLSC-R for groups of black and white children from the WISC-R standardization sample. This study is particularly important to examine in determining the construct validity of the WISC-R across races, because of the sample employed in the investigation. The sample included 1,868 white and 305 black children obtained in a stratified random sam-

pling procedure designed to mimic the 1970 U.S. census data on the basis of age, sex, race, SES, geographic region of residence, and community size. Similarity of the WISC-R factor structure across race was investigated by comparing the black and white groups for the two- and three-factor solutions on (1) the magnitude of unique variances, (2) the pattern of subtest loadings on each factor, (3) the portion of total variance accounted for by common factor variance, and (4) the percentage of common factor variance accounted for by each factor. Coefficients of congruence comparing the unique variances, the g factor, the two-factor solutions, and the three-factor solutions across races all achieved a value of .99. The portion of total variance accounted for by each factor was the same in both the two- and three-factor racial groups. Gutkin and Reynolds concluded that for white and black children the WISC-R factor structure was essentially invariant, and that no evidence of single-group or differential construct validity could be found.

Subsequent studies comparing the WISC-R factor structure for referral populations of white and Mexican American children have also strongly supported the construct validity of the WISC-R across races. Dean (1979b) compared three-factor WISC-R solutions across races for whites and Mexican Americans referred because of learning problems in the regular classroom. Analyzing the 10 regular WISC-R subtests, Dean reported coefficients of congruence between corresponding factors of .84 for factor 1 (Verbal Comprehension), .89 for factor 2 (Perceptual Organization), and .88 for factor 3 (Freedom from Distractibility). Although not quite reaching the typical value of .90 required to indicate equivalent factors, Dean's results do indicate a high degree of similarity. The relative strength of the various factors was also highly consistent across races.

Gutkin and Reynolds (1980) also compared two- and three-factor principal-factor solutions to the WISC-R across race for referral populations of white and Mexican American children. Gutkin and Reynolds made additional comparisons of the factor solutions derived from their referral sample to solutions derived by Reschly (1978; personal communication, 1979), and also to solutions from the WISC-R standardization sample. Coefficients of congruence for the Gutkin and Reynolds two-factor solutions for whites and Mexican Americans were .98 and .91, respectively. The g factor showed a coefficient of congruence value of .99 across races. When Gutkin and Reynolds compared their solutions with those derived by Reschly (1978) for nonexceptional white, black, Mexican American, and Papago children, and with results based on the WISC-R standardization sample, the coefficients of congruence all exceeded .90. When three-factor solutions were compared, the results were more varied, but also supported the consistent similarity of WISC-R factor-analytic results across race.

DeFries and colleagues (1974) administered 15 mental tests to large samples of Americans of Japanese ancestry and Americans of Chinese ancestry. After examining the pattern of intercorrelations among the 15 tests for each of these two ethnic groups, DeFries and colleagues concluded that the cognitive organization of the two groups was virtually identical. In reviewing this study, Willerman (1979) concluded that "The similarity in factorial structure [between the two groups] suggests that the manner in which the tests are constructed by the subjects is similar regardless of ethnicity and that the tests are measuring the same mental abilities in the two groups" (p. 468).

At the adult level, Kaiser (1986) and Scholwinski (1985) have analyzed the Wechsler Adult Intelligence Scale—Revised (WAISR; Wechsler, 1981) and reported substantial similarity between factor structures for black and white samples obtained from the WAISR standardization data. Kaiser completed separate hierarchical analyses for all black subjects (n = 192) and white subjects (n = 1,664) in the WAIS-R standardization sample and calculated coefficients of congruence of .99 for the g factor, .98 for the Verbal factor, and .97 for the Performance or nonverbal factor. Scholwinski selected 177 black and 177 white subjects from the standardization sample, closely matched on the basis of age, sex, and Full Scale IQ. Separate factor analyses again showed that structures generated from the Wechsler format showed strong similarity

across black–white groups beyond childhood and adolescent levels of development.

At the preschool level, factor-analytic results also tend to show consistency of construct validity across races, though the results are less clear-cut. In a comparison of separate factor analyses of the McCarthy Scales of Children's Abilities (McCarthy, 1972) for groups of black and white children, Kaufman and DiCuio (1975) concluded that the McCarthy Scales showed a high degree of factorial similarity between the two races. The conclusion was not straightforward, however. Four factors were found for the blacks and three for the whites. Kaufman and DiCuio based their conclusion of factorial similarity on the finding that each "white" factor had a coefficient of congruence of .85–.93 with one "black" factor. One black factor on the McCarthy Scales had no white counterpart with a coefficient of congruence beyond .74 (the Memory factor), and the black and white Motor factors showed a coefficient of congruence of only .85.

When investigating the factor structure of the WPPSI across race, Kaufman and Hollenbeck (1974) found much "cleaner" factors for blacks and whites than with the McCarthy Scales. The two factors, essentially mirroring Wechsler's Verbal and Performance scales, were virtually identical between the races. Both factors also appear closely related to the hierarchical factor solution presented by Wallbrown and colleagues (1973) for blacks and whites on the WPPSI. When comparing factor analyses of the Goodenough–Harris Human Figure Drawing Test scoring item, Merz (1970) found highly similar factor structures for blacks, whites, Mexican Americans, and Native Americans.

Other investigators have found differences across races in the factor structures of several tests designed for preschool and primary-grade children. Goolsby and Frary (1970) factor-analyzed the Metropolitan Readiness Test (MRT) together for separate groups of blacks and whites, finding differences in the factor structure of this grouping of tests across races. When evaluating the experimental edition of the Illinois Test of Psycholinguistic Abilities, Leventhal and Stedman (1970) noted differences in the factor structure of this battery for blacks and whites. Two more recent studies have clarified somewhat the issue of differential construct validity of preschool tests across race.

The MRT (Hildreth, Griffith, & McGauvran, 1969) is one of the most widely employed of all preschool screening measures, and its 1969 version is composed of six subtests: Word Meaning, Listening, Matching, Letter Naming, Numbers, and Copying. Reynolds (1979a) had previously shown this to be essentially a one-factor (General Readiness) instrument. In a subsequent study, Reynolds (1979b) compared the general factor making up the MRT across races (blacks and whites) and genders. Substantial congruence was noted: Coefficients of congruence across each pair of race–sex groupings ranged only from .92 to .99, with the lowest coefficient derived from the intraracial comparison for white females and white males. Eigenvalues, and subsequently the proportion of variance accounted for by the factor, were also highly similar for the race–sex groupings. Reynolds (1979b) concluded that these findings supported the presence of a single General Readiness factor and the construct validity of the MRT across race and sex; that is, the results indicated that the MRT measures the same abilities in the same manner for blacks, whites, males, and females. The lack of differential or single-group construct validity across sex has also been demonstrated with aptitude tests for school-age children (Reynolds & Gutkin, 1980b).

In a more comprehensive study employing seven major preschool tests (the McCarthy Draw-A-Design and Draw-A-Child subtests, the Lee–Clark Reading Readiness Tests, the Tests of Basic Experiences Language and Mathematics subtests, the Preschool Inventory—Revised Edition, and the MRT), Reynolds (1980a) reached a similar conclusion. A two-factor solution was determined with this battery for each of the four race–sex groups as above. Coefficients of congruence ranged only from .95 to .99 for the two factors, and the average degree of intercorrelation was essentially the same for all groups, as were eigenvalues and the percentage of variance accounted for by the factors. Reynolds again concluded that the abilities being measured were invariant across race, and that there was no evidence of differential or single-group construct va-

lidity of preschool tests across races or genders. The clear trend in studies of preschool tests' construct validity across race (and sex) is to uphold validity across groups. Such findings add support to the use of existing preschool screening measures with black and white children of both sexes in the very necessary process of early identification (Reynolds, 1979c) of potential learning and behavior problems.

As is appropriate for studies of construct validity, comparative factor analysis has not been the only method of determining whether single-group or differential validity exists. Another method of investigation involves comparing internal-consistency reliability estimates across groups. Internal-consistency reliability is determined by the degree to which the items are all measuring a similar construct. To be unbiased with regard to construct validity, internal-consistency estimates should be approximately equal across races. This characteristic of tests has been investigated with blacks, whites, and Mexican Americans for a number of popular aptitude tests.

With groups of black and white adults, Jensen (1977) calculated internal-consistency estimates (using the Kuder–Richardson 21 formula) for the Wonderlic Personnel Test (a frequently used employment/aptitude test). Kuder–Richardson 21 values of .86 and .88 were found, respectively, for blacks and whites. Using Hoyt's formula, Jensen (1974) determined internal-consistency estimates of .96 on the PPVT for each of three groups of children: blacks, whites, and Mexican Americans. When children were categorized by gender within each racial grouping, the values ranged only from .95 to .97. On Raven's Progressive Matrices (colored), internal-consistency estimates were also quite similar across race and sex, ranging only from .86 to .91 for the six race–sex groupings. Thus Jensen's (1974, 1977) research with three popular aptitude tests shows no signs of differential or single-group validity with regard to homogeneity of test content or consistency of measurement across groups.

Sandoval (1979) and Oakland and Feigenbaum (1979) have extensively investigated internal consistency of the various WISC-R subtests (excluding Digit Span and Coding, for which internal-consistency analysis is inappropriate) for whites, blacks, and Mexican Americans. Both of these studies included large samples of children, with Sandoval's including over 1,000. Sandoval found internal-consistency estimates to be within .04 of one another for all subtests except Object Assembly. This subtest was most reliable for blacks (.95), while being about equally reliable for whites (.79) and Mexican Americans (.75). Oakland and Feigenbaum reported internal-consistency estimates that never differed by more than .06 among the three groups, again with the exception of Object Assembly. In this instance, Object Assembly was most reliable for whites (.76), with about equal reliabilities for blacks (.64) and Mexican Americans (.67). Oakland and Feigenbaum also compared reliabilities across sex, finding highly similar values for males and females. Dean (1977) examined the internal consistency of the WISC-R for Mexican American children tested by white examiners. He reported internal-consistency reliability estimates consistent with, although slightly exceeding, values reported by Wechsler (1974) for the predominantly white standardization sample. The Bender–Gestalt Test has also been reported to have similar internal-consistency estimates for whites (.84), blacks (.81), and Mexican Americans (.72), and for males (.81) and females (.80) (Oakland & Feigenbaum, 1979).

Several other methods have also been used to determine the construct validity of popular psychometric instruments across races. Since intelligence is considered a developmental phenomenon, the correlation of raw scores with age has been viewed as one measure of construct validity for intelligence tests. Jensen (1976) reported that the correlations between raw scores on the PPVT and age were .79 for whites, .73 for blacks, and .67 for Mexican Americans. For Raven's Progressive Matrices (colored), correlations for raw scores with age were .72 for whites, .66 for blacks, and .70 for Mexican Americans. Similar results are apparent for the K-ABC (Kamphaus & Reynolds, 1987). Thus, in regard to increase in scores with age, the tests behave in a highly similar manner for whites, blacks, and Mexican Americans.

Construct validity of a large number of popular psychometric assessment instruments has been investigated across races and genders with a variety of populations of minority and white children and with a divergent set of methodologies (see Reynolds, 1982, for a review of methodologies). All roads have led to Rome: No consistent evidence of bias in construct validity has been found with any of the many tests investigated. This leads to the conclusion that psychological tests (especially aptitude tests) function in essentially the same manner, that test materials are perceived and reacted to in a similar manner, and that tests measure the same construct with equivalent accuracy for blacks, whites, Mexican Americans, and other American minorities of both sexes and at all SES levels. Single-group validity and differential validity have not been found and probably do not exist with regard to well-constructed and well-standardized psychological and educational tests. This means that test score differences across race are real and not an artifact of test bias; that is, the tests are measuring the same constructs across these variables. These differences cannot be ignored. As Mille (1979) has succinctly stated, "If this . . . difference [in test scores] is the result of genetic factors, acceptance of the cultural bias hypothesis would be unfortunate. If the difference is the result of environmental factors, such acceptance would be tragic" (p. 162).

Bias in Predictive or Criterion-Related Validity

Evaluating bias in predictive validity of educational and psychological tests is less closely related to the evaluation of group mental test score differences than to the evaluation of individual test scores in a more absolute sense. This is especially true for aptitude (as opposed to diagnostic) tests, where the primary purpose of administration is the prediction of some specific future outcome or behavior. Internal analyses of bias (such as in content and construct validity) are less confounded than analyses of bias in predictive validity, however, because of the potential problems of bias in the criterion measure. Predictive validity is also strongly influenced by the reliability of criterion measures, which frequently is poor. The degree of relationship between a predictor and a criterion is restricted as a function of the square root of the product of the reliabilities of the two variables.

Arriving at a consensual definition of bias in predictive validity is also a difficult task, as has already been discussed. Yet, from the standpoint of the practical applications of aptitude and intelligence tests, predictive validity is the most crucial form of validity in relation to test bias. Much of the discussion in professional journals concerning bias in predictive validity has centered around models of selection. These issues have been discussed previously in this chapter and are not reiterated here. Since this section is concerned with bias in respect to the test itself and not the social or political justifications of any one particular selection model, the Cleary and colleagues (1975) definition, slightly rephrased here, provides a clear and direct statement of test bias with regard to predictive validity.

> A test is considered biased with respect to predictive validity if the inference drawn from the test score is not made with the smallest feasible random error or if there is constant error in an inference or prediction as a function of membership in a particular group.

This definition is a restatement of previous definitions by Cardall and Coffman (1964), Cleary (1968), and Potthoff (1966), and has been widely accepted (though certainly not without criticism; e.g., Bernal, 1975; Linn & Werts, 1971; Schmidt & Hunter, 1974; Thorndike, 1971).

Oakland and Matuszek (1977) examined procedures for placement in special education classes under a variety of models of bias in prediction, and demonstrated that the smallest number of children are misplaced when the Cleary and colleagues (1975) conditions of fairness are met. (However, under legislative "quota" requirements, Oakland and Matuszek favor the Thorndike [1971] conditions of selection.) The Cleary and colleagues definition is also apparently the definition espoused in government guidelines on testing and has been held in at least one recent court decision (*Cortez v. Rosen*, 1975) to be the only historically, legally, and logically required condition of test fairness (Ramsay, 1979), although apparently the judge in the *Larry P. v. Riles* (1979) decision adopted the

"mean score differences as bias" approach. A variety of educational and psychological personnel have adopted the Cleary and colleagues regression approach to bias, including (1) noted psychological authorities on testing (Anastasi, 1986; Cronbach, 1970; Humphreys, 1973); (2) educational and psychological researchers (Bossard, Reynolds, & Gutkin, 1980; Kallingal, 1971; Pfeifer & Sedlacek, 1971; Reynolds & Hartlage, 1978, 1979; Stanley & Porter, 1967; Wilson, 1969); (3) industrial/organizational psychologists (Bartlett & O'Leary, 1969; Einhorn & Bass, 1971; Gael & Grant, 1972; Grant & Bray, 1970; Ramsay, 1979; Tenopyr, 1967); and (4) even critics of educational and psychological testing (Goldman & Hartig, 1976; Kirkpatrick, 1970; Kirkpatrick, Ewen, Barrett, & Katzell, 1968).

The evaluation of bias in prediction under the Cleary and colleagues (1975) definition (the regression definition) is quite straightforward. With simple regression, predictions take the form of $Y_i = aX_i + b$, where a is the regression coefficient and b is a constant. When this equation is graphed (forming a regression line), a represents the slope of the regression line and b the Y intercept. Since our definition of fairness in predictive validity requires errors in prediction to be independent of group membership, the regression line formed for any pair of variables must be the same for each group for whom predictions are to be made. Whenever the slope or the intercept differs significantly across groups, there is bias in prediction if one attempts to use a regression equation based on the combined groups. When the regression equations for two (or more) groups are equivalent, prediction is the same for all groups. This condition is referred to variously as "homogeneity of regression across groups, "simultaneous regression," or "fairness in prediction." Homogeneity of regression across groups is illustrated in Figure 22.1. In this case, the single regression equation is appropriate with all groups, any errors in prediction being random with respect to group membership (i.e., residuals uncorrelated with group membership). When homogeneity of regression does not occur, for "fairness in prediction" to occur, separate regression equations must be used for each group.

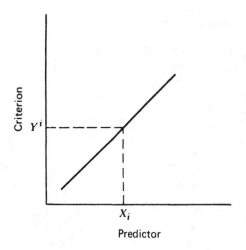

FIGURE 22.1. Equal slopes and intercepts result in homogeneity of regression that causes the regression lines for group *a*, group *b*, and the combined group *c* to be identical.

In actual clinical practice, regression equations are seldom generated for the prediction of future performance. Instead, some arbitrary or perhaps statistically derived cutoff score is determined, below which "failure" is predicted. For school performance, IQs two or more standard deviations below the test mean are used to infer a high probability of failure in the regular classroom if special assistance is not provided for the student in question. Essentially, then, clinicians are establishing mental prediction equations that are assumed to be equivalent across races, genders, and so on. Although these mental equations cannot be readily tested across groups, the actual form of criterion prediction can be compared across groups in several ways. Errors in prediction must be independent of group membership. If regression equations are equal, this condition is met. To test the hypothesis of simultaneous regression, slopes and intercepts must both be compared. An alternative method is the direct examination of residuals through ANOVA or a similar design (Reynolds, 1980c).

In the evaluation of slope and intercept values, two basic techniques have been most often employed in the research literature. Gulliksen and Wilks (1965) and Kerlinger (1973) describe methods for separately testing regression coefficients and intercepts for significant differences across groups. Using

separate, independent tests for these two values considerably increases the probability of a decision error and unnecessarily complicates the decision-making process. Potthoff (1966) has described a useful technique that allows one to test simultaneously the equivalence of regression coefficients and intercepts across K independent groups with a single F ratio. If a significant F results, the researcher may then test the slopes and intercepts separately if information concerning which value differs is desired. When homogeneity of regression does not occur, there are three basic conditions that can result: (1) Intercept constants differ, (2) regression coefficients (slopes) differ, or (3) slopes and intercepts differ. These conditions are depicted pictorially in Figures 22.2, 22.3, and 22.4, respectively.

The regression coefficient is related to the correlation coefficient between the two variables and is one measure of the strength of the relationship between two variables. When intercepts differ and regression coefficients do not, a situation such as that shown in Figure 22.2 results. Relative accuracy of prediction is the same for the two groups (a and b); yet the use of a regression equation derived by combining the two groups results in bias that works against the group with the higher mean criterion score. Since the slope of the regression line is the same for all groups, the degree of error in prediction remains constant and does not fluctuate as a function of an individual's score on the independent variable. That is, regardless of a member of group *b*'s score on the predictor,

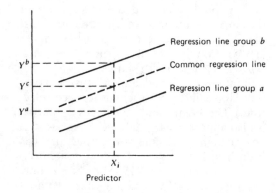

FIGURE 22.2. Equal slopes with differing intercepts result in parallel regression lines and a constant bias in prediction.

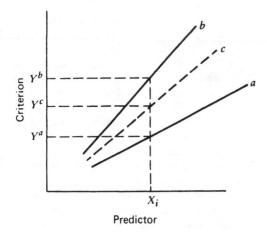

FIGURE 22.3. Equal intercepts and differing slopes result in nonparallel regression lines, with the degree of bias dependent on the distance of the individual's score (X_i) from the origin.

the degree of underprediction in performance on the criterion is the same. As illustrated in Figure 22.2, the use of the common score of Y_c for a score of X overestimates how well members of group a will perform and underestimates the criterion performance of members of group b.

In Figure 22.3, nonparallel regression lines illustrate the case where intercepts are constant across groups but the slope of the line is different for each group. Here, too, the performance of the group with the higher mean criterion score is typically underpredicted when a common regression equation is applied. The amount of bias in prediction that results from using the common regression line is the distance of the score from the mean. The most difficult, complex case of bias is represented in Figure 22.4. Here we see the result of significant differences in slopes and intercepts. Not only does the amount of bias in prediction accruing from the use of a common equation vary in this instance; the actual direction of bias can reverse, depending on the location of the individual's score in the distribution of the independent variable. Only in the case of Figure 22.4 do members of the group with the lower mean criterion score run the risk of having their performance on the criterion variable underpredicted by the application of a common regression equation.

A considerable body of literature has de-

veloped regarding the differential predictive validity of tests across races for employment selection and college admissions. In a recent review of 866 black–white test validity comparisons from 39 studies of test bias in personnel selection, Hunter and colleagues (1979) concluded that there was no evidence to substantiate hypotheses of differential or single-group validity with regard to the prediction of job performance across races for blacks and whites. A similar conclusion was reached by O'Conner, Wexley, and Alexander (1975). A number of studies have also focused on differential validity of the Scholastic Aptitude Test (SAT; now known as the Scholastic Assessment Tests) in the prediction of college performance (typically measured by grade point average of GPA). In general, these studies have found either no differences in the prediction of criterion performance for blacks and whites or a bias (underprediction of the criterion) against whites (Cleary, 1968; Cleary et al., 1975; Goldman & Hewitt, 1976; Kallingal, 1971; Pfeifer & Sedlacek, 1971; Stanley, 1971; Stanley & Porter, 1967; Temp, 1971). When bias against whites has been found, the differences between actual and predicted criterion scores, although statistically significant, have a been quite small.

Reschly and Sabers (1979) evaluated the validity of WISC-R IQs in the prediction of

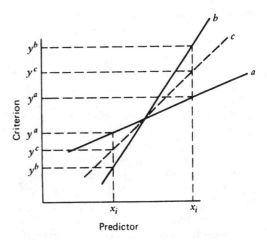

FIGURE 22.4. Differing slopes *and* intercepts result in the complex condition where the amount and the direction of the bias are functions of the distance of an individual's score from the origin.

Metropolitan Achievement Tests (MAT) performance (Reading and Math subtests) for whites, blacks, Mexican Americans, and Native American Papagos. The choice of the MAT as a criterion measure in studies of predictive bias in particularly appropriate, since item analysis procedures were employed (as described earlier) to eliminate racial bias in item content during the test construction phase. Anastasi (1986) has described the MAT as an excellent model of an achievement test designed to reduce or eliminate cultural bias. Reschly and Sabers's comparison of regression systems indicated bias in the prediction of the various achievement scores. Again, however, the bias produced generally significant underprediction of white performance when a common regression equation was applied. Achievement test performance of the Native American Papago group showed the greatest amount of overprediction of all nonwhite groups. Though some slope bias was evident, Reschly and Sabers typically found intercept bias resulting in parallel regression lines. Using similar techniques, but including teacher ratings, Reschly and Reschly (1979) also investigated the predictive validity of WISC-R factor scores with the samples of white, black, Mexican American, and Native American Papago children. A significant relationship occurred between the three WISC-R factors first delineated by Kaufman (1975) and measures of achievement for the white and nonwhite groups, with the exception of the Papagos. Significant correlations occurred between the WISC-R Freedom from Distractibility factor (Kaufman, 1975) and teacher ratings of attention for all four groups. Reschly and Reschly concluded that "These data also again confirm the relatively strong relationship of WISC-R scores to achievement for most non-Anglo as well as Anglo groups" (1979, p. 239).

Reynolds and Hartlage (1979) investigated the differential validity of Full Scale IQs from the WISC-R and its 1949 predecessor, the WISC, in predicting reading and arithmetic achievement for black and white children who had been referred by their teachers for psychological services in a rural Southern school district. Comparisons of correlations and a Potthoff (1966) analysis to test for identity of regression lines revealed no significant differences in the abili-

ty or function of the WISC and WISC-R to predict achievement for these two groups. Reynolds and Gutkin (1980a) replicated this study for the WISC-R with large groups of white and Mexican American children from the Southwest. Reynolds and Gutkin contrasted regression systems between WISC-R Verbal, Performance, and Full Scale IQs and the "academic basics" of reading, spelling, and arithmetic. Only the regression equation between the WISC-R Performance IQ and arithmetic achievement differed for the two groups. The difference in the two equations was due to an intercept bias that resulted in the overprediction of achievement for the Mexican American children. Reynolds, Gutkin, Dappen, and Wright (1979) also failed to find differential validity in the prediction of achievement for males and females with the WISC-R.

In a related study, Hartlage, Lucas, and Godwin (1976) compared the predictive validity of what they considered to be a relatively culture-free test (Raven's Progressive Matrices) with a more culture-loaded test (the 1949 WISC) for a group of low-SES, disadvantaged rural children. Harlage and colleagues found that the WISC had consistently larger correlations with measures of reading, spelling, and arithmetic than did Raven's Matrices. Although it did not make the comparison with other groups that is necessary for the drawing of firm conclusions, the study does support the validity of the WISC, which has been the target of many of the claims of bias in the prediction of achievement for low-SES, disadvantaged rural children. Henderson, Butler, and Goffeney (1969) also reported that the WISC and the Bender–Gestalt Test were equally effective in the prediction of reading and arithmetic achievement for white and nonwhite groups, though their study had a number of methodological difficulties, including heterogeneity of the nonwhite comparison group. Reynolds, Willson, and Chatman (1985) evaluated the predictive validity of the K-ABC for blacks and for whites. Occasional evidence of bias was found in each direction, but mostly in the direction of overprediction of the academic attainment levels of blacks. However, for most of the 56 Potthoff comparisons of regression lines, no evidence of bias was revealed.

A study by Goldman and Hartig (1976) produced quite different results with the 1949 WISC. These researchers reported that when validities were calculated for the prediction of achievement separately for whites, blacks, and Mexican Americans, the predictive validity of the WISC was good for white children but near zero for the nonwhite groups. A closer examination of the methodology of the study gives considerable insight into this unusual finding. The criterion measure, academic CPA, showed considerable restriction of range for the black and Mexican American groups. In addition, calculation of the academic CPA inexplicably included, in addition to traditional academic subjects, grades from music, health, art, instrumental music, and physical education, where very high grades approaching zero variance were common. It is clearly inappropriate to include inflated grades from such school activities in the calculation of "academic GPA."

The use of academic CPA, especially in presecondary settings, is fraught with other problems, including unreliability, questionable validity, and the lack of constant scaling. Teachers may be grading on some absolute scale of achievement; relative to other children in the classroom; relative to how well teachers believe children should be performing; or on the basis of effort, motivation, or even attractiveness. Some parents will even demand stricter or more lenient grading standards for their children than for others. To confound the problems of academic CPA as a criterion, grading practices vary not only among classrooms and schools, but within classrooms as well (the Goldman and Hartig children came from 14 different schools). When groups are to be combined across schools, and homogeneity of the new group is then to be assumed, the equivalence of the schools regarding environments, academic standards, and grading practices must first be demonstrated empirically (Jensen, 1980). Reading the Goldman and Hartig (1976) paper leads one to question whether the researchers had not decided on the outcome a priori and then set out to prove it! The predictive validities reported for white children in this study are also considerably lower than are typically reported for the WISC. Thus the contradictory nature of this study, as compared to a

large number of other studies, must certainly be called into question. Studies with a number of other aptitude tests also contradict Goldman and Hartig.

Bossard and colleagues (1980) published a regression analysis of test bias on the 1972 Stanford–Binet Intelligence Scale for separate groups of black and white children. Neither progression system nor correlations differed at $p < .05$ for the prediction of the basic academic skills of reading, spelling, and arithmetic achievement for these two groups of referred children. An earlier study by Sewell (1979), a black opponent of testing, did not compare regression systems, but also found no significant differences in validity coefficients for Stanford–Binet IQs predicting California Achievement Test (CAT) scores for black and white first-grade children.

A series of studies comparing the predictive validity of group IQ measures across races has been reviewed by Jensen (1980) and Sattler (1974). Typically, regression systems have not been compared in these studies; instead, researchers have compared only the validity coefficients across races—a practice that tells only whether the magnitude of the relationships is similar, not whether the test is actually nonbiased. The comparison of validity coefficients is nevertheless relevant, since equivalence in predictive validities is a first step in evaluating differential validity. That is, if predictive validities differ, then regression systems must differ; the reverse is not necessarily true, however, since the correlation between two variables is a measure of the strength or magnitude of a relationship and does not dictate the form of a relationship. Although the number of studies evaluating group IQ tests across races is small, they have typically employed extremely large samples. The Lorge–Thorndike verbal and nonverbal IQs have been most often investigated. Jensen and Sattler concluded that the few available studies suggest that standard IQ tests in current use have comparable validities for black and white children at the elementary school level.

Guterman (1979) reported on an extensive analysis of the predictive validity of the Ammons and Ammons Quick Test (QT; a measure of verbal IQ) for adolescents of different social classes. Social class was determined by a weighted combination of Duncan s SES index and the number of years of education of each parent. Three basic measures of scholastic attainment were employed as criterion measures: (1) the Vocabulary subtest of the General Aptitude Test Battery (GATB); (2) the test of Reading Comprehension from the Gates Reading Survey; and (3) the Arithmetic subtest of the GATB. School grades in academic subjects for 9th, 10th, and 12th grades were also used to examine for bias in prediction. Guterman reached similar conclusions with regard to all criterion measures across all social classes: Slopes and intercepts of regression lines did not differ across social class for the prediction of any of the criterion measures by the IQ derived from the QT. Several other social knowledge criterion measures were also examined. Again, slopes were constant across social class, and, with the exception of sexual knowledge, intercepts were also constant. Guterman concluded that his data provide strong support for equivalent validity of IQ measures across social class. In reanalyzing the Guerman study, Gordon and Rudert (1979) reached even stronger conclusions. By analyzing the Guterman data by race within the various SES categories through a method of path analysis, Gordon and Rudert demonstrated that the QT was also not biased across race in the prediction of academic attainment, and that IQ (as determined by the QT) plays the same role in status attainment models for blacks and whites and has stronger direct effects on later status attainment than does SES. Certainly with school-age children and adults, there is compelling evidence that differential and single-group predictive validity hypotheses must be rejected.

As with construct validity, at the preschool level the evidence is less clear and convincing but points toward a lack of bias against minorities. Because of doubts expressed about the usefulness of customary readiness tests with students of certain racial and ethnic backgrounds and with low-SES children, Mitchell (1967) investigated the predictive validity of two preschool readiness tests used in the U.S. Office of Education Cooperative First-Grade Reading Study of 1964–1965. Chosen for study were the MRT, Form A (1964–1965 revision) and the Murphy–Durrell Reading Readiness Analysis (1964 revision). Mitchell's sample included 7,310 whites, 518 blacks, and 39 Mexican Americans. Criterion measures chosen were the Stanford Achievement Test (1963 revision) and the Primary I Reading and Spelling subtests. Mitchell's results do not support a hypothesis of lower predictive validity for nonwhites than for whites on either readiness scale. Although some significant differences occurred in the obtained correlations with achievement for blacks and whites, 26 correlations were higher for blacks. Mitchell concluded that the two readiness tests performed their functions as well with black as with white children, and that the general level of predictive validity was similar. This overstates the case somewhat, since only validity coefficients and not regression systems were compared, but Mitchell's study does support the predictive validity of these readiness tests across race.

Oakland (1978) assessed the differential predictive validity of four readiness tests (the MRT, the Tests of Basic Experiences battery, the Slosson Intelligence Test, and the Slosson Oral Reading Test) across races (black, white, and Mexican American) for middle- and lower-SES children. The MAT, the CAT, and the California Test of Mental Maturity (CTMM) served as criterion variables. Since the CTMM is an IQ test, prediction of CTMM scores by the various readiness tests is excluded from the following discussion. Although Oakland did not use any test of statistical significance to compare the correlations between the independent and dependent variable pairs across races and SES, a clear pattern was found, showing higher levels of prediction for white as opposed to nonwhite groups. Oakland also did not compare regression systems, limiting his study to the report of the various validity coefficients for each race–SES grouping. Oakland's results clearly indicate potential bias in the prediction of early school achievement by individual readiness or screening tests. The lower correlations for nonwhite groups, however, given their lower mean criterion scores, lead to anticipation of bias favoring nonwhites in the prediction of early school achievement.

To investigate this possibility, Reynolds (1978) conducted an extensive analysis of predictive bias for seven major preschool tests (the Draw-A-Design and Draw-A-Child subtests of the McCarthy Scales; the Mathematics and Language subtests of the Tests of Basic Experiences; the MRT; the preschool Inventory—Revised Edition; and the Lee–Clark Reading Readiness Test) across races and genders for large groups of blacks and whites. For each preschool test, validity coefficients, slopes, and intercepts were compared, with prediction of performance on four subtests of the MAT (Word Knowledge, Word Discrimination, Reading, and Arithmetic) as the criterion measure. The general advantage of the MAT as a criterion in external studies of bias has previously been pointed out. In the Reynolds study, the MAT had the added advantage of being chosen by the teachers in the district: Data were gathered on a large number of early achievement tests, and the teachers selected the MAT as the battery most closely measuring what was taught in their classrooms. Regression systems and validity coefficients were compared for each independent–dependent variable pair for white females (WF) versus white males (WM), black females (BF) versus black males (BM), WF versus BF, and WM versus BM, resulting in 112 comparisons of validity coefficients and 112 comparisons of regression systems. Mean performance on all criterion measures was in the following rank order: WF > WM > BF > BM. The mean validity coefficients (by Fisher z-transformation) between the independent and dependent variables across the 12-month period from pre- to posttest were .59 for WF, .50 for WM, .43 for BF, and .30 for BM. Although the mean correlations were lower for blacks, the 112 comparisons of pairs of correlations revealed only three significant differences, a less-than-chance occurrence with this number of comparisons (Sakoda, Cohen, & Beall, 1954). Using the Potthoff (1966) technique for comparing regression lines produced quite different results. Of the 112 comparisons of regression lines, 43 (38.4%) showed differences. For comparisons with race as the major variable (and sex controlled), 31(55.2%) of the 56 comparisons showed significantly different regression lines. Clearly, racial bias was significantly more prevalent than sex bias ($p < .01$) in prediction. In comparing the various

pretests, bias occurred most often with the Preschool Inventory and the Lee–Clark, whereas none of the comparisons involving the MRT showed bias. Though race clearly influenced homogeneity of regression across groups, the bias in each case acted to overpredict performance of lower-scoring groups; thus the bias acted against whites and females and in favor of blacks and males. A follow-up study (Reynolds, 1980c) has indicated one potential method for avoiding bias in the prediction of early school achievement with readiness or screening measures.

Brief screening measures, especially at the preschool level, typically do not have the high level of reliability obtained by such instruments as the WISC-R or the Stanford–Binet. As previously discussed, Linn and Werts (1971) have convincingly demonstrated that poor reliability can lead to bias in prediction. Early screening measures, as a rule, also assess a very limited area of functioning, rather than allowing the child to demonstrate his or her skills in a variety of areas of cognitive functioning. The one well-researched, reliable, broad-based readiness test, the MRT, has failed to show bias with regard to internal or external criteria. Comprehensive and reliable individual preschool instruments such as the WPPSI and the McCarthy Scales, while showing no internal evidence of test bias, have not been researched with regard to predictive bias across race. Reynolds (1980c) examined the predictive validity of the seven preschool measures described previously when these were combined into a larger battery, thus increasing the scope and reliability of the assessment.

Since our definition of predictive bias requires that errors in prediction be independent of group membership, Reynolds (1980c) directly examined residuals (a "residual term" is the remainder when the predicted score for an individual is subtracted from the individual's obtained score) across races and genders when the seven-test battery was used to predict MAT scores in a multiple-regression formula. Subtests of the seven-test battery were also examined. Results of a race × sex ANOVA of residuals for each of the MAT subtests when the seven-test battery was employed revealed no significant differences in residuals across races and genders, and no significant inter-actions occurred. When a subset of the larg-er battery was submitted to the same analy-sis, racial bias in prediction did not occur; however, a significant F resulted for sex ef-fects in the prediction of two of the four MAT subscores (Word Discrimination and Word Knowledge). Examination of the residuals for each group showed that the bias in prediction was again against the group with the higher in mean criterion scores: There was a consistent underpredic-tion of performance for females. The magni-tude of the effect was small, however, being on the order of 0.13 to 0.16 standard devia-tion. Thus, at the preschool level, the only convincing evidence of bias in predictive va-lidity is a sex effect, not a race effect. Al-though females tend to be slightly overiden-tified through early screening, it is interesting to note that while special educa-tion classes are more blatantly sexist than racist in composition, it is boys who out-number girls at a ratio of about 3.5:1 to 4:1. Few, if any, would argue that this dispro-portionate representation of males in special education is inappropriate or due to "test bias."

Kamphaus and Reynolds (1987) reviewed the available literature on predictive bias with the K-ABC and concluded that over-prediction of black children's performance in school is more common with the K-ABC, particularly the K-ABC Sequential Process-ing scale, than with other tests. The effects are small, however, and are mitigated in large part by using the K-ABC Mental Pro-cessing Composite. Some bias also occurs against blacks, but when the extensive na-ture of the bias research with the K-ABC is considered, results with the K-ABC are not substantially different from the results with the WISC-R (with the exception of overpre-diction of black academic performance by the K-ABC Sequential Processing scale).

With regard to bias in predictive validity, the empirical evidence suggests conclusions similar to those regarding bias in content and construct validity. There is no strong evidence to support contentions of differen-tial of single-group validity. Bias occurs in-frequently and with no apparently observ-able pattern, except when instruments of poor reliability and high specificity of test content are examined. When bias occurs, it

is most often in the direction of favoring low-SES, disadvantaged ethnic minority children, or other low-scoring groups. Clearly, bias in predictive validity cannot account for the disproportionate number of minority group children diagnosed and placed in settings for "EMR" and "emo-tionally disturbed" children.

CONCLUSION

There is little question that the issue of bias in mental testing is an important one with strong historical precedence in the social sci-ences and, ultimately, formidable social con-sequences. Because the history of mental measurement has been closely wed from the outset to societal needs and expectations, testing in all forms has remained in the lime-light, subjected to the crucible of social in-spection, review, and (at times) condemna-tion. However, the fact that tests and measures of human aptitude and achieve-ment continue to be employed in most mod-ern cultures indicates strongly that the prac-tice has value, despite the recurring storms of criticism over the years. The ongoing controversy related to test bias and the "fair" use of measures will undoubtedly re-main with the social sciences for at least as long as we intertwine the nature–nurture question with these issues and affirm differ-ences between/among groups in mean per-formance on standardized tests. Numerous scholars in the field of psychometrics have been attempting to separate the nature–nur-ture issue and data on mean score differ-ences from the more orderly, empirically driven specialty of bias investigation, but the separation will undoubtedly not be a clean one. A sharp distinction has developed between the popular press and scientific lit-erature with regard to the interpretation of mental measurement research. The former all too often engenders beliefs that biased measures are put into use for socially perni-cious purposes (e.g., Gould, 1981); the lat-ter has attempted to maintain balanced sci-entific analysis and inquiry in fields (i.e., psychology and education) often accused of courting political, social, and professional ideologies. The former appears to have cre-ated confusion in public opinion concerning the possibility of "fair" testing, to say the least. The latter—reported in this chapter—has been demonstrating through a rather sizable body of data that the hypothesis of cultural bias on tests is not a particularly strong one at present. In any event, societal scrutiny and ongoing sentiment about testing have without question served to force the psychometric community to refine its definition of bias further, to inspect practices in the construction on nonbiased measures, and to develop statistical procedures to detect bias when it is occurring. We can argue whether the social sciences have from the outset overstepped their bounds in implementing testing for social purposes before adequate data and methods were developed, but the resulting advances made in bias technology in response to ongoing public inspection are undeniable.

Data from the empirical end of bias investigation do suggest several guidelines to follow in order to insure equitable assessment. Points to consider include (1) investigation of possible referral source bias, as there is evidence that persons are not always referred for services on the basis of impartial, objective rationales; (2) inspection of test developers' data for evidence that sound statistical analyses for bias across groups to be evaluated with the measure have been completed; (3) assessment with the most reliable measure available; and (4) assessment of multiple abilities with multiple methods. In other words, psychologists need to view multiple sources of accurately derived data prior to making decisions concerning children. We may hope that this is not too far afield from what has actually been occurring in the practice of psychological assessment, though one continues to hear isolated stories of grossly incompetent placement decisions being made (e.g., Mason, 1979). This does not mean that psychologists should ignore a child's environmental background. Information concerning the home, community, and school environment must all be evaluated in the individualized decision-making process. Exactly how this may be done is addressed in other chapters of this volume. Neither, however, can the psychologist ignore the fact that low-IQ, disadvantaged children from ethnic minority groups are just as likely to fail academically as are white middle-class low-IQ children, provided that their environmental circum-

stances remain constant. Indeed, it is the purpose of the assessment process to beat the prediction—to provide insight into hypotheses for environmental interventions that will prevent the predicted failure.

A philosophical perspective is emerging in the bias literature that is requiring test developers not only to demonstrate whether their measures demonstrate differential content, construct, and predictive validity across groups prior to publication, but also to incorporate in some form content analyses by interested groups to insure that offensive materials are omitted. Although there are no sound empirical data to suggest that persons can determine bias upon surface inspection, the synergistic relationship between test use and pure psychometrics must be acknowledged and accommodated in orderly fashion before tests gain greater acceptance within society. Ideally, a clear consensus on "fairness" (and steps taken to reach this end) is needed between those persons with more subjective concerns and those interested in gathering objective bias data during the after test construction. Accommodation along this line will ultimately insure that all parties interested in any given test believe that the measure in question is nonbiased and that the steps taken to achieve "fairness" can be held up to public scrutiny without reservation. Given the significant and reliable methods developed over the last several decades in bias research, it is untenable at this point to abandon statistical analyses in favor of "armchair" determinations of bias. Test authors and publishers need to demonstrate factorial invariance across all groups for whom the test is designed in order to make the instrument more readily interpretable. Comparisons of predictive validity across races and genders during the test development phase are also needed. With the exception of some recent achievement tests, this has not been common practice, yet it is at this stage that tests can be altered through a variety of item analysis procedures to eliminate any apparent racial and sexual bias.

A variety of criteria must be explored further before the question of bias is empirically resolved. Many different achievement tests and teacher-made, classroom-specific tests need to be employed in future studies of predictive bias. The issues of differential validity of tests in the affective domain are important but have been subjected to far less research than tests in the cognitive domain. This is an important area for examination as more objective determinations of emotional disturbance are required. It will also be important to stay abreast of metholodological advances that may make it possible to resolve some of the current issues and to identify common characteristics among the (now seen by irregular or random and infrequent) findings of bias.

REFERENCES

Alley, C., & Foster, C. (1978). Nondiscriminatory testing of minority and exceptional children. *Focus on Exceptional Children, 9,* 1–14.

Anastasi, A. (1986). *Psychological testing* (4th ed.). New York: Macmillan.

American Psychological Association. (1970). Psychological assessment and public policy. *American Psychologist, 31,* 264–266.

Angoff, W. H. (1976). Group membership as a predictor variable: A comment on McNemar. *American Psychologist, 31,* 612.

Angoff, W. H., & Ford, S. R. (1973). Item–race interaction on a test of scholastic aptitude. *Journal of Educational Measurement, 10,* 95–106.

Auerbach, A. C. (1971). The social control of learning disabilities. *Journal of Learning Disabilities, 4,* 25–34.

Bartlett, C. J., & O'Leary, B. S. (1969). A differential prediction model to moderate the effect of heterogeneous groups in personnel selection. *Personnel Psychology, 22,* 1–18.

Bass, A. R. (1976). The "equal risk" model: A comment on McNemar. *American Psychologist, 31,* 611–612.

Bayley, N. (1969). *Bayley Scales of Infant Development.* New York: Psychological Corporation.

Beauchamp, D. P., Samuels, D. D., & Criffore, R. J. (1979). WISC-R Information and Digit Span scores of American and Canadian children. *Applied Psychological Measurement, 3,* 231–236.

Berk, R. A. (Ed.). (1982). *Handbook of methods for detecting test bias.* Baltimore: Johns Hopkins University Press.

Bernal, E. M. (1975). A response to "Educational uses of tests with disadvantaged students." *American Psychologist, 30,* 93–95.

Binet, A., & Simon, T. (1905). Methodes nouvelles pour le diagnostic do niveau intellectuel des anormaux. *L'Année Psychologique, 11,* 191–244.

Blaha, J., Wallbrown, F., & Wherry, R. J. (1975). The hierarchial factor structure of the Wechsler Intelligence Scale for Children. *Psychological Reports, 35,* 771–778.

Bogen, J. E., DeZure, R. Tenhouten, N., & Marsh, J. (1972). The other side of the brain: IV. The A/P ra-

tio. *Bulletin of the Los Angeles Neurological Society, 37,* 49–61.

Bond, L. (1981). Bias in mental tests. In B. F. Green (Ed.), *Issues in testing: Coaching, disclosure, and ethnic bias.* San Francisco: Jossey-Bass.

Bossard, M. D., Reynolds, C. R., & Gutkin, T. B. (1980). A regression analysis of test bias on the Stanford–Binet Intelligence Scale. *Journal of Clinical Child Psychology.*

Bower, E. M. (1974). The three-pipe problem: Promotion of competent human beings through a preschool, kindergarten, program and other sundry elementary matters. In G. J. Williams & S. Gordon (Eds.), *Clinical child psychology: Current practices and future perspectives.* New York: Behavioral.

Burrill, L. (1975). *Statistical evidence of potential bias in items and tests assessing current educational status.* Paper presented at the annual meeting of the Southeastern Conference on Measurement in Education, New Orleans, LA.

Cancro, R. (1971). Genetic contributions to individual differences in intelligence: An introduction. In R. Camcro (Ed.), *Intelligence: Genetic and environmental influences.* New York: Grune & Stratton.

Cardall, C., & Coffman, W. E. (1964). *A method of comparing the performance of different groups on the items in a test* (Research Bulletin No. 64–61). Princeton, NJ: Educational Testing Service.

Cattell, R. B. (1979). Are culture fair intelligence tests possible and necessary? *Journal of Research and Development in Education, 12,* 3–13.

Chinn, P. C. (1979). The exceptional minority child: Issues and some answers. *Exceptional Children, 46,* 532–536.

Cleary, T. A. (1968). Test bias: Prediction of grades of Negro and white students in integrated colleges. *Journal of Educational Measurement, 5,* 118–124.

Cleary, T. A., & Hilton, T. L. (1968). An investigation of item bias. *Educational and Psychological Measurement, 28,* 61–75.

Cleary, T. A., Humphreys, L. G., Kendrick, S. A., & Wesman, A. (1975). Educational uses of test with disadvantaged students. *American Psychologist, 30,* 15–41.

Cortez v. Rosen, United States District Court of Northern District of California (not reported in FEP) (1975).

Council for Exceptional Children. (1978). Minorities position policy statements. *Exceptional Children, 45,* 57–64.

Critchley, D. L. (1979). The adverse influence of psychiatric diagnostic labels on the observation of child behavior. *American Journal of Orthopsychiatry, 49,* 157–160.

Cronbach, L. J. (1970). *Essentials of psychological testing.* New York: Harper & Row.

Cronbach, L. J. (1976). Equity in selection—where psychometrics and political philosophy meet. *Journal of Educational Measurement, 13,* 31–42.

Cronbach, L. J. (1980). Validity on parole: How can we go straight? In W. B. Schraeder (Ed.), *New directions for testing and measurement: Vol. 5. Measuring achievement: Progress over a decade.* San Francisco: Jossey-Bass.

Darlington, R. B. (1971). Another look at "cultural fairness. "*Journal of Educational Measurement, 8,* 71–82.

Darlington, R. B. (1976). A defense of rational personnel selection, and two new methods. *Journal of Educational Measurement, 13,* 43–52.

Darlington, R. B. (1978). Cultural test bias: Comments on Hunter and Schmidt. *Psychological Bulletin, 85,* 673–674.

Dean, B. S. (1977). Reliability of the WISC-R with Mexican American children, *Journal of School Psychology, 15,* 267–268.

Dean, R. S. (1979a). Distinguished patterns for Mexican American children on the WISC-R. *Journal of Clinical Psychology, 35,* 790–794.

Dean, R. S. (1979b, September). *WISC-R factor structure for Anglo and Hispanic children.* Paper presented at the annual meeting of the American Psychological Association, New York.

DeFries, J. C., Vandenberg, S. G., McClearn, G. E., Kuse, A. R., Wilson, J. C., Ashton, G. C., & Johnson, R. C. (1974). Near identity of cognitive structure in two ethnic groups. *Science, 183,* 338–339.

Dershowitz, Z., & Frankel, Y. (1975). Jewish culture and the WISC and WAIS test patterns. *Journal of Consulting and Clinical Psychology, 43,* 126–134.

Diana v. State Board of Education, CA. No. C-70-37 (N.D. Cal. 1970).

Dworkin, N., & Dworkin, Y. (1979). The legacy of Pygmalion in the classrooms. *Phi Delta Kappan, 61,* 712–715.

Ebel, R. L. (1979). Intelligence: A skeptical view. *Journal of Research and Development in Education, 12,* 14–21.

Eells, K., Davis, A., Havighurst, R. J., Herrick, V. E., & Typer, R. W. (1951). *Intelligence and culture differences.* Chicago: University of Chicago Press.

Einhorn, H. J., & Bass, A. B. (1971). Methodological considerations relevant to discrimination in employment testing. *Psychological Bulletin, 75,* 261–269.

Fancher, R. E. (1979). *Pioneers of psychology.* New York: Norton.

Flaugher, R. L. (1978). The many definitions of test bias. *American Psychologist, 33,* 671–679.

Flaugher, B. L., & Schrader, W. B. (1978). *Eliminating differentially difficult times as an approach to test bias* (Research Bulletin No. 78-4). Princeton, NJ: Educational Testing Service.

Foster, G., & Ysseldyke, J. (1976). Expectancy and halo effects as a result of artificially induced teacher bias. *Contemporary Educational Psychology, 1,* 37–45.

Frame, R. (1979, September). *Diagnoses related to school achievement, client's race, and socioeconomic status.* Paper presented at the annual meeting of the American Psychological Association, New York.

Freeman, F. N. (1926). *Mental tests: Their history, principles and applications.* Boston: Houghton Muffin.

Gael, S., & Grant, D. L. (1972). Employment test validation for minority and non-minority telephone company service representatives. *Journal of Applied Psychology, 56,* 135–139.

Gerber, M., & Dean, R. F. (1957). Gesell tests on African children. *Pediatrics, 20,* 1055–1065.

Goldman, R. D., & Hartig, (1976). The WISC may not be a valid predictor of school performance for primary-grade minority children. *American Journal of Mental Deficiency, 80,* 583–587.

Goldman, R. D., & Hewitt, B. N. (1976). Predicting the success of black, Chicano, Oriental, and white college students. *Journal of Educational Measurement, 13,* 107–117.

Goolsby, T. M., & Frary, R. B. (1970). Validity of the Metropolitan Readiness Test for white and Negro students in a Southern city. *Educational and Psychological Measurement, 30,* 443–450.

Gordon, R. A. (1984). Digits backward and the Mercer–Kamin law: An empirical response to Mercer's treatment of internal validity of IQ tests. In C. R. Reynolds & B. T. Brown (Eds.), *Perspectives on bias in mental testing,* New York: Plenum Press.

Gordon, R. A., & Rudert, E. E. (1979). Bad news concerning IQ tests. *Sociology of Education, 52,* 174–190.

Gould, S. J. (1981). *The mismeasure of man.* New York: Norton.

Grant, D. L., & Bray, D. W. (1970). Validation of employment tests for telephone company installation and repair occupations. *Journal of Applied Psychology, 54,* 7–14.

Griggs v. Duke Power Co., 401 U.S. 424 (1971).

Gross, A. L., & Su, W. (1975). Defining a "fair" or "unbiased" selection model. *Journal of Applied Psychology, 60,* 345–351.

Gross, M. (1967). *Learning readiness in two Jewish groups.* New York: Center for Urban Education.

Gulliksen, H., & Wilkin, S. S. (1965). Regression tests for several samples. *Psychometrika, 15,* 91–114.

Guterman, S. S. (1979). IQ tests in research on social stratification: The cross-class validity of the tests as measures of scholastic aptitude. *Sociology of Education, 52,* 163–173.

Gutkin, T. B., & Reynolds, C. R. (1980). Factorial similarity of the WISC-R for Anglos and Chicanos referred for psychological services. *Journal of School Psychology, 18,* 34–39.

Gutkin, T. B., & Reynolds, C. R. (1981). Factorial similarity of the WISC-R for white and black children from the standardization sample. *Journal of Educational Psychology, 73,* 227–231.

Gutkin, T. B., & Tieger, A. G. (1979). Funding patterns for exceptional children: Current approaches and suggested alternatives. *Professional Psychology, 10,* 670–680.

Harman, H. (1976). *Modern factor analysis* (2nd ed.). Chicago: University of Chicago Press.

Harrington, G. M. (1968a). Genetic–environmental interaction in "intelligence": I. Biometric genetic analysis of maze performance of *Rattus norvegicus. Developmental Psychobiology, 1,* 211–218.

Harrington, G. M. (1968b). Genetic–environmental interaction in "intelligence": II. Models of behavior, components of variance, and research strategy. *Developmental Psychobiology, 1,* 245–253.

Harrington, G. M. (1975). Intelligence tests may

favour the majority groups in a population. *Nature, 258,* 708–709.

Harrington, G. M. (1976, September). *Minority test bias as a psychometric artifact: The experimental evidence.* Paper presented at the annual meeting of the American Psychological Association, Washington, DC.

Harrington, G. M. (1984). An experimental model of bias in mental testing, In C. R. Reynolds & R. T. Brown (Eds.), *Perspectives on bias in mental testing.* New York: Plenum Press.

Hartlage, L. C., Lucas, T., & Godwin, A. (1976). Culturally biased and culture fair tests correlated with school performance in culturally disadvantaged children. *Journal of Clinical Psychology, 32,* 235–237.

Heidbreder, E. (1933). *Seven psychologies.* Englewood Cliffs, NJ: Prentice-Hall.

Henderson, N. B., Butler, B. B., & Goffeney, B. (1969). Effectiveness of the WISC and Bender–Gestalt test in predicting arithmetic and reading achievement for white and non-white children. *Journal of Clinical Psychology, 25,* 268–271.

Hickman, J. A., & Reynolds, C. R. (1986). Race differences on mental tests: A test of Harrington's experimental model. *Journal of Special Education, 20,* 409–430.

Hildreth, G. H., Griffiths, N. L., & McGauvran, M. E. (1969). *Metropolitan Readiness Tests.* New York: Harcourt Brace Jovanovich.

Hilliard, A. G. (1979). Standardization and cultural bias as impediments to the scientific study and validation of "intelligence." *Journal of Research and Development in Education, 12,* 47–58.

Hobbs, N. R. (1975). *The future of children.* San Francisco: Jossey-Bass.

Hobson v. Hansen, 269 F. Supp. 401 (D.C. 1967).

Humphreys, L. G. (1973). Statistical definitions of test validity for minoriity groups. *Journal of Applied Psychology, 58,* 1–4.

Hunter, J. E. (1975, December). *A critical analysis of the use of item means and item–test correlations to determine the presence or absence of content bias in achievement test items.* Paper presented at the National Institute of Education Conference on Test Bias, Annapolis, MD.

Hunter, J. E., & Schmidt, F. L. (1976). Critical analysis of the statistical and ethical implications of various definitions of test bias. *Psychological Bulletin, 83,* 1053–1071.

Hunter, J. E., & Schmidt, F. L. (1978). Bias in defining test bias: Reply to Darlington. *Psychological Bulletin, 85,* 675–676.

Hunter, J. E., Schmidt, F. L., & Hunter, R. (1979). Differential validity of employment tests by race: A comprehensive review and analysis. *Psychological Bulletin, 86,* 721–735.

Hunter, J. E., Schmidt, F. L., & Rauschenberger, J. (1984). Methodological, statistical, and ethical issues in the study of bias in psychological tests. In C. R. Reynolds & R. T. Braun (Eds.), *Perspectives on bias in mental testing.* New York: Plenum Press.

Jackson, G. D. (1975). Another psychological view from the Association of Black Psychologists. *American Psychologist, 30,* 88–93.

Jacobs, W. R. (1978). The effect of the learning disability label on classroom teachers' ability objectively to observe and interpret child behaviors. *Learning Disability Quarterly, 1,* 50–55.

Jensen, A.R. (1969). How much can we boost IQ and scholastic achievement? *Harvard Educational Review, 39,* 1–123.

Jensen, A. R. (1974). How biased are culture-loaded tests? *Genetic Psychology Monographs, 90,* 185–224.

Jensen, A. R. (1976). Test bias and construct validity. *Phi Delta Kappan, 58,* 340–346.

Jensen, A. R. (1977). An examination of culture bias in the Wonderlic Personnel Test. *Intelligence, 1,* 51–64.

Jensen, A. R. (1980). *Bias in mental testing.* New York: Free Press.

Jensen, A. R. (1985). The nature of the black–white difference on various tests: Spearman's hypothesis. *Behavioral and Brain Sciences, 8,* 193–263.

Jenson, A. R., & Figueroa, R. A. (1975). Forward and backward Digit Span interaction with race and IQ. *Journal of Educational Psychology, 67,* 882–893.

Jensen, A. R., & Reynolds, C. R. (1982). Race, social class, and ability patterns of the WISC-R. *Personality and Individual Differences, 3,* 423–438.

Jöreskog, K. G. (1969). A general approach to confirmatory maximum likelihood factor analysis. *Psychometrika, 34,* 183.

Jöreskog, K. G. (1971). Simultaneous factor analysis in several populations. *Psychometrika, 36,* 409–426.

Kaiser, S. M. (1986). *Ability patterns of black and white adults on the Wechsler Adult Intelligence Scale—Revised independent of general intelligence and as a function of socioeconomic status.* Unpublished doctoral dissertation, Texas A&M University.

Kallingal, A. (1971). The prediction of grades for black and white students at Michigan State University. *Journal of Educational Measurement, 8,* 263–265.

Kamphaus, R. W., & Reynolds, C. R. (1987). *Clinical and research application of the K-ABC.* Circle Pines, MN: American Guidance Service.

Katzenmeyer, W. G., & Stenner, A. J. (1977). Estimation of the invariance of factor structures across sex and race with implications for hypothesis testing. *Educational and Psychological Measurement, 37,* 111–119.

Kaufman, A. S. (1975). Factor analysis of the WISC-R at 11 age levels between 6½ and 16½ years. *Journal of Consulting and Clinical Psychology, 43,* 135–147.

Kaufman, A. S. (1979, October). *The future of psychological assessment and its relationship to school psychology.* Invited address to the Fourth Annual Midwestern Conference on Psychology in the Schools, Boys Town, NE.

Kaufman, A. S., & DiCuio, R. (1975). Separate factor analyses of the McCarthy Scales for groups of black and white children. *Journal of School Psychology, 13,* 10–18.

Kaufman, A. S., & Hollenbeck, G. P. (1974). Comparative structure of the WPPSI for blacks and whites. *Journal of Clinical Psychology, 30,* 316–319.

Kennedy, D. A. (1978). Rationality, emotionality, and testing. *Journal of School Psychology, 16*, 16–24.

Kerlinger, F. N. (1973). *Foundations of behavioral research.* New York: Holt, Rinehart & Winston.

Kirkpatrick, J. J. (1970, September). *The psychological testing establishment: Vested interest versus responsibility.* Paper presented at the annual meeting of the American Psychological Association, Miami Beach, FL.

Kirkpatrick, J. J., Ewen, H. G., Barrett, H. S., & Katzell, H. A. (1968). *Testing and fair employment.* New York: New York University Press.

Kohs, S. C. (1923). *Intelligence measurement.* New York: Macmillan.

Larry P. v. Riles, 495 F. Supp. 926 (ND. Cal. 1979).

Leiderman, P. H., Babu, B., Kagia, J., Kraemer, H. C., & Leiderman, F. G. (1973). African infant precocity and some social influences during the first year. *Nature, 242*, 247–249.

Leventhal, D. S., & Stedman, D. J. (1970). A factor analytic study of the Illinois Test of Psycholinguistic Abilities. *Journal of Clinical Psychology, 26*, 473–477.

Lewis, D. O., Balla, D. A., & Shanok, S. S. (1979). Some evidence of race bias in the diagnosis and treatment of the juvenile offender. *American Journal of Orthopsychiatry, 49*, 53–61.

Lewontin, R. C. (1970). Race and intelligence. *Bulletin of the Atomic Scientists, 26*, 2–8.

Lindsey, J. (1967). *The factorial organization of intelligence in children as related to the variables of age, sex, and subculture.* Unpublished doctoral dissertation, University of Georgia.

Linn, R. L. (1976). In search of fair selection procedures. *Journal of Educational Measurement, 13*, 53–58.

Linn, R. L., & Werts, C. E. (1971). Considerations for studies of test bias. *Journal of Educational Measurement, 8*, 1–4.

Loehlin, J., Lindzey, C., & Spuhler, J. N. (1975). *Race differences in intelligence.* San Francisco: W. H. Freeman.

Lord, F. M. (1977). A study of item bias, using item characteristic curve theory. In Y. H. Poortinga (Ed.), *Basic problems in cross-cultural psychology.* Amsterdam: Swets & Zeitlinger.

MacArthur, R. S. (1968). Some differential abilities of northern Canadian youth. *International Journal of Psychology, 3*, 43–51.

MacMillan, D. L., Jones, R. L., & Aloia, G. F. (1974). The mentally retarded label: A theoretical analysis and review of research. *American Journal of Mental Deficiency, 79*, 241–261.

Marjoribanks, K. (1972). Ethnic and environmental influences on mental abilities. *American Journal of Sociology, 78*, 323–337.

Mason, E. J. (1979). A blessing dressed up like the plague? *The School Psychologist, 35*, 6.

Matuszek, P., & Oakland, T. (1979). Factors influencing teachers' and psychologists' recommendations regarding special class placement. *Journal of School Psychology, 17*, 116–125.

McCarthy, D. (1972). *McCarthy Scales of Children's Abilities.* New York: Psychological Corporation.

McCoy, S. A. (1976). Clinical judgements of normal childhood behaviors. *Journal of Consulting and Clinical Psychology, 44*, 710–714.

McGurk, F. V. J. (1951). *Comparison of the performance of Negro and white high school seniors on cultural and noncultural psychological test questions.* Washington, DC: Catholic University Press.

McNemar, Q. (1975). On so-called test bias. *American Psychologist, 30*, 848–851.

Mercer, J. B. (1971). The meaning of mental retardation. In R. Koch & J. Dobson (Eds.), *The mentally retarded child and his family: A multidisciplinary handbook.* New York: Brunner/Mazel.

Mercer, J. R. (1976, August). *Cultural diversity, mental retardation, and assessment: The case for nonlabeling.* Paper presented at the Fourth International Congress of the International Association for the Scientific Study of Mental Retardation, Washington, DC.

Mercer, J. R. (1979). In defense of racially and culturally nondiscriminatory assessment. *School Psychology Digest, 8*, 89–115,

Merz, W. A. (1970). *Factor analysis of the Goodenough–Harris drawing test items across four ethnic groups.* Ann Arbor, MI: University Microfilms. (No. 10–19, 714)

Meyers, C. E., MacMillan, D. L., & Yoshida, R. K. (1978). Validity of psychologists' identification of EMR students in the perspective of the California decertification experience. *Journal of School Psychology, 16*, 3–15.

Mille, F. (1979). Cultural bias in the WISC. *Intelligence, 3*, 149–164.

Minton, H, L., & Schneider, F. W. (1980). *Differential psychology.* Monterey, CA: Brooks/Cole.

Mitchell, B. C. (1967). Predictive validity of the Metropolitan Readiness Tests and the Murphy–Durrell Reading Analysis for white and for Negro pupils. *Educational and Psychological Measurement, 27*, 1047–1054.

Nalven, F. B., Hoffman, L. J., & Bierbryer, B. (1969). The effects of subject's age, sex, race, and socioeconomic status on psychologists' estimates of "true IQ" from WISC scores. *Journal of Clinical Psychology, 25*, 271–274.

Nichols, R. C. (1978). Policy implications of the IQ controversy. In L. S. Schulman (Ed.), *Review of research in education* (Vol. 6). Itasca, IL: F. E. Peacock.

Novick, M. R., & Petersen, N. S. (1976). Towards equalizing educational and employment opportunity. *Journal of Educational Measurement, 13*, 77–88.

Oakland, T. (1978). Predictive validity of readiness tests for middle and lower socioeconomic status Anglo, black and Mexican American children. *Journal of Educational Psychology, 70*, 574–582.

Oakland, T., & Feigenbaum, D. (1979). Multiple sources of test bias on the WISC-R and the Bender–Gestalt Test. *Journal of Consulting and Clinical Psychology, 47*, 968–974.

Oakland, T., & Matuszek, P. (1977). Using tests of nondiscriminatory assessment. In T. Oakland (Ed.), *Psychological and educational assessment of minority group children.* New York: Brunner/Mazel.

O'Conner, E. J., Wexley, K. N., & Alexander, R. A. (1975). Single group validity: Fact or fallacy? *Journal of Applied Psychology, 60,* 352–355.

Petersen, N. S., & Novick, M. R. (1976). An evaluation of some models for culture fair selection. *Journal of Educational Measurement, 13,* 3–29.

Pfeifer, C. M., & Sedlacek, W. E. (1971). The validity of academic predictors for black and white students at a predominately white university. *Journal of Educational Measurement, 8,* 253–261.

Pintner, R. (1923). *Intelligence testing.* New York: Henry Holt.

Pintner, R., & Keller, R. (1922). Intelligence tests of foreign children, *Journal of Educational Psychology, 13,* 214–222.

Plake, B., & Hoover, H. (1979, September). *A methodology for identifying biased achievement test items that removes the confounding in a items by groups interaction due to possible group differences in instructional level.* Paper presented at the annual meeting of the American Educational Research Association, Toronto.

Potthoff, R. F. (1966). *Statistical aspects of the problem of biases in psychological tests.* (Institute of Statistics Mimeo Series No. 479). Chapel Hill: University of North Carolina, Department of Statistics.

Pressey, S. L., & Pressey. L. L. (1922). *Introduction to the use of standardized tests.* Yonkers, NY: World.

Ramsey, B. T. (1979). *The testing manual: A guide to test administration and use.* Pittsburgh, PA: Author.

Reschly, D. J. (1978). WISC-R factor structures among Anglos, blacks, Chicanos, and Native American Papagos. *Journal of Consulting and Clinical Psychology, 46,* 417–422.

Reschly, D. J. (1980). Concepts of bias in assessment and WISC-R research with minorities. In H. Vance & F. Wallbrown (Eds.), *WISC-R: Research and interpretation.* Washington, DC: National Association of School Psychologists.

Reschly, D. J., & Reschly, J. E. (1979). Validity of WISC-R factor scores us predicting achievement and attention for four sociocultural groups. *Journal of School Psychology, 17,* 355–361.

Reschly, D. J., & Sabers, D. (1979). Analysis of test bias in four groups with the regression definition. *Journal of Educational Measurement, 16,* 1–9.

Reynolds, C. R. (1978). *Differential validity of several preschool assessment instruments for blacks, whites, males, and females.* Unpublished doctoral dissertation, University of Georgia.

Reynolds, C. R. (1979a). A factor analytic study of the Metropolitan Readiness Test. *Contemporary Educational Psychology, 4,* 315–317.

Reynolds, C. R. (1979b). The invariance of the factorial validity of the Metropolitan Readiness Tests for blacks, whites, males and females. *Educational and Psychological Measurement, 39,* 1047–1052.

Reynolds, C. R. (1979c). Should we screen preschoolers? *Contemporary Educational Psychology, 4,* 175–181.

Reynolds, C. R. (1980a). Differential construct validity of a preschool battery for blacks, whites, males and females. *Journal of School Psychology, 18,* 112–125.

Reynolds, C. R. (1980b, April). *Differential predictive validity of a preschool battery across race and sex.* Paper presented to the annual meeting of the American Educational Research Association, Boston.

Reynolds, C. R. (1980c). A examination for test bias in a preschool battery across race and sex. *Journal of Educational Measurement, 17,* 137–146.

Reynolds, C. R. (1982). Methods for the detecting construct and predictive bias. In R. A. Berk (Ed.), *Handbook of methods of detecting test.* Baltimore: John Hopkins University Press.

Reynolds, C. R., Bossard, M. D., & Gutkin, T. B. (1980, April). *A regression analysis of test bias on the Stanford–Binet Intelligence Scale.* Paper presented at the annual meeting of the American Educational Research Association, Boston.

Reynolds, C. R., & Brown, R. T. (Eds.). (1984). *Perspectives on bias in mental testing.* New York: Plenum.

Reynolds, C. R., & Clark, J. H. (1986). Profile analysis of standardized intelligence test performance on very high functioning individuals. *Psychology in the Schools, 23,* 5–12.

Reynolds, C. R., & Gutkin, T. B. (1979). Predicting the premorbid intellectual status of children using demographic data. *Clinical Neuropsychology, 1,* 36–38.

Reynolds, C. R., & Gutkin, T. B. (1980a). A regression analysis of test bias on the WISC-R for Anglos and Chicanos referred to psychological services. *Journal of Abnormal Child Psychology, 8,* 237–243.

Reynolds, C. R., & Gutkin, T. B. (1980b). Stability of the WISC-R factor structure across sex at two age levels. *Journal of Clinical Psychology, 36,* 775–777.

Reynolds, C. R., & Gutkin, T. B. (1980c, September). *WISC-R performance of blacks and whites matched on four demographic variables.* Paper presented at the annual meeting of the American Psychological Association, Montreal.

Reynolds, C. R., Gutkin, T. B., Dappen, L., & Wright, D. (1979). Differential validity of the WISC-R for boys and girls referred for psychological services. *Perceptual and Motor Skills, 48,* 868–879.

Reynolds, C. R., & Harding, B. E. (1983). Outcome in two large sample studies of factorial similarity under six methods of comparison. *Educational and Psychological Measurement, 43,* 723–728.

Reynolds, C. R., & Hartlage, L. C. (1978, March). *Comparison of WISC and WISC-R racial regression lines.* Paper presented at the annual meeting of the Southeastern Psychological Association, Atlanta, GA.

Reynolds, C. R., & Hartlage, L. C. (1979). Comparison of WISC and WISC-R regression lines for academic prediction with black and with white referred children. *Journal of Consulting and Clinical Psychology, 47,* 589–591.

Reynolds, C. R., & Jansen, A. B. (1983). WISC-R subscale patterns of abilities of blacks and whites matched on Full Scale IQ. *Journal of Educational Psychology, 75,* 207–214.

Reynolds, C. R., McBride, R. D., & Gibson, L. J. (1979, March). *Black–white IQ discrepancies may be related to differences in hemisphericity.* Paper presented at the annual meeting of the National Association of School Psychologists, San Diego, CA.

Reynolds, C. R., Willson, V. L., & Chatman, S. P. (1984). Item bias on the 1981 revision of the Peabody Picture Vocabulary Test using a new technique for detecting bias. *Journal of Psychoeducational Assessment, 2,* 219–227.

Reynolds, C. H., Willson, V. L., & Chatman, S. P. (1985). Regression analyses of bias on the Kaufman Assessment Battery for Children. *Journal of School Psychology, 23,* 195–204.

Rosenthal, D. (1975). Heredity in criminality. *Criminal Justice and Behavior, 2,* 3–21.

Ross, A. O. (1974). A clinical child psychologist "examines retarded children. In G. J. Williams & S. Gordon (Eds.), *Clinical child psychology: Current trends and future perspectives.* New York: Behavioral.

Ross, A. O. (1976). *Psychological aspects of learning disabilities and reading disorders.* New York: McGraw-Hill.

Sakoda, J. M., Cohen, B. H., & Beall, G. (1954). Test of significance for a series of statistical tests. *Psychological Bulletin, 51,* 172–175.

Sandoval, J. (1979). The WISC-R and internal evidence of test bias with minority groups. *Journal of Consulting and Clinical Psychology, 47,* 919–927.

Sandoval, J., & Mille, M. (1979, September). *Accuracy judgements of WISC-R item difficulty for minority groups.* Paper presented at the annual meeting of the American Psychological Association, New York.

Sattler, J. M. (1974). *Assessment of children's intelligence.* Philadelphia: W. B. Saunders.

Sawyer, R. L., Cole, N. S., & Cole, J. W. (1976). Utilities and the issue of fairness in a decision theoretic model for selection. *Journal of Educational Measurement, 13,* 59–76.

Scheuneman, J. D. (1987). An experimental, exploratory study of causes of bias in test items. *Journal of Educational Measurement, 29,* 97–118.

Schmidt, F. L., & Hunter, J. E. (1974). Racial and ethnic bias in psychological tests: Divergent implications of two definition of test bias. *American Psychologist, 29,* 1–8.

Schmidt, W. H. (1983). Content biases in achievement tests. *Journal of Educational Measurement, 20,* 165–178.

Scholwinski, E. J. (1985). *Ability patterns of white and black adults as determined by the subscales on the Wechsler Adult Intelligence Scale—Revised.* Unpublished doctoral dissertation, Texas A&M University.

Semler, I., & Iscoe, I. (1966). Structure of intelligence in Negro and white children. *Journal of Educational Psychology, 57,* 326–336.

Sewell, T. E. (1979). Intelligence and learning tasks as predictors of scholastic achievement in black and white first-grade children. *Journal of School Psychology, 17,* 325–332.

Shepard, L. A. (1982). Definitions of bias. In B. A. Berk (Ed.), *Handbook of methods for detecting test bias.* Baltimore: Johns Hopkins University Press.

Shuey, A. M. (1966). *The testing of Negro intelligence* (2nd ed.). New York: Social Science Press.

Silverstein, A. B. (1973). Factor structure of the Wechsler Intelligence Scale for Children for three ethnic groups. *Journal of Educational Psychology, 65,* 408–410.

Stanley, J. C. (1969). Plotting ANOVA interactions for ease of visual interpretation. *Educational and Psychological Measurement, 29,* 793–797.

Stanley, J. C. (1971). Predicting college success of the educationally disadvantaged. *Science, 171,* 640–647.

Stanley, J. C., & Porter, A. C. (1967). Correlation of scholastic aptitude test scores with college grades for Negroes vs. whites. *Journal of Educational Measurement, 4,* 199–218.

Sternberg, R. J. (1985). The black–white differences and Spearman's g: Old wine in new bottles that still doesn't taste good. *Behavioral and Brain Sciences, 8,* 244.

Temp, G. (1971). Validity of the SAT for blacks and whites in thirteen integrated institutions. *Journal of Educational Measurements, 8,* 245–251.

Tenopyr, M. L. (1967, September). *Race and socioeconomic status as moderators in predicting machine-shop training success.* Paper presented at the annual meeting of the American Psychological Association, Washington, DC.

Thorndike, R. L. (1968). [Review of *Pygmalion in the classroom* by R. Rosenthal and L. Jacobsen]. *American Educational Research Journal, 5,* 708–711.

Thorndike, R. L. (1971). Concepts of culture-fairness. *Journal of Educational Measurement, 8,* 63–70.

Tittle, C. K. (1975). Fairness in educational achievement testing. *Education and Urban Society, 8,* 86–103.

Tittle, C. K. (1982). Use of judgemental methods in item bias studies. In B. A. Berk (Ed.), *Handbook of methods for detecting test bias.* Baltimore: John Hopkins University Press.

Tomlinson, J. R., Acker, N., Canter, A., & Lindborg, S. (1977). Minority status, sex, and school psychological services. *Psychology in the Schools, 14,* 456–460.

Torrance, E. P. (1980). Psychology of gifted children and youth. In W. M. Cruickshank (Ed.), *Psychology of exceptional children and youth.* Englewood Cliffs, NJ: Prentice-Hall.

Tyler, L. E. (1965). *The psychology of human differences.* (2nd ed.). New York: Appleton-Century-Crofts.

Vance, H. B., Hankins, N., & McGee, H. (1979). A preliminary study of black and white differences on the Revised Wechsler Intelligence Scale for Children. *Journal of Clinical Psychology, 35,* 815–819.

Vance, H. B., Huelsman, C. B., & Wherry, R. J. (1976). The hierarchical factor structure of the Wechsler Intelligence Scale for Children as it relates to disadvantaged white and black children. *Journal of General Psychology, 95,* 287–293.

Vance, H. B., & Wallbrown, F. H. (1978). The structure of intelligence for black children: A hierarchical approach. *Psychological Record, 28,* 31–39.

Veale, J. R., & Foreman, D. I. (1983). Assessing cultural bias using foil response data: Cultural variation. *Journal of Educational Measurement, 20,* 249–258.

Waits, C., & Richmond, B. O. (1978). Special education—who needs it? *Exceptional Children, 44,* 279–280.

Wallbrown, F. H., Blabs, J., Wallbrown, J., & Engin, A. (1974). The hierarchical factor structure of the Wechsler Adult Intelligence Scale. *British Journal of Educational Psychology, 44,* 47–65.

Wallbrown, F. H., Blabs, J., & Wherry, R. J. (1973). The hierarchical factor structure of the Wechsler Preschool and Primary Scale of Intelligence. *Journal of Consulting and Clinical Psychology, 41,* 356–362.

Warren, N. (1972). African infant precocity. *Psychological Bulletin, 78,* 535–367.

Wechsler, D. (1949). *Wechsler Intelligence Scale for Children.* New York: Psychological Corporation.

Wechsler, D. (1974). *Wechsler Intelligence Scale for Children—Revised.* New York: Psychological Corporation.

Wechsler, D. (1981). *Wechsler Adult Intelligence Scale—Revised.* New York: Psychological Corporation.

Wherry, R. J., & Wherry, R. J., Jr. (1969). WHEWH program. In B. J. Wherry (Ed.), *Psychology department computer programs.* Columbus: Ohio State University, Department of Psychology.

Willerman, L. (1979). *The psychology of individual and group differences.* San Francisco: W. H. Freeman.

Williams, R. L. (1970). Danger: Testing and dehumanizing black children. *Clinical Child Psychology Newsletter, 9,* 5–6.

Williams, R. L. (1972, September). *The BITCH-100: A culture specific test.* Paper presented at the annual meeting of the American Psychological Association, Honolulu.

Williams, R. L. (1974). From dehumanization to black intellectual genocide: A rejoinder. In G. J. Williams & S. Gordon (Eds.), *Clinical child psychology: Current practices and future perspectives.* New York: Behavioral.

Wilson, K. M. (1969). *Black students entering CRC colleges: Their characteristics and their first year academic performance* (Research Memo No. 69–1). Poughkeepsie, NY: College Research Center.

Wright, B. J., & Isenstein, V. R. (1977). *Psychological tests and minorities* (DHEW Publication No. ADM 78-482). Washington, DC: U.S. Government Printing Office.

23

Assessment of Culturally and Linguistically Diverse Children

SALVADOR HECTOR OCHOA

Demographic data clearly illustrate that the number of students from diverse linguistic backgrounds in U.S. schools is increasing. In 1990, children (ages 5–17) from non-English-speaking backgrounds constituted 13% of the school-age population (Chapa, 1990). There was a 49% increase in the number of students from linguistically diverse backgrounds from 1979 to 1988 (Chapa, 1990). Reports vary as to the number of children with limited English proficiency (LEP) in the United States. Chapa (1990) reported that there were 5.7 million students with LEP, whereas Gonzalez, Brusca-Vega, and Yawkey (1997) indicated that there were 6.3 million such students in the United States. Lopez (1997) states that figures associated with the number of students with LEP will differ as a result of "inconsistencies in the implementation of definitions, methods, and criteria found throughout the country" (p. 504). Many different language groups make up the school-age population with LEP.

Children from Spanish-speaking backgrounds are the largest group (Gonzalez et al., 1997). Spanish-speaking children constitute approximately two-thirds (McLeod, 1994) to 73% (Gonzalez et al., 1997) of the student population with LEP in the United

States. Ochoa, Gonzalez, Galarza, and Guillemard's (1996) survey of school psychologists from Arizona, California, Colorado, Florida, New Jersey, New Mexico, New York, and Texas indicated that the most common non-English-language group assessed was overwhelmingly Spanish-speaking. This survey also revealed that school psychologists in the aforementioned states assessed children from 84 additional low-incidence language groups. After Spanish, languages spoken by Asian and Pacific Islanders were most common. In order of frequency, these languages included Vietnamese, Cambodian, Chinese, and Japanese.

Given the demographic and assessment practice trends just described, many school psychologists will be faced with assessing linguistically diverse students. Ochoa, Gonzalez, and colleagues (1996) found that 57% of the school psychologists who responded to their survey indicated that they had assessed linguistically diverse students. The assessment of such students is complex and difficult. In order to assist school psychologists in this area, this chapter addresses many issues associated with the psychoeducational assessment of linguistically diverse pupils. These issues include (1) definitions; (2) critical issues that affect practice; (3) second-language acquisition and dual-language instruction factors; (4) reasons given for, and factors that need to be addressed during, referral; (5) assessment of language proficiency; (6) academic assessment; and (7) intellectual assessment. The chapter is limited to discussion of assessing school-age children. Individuals interested in the assessment of culturally and linguistically diverse preschoolers are referred to the following references: Barona (1991), Barona and Santos de Barona (2000); and Li, Walton, and Nuttall (1999).

DEFINITIONS

Many students who are linguistically diverse are often referred to or described as having "LEP" (see above) and/or as "bilingual." LEP is defined as "the lack of facility, fluency, or linguistic competence in English as a second language relative to a normal native speaker–listener of the language" (Kretschmer, 1991, p. 5). Students who are bilingual will have varying degrees of proficiency in their first (native) language and in their second (English) language. Valdes and Figueroa (1996) state that "it is important to view bilingualism as a continuum and bilingual individuals as falling along this continuum at different points to each other, depending on the varying strength and cognitive characteristics of their two languages" (p. 8). Hamayan and Damico (1991a) state that the majority of bilingual children will vary in their ability to listen, speak, read, and write across two languages. Being stronger in each of these four areas in one language is referred to as "nonbalanced bilingualism," whereas being stronger in one or more of the domains in one language and yet stronger in other domain(s) in the other language is called "mixed dominance" (Hamayan & Damico, 1991, p. 42). Having commensurate levels of proficiency across all four domains in both one's first and second languages is referred to as "balanced bilingualism" (Hamayan & Damico, 1991, p. 42).

Other constructs have been used to differentiate types of bilingualism. Valdes and Figueroa (1996) differentiate between "si-multaneous" versus "sequential" bilingualism and "elective" versus "circumstantial" bilingualism. Children with sequential bilingualism are students who have been exposed to their first language since birth and were later exposed to a second language. Such children may have been exposed to English (Hamayan & Damico, 1991a); however, they generally do not use it until entering school. Children with simultaneous bilingualism are individuals who were exposed to and learned two languages at the same time. Valdes and Figueroa also stress the importance of recognizing the difference between elective and circumstantial bilingualism. Persons with elective bilingualism are individuals who want to acquire a second language. Those with circumstantial bilingualism "are individuals who because of their circumstances, find that they must learn another language in order to survive. . . . [T]hese individuals find themselves in a context which their ethnic language is not the majority, prestige, or national language" (Valdes & Figueroa, 1996, p. 12).

The overwhelming majority of linguistically diverse children whom school psychologists will assess will have nonbalanced or mixed balanced bilingualism, sequential bilingualism and/or circumstantial bilingualism. Such children will have varying degrees of language proficiency in both their first language and English.

CRITICAL ISSUES THAT AFFECT PRACTICE

Historically, minority school-age children have been disproportionately represented in special education (Chinn & Hughes, 1987: Figueroa & Artiles, 1999; Mercer, 1973; Ortiz & Yates, 1983; Wright & Cruz, 1983). The most notable case in the assessment of linguistically diverse students was *Diana v. State Board of Education* (1970). This California case claimed that elementary-age Mexican American students were misdiagnosed as having mental retardation, as a result of being administered biased intelligence tests in English. While this case was settled out of court, testing safeguards were outlined during the settlement process. The most significant safeguard required that bilingual students be assessed in their native language. The impact of this case was clearly noted in the testing requirements outlined in Public Law (PL) 94-142, the Education for All Handicapped Children Act of 1975.

Minorities continue to be overrepresented in special education (Artiles & Trent, 1994; Daughtery, 1999; National Research Council, 2002; Parrish, 2002). The "U.S. Office of Special Education Programs (OSEP) and the U.S. Office of Civil Rights (OCR) view the issue of disproportionate placement as an ongoing national problem that varies from district to district, from state to state, and from region to region" (Daugherty, 1999, p. 16). Ochoa, Morales, and Hernandez (1997) found that misdiagnosis/overidentification was the fourth most-cited concern of school psychologists about conducting bilingual psychoeducational assessment.

Many critical factors can impede or facilitate improvement with respect to the disproportionality problem. These factors include (1) lack of bilingual school psychologists resulting in the use of interpreters; (2) lack of training; (3) referral practices; (4) federal regulations; and (5) ethical guidelines and professional standards.

Lack of Bilingual School Psychologists, Resulting in the Use of Interpreters

The ideal situation for assessing a child learning a second language is to have a school psychologist who speaks the same language as the child (Kamphaus, 1993). There is, however, a shortage of bilingual school psychologists (Nuttall, 1987; Rosenfield & Esquivel, 1985). One study (Ochoa, Rivera, & Ford, 1994) revealed that approximately 75% of school psychologists believe there is a significant shortage of bilingual school psychologists. This shortage will probably become more severe when one considers recent demographic trends indicating a large increase of students with LEP in the United States.

When a bilingual examiner is not available, common practice is to utilize an interpreter (Figueroa, 1989). Ochoa, Gonzalez, and colleagues (1996) found that over half of the school psychologists we surveyed used interpreters when assessing bilingual students. Unfortunately, an untrained person serves as an interpreter in most cases.

Ochoa, Gonzalez, and colleagues also found that

> [77%] of the school psychologists who reported using an interpreter had received no or very little training to do so. Only 37% of the school psychologists reported that their interpreter had received formal training. In only 7% of the cases reported were both school psychologists and interpreters trained in the interpretation process. (p. 19)

The use of an untrained interpreter can result in many errors (Caterino, 1990; Figueroa, Sandoval, & Merino, 1984; Holtzman & Wilkinson, 1991) and affect the validity of assessment data (Figueroa, 1990b).

Lopez (1995) states that interpreters should only be utilized as "the absolute last resort" (p. 1119). The 1999 *Standards for Educational and Psychological Testing* volume by the American Educational Research Association (AERA), the American Psychological Association (APA), and the National Council on Measurement in Education (NCME) stresses the importance of using a "fully qualified interpreter" (p. 95). This volume (AERA et al., 1999) includes the following standard (Standard 9.11) pertaining to the use of interpreters:

> When an interpreter is used in testing, the interpreter should be fluent in both the language of the test and the examinee's native language, should have expertise in translating, and should have a basic understanding of the assessment process. (p. 100)

An interpreter should be trained in many areas, including (1) the interpretation process (AERA et al., 1999; Chamberlain & Medinos-Landurand, 1991; Scribner, 1993; Wilen & Sweeting, 1986); (2) the assessment process (AERA et al., 1999; Medina, 1982, Miller & Abudarham, 1984; Scribner, 1993); and (3) ethical conduct (Medina, 1982). Several guidelines pertaining to the use of interpreters have also been developed (Chamberlain & Medinos-Landurand, 1991; Fradd & Wilen, 1990; Medina, 1982; Miller & Aburdarham, 1984; Scribner, 1993; Wilen & Sweeting, 1986). Moreover, Figueroa and colleagues (1984) specify the training that school psychologists need to have in order to work with interpreters. Although the aforementioned training areas for both interpreters and school psychologists have been identified, "[t]here is no empirically validated model for training or using an interpreter" (Figueroa, 1989, cited in Kamphaus, 1993, pp. 458–459).

Lack of Training

Research indicates that school psychologists have not been trained to assess children learning a second language. One study (Ochoa, Morales, & Hernandez, 1997) found that inadequate or lack of preservice or in-service training was the concern most often cited by school psychologists about conducting bilingual psychoeducational assessment. Rogers, Ponterotto, Conoley, and Wiese (1992) found that 40% of school psychology programs did not offer multicultural coursework. Rogers and colleagues also found that approximately 60% of school psychology programs incorporated multicultural content from 0% to 15% of the time into existing assessment courses. Rogers, Martin, and Druckman's (1994) study revealed that only 6 of the 17 school psychology programs that were judged to be "model" multicultural programs offered a bilingual assessment course. Ochoa, Rivera, and Ford (1997) found that approximately "83% of the school psychologists actually conducting bilingual assessment described their training as less than adequate. Moreover, 56% stated that they had received no or very little training on interpreting results of bilingual assessment" (p. 341). Based on their findings, Ochoa, Rivera, and Ford concluded:

> These figures raise serious questions about the validity of test results when LEP students are assessed. The implications of these findings regarding the eligibility decisions of culturally and linguistically diverse students [are] frightening. The field of school psychology must ask itself whether the lack of adequate training by approximately 80% school psychologists conducting bilingual psychoeducational assessment has any bearing on the overrepresentation of minority children in special education. (p. 341)

In order to help better prepare school psychologists, several groups of researchers (Figueroa et al., 1984; Ochoa, Rivera, & Ford, 1997; Rogers et al., 1999) have identified the competencies that school psychologists should possess in order to assess students with LEP. Moreover, school psychologists should review (1) guidelines and (2) practical, theoretical, and research considerations available in the literature (AERA et al., 1999; APA, 1990; Barona & Santos de Barona, 1987; Caterino, 1990; Educational Testing Service [ETS], 2000; Esquivel, 1988; Figueroa, 1990b; Hamayan & Damico, 1991b; Lopez, 1995, 1997; McGrew, Flanagan, & Ortiz, 1998; Ochoa, Galarza, & Gonzalez, 1996; Ochoa, Powell, & Robles-Pina, 1996; Valdes & Figueroa, 1996; Wilen & Sweeting, 1986).

Referral Practices

Reynolds and Kaiser (1990) state that one should consider the possibility of "referral source bias, . . . [because] there is evidence that persons are not always referred for services on the basis of impartial, objective rationales" (p. 646). Several studies (Ochoa, Robles-Pina, Garcia, & Breunig, 1999; Ortiz & Polyzoi, 1986; Rueda, Cardoza, Mercer, & Carpenter, 1985) have examined why linguistically diverse students are referred to special education. Ochoa and colleagues (1999) found that the most common reasons why such students were referred included (1) poor achievement, (2) reading problems, (3) behavioral problems, and (4) oral-language-related factors. We also reported that 8 of the 17 most common referral reasons, which consisted of 54% of the total responses, "have a plausible linkage with language and/or culture" (Ochoa et al., 1999, p. 7).

The prereferral process is an important step that should be undertaken in order to insure that language and culture factors are carefully reviewed and considered as potential contributing variables on the bilingual student's academic difficulties. Ortiz and Polyzoi (1986) recommend that at least one person on the prereferral committee have expertise or training in educating children learning a second language. Ochoa and colleagues (1999) found that the presence of someone with this type of expertise on prereferral committees occurred about 50% of the time. School psychologists should review various prereferral guidelines/procedures developed for children learning a second language (Garcia & Ortiz, 1988; Garcia & Yates, 1986; Hoover & Collier, 1985; Ortiz & Wilkinson, 1991). Research (Ortiz, 1990) has revealed that when school personnel are trained to understand and deal with second-language acquisition factors, the number of bilingual students referred to special education is significantly reduced.

Federal Guidelines

The first federal guideline to address the issue of appropriate assessment of linguistically diverse students was PL 94-142 in 1975. This law required that nondiscriminatory assessment be conducted and that students be assessed in their native language unless it was clearly unfeasible. The same requirements were included in the two subsequent laws amending PL 94-142: the Individuals with Disabilities Education Act (IDEA) of 1990 (PL 101-476), and the 1997 reauthorization of IDEA (PL 105-17).

Sections of PL 105-17 clearly indicate Congress's concern about the issue of misidentification/disproportionate minority representation in special education and include additional requirements concerning the assessment of ethnically diverse students. The concerns noted by Congress can be found in PL 105-17, sections 601(c) (8) (a & b): "Greater efforts are needed to prevent the intensification of problems connected with mislabeling minority children with disabilities," and "More minority children continue to be served in special education than would be expected given the percentage of minority students in the general population."

Two new requirements are included in PL 105-17 that have significant implications for school psychologists who assess linguistically diverse students. These two requirements are in section 614 (b)(5) of this law: "In making a determination of eligibility under paragraph 4(A), a child shall not be determined to be a child with disability if the determinant factor for such determination is lack of instruction in reading or math or limited English proficiency." As Kovaleski and Prasse (1999) have commented,

the authors of IDEA '97 believed that students were being incorrectly identified as having a

disability (typically learning disability) because they displayed academic difficulties that were a direct result of ineffective instruction or the lack of opportunity to receive effective instruction. To prevent these students from being over-identified, the "lack of instruction" requirement was added to the law. (p. 24)

School psychologists will need to have knowledge about the second-language acquisition process and dual-language instruction in order to address these two requirements. Very few school psychologists who conduct bilingual evaluations have knowledge in these areas. In one study (Ochoa, Rivera, & Ford, 1997), approximately 79% of school psychologists who assessed bilingual students and/or students with LEP indicated that they had received less than adequate training from their school psychology program about second-language acquisition factors and their relationship to assessment. Given these new requirements, issues associated with second-language acquisition and dual-language instruction (e.g., bilingual education) are discussed later in this chapter.

Another important requirement in this area that was included in PL 94-142, IDEA, and the 1997 reauthorization of IDEA, but that has not received much attention in the best-practice and research literature, is the exclusionary clause. The exclusionary clause stipulates that a student should not be identified as learning disabled if the "discrepancy between ability and achievement is primarily the result of environmental, cultural, or economic disadvantage" (U.S. Office of Education, 1997, p. 65083). The exclusionary clause is an important factor that should be given due consideration in assessing and making eligibility decisions about linguistically diverse students (Ochoa, Rivera, & Powell, 1997). Harris, Gray, Davis, Zaremba, and Argulewicz's (1988) study revealed that fewer than 50% of school psychologists complied with the exclusionary-clause provision on a regular basis. Ochoa, Rivera, and Powell (1997) researched how school psychologists applied the exclusionary clause with bilingual students. Although this study identified 36 factors used by school psychologists to comply with the exclusionary clause, only the following five factors were reported to be used by more than 10% of such psychologists:

(1) "review of sociological information and family history" (used by 25%); (2) "parent interview and information" (used by 18%); (3) "length of time or numbers of years the student has lived in the U.S." (used by 15%); (4) "past educational history or educational opportunity background" (used by 14%); and (5) "district-wide and/or individual language assessment data: dominance or proficiency" (used by 11%) (p. 164). Moreover, Ochoa, Rivera, and Powell (1997) recommended an additional 17 factors that school psychologists need to consider when attempting to comply with the exclusionary clause with linguistically diverse students. We stated that the 53 factors identified and discussed in their article can serve as "beginning criteria or guidelines in helping special educators and school psychologists meet the egalitarian intent of the exclusionary clause" (Ochoa, Rivera, & Powell, 1997, p. 166).

Ethical Guidelines and Professional Standards

In order to provide direction to both practitioners and test developers in this area, guidelines and professional standards have been established by key professional organizations. These organizations include the National Association of School Psychology (NASP, 1997); AERA, APA, and NCME (1999); and ETS (2000). With respect to assessment practices used with culturally and linguistically diverse populations, the following standards should be considered and implemented by school psychologists.

1. The NASP (1997) principles for professional ethics (Section IV. B. 1) state:

School psychologists will maintain the highest standard for educational and psychological assessment. a.) In conducting psychological, educational, or behavioral evaluations ... due consideration will be given to individual integrity and individual differences. b.) School psychologists respect differences in age, gender, sexual orientation, and socioeconomic, cultural and ethnic backgrounds. They select and use appropriate assessment or treatment procedures, techniques, and strategies. (p. 11)

2. The NASP (1997) standards for the provision of school psychological services

(Sections 3.5.3.1–3.5.3.3, Non-Biased Assessment Techniques) state:

3.5.3.1. Assessment procedures and program recommendations are chosen to maximize the student's opportunities to be successful in the general culture, while respecting the student's ethnic background.
3.5.3.2. Multifaceted assessment batteries are used that include a focus on the student's strengths.
3.5.3.3. Communications are held and assessments are conducted in the client's dominant spoken language or alternative communication system. All student information is interpreted in the context of the student's sociocultural background and the setting in which she/he is functioning. (p. 62)

3. The AERA and colleagues (1999) *Standards for Educational and Psychological Testing* volume (Standards 9.1, 9.3, 9.10, and 9.11) states:

9.1. Testing practice should be designed to reduce threats to reliability and validity of test score inferences that may arise from language difference. . . .
9.3. When testing an examinee proficient in two or more languages for which the test is available, the examinee's relative language proficiencies should be determined. The test generally should be administered in the test taker's most proficient language, unless proficiency in the less proficient language is part of the assessment. . . .
9.10. Inferences about test takers' general language proficiency should be based on tests that measure a range of language features, and not a single skill.
9.11. When an interpreter is used in testing, the interpreter should be fluent in both the language of the test and the examinee's native language, should have expertise in translating, and should have a basic understanding of the assessment process. (pp. 97–100)

In addition, test developers should incorporate the following guidelines when developing a test for, and/or recommending a test be used with, culturally and linguistically diverse students.

1. The AERA and colleagues (1999) *Standards for Educational and Psychologi-*

cal Testing volume (Standards 9.2, 9.4, 9.5, 9.6, 9.7, and 9.9) states:

9.2. When credible research evidence reports that test scores differ in meaning across subgroups of linguistically diverse test takers, then to the extent feasible, test developers should collect for each linguistic subgroup studied the same form of validity evidence collected for the examinee population as a whole. . . .

9.4. Linguistic modifications recommended by test publishers, as well as the rationale for the modifications, should be described in detail in the test manual.

9.5. When there is credible evidence of score comparability across regular and modified tests or administrators, no flag should be attached to a score. When such evidence is lacking, specific information about the nature of the modification should be provided, if permitted by law, to assist test users properly to interpret and act on test scores.

9.6. When a test is recommended for use with linguistically diverse test takers, test developers and publishers should provide the information necessary for appropriate test use and interpretation.

9.7. When a test is translated from one language to another, the methods used in establishing the adequacy of the translation should be described, and empirical and logical evidence should be provided for score reliability and the validity of the translated test's score inferences for the uses intended in the linguistic groups to be tested. . . .

9.9. When multiple language versions of a test are intended to be comparable, test developers should report evidence of test comparability. (pp. 97–99)

2. The ETS (2000) publication *ETS Standards for Quality and Fairness* (Standards 4.7 and 6.4) states:

Standard 4.7. Consider the needs of nonnative speakers of English in the development and use of products or services. For assessments, reduce threats to validity that may arise from language differences. Take the following actions, as appropriate for the product or service. State the suitability of the product or service for people with limited English proficiency. If a product . . . is recommended for use with a linguistically diverse population, provide the information necessary for appropriate use with nonnative speakers of English. If a translation is made, describe the

process and evaluate the outcome and its comparability to the original version. If linguistic modifications are recommended, describe the modifications in a document available to the public. . . . When sufficient relevant data are available, provide information on the validity and interpretation of assessment results for linguistically diverse groups. (p. 21)

Standard 6.4. Obtain and document the logical and/or empirical evidence that the assessment will meet its intended purpose(s) and support the intended interpretation(s) of assessment results for the intended population(s). (p. 29)

The implementation of these guidelines and standards from both a practitioner's and a test developer's perspective would significantly improve current assessment practices for bilingual students and/or students with LEP. Moreover, it might help address the disproportionality problem that has plagued our profession for nearly 30 years.

SECOND-LANGUAGE ACQUISITION AND DUAL-LANGUAGE INSTRUCTION FACTORS

There are several reasons why school psychologists who assess linguistically diverse students should have knowledge about second-language acquisition and dual-language instruction factors. First, among the main reasons why such children are referred for testing are oral-language-related problems (i.e., acquisition and/or delay) (Ochoa et al., 1999; Ortiz & Polyzoi, 1986; Rueda et al., 1985). Second, children with LEP often display behavioral characteristics similar to those of students with learning disabilities (Hoover & Collier, 1985; Ortiz & Maldonado-Colon, 1986). School psychologists who are unaware of the similarities may make incorrect assumptions about a student's difficulty. Moreover, they may fail to recognize the importance of differentiating between a bilingual student with a disability and a linguistically diverse pupil who is experiencing common problems associated with second-language acquisition (Ochoa et al., 1999). Third, the academic difficulties of students with LEP have been associated with dual-language instructional programs that fail to adequately facilitate the development of the children's first language, which in turn has a negative impact on their second-language development (Cziko, 1992; Ramirez, 1992; Thomas & Collier, 1996, 1997). Cummins (1983) states that "many (but by no means all) of the difficulties minority students experience in school are the result of both inappropriate pedagogy and misconceptions about the nature and effects of bilingualism among educational professionals" (p. 384). Fourth, the new regulations included in PL 105-17 stipulate that lack of instruction or LEP cannot be the determining factor of a child's academic difficulties. In order for school psychologists to reach this conclusion, they will need to understand the second-language acquisition process and dual-language instruction. Fifth, it is important to recognize the impact that bilingualism can have on test performance (Valdes & Figueroa, 1996). Valdes and Figueroa (1996) state that "without an understanding of the nature of bilingualism itself, the problems encountered by bilingual individuals on such tests will continue to be misunderstood" (p. 2).

Second-Language Acquisition

A critical factor that school psychologists need to be aware of when assessing children learning a second language is the difference between basic interpersonal communication skills (BICS) and cognitive academic language proficiency (CALP) (Cummins, 1984). BICS is the type of language that one uses in social conversational settings; CALP is the type of language that one needs to possess in order to experience success in academic situations (Cummins, 1984). The existence of these two types of language proficiencies has been supported by the research literature (Collier, 1987, 1989; Cummins, 1992). Cummins (1984) states that it will take students with LEP approximately 2–3 years to acquire BICS and 5–7 years to acquire CALP.

Cummins (1984) states that in order for linguistically diverse students to acquire CALP in their second language, they need to achieve a minimum threshold level (i.e., at least CALP) in their first language. Thus students who fail to achieve CALP in their first language will have a difficult time acquiring CALP in English. This in turn has a negative impact on their ability to succeed

in academic settings in which only English is used.

The constructs of BICS and CALP have important implications for assessing children learning a second language. School psychologists who are unaware of these constructs can make inappropriate conclusions about the English-language proficiency of a child with LEP. If a school psychologist is able to have a social conversation with such a child in English, he or she might conclude that this child has sufficient English-language proficiency to be assessed in English. Cummins's (1984) research noted that psychologists frequently do not consider the BICS and CALP constructs. Based on the work of Cummins, Ochoa, Gonzalez, and colleagues (1996) have stated: "In these situations, the school psychologist should be careful not to make the assumption that the demonstrated BICS proficiency provides an accurate representation of CALP" (p. 22). Moreover, Chapter 9 of the AERA and colleagues (1999) *Standards for Educational and Psychological Testing* volume provides the following cautions for examiners: "Test use with individuals who have not sufficiently acquired the language of the test may introduce construct-irrelevant components to the testing process. In such instances, test results may not reflect accurately the qualities and competencies intended to be measured" (p. 91).

Dual-Language Instruction Factors

Much controversy surrounds bilingual education in the United States. Krashen (1996) provides an excellent summary of critical issues raised about bilingual education. Many linguistically diverse students in the United States do not receive dual-language instructional programs (Council of Chief State School Officers, cited in McLeod, 1994). When bilingual education is available, one of the following types is usually provided: English as a second language (ESL), transitional bilingual education, maintenance bilingual education, and two-way/dual bilingual education. An ESL program uses English as the language of instruction. This program, however, uses teaching strategies that will help students facilitate the understanding of English. Transitional programs initially use children's native language as the medium of instruction, but eventually switch to English. Transitional programs are usually offered for 2–3 years. In such a program, students are expected to learn English at the expense of their first language and usually exit the program by second or third grade. Maintenance programs use both children's native language and English for instructional purposes. Initially, the ratio of the first language to English is usually 90:10 or 80:20. As students proceed through elementary grades, the amount of instruction in the native language decreases while the amount of instruction in English increases. Usually by third grade, the ratio is 50:50. Students enrolled in maintenance programs learn English, but also maintain their first language. In a two-way/dual bilingual education program, approximately 50% of the students speak a non-English language and 50% speak English. In this program, the non-English language and English are equally valued. The amount of instruction provided in English and the non-English language is approximately equal. This type of program usually lasts from 5 to 6 years. It should be noted that ESL and transitional programs are much more often implemented than maintenance and two-way/dual bilingual education programs.

Ascertaining the type of bilingual education program offered is critical for two reasons. First, "students with LEP are often removed from bilingual [i.e., transitional] and/or English-as-a-second-language (ESL) program prior to achieving CALP in their first language" (Ochoa, Gonzalez, et al., 1996, p. 22). When this removal occurs, such a student may begin to experience academic failure in an English-only instructional setting. Although school officials may attribute this failure to a within-child deficit (Cummins, 1984), "the impact of the early exit, however, needs to be given equal consideration in terms of its influence on the pupil's academic failure" (Ochoa, Gonzalez, et al., 1996, p. 22). Cummins (1984) states:

Minority language students are frequently transferred from bilingual to English-only classrooms when they have developed superficially fluent English communicative skills. Despite being classified as "English proficient" many such students fall progressively further behind grade norms in the development of English academic skills. (p. 131)

A second reason to examine the type of bilingual education program offered is that research indicates variability in terms of educational outcomes. Much research has examined the effectiveness of bilingual education (Baker & de Kanter, 1981, 1983; Ramirez, 1992; Thomas & Collier, 1996, 1997, 2002; Troike, 1978; U.S. General Accounting Office, 1987; Willig, 1985; Zappert & Cruz, 1977) (see Cziko, 1992, and Weaver & Padron, 1999, for thorough reviews). Research has shown very positive student academic outcomes when students have been enrolled in maintenance programs (Ramirez, 1992; Thomas & Collier, 1996, 1997) and dual-language programs (Thomas & Collier, 1996, 1997, 2002). These same studies have found significantly lower academic outcomes for students enrolled in ESL and transitional programs. Thomas and Collier (1997) state that the amount of native-language instruction was the most powerful predictor of students' having positive outcomes. Given this research highlighting significant differences in educational outcomes by type of bilingual program, school psychologists need to consider whether the academic difficulties of a student with LEP might be pedagogically induced.

ASSESSMENT OF LANGUAGE PROFICIENCY

Assessing linguistically diverse students' language proficiency in both their native and second languages is a critical component of assessment that is often not given sufficient consideration by school psychologists. Ochoa, Galarza, and Gonzalez (1996) provide several reasons why language proficiency assessment needs to be conducted with such students. First, there are legal requirements (PL 105-17) and guidelines (AERA et al., 1999, Standards 9.3 and 9.10) that have been previously discussed in this chapter. Second, language proficiency assessment can help the school psychologist ascertain whether a child is in the appropriate educational environment (i.e., bilingual/ESL setting vs. English-only setting). If data obtained from the language proficiency assessment indicate that the child is not placed in the appropriate educational environment for his or her language abilities, one must consider the impact of this inappropriate educational placement on the student's academic difficulties. It is not uncommon to find children with LEP being educated in English-only educational settings because the school does not have bilingual education programs. Third, language proficiency data will help school psychologists "to determine the language in which testing . . . should be done" (Figueroa, 1990b, p. 97). Fourth, language proficiency assessment data can shed light on whether a bilingual child's academic problems stem from the second-language-learning process or a genuine inherent disability (Chamberlain & Medinos-Landurand, 1991; Willig, 1986). It is critical to note that

> a true disability must be apparent in both languages. If there is no disability in the child's dominant language, there can be no disability. Any symptoms of disability must then be manifestations of the process of second language acquisition. (Willig, 1986, p. 164)

The Ochoa, Galarza, and Gonzalez (1996) study revealed that many school psychologists failed to implement all of the following recommended practices in this area: "(a) conducting their own testing rather than relying on external sources, (b) obtaining information about the child's CALP level, and (c) utilizing informal language assessment methods such as language samples and/or interviews" (p. 33). To the extent possible, school psychologists should conduct their own language proficiency assessments. In the event that information used is collected by outside sources (e.g., bilingual education program personnel, other teachers, or paraprofessionals) before the assessment, it is critical to ascertain (1) whether the examiner had training in assessment and scoring procedures (Ochoa, Galarza, & Gonzalez, 1996) and (2) how current the data are. Ortiz and Polyzoi (1986) recommend that language proficiency data be used only if they are less than 6 months old. Thus school psychologists should refrain from using language proficiency data older than 6 months from external sources.

School psychologists should use both formal and informal language methods to assess language proficiency (Figueroa, 1990b; Lopez, 1995; Willig, 1986). Both formal

(Barona & Santos de Barona, 1987; Damico, 1991; Lopez, 1997) and informal (Lopez, 1997) language assessment methods have limitations. Moreover, both receptive and expressive skills should be assessed (Barona & Santos de Barona, 1987; Lopez, 1997). One study (Ochoa, Galarza, & Gonzalez, 1996) found that school psychologists commonly used formal language proficiency measures in both English and Spanish that assessed very limited aspects of language. This practice violates AERA and colleagues (1999) Standard 9.10, as noted above. School psychologists should use both formal and informal methods to assess a bilingual child's CALP capabilities in particular. Currently, there is only one formal language proficiency measure (the Woodcock–Muñoz Language Survey; Woodcock & Muñoz-Sandoval, 1993) that provides data about a child's CALP level via a broad view of language (oral language, reading/writing, and broad skills) in both English and Spanish. The Woodcock–Muñoz Language Survey manual provides five different CALP levels: 1= negligible, 2 = very limited, 3 = limited, 4 = fluent, and 5 = advanced. According to the test authors, a student must have at least a CALP score of 4 in order to be considered to have CALP in a given language. Information obtained from the Woodcock–Muñoz Language Survey can be corroborated by informal language proficiency procedures. Lopez (1997) states that CALP can be assessed informally by observing a student with LEP verbally interacting with peers and his or her teacher via classroom instructional activities in both his native language and English. Lopez also recommends that samples of such a student's written work in the native language and English be produced. Moreover, Lopez states that a school psychologist can assess a child's BICS via language samples by observing him or her verbally interacting with friends and family members in nonacademic settings. School psychologists should refer to Damico (1991) and Prutting (1983) for further discussions of how to obtain and conduct language samples. Moreover, the use of other informal language assessment methods, such as the Qualitative Use of English and Spanish Tasks (Gonzalez, 1991, 1994, 1995; Gonzalez et al., 1997), may provide additional information about the linguistic abilities of a child with LEP.

ACHIEVEMENT ASSESSMENT

Overview of Historical and Current Research Pertaining to Achievement Testing

Figueroa (1990a) and Valdes and Figueroa (1996) provide excellent historical reviews of the empirical research literature pertaining to the achievement testing of bilingual students. Their reviews state that the achievement outcomes for linguistically diverse learners have traditionally been significantly below those of English-speaking white children. Figueroa states, "Unlike the early research literature on intelligence, the early achievement studies on linguistic minority pupils gave more attention to the complex background variables possibly affecting academic achievement: SES, language proficiency, and schooling" (pp. 677–678). Figueroa, however, states that while the low socioeconomic levels of linguistically diverse students were described in studies, they were not controlled for; the same pattern was noted for language proficiency. Figueroa, noting that studies also described the unfavorable schooling conditions of bilingual children, observes that: "Inherently, achievement tests evaluate not only what a student has learned, but also what a school system provides" (p. 679). More recent research studies have continued to ignore the impact that different levels of English-language proficiency have on achievement test results (Figueroa, 1990a). Valdes and Figueroa's review of the empirical literature found that achievement tests had appropriate psychometric properties with linguistically diverse children; the studies they reviewed, however, did not account for different levels of language proficiency. Valdes and Figueroa also note that based on a review of empirical studies, "achievement tests are open to criticism with respect to predictive validity" (p. 112).

Current Practice

Ochoa, Powell, and Robles-Pina (1996) examined the assessment practices of school psychologists who evaluated linguistically diverse students. We found that the most commonly used formal measures to assess achievement of such students in English and Spanish were the Woodcock–Johnson or Woodcock–Johnson—Revised and the Bateria Woodcock Psico-Educativa en Espanol, respectively. These two instruments were used by 77% and 79% of the school psychologists surveyed, respectively. Moreover, they were the most preferred formal measures. In addition, the Spanish version of Brigance Diagnostic Assessment of Basic Skills was utilized by nearly half of the school psychologists to assess achievement. Curriculum-based assessment was used by approximately two-thirds of the school psychologists to assess academic achievement. Ochoa, Powell, and Robles-Pina also noted that "interestingly, many more school psychologists reported how they assessed achievement in English but failed to provide the same information for Spanish" (p. 268). We concluded that this might be a result of school psychologists' assessing achievement in English only.

Caution should be exercised in using formal standardized achievement measures with bilingual students, for several reasons other than just psychometric issues. First, the impact of level of language proficiency should be considered. "Achievement tests can become measures of English-language proficiency, especially when an analysis of their instructions, content, and format clearly shows that these rest on linguistic skills commensurate with those of monolingual pupils (idioms, facts, CALP, etc)." (Figueroa, 1990a, p. 688). Second, the context in which these students are taught must also be considered.

> Valid tests in the ethnic language are relevant for children in the United States if the educational experiences of the norming samples are congruent with curricula in bilingual education programs. But even in these special circumstances, the tests should reflect the unique academic learning and classroom information processing of children in classes where two language systems are appropriately used. (Valdes & Figueroa, 1996, p. 114)

Alternative Methods of Assessment and Future Directions

The use of alternative assessment methods to assess the academic performance of linguistically diverse students is warranted, given the previously noted concerns. Some of these methods include observations, rating scales, checklists, performance assessments, (Barona & Santos de Barona, 1987; Gonzalez et al., 1997), work samples (Barona & Santos de Barona, 1987; de Valenzuela & Cervantes, 1998), student interviews (Barona & Santos de Barona, 1987), criterion-referenced tests, and curriculum-based measurements (Barona & Santos de Barona, 1987; Lopez, 1995). In addition, Caterino (1990) recommends developing local norms. Developing local norms with curriculum-based measurements in both the native language and English would help to address the two concerns noted about formal measures. This alternative method would allow a school psychologist to compare the academic performance of a child with LEP to that of other such students who have been provided a similar instructional arrangement (e.g., bilingual education). If the child in question is performing significantly below his peers with LEP, this might provide a clinical indication that this child's academic problems could stem from factors other than second-language acquisition. Moreover, the school psychologist can compare the child's performance across both languages. The school psychologist should also determine whether the data obtained from curriculum-based measurement seem to corroborate information obtained from formal academic measures, as well as information about the child's CALP reading/writing score obtained during language proficiency assessment.

Moreover, the school psychologists should examine the school records of the child with LEP, especially grades. The school psychologist should examine whether the child was able to perform adequately while in bilingual education. If the child in question has been removed from a bilingual education program and is now in an English-only instructional setting, the school psychologist can compare the child's performance when native-language support is and is not provided. If the student's academic performance appeared to decline once native-language instructional support was dropped, the psychologist needs to examine whether this might have caused the child's failure. Second, some states require that students with LEP who are in bilingual educa-

tion be assessed with a state-administered, criterion-referenced test in their native language (e.g., the Texas Assessment of Academic Skills). Data obtained from this type of test will help the school psychologist to ascertain what skills a child has and has not mastered. Moreover, a comparison of the child's performance to that of other same-grade students with LEP who have had the same type of bilingual education instructional opportunities should also be conducted.

One future direction that merits consideration in this area is to incorporate Cummins's (1984) work in the area of CALP (Valdes & Figueroa, 1996). Valdes and Figueroa (1996) state:

> Using the most popular model for bilingual academic learning (Cummins, 1984) . . . these criteria might include norms in the ethnic and societal language that would covary directly with Cognitive Language Academic Proficiency (CALP) in the ethnic language and with the development of a common underlying proficiency that would be accessible in both languages only after reaching a critical stage in bilingual language proficiency. . . . The bilingual learner and the manner in which he or she "achieves" [are] currently not addressed in tests that are available in the ethnic language and societal languages. . . . The process of academic learning for these students is far more complicated than for a monolingual learner. (pp. 114–115)

INTELLECTUAL ASSESSMENT

Historical Overview of Research

Figueroa (1990a) and Valdes and Figueroa (1996) also provide excellent historical reviews of the empirical research literature pertaining to the intellectual assessment of bilingual students. Figueroa (1990a) has identified the following four major themes in the literature:

> 1. Nonverbal test scores were consistently higher than verbal test scores for virtually all language groups. . . . 2. Most studies ignored the effects of a second language on test scores. . . . 3. The design of most studies was typically inadequate. . . . 4. National chauvinism and "genetic" attributions about mental ability permeated the studies on "race psychology." (pp. 674–676)

With respect to the second point noted, Valdes and Figueroa state that the research literature viewed bilingualism as a "language handicap" that had a negative impact on verbal IQ scores and students' ability to acquire English. These authors question the designs of studies because they failed to consider the effects of socioeconomic status, poor schooling, and English-language proficiency in student test results. Valdes and Figueroa state that

> psychometric properties, by and large, came to be seen as robust indices of test appropriateness for use with circumstantial bilingual populations. Reliabilities were universally as good for monolingual English speakers and for speakers of other languages. The same applied to most measures of validity. The one unattended and occasional exception was predictive validity. Its record was not universally consistent. (p. 90)

Overview of Current Research

Upon reviewing the research literature to 1990 on statistical test bias, Reynolds and Kaiser (1990) concluded that tests of intelligence were not biased against minority English-speaking students. Reynolds and Kaiser have discussed three types of bias that need to be reviewed: content bias, construct bias, and predictive bias. Moreover, they caution against using expert judgment of bias: "Given the significant and reliable methods developed over the last several decades in bias research, it is untenable at this point to abandon statistical analysis in favor of 'armchair' determinations of bias" (p. 647).

With respect to content bias, Valdes and Figueroa's (1996) review of the empirical literature failed to reveal ethnic differences between Hispanics and whites with respect to item difficulty values. With respect to construct bias, Valdes and Figueroa's review also found no ethnic differences with respect to test reliability and test factor structures. The research literature, however, is not as conclusive with respect to predictive bias. Reynolds and Kaiser's (1990) definition of predictive bias, which is rephrased from Cleary, Humphreys, Kendrick, and Wesman's (1975) definition, is as follows:

> A test is considered biased with respect to predictive validity if the inference drawn from the test score is not made with the smallest feasible random error or if there is constant error in an inference for prediction as a function of membership in a particular group. (p. 638)

Thus the issue with predictive validity is not whether one group scores lower than another; rather, it is whether the test predicts with the same degree of accuracy for both groups (Valdes & Figueroa, 1996). In their review of the research literature, Valdes and Figueroa state that "predictive validity is not consistently found when language proficiency is controlled for . . ." (p. 102).

Current Practice

Ochoa, Robles-Pina, and Powell (1996) investigated how school psychologists assessed the intellectual functioning of linguistically diverse students. They noted five assessment trends. First, the school psychologists surveyed were using more than one instrument to assess the cognitive functioning of bilingual students. The most commonly used measure to assess such pupils was the Wechsler Intelligence Scale for Children—Revised (WISC-R) or WISC-III in English only. This measure was utilized by 52% of the school psychologists surveyed. Second, nonverbal measures were frequently utilized. The following four nonverbal measures or methods ranked among the top six instruments utilized: the Draw-A-Person (47%), the Leiter International Performance Scale (40%), the WISC-R or WISC-III Performance scale only (38%), and the Test of Nonverbal Intelligence (TONI) or TONI-2 (36%). Third, formally and informally translated intelligence measures were not frequently used. Fourth, intermixing or switching languages while administering a test was not a frequently employed practice. Fifth, the use of alternative or dynamic assessment was rare.

Use of More than One Instrument, and Testing in English Only

A review of these assessment trends merits discussion. In regard to the first practice, the use of several measures to assess the intellectual abilities of children with LEP is viewed positively. Upon reviewing the empirical literature of test bias, Reynolds and Kaiser recommend that "assessment of multiple abilities with multiple methods" is one guideline "to follow in order to insure equitable assessment" (p. 646).

Experts in the area of bilingual assessment raise several concerns about using IQ measures in English with linguistically diverse students. Lopez (1997) cautions against using intelligence measures in English with this population. Figueroa (1990b) states that assessing such students only in English will not provide a valid picture of the children's intellectual abilities. Barona and Santos de Barona (1987) state, "Since limited English proficient students generally are not included in the standardization sample, comparisons to the norm reference group are not appropriate" (p. 196). Chamberlain and Medinos-Landurand (1991) add:

> If the purpose of testing is to diagnose a learning disability, both languages must be used. . . . If LEP students suspected of having disabilities are assessed in English only, the result will be an incomplete profile no matter how excellent the assessment. When assessing in only one language, a disability cannot be accurately distinguished from limited English proficiency. (p. 133)

Given these issues/concerns, school psychologists should proceed with extreme caution when assessing linguistically diverse students with IQ measures in English.

Given that the WISC-R or WISC-III is the instrument most commonly used with linguistically diverse students, additional discussion of this instrument is warranted. Cummins (1984) has expressed reservations about interpreting the scores as a true picture of such a child's intelligence when this test is administered in English, although he notes that "the pattern of scores may suggest diagnostic clues if the individual student's scores are interpreted in relation to the typical pattern" noted for students with LEP (p. 57). Flanagan, McGrew, and Ortiz (2000) state that "dual-language learners or bilingual pupils tend not to be systematically included or accommodated in the design and norming of any of the currently available Wechsler Scales (or any other test of intelligence or cognitive ability)" (p. 303). Also according to Flanagan and colleagues,

> In sum, professionals engaged in the assessment of culturally and linguistically diverse individuals with the Wechsler Scales (or other standardized, norm-referenced instruments) should recognize three essential points: (1) the Wechsler Scales are culturally loaded and tend to reflect the values, beliefs, and knowledge that are deemed important for success in the culture in which the test were developed—that is, U.S. mainstream culture; (2) the Wechsler Scales require language (or communication) on both the part of the examiner and the examinee and . . . linguistic factors can affect administration, comprehension, and performance on virtually all tests including the performance tests, such as Block Design; and (3) the individual Wechsler subtests vary on both dimensions, that is, the degree to which they are culturally loaded and require language. (p. 304)

Flanagan and colleagues, however, contend:

> When the Wechsler Scales are used within a selective cross-battery framework that also accommodates cultural and linguistic elements, they can be used to provide a defensible method that may lead to increases in specificity and validity with concomitant reductions in diagnostic and interpretive bias for diverse populations. (p. 295)

I myself believe that the use of the WISC-III in English only can be construed as appropriate practice only if a student has achieved CALP in English. Even in these cases, one would need to address the first and third factors previously noted by Flanagan and colleagues via the cross-battery approach they have developed.

Use of Nonverbal Measures

The use of nonverbal measures to assess the intellectual abilities of linguistically diverse students is generally regarded as an acceptable or promising practice (Caterino, 1990; Clarizio, 1982; Esquivel, 1988; Figueroa, 1990b; Wilen & Sweeting, 1986). Figueroa (1990b), Holtzman and Wilkinson (1991), and Lopez (1997) delineate the limitations of using nonverbal measures. Figueroa states that nonverbal measures "are often not good predictors of academic achievement" (p. 102). Holtzman and Wilkinson note that "only a partial measure of student's intellectual ability is obtained and no measure . . . of verbal abilities can be calculated" (p. 265). Lopez adds that many nonverbal measures do not include bilingual children in their norms.

One recently developed measure, the Universal Nonverbal Intelligence Test (UNIT; Bracken & McCallum, 1998), appears to address some of the aforementioned concerns associated with nonverbal tests. According to Bracken and McCallum (1998), "Although its administration and response formats are entirely nonverbal, the UNIT is designed to provide a comprehensive assessment of general intelligence" (p. 1). The UNIT provides a Full Scale IQ and the following four quotient scores: Memory, Reasoning, Symbolic (verbal), and Nonsymbolic. In particular, it should be noted that the Symbolic Quotient "is an index of an individual's ability to solve problems that involve meaningful material and whose solutions lend themselves to internal verbal mediation, including labeling, organizing, and categorizing" (p. 4). The sample did include "students receiving English as a second language (ESL) and bilingual education" (Bracken & McCallum, 1998, p. 1).

Bracken and McCallum (1998) obtained the following corrected correlations between the UNIT Extended Battery Full Scale IQ and the reading scales of the Spanish Woodcock Language Proficiency Battery—Revised with a sample of students being served in bilingual education: .17 with Basic Reading Skills, .55 with Reading Comprehension, and .39 with Broad Reading. Moreover, the corrected correlations obtained between the Symbolic Quotient (verbal) of the UNIT Extended Battery and the reading scales of the Spanish Woodcock Language Proficiency Battery—Revised with a sample of students being served in bilingual education were .30 with Basic Reading Skills, .57 with Reading Comprehension, and .50 with Broad Reading. Bracken and McCallum also conducted fairness studies with students in bilingual and ESL programs. These students were matched with English-speaking students from the standardization sample with respect to age, gender, and parental educational level. The Full Scale IQ score (mean = 100, standard deviation = 15) differences between these two groups were 2.82, 3.56, and 3.73 on the Abbreviated Battery, Standard Battery, and Extended Battery, respectively. The English-speaking group scored higher than the linguistically diverse students on all three batteries.

Flanagan and colleagues (2000) raise a factor that one should consider before using a nonverbal measure to assess the intellectual functioning of linguistically diverse students. They suggest that the use of some nonverbal measures will reduce a significant amount of or all "oral (expressive or receptive) language requirements" (p. 301). They also point out that test performance in these situations is still "dependent on" accurate nonverbal communication between the psychologist and child, and that "nonverbal measures do not necessarily eliminate the influence of culture either" (p. 302).

Formally and Informally Translated Tests

The use of formally translated IQ measures with linguistically diverse students has many limitations (Barona & Santos de Barona, 1987; Esquivel, 1988; Figueroa, 1990b, Lopez, 1997; Valdes & Figueroa, 1996; Wilen & Sweeting, 1986). An example of a formally translated test is the Escala de Inteligencia Wechsler para Ninos—Revisada. The use of formally translated measures is not appropriate practice, unless a translation has been *independently* standardized, normed, and validated (which is rarely the case). Moreover, the use of informally translated IQ measures is not valid (Figueroa, 1990b). According to Figueroa (1990b), "this is one instance when confession does not absolve" (p. 98). "A translated test is a different test, an unknown test, an unfair test" (Valdes & Figueroa, 1996, p. 106).

Intermixing or Switching between Languages

The practice of intermixing or switching between a child's first and second languages when administering an IQ measure is also not appropriate practice, unless the IQ measure has been developed and normed in this fashion. Most IQ tests, however, have not been developed and normed in a manner that incorporates simultaneous administration in two languages.

One might argue from a theoretical perspective, however, that it is appropriate to intermix and switch languages during testing, because this allows a child to use both language registers to tackle the problem at hand. When linguistically diverse children attempt to solve tasks in the real world, they use all of the dual-language skills at their disposal. Such students may be able to complete a task successfully in one language but not in the other language or vice versa, depending on the type of dual-language instructional program they have received and their CALP level in each language. When these students are assessed in separate languages in a sequential manner (e.g., entirely in Spanish only, and then entirely in English only, or vice versa), this might result in an underestimate of their abilities. Valdes and Figueroa (1996) state:

> When a bilingual individual confronts a monolingual test, developed by monolingual individuals, and standardized and normed on a monolingual population, both the test taker and test are asked to do something that they cannot. The bilingual test taker cannot perform like a monolingual. The monolingual test can't "measure' in the other language. (p. 172)

One recently developed IQ test, the Bilingual Verbal Ability Test (BVAT; Munoz-Sandoval, Cummins, Alvarado, & Ruef, 1998), appears to address both the psychometric and theoretical concerns about using two languages simultaneously. The BVAT is first administered in English. Once an appropriate basal and ceiling are established in each subtest in English, the student is then read-ministered those items missed in English in his or her native language (e.g., Spanish) and given additional items, if appropriate, in order to establish a new ceiling in the second language. The additional items answered in the second language are added in order to obtain a gain score. The BVAT provides a Verbal IQ that incorporates both of the child's languages by adding the correct items in English and the gain score obtained in the second language. Thus the examiner can obtain information about how the child's Verbal IQ is affected when the student is allowed to use both languages. The BVAT is available in the following 15 languages: Arabic, Chinese (Simplified and Traditional), French, German, Haitian Creole, Hindi, Japanese, Korean, Polish, Portuguese, Russian, Spanish, Turkish, and Vietnamese.

Use of Alternative or Dynamic Assessment

Ochoa, Robles-Pina, and Powell's (1996) found that alternative or dynamic assessment practices—such as the Learning Potential Assessment Device (LPAD; Feuerstein, 1979) and the System of Multicultural Pluralistic Assessment (SOMPA; Mercer, 1979)—were rarely used, and then only by less than 1% of the sample we surveyed. The LPAD lacks psychometric support (Frisby & Braden, 1992) and has other limitations (Glutting & McDermott, 1990). Kamphaus (1993) points out similar problems with the SOMPA. Ochoa, Robles-Pina, and Powell (1996) and Lopez (1997) suggest that additional research is needed in this area.

FUTURE DIRECTIONS

The assessment of culturally and linguistically diverse students is quite complex and plagued with many problems. According to Valdes and Figueroa (1996), the following three options are available to those in the testing profession:

> Option 1 [would be to] attempt to minimize the potential harm of using existing tests, Option 2 [would be to] temporarily ban all testing of circumstantial bilinguals until psychometrically valid tests can be developed for this population, or Option 3 [would be to] develop alternative approaches to testing and assessment. (p. 172)

Valdes and Figueroa recommend the second option. During this test-banning period, Valdes and Figueroa advocate "funding and support of basic research on circumstantial bilingualism and the funding and support of the development of both a theory and a practice of bilingual testing" (p. 187).

With regard to the first option, Valdes and Figueroa state: "In spite of best intentions, it is doubtful that existing instruments can actually be used either equitably or meaningfully to make important decisions about circumstantial bilingual individuals" (p. 174). Thus they do not endorse this option.

However, a recent model developed by Flanagan and colleagues (2000) attempts to limit bias in the assessment of culturally and linguistically diverse learners, and thus in essence incorporates Valdes and Figueroa's (1996) first option. Flanagan and colleagues' model uses the Gf-Gc theoretical framework. Moreover, this model classifies subtests of existing measures along two additional factors. The first factor, "degree of cultural loading" (p. 305), "represents the degree to which subtests require specific knowledge of and experience with mainstream U.S. culture" (p. 305). The second factor is "degree of linguistic demand" (p. 305). Flanagan and colleagues classified subtests of existing measures along these two factors within the Gf-Gc theoretical framework. Subtests of existing measures were identified as being at one of three levels in regard to both factors: high, moderate, or low. Flanagan and colleagues acknowledge that the classification of subtests into particular levels across both linguistic-demand and cultural-loading factors needs much additional empirical study. They make the following statements about their framework:

> Although the classifications are insufficient, by themselves, to establish a comprehensive basis for assessment of diverse individuals, they are, nevertheless, capable of greatly supplementing the assessment process in both the diagnostic and interpretive arenas. . . . These classifications may also serve as a starting point for researchers and practitioners to establish empirically supportable standards of practice with respect to test selection. (pp. 311, 313)

Flanagan and colleagues' model is innovative and warrants serious consideration by researchers.

With respect to Valdes and Figueroa's (1996) third option, one factor that needs to be seriously considered in developing alternative approaches is the extent of a child's linguistic abilities across both languages. Valdes and Figueroa note that "Limited English speakers are not included in the norms [of most existing instruments] and the continua of bilingual skills [are] not controlled for in norm tables" (p. 191). Future research should examine the impact of children's varying CALP levels in both their native language and in English on assessment outcomes. This line of research should be pursued in examining for statistical bias.

Valdes and Figueroa state that many studies have not controlled for varying degrees of language proficiency in examining for bias. Research needs to examine whether bias exists, does not exist, or varies according to a student's CALP level both in his or her native language and in English. This should be done across the following methods of assessment used with bilingual students: (1) nonverbal measures, (2) testing in English, (3) testing in a student's native language, and (4) testing in both English and the native language simultaneously.

The use of the Woodcock–Munoz Language Survey (Woodcock & Muñoz-Sandoval, 1993) might enable researchers to identify the many different types of circumstantial bilingualism, and thus allow them to conduct statistical bias studies. As noted earlier, the Woodcock–Munoz Language Survey classifies the linguistic abilities of students with LEP into five different CALP levels: 1= negligible, 2 = very limited, 3 = limited, 4 = fluent, and 5 = advanced. Students receive a CALP level in English and in Spanish. Thus there are 25 different types of bilingualism (e.g., each CALP level in English crossed with each CALP level in Spanish) that can be obtained from the Woodcock–Muñoz Language Survey. Each of these types of bilingualism should be examined. This line of research would help the field to examine whether norms should control for students' varying degrees of proficiency in their first language and in English, as discussed by Valdes and Figueroa. Results from this line of research could have significant implications for practice. For example, if a student with circumstantial bilingualism has not achieved CALP in either language (e.g., CALP level of 2 in Spanish and CALP level of 1 in English), would it be more appropriate to administer a nonverbal measure (e.g., the UNIT) or to assess the student in both languages simultaneously (e.g., the BVAT) than to assess the child in Spanish, even if he or she is more proficient in this language? How should practice differ if the student has achieved CALP in his or her first language but not in English (e.g., CALP level of 4 in Spanish and CALP level of 2 in English)? Moreover, how should one assess a bilingual student who has achieved CALP in both languages (e.g., CALP levels of 4 in both Spanish and English)? What should be done when a student with LEP has few or almost no language abilities in either his or her native language or English (e.g., CALP levels of 1 in both Spanish and English)? Similar questions could be asked for each of the other types of bilingualism.

I believe that practitioners should continue to proceed along the first option with extreme caution, and should acknowledge many of the limitations and issues raised in this chapter when interpreting results and making eligibility decisions. Given ethical guidelines, professional standards, and legal mandates, university trainers need to make sure that their students are exposed to and fully comprehend the issues associated with assessing linguistically diverse children. Moreover, state and national associations should make sure that this information is available to practitioners via continuing education requirements. Proceeding with the first option is justifiable as long as the field begins to proceed with the third option, along with the research advocated in regard to the second option by Valdes and Figueroa (1996). Given the issues raised with disproportionate representation, the field can ill afford to maintain the current status quo.

REFERENCES

American Educational Research Association (AERA), American Psychological Association (APA), & National Council on Measurement in Education (NCME). (1999). *Standards for educational and psychological testing*. Washington, DC: American Educational Research Association.

American Psychological Association APA. (1990). *Guidelines for providers of psychological services to ethnic, linguistic, and culturally diverse populations*. Washington, DC: Author.

Artiles, A. J., & Trent, S. C. (1994). Overrepresentation of minority students in special education: A continuing debate. *Journal of Special Education, 27,* 410–437.

Baker, K., & de Kanter, A. (1981). *Effectiveness of bilingual education: A review of the literature*. Washington, DC: U.S. Department of Education, Office of Planning, Budget, and Evaluation.

Baker, K., & de Kanter, A. (1983). Federal policy and the effectiveness of bilingual education. In K. Baker & A. de Kanter (Eds.), *Bilingual education: A reappraisal of federal policy* (pp. 33–86). Lexington, MA: Heath.

Barona, A. (1991). Assessment of multicultural preschool children. In B. Bracken (Ed.), *The psychoeducational assessment of preschool children*

(2nd ed., pp. 379–391). Needham Heights, MA: Allyn & Bacon.

Barona, A., & Santos de Barona, M. (1987). A model for the assessment of limited English proficient students referred for special education services. In S. H. Fradd & W. J. Tikunoff (Eds.), *Bilingual education and bilingual special education* (pp. 183–210). Boston: College-Hill Press.

Barona, A., & Santos de Barona, M. (2000). Assessing multicultural preschool children. In B. Bracken (Ed.), *The psychoeducational assessment of preschool children* (3rd ed., pp. 282–297). Needham Heights, MA: Allyn & Bacon.

Bracken, B., & McCallum, R. S. (1998). *Universal Nonverbal Intelligence Test: Examiner's manual*. Itasca, IL: Riverside.

Caterino, L. C. (1990). Step-by-step procedures for the assessment of language minority children. In A. Barona & E. E. Garcia (Eds.), *Children at risk: Poverty, minority status, and other issues in educational equity* (pp. 269–282). Washington DC: National Association of School Psychologists.

Chamberlain, P., & Medinos-Landurand, P. (1991). Practical considerations in the assessment of LEP students with special needs. In E. V. Hamayan & J. S. Damico (Eds.), *Limiting bias in the assessment of bilingual students* (pp. 111–156). Austin, TX: Pro-Ed.

Chapa, J. (1990). Limited English proficient student demographics. In *Proceedings of the first research symposium on limited English proficient students' issues* (pp. 85–112). Washington, DC: Office of Bilingual Education and Minority Students.

Chinn, P. C., & Hughes, S. (1987). Representation of minority students in special education classes. *Remedial and Special Education, 8,* 41–46.

Clarizio, H. F. (1982). Intellectual assessment of Hispanic children. *Psychology in the Schools, 19*(1), 61–71.

Cleary, T. A., Humphreys, L. G., Kendrick, S. A., & Wesman, A. (1975). Educational uses of tests with disadvantaged students. *American Psychologist, 30,* 15–41.

Cummins, J. (1983). Bilingualism and special education: Program and pedagogical issues. *Learning Disability Quarterly, 6,* 373–386.

Cummins, J. (1984). *Bilingual special education issues in assessment and pedagogy*. San Diego, CA: College-Hill Press.

Cummins, J. (1992). Bilingual education and English immersion: The Ramirez report in theoretical perspective. *Bilingual Research Journal, 16,* 91–104.

Cziko, G. (1992). The evaluation of bilingual education: From necessity and probability to possibility. *Educational Researcher, 21*(2), 10–15.

Damico, J. S. (1991). Descriptive assessment of communicative ability in limited English proficient students. In E. V. Hamayan & J. S. Damico (Eds.), *Limiting bias in the assessment of bilingual students* (pp. 157–217). Austin, TX: Pro-Ed.

Daughtery, D. W. (1999). Disproportionality issues in the implementation of IDEA '97. *National Association of School Psychologists Communique, 28*(4), 16–18.

de Valenzuela, J. S., & Cervantes, H. T. (1998). Procedures and techniques for assessing the bilingual exceptional child. In L. M. Baca & H. T. Cervantes (Eds.), *The bilingual special education interface* (3rd ed., pp. 168–187). Columbus, OH: Merrill.

Diana v. State Board of Education, C.A. No. C-70-37 (N.D. Cal. 1970) (settled by consent decree).

Education for All Handicapped Children Act of 1975, PL 94-142, 20 U.S.C. § 1401 (1975).

Educational Testing Service (ETS). (2000). *ETS standards for quality and fairness*. Princeton, NJ: Author.

Esquivel, G. B. (1988). Best practices in the assessment of limited English proficient and bilingual children. In A. Thomas & J. Grimes (Eds.), *Best practices in school psychology* (pp. 113–123). Washington, DC: National Association of School Psychologists.

Feuerstein, R. (1979). *The dynamic assessment of retarded performers*. Baltimore: University Park Press.

Figueroa, R. A. (1989). Psychological testing of linguistic-minority students: Knowledge gaps and regulations. *Exceptional Children, 56,* 145–152.

Figueroa, R. A. (1990a). Assessment of linguistic minority group children. In C. R. Reynolds & R. W. Kamphaus (Eds.), *Handbook of psychological and educational assessment of children: Intelligence and achievement* (pp. 671–696). New York: Guilford Press.

Figueroa, R. A. (1990b). Best practices in the assessment of bilingual children In A. Thomas & J. Grimes (Eds.), *Best practices in school psychology II* (pp. 93–106). Washington, DC: National Association of School Psychologists.

Figueroa, R. A., & Artiles, A. (1999). Disproportionate minority placement in special education programs: Old problems, new explanations. In A. Tashakkori & S. H. Ochoa (Eds.), *Reading on equal education: Vol. 16. Education of Hispanics in the United States: Politics, policies, and outcomes* (pp. 93–118). New York: AMS Press.

Figueroa, R. A., Sandoval, J., & Merino, B. (1984). School psychology and limited English-proficient (LEP) children: New competencies. *Journal of School Psychology, 22,* 131–143.

Flanagan, D. P., McGrew, K. S., & Ortiz, S. O. (2000). *The Wechsler intelligence scales and Gf-Gc theory: A contemporary approach to interpretation.* Needham Heights, MA: Allyn & Bacon.

Fradd, S. H., & Wilen, D. K. (1990). *Using interpreters and translators to meet the needs of handicapped language minority students and their families.* Washington, DC: National Clearinghouse for Bilingual Education. (ERIC Document Reproduction Service No. ED 332540)

Frisby, C. L., & Braden, J. P. (1992). Feuerstein's dynamic assessment approach: A semantic, logical, and empirical critique. *Journal of Special Education, 26*(3), 281–301.

Garcia, S. B., & Ortiz, A. A. (1988). *Preventing inappropriate referrals of language minority students to special education* (Occasional Papers in Bilingual Education No. 5). Wheaton, MD: National Clearinghouse for Bilingual Education.

Garcia, S. B., & Yates, J. (1986). *Policy issues associated with serving bilingual exceptional children.* Washington, DC: National Clearinghouse for Hand-

icapped and Gifted Children. (ERIC Document Reproduction Service No. ED 261-524)

Glutting, J. J., & McDermott, P. A. (1990). Principles and problems in learning potential. In C. R. Reynolds & R. W. Kamphaus (Eds.), *Handbook of psychological and educational assessment of children: Intelligence and achievement* (pp. 296–347). New York: Guilford Press.

Gonzalez, V. (1991). *A model of cognitive, cultural, and lingusitic variables affecting bilingual Spanish/English children's development of concepts and language.* Doctoral dissertation, University of Texas at Austin. (ERIC Document Reproduction Service No. ED 345 562)

Gonzalez, V. (1994). A model of cognitive, cultural, and linguistic variables affecting bilingual Spanish/English children's development of concepts and language. Hispanic *Journal of Behavioral Sciences, 16*(4), 396–421.

Gonzalez, V. (1995). *Cognition, culture, and language in bilingual children: Conceptual and semantic development.* Bethesda, MD: Austin & Winfield.

Gonzalez, V., Brusca-Vega, R., & Yawkey, T. (1997). *Assessment and instruction of culturally and linguistically diverse students with or at risk of learning problems.* Boston: Allyn & Bacon.

Hamayan, E. V., & Damico, J. S. (1991a). Developing and using a second language. In E. V. Hamayan & J. S. Damico (Eds.), *Limiting bias in the assessment of bilingual students* (pp. 39–76). Austin, TX: Pro Ed.

Hamayan, E. V., & Damico, J. S. (Eds.). (1991b). *Limiting bias in the assessment of bilingual students.* Austin, TX: Pro-Ed.

Harris, J. D., Gray, B. A., Davis, J. E., Zaremba, E. T., & Argulewicz, E. N. (1988). The exclusionary clause and the disadvantaged: Do we try to comply with the law? *Journal of Learning Disabilities, 21,* 581–583.

Holtzman, W. H., Jr., & Wilkinson, C. Y. (1991). Assessment of cognitive ability. In E. V. Hamayan & J. S. Damico (Eds.), *Limiting bias in the assessment of bilingual students* (pp. 111–156). Austin, TX: Pro-Ed.

Hoover, J. J. & Collier, C. (1985). Referring culturally different children: Sociocultural considerations. *Academic Therapy, 20,* 503–509.

Individuals with Disabilities Education Act (IDEA) of 1990, PL 101-476, 20 U.S.C. § 1400 (1990).

Individuals with Disabilities Education Act (IDEA) Amendments of 1997, PL 105-17, 20 U.S.C. § 1400 et seq. (West, 1997).

Kamphaus, R. W. (1993). *Clinical assessment of children's intelligence: A handbook for professional practice.* Boston: Allyn & Bacon.

Kovaleski, J. F., & Prasse, D. P. (1999). Assessing lack of instruction. *National Association of School Psychologists Communique , 28*(4), 24–25.

Krashen, S. D. (1996). *Under attack: The case against bilingual education.* Culver City, CA: Language Education Associates.

Kretschner, R. E. (1991). Exceptionality and the limited-English-proficient student: Historical and practical contexts. In E. V. Hamayan & J. S. Damico (Eds.), *Limiting bias in the assessment of bilingual students* (pp. 1–38). Austin, TX: Pro-Ed.

Li, C., Walton, J. R., & Nuttall, E. V. (1999). Preschool evaluation of culturally and linguistically diverse children. In E. Vasquez Nuttall, I. Romero, & J. Kalesnik (Eds.), *Assessing and screening preschoolers: Psychological and educational dimensions* (pp. 296–317). Needham Heights, MA: Allyn & Bacon.

Lopez, E. C. (1995). Best practices in working with bilingual children. In A. Thomas & J. Grimes (Eds.), *Best practices in school psychology III* (pp. 1111–1121). Washington, DC: National Association of School Psychologists.

Lopez, E. C. (1997). Cognitive assessment of LEP and bilingual children. In D. P. Flanagan, J. L. Genshaft, & P. L. Harrison (Eds.), *Contemporary intellectual assessment: Theories, tests and issues* (pp. 503–516). New York: Guilford Press.

McGrew, K. S., Flanagan, D. P., & Ortiz, S. O. (1998). Gf-Gc cross-battery interpretation and selective cross-battery assessment: Referral concerns and the needs of culturally and linguistically diverse populations. In K. S. McGrew & D. P. Flanagan (Eds.), *The intelligence test desk reference: Gf-Gc cross-battery assessment* (pp. 401–444). Needham Heights, MA: Allyn & Bacon.

McLeod, B. (1994). Linguistic diversity and academic achievement. In B. McLeod (Ed.), *Language and learning* (pp. 9–44). Albany: State University of New York Press.

Medina, V. (1982). *Issues regarding the use of interpreters and translators in a school setting.* Washington, DC: National Clearinghouse for Handicapped and Gifted Children. (ERIC Document Reproduction Service No. ED 239454)

Mercer, J. R. (1979). *System of multicultural pluralistic assessment: Conceptual and technical manual.* New York: Psychological Corporation.

Miller, N., & Abudarham, S. (1984). Management of communication problems in bilingual children. In N. Miller (Ed.), *Bilingualism and language disability: Assessment and remediation* (pp. 177–198). San Diego, CA: College-Hill Press.

Munoz-Sandoval, A. F., Cummins, J., Alvarado, C. G., & Ruef, M. L. (1998). *Bilingual Verbal Ability Test.* Itasca, IL: Riverside.

National Association of School Psychologists (NASP). (1997). *Professional conduct manual for school psychologists containing the principles for professional ethics and the standards for the provision of school psychological services.* Bethesda, MD: Author.

National Research Council. (2002). *Minority students in special and gifted education* (M. S. Donovan & C. T. Cross, Eds.). Washington, DC: National Academy Press.

Nuttall, E. V. (1987). Survey of current practices in the psychological assessment of limited-English proficient handicapped children. *Journal of School Psychology, 25,* 53–61.

Ochoa, S. H., Galarza, A., & Gonzalez, D. (1996). An investigation of school psychologists' assessment practices of language proficiency with bilingual and limited-English-proficient students. *Diagnostique, 21*(4), 17–36.

Ochoa, S. H., Gonzalez, D., Galarza, A., & Guille-

mard, L. (1996). The training and use of interpreters in bilingual psycho-educational assessment: An alternative in need of study. *Diagnostique, 21*(3), 19–40.

Ochoa, S. H., Morales, P., & Hernandez, M. (1997, April). *School psychologists' concerns about assessing culturally and linguistically diverse pupils.* Paper presented at the 29th Annual Convention of the National Association of School Psychologists Anaheim, CA.

Ochoa, S. H., Powell, M. P., & Robles-Pina, R. (1996). School psychologists' assessment practices with bilingual and limited-English-proficient students. *Journal of Psychoeducational Assessment, 14,* 250–275.

Ochoa, S. H., Rivera, B., & Ford, L. (1994, August). *School psychology training pertaining to bilingual psychoeducational assessment.* Paper presented at the 102nd Annual Convention of the American Psychological Association, Los Angeles, CA.

Ochoa, S. H., Rivera, B. D., & Ford, L. (1997). An investigation of school psychology training pertaining to bilingual psycho-educational assessment of primarily Hispanic students: Twenty-five years after *Diana v. California. Journal of School Psychology, 35*(4), 329–349.

Ochoa, S. H., Rivera, B., Powell, M. P. (1997). Factors used to comply with the exclusionary clause with bilingual and limited-English-proficient pupils: Initial guidelines. *Learning Disabilities Research and Practice, 12*(3), 161–167.

Ochoa, S. H., Robles-Pina, R., Garcia, S. B., & Breunig, N. (1999). School psychologists' perspectives on referrals of language minority students. *Multiple Voices for Ethnically Diverse Exceptional Learners, 3*(1), 1–14.

Ortiz, A. A. (1990). Using school-based problem-solving teams for prereferral intervention. *Bilingual Special Education Perspective, 10*(1), 3–5.

Ortiz, A. A., & Maldonado-Colon, E. (1986). Recognizing learning disabilities in bilingual children: How to lessen inappropriate referrals of language minority students to special education. *Journal of Reading, Writing, and Learning Disabilities International, 2,* 43–56.

Ortiz, A. A., & Polyzoi, E. (1986). *Characteristics of limited English proficient Hispanic students in programs for the learning disabled: Implications for policy, practice and research. Part I. Report Summary.* Austin: University of Texas at Austin. (ERIC Document Reproduction Service No. ED 267578)

Ortiz, A. A., & Wilkinson, C. Y. (1991). Assessment and intervention model for bilingual exceptional students (Aim for the BESt). *Teacher Education and Special Education, 14,* 35–42.

Ortiz, A. A., & Yates, J. (1983). Incidence of exceptionality among Hispanics: Implications for manpower planning. *National Association of Bilingual Education Journal, 7,* 41–54.

Parrish, T. (2002). Disparities in the identification, funding, and provision of special education. In D. J. Losen & G. Orfield (Eds.), *Racial inequity in special education* (pp. 15–38). Cambridge, MA: Harvard University Press.

Prutting, C. A. (1983). Assessing communicative behavior using a language sample. In D. R. Omark & J. G. Erickson (Eds.), *The bilingual exceptional child* (pp. 89–99). San Diego, CA: College-Hill Press.

Ramirez, J. D. (1992). Executive summary of volumes I and II of the final report: Longitudinal study of structured English immersion strategy, early-exit, and late-exit transitional bilingual education programs for language-minority children. *Bilingual Research Journal, 16,* 1–62.

Reynolds, C. R., & Kaiser, S. M. (1990). Bias in assessment of aptitude. In C. R. Reynolds & R. W. Kamphaus (Eds.), *Handbook of psychological and educational assessment of children: Intelligence and achievement* (pp. 611–653). New York: Guilford Press.

Rogers, M. R., Ingraham, C. L., Bursztyn, A., Cajigas-Segredo, N., Esquivel, G., Hess, R., Nahari, S. G., & Lopez, E. (1999). Providing psychological services to racially, ethnically, culturally, and linguistically diverse individuals in the schools: Recommendations for practice. *School Psychology International, 20*(3), 243–264.

Rogers, M. R., Martin, J., & Druckman, L. (1994, March). *Model multicultural training programs in school psychology: An examination of program philosophies and characteristics.* Paper presented at the 26th Annual Convention of the National Association of School Psychologists, Seattle, WA.

Rogers, M. R., Ponterotto, J. G., Conoley, J. C., & Wiese, M. J. (1992). Multicultural training is school psychology: A national survey. *School Psychology Review, 21,* 603–616.

Rosenfield, S., & Esquivel, G. B. (1985). Educating school psychologists to work with bilingual/bicultural populations. *Professional Psychology: Research and Practice, 16,* 199–208.

Rueda, R., Cardoza, D., Mercer, J., & Carpenter, L. (1985). *An examination of special education decision making with Hispanic first-time referral in large urban school districts.* Los Alamitos, CA: Southwest Regional Laboratory for Educational Research and Development. (Eric Document Reproduction Service No. ED 312 810)

Scribner, A. P. (1993). The use of interpreters in the assessment of language minority students. *Bilingual Special Education Perspective, 12,* 2–6.

Thomas, W., & Collier, V. (1996). *Language minority student achievement and program effectiveness.* Fairfax, VA: Center for Bilingual/Multicultural/ESL Education, George Mason University.

Thomas, W. P., & Collier, V. (1997). *School effectiveness for language minority students.* Washington, DC: National Clearinghouse for Bilingual Education.

Thomas, W. P., & Collier, V. (2002). *A national study of school effectiveness for language minority students' long-term academic achievement* [Online]. Available: www.crede.uscu.edu/research/llaa1.html

Troike, R. (1978). Research evidence for the effectiveness of bilingual education. *NABE Journal, 3,* 13–24.

U.S. General Accounting Office. (1987, March). *Bilingual education: A new look at the research evidence.* Washington, DC: Author.

U.S. Office of Education. (1997). Assistance to states for education of handicapped children: Procedures for evaluating specific learning disabilities. *Federal Register, 42,* 65083.

Valdes, G., & Figueroa, R. A. (1996). *Bilingualism and testing: A special case of bias.* Norwood, NJ: Ablex.

Weaver, L., & Padron, Y. (1999). Language of instruction and its impact on educational access and outcomes. In A. Tashakkori & S. H. Ochoa (Eds.), *Reading on equal education: Vol. 16. Education of Hispanics in the United States: Politics, policies, and outcomes* (pp. 75–92). New York: AMS Press.

Wilen, D. K., & Sweeting, C. V. M. (1986). Assessment of limited English proficient Hispanic students. *School Psychology Review, 15,* 59–75.

Willig, A. (1985). A meta-analysis of selected studies on the effectiveness of bilingual education. *Review of Educational Research, 55*(3), 269–317.

Willig, A. (1986). Special education and the culturally and linguistically different child: An overview of issues and challenges. *Reading, Writing, and Learning Disabilities, 2,* 161–173.

Woodcock, R., & Muñoz-Sandoval, A. (1993). *Woodcock–Muñoz Language Survey.* Chicago: Riverside.

Wright, P., & Cruz, R. S. (1983). Ethnic composition of special education programs in California. *Learning Disability Quarterly, 6,* 387–394.

Zappert, L., & Cruz, B. (1977). *Bilingual education: An appraisal of empirical research.* Berkeley, CA: Bay Area Bilingual Education League.

24

Assessment of Creativity in Children and Adolescents

E. PAUL TORRANCE
PATRICIA A. HAENSLY

Many of the leading creativity scholars and practitioners believe that the essential source of creativity is the irrational, suprarational, preconscious—something other than the rational, logical mind. Alex F. Osborn (1963), who originated one of the most widely taught of the disciplined, systematic procedures of creative problem solving, used the terms "critical intelligence" and "creative intelligence." He argued that these two kinds of intelligence cannot function optimally at the same time, and he pioneered training methods for calling into play whichever kind of intelligence or information processing is needed. He invented various kinds of technology for facilitating the shift from one kind of "intelligence" to another. What Osborn described as "critical intelligence" appears to be essentially what has been described as the specialized functioning of the left hemisphere, and what he labeled as "creative intelligence" seems to fit what is now described as the specialized functioning of the right hemisphere. For example, Osborn's rules for brainstorming were designed to aid in suspending left-hemisphere functioning and in activating right-hemisphere functioning. After the brainstorming has been done, there is an

evaluation phase in which criteria are formulated and applied in judging the alternatives produced through brainstorming. This phase is designed to activate the left-hemisphere functions. The entire process (Parnes, Noller, & Biondi, 1971) may be described as one of alternating shifts between right- and left-hemisphere functioning.

Other creativity theorists and developers of creative problem-solving models and technology have considered these two different kinds of information processing, although they have not used the right- and left-hemisphere labels in describing them. Edward de Bono (1970) used the term "lateral" and "vertical" thinking. Essentially, his lateral thinking seems to involve left-hemisphere functions. Rollo May (1975) used the terms "rational" and "suprarational." His rational thinking would seem to involve the specialized cerebral functions of the left hemisphere, and his suprarational thinking seems to call for the specialized functions of the left and right hemispheres, respectively. Gordon's (1961) position was that in creative thinking the irrational, emotional aspects of mental functioning are more important than the intellectual. Once creative ideas are produced, they must be subjected to the tests of logic, but such ideas do not occur as the result of logical processes.

Though we recognize the complexity of creativity and the elusiveness (as yet) of its essential constituency, we should not be deterred from trying to identify individuals with outstanding creative potential by using whatever information is available to us. Despite conceptual limitations regarding what is to be measured in creativity assessment, and an inadequate data base for reliability and validity studies (Brown, 1989), evidence of a relationship between test behavior and real-life creative achievement has been accumulating. Longitudinal studies, spanning several decades, of individuals who as high school students and elementary school pupils had been administered the Torrance Tests of Creative Thinking (TTCT; Cramond, Matthews-Morgan, & Torrance, 2001; Plucker, 1999; Torrance, 1966, 1972a, 1972b, 1981, 1982, 1993) indicate a moderate capability of the TTCT to predict quantity and quality of creative achievements. These studies have also produced information that will permit educators and psychologists to extend creative potential and increase life satisfaction by constructing personal and material environments to facilitate creative expression and reduce inhibitive factors.

It is especially critical that we recognize during the early years of schooling the capability of very young children to express or produce creative work. Delaying attempts at assessment, incomplete as it may be, may jeopardize the chances of these children for receiving instruction in the creativity-relevant skills that will permit their creative potential to flourish (e.g., Amabile, 1983a; Bloom, 1985; Brown, 1989; Feldman, 1986).

An overview of the definitions of creativity that have evolved as investigators have attempted to extract measurable elements follows, along with special emphasis on the implications of these definitions for assessment. The overview includes a general description of (1) characteristics of creativity; (2) its complex origin (i.e., wherein does creativity reside—the process, person, product, or environment?) and the implications its origin has for investigation and assessment; and (3) the notion of levels of creative endeavor—an idea that is especially critical to our assessment of creative ability in children and adolescents, where less advanced levels of creative product and performance are more likely to be found. The purpose of such an extended introduction to assessment of creativity is to insure that those who use the instruments to be described later understand the framework within which assessment results must be interpreted. Creativity assessment data used superficially, carelessly, or with incorrect assumptions can hinder progress toward freeing potential and creating receptive environments.

The next section of the chapter focuses on how and when creativity should be assessed, with reference to instruments most commonly used, their source, and their technical quality. This section is organized according to the categories of person, process, and product mentioned above. Considerations regarding interpretation, or "making sense of assessment," and appropriate application of assessment conclude the chapter.

CREATIVITY AS A PHENOMENON FOR ASSESSMENT

Current Views

Guilford, in his frequently cited presidential address to the American Psychological Association (Guilford, 1950), admonished psychologists for their lack of attention to college graduates' inability to solve problems in which old information was nonproductive and new solutions had to be found. Guilford's interest in this area of endeavor originated in his earlier work as a graduate student engaged in the administration of IQ tests to children, where he experienced great frustration with the inability of intelligence tests to assign worth to children's "ingenuity, inventiveness, and originality of thinking" (Guilford, 1976, p. 8). Guilford (1950) introduced his American Psychological Association audience to the complexity of the task of the assessment of the phenomenon with this circular and not very specific definition:

> In its narrow sense, creativity refers to the abilities that are most characteristic of creative people. Creative abilities determine whether the individual has the power to exhibit cre-

ative behavior to a noteworthy degree. Whether or not the individual who has the requisite abilities will actually produce results of a creative nature will depend upon his motivational and temperamental traits. (p. 444)

Guilford later went on to elaborate on the problem of defining creative traits and the creative personality. The questions he posed at that time remain with us today and have definite implications for assessment results: "(1) How can we discover creative promise in our children and our youth? And (2) How can we promote the development of creative personalities?" (Guilford, 1976, p. 3).

In an attempt to organize the definitions of creativity that subsequently proliferated, Taylor (1960, reported in Taylor, 1988) used the main themes of the approximately six different definitions he had encountered to establish six classes of definitions. These classes include (1) "aesthetic or expressive" (i.e., focusing on the individual's expression of ideas or work, unique to self); (2) "psychoanalytic or dynamic" (focusing on the preconscious or unconscious); (3) "Gestalt or perception" (focusing on any recombination of ideas); and (4) "Varia" (focusing on somewhat nebulous new-knowledge production). Although the foregoing definitions do not lend themselves well to assessment, Taylor's other two definitions focus on (5) ideas and objects useful or applicable to some group at some point in time; and (6) "solution thinking," or any of the many specific processes that contribute to solving problems in new ways.

Discussants over the past several decades have debated, at length, the existence of creativity as a legitimate ability. In particular, investigators have been unable to agree on the source of creativity, whether it is in the process, product, person, or environment. Investigators have alternately dwelled on creativity as a *specific mental process* (differentiated from intelligence and other mental processes), as a definable cluster of *personality characteristics* that results in creative behavior, and as a unique kind of *product*; they have also differed on the type of particular *environments* needed for creative expression. Concurrently, investigators have also grappled with the task of identifying who and what is creative, and where

and when we may unequivocally designate some performance or product of performance as creative.

Howard Gardner (1983, 1993) has complicated this problem by his theory of multiple intelligences. His concept has caught the attention of educators, psychologists, and the public at large. Although many investigators, such as Getzels and Jackson (1962), Guilford (1950, 1967, 1986), MacKinnon (1978), and Torrance (1979b), had been finding that there are numerous kinds of mental abilities, it was not until Gardner's (1983) *Frames of Mind* came along that this concept received widespread attention. Gardner argues that human beings have evolved to be able to carry out at least seven separate forms of analysis:

1. Linguistic intelligence (as a poet or other type of writer or speaker).
2. Logical/mathematical intelligence (as in a scientist).
3. Musical intelligence (as in a composer).
4. Spatial intelligence (as in a sculptor or airplane pilot).
5. Bodily/kinesthetic intelligence (as in an athlete or dancer).
6. Interpersonal intelligence (as in a salesperson or teacher).
7. Intrapersonal intelligence (exhibited by individuals with accurate views of themselves).

More recently, Gardner has proposed three additional intelligences: "naturalist," "spiritual," and "existential." Educators have rushed to develop educational material of naturalist intelligence (Glock, Werts, & Meyer, 1999), but thus far, no such implementation has been offered on spiritual and existential intelligences.

At this writing, no one has proposed anything regarding the measurement of these intelligences. However, Lazear (1994) has written about the "assessment" of the original seven intelligences. Lazear's efforts have only included observations, not quantification.

Although Gardner has virtually ignored the measurement of his multiple intelligences and denied the possibility or desirability of measuring creative thinking abilities, others have been considering the possibility of measuring creative thinking ability as related to each of the intelligences. Widely used tests of creativity all largely tie into the linguistic and spatial (figural) categories, although there have been developments in the bodily/kinesthetics and logical/mathematics area. Just as the verbal and figural creativity tests identified different groups of gifted individuals than general intelligence tests did, measures of Gardner's intelligences would differ from measures of creativity in the same modalities. It is likely that we will see developments in this area.

Defining the Concept

The fact that we cannot precisely define creativity should not overly disturb us. It should in fact remind us that, by the very nature of this phenomenon, creativity involves more than the semantic world. It encompasses all of our senses and is expressed through and for all modalities. Examples of the richness of imagery in expressing the attributes of creativity, along with numerous visual analogies (Torrance, 1988, pp. 49–57), demonstrate the value of accessing symbol systems other than semantic to enlarge our understanding of creativity. It quite possibly may be beyond our powers to analyze through logic or delimit with semantic boundaries, as well as beyond our own finite capability to understand, a phenomenon that is produced and realized in every conceivable modality through processes that transcend our conscious world. This inability on our part to concretize creativity will perhaps keep us honest and humble enough to remind us that assessment of creative potential, as of other characteristics, can never be absolute.

In order to extract variables we might validly use in the assessment of creativity, as well as to appreciate the limitations that any one type of variable may place on accurate assessment of creativity, we believe it helpful to examine how creativity has been perceived by investigators in the field.

Characteristics of Creativity

Definitions focused on the primary characteristics of creativity, whether ability, product, or process, have consis-tently referred to newness. "Every-person" definitions see the novelty that results from a sudden closure in a solu-tion to a problem as available to the

thinker in any domain (Thurstone, 1952), even if the idea was produced by someone else earlier (Stewart, 1950). Guilford's (1956, 1959, 1960, 1976, 1986) conceptualization of creativity limits this every-person category, to the extent that sensitivity to problems and the ability to redefine and transform meanings, uses, or functions of an object must precede or accompany the operation of divergent production. This sensitivity in itself may constitute a special ability. Guilford also states that the prerequisite for fluent transformation is freedom from functional fixedness, a condition that seems related to nonconformity. Nonconformity versus con-formity likewise could reasonably be construed as novelty available to all, and includes new ways of looking at problems (Bartlett, 1958; Crutchfield, 1962; de Bono, 1967), as well as the freedom to conform or not to conform to produce something individually pleasing (Starkweather, 1976). Perceptions that creativity demands absolute novelty to the culture would severely limit its appearance to a few individuals throughout history.

Additional attributes of creative contributions that have been proposed are that they be true or verifiable, surprising in light of what was known at the time (Selye, 1962), although Anderson (1959) allowed that the truth may be as the *individual* understands it. Jackson and Messick (1967) described the requisite characteristics of creative responses as unusualness versus commonality; appropriateness or goodness of fit with the program; transformation in form; and condensation. This last criterion refers to the bringing together of a set of ideas in such a simple way as to pro-duce a sense of "Why didn't I think of that before? It is so clearly fortuitous"—comp1exity conveyed with such sim-plicity as to generate new understanding. The personal impact on others produced by each of these characteristics helps clarify their meaning: surprise to the criterion of unusualness; satisfaction to appropriateness; stimulation of ideas to transformation; and savoring or pondering to condensation.

Creativity's Origin: The Process?

The complexity of precisely what we might measure in our assessment of creative ability is compounded not only by the fact that there is disagreement about valid criteria for creative product and performance, but also by the fact that each of the many theoretical approaches to creativity assumes different origins, factors, and processes as critical to the development of a creative product (Brown, 1989). Assessment thus might center either on what the individual does to produce creatively, or on the typical traits and personality characteristics of the person, or on the evaluation of the products of that process—or it might identify elements of the environment in which the individual functions to determine how and why creativity has or has not occurred.

Definitions focusing on process range from the very amorphous to the highly specific. Representative of the possible such definitions are the following: Ghiselin (1952) speaks of the emergence of insight to produce a new configuration; Kubie (1958) of scanning the preconscious at higher speeds than possible in conscious thought, in order to find relationships; Barchillon (1961) of shaking up one's information storage and throwing things together in new ways; Sternberg (1988) of flashes of insight; Guilford (1956) of being sensitive to problems; Spearman (1930) of recognizing and generating relationships; Ribot (1906) of generating relationships by emphasizing analogy formation; Wittrock (1974) of generative processing through adding new pieces to stored mental schemes, and thus constructing new schemes; and Simonton (1988) of chance permutation of elements.

The process definitions that have been used to the greatest extent in assessment to date have focused on "divergent production"—a concept formally introduced through Guilford's (1956) structure-of-intellect model. In Guilford's hypothesizing about what creative ability might include, as a prerequisite to conducting a research program on creativity (Guilford, 1959), he determined that first of all, the ability to sense problems that call for solution would result in increased opportunities to work on such problems and an increased probability of coming up with solutions. He also concluded that the higher the fluency or rate of producing (1) words, (2) ideas, (3) associations, or (4) ways of expressing oneself (i.e., one's fluency), the more likely one would be to arrive at an original and workable solution. The greater the variety of ideas produced (flexibility), the greater also the likelihood of arriving at a clever or less commonplace solution. Guilford further proposed that the greater one's ability to analyze, synthesize, redefine, and transform ideas, objects, and functions of objects, the greater one's likelihood of arriving at an unusual and useful solution.

Critical to our understanding of the limitations of assessment, our construction of valid plans for assessment, and our interpretation of the results of assessment is the realization that divergent production in itself is insufficient for creative endeavor. Although Guilford specified that creative performance in life cannot be accounted for solely by these abilities, he felt sure that they are essential and contribute extensively to the creative performance. In addition, Guilford viewed the ability to sense problems that call for solution—a prerequisite for creativity (as stated above)—as reflecting the evaluation operation, not the operating of divergent production. Thus Guilford did not limit creative performance solely to divergent production, but extended it to the application, as it were, of divergent production.

Brown (1989) and others have expressed concern that tests of divergent thinking measure only a very specific area of creative behavior. Brown suggests that in all likelihood, high divergent-thinking response frequency may be supported as much by training and preparation in a domain, specific ability in that area, and experiences as it is by the creativity-associated traits of tolerance of ambiguity and resistance to premature closure. Thus divergent thinking is only one small part of the complex predictive equation for creative productivity.

Recognition of this limitation is evident in the TTCT (Torrance, 1966, 1974), which have also operationalized creativity through fluency and flexibility counts, and added originality and elaboration counts. However, a critical extension to this operationalized definition has been a process definition of creativity developed for research purchases (Torrance, 1967) and for the eventual construction of the creativity tests. It conveys an idea somewhat similar to Guilford's constructive responses to existing or new situations, as follows:

. . . the process of becoming sensitive to problems, deficiencies, gaps in knowledge, missing elements, disharmonies, and so on; identifying the difficulties; searching for solutions, making guesses, or formulating hypotheses and possibly modifying them and retesting them; and finaIIy communicating the results. (Torrance, 1967, pp. 73–74)

Construction of the TTCT wove the already described and defined processes into a test battery made up of situations for demonstrating the ability to exhibit these processes, with responses to the situations representing a component ability assessed by quantity (fluency) and quality (flexibility, originality, and elaboration) of particular responses. The contrivance of artificial situations to elicit creative responses parallels the approach used by most if not all those who have constructed tests for the assessment of intelligence, as well as of other specific abilities. Personalizing the tests and gathering of information on the person and environment variables that affect responses on these tests are described elsewhere (Torrance, 1988).

Torrance's (1988) "survival" definition of creativity reflects the realization that greater reality in the situations used for assessment brings us closer to representing the true creative ability or potential of individuals, adding validity and reliability to our assessment. The survival definition arose out of research on U.S. Air Force survival training (Torrance, 1955, 1957). Thus, in air crew survival situations, creative solutions required imaginatively gifted recombination of old elements (information about how Native Americans and pioneers lived off the land, how the early explorers survived under Arctic conditions, etc.) into new configurations to fit the current situation and need for survival. A parallel with Sternberg's position on the difference between practical intelligence and the "intelligence" measured on IQ tests (Sternberg & Wagner, 1986) should be evident. But the usefulness of using particular abilities to assist in the assessment of creative potential, even though they give us only a partial picture of potential, should also be evident.

A view of process involving four particular steps—preparation through information gathering, incubation of ideas, illumination, and verification, all preceded by a sense of need or deficiency in the problem area (Wallas, 1926)—has been explicated as creative problem solving by numerous investigators (e.g., Parnes, 1962; Parnes et al., 1971). Although some of the assessment of creativity in children and adolescents, especially with regard to responsiveness in the classroom, has involved the evaluation of responses in creative problem solving, much of this level of assessment has depended upon the quite specific measurement of divergent production through responses quantified for their fluency, flexibility, and originality (Guilford, 1976).

Creativity's Origin: The Person?

The Torrance research agenda on creativity has proceeded from a focus on process to the identification of what kind of person one must be to engage in the process successfully, what kinds of environments will facilitate it, and what kind of product will result from successful operation of the process (Torrance, 1965). After a lifetime of studies carrying out this agenda, the conclusion that has been reached and repeatedly supported—especially with data from the 22-year study of elementary school children first tested with the TTCT in 1958 (Torrance, 1981, 1982)—is that the salient characteristic of the creative person is "being in love with what one is doing" (see Torrance, 2000). This characteristic appears to make possible all the other personality characteristics associated with creative persons: dependence of thought and judgment, perseverance, curiosity, willingness to take risks, courage to be different, and willingness to tackle difficult tasks. Assessment of creativity through personality inventories, rating scales, and the like may be a psychological anachronism, although the information provided to the individual may be self-revealing and in this way may assist the individual to improve personal attitudes, thus enhancing creative potential. An example of this application is the finding that an important part of Air Force survival training was practicing means of self-discovery and self-discipline to complement the acquisition of specific information about survival situations (Torrance, 1955, 1957).

Many investigators have focused consistently over the years on a search for the characteristics of "creative persons," compiling lists that in turn might be used to identify individuals with creative potential (e.g., Barron, 1969, 1978; Davis, 1975; MacKinnon, 1976, 1978; Roe, 1951, 1953). Taken singly, identified characteristics cannot add significantly to the power of a creativity prediction equation. However, the importance of characteristics appears to lie in the interaction between the set that refers in some way to creative process (such as tolerance of ambiguity and resistance to premature closure) and the set that refers in some way to motivation for creative endeavor (such as independence of thought, persistence, courage). Nevertheless, biographical inventories may provide valuable information for assessment of creative potential. Whiting (1976) gives validity information of their use with adults in several research and development fields, linking biographical data with creative job performance. The Torrance longitudinal studies (Torrance, 1972a, 1972b, 1981, 1982, 1993) have identified particular characteristics in children and adolescents that persisted into adulthood and were consistently related to school and postschool creative achievements.

Creativity's Origin: The Product?

Assessment of the creativity of individuals' products is logically limited to some type of consensual process by judges who are particularly qualified in the domain and specific field of productivity. That is, scientists can hardly be expected to assess the originality and transformation characteristics or quality of a musical composition, any more than most artists would be qualified judges of creative contributions in biochemistry. Once again, the Torrance longitudinal studies (Torrance, 1972a, 1972b, 1981, 1982, 1993) provide moderately strong predictive validity data on the relationship between high school creative achievements and achievements after high school. This type of information on the quantity and quality of products and performances during childhood years may in this way be useful in the prediction of future performance, as well as in concurrent assessment of creative ability in children and adolescents. The notion of levels of creativity and performances is rele-

vant here and is discussed in the next section.

Levels of Creativity

It seems appropriate in any discussion of assessment of creativity to consider the questions of differences in levels of creativity exhibited or expressed. I. A. Taylor (1959) suggested the following five levels: (1) expressive (spontaneous, as in the drawings of children); (2) productive (where free play is somewhat contained by restrictions of the field); (3) inventive (technical contributions to solve practical problems); (4) innovative (based on coneptualization); and (5) emergentative, the highest level (involving an entirely new principle or assumption). Ghiselin (1963) differentiated between secondary-level creativity, which extends a concept into a new application, and higher-level or primary-level creativity, which radically alters what has gone before.

Jackson and Messick (1967) imply the notion of levels through four increasingly complex criteria for creative products, relating these criteria to characteristics of creators and to the responses of audiences toward the products. However, one might also reason that without all of these four criteria—novelty, appropriateness, transformation, and condensation—the product is not truly creative. These criteria may be used to judge effectively the quality of contribution in all domains, but may also appropriately be applied at any level of expertise within a domain. Expanding on this idea, one may propose that judgment of level of creativity must also recognize the contributor's level of intelligence and his or her training and expertise within the particular domain (Haensly & Reynolds, 1989).

One last point about definitions and assessment needs to be made here. As in all psychological assessment, we may observe and measure responses that reflect the component abilities of creative process, evaluate products of creative ability, and link abilities with products, thus documenting the potential to produce; however, we cannot prove the absence of potential. Thus, to a degree, we may reliably predict the recurrence of this kind of response *given the appropriate conditions,* supporting our hypotheses about facilitation and/or obstruction of this ability. Information gained from assessment and the conditions under which measurements were made can then inform us regarding the environments within which individuals act creatively. Acting on this information, we are more likely to insure that creative potential will surface at some level for all individuals. Such a purposeful and dynamic agenda is what makes assessment of creative ability stand apart from the more static relationship between assessment and use of assessment data that may exist for many other abilities. In terms of medical models, we may in this way be able, to assume a problem-preventative stance for healthful self-actualization early in life through creative expression, rather than a pathological treatment approach for individuals who have become isolated or nonproductively deviant in order to express their creative potential.

ASSESSMENT OF CREATIVITY: HOW AND WHEN

Procedural Considerations

General Psychometric Concerns

Defensible procedure in psychological assessment demands concern for the specificity of procedures in testing, and the assessment of creativity is no exception. Questions of validity and reliability of the instruments; establishment of personal rapport and a material environment that will elicit the behaviors under study; and procedures that are sufficiently standardized to insure that data can be compared among individuals and test administrators are all legitimate concerns. The nature of the phenomenon we are addressing often seems to encourage greater laxness than is defensible, perhaps because those who are more likely to use creativity tests may be those who view restrictions as inhibiting creative expression. Misunderstandings and questionable procedures are common in practice as well as in the research literature. Keeping a clear purpose in mind for the particular test administration will facilitate sound decision making. If the purpose is to make judgments about relative ability in comparison to a defined normative group, one

must follow the standardized procedures rigorously. However, experimentation with procedure may be desirable when one wishes to learn more about factors that inhibit or facilitate creative expression, or when creativity tests are being used to stimulate growth in the component abilities of creativity.

In applied settings, the purpose of creativity testing is frequently identification of students to be considered for special programs—for example, gifted programs in schools, special talent development instruction, or specific endeavors especially requiring creative thinking. Another purpose may be the evaluation of instructional treatments or programs. In either case, the ability to generate accurate comparisons will be essential. By contrast, in order to test hypotheses about effective, reasonable (or valid), and reliable assessment of creative functioning, experimentation with different testing conditions and procedures will be necessary, just as it has been in the study of abilities other than creativity.

A third use of creativity tests—training or facilitation of creative functioning—sometimes requires additional justification to critics who would categorize this with "teaching to tests." Yet, as a critical component of educational goals and of life outside the classroom, creative functioning must be taught in as many ways as possible. When test performances have analogues in classroom performance, and/or analogues in performance in the everyday world of work, play, human interaction, and service, it makes great sense to use them in this manner. This use of creativity tests actually falls outside the realm of assessment, but it must be mentioned so that the novice user of creativity tests and the expert psychologist alike will respect the line of demarcation between standardized procedure and "creative" use. However, one assessment extension of a nonstandardized procedure with creativity tests must be mentioned. Testing the limits, as described by Sattler (1974) and Kaufman (1979), parallels the procedure used with intelligence tests. That is, children or students may be encouraged strongly and persistently to continue with the production of ideas, in order to test a hypothesis that the test takers are more capable than they are allowing themselves to demonstrate or than some external variable is allowing.

Specific Creativity Test Guidelines

Practical guidelines for the training of creativity test administrators and scorers, reprinted from the *Journal of Creative Behavior*, have been compiled in a manual published by Scholastic Testing Service, Inc. (Torrance, 1987a). Variations in administration of creativity tests, with documented results from the use of these variations, are also included in this manual. These guidelines would seem just as applicable to any assessment of creativity, although they are particularly relevant to the TTCT.

Admonitions to test administrators include those that are similar for the use of other psychological instruments, such as (1) close adherence to the printed directions, with accurate description and recording of deviations that occur; (2) strict adherence to time limits where recommended; and (3) use of clearly marked booklets with clear directions by test administrators. Directions for motivating the performance of students are specified and include allowance of oral administration of the tests with dialect, colloquial, or conversational language, as well as a lengthy list of examples of positive verbal reinforcement that may be used with the verbal form of the TTCT.

In the above-mentioned manual (Torrance, 1987a), scorers are also provided with standard procedures that include training, establishment of intra- and interscorer reliability, establishment of decision rules for special cases, and ways of keeping students from working so long at the task that fatigue and carelessness occur.

What has been demonstrated clearly is that test administration and testing conditions influence performance on creativity tests. The TTCT have perhaps been subjected to more experiments on ways to administer them than any other tests in the history of educational and psychological testing. We know from the results of extensive experimentation many of the factors that enhance, facilitate, or hinder creative thinking. These factors—tabulated from 36 different experiments on both the TTCT and the Wallach and Kogan (1965) measure, and published between 1968 and 1972 (see Torrance, 1987a, 1987b, 1988)—include such things as type, quality, and length of warm-up provided prior to the test administration; timing; stimuli in the testing setting; reinforcement; evaluation; and group versus individual administration. The clear trends indicate that psychological warm-up for the tasks results in small but consistent and statistically significant gains; however, warm-up that lasts too long or is given too far in advance is ineffective in increasing creative responding.

Creativity Tests

Psychologists and educators have been developing measures of creativity for as long as they have been trying to develop measures of the development of intelligence (Whipple, 1915/1973). At the time we wrote the chapter for the first edition of this book (Haensly & Torrance, 1990), Torrance had assembled a collection of 225 such tests. Although he has not kept this collection, Puccio and Murdock (1999) have published a compendium that fulfills a similar purpose. Rather than analyze these tests, we concentrate primarily on the TTCT, the most widely used and researched such tests. The most recent cumulative bibliography on the TTCT battery cites over 2,000 publications describing some uses of this battery.

Process: Fluency and So Forth

The Torrance Creativity Tests include four batteries or groups of tests that are primarily concerned with fluency, flexibility, and originality of idea production; they are available through Scholastic Testing Service. The first of these is a general all-purpose battery, known as the TTCT. It contains a verbal test (Thinking Creatively with Words) with seven subtests and a figural test (Thinking Creatively with Pictures) with three subtests, all of which represent the elements of the Torrance research/process definition of creativity described earlier, and are timed for either 5- or 10-minute limits. The verbal subtests include Asking (which requires the respondent to list all of the questions that can be thought of about nonobvious events in a provided picture); Guessing Causes (of the events in the picture); and

Guessing Consequences (of the events). These are followed by Product Improvement, in which the respondent lists all the improvements that could be made on a stuffed toy monkey or elephant pictured in the booklet to make it more fun to play with; Unusual Uses, in which uses for cardboard boxes or tin cans are listed; Unusual Questions, in which questions about the boxes or cans are listed as fluently as possible; and Just Suppose, in which the test taker poses as many ideas as possible about what would happen if an unlikely event (as pictured) occurred. For each of the three subtests of Thinking Creatively with Pictures, the respondent is asked to complete a drawing, having been presented with (1) a kidney-shaped form (a teardrop shape, in the alternate form) to be used as the basis for an entire picture; (2) 10 incomplete figures to complete and label; and (3) two pages of circles or parallel lines to be completed and/or joined into a meaningful drawing.

Two forms of the entire battery of subtests are available, contributing to their usefulness for pre- and posttests. The subtests are scored for fluency, flexibility, and originality (based upon statistical-infrequency norms); the figural subtests are also scored for elaboration (based on the number of details added to the figure or boundary or surrounding space). Scoring is time-consuming, or expensive if returned to trained scorers at Scholastic Testing Service, and sometimes difficult when decisions about the originality of ambiguous responses must be made. The technical–norms manual (Torrance, 1974) provides reliability and validity data derived from over 1,500 studies using the TTCT. The interscorer reliability coefficients range from about .90 to .99 (as do the fluency scores). The majority of test–retest reliability coefficients are in the .60 to .80 range. Validity data have been derived from correlation studies of "person" characteristics, such as preferences for open-structure activities or aesthetic-related careers, originality in the classroom, humor, wild ideas produced, and lack of rigidity, as rated by both peers and teachers. Product-related validity data have been derived from longitudinal studies of elementary and high school students over periods as long as 40 years (Torrance, 1972a, 1972b, 1981, 1982;

Torrance & Wu, 1981). Creative achievements, higher quality of creative achievements, and a higher level of creative aspirations as young adults have been shown to characterize individuals who score high as opposed to low on creativity; these characteristics appear to increase over time for those scoring high, but remain the same for those scoring low.

Over the last few decades, Torrance has been developing and validating a method for the "streamlined" scoring of the TTCT. Manuals (Torrance & Ball, 1984) for the figural forms have now been published, and some of the validity studies have been completed for the verbal forms but not published. Torrance tells how the 5 norm-referenced and 13 criterion-referenced variables have been developed in the following words:

I initially sought clues in the biographies and other accounts of history's greatest inventors, scientific discoverers, and artists. All along, I was also searching for clues in the everyday creative behaviors and achievements of children, youth, and adults. I also looked at the variables that other investigators had assessed (e.g., Broadley, 1943; Guilford, 1967; Whipple, 1915/1973). Recently, I (Torrance, 1979b) have sought clues in the leading technologies for teaching creative problem-solving skills, inventing and similar activities. In each of these systems, I have tried to determine what creative skills are activated and practiced. I have included the leading technologies in the United States, England, and Japan. . . . In *The Search for Satori and Creativity,* I tried to show how each of these technologies attempts to activate and make use of each test variable used in the present scoring system of the Torrance Tests of Creative Thinking TTCT) (Torrance, 1979b).

In summary, I tried to be certain that each of the test variables selected had been important in the great creative achievements in history; was observable and important in the everyday creativity of children, youth, and adults; had been identified as important in the creativity research of the past; and had been found to be teachable through the major technologies used in the United States, England, and Japan. I also required that each test indicator I selected meet the following criteria: clear manifestation in test performances; adequate frequency of occurrence; developmental characteristics; amenability to improvement through instruction, training, and practice; and satisfactory connection between test performances in elementary, high school, and adult creative achievements as demonstrated through longitudinal studies of predictive validity (Torrance & Ball, 1984). (Torrance, 1987a, p. 3)

Thus the figural batteries are scored for each of the following variables, which are defined and discussed elsewhere (Torrance, 1979b, 1987a):

• Finding the problem
• Producing alternatives (fluency)
• Originality
• Abstracting (highlighting the essence)
• Elaborating
• Telling a story articulately
• Keeping open
• Being aware of and using emotions
• Putting ideas in context
• Combining and synthesizing
• Visualizing richly and colorfully
• Fantasizing
• Using movement and sound
• Looking at things from a different perspective
• Visualizing things internally
• Extending boundaries
• Humor
• Respect for infinity

The TTCT are appropriate for kindergarten children through graduate school students and have been translated for use in a wide variety of cultures around the world. The Torrance tests have been translated into more than 32 languages. Children who cannot yet read or for whom writing would be difficult may be given the TTCT orally, with administrators recording their responses. High school students are as likely to find the TTCT a fascinating and enjoyable experience as are younger students. Test administrators are expected to provide a climate for creative responsiveness within the standardized format by encouraging playfulness, production of as many ideas as possible, and so forth.

The second Torrance battery, Thinking Creatively in Action and Movement, was developed for use with preschool children and others with limited verbal and drawing skills, including students with disabilities (e.g., emotional disturbances or deafness) (Torrance, 1987b). Responses to the four subtests may be given in action and move-

ment or in words; are scored for fluency, originality, and imagination; and are untimed. The battery usually takes between 10 and 30 minutes. The subtests are How Many Ways? (to walk or run), scored for fluency and originality; Can You Move Like? (six situations, such as a tree in the wind and different animals), scored for imagination; and What Other Ways? (to put a paper cup in a wastebasket) and What Can You Do With a Paper Cup?, both scored for fluency and originality.

Interscorer reliabilities are about .99 for fluency and .96 for originality. Test–retest reliability coefficients of .84 for the total test and of .58 to .79 for the subtests have been documented. Validity criteria at this time are limited to teacher-observed creative behavior and children's joke humor.

The third battery, Thinking Creatively with Sounds and Words, jointly developed (Khatena & Torrance, 1973), uses a quite different stimulus for response: Two long-playing records are used to present four abstract sounds (Sounds and Images) and five onomatopoetic words (Onomatopoeia and Images). The respondent describes the mental images stimulated by the sounds and by the words; each set of stimuli is presented three times to generate more and more original associations. The responses are scored for originality based on frequency of responses; from 0 to 4 points are assigned to each of the 12 responses. The battery is available in two forms, one for adults and one for children.

Interscorer reliabilities range from .88 to .99 (Torrance, 1982). Alternate-forms reliabilities range from .36 to .92. The test's predictive validity varies greatly (.13 to .45) as derived from over 80 research studies, although it has not as yet been used widely enough to arrive at more stable validity coefficients or appropriate criteria. This battery may be used with children and youths from 3rd to 12th grades; with students in college, graduate school, and professional schools; and with adults. It has been found to be especially useful for individuals who are blind.

Sounds and Images appears to be one of the best measures of general creativity. This can be expected because imagery seems to be basically involved in all kinds of creative performance. However, it has not been widely accepted because it lacks the face validity represented by the TTCT, figural and verbal forms. However, a new and updated manual has been published recently (Khatena & Torrance, 1998b).

Process: Divergent Thinking

Guilford developed a number of creativity tests suitable for use in schools and based on his structure-of-intellect model. The activity of the divergent-production operation, assumed to represent the creative component of cognitive ability, became the basis of the Guilford creativity tests, measuring 24 different divergent productive abilities (6 products × 4 contents). A battery of these tests, Creativity Tests for Children (CTC), was published by the Sheridan Psychological Services in 1971 (Guilford, 1971). All of these tests of divergent production are described by Guilford (1967, 1977) and include such items as asking the respondent to list as many words as possible that are similar to a given word (associational fluency—i.e., relations between words), or to find a way to remove four matchsticks from a six-square rectangle and leave only three squares (figural transformation). The problem of relating divergent production measured in this way to real-world creative productivity has not been resolved. Meeker, Meeker, and Roid (1985) have continued, however, to develop new tests and norms.

The Test of Creative Potential (TCP; Hoepfner & Hemenway, 1973) has built on Guilford's work and is available from Monitor Publishers in two forms for use in 2nd through 12th grades. The TCP consists of three subtests: Writing Words, Picture Decorations, and License Plate Words, respectively measuring divergent production of semantic units and classes, figural units and implications, and symbolic units and transformations. Writing Words requires word responses that are similar to a given word and is scored for associational fluency and spontaneous flexibility; Picture Decorations requires decorations of three different pictures, yielding a design element score and a pictorial element score; License Plate Words requires creation of words from sets of three letters and is scored for word fluency and originality. The TCP has a standardized administration and scoring guide, and each of the parts of the subtests is timed. The test

may be used with children as young as age 7 and is also appropriate for adolescents and adults. Interscorer reliabilities range from .94 to .99. When children ages 7–9 retook the test 3 months later using the alternate form (a mixed form of reliability), two reliability coefficients obtained were .62 and .67. Validity data were not available.

The Ingenuity Test, developed by Flanagan and published by Science Research Associates, is part of Flanagan's Aptitude Classification Tests (see Flanagan, 1963), used in the nationwide PROJECT TALENT. This test is suitable for use with high school students and has a multiple-choice format in which the options are incomplete; that is, only the first and last letters are provided. The items in which problems are presented are said to test "the ability to invent or discover a solution which represents an unusually neat, clever, or surprising way of solving an existing problem" (Flanagan, 1976, p. 118). Although it appears to offer opportunities for divergent production, a limited number of possibilities are already in place in the options, and arrayed in "guess what falls between these letters" choices. Students tested in the project are being followed after completion of high school, but no validity data are currently available, with this exception: The 1-year follow-ups indicate that individuals who scored high are typically found in art, architecture, and science careers.

A somewhat different view of divergent thinking forms the basis of the Starkweather creativity instruments for preschool children. Starkweather's goal in the construction of tests for identification of creative potential in a very young child was the "development of a game which the child would want to play" (Starkweather, 1976, p. 81). Using the child's response to the game, the researcher would be able to ascertain compulsive conformity or nonconformity versus choices made freely to suit one's own preference, willingness to try difficult tasks, and originality. In the Starkweather Form Boards Test, the administrator uses four colored formboards in which the colored picture pieces depict a tree, house, playground, and barnyard, to he inserted against a background of black-and-white line drawings on the formboard. Measures of conformity require two sessions with the child. For example, using the tree form-board, the child chooses between a rabbit and flowers, although the line drawing model depicts a rabbit; in the second session, the child again chooses between a rabbit and flowers, but the line drawing model depicts flowers. Starkweather determined that either conforming over the two sessions by choosing the pictures corresponding to the line drawing provided, or nonconforming by not using the model each time, reflects rigidity. The child who is free or willing to be different will choose a personally preferred picture, which will correspond to the drawing provided 50% of the time (Starkweather & Cowling, 1963).

A second test of conformity, the Starkweather Social Conformity Test, is based on the same principle of rigidity versus the freedom to conform or not to conform. The child is provided with an opportunity to select colored place cards for a table setting for his or her mother, father, and self, after what colors the child likes and dislikes are determined.

The Starkweather (1976) Target Game consists of a box with a target, which, when the bull's eye is hit, releases a lid and discloses a surprise picture. Difficulty of the game is adjusted through a pretest to a 50% chance of success for each child by assessing the child's accuracy at rolling the ball from different target distances. The measured variable consists of choices made during the game between an easy distance and a hard distance. For preschool children, the game contains an element of a surprise picture as a motivating force to continue the game. For first- and second-grade children, success in hitting the target retains the children's attention and effort. This game cannot be used for older children because of the difficulty of adjusting for an individual child's skill level.

The Starkweather (1976) Originality Test consists of 40 plastic foam pieces of four different shapes (each shape comes in four different colors). In a warm-up pretest, the administrator encourages the child to think of as many different things a piece from a smaller subset of pieces may be. For the test itself, the administrator puts out a box of 20 pieces and directs the child to take one piece at a time and tell what the piece might be; the same procedure is followed for the second box of 20 pieces. Thus each of the four

shapes generates four responses scored in order, with credit given for each response that is different from previous responses. Validity for this test was determined by comparing teachers' judgments of the children's originality with the children's test scores; validity was also demonstrated by comparing the children's test scores with their freedom of expression when playing alone with simple toys. Correlations with scores on the Peabody Picture Vocabulary Test (PPVT) were not significant, indicating independence of the type of verbal ability demonstrated through the correct labeling responses required in the PPVT. Interrater reliability in scoring was determined by comparing the scoring of judges familiar with the test to that of a judge naive to the test. The materials for this test must be constructed by the user.

Process: Association

The ability to produce many verbal responses or ideas to a given stimulus word and to associate diverse elements in relevant ways has been viewed as still another measure of creative process. The Remote Associates Test (RAT; Mednick & Mednick, 1967) is published by Houghton Mifflin. This objective-type measure consists of items in which three words are given and the respondent must find a fourth word that links the three or could be associated with all of them. The combination must meet the experimenter-imposed criteria; that is, only "correct" answers add to one's score. There is a .40 to .60 correlation between RAT scores and verbal intelligence scores. Mednick and Mednick (1967) report Spearman–Brown reliabilities of .91 and .92 on samples of 215 and 289 college students, respectively. The RAT is suitable for use with older high school students and college students. It would appear that the RAT may require more convergency in responses than divergency.

The Person: Personality, Attitude, and Interest Inventories

As stated earlier, determining what kind of person one must be to engage successfully in the creative process was one objective of the Torrance (1963) creativity research agenda. Much information in this regard was obtained from the 22-year study of elementary school children first tested with the TTCT in 1958 (Torrance, 1981, 1982). Biographical inventories, often based on the work of such individuals as Barron (1969, 1978), MacKinnon (1976, 1978), and Roe (1951, 1953), have added much to our knowledge about the personality characteristics most frequently associated with the creative process. However, even if it could be assumed that such lists define who might become creative if given the opportunity and reinforcement (creative potential), it would not be feasible to reference all of the inventories and checklists that resulted from these searches. Nevertheless, many trait characteristics seem common enough among creative individuals that the lists may be useful for identifying characteristics that ought to he recognized and reinforced in order to facilitate creative growth, if not for identifying creativity outright. This may be particularly relevant to our concern in this handbook on assessment of children and adolescents, especially if we can locate instruments with good validity and high reliability. The instruments described here have respectable psychometric qualities, are designed particularly for pupils in preschool through high school (sometimes on into the college years), and are both readily available and usable.

One frequently used instrument for assessing the creative person is the Khatena–Torrance Creative Perception Inventories battery (Khatena & Torrance, 1976, 1998a). This battery consists of two separate tests, which may be used separately or in combination. What Kind of Person Are You? (WKOPAY?) and Something About Myself (SAM). The WKOPAY? and SAM are measures of relatively different aspects of personality. The WKOPAY? was originally created and developed by Torrance (1971) and uses a forced-choice type of response. Subjects are asked to choose, of two characteristics, the one that best describes the respondent. The characteristics were judged by a panel of raters (who were judged to be expert in the study of the creative personality) in order of importance and ordered accordingly. One point is scored for each "correct" response—the characteristic rated higher in importance by the panel of judges. The SAM is biographi-

cal and results in a list of creative achievements and interests. Extensive reliability data are presented in the technical–norms manual (Khatena & Torrance, 1998a). This source cites 90 publications that bear upon the reliability and validity in these measures.

A series of inventories spanning the entire age group described above has been developed by Gary Davis and Sylvia Rimm and is available through Educational Assessment Service. Each is somewhat different in the trait characteristics for which scores are available—apparently an attempt to identify characteristics particularly relevant at the specifically targeted age group. The Group Inventory for Finding Talent (GIFT; Rimm, 1976; Rimm & Davis, 1976, 1980) is a self-report instrument that assesses the traits of independence, flexibility, curiosity, perseverance, and breadth of interests, and identifies past creative activities and hobbies. The GIFT is available in three forms—Primary for first and second grades, Elementary for third and fourth grades, and Upper Elementary for fifth and sixth grades—which differ in the size of print and in about one-fourth of the items All forms are brief, containing 25 yes–no items common to all grade levels, and 7, 9, and 8 items respectively that are specific to each grade level. In addition to a total score, subscale scores for Imagination, Independence, and Many Interests are obtained. Validity coefficients using teacher ratings plus ratings of stories produced by the children as a criterion range from about .25 to .45 (Davis, 1986). Internal-consistency reliabilities of .80, .86, and .88 are reported for the Primary, Elementary, and Upper Elementary forms. The items are sufficiently broad to be useful with many different groups of children: white, black, and Hispanic-surnamed groups of children; children of high and low socioeconomic status (SES); urban, suburban, and rural children; and Israeli, French, and Australian children. Sample items include "I ask a lot of questions," "I like things that are hard to do," and "I like to make up my own songs."

The Group Inventory for Finding Interests I (GIFFI I; Davis & Rimm, 1982; Rimm & Davis, 1979, 1983) is similarly a self-report instrument, but requires rating 60 items on a 5-point scale from "no" to "definitely." It is designed for students from sixth through ninth grades, and produces a total creativity score with subscale scores for Confidence, Challenge–Inventiveness, Imagination, Creative Arts and Writing, and Many Interests. Internal-consistency reliability coefficients are above .90, and validity coefficients, again determined according to a combined criterion of teacher ratings of creativeness and a creativity rating for a produced story, range from low-moderate to high-moderate. The Group Inventory for Finding Interests II (GIFFI II; Davis & Rimm, 1980, 1982; Rimm & Davis, 1983) is similar to the GIFFI I, but was developed for 9th through 12th grades. The items are designed to measure independence, self-confidence, risk taking, energy, adventurousness, curiosity, reflectiveness, sense of humor, and artistic interests, as well as to identify creative activities and hobbies. Internal-consistency reliabilities range from .91 to .96, reflecting that the items are measuring a single characteristic. The instrument has been validated with many ethnic groups and all SES levels, as well as in urban, suburban, and rural areas. As in the remainder of the series, the criterion used for validity studies is a combination of teacher ratings of individual creativity with creativity ratings for a produced story, producing a median coefficient of .45 (see Davis, 1986, p. 182, for the range of coefficients obtained).

An alternative that is less psychometrically sound than the Davis and Rimm instruments, but that considers some highly different interests, is the Creativity Attitude Survey (CAS; Schaefer, 1971), for children from fourth to sixth grades. The CAS is a self-report, 32-item, yes–no instrument designed to measure such things as imagination, humor, interest in art and writing, appreciation of fantasy and wild ideas, and attraction to the magical. Internal-consistency reliabilities of .75 and .81, and a 5-week test–retest reliability of .61, have been reported. The primary criterion used in validity studies has been the test itself given after creativity training, although one study of 35 fifth-grade students reported teacher evaluation of "concrete evidence of creativity" related to CAS scores.

Davis (1973) has developed another inventory for assessing attitudes, motivations, interests, values, beliefs, and other creativi-

ty-relevant concerns, the How Do You Think (HDYT). Although this inventory was constructed with college students in mind, there seems no reason why the items would not prove equally valid for older high school students as well, even though much more attention is given to creative accomplishments than in the GIFFI instruments. Form B of the HDYT is a 102-item, 5-point rating scale with responses ranging from "agree" to "disagree." Its high internal consistency (a reliability coefficient of .93), and its strong validity in predicting the creativeness of an assigned writing project, an art or handicraft project, ideas for two inventions, and ideas for a creative teaching project (a correlation of .42 between the HDYT and the creative projects), warrant additional study. The test is available from its author.

Rating Scales

Although both self-report instruments and scales rated by those individuals purporting to know an index person's characteristics may be confounded by bias and lack of objectivity, checklists and inventories to be completed by individuals who should know a great deal about the person abound. A parent rating scale, produced on the same theoretical assumptions about the characteristics of creative individuals as the GIFT and GIFFI inventories, but constructed for preschool and kindergarten children ages 3–6, is the Preschool and Kindergarten Interest Descriptor (PRIDE; Rimm, 1983). This questionnaire, available through Educational Assessment Service, consists of 50 items rated on a 5-point scale and purports to measure the same kinds of traits addressed in the GIFT and GIFFI instruments. The PRIDE requires about 2–5 minutes to complete; it produces a total creativity score and subscale scores for Many Interests, Independence–Perseverance, Imagination–Playfulness, and Originality, and shows an internal-consistency reliability of .92. Validity coefficients of .38, .50, and .32 have been obtained, again using the criterion of combined teacher ratings of creativeness with experimenter ratings of the creativeness of children's pictures and short stories (both determined from a 5-point rating scale).

A rating scale that is perhaps the most

widely known and widely used among teachers in gifted programs throughout schools for all age levels is the Scale for Rating the Behavioral Characteristics of Superior Students (SRBCSS; Renzulli, 1983; Renzulli & Hartman, 1971). The Creativity subscale is only one of five subscales; is composed of 10 items rated on a scale of 1–4; and assesses such characteristics as curiosity, fluency of idea production, risk taking, humor and intellectual playfulness, emotional and aesthetic sensitivity, nonconformity, and critical evaluation. Its validity is thought to be in its ability to identify creative students who should be included in programs for gifted children.

Products

The use of products to assess creative potential and current creativity among children is widespread and is one means of identifying candidates for qualitatively sound gifted programs in schools. School district personnel concerned with gifted programs most often develop their own rating scales for such products or portfolios of accomplishments in a variety of fields. Some states, such as Louisiana, have focused extensively on the development of statewide rating scales for the many different areas of artistic endeavor and performance, and have implemented statewide guidelines for the evaluation of products and performances (Dial, 1975). Assumed with most such rating scales is that experts in the field of the product or performance will do the rating, and that a consensus approach with multiple judges will be used.

Based on a model for analyzing a product's creativity by Besemer and Treffinger (1981), Besemer and O'Quin (1986) developed a bipolar semantic scale to be used as a judging instrument. The 80-item Creative Product Semantic Scale has three subscales: Novelty, characterizing originality, surprise effect, and germinal quality; Resolution, characterizing the value, logic, and usefulness of the product; and Elaboration and Synthesis, characterizing the product's organicity, elegance, complexity, capability to be understood, and degree of crafting. At this time, this instrument is still in the process of development.

Another example of an instrument currently in the process of development is the Creative Processes Rating Scale (Kulp & Tarter, 1986) for measuring the creative process of' children in the visual arts. Uniqueness, rearrangements, magnification and variation, and generation of ideas in transformation of basic shapes in response to five given basic shapes are the elements assessed on a 5-point rating scale by an art expert. Its authors believe that the scale provides a visible alternative for measurement of the child's creative process, thus allowing early recognition of the potentially highly creative child: "The existence of an objective instrument to measure the complex and abstract concepts of visual creativity should provide assistance to both researchers and practitioners in the identification and instruction of visual art practices" (Kulp & Tarter, 1986, p. 170).

A third example of an instrument for evaluating creative products—one that is still in the process of development—is the Test for Creative Thinking–Drawing Production (TCT-DP; Jellen & Urban, 1986). This paper-and-pencil instrument designed for most age and ability groups focuses on drawing products resulting when respondents are presented with a given group of figural stimuli; thus it is not a direct measure of product creativity. However, it allows respondents to interpret what they consider to be significant in the development of a creative product and to complete this interpretation through their own creative drawing production. The assumption by the instrument developers is that this interpretation of what would be creative in the test-drawing situation should generalize to naturally produced drawings and should thus serve as a valid predictor of creativity in an individual's drawings.

The test drawings are evaluated according to a specific point list for each of II criteria. The authors describe the 11 criteria or "key elements" as linked with the six components of creative thought—that is, with fluency, flexibility, originality, elaboration, risk taking, and composition, all applied to characteristics of the drawing product. The 11 criteria are completion, additions, new elements, connections made with a line, connections made to produce a theme, boundary breaking that is fragment-dependent, boundary breaking that is fragment-independent, perspective (any breaking away from two-dimensionality), humor, unconventionality, and speed. In the TCT-DP, six figural fragments are irregularly placed within a square frame presented on a sheet of paper. Respondents are allowed 15 minutes for the testing procedure. Evaluation of each case requires approximately 3–5 minutes. In addition to belief in the TCT-DP's conceptual soundness for linkage between creative abilities and a visible product, the authors claim as advantages of this instrument the low cost for test material, minimal time required for administration and evaluation, and ease of training for use of the test (Jellen & Urban, 1986). Interrater reliability is reported as ranging between .89 and .97, based on approximately 100 cases. The authors suggest that the criteria of the TCT-DP could be applicable with minor modification to creative acts in music, dance, writing, and dramatics. They also suggest its possibilities as a psychiatrically relevant clinical instrument for interpretation of schizophrenic or primitive thinking.

MAKING SENSE OF OBSERVATIONS AND MEASUREMENTS

A major problem in the assessment of creativity has been deciding what creative abilities/skills are most worth assessing and what sense can be made of the assessment data. In the operational situations of schools, colleges, businesses, and the like, it would not be practical to assess all of these abilities and skills; nor would it necessarily be useful. The abilities and skills assessed through tests must have their analogues in classroom performances, and in turn in real-life creative achievements. That linkage or lack of it (as the case may be) is at the heart of controversies over whether creative functioning should be a core concern in education and eventually in society at large, or an after-the-fact concern, nice but not essential.

As elaborated throughout the preceding text, we continue to be dependent on assessing only the elements of performance that might lead to full-blown creative contributions, rather than creativity as a "Gestalt."

We need, then, to ask where information may be obtained to substantiate the priority we give to particular elements in verifying creative acts and in increasing our ability to predict productive outcome. Biographies and other accounts of history's greatest inventors, scientific discoverers, and artists have provided such information. Clues have also been located in the everyday creative behaviors and achievements of children, youths, and adults who were at early ages displaying creative performance in their familiar contexts and at levels reflecting their experience and training. Longitudinal studies of children in the process of development (Albert, 1983; Feldman, 1986) provide additional clues about the elements involved in their precocious performance. As stated earlier, the approaches used by leading technologies in the United States, England, and Japan to teach creative problem-solving skills, inventing, and other similar activities have provided further valuable information on the relative necessity of various abilities (Torrance, 1979b). And, throughout each of these searches, it has become obvious that creativity test indicators must meet reasonable criteria of clear and frequent manifestation in test performance; must possess the potential for development and improvement through instruction and training; and must demonstrate linkage to creative performance later in life.

Although accurate forecasting of future behavior is considered a desirable goal of psychological assessment, and valid predictions of later behavior can verify the theoretical construct from which a particular assessment instrument evolved, we are reminded of an additional value of such assessment (Heist, 1968). Psychological assessment has often been much more successful at enhancing current knowledge about individuals than at specifying what they will achieve or accomplish in the future. When such information is interpreted wisely and used appropriately, it serves educators and students alike in the attempts to individualize the teaching learning process. Heist (1968) focused on the postadolescent and college levels in the consideration of identification of creative potential, but his ideas are applicable in the earlier years of schooling as well. Furthermore, he limited this identification to the assessment of traits that appear to be part of the complex of creative behavior, rather than to tests that might reflect creative products or process. Thus the inventories he described assess values (the Study of Values; Allport, Vernon, & Lindzey, 1960), personal preferences (the Edwards Personal Preference Schedule; Edwards, 1957), academic motivation and intellectual concerns (the California Psychological Inventory; Gough, 1957), the behavioral syndromes associated with creative individuals (the Omnibus Personality Inventory; Heist, McConnell, Webster, & Yonge, 1968), and attitudes toward one's cognitive and perceptual environment (the Myers–Briggs Type Indicator; Myers & Briggs, 1957). In Amabile's (1983b) and Brown's (1989) componential models for creative behavior, these inventories address both the creativity-relevant skills component and the task motivation component, both of which are believed to originate from traits, training, experience, and perceptions of that experience. In the Amabile and Brown models, creative behavior is expressed as a coalescence of these two components with domain-relevant skills (knowledge, skills, and talent), which are dependent upon inherent ability and education, focused through interest in the domain.

Various researchers have sharply criticized the use of creativity tests that assess the processes of fluency, flexibility, originality, and elaboration; the implication is that these latter are not creative abilities. The relationship of these abilities to creativity and the supporting rationale for identifying and teaching them have been elaborated elsewhere, but they must be reaffirmed here. Possession of these abilities will not guarantee creative behavior, just as a high degree of measured intelligence does not guarantee intelligent behavior. Although these somewhat unitary abilities do not make up the entire constellation of abilities needed to perform creatively, assessment should not be avoided. And, subsequently, we should not be deterred from fostering specific creativity-relevant skills in children and adolescents in order to increase the probability of creative performance by these individuals, given the opportune situation and time.

APPROPRIATE APPLICATION OF ASSESSMENT RESULTS

It probably goes without saying that all psychometric and clinical assessment devices and procedures should help teachers, counselors, psychologists, and others who use assessment data do a better job. If test performances are to have their analogues in classroom performances, and subsequently in life outside the classroom, the most obvious and direct application of the results of assessment of creativity in children and adolescents may be in planning lessons and other curricular and extracurricular experiences that support creative responses, and in evaluating outcomes of instruction without bias against creative strengths.

The assessment of creativity in children and adolescents will be pointless, however, if it serves to exclude them from opportunity—that is, to keep them out of special programs where they might begin to learn how to express their ideas and feelings creatively. Assessment data must be more appropriately used to plan instruction that takes advantage of identified creative potential already bubbling forth, and works to release that potential when it has been inhibited and obstructed in its natural development.

Assessment data should have as a primary goal to accomplish the following specific outcomes if they are to help teachers do a better job:

- Awareness among teachers, psychologists, students, and parents of the creative abilities and skills that should be developed and practiced, as well as the personality characteristics, attitudes, and values that support creative responsiveness.
- Awareness of the individual student's strengths for creative learning and problem solving.
- Awareness of gaps or deficits in the student's repertoire of creative abilities and skills.
- Provision of a basis for generating appropriate learning activities and planning instruction.
- Provision of a basis for generating evaluation procedures that assess not only the traditionally tested types of outcomes,

but also some of the more elusive objectives of education.

Assessment data as discussed above can be useful in designing individual education programs (IEPs) or in working with an entire class or group of classes. Though assessment will demonstrate considerable variability among students on any of the creativity indicators, it will quite often be possible to identify common strengths and weaknesses in a class or even in a school population. Cultural homogeneity will often result in an unusually high level of a specific creativity indicator, or sometimes an unusually low level of a specific indicator, For example, in one school system (kindergarten through 12th grade) of Native American children, imagery and boundary extension were strengths, appearing much more frequently than among the larger norm sample. On the other hand, fantasy, expression of feeling and emotion, humor, and putting things in context were significantly less frequent. Direct teaching or encouragement of these skills may be necessary in such cases before creative abilities can be adequately expressed.

An instructional model for integrating the teaching of creative thinking skills into the teaching of reading and social studies, described and illustrated in *Encouraging Creativity in the Classroom* (Torrance, 1970; see also Torrance, 1979a), focuses on the things that can be done before, during, and after a lesson to enhance incubation and creative thinking and action. Both anticipatory and participatory learning are emphasized, calling into play creative thinking skills. Heightening anticipation and expectations creates a desire to know or to find out, fostering curiosity and making room for creative responses (Botkin, Elmandjra, & Malitza, 1979). Other creativity-relevant skills may be fostered during and after the lesson, again using current levels of functioning via assessment data to guide the extent to which skills must be introduced through direct instruction, nurtured through gentle encouragement, or simply allowed to be practiced and to soar when already at a high level. Bogner (1981) has used psychometric data from the TTGT not only to write IEPs for her gifted students, but to encourage them to write their own

IEPs. Some of her students used the checklist of creativity indicators to evaluate their own creative productions, much as in the TCT-DP instrument developed by Jellen and Urban (1986), described earlier.

Perhaps one of the most significant uses of creativity assessment data has been to identify areas of strength among children from racial groups and SES levels who have previously been denied access to special or even ordinary educational opportunities on the basis of weaknesses identified through intelligence tests and/or school achievement data. Results of 16 different studies in different parts of the United States (Torrance, 1971, 1975) indicated no racial or economic differences on either the verbal or figural TTCT. In some cases, black children excelled over white children on certain tasks; since children may respond to tests such as these in terms of their own life experiences, and tasks are open-ended, children are not penalized for lack of academically intellectual experiences.

Through focusing on strengths in creative thinking abilities, Carlson (1975) was able to demonstrate gains by a child with a learning disability in specific behaviors related to academic and social performance. This child's strengths were dependable fluency of ideas and elaboration, as well as original or unique behavior; however, her ability to shift categories and classifications was not a strength. Although gains were achieved by Carlson in a one-to-one setting, others have achieved gains in a similar fashion with an entire class of underachieving children at about the fifth- or sixth-grade level (Carlson, 1975). Using creativity assessment data and the model of creative strengths in a fashion similar to Carlson's approach, a teacher in another district not only demonstrated increased academic achievement in reading, arithmetic, and other areas over that in comparable classes, but also found improvement in health (or attitude) as measured in significantly decreased visits to the school nurse (Torrance, 1987b).

Creativity tests themselves may be used creatively, as demonstrated by one teacher who used them to reduce test-taking phobia (Torrance, 1987b). Children who had been exhibiting anger, frustration, and helplessness about regular achievement tests were given the opportunity to take the TTCT several times, to take it at home, to correspond with the test author, and generally to defuse their anxiety about the test-taking process. Subsequent exposure 3 months later to the standardized achievement testing situation revealed an increased functional attitude by these students, culminating in academic performance growth of about 2 years—much more than might have been expected through academic instruction alone.

Finally, it must be pointed out that even though teachers, educational planners/decision makers, psychologists and other clinicians, and sometimes parents seek objective data to assure themselves that particular children have creative ability and the potential for creative productivity, this kind of ability will always be evident to attentive educators at all levels, The assessment instrument through which this ability becomes evident is sensitive observation of children at work and play. Some facets of this complex phenomenon may be more readily apparent than others. The 4-year-old boy in a program for gifted preschoolers who, oblivious of others, has figuratively transformed his body into the fluid movements of the aquarium fish he is observing intently; the 3-year-old girl who states that the ants are guests at her picnic; and the boy who with great facility transforms the blob of paint that has emerged on his paper into a crab with six "legs," one of which is explained by him to be "detached but the crab will grow it again," are all reflecting creative potential. Their fluid responses to the reality of facts, information, and materials they have encountered are spontaneous indicators of productivity yet to come if such responses are allowed, nurtured, and reinforced. Nontest indicators may be found in regular classroom activities, as well as in classroom situations that have been especially designed to evoke creative behavior. The third-grader who consistently suggests an alternative ending for stories in reading; the eighth-grader who insists that the Yalta agreements have been misconstrued because of facts A, B, and C; and the trigonometry student who chooses to arrive at problem solutions through nonclassical procedure variants are all demonstrating their creative potential in what should be highly acceptable ways in the classroom.

However, the effects of suppressive versus facilitative environments on creative expression will also have to be acknowledged if one is to observe creative potential. The misplaced construction of humor inappropriately applied by an adolescent in a rigid class setting may reflect creative potential struggling to express itself. Graffiti, often assumed to be the work of illiterate and uneducated individuals who have a crude sense of societal propriety, speaks for people who seek an audience, legitimate or otherwise. On occasions, graffiti has come to be viewed as a form of creative expression for the social conscience and an art form in its own right, with a recognized audience; it has even found its way into art museums.

Although entrance into programs or recognition for appropriate educational services will continue to be dependent upon the documented data from proven assessment instruments, the day-to-day response of parents, teachers, and other types of educators to the creativity their children or students spontaneously emit will continue to be critical to the transformation of creative potential into creative productivity. Such levels of assessment in no way deny the contribution of specific domain-related abilities, creativity-relevant abilities (inherent or trained), and the domain-specific acquisition of foundation knowledge that will affect the eventual direction and substance of creative production.

SUMMARY

In summary, we have presented in this chapter an overview of current views of the creativity phenomenon as we believe they apply to assessment—specifically, to the assessment of creativity in children and adolescents. Thus we have not addressed the vast amount of work concerned with understanding, evaluating, and predicting creative productivity that emerges in adulthood, in industrial and corporate settings, in the various scientific fields, or in the aesthetic domains. However, in order to establish an overarching perspective, we have examined an array of definitions and suggested an integrated dimension that takes into account the contribution of processes, personal characteristics/attributes, and types of products that are involved in creative endeavor.

A description of instruments currently available to assess creativity as it is present in process, person, and product provides readers with a wide variety of ways to sensibly conduct assessments of creativity with children and adolescents—assessments that will find meaningful application. Furthermore, we have recommended applications of assessment results that we consider to have been fruitful in the past and that seem most closely attuned to the most advanced current understanding of creativity. We particularly advocate the use of such data to structure (or modify when necessary) instruction and the environment in our schools and society, in order to facilitate the emergence and maximization of creative potential for all the children and adolescents who are our concern in this handbook.

REFERENCES

Albert, R. S. (Ed.). (1983). *Genius and eminence.* New York: Pergamon Press.

Allport, G. W., Vernon, P. E., & Lindzey, C. (1960). *Study of values* (3rd ed.). Boston: Houghton Mifflin.

Amabile, T. M. (1983a). *The social psychology of creativity.* New York: Springer.

Amabile, T. M. (1983b). The social psychology of creativity: A componential conceptualization. *Journal of Personality and Social Psychology, 45,* 357–376.

Anderson. H. H. (Ed.). (1959). *Creativity and its cultivation.* New York: Harper & Row.

Barchillon. J. (1961). *Personality dimensions of creativity.* New York: Lincoln Institute of Psychotherapy.

Barron, F. (1969). *Creative person and creative process.* New York: Holt, Rinehart & Winston.

Barron. F. (1978). An eye more fantastical. In G. A. Davis & J. A. Scott (Eds.), *Training creative thinking* (pp. 181–193). Melbourne, FL: Krieger.

Bartlett, F. (1958). *Thinking.* New York: Basic Books.

Besemer, S. P., & O'Quin, K. (1986). Analyzing creative products: Refinement and test of a judging instrument. *Journal of Creative Behavior, 20,* 115–126.

Besemer, S. P., & Treffinger, D. J. (1981). Analysis of creative products: Review and synthesis. *Journal of Creative Behavior, 15,* l58–178.

Bloom, B. (1985). *Developing talent in young children.* New York: Ballantine.

Bogner, D. (1981). Creative individual education programs (IEP's) from creativity tests. *Creative Child and Adult Quarterly, 6,* 160–162.

Botkin, J. W., Elmandjra, M., & Malitza, M. (1979). *No limits to learning.* New York: Pergamon Press.

Broadley, M. E. (1943). *Square pegs in square holes.* Garden City, NY: Doubleday.

Brown, R. T. (1989). Creativity: What are we to measure? In J. A. Glover, R. Ronning, & C. R. Reynolds (Eds.), *A handbook of creativity: Assessment, research, and theory.* New York: Plenum Press.

Carlson, N. A. (1975). Using the creative strengths of a learning disabled child to increase evaluative effort and academic achievement (Doctoral dissertation, Michigan State University, 1974). *Dissertation Abstracts International, 35,* 5962A. (University Microfilms No. 75-07135)

Cramond, B., Matthews-Morgan, J., & Torrance, E. P. (2001). The forty-year follow-up on the Torrance Tests of Creative Thinking. *Journal of Creative Behavior.*

Crutchfield, R. S. (1962). Conformity and creative thinking. In H. E. Gruber, C. Terrell, & M. Wertheimer (Eds.), *Contemporary approaches to creative thinking* (pp. 120–140). New York: Atherton Press.

Davis, G. A. (1973). *Psychology of problem solving.* New York: Basic Books.

Davis. G. A. (1975). In frumious pursuit of the creative person. *Journal of Creative Behavior, 9,* 75–87.

Davis, G. A. (1986). *Creativity is forever* (2nd ed.). Dubuque, IA: Kendall/Hunt.

Davis, G. A., & Rimm. S. (1980). *Group inventory for finding interests II.* Watertown, WI: Educational Assessment Service.

Davis, G. A., & Rimm, S. (1982). Group Inventory for Finding Interests (GIFFI) I and II: Instruments for identifying creative potential in the junior and senior high school. *Journal of Creative Behavior, 16,* 50–57.

de Bono, E. (1967). *New think: The use of lateral thinking in the generation of new ideas.* New York: Basic Books.

de Bono, E. (1970). *Lateral thinking: Creativity step by step.* New York: Harper & Row.

Dial, P. C. (1975). *Identifying and serving the talented student in Louisiana Schools.* Baton Rouge: Louisiana Department of Education, Gifted and Talented Programs.

Edwards, A. L. (1957). *Edwards Personal Preference Schedule.* New York: Psychological Corporation.

Feldman, D. H. (1986). *Nature's gambit.* New York: Basic Books.

Flanagan, J. C. (1963). The definition and measurement of ingenuity. In C. W. Taylor & F. Barron (Eds.), *Scientific creativity: Its recognition and development* (pp. 89–98). New York: Wiley.

Flanagan, J. C. (1976). Ingenuity Test. In A. M. Biondi & S. J. Parnes (Eds.), *Assessing creative growth: The tests and measured changes* (pp. 117–119). Buffalo, NY: Bearly.

Gardner, H. (1983). *Frames of mind: The theory of multiple intelligences.* New York: Basic Books.

Gardner, H. (1993). *Multiple intelligences: The theory in practice.* New York: Basic Books.

Getzels, J. W., & Jackson, D. W. (1962). *Creativity and intelligence.* New York: Wiley.

Ghiselin, B. (Ed.). (1952). *The creative process.* New York: Mentor.

Ghiselin, B. (1963). Ultimate criteria for two levels of creativity. In C. W. Taylor & F. Barron (Eds.), *Sci-*

entiftc creativity: Its recognition and development (pp. 30–43). New York: Wiley.

Glock, J., Wertz, S., & Meyer, M. (1999). *Discovering the naturalist intelligence.* Tucson, AZ: Zephyr Press.

Gordon, W. J. J. (1961). *Synectics.* New York: Harper & Row.

Gough, H. C. (1957). *The California Psychological Inventory.* Palo Alto, CA: Consulting Psychologists Press.

Guilford, J. P. (1950). Creativity. *American Psychologist, 5,* 444–454.

Guilford, J. P. (1956). Structure of intellect. *Psychological Bulletin, 53,* 267–293.

Guilford, J. P. (1959). *Personality.* New York: McGraw-Hill.

Guilford, J. P. (1960). Basic conceptual problems of the psychology of thinking. *Annals of the New York Academy of Sciences, 91,* 6–21.

Guilford, J. P. (1967). *The nature of human intelligence.* New York: McGraw-Hill.

Guilford, J. P. (1971). *Creativity Tests for Children (CTC).* Orange, CA: Sheridan Psychological Services.

Guilford, J. P. (1976). Creativity: Its measurement and development. In A. Biondi & S. J. Parnes (Eds.), *Assessing creative growth: The tests and measured changes* (pp. 2–26). Buffalo, NY: Bearly.

Guilford, J. P. (1977). *Way beyond the IQ.* Buffalo, NY: Bearly.

Guilford, J. P. (1986). *Creative talents: Their nature, uses, and development.* Buffalo, NY: Bearly.

Haensly, P. A., & Reynolds, C. R. (1989). Creativity and intelligence. In J. A. Glover, R. R. Ronning, & C. R. Reynolds (Eds.), *A handbook of creativity: Assessment, research, and theory.* New York: Plenum Press.

Haensly, P. A., & Torrance, E. P. (1990). Assessment of creativity in children and adolescents. In C. R. Reynolds & R. A. Kamphaus (Eds.), *Handbook of psychological and educational assessment of children: Intelligence and achievement* (pp. 697–722). New York: Guilford Press.

Heist, P. (1968). Considerations in the assessment of creativity. In P. Heist (Ed.), *The creative college student: An unmet challenge* (pp. 208–223). San Francisco: Jossey-Bass.

Heist, P., McConnell, T. R., Webster, H., & Yonge, G. (1968). *The Omnibus Personality Inventory* (rev. version). Berkeley: University of California, Center for Research and Development in Higher Education.

Hoepfner, R., & Hemenway, J. (1973). *Test of Creative Potential (TCP).* Hollywood, CA: Monitor.

Jackson, P. W., & Messick, S. (1967). The person, the product, and the response: Conceptual problems in the assessment of creativity. In J. Kagan (Ed.), *Creativity and learning* (pp. 1–19). Boston: Houghton Mifflin.

Jellen, H. G., & Urban, K. K. (1986). The TCT-DP (Test for Creative Thinking–Drawing Production): An instrument that can be applied to most age and ability groups. *Creative Child and Adult Quarterly, 11,* 138–155.

Kaufman, A. S. (1979). *Intelligent testing with the WISC-R.* New York: Wiley.

Khatena, J., & Torrance, E. P. (1973). *Thinking Creatively with Sounds and Words.* Bensenville, IL: Scholastic Testing Service.

Khatena, J., & Torrance, E. P. (1976). *Khatena–Torrance Creative Perception Inventories.* Chicago: Stoelting.

Khatena, J., & Torrance, E. P. (1998a). *Khatena–Torrance Creative Perception Inventories: Instruction manual.* Bensenville, IL: Scholastic Testing Service.

Khatena, J., & Torrance, E. P. (1998b). *Thinking Creatively with Sounds and Words (TCSW): Norms–technical manual.* Bensenville, IL: Scholastic Testing Service.

Kubie, L. S. (1958). *The neurotic distortion of the creative process.* Lawrence: University of Kansas Press.

Kulp, M., & Tarter, B. J. (1986). The Creative Process-es Rating Scale. *Creative Child and Adult Quarterly, 11,* 163–173, 176.

Lazear, D. (1994). *Multiple intelligences approach to assessment: Solving the assessment conundrum.* Phoenix, AZ: Zephyr Press.

MacKinnon, D. W. (1976). Architects, personality types, and creativity. In A. Rothenberg & C. R. Hausman (Eds.), *The creativity question* (pp. 175–179). Durham, NC: Duke University Press.

MacKinnon, D. W. (1978). Educating for creativity: A modern myth? In G. A. Davis & J. A. Scott (Eds.), *Training creative thinking* (pp. 194–207). Melbourne, FL: Krieger.

May, R. (1975). *The courage to create.* New York: Norton.

Mednick, S. A., & Mednick, M. T. (1967). *Remote Associates Test.* Boston: Houghton Mifflin.

Meeker, M., Meeker, R., & Roid, G. H. (1985). *Structure of Intellect Learning Abilities Test (SOI-LAT) manual.* Los Angeles, CA: Western Psychological Services.

Myers, I. B., & Briggs, K. C. (1957). *The Myers–Briggs Type Indicator.* Princeton, NJ: Educational Testing Service.

O'Connor, J. (1945). *Square pegs in square holes.* Garden City, NY: Doubleday.

Osborn, A.F. (1963). *Applied imagination* (3rd ed.). New York: Scribner.

Parnes, S. J. (1962). Can creativity be increased? In S. J. Parnes & H. F. Harding (Eds.), *A source book for creative thinking* (pp. 185–191). New York: Scribner.

Parnes, S. J., Noller, R, B., & Biondi, A. M. (1971). *Guide to creative action.* New York: Scribner.

Plucker, J. A. (1999). Is the proof in the pudding?: Reanalyses of Torrance's data (1958–1980) longitudinal study. *Creativity Research Journal, 12,* 103–114.

Puccio, G. J., & Murdock, M. C. (Eds.). (1999). *Creativity assessment: Readings and resources.* Buffalo, NY: Creative Education Press.

Renzulli, J. S. (1983, September–October). Rating the behavioral characteristics of superior students. *G/C/T,* pp. 30–35.

Renzulli, J. S., & Hartman, R. K. (1971). Scale for Rating Behavioral Characteristics of Superior Students. *Exceptional Children, 38,* 243–359.

Ribot, T. (1906). *Essays on the creative imagination*. London: Routledge & Kegan Paul.

Rimm, S. (1976). *GIFT: Group Inventory for Finding Talent*. Watertown, WI: Educational Assessment Service.

Rimm, S. (1983). *Preschool and Kindergarten Interest Descriptor*. Watertown, WI: Educational Assessment Service.

Rimm, S., & Davis, G. A. (1976). GIFT: An instrument for the identification of creativity. *Journal of Creative Behavior, 10*, 178–182.

Rimm, S., & Davis, G. A. (1979). *Group Inventory for Finding Interests I*. Watertown, WI: Educational Assessment Service.

Rimm, S., & Davis, G. A. (1980). Five years of international research with GIFT: An instrument for the identification of creativity. *Journal of Creative Behavior, 14*, 35–46.

Rimm, S., & Davis, G. A. (1983, September–October). Identifying creativity, Part II. *G/C/T*, pp. 19–23.

Roe, A. (1951). A psychological study of physical scientists. *Genetic Psychology Monographs, 43*, 121–235.

Roe, A. (1953). A psychological study of eminent psychologists and anthropologists and a comparison with biological and physical scientists. *Psychological Monographs, 67*(2, Whole No. 352).

Sattler, J. M. (1974). *Assessment of children's intelligence* (rev. ed.). Philadelphia: Saunders.

Schaefer, C. E. (1971). *Creativity attitude survey*. Jacksonville, IL: Psychologists and Educators.

Selye, H. (1962). The gift for basic research. In G. Z. F. Bereday & J. A. Lauwerys (Eds.), *The gifted child: The yearbook of education* (pp. 339–408). New York: Harcourt, Brace & World.

Simonton, D. K. (1988). Creativity, leadership and chance. In R. Sternberg (Ed.), *The nature of creativity* (pp. 386–426). Cambridge, England: Cambridge University Press.

Spearman, C. E. (1930). *Creative mind*. Cambridge, England: Cambridge University Press.

Starkweather, E. K. (1976). Creativity research instruments designed for use with preschool children. In A. M. Biondi & S. J. Parnes (Eds.), *Assessing creative growth: The tests and measured changes* (pp. 79–90). Buffalo, NY: Bearly.

Starkweather, E. K., & Cowling, F. G. (1963). The measurement of conforming and nonconforming behavior in preschool children. *Proceedings of the Oklahoma Academy of Science, 44*, 168–180.

Sternberg, R. J. (1988). A three-facet model of creativity. In R. Sternberg (Ed.), *The nature of creativity* (pp. 125–147). Cambridge, England: Cambridge University Press.

Sternberg, R. J., & Wagner, R. K. (1986). *Practical intelligence: Nature and origins of competence in the everyday world*. Cambridge, England: Cambridge University Press.

Stewart, G. W. (1950). Can productive thinking be taught? *Journal of Higher Education, 21*, 411–414.

Taylor, I. A. (1959). The nature of the creative process. In P. Smith (Ed.), *Creativity* (pp. 51–82). New York: Hastings House.

Taylor, C. W. (1988). Various approaches to the definitions of creativity. In R. J. Sternberg (Ed.), *The nature of creativity* (pp. 99–121). Cambridge, England: Cambridge University Press.

Thurstone, L. L. (1952). Creative talent. In L. L. Thurstone (Ed.), *Applications of psychology* (pp. 18–37). New York: Harper & Row.

Torrance, E. P. (1955). Techniques for studying individual and group adaptation in emergencies and extreme conditions. In *Air Force human engineering personnel and training research* (pp. 286–297). Washington, DC: National Academy of Sciences/National Research Council.

Torrance, E. P. (1957). *Psychology of survival*. Unpublished manuscript, Air Force Personnel Research Center, Lackland Air Force Base, TX.

Torrance, E. P. (1963). *Education and the creative potential*. Minneapolis: University of Minnesota Press.

Torrance, E. P. (1965). *Rewarding creative behavior*. Englewood Cliffs, NJ: Prentice-Hall.

Torrance, E. P. (1966). *The Torrance Tests of Creative Thinking: Technical–norms manual* (research ed.). Princeton, NJ: Personnel Press.

Torrance, E. P. (1967). Scientific views of creativity and factors affecting its growth. In J. Kagan (Ed.), *Creativity and learning* (pp. 73–91). Boston: Houghton Mifflin.

Torrance, E. P. (1970). *Encouraging creativity in the classroom*. Dubuque, IA: William C. Brown.

Torrance, E. P. (1971). Are the Torrance Tests of Creative Thinking biased against or in favor of disadvantaged groups? *Gifted Child Quarterly, 15*, 75–80.

Torrance, E. P. (1972a). Career patterns and peak creative experiences of creative high school children 12 years later. *Gifted Child Quarterly, 16*, 75–88.

Torrance, E. P. (1972b). Predictive validity of the Torrance Tests of Creative Thinking. *Journal of Creative Behavior, 9*, 182–192.

Torrance, E. P. (1974). *The Torrance Tests of Creative Thinking: Technical–norms manual*. Bensenville, IL: Scholastic Testing Service.

Torrance, E. P. (1975). Sociodrama as a creative problem solving approach to studying the future. *Journal of Creative Behavior, 9*, 182–195.

Torrance, E. P. (1979a). An instructional model for enhancing incubation. *Journal of Creative Behavior, 13*, 23–35.

Torrance, E. P. (1979b). *The search for satori and creativity*. Buffalo, NY: Bearly.

Torrance, E. P. (1981). Predicting the creativity of elementary school children (1958–1980)—and the teachers who made a "difference." *Gifted Child Quarterly, 25*, 55–62.

Torrance, E. P. (1982). Sounds and images productions of elementary school pupils as predictors of the creative achievement of young adults. *Creative Child and Adult Quarterly, 7*, 8–14.

Torrance, E. P. (1987a). *Guidelines for administration and scoring/comments on using the Torrance Tests of Creative Thinking*. Bensenville, IL: Scholastic Testing Service.

Torrance, E. P. (1987b). *Survey of the uses of the Torrance Tests of Creative Thinking*. Bensenville, IL: Scholastic Testing Service.

Torrance, E. P. (1988). The nature of creativity as manifested in its testing. In R. J. Sternberg (Ed.), *The nature of creativity* (pp. 43–75). Cambridge, England: Cambridge University Press.

Torrance, E. P. (1993). The beyonders in a thirty year longitudinal of creative achievement. *Roeper Review: A Journal of Gifted Education, 15,* 131–134.

Torrance, E. P. (2000). *Research review for the Torrance Tests of Creative Thinking: Figural and verbal forms A and B.* Bensenville, IL: Scholastic Testing Service.

Torrance, E. P., & Ball, O. E. (1984). *Torrance Tests of Creative Thinking: Streamlined (revised) manual, figural forms A and B.* Bensenville, IL: Scholastic Testing Service.

Torrance, E. P., & Wu, T. H. (1981). A comparative longitudinal study of the adult creative achievements of elementary school children identified as highly creative. *Creative Child and Adult Quarterly, 6,* 71–76.

Wallach, M. A., & Kogan, N. (1965). *Modes of thinking in young children.* New York: Holt.

Wallas, G. (1926). *The art of thought.* New York: Harcourt, Brace & World.

Whipple, G. M. (1973). *Manual for mental and physical tests.* New York: Arno Press. (Original work published 1915)

Wittrock, M. C. (1974). Learning as a generative process. *Educational Psychologist, 11,* 87–95, 20.

25

Cognitive Abilities and Assessment of Children with Language Impairment

JUDITH M. KROESE

The purpose of this chapter is to describe the population of children who exhibit significant oral language problems and to summarize pertinent information regarding assessment. Testing cognitive functioning in individuals with these language problems—or, as such problems are called in this chapter, "specific language impairment" (SLI)—entails far more than simply using a test with nonverbal content and directions. Although many of these children have nonverbal cognitive abilities within the average range, others do not. Nonverbal cognitive difficulties, along with oral language deficits, can affect the assessment results and the outcomes of assessment for these children.

This chapter reviews the characteristics of this population and provides pertinent information regarding the etiology, prevalence, and course of SLI. The chapter begins with a description of some of the problems evidenced by these individuals. Then factors to consider in the selection, administration, and interpretation of assessment instruments are presented. In the next section, several instruments for assessing cognitive functioning are summarized briefly, accompanied by pertinent validity information with this population.

WHAT IS SLI?

The heterogeneity of children with SLI has been noted by many researchers and clinicians (e.g., Bishop, 1992; Leonard, 1998; Stromswold, 2000). However, there are also many similarities, as described in the following sections.

Definition

SLI has been categorized by many labels during the past 40 years including "language disorder," "language delay," "language impairment," "aphasia," and "language-learning disability" (Kamhi, 1998). During the past 10 years or more, the label most often used in the literature has been "SLI" (see above), although from a clinical perspective, many of the terms just mentioned continue in common use. The definition of SLI in the literature also differs from and is narrower than the definition of language impairment used clinically. Leonard (1998) notes that it is relatively easy to make a diagnosis of a language impairment, but that it is sometimes difficult to distinguish it from other disorders of which a language problem is only one feature. This chapter uses the term "SLI" to refer to this condition, but will define it as including the "clinical" and broader meaning rather than the narrower, research meaning.

Similar to definitions of a learning disability, definitions of SLI often characterize it by what it is *not* rather than what it is (Watkins, 1994). It is a disorder of oral language, either expressive and/or receptive, not associated with, or in excess of, an impairment in intellectual capacity. It is also not associated with a sensory or speech–motor deficit, neurological insult or disorder, or social–emotional problem (American Psychiatric Association, 1994). The language deficit has to be verified by one or more individualized, standardized tests of oral language. However, Leonard (1998) notes that standardized language results do not cover either the breadth or the depth of language difficulties these children have.

Criteria for Diagnosing SLI

Stark and Tallal (1981) were the first to delineate criteria for applying a diagnosis of SLI. Since that time, several variations of their criteria have been used (Stromswold, 2000). Currently, the criteria generally include language test results at least 1.25 standard deviations below average; nonverbal intellectual functioning (nonverbal or Performance IQ) of 85 or above; normal hearing sensitivity; no recent history of middle-ear infections; no evidence of a neurological problem; no obvious problems with oral structures or function; and no symptoms of social difficulties in interactions with others (Leonard, 1998).

Including the criterion of normal nonverbal intelligence in the definition of SLI has been a hotly debated issue (e.g., Casby, 1992; Cole, Dale, & Mills, 1992; Cole, Schwartz, & Notari, 1995; Fey, Long, & Cleave, 1994; Francis, Fletcher, Shaywitz, Shaywitz, & Rourke, 1996; Kamhi, 1998; Krassowski & Plante, 1997; Lahey, 1990; Restrepo, Swisher, Plante, & Vance, 1992). Lahey (1990) noted that traditional intelligence tests do not measure the type of cognitive development that most often has been investigated in studies of language development. She further noted that there are no theoretical reasons for assuming that an intelligence test score should predict current or future levels of language functioning. Therefore, she recommended that language performance should be compared to a child's chronological age, rather than to a child's performance on a standardized intelligence test.

Following the comments made by Lahey (1990), several other language researchers/practitioners noted other difficulties with a discrepancy definition of SLI. Restrepo and colleagues (1992) found that relationships among cognitive and language variables differed between children with normal language and children with SLI, indicating that there are qualitative differences rather than quantitative differences between these two groups. Krassowski and Plante (1997) found that the average mean Performance IQ on the Wechsler Intelligence Scale for Children—Revised (WISC-R; Wechsler, 1974) changed significantly over a 3-year period for children diagnosed with SLI (increasing for some and decreasing for others, but resulting in a significantly higher Performance IQ score overall). They further noted that 32% of these children's Performance IQ scores changed by 10 points or more within that 3-year period. These changes in IQ scores could have resulted in substantial changes in eligibility for special education programs for children with SLI. Stability of the measured discrepancy between IQ scores and language scores was the goal of research by Cole and colleagues (1992, 1995). They found that the absolute difference between language and cognitive measures was not stable over time, and that the differences varied relative to the psychometric measures used. Thus eligibility for SLI treatment programs would also vary. Fey and colleagues (1994) found that children with below-average language abilities improved significantly following treatment, whether their Performance IQ scores were within the average range or not; this finding indicated that scores on tests of nonverbal intellectual functioning apparently were not related to improvement following therapy. Casby (1992) noted that some state and local school districts may employ the discrepancy criteria in order to limit special education costs, although these regulations are inconsistent with appropriate practice for eligibility for language treatment, as defined by the American Speech–Language–Hearing

Association (1989). Francis and colleagues (1996) further delineated the conceptual and psychometric problems regarding using discrepancy criteria in the definition of language and learning disabilities; they noted that, unfortunately, these criteria are currently firmly established in our laws and in clinical practice.

Finally, Kamhi (1998) attempted to bring closure to this issue by noting that researchers and clinicians are naturally going to define "developmental language disorders" differently, because they have different objectives. He pointed out that SLI as defined by researchers is a much narrower concept than that used by clinicians. Researchers attempt to reduce the heterogeneity of this condition by imposing restrictions on the range of cognitive abilities, whereas clinicians attempt to treat a language impairment no matter what other conditions accompany it (e.g., recurrent otitus media, nonverbal or Performance IQ below 85, etc.).

There is clearly a difference between a *diagnosis* of SLI and *eligibility* for services. In the private sector, the discrepancy criteria is probably much less of an issue than in the public schools, where the costs of education must be considered in establishing special education regulations. More importantly, assessment of cognitive functioning, although important in painting a complete picture of an individual child, may not be a critical factor in determining whether the child has SLI and may only be an issue because of current laws and practices in the public schools.

Linguistic Characteristics

Leonard (1998) reviewed and highlighted the significant language findings relative to SLI. Although a good percentage of these youngsters show both language comprehension and production problems, at least half have obvious problems with language production only. Children with SLI are almost always late in starting to talk, although a good percentage of children who begin talking late eventually develop normal language abilities (Paul, 1996). Leonard notes that research findings indicate that children with SLI seem to learn and use a more limited variety of verbs than other children do. Many

also seem to evidence word-finding problems (i.e., problems retrieving specific words from long-term memory), although Leonard believes that these problems are related to a lack of depth and breadth of word meanings, rather than to a problem with actually retrieving the words (Kail & Leonard, 1986). Problems in this area are indicated by frequent pauses in production, many circumlocutions, and frequent use of nonspecific nouns and pronouns (e.g., "thing" or "stuff"). Both semantic and phonological substitutions are also common (e.g., "socks" for "shoes" or "telescope" for "stethoscope"). Almost all of these individuals have difficulty learning syntactic structure (i.e., learning how to put words together to form sentences) and grammatical morphemes (i.e., learning the rules for combining morphemes with words, such as "-ed" for past tense and "-s" or "-es" for plural). These individuals also almost always have difficulty with learning the phonological system (i.e., the speech sound system), although some of these difficulties are subtle and less obvious than the grammatical and syntactical problems. Subtle difficulties with language pragmatics are also present, such as difficulties with verbally resolving conflicts and providing ample details in narratives. In older individuals with SLI, problems with understanding figurative language such as idioms, proverbs, and metaphors are also apparent. There is considerable evidence that SLI exists in all languages; however, the characteristics of the linguistic deficits vary across languages (Leonard, 1998, 2000).

Nonlinguistic Characteristics

Not only do children with SLI have characteristic linguistic deficits, but they show specific deficits in some nonverbal cognitive abilities as well, in spite of average performance on tests of nonverbal intellectual functioning. Johnston (1994) describes the development of thought and the development of language as being "out of phase" in these children (p. 107); Swisher, Plante, and Lowell (1994) describe "pockets of nonverbal cognitive deficits" (p. 239); and Thal (1991) notes that relationships between developing linguistic and nonlinguistic cognitive abilities are different at different points in time.

Numerous studies have investigated the types of cognitive deficits that are represented in this population (Leonard, 1998). Deficits in symbolic representation have been noted (e.g., Kamhi, 1981; Snyder, 1987), as well as difficulties with "anticipatory imagery" (e.g., Johnston & Ramstad, 1983; Savich, 1984; Snyder, 1987). Anticipatory imagery is the ability to predict future change in the form or position of an object or an internal representation of that object (Savich, 1984). There is also evidence that individuals with SLI have difficulties with dimensional thinking. These difficulties are particularly obvious relative to judging size versus color, since size changes along an ordinal dimension, while color is nominally different (Johnston & Smith, 1989). Nippold, Erskine, and Freed (1988) found that children with SLI had difficulty with analogical reasoning (e.g., matrices), while Masterson (1993) and Nelson, Kamhi, and Appel (1987) found that such children had difficulty with rule abstraction (e.g., difficulties with the Concept Formation test of the Woodcock–Johnson Psycho-Educational Battery—Revised, Tests of Cognitive Ability; Woodcock, 1997).

The most robust findings relative to cognitive deficits in children with SLI are related to their slow processing abilities (e.g., Bishop, 1992; Johnston & Weismer, 1983; Kail, 1994; Lahey & Edwards, 1996; Miller, Kail, Leonard, & Tomblin, 2001; Nelson et al., 1987; Sininger, Klatzky, & Kirchner, 1989) and capacity limitations (e.g., Hanson & Montgomery, 2002; Johnston & Smith, 1989; Kamhi, Catts, Mauer, Appel, & Gentry, 1988; Kirchner & Klatzky, 1985; Kushnir & Blake, 1996; Maillart & Schelstraete, 2002; Montgomery, 2000; Nelson et al., 1987). Further robust findings highlight their difficulties with processing extremely short linguistic and nonlinguistic stimuli through both auditory and visual channels, as well as difficulties with processing such stimuli when the interval between stimuli is short (Leonard, 1998; Sininger et al., 1989; Tallal, Stark, Kallman, & Mellits, 1981). Leonard (1998) offers convincing arguments for why these latter findings are possibly related to the difficulties with capacity and rate of processing.

With regard to performance on tests of nonverbal intellectual functioning that are purportedly tapping general cognitive abilities, it has been found that children with SLI perform within the average range (Johnston, 1994; Leonard, 1998). However, two studies analyzed the content of three nonverbal intelligence tests—the original Leiter International Performance Scale (Leiter; Arthur, 1952), the original Test of Nonverbal Intelligence (TONI; Brown, Sherbenou, & Johnsen, 1982), and the Columbia Mental Maturity Scale (CMMS; Burgemeister, Blum, & Lorge, 1972)—frequently used for children with SLI (Johnston, 1982; Kamhi, Minor, & Mauer, 1990). It was noted that the items on which young children (both nonexceptional children and those with SLI) scored well were primarily items requiring perceptual judgments rather than conceptual reasoning.

If children with SLI indeed have the types of disabilities noted in the research cited above, then one might anticipate that as they get older, their scores on tests of nonverbal intellectual functioning might become lower as they are required to respond correctly to more conceptual and challenging items. Although this in fact has been found in several research studies (e.g., Aram, Ekelman, & Nation, 1984; Tomblin, Freese, & Records, 1992), evidence has also been found to the contrary (e.g., Krassowski & Plante, 1997).

Thus it is obvious that nonlinguistic deficits are present in individuals with SLI. These include problems with symbolic representation, anticipatory imagery, dimensional thinking, analogical reasoning, rule abstraction, rate of processing, processing capacity, and processing of rapidly presented short stimuli (especially through the auditory channel). It is important to consider such deficits in assessing the nonverbal cognitive abilities of individuals with SLI. It is likely that tests that involve one or more of these problem areas will result in lower scores than tests that do not include these areas of functioning.

Prevalence

Depending on the method used to define SLI, prevalence estimates vary. The American Psychiatric Association (1994) reports an estimate of 5% of expressive-only language problems and 3% for combined receptive–expressive deficits among school-age children. This combined 8% estimate is comparable to prevalence rates found in a large-scale study by Tomblin and colleagues (1997) of over 6,000 children age 5. These investigators found a prevalence rate of 7.4% for children displaying well-documented language problems and normal nonverbal intelligence (i.e., IQ of 85 or over on a standardized test of nonverbal intellectual functioning). Even though there were slightly more males than females diagnosed with SLI in this study, the difference was not statistically significant.

Etiology

In discussing the genetic basis of SLI, Leonard (1998) cites several studies documenting its apparent propensity to occur in families. Studies of children with SLI indicate that approximately 20%–30% of their first-degree relatives also have a language problem. In studies where a history of a reading problem is also included, the percentage of affected family members is even higher (38%–75%). However, studies also show that not all children with SLI have family members who exhibit the same types of problems. In fact, research indicates that 30%–35% of children with SLI do not have a family history of a language problem. The heterogeneity of individuals with SLI may indicate that some types of SLI are inherited, while others are not (see also Stromswold, 2000; Tallal, Hirsch, Realpe-Bonilla, Miller, & Brzustowicz, 2001).

There are indications in the literature of differences in the brain structures responsible for language in individuals with SLI and in their relatives. Plante and colleagues have found structural differences in the perisylvian areas of the brain (i.e., the area most related to language function) of children and adults with language problems and in their first-degree relatives (Clark & Plante, 1998; Plante, 1991; Plante, Swisher, Vance, & Rapcsak, 1991). Gauger, Lombardino, and Leonard (1997) found differences between children with SLI and control children on measurements of the language area in the frontal lobe of the brain. Thus, although this type of research is in its infancy, there is ample evidence to suggest anatomical correlates to the behavioral deficits seen in children with SLI (Ahmed, Lombardino, & Leonard, 2001; Bishop, 2000). These differences in brain structure may account for at least a portion of the differences seen in their language and other cognitive abilities. As yet, the causes of these brain differences have not been identified.

There are few indications in the literature that SLI is learned behavior, despite a respectable amount of research attempting to document this possibility. Although it has been established that the language these children hear is often different from the language heard by children with normal language abilities, most of the research indicates that this "different language" is a result of, not the cause of, the language used by the children with SLI (Leonard, 1998). Thus the etiology of SLI does not seem to be related to environmental causes—at least not to those that are present in the learning environment.

Course

The long-term outlook for children with SLI depends on the depth and breadth of the language disorder, on the treatment received, and on the children's overall cognitive abilities. Aram and colleagues (1984) assessed language, intelligence, academic achievement, and behavioral adjustment in a group of 20 adolescents who had been diagnosed with SLI 10 years earlier. Of the 20, 5 were in special education classes for children with mild mental retardation, while another 11 had required additional support services (e.g., outside tutoring, placement in a program for students with learning disabilities, or grade retention). Of the 16 students who had continued to have problems, all were rated by their parents as being less socially competent than their peers.

In two studies of the same cohort of children diagnosed with SLI, these children were examined over a period of $1\frac{1}{2}$ years (Bishop & Edmundson, 1987) and then retested 10 years later (Stothard, Snowling, Bishop, Chipchase, & Kaplan, 1998). During the first study, 87 children were seen for assessment at ages 4, $4\frac{1}{2}$, and $5\frac{1}{2}$. In 37% of these children, the language disorder had resolved itself by the age of $5\frac{1}{2}$. In another 7%, generally low cognitive abilities were diagnosed. When 71 of these same individuals were seen for assessment approximately 10 years later, they were divided into three groups on the basis of their status at $5\frac{1}{2}$ years: those with "general delay" (i.e., nonverbal intellectual functioning below the average range; $n = 15$); those whose language problems had resolved (resolved SLI; $n = 26$); and those with persistent SLI ($n = 30$). On tests of vocabulary and language comprehension, the group with resolved SLI did not differ from the normal control group; however, this group did perform significantly more poorly on tests of phonological processing and literacy skills. The group with persistent SLI continued to have problems in all aspects of oral and written language, as did the children with general delay. These researchers noted that although none of the children with resolved SLI was diagnosed as having dyslexia, their literacy skills were significantly weaker than those of their normal peers. Thus early spoken language deficits appeared to be related to later weaknesses in reading abilities.

Studies by Kamhi, Lee, and Nelson (1985) and Kamhi and Catts (1986) confirm the presence of phonological processing deficits in children with SLI, and verify that these problems are similar in these children and in children with reading impairment. In studies assessing early oral language development in children who later became poor readers, problems have been noted as well (e.g., Catts, 1991; Scarborough, 1990, 1991; Scarborough & Dobrich, 1990). In general, many of these children displayed early problems with syntax and phonological production, but the syntactical problems had resolved by age 5, before they began encountering difficulties with learning in school.

With regard to treatment efficacy, Leonard (1998) cites numerous studies of well-documented treatment gains following therapy designed to improve the syntax, morphology, and phonological production abilities of children with SLI. He does point out, however, that although treatment accelerates language learning in many such children, there are many children with SLI, who improve but do not achieve normal language functioning. In one study, Paul, Murray, Clancy, and Andrews (1997) found that 16% of children who were initially late in talking did not achieve normal language functioning by second grade. These children then sustained repercussions evident in their social adjustment and academic learning.

FACTORS IMPORTANT IN COGNITIVE ASSESSMENT OF CHILDREN WITH SLI

Because both verbal and nonverbal cognitive deficits are present in individuals with SLI, the selection of nonverbal intelligence tests is more complicated than just insuring that the directions and the required responses are nonverbal. Following are some suggestions for selecting and using current intelligence tests:

1. Evidence of slow processing in individuals with SLI is strong; therefore, using tests that include time limits in either the administration or scoring of items may result in lower scores than those obtained on tests with no timing factors. Examples of tests that might emphasize the timing aspect include the Wechsler Intelligence Scale for Children—Third Edition (WISC-III; Wechsler, 1991) and the Wechsler Preschool and Primary Scale of Intelligence—Revised (WPPSI-R; Wechsler, 1989), which place a heavy emphasis on time in their scoring procedures. In addition, there are time limits involved in exposure of test items on the Differential Ability Scales (DAS) Recall of Designs subtest (Elliott, 1990) and on the new Universal Nonverbal Intelligence Test (UNIT; Bracken & McCallum, 1998). Memory tests. Since timing elements are present on other nonverbal tests, the examiner should be aware of the effect this may have on the obtained score.

Slow processing may also have important effects on overall scores on intelligence tests. Ottem (2002) found that composite scores obtained on the WPPSI and the WISC-R were significantly affected by the uneven pattern of scores obtained by SLI children on the subtests comprising the composites. He proposed that information processing weaknesses of SLI children affected their performance on several subtests, primarily on the performance scales. This in turn had a significant negative effect on the Performance IQ, diminishing the Verbal–Performance IQ split that might be anticipated in these children.

2. Due to the obvious difficulties that many children with SLI have with understanding spoken language, use of nonverbal tests with oral directions should be weighed carefully. Flanagan, Alfonso, Kaminer, and Rader (1995) investigated the presence and frequency of basic concepts in the directions of several intelligence tests, some of which have nonverbal portions or may be used to assess children with SLI: namely, the WPPSI-R, the DAS, and the Bayley Scales of Infant Development—Second Edition (BSID-II; Bayley, 1993). They found a rather large proportion of basic concepts in the directions of these tests that are frequently unknown to normal preschoolers; obviously, these concept-loaded directions are of even more concern for children who have difficulty understanding language. If an estimate of *nonverbal* intellectual functioning is the goal of the assessment, then using a test with difficult verbal instructions is not appropriate.

3. Problems with anticipatory imagery and symbolic representation may interfere with performance on several subtests of the various nonverbal intelligence measures. For example, the symbolic tests of the UNIT may be more difficult for them, as well as the higher-level reasoning subtests on all of the batteries. Of course, since such problems are in fact among the deficits seen in SLI, then lower performance on these tasks is to be expected.

4. Although gestures may be lower-level communicative acts than oral language, they are still *symbolic*; as such, they may also be difficult for children with SLI to interpret, considering their difficulties with symbolic representation. Some gestures are more ideographic (i.e., represent the thing to be communicated more pictorially) than others. Therefore, using ideographic gestures may be helpful in conveying instructions for individuals with SLI.

5. Most importantly, the goal of cognitive assessment of a youngster with SLI should be paramount in determining the instrument used. If the assessment of cognitive abilities is being done to determine eligibility for a program in the public schools, then the examiner may want to choose an instrument that will show the child's nonlinguistic cognitive strengths. On the other hand, if the goal of the assessment is to assist in de-termining strengths and weaknesses in a child's cognitive abilities to help in describing the child to parents, teachers, and other related professionals, and to help plan appropriate treatment, then an assessment instrument that would display all cognitive characteristics should be the instrument of choice.

TESTS TO USE IN COGNITIVE ASSESSMENT OF CHILDREN WITH SLI

Following is a discussion of tests that either are nonverbal or include a nonverbal scale. The tests are briefly described, followed by any validity data available on individuals with SLI. Some of the tests are so new that little validity information is available. All tests are listed in Table 25.1, with a summary of the pertinent information relative to individuals with SLI.

Bayley Scales of Infant Development— Second Edition

The BSID-II assesses the cognitive ability of infants and toddlers between the ages of 1 and 42 months. It represents a major change from its predecessor, the original BSID, in that over 100 items were added to or deleted from the original version. The items on the BSID-II cover cognitive, language, motor, and personal/social areas. Although expressive language demands are minimal (requiring only one-word answers), gestures are not acceptable responses. Administration does allow for examiner demonstration, and there is frequent use of multiple trials on items, which should be helpful in testing children with language impairments (Alfonso & Flanagan, 1999). It should be noted that the BSID-II item directions do contain many basic concepts that are frequently not understood by young children (Flanagan et al., 1995), particularly if they have language impairments.

Technical characteristics of the BSID-II are excellent (Alfonso & Flanagan, 1999; Bracken & Walker, 1997; Flanagan & Alfonso, 1995). However, findings of one study indicated that overall composite scores can vary considerably depending on the item set administered, at least at the 12-month level (Gauthier, Bauer, Messinger, &

TABLE 25.1. Summary of Information on Nonverbal Tests of Intelligence

Test[a]	Year of publication	Pantomime or gestures[b]	Validity with SLI	Considerations with SLI	Age range[c]
BSID-II	1993	No	Earlier version	Verbal directions	1 month to 42 months
CMMS	1972	No	Yes	"Odd-one-out" format	3-6 to 9-11
CTONI	1997	Yes	No	Analogy items	6-0 to 90-11
DAS Nonverbal	1990	No	Yes	Verbal directions; 5-second stimulus exposures	Preschool: 2-6 to 5-11; School-Age: 6-0 to 17-11
K-ABC Nonverbal	1983	Yes	Yes	Matrix Analogies subtest	2-6 to 12-5
Leiter-R	1997	Yes	Yes	Anticipatory imagery (e.g., paper folding)	2-0 to 20-11
TONI-3	1997	Yes	Earlier versions	See discussion	6-0 to 89-11
UNIT	1998	Yes	Yes	Symbolic tests; Analogy test; 5-second exposures	5-0 to 17-11
WISC-III Performance	1991	No	Yes	Verbal directions; timed subtests	6-0 to 16-11
WPPSI-R Performance	1989	No	Yes	Verbal directions; timed subtests	3-0 to 7-3

[a]BSID-II, Bayley Scales of Infant Development—Second Edition; CMMS, Columbia Mental Maturity Scale; CTONI, Comprehensive Test of Nonverbal Intelligence; DAS, Differential Ability Scales; K-ABC, Kaufman Assessment Battery for Children; Leiter-R, Leiter International Performance Scale—Revised; TONI-3, Test of Nonverbal Intelligence—Third Edition; UNIT, Universal Nonverbal Intelligence Test; WISC-III, Wechsler Intelligence Scale for Children—Third Edition; WPPSI-R, Wechsler Preschool and Primary Scale of Intelligence—Revised.
[b]Examiners can pantomime and/or use gestures to the exclusion of any verbal instructions.
[c]Ages in years and months are given as, say, "3-6" for "3 years, 6 months."

Closius, 1999). Although the BSID-II does not contain a nonverbal scale, Vandermeulen, Smrkovsky, LeCoultre-Martin, and Wijnberg-Williams (1994) extracted items from the earlier version to create a normed, nonverbal scale administered through gestures and pantomime. Their experience suggests that it would be possible to produce such a version based on the current test. Bradley-Johnson (2001) noted that a "nonvocal" score would be very helpful.

Columbia Mental Maturity Scale

Although the normative data on the CMMS are considerably outdated (Kamphaus, 1993; Naglieri & Prewett, 1990), it is being reviewed for this chapter because of its long use for children with SLI, particularly in research settings (e.g., Cole, Mills, & Kelley, 1994; Fazio, Naremore, & Connell, 1996; Johnston & Weismer, 1983; Kamhi et al.,

1988; Wren, 1981). The CMMS consists of 92 items, each of which requires a child to select the one drawing among three to five drawings that "does not belong." The test can be administered to children between the ages of 3 years, 6 months and 9 years, 11 months; it was originally designed for special populations, including "speech-impaired" children. The sample on which it was standardized was excellent although considerably outdated (Kamphaus, 1993), but it has inadequate subtest item gradients, and there is inadequate stability information (Flanagan, Sainato, & Genshaft, 1993). Generally, this test is regarded as a screening instrument rather than an in-depth assessment of cognitive abilities (Kamphaus, 1993; Naglieri & Prewett, 1990).

The CMMS has frequently been used to establish normal intellectual functioning in children with SLI in research studies (e.g., Johnston & Weismer, 1983; Kamhi et al.,

1985; Nelson et al., 1987; Wren, 1981). In a study that compared the performance of children with SLI on various tests of language and cognitive abilities, Cole and colleagues (1994) compared performance on the CMMS and the McCarthy Scales of Children's Abilities (MSCA; McCarthy, 1972). Although all children in this study had language delay, 50% of them also were being seen for cognitive delay, 20% for social–emotional delay, and 20% for motor delay. Significant differences were found among all three of the following composite score means: CMMS, MSCA General Cognitive Index, and MSCA Perceptual–Performance Index. The means for these three composite scores were all significantly below the average range, perhaps because these children had multiple disabilities with associated language impairments.

In a unique look at the CMMS, Kamhi and colleagues (1990) analyzed the types of items constituting the test, dividing them into perceptual and conceptual items. Although they noted that all items require some type of classificatory ability, they do not all require prior conceptual knowledge; some items could be answered correctly on the basis of perception alone. Their judgments were made on the basis of whether a child could solve the item by noting physical similarity. In this manner, 39% of the items were classified as perceptual, and 61% were classified as conceptual. The researchers then compared the performance of 22 children with SLI to the performance of 28 nondisabled control children, ranging in age from 3 years, 2 months to 7 years, 0 months, on the individual items of the CMMS. Both the control children and the children with SLI earned scores within the average range. They all correctly answered the perceptual-type items, which tend to occur in the earlier portion of the test. The children with SLI performed as well on the conceptual-type items as the control children. The conceptual-type items became predominant at about the 5-year level. These researchers noted that in their clinical experience they had assessed several preschool-age children with SLI who could not perform on the CMMS but could do well on the Leiter International Performance Scale. This observation suggested that these particular youngsters had difficulty with the "odd-one-out" format of the

CMMS (i.e., "Which one does not belong?").

Comprehensive Test of Nonverbal Intelligence

The Comprehensive Test of Nonverbal Intelligence (CTONI; Hammill, Pearson, & Wiederholt, 1997a) is a nonverbal measure of intelligence appropriate for individuals between the ages of 6 years, 0 months and 90 years, 11 months. It measures analogical reasoning, categorical classifications, and sequential reasoning, utilizing pictures of objects and geometric designs. Either spoken or pantomimed instructions may be used, and pointing responses are required. The CTONI yields three composite scores: a Nonverbal Intelligence Quotient (combining analogical reasoning, categorical classifying, and sequential reasoning); a Pictorial Nonverbal Intelligence Quotient (measuring problem solving and reasoning using pictured objects); and a Geometric Nonverbal Intelligence Quotient (using unfamiliar designs to measure problem solving and reasoning).

The examiner's manual for the CTONI provides a helpful array of normative data, as well as reliability and validity data (Hammill, Pearson, & Wiederholt, 1997b). Approximately 1% of the school-age norming sample and 4% of the adult sample exhibited a speech–language disorder. Although it is not clearly stated in the examiner's manual, it appears that the normative data were obtained using oral, rather than pantomimed, instructions. The authors did do two assessments 1 month apart on a sample of 33 children in 3rd grade and 30 adolescents in 11th grade, first using pantomime and then using oral instructions. Test–retest reliabilities ranged from .79 to .89 on the subtest scores and from .87 to .94 on the composite scores. Although there are 11 subgroups for which data are provided in the manual, speech–language impairment is not among them. There are also no current data in the literature regarding the validity of using the CTONI with individuals who have SLI.

Differential Ability Scales

The DAS has Preschool and School-Age forms, both of which have a Special Nonverbal Composite (SNC) score. The SNC at the Lower Preschool Level (2 years, 6 months to 3 years, 5 months) consists of two subtests: Block Building and Picture Similarities. At the Upper Preschool Level (3 years, 6 months to 5 years, 11 months), the SNC consists of three subtests: Picture Similarities, Pattern Construction, and Copying. The SNC at the School-Age Level consists of two clusters: Nonverbal Reasoning Ability (comprising Matrices and Sequential and Quantitative Reasoning) and Spatial Ability (comprising Recall of Designs and Pattern Construction). Directions are given orally, which may cause problems for youngsters with SLI, and there are no norms based on a nonverbal administration of the nonverbal scales (Alfonso & Flanagan, 1999; Harrison, Flanagan, & Genshaft, 1997). However, test administration does include demonstration and teaching items, which may partially offset any difficulties arising from using the oral directions. Elliott (1990) notes that verbal mediation is probably necessary for solving the problems presented on the Matrices subtest, which may also affect the performance of individuals with SLI.

Several authors have noted that the psychometric properties of the DAS are excellent (Alfonso & Flanagan, 1999; Bracken & Walker, 1997; Flanagan & Alfonso, 1995; Kamphaus, 1993), although there is some disagreement about its subtest floors. Alfonso and Flanagan (1999) indicate that its subtest floors are not adequate, especially at the lower end of the preschool range (2 years, 6 months to 3 years, 5 months); Bracken and Walker (1997) note excellent subtest floors for this age range, with the exception of a few subtests that are not included in the SNC. The norming sample included children with impairments, with the exception of those with severe disabilities. One potential problem in using this instrument for youngsters with SLI is that there is a high percentage of use of basic concepts in the test directions (Flanagan et al., 1995).

One study used the SNC of the DAS to assess children with SLI. Riccio, Ross, Boan, Jemison, and Houston (1997) administered the DAS to a group of 100 children ranging in age from 3 years to 6 years. The sample consisted of 23 children with SLI; 14 children with deafness or hearing impairment (D/HI); 19 children with developmental de-

lay (DD); 10 children learning English as a second language (ESL); and 34 control children. The youngsters with SLI and D/HI obtained SNC scores significantly lower than those of children in the control and ESL groups, but significantly higher than those of youngsters in the DD group. Although the mean SNC score obtained by the children with SLI was within the average range (standard score = 90.18), the investigators noted that the influence of language delay on their performance could not be ruled out.

Kaufman Assessment Battery for Children

The Kaufman Assessment Battery for Children (K-ABC; Kaufman & Kaufman, 1983) is another test on which the norms are outdated, according to the criteria of Kamphaus (1993); however, it has been used in several studies of children with SLI (Kennedy & Hiltonsmith, 1988; Swisher & Plante, 1993; Swisher et al., 1994; Williams, Voelker, & Ricciardi, 1995). Therefore, it is included here. The Nonverbal scale of the K-ABC consists of subtests that can be administered using pantomime and can be responded to motorically. The subtests making up this composite scale differ somewhat at various age levels: at 4 years, Faces and Places, Hand Movements, and Triangles; at 5 years, the latter two subtests plus Matrix Analogies and Spatial Memory; and at 6 through 12 years, the latter four subtests and Photo Series. Although the technical adequacy of the K-ABC is excellent in most respects, problems with inadequate floors and ceilings have been noted (Bracken, 1987; Flanagan et al., 1993; Kamphaus, 1993). In addition, the Nonverbal scale uses norms that were obtained through verbal administration (Harrison et al., 1997; McCallum & Bracken, 1997).

The concurrent validity of the K-ABC Nonverbal scale in comparison to the Pictorial Test of Intelligence (PTI; French, 1964) and the Hiskey–Nebraska Test of Learning Aptitude (HNTLA; Hiskey, 1966) was investigated in 30 children by Kennedy and Hiltonsmith (1988). The children ranged in age from 4 to 5 years and were determined to have an expressive communication disorder, such as stuttering, impaired articulation, language impairment, or voice impairment (receptive language was noted to be intact). The K-ABC Nonverbal scale yielded the lowest mean score for this group of mixed expressive communication problems in comparison to the other two tests, resulting in an average score of 103.2. Pearson correlations with the K-ABC Nonverbal scale were .65 for the PTI and .72 for the HNTLA. Part of the difference in scores on the three instruments, with the K-ABC being the lowest, may relate to the newer norms on the K-ABC. The PTI and the HNTLA were normed in the early 1960s, whereas the K-ABC was normed in the early 1980s. Flynn (1984, cited in Kamphaus, 1993) found that intelligence test norms increase in difficulty by approximately 3 standard-score points every decade. Even though this study was completed on children with communication impairments, it is unclear how many of them fit the diagnosis of language impairment only.

Williams and colleagues (1995) examined the predictive validity of the K-ABC Global scales (including the Mental Processing Composite, Sequential Processing, Simultaneous Processing, and Achievement, but not the Nonverbal scale) on 39 children, of whom 10 were diagnosed with SLI, 13 had behavior problems, and 16 were nondisabled controls. They found that the relationship between the initial K-ABC scores (given while they were preschoolers) and later K-ABC, language, and achievement measures (given at a mean age of 9 years, 9 months) was weak, suggesting that the Global scales of the K-ABC were not helpful in predicting later cognitive and achievement scores in children with SLI. It should be noted, however, that this was a small sample and that the Nonverbal scale of the K-ABC was not utilized.

In two studies (Swisher & Plante, 1993; Swisher et al., 1994) on children with SLI and nonexceptional children, *patterns* of performance between the groups were found to differ on the K-ABC as well as on other nonverbal measures of intellectual functioning (i.e., the Leiter International Performance Scale and the Matrix Analogies Test [MAT; Naglieri, 1985]). Mean standard scores for the children with SLI groups were significantly lower than scores obtained for the nonexceptional children (which may have been related to participant selection procedures) on all three measures. However, in all cases, mean standard scores were within the average range for the children with SLI on all three measures. The average scores obtained on the Nonverbal scale of the K-ABC were lower than those obtained on the Leiter and on the MAT (again, possibly reflecting the difference in the age of the normative data; Kamphaus, 1993).

Allen, Lincoln, and Kaufman (1991) investigated the performance of 20 children diagnosed with autism and 20 children diagnosed with SLI, ranging in age from 6 to 12 years, on the K-ABC Simultaneous Processing, Sequential Processing, and Mental Processing Composite scores. The children with SLI scored higher than the children with autism on all composites and subtests, with the exception of the Triangles subtest. Fifteen children with SLI had higher scores on Simultaneous Processing than on Sequential Processing. Although not unexpected in view of their noted difficulties with processing capacity and speed (Bishop, 1992; Kail, 1994; Lahey & Edwards, 1996), Kamphaus (1993) points out that two of the three Sequential Processing subtests have language content (Number Recall, Word Order), whereas only one of the five Simultaneous Processing subtests has language content (Gestalt Closure). Thus, for children with SLI, it is difficult to separate the language requirements from the processing requirements on this test. The Overall Mental Processing Composite on the K-ABC (88.45) for the children with SLI was comparable to their Full Scale IQ on the WISC-R (88); however, the Nonverbal scale (89.65) was lower than the WISC-R Performance IQ (97.10). Part of the differences in scores may be attributable to the difference in time of standardization (the early 1970s for the WISC-R; the early 1980s for the K-ABC).

Leiter International Performance Scale—Revised

The Leiter International Performance Scale —Revised (Leiter-R; Roid & Miller, 1997a) is a major revision of the original Leiter. It is designed to assess individuals between the ages of 2 years, 0 months and 20 years, 11 months. It is based on hierarchical factor models, including Carroll's three-stratum model of cognitive abilities (Carroll, 1993) and Gustafsson's hierarchical model of cognitive abilities (cited in Roid & Miller, 1997b). The 20 subtests of the Leiter-R are split evenly between the Visualization and Reasoning Battery and the Attention and Memory Battery. Not all subtests are administered at each age level. Full Scale IQ scores composed of six subtests are available for preschool and school-age individuals and are deviation IQ scores based on the sums of the subtest scaled scores ($M = 100$; $SD = 15$). Composite scores are also available on the Visualization and Reasoning Battery for Fluid Reasoning, Fundamental Visualization, and Spatial Visualization. There are also various composite scores available for the Attention and Memory Battery. The test is administered through pantomiming that includes a combination of hand and head movements, facial expressions, and demonstration. The test was normed with nonverbal instructions. Every subtest includes a teaching item at the beginning.

The authors of the Leiter-R matched each of the items of the original Leiter to "documented cognitive abilities" as outlined by Carroll (1993). Then these sets of items were "reformatted" and expanded to better cover each of the dimensions on the revised test (Roid & Miller, 1997b). The response mode is quite similar to that of the original Leiter, but the wooden blocks of the original test have been replaced with colorful "playing cards" and foam rubber manipulatives. Thus the Leiter-R appears to be substantially different from the original version, even though it has retained many of the same items and uses the same response mode.

The original Leiter has been used frequently in research studies of children with SLI (e.g., Aram et al., 1984; Bishop & Edmundson, 1987; Johnston, 1982; Johnston & Smith, 1989; Kushnir & Blake, 1996; Weiner, 1971; Wren, 1981); however, because the Leiter-R represents a major revision, findings in these studies would not necessarily apply to the new version. One validity study with adolescents who were "speech-impaired" has been completed using the Leiter-R. Flemmer and Roid (1997) analyzed data from the standardization sample to compare performance of 21 individuals with speech impairment to 203 persons without such impairment (age range of 11 to 15 years). "Speech impairment" was defined according to American Psychiatric Association (1994) categories, which included phonological disorder, expressive or mixed expressive–receptive language disorder, stuttering, and communication disorder not otherwise specified. Six of the 10 subtests of the Visualization and Reasoning Battery were significantly lower for the group with speech impairment (Repeated Patterns, Sequential Order, Figure Ground, Design Analogies, Figure Rotation, and Paper Folding), whereas the other four subtests were not significantly different between the two samples (Matching, Picture Context, Classification, and Form Completion). The authors noted that the latter subtests are more "visual" in quality. It was also noted that this heterogeneous population of individuals with communication impairments obtained a significantly lower score on the brief IQ screener from this test (87), in comparison to the standard score obtained by the unimpaired sample of 100.

Farrell and Phelps (2000) administered the Leiter-R (along with the UNIT) to 43 children with severe SLI. The students ranged in age from 6.1 to 12.5 years, were from several different school districts, and were in a central Language Development Program paid for by their home school districts. Seven subtests from the Fluid Reasoning Scale and the Full Scale IQ were appropriate at this age level and were administered. Results of the testing were substantially below average with all subtest score means falling 1–2 standard deviations below the mean of the standardization sample. Composite scores on Fluid Reasoning and Visualization and Reasoning Full Scale IQ were 65.07 and 66.33, respectively. All correlations between the Leiter-R and the UNIT were significant, indicating good concurrent validity between these two tests. Farrell and Phelps also note that the significantly low scores obtained by this sample of children may have in part been related to the severity of their language disorder. (These children were all sent to this intervention setting because their respective school districts were unable to successfully educate them locally.) Furthermore, they noted that it was possible that these children had other cognitive problems in addition to language.

It appears that this nonverbally administered test of intellectual functioning has the potential to offer a comprehensive measure of cognitive abilities in individuals with SLI. However, validity studies with this population are needed to verify its use. Farrell and Phelps (2000) note that assessment of children with mild-to-moderate SLI would be particularly helpful.

Test of Nonverbal Intelligence—Third Edition

The TONI-3 (Brown, Sherbenou, & Johnsen, 1997b) is a nonverbal screening test of cognitive abilities appropriate for testing individuals ranging in age from 6 years, 0 months to 89 years, 11 months. It is a 45-item test, shorter than its previous versions (TONI and TONI-2; Brown, Sherbenou, & Johnsen, 1982, 1990), and measures nonverbal intellectual functioning by having individuals solve or reason through figures or matrices. There are two equivalent forms, and the normative data have been updated and expanded. The sample included children with disabilities who were attending regular education classes. Approximately 3% of the sample had a "speech–language disorder" (Brown, Sherbenou, & Johnsen, 1997a). The directions can be pantomimed, and a pointing response is usually the required response.

The manual for the TONI-3 lists an impressive array of normative data, as well as reliability and validity information. However, no studies of children with SLI were included. The manual does note that the test is appropriate for individuals with "acquired or developmental aphasia or other severe spoken language disorders" (Brown et al., 1997a p. 31). Although previous versions of the TONI have been used to select/match participants in research studies of SLI (e.g., Kamhi & Catts, 1986; Kamhi et al., 1988; Lahey & Edwards, 1996; Masterson, 1993), no current research was found in which the TONI-3 was used. One interesting validity study of a referred population by D'Amato, Lidiak, and Lassiter (1994) found that correlations between the original TONI and the Verbal, Performance, and Full Scale IQ scores of the

WISC-R were .55, .58 and .59, respectively, which do not support the TONI as a nonverbal measure of intelligence. These correlations are consistent with those reported in the manual for the Leiter-R and the WISC-III.

A study completed by Kamhi and colleagues (1990) analyzed the types of items on the original TONI according to whether they were perceptual or conceptual (see the earlier discussions of this study in the "Nonlinguistic Characteristics" section and the section on the CMMS). These investigators found that 30% of the 50 items on the TONI were perceptual, while the remaining were conceptual. More importantly, the first 13 items on the test were perceptual, allowing a child to obtain an IQ score within the average range by answering correctly only perceptual items until the age of 11 years. Although the TONI-3 may be different in this respect, this is an important dimension to think about when considering its use as a screening test of intellectual functioning.

Universal Nonverbal Intelligence Test

The UNIT (Bracken & McCallum, 1998) appears to have good potential for individuals with SLI. It has entirely nonlanguage administration and response formats, and is appropriate for ages 5 years, 0 months to 17 years, 11 months. The UNIT consists of six subtests that assess abilities in two areas: memory and reasoning. These areas are organized into symbolic and nonsymbolic mediation. The Memory subtests include Spatial Memory (Nonsymbolic) and Symbolic Memory and Object Memory (Symbolic). The Reasoning subtests include Cube Design (Nonsymbolic) and Analogic Reasoning and Mazes (Symbolic). The composite scores available from the UNIT include a Full Scale score, as well as a Memory Quotient, Reasoning Quotient, Symbolic Quotient, and Nonsymbolic Quotient. There are 5-second exposure times for the stimuli on the Memory subtests, and "liberal" time limits on responses for the Cube Design and Mazes subtests (Bracken & McCallum, 1998; McCallum & Bracken, 1997).

As part of the norming sample, 57 youngsters with speech/language impairments were assessed with the UNIT. These children had an average age of 7.84 years and were diagnosed according to the American Psychiatric Association (1994) DSM-IV criteria mentioned in the section on the Leiter-R. They were all being served in special education for speech/language difficulties for an average of 10.02 hours per week. These individuals earned Full Scale IQs 6.81 and 8.72 points lower than a matched control group on the Standard and Extended Batteries, respectively. All mean scores were lower for the group of children with SLI than for the control group, although all scores for both groups were within the average range (e.g., composite scores ranged from 90.42 [Reasoning Quotient] to 94.81 [Memory Quotient] for the group with SLI) (Bracken & McCallum, 1998; McCallum et al., 2001).

Farrell and Phelps (2000) assessed children with severe SLI with both the Leiter-R and the UNIT. All six of the subtests of the UNIT were administered to the 43 children. Finding for the UNIT were similar to those of the Leiter-R. All subtest means were 1–2 standard deviations below the mean of the standardization group; composite scores for the Memory, Reasoning, Symbolic, and Nonsymbolic Quotients and the Full Scale IQ ranged from 66.71 to 70. Correlations between the subtest and composite scores for the UNIT and the Leiter-R were all statistically significant, indicating good concurrent validity between the two tests.

The UNIT has many good technical qualities (Bracken & McCallum, 1998; McCallum & Bracken, 1997), and individuals with SLI were part of the norming sample (Bracken & McCallum, 1998; McCallum, Bracken, & Wasserman, 2001). Although it appears to have good potential for use with such individuals, more validity data are needed to substantiate its use with this population.

Wechsler Intelligence Scale for Children—Third Edition

The WISC-III and its predecessor, the WISC-R, have been used to assess children with SLI both clinically (Ganschow, Sparks, & Helmick, 1992; Sparks, Ganschow, & Thomas, 1996) and in research studies (e.g., Allen et al., 1991; Aram et al., 1984; Scarborough & Dobrich, 1990; Sininger et al., 1989). Therefore, a description of the WISC-III and its appropriateness for youngsters with SLI is included.

The Performance scale of the WISC-III consists of five subtests: Picture Completion, Picture Arrangement, Block Design, and Object Assembly (constituting the Perceptual Organization Index), plus Coding (which, along with the optional Symbol Search subtest, constitutes the Processing Speed Index). Although no verbal responses are required on this scale, all of these subtests are scored for both correctness and speed of response, a particular problem for the population with SLI (Kail, 1994; Lahey & Edwards, 1996; Windsor & Hwang, 1999). In addition, the directions are oral and quite wordy (Kamphaus, 1993). Furthermore, there are no allowances in the administration procedures to help a child learn the tasks.

Even though the WISC-III Performance IQ appears to be a poor choice for assessing a child with SLI, it is certainly preferable to basing the estimate of such a child's intellectual functioning on the Verbal IQ or Full Scale IQ of the WISC-III, since those composite scores include measurement of the child's deficit areas. In a child whose oral language problems may be subtle, and therefore, difficult for a non-language-trained professional to note, use of the Verbal scale of the WISC-III may be helpful in deciding whether the child should be referred for more in-depth language assessment (Sparks et al., 1996). Therefore, a profile of Verbal IQ < Performance IQ with a significant discrepancy between the two scores might be helpful in determining when to refer a child to a speech–language pathologist (Ganschow et al., 1992; Sparks et al., 1996). The Verbal IQ score, however, should not be considered a measure of a child's language skills, since it does not assess syntax, morphology, phonological production, or phonological processing—the areas most problematic for children with SLI (Kamhi & Catts, 1989; Leonard, 1998). Therefore, even if a child obtains a Verbal IQ score within the average range and/or not significantly lower than the Performance IQ, this should not be considered as conclusive evidence that there is no language impairment.

Although only two studies of the WISC-III for children with SLI are reported in the literature (Doll & Boren, 1993; Phelps, 1993, cited in Phelps, 1998), numerous research endeavors have utilized the WISC-R with such children (e.g., Johnston & Ramstad, 1983; Scarborough & Dobrich, 1990; Stark, Tallal, Kallman, & Mellits, 1983). Three of those investigations are highlighted here. In a longitudinal study of 20 adolescents diagnosed with SLI 10 years earlier, Aram and colleagues (1984) found that on the WISC-R the mean Performance IQ score (89.15), Verbal IQ score (83.10), and Full Scale IQ score (84.70) were all within the low average range. However, considerable range of individual scores was observed (<45 to 129 on the Performance scale, <45 to 123 on the Verbal scale, and <40 to 126 on the Full Scale). Furthermore, 15 of the 20 individuals exhibited Performance IQ scores greater than Verbal IQ scores.

In a study comparing performance on the WISC-R in two clinical groups and one control group (21 children with SLI, 30 children with learning disabilities, and 12 unimpaired children), Rose, Lincoln, and Allen (1992) found that there was an atypical correlation of subtest scale scores for the group with SLI in comparison to the other two groups, consistent with findings by Restrepo and colleagues (1992) and Swisher and Plante (1993) that cognitive abilities in SLI children do not seem to follow a normal pattern. Finally, as reported in the section on "Criteria for Diagnosing SLI," the stability of WISC-R IQ scores in children with SLI over a 3-year period was investigated by Krassowski and Plante (1997). In addition to the previously reported findings, these investigators found that differences in IQ scores of one standard deviation (15 points) or more occurred in 16%–27% of this population sample.

Wechsler Preschool and Primary Scale of Intelligence—Revised

The Performance scale of the WPPSI-R consists of five subtests: Object Assembly, Geometric Design, Block Design, Mazes, and Picture Completion. In general, the technical characteristics of the WPPSI-R are good (Alfonso & Flanagan, 1999; Kamphaus, 1993); however, none of these subtests can be administered with pantomime or ges-

tures, and the level of receptive and expressive language required is quite high (Alfonso & Flanagan, 1999; Flanagan et al., 1995). In addition, because the test is so long, normal preschoolers have difficulty attending (Kamphaus, 1993); therefore, expecting children with language impairments to attend to directions that may be difficult for them to understand may be even more challenging.

Prior to the publication of the WPPSI-R, its predecessor, the WPPSI (Wechsler, 1967) (which also enjoyed generally good technical adequacy; Bracken, 1987) was used in several investigations of children with SLI. Stark, Tallal, and colleagues have used the Performance IQ of the WPPSI (i.e., >85) as one of the criteria for inclusion of children with SLI in several studies (Stark et al., 1983, 1984; Stark & Tallal, 1981); it was also used to document cognitive abilities in children with SLI by Beitchman and colleagues (Beitchman et al., 1989; Beitchman, Wilson, Brownlie, Walters, & Lancee, 1996). In addition, children with SLI have been assessed with the WPPSI in two validity studies (Field, 1987; Stark et al., 1983). Stark and colleagues (1983) used the WPPSI and the WISC-R to assess 38 children with SLI and 34 nonexceptional control children with an age range of 5 years, 0 months to 8 years, 6 months. Inclusion in both groups was based on normal Performance IQ scores (mean Performance IQ scores were as follows: controls = 103, children with SLI = 100) on either the WPPSI or the WISC-R (approximately half of the children took each test). However, both Verbal IQ (controls = 108; children with SLI = 82) and Full Scale IQ (controls = 106; children with SLI = 90) scores for the group with SLI were significantly lower than for the control group; the average Verbal IQ for the group with SLI fell significantly below the average range. Furthermore, there were significant differences between the two groups on each of the Verbal subtests but no significant differences between the two groups on any of the Performance subtests. Profiles of the Verbal subtests were different for children with SLI in comparison to the control group, in that the scores obtained on the Vocabulary and Digit Span subtests were significantly lower than scores on other subtests for the group with SLI, while these same subtest scores for the control group (plus Comprehension) were significantly higher than other subtest scores.

Field (1987) compared the performance of preschool children on the original Leiter and the Stanford–Binet Scale of Intelligence: Third Revision, Form L-M (Binet; Terman & Merrill, 1972) to later performance on the WPPSI. Twenty-six children (of which 21 were diagnosed with SLI) were approximately 48 months of age at initial testing and 64 months when given the WPPSI. They had originally been given the Binet, but had also been given the Leiter if an experienced psychologist had believed that their low scores on the Binet had been an "incomplete reflection of their cognitive abilities" (Field, 1987, p. 113). The WPPSI Verbal IQ correlated significantly with the Binet (.66); the WPPSI Performance IQ correlated significantly with the Leiter (.60); and the Full Scale IQ on the WPPSI was significantly correlated with both the Leiter (.59) and the Binet (.64).

CONCLUSIONS

Children with SLI exhibit problems in both language and nonlanguage cognitive abilities. Their strengths as well as their deficits should be considered when examiners are selecting assessment instruments in the area of intellectual functioning. Although many nonverbal tests of cognitive abilities and a number of new instruments appear promising, little validity information is available on these tests with this population. Therefore, research to validate their use with children with significant language deficits is needed. In the meantime, cognitive assessment of children with SLI should be based on a thorough understanding of the characteristics of this population in conjunction with the stated purpose of the evaluation. Relying on one score, particularly if this score has been obtained on a "screening" instrument, is clinically unsound and not in the best interests of these children.

REFERENCES

Ahmed, S. T., Lombardino, L. J., & Leonard, C. M. (2001). Specific language impairment: Definitions, causal mechanisms and neurobiological factors.

Journal of Medical Speech-Language Pathology, 9, 1–15.

Alfonso, V. C., & Flanagan, D. P. (1999). Assessment of cognitive functioning in preschoolers. In E. V. Nuttall, I. Romero, & J. Kalesnik (Eds.), *Assessing and screening preschoolers: Psychological and educational dimensions* (pp. 186–217). Boston: Allyn & Bacon.

Allen, M. H., Lincoln, A. J., & Kaufman, A. S. (1991). Sequential and simultaneous processing abilities of high-functioning autistic and language-impaired children. *Journal of Autism and Developmental Disorders, 21,* 483–502.

American Psychiatric Association. (1994). *Diagnostic and statistical manual of mental disorders* (4th ed.), Washington, DC: Author.

American Speech–Language–Hearing Association (ASHA), Committee on Language Learning Disorders. (1989). *Report on issues in determining eligibility for language intervention.* Rockville, MD: ASHA.

Aram, D. M., Ekelman, B. L., & Nation, J. E. (1984). Preschoolers with language disorders: 10 years later. *Journal of Speech and Hearing Research, 27,* 232–244.

Arthur, G. (1952). *The Arthur adaptation of the Leiter International Performance Scale.* Chicago: Stoelting.

Bayley, N. (1993). *Bayley Scales of Infant Development—Second Edition.* San Antonio, TX: Psychological Corporation.

Beitchman, J. H., Hood, J., Rochon, J., Peterson, M., Mantini, T., & Majumdar, S. (1989). Empirical classification of speech/language impairment in children: I. Identification of speech/language categories. *Journal of the American Academy of Child and Adolescent Psychiatry, 28,* 112–117.

Beitchman, J. H., Wilson, B., Brownlie, E. B., Walters, H., & Lancee, W. (1996). Long-term consistency in speech/language profiles: Developmental and academic outcomes. *Journal of the Americal Academy of Child and Adolescent Psychiatry, 35,* 804–814.

Bishop, D. V. M. (1992). The underlying nature of specific language impairment. *Journal of Child Psychology and Psychiatry, 33,* 3–66.

Bishop, D. V. M. (2000). How does the brain learn language? Insights from the study of children with and without language impairment. *Developmental Medicine and Child Neurology, 42,* 133–142.

Bishop, D. V. M., & Edmundson, A. (1987). Language-impaired 4-year-olds: Distinguishing transient from persistent impairment. *Journal of Speech and Hearing Disorders, 52,* 156–173.

Bracken, B. A. (1987). Limitations of preschool instruments and standards for minimal levels of technical adequacy. *Journal of Psychoeducational Assessment, 4,* 313–326.

Bracken, B. A., & McCallum, S. (1998). *Universal Nonverbal Intelligence Test.* Itasca, IL: Riverside.

Bracken, B. A., & Walker, K. C. (1997). The utility of intelligence tests for preschool children. In D. P. Flanagan, J. L. Genshaft, & P. L. Harrison (Eds.), *Contemporary intellectual assessment* (pp. 484–502). New York: Guilford Press.

Bradley-Johnson, S. (2001). Cognitive assessment for

the youngest children: A critical review of tests. *Journal of Psychoeducational Assessment, 19,* 19–44.

Brown, L., Sherbenou, R. J., & Johnsen, S. K. (1982). *Test of Nonverbal Intelligence.* Austin, TX: Pro-Ed.

Brown, L., Sherbenou, R. J., & Johnsen, S. K. (1990). *Test of Nonverbal Intelligence, Second Edition.* Austin, TX: Pro-Ed.

Brown, L., Sherbenou, R. J., & Johnsen, S. K. (1997a). *Examiner's manual: Test of Nonverbal Intelligence—Third Edition.* Austin, TX: Pro-Ed.

Brown, L., Sherbenou, R. J., & Johnsen, S. K. (1997b). *Test of Nonverbal Intelligence—Third Edition.* Austin, TX: Pro-Ed.

Burgemeister, B. B., Blum, L. H., & Lorge, I. (1972). *Columbia Mental Maturity Scale.* New York: Psychological Corporation.

Carroll, J. B. (1993). *Human cognitive abilities: A survey of factor-analytic studies.* New York: Cambridge University Press.

Casby, M. W. (1992). The cognitive hypothesis and its influence on speech–language services in schools. *Language, Speech, and Hearing Services in Schools, 23,* 198–202.

Catts, H. W. (1991). Early identification of dyslexia: Evidence from a follow-up study of speech–language impaired children. *Annals of Dyslexia, 41,* 163–177.

Clark, M. M., & Plante, E. (1998). Morphology of the inferior frontal gyrus in developmentally language-disordered adults. *Brain and Language, 61,* 288–303.

Cole, K. N., Dale, P. S., & Mills, P. E. (1992). Stability of the intelligence quotient–language quotient relation: Is discrepancy modeling based on a myth? *American Journal on Mental Retardation, 97,* 131–143.

Cole, K. N., Mills, P. E., & Kelley, D. (1994). Agreement of assessment profiles used in cognitive referencing. *Language, Speech, and Hearing in Schools, 25,* 25–31.

Cole, K. N., Schwartz, I. S., & Notari, A. R. (1995). Examination of the stability of two methods of defining specific language impairment. *Applied Psycholoinguistics, 16,* 103–123.

D'Amato, R. C., Lidiak, S. E., & Lassiter, K. S. (1994). Comparing verbal and nonverbal intellectual functioning with the TONI and WISC-R. *Perceptual and Motor Skills, 78,* 701–702.

Doll, B., & Boren, R. (1993). Performance of severely language-impaired students on the WISC-III, language scales, and academic achievement measures. *Journal of Psychoeducational Assessment Monograph Series, 11,* 77–86.

Elliott, C. D. (1990). *Differential Ability Scales.* San Antonio, TX: Psychological Corporation.

Farrell, M. M., & Phelps, L. (2000). A comparison of the Leiter-R and the Universal Nonverbal Intelligence Test (UNIT) with children classified as language impaired. *Journal of Psychoeducational Assessment, 18,* 268–274.

Fazio, B. B., Naremore, R. C., & Connell, P. J. (1996). Tracking children from poverty at risk for specific language impairment: A 3-year longitudinal study. *Journal of Speech and Hearing Research, 39,* 611–624.

Fey, M. E., Long, S. H., & Cleave, P. L. (1994). Reconsideration of IQ criteria in the definition of specific language impairment. In R. V. Watkins & M. L. Rice (Eds.), *Specific language impairments in children* (Vol. 4, pp. 161–178). Baltimore: Brookes.

Field, M. (1987). Relation of language-delayed preschoolers' Leiter scores to later IQ. *Journal of Clinical Child Psychology, 16,* 111–115.

Flanagan, D. P., & Alfonso, V. C. (1995). A critical review of the technical characteristics of new and recently revised intelligence tests for preschool children. *Journal of Psychoeducational Assessment, 13,* 66–90.

Flanagan, D. P., Alfonso, V. C., Kaminer, T., & Rader, D. E. (1995). Incidence of basic concepts in the directions of new and recently revised American intelligence tests for preschool children. *School Psychology International, 16,* 345–364.

Flanagan, D. P., Sainato, D. M., & Genshaft, J. L. (1993). Emerging issues in the assessment of young children with disabilities: The expanding role of school psychologists. *Canadian Journal of School Psychology, 9,* 192–203.

Flemmer, D. D., & Roid, G. H. (1997). Nonverbal intellectual assessment of Hispanic and speech-impaired adolescents. *Psychological Reports, 80,* 1115–1122.

Francis, D. J., Fletcher, J. M., Shaywitz, B. A., Shaywitz, S. E., & Rourke, B. P. (1996). Defining learning and language disablities: Conceptual and psychometric issues with the use of IQ tests. *Language, Speech, and Hearing Services in Schools, 27,* 132–143.

French, J. L. (1964). *Pictorial Test of Intelligence.* Boston: Houghton Mifflin.

Ganschow, L., Sparks, R., & Helmick, M. (1992). Speech/language referral practices by school psychologists. *School Psychology Review, 21,* 313–326.

Gauger, L. M., Lombardino, L. J., & Leonard, C. M. (1997). Brain morphology in children with specific language impairment. *Journal of Speech, Language, and Hearing Research, 40,* 1272–1284.

Gauthier, S. M., Bauer, C. R., Messinger, D. S., & Closius, J. M. (1999). The Bayley Scales of Infant Development II: Where to start? *Journal of Developmental and Behavioral Pediatrics, 20,* 75–79.

Hammill, D. D., Pearson, N. A., & Wiederholt, J. L. (1997a). *Comprehensive Test of Nonverbal Intelligence.* Austin, TX: Pro-Ed.

Hammill, D. D., Pearson, N. A., & Wiederholt, J. L. (1997b). *Examiner's manual: Comprehensive Test of Nonverbal Intelligence.* Austin, TX: Pro-Ed.

Hanson, R. A., & Montgomery, J. W. (2002). Effects of general processing capacity and sustained selective attention on temporal processing performance of children with specific language impairment. *Applied Psycholinguistics, 23,* 75–93.

Harrison, P. L., Flanagan, D. P., & Genshaft, J. L. (1997). An integration and synthesis of contemporary theories, tests, and issues in the field of intellectual assessment. In D. P. Flanagan, J. L. Genshaft, & P. L. Harrison (Eds.), *Contemporary intellectual assessment* (pp. 533–561). New York: Guilford Press.

Hiskey, M. (1966). *Hiskey–Nebraska Test of Intelligence*. Lincoln, NE: Union College Press.

Johnston, J. R. (1982). Interpreting the Leiter IQ: Performance profiles of young normal and language-disordered children. *Journal of Speech and Hearing Research, 25,* 291–296.

Johnston, J. R. (1994). Cognitive abilities of children with language impairment. In R. V. Watkins & M. L. Rice (Eds.), *Specific language impairments in children* (Vol. 4, pp. 107–121). Baltimore: Brookes.

Johnston, J. R., & Ramstad, V. (1983). Cognitive development in pre-adolescent language-impaired children. *British Journal of Disorders of Communication, 18,* 49–55.

Johnston, J. R., & Smith, L. B. (1989). Dimensional thinking in language-impaired children. *Journal of Speech and Hearing Research, 32,* 33–38.

Johnston, J. R., & Weismer, S. E. (1983). Mental rotation abilities in language-disordered children. *Journal of Speech and Hearing Research, 26,* 397–403.

Kail, R. (1994). A method for studying the generalized slowing hypothesis in children with specific language impairment. *Journal of Speech and Hearing Research, 37,* 418–421.

Kail, R., & Leonard, L. (1986). Word-finding abilities in language-impaired children. *ASHA Monographs, 25,* 1–35.

Kamhi, A. G. (1981). Nonlinguistic symbolic and conceptual abilities of language-impaired and normally developing children. *Journal of Speech and Hearing Research, 24,* 446–453.

Kamhi, A. G. (1998). Trying to make sense of developmental language disorders. *Language, Speech, and Hearing in Schools, 29,* 35–44.

Kamhi, A. G., & Catts, H. W. (1986). Toward an understanding of developmental language and reading disorders. *Journal of Speech and Hearing Disorders, 51,* 337–347.

Kamhi, A. G., & Catts, H. W. (1989). *Reading disabilities: A developmental language perspective.* Boston: Little, Brown.

Kamhi, A. G., Catts, H. W., Mauer, D., Apel, K., & Gentry, B. F. (1988). Phonological and spatial processing abilities in language- and reading-impaired children. *Journal of Speech and Hearing Disorders, 53,* 316–327.

Kamhi, A. G., Lee, R. F., & Nelson, L. K. (1985). Word, syllable, and sound awareness in language-disordered children. *Journal of Speech and Hearing Disorders, 50,* 207–212.

Kamhi, A. G., Minor, J. S., & Mauer, D. (1990). Content analysis and intratest performance profiles on the Columbia and the TONI. *Journal of Speech and Hearing Research, 33,* 375–379.

Kamphaus, R. W. (1993). *Clinical assessment of children's intelligence.* Boston: Allyn & Bacon.

Kaufman, A. S., & Kaufman, N. L. (1983). *Kaufman Assessment Battery for Children.* Circle Pines, MN: American Guidance Service.

Kennedy, M. H., & Hiltonsmith, R. W. (1988). Relationship among the K-ABC Nonverbal scale, the Pic-

torial Test of Intelligence, and the Hiskey–Nebraska Test of Learning Aptitude for speech- and language-disabled preschool children. *Journal of Psychoeducational Assessment, 6,* 49–54.

Kirchner, D. M., & Klatzky, R. L. (1985). Verbal rehearsal and memory in language-disordered children. *Journal of Speech and Hearing Research, 28,* 556–565.

Krassowski, E., & Plante, E. (1997). IQ variability in children with SLI: Implications for use of cognitive referencing in determining SLI. *Journal of Communication Disorders, 30,* 1–9.

Kushnir, C. C., & Blake, J. (1996). The nature of the cognitive deficit in specific language impairment. *First Language, 16,* 21–40.

Lahey, M. (1990). Who shall be called language disordered?: Some reflections and one perspective. *Journal of Speech and Hearing Disorders, 55,* 612–620.

Lahey, M., & Edwards, J. (1996). Why do children with specific language impairment name pictures more slowly than their peers? *Journal of Speech and Hearing Research, 39,* 1081–1098.

Leonard, L. B. (1998). *Children with specific language impairment.* Cambridge, MA: MIT Press.

Leonard, L. B. (2000). Specific language impairment across languages. In D. V. M. Bishop & L. B. Leonard (Eds.), *Speech and language impairments in children: Causes, characteristics, intervention and outcome* (pp. 115–129). Philadelphia: Psychology Press.

Maillart, C., & Schelstraete, M. A. (2002). Morphosyntactic problems in children with specific language impairment: Grammatical SLI or overload in working memory? In F. Windsor & L. M. Kelly (Eds.), *Investigations in clinical phonetics and linguistics* (pp. 85–97). Mahwah, NJ: Erlbaum.

Masterson, J. J. (1993). The performance of children with language-learning disabilities on two types of cognitive tasks. *Journal of Speech and Hearing Research, 36,* 1026–1036.

McCallum, R. S., & Bracken, B. A. (1997). The Universal Nonverbal Intelligence Test. In D. P. Flanagan, J. L. Genshaft, & P. L. Harrison (Eds.), *Contemporary intellectual assessment* (pp. 268–280). New York: Guilford Press.

McCallum, S. R., Bracken, B. A., & Wasserman, J. D. (2001). *Essentials of nonverbal assessment.* New York: Wiley.

McCarthy, D. (1972). *McCarthy Scales of Children's Abilities.* New York: Psychological Corporation.

Miller, C. A., Kail, R., Leonard, L. B., & Tomblin, B. J. (2001). Speed of processing in children with specific language impairment. *Journal of Speech, Language, and Hearing Research, 44,* 416–433.

Montgomery, J. W. (2000). Verbal working memory and sentence comprehension in children with specific language impairment. *Journal of Speech, Language, and Hearing Research, 43,* 293–308.

Naglieri, J. A. (1985). *Matrix Analogies Test—Short Form.* New York: Psychological Corporation.

Naglieri, J. A., & Prewett, P. N. (1990). Nonverbal intelligence measures: A selected review of instruments and their use. In C. R. Reynolds & R. W. Kamphaus (Eds.), *Handbook of psychological and educational assessment of children: Intelligence and achievement* (pp. 348–370). New York: Guilford Press.

Nelson, L. K., Kamhi, A. G., & Apel, K. (1987). Cognitive strengths and weaknesses in language-impaired children: One more look. *Journal of Speech and Hearing Disorders, 52,* 36–43.

Nippold, M. A., Erskine, B. J., & Freed, D. B. (1988). Proportional and functional analogical reasoning in normal and language-impaired children. *Journal of Speech and Hearing Disorders, 53,* 433–440.

Oteem, E. (2002). Do the Wechsler scales underestimate the difference between verbal and performance abilities in children with language-related disorders? *Scandinavian Journal of Psychology, 43,* 291–298.

Paul, R. (1996). Clinical implications of the natural history of slow expressive language development. *American Journal of Speech–Language Pathology, 5*(2), 5–21.

Paul, R., Murray, C., Clancy, K., & Andrews, D. (1997). Reading and metaphonological outcomes in late talkers. *Journal of Speech, Language, and Hearing Research, 40,* 1037–1047.

Phelps, L. (1998). Utility of the WISC-III for children with language impairments. In A. Prifitera & D. H. Saklofske (Eds.), *WISC-III clinical use and interpretation* (pp. 157–174). San Diego, CA: Academic Press.

Plante, E. (1991). MRI findings in the parents and siblings of specifically language-impaired boys. *Brain and Language, 41,* 67–80.

Plante, E., Swisher, L., Vance, R., & Rapcsak, S. (1991). MRI findings in boys with specific language impairment. *Brain and Language, 41,* 52–66.

Restrepo, M. A., Swisher, L., Plante, E., & Vance, R. (1992). Relations among verbal and nonverbal cognitive skills in normal language and specifically language-impaired children. *Journal of Communication Disorders, 25,* 205–219.

Riccio, C. A., Ross, C. M., Boan, C. H., Jemison, S., & Houston, F. (1997). Use of the Differential Ability Scales (DAS) Special Nonverbal Composite among young children with linguistic differences. *Journal of Psychoeducational Assessment, 15,* 196–204.

Roid, G., & Miller, L. (1997a). *Leiter International Performance Scale—Revised.* Wood Dale, IL: Stoelting.

Roid, G. H., & Miller, L. (1997b). *Technical manual: Leiter International Performance Scale—Revised.* Wood Dale, IL: Stoelting.

Rose, J. C., Lincoln, A. J., & Allen, M. H. (1992). Ability profiles of developmental language disordered and learning disabled children: A comparative analysis. *Developmental Neuropsychology, 8,* 413–426.

Savich, P. A. (1984). Anticipatory imagery ability in normal and language-disabled children. *Journal of Speech and Hearing Research, 27,* 494–501.

Scarborough, H. S. (1990). Very early language deficits in dyslexic children. *Child Development, 61,* 1728–1748.

Scarborough, H. S. (1991). Antecedents to reading disability: Preschool language development and literacy experiences of children from dyslexic families. *Read-*

ing and Writing: An Interdisciplinary Journal, 3, 219–233.

Scarborough, H. S., & Dobrich, W. (1990). Development of children with early language delay. *Journal of Speech and Hearing Research, 33,* 70–83.

Sininger, Y. S., Klatzky, R. L., & Kirchner, D. M. (1989). Memory scanning speed in language-disordered children. *Journal of Speech and Hearing Research, 32,* 289–297.

Snyder, L. S. (1987). Symbolization in language impaired children. In D. Cicchetti & M. Beeghly (Eds.), *New directions for child development: Vol. 36. Symbolic development in atypical children* (pp. 87–108). San Francisco: Jossey-Bass.

Sparks, R., Ganschow, L., & Thomas, A. (1996). Role of intelligence tests in speech/language referrals. *Perceptual and Motor Skills, 83,* 195–204.

Stark, R. E., Bernstein, L. E., Condino, R., Bender, M., Tallal, P., & Catts, H. C., III. (1984). Four-year followup study of language impaired children. *Annals of Dylexia, 34,* 49–68.

Stark, R. E., & Tallal, P. (1981). Selection of children with specific language deficits. *Journal of Speech and Hearing Disorders, 46,* 114–122.

Stark, R. E., Tallal, P., Kallman, C., & Mellits, E. D. (1983). Cognitive abilities of language-delayed children. *Journal of Psychology, 114,* 9–19.

Stothard, S. E., Snowling, M. J., Bishop, D. V. M., Chipchase, B. B., & Kaplan, C. A. (1998). Language-impaired preschoolers: A follow-up into adolescence. *Journal of Speech, Language, and Hearing Research, 41,* 407–418.

Stromsvold, K. (2000). Specific language impairments. In M. J. Farah & T. E. Feinberg (Eds.), *Patient-based approaches to cognitive neuroscience* (pp. 217–234). Cambridge, MA: MIT Press.

Swisher, L., & Plante, E. (1993). Nonverbal IQ tests reflect different relations among skills for specifically language-impaired and normal children: Brief report. *Journal of Communication Disorders, 26,* 65–71.

Swisher, L., Plante, E., & Lowell, S. (1994). Nonlinguistic deficits of children with language disorders complicate the interpretation of their nonverbal IQ scores. *Language, Speech, and Hearing Services in Schools, 25,* 235–240.

Tallal, P., Hirsch, L. S., Realpe-Bonilla, T., Miller, S., & Brzustowicz, L. M. (2001). Familial aggregation in specific language impairment. *Journal of Speech, Language, and Hearing Research, 44,* 1172–1182.

Tallal, P., Stark, R., Kallman, C., & Mellits, D. (1981). A reexamination of some nonverbal perceptual abilities of language-impaired and normal children as a function of age and sensory modality. *Journal of Speech and Hearing Research, 24,* 351–357.

Terman, L. M., & Merrill, M. A. (1972). *Stanford–Binet Scale of Intelligence: Third Revision, Form L-M.* Chicago: Riverside.

Thal, D. J. (1991). Language and cognition in normal and late-talking toddlers. *Topics in Language Disorders, 11,* 33–42.

Tomblin, J. B., Freese, P. R., & Records, N. L. (1992). Diagnosing specific language impairment in adults for the purpose of pedigree analysis. *Journal of Speech and Hearing Research, 35*, 832–843.

Tomblin, J. B., Records, N. L., Buckwalter, P., Zhang, X., Smith, E., & O'Brien, M. (1997). Prevalence of specific language impairment in kindergarten children. *Journal of Speech and Hearing Research, 40*, 1245–1260.

Vandermeulen, B. F., Smrkovsky, M., LeCoultre-Martin, P., & Wijnberg-Williams, B. J. (1994). A nonverbal version of the Bayley Scales of Infant Development. *Psychologica Belgica, 34*, 141–152.

Watkins, R. V. (1994). Specific language impairments in children: An introduction. In R. V. Watkins & M. L. Rice (Eds.), *Specific language impairments in children* (Vol. 4, pp. 1–15). Baltimore: Brookes.

Wechsler, D. (1967). *Wechsler Preschool and Primary Scale of Intelligence*. New York: Psychological Corporation.

Wechsler, D. (1974). *Wechsler Intelligence Scale for Children—Revised*. New York: Psychological Corporation.

Wechsler, D. (1989). *Wechsler Preschool and Primary Scale of Intelligence—Revised*. San Antonio, TX: Psychological Corporation.

Wechsler, D. (1991). *Wechsler Intelligence Scale for Children—Third Edition*. San Antonio, TX: Psychological Corporation.

Weiner, P. S. (1971). Stability and validity of two measures of intelligence used with children whose language development is delayed. *Journal of Speech and Hearing Research, 14*, 254–261.

Williams, J. M., Voelker, S., & Ricciardi, P. W. (1995). Predictive validity of the K-ABC for exceptional preschoolers. *Psychology in the Schools, 32*, 178–185.

Windsor, J., & Hwang, M. (1999). Testing the generalized slowing hypothesis in specific language impairment. *Journal of Speech, Language, and Hearing Disorders, 42*, 1205–1218.

Woodcock, R. W. (1997). The Woodcock–Johnson Tests of Cognitive Ability—Revised. In D. P. Flanagan, J. L. Genshaft, & P. L. Harrison (Eds.), *Contemporary Intellectual Assessment* (pp. 230–246). New York: Guilford Press.

Wren, C. T. (1981). Identifying patterns of syntactic disorder in six-year-old children. *British Journal of Disorders of Communication, 16*, 101–109.

26

Computerized Assessment

C. SUE MCCULLOUGH
DANIEL C. MILLER

Computerized assessment has been enhanced by significantly faster, more powerful, and more widely available personal computers, along with the rapid growth and improved technical capacity of the Internet or World Wide Web. Computerized assessment has been further affected by the fact that today's children interact quite naturally with rapidly changing technology in all its forms, including video games, VCRs, calculators, and personal computers, making technology inextricably linked to children's acquisition of knowledge. Computers are now used in over 95% of American classrooms and have transformed instructional and assessment practices.

"Computerized assessment," as defined by this chapter, includes all those procedures that incorporate computer assistance to assess the progress of children or adolescents in meeting educational or behavioral goals. This definition includes systems such as traditional or nontraditional psychological tests, questionnaires, or interviews directly administered on the computer; automated test scoring, analysis, and interpretation; computer-adapted testing; instructional delivery systems; assistive technology; computer simulations; electronic portfolios; cogni-

tive mapping; automated data recording and retrieval of directly observed behavior; and other procedures possible only since the advent of the personal computer.

Technology has transformed assessment practices through changes in test design, item generation, task presentation, scoring, testing purpose, location, and practitioner and client roles (Bennett, 1999; Groth-Marnat, 2000). However, assessment innovations may have negative, unintended, and unpredictable consequences (Groth-Marnat, 2000; Madaus, 1994; Sutton, 1991), especially related to equity, test bias, and client confidentiality. Yet computerized versions of high-stakes tests such as the Graduate Record Examination (GRE) and Praxis I: Academic Skills Assessment are in widespread use. In addition, computerized versions of mandated, large-scale, high-stakes basic skills tests in states such as Texas are under development (Texas Education Agency, personal communication, 2000).

The focus of this chapter is on reviewing computerized assessment procedures and addressing issues raised by computer use and published research. The chapter is organized into five main sections. The first of these is a brief history of computerized assessment.

The second one covers selected applications including general background information and research findings. Third, issues related to computerized assessment are discussed. Fourth, changing data or information management paradigms are presented. The fifth section discusses future trends.

A BRIEF HISTORY OF COMPUTERIZED ASSESSMENT

The potential for computer utilization in traditional assessment practices has long been recognized. In 1968, Green predicted "the inevitable computer conquest of testing" (Green, 1970, p. 194). Until the mid–1980s, the predicted revolution was slow but deliberate, as psychological and educational measurement changed under the influence of technology. Beginning in 1930, scoring machines that processed over 1,200 Hollerith cards for each protocol scored the Strong Vocational Interest Blank (SVIB). In 1946, an analog computer began scoring and profiling the SVIB. This technology was also adapted a year later to score the Minnesota Multiphasic Personality Inventory (MMPI). Computer-based test interpretation (CBTI) systems emerged in the late 1950s, primarily focused on the MMPI and operated from centralized test-scoring businesses. Digital computers and optical scanners in the early 1960s permitted the processing of large amounts of data and the analysis of psychometric data in ways never possible before by using punch cards and batch processing (Moreland, 1991). Latent-trait theory, computer-adapted testing, and computerized assessment, hypothesized years earlier (Cowden, 1946) but not possible prior to the existence of high-speed digital computers, became practical (Weiss, 1983). As data storage, computer memory, and operating speed improved, mainframe computers were supplanted by minicomputers, microcomputers, portable computers, hand-held computers or personal digital assistants (PDAs), and other information appliances (e.g., smart cards). The power of interactive computing became increasingly practical and affordable in research laboratories, and finally in applied settings such as schools, clinics, and homes.

During the 2001–02 school year, U.S. public school districts spent $6.45 billion on technology, and it was projected that $7.185 billion would be spent in the 2002–2003 school year (Quality Education Data, 2002b). Internet access has become the rule in K–12 education, with 96% of K–12 teachers in public schools reporting that they used the Internet as a teaching resource, up from 90% in 2001 and 86% in 2000 (Quality Education Data, 2002a). The number of public schools in America that are connected to the Internet was 99% in 2002, up from 97% in 2001 and 91% of public school classrooms are connected to the Internet, up from 84% in 2001 (Quality Education Data, 2002a). Internet access in schools continues to present limitations for computerized assessment applications, however, as virtual firewalls erected to limit access of children to the Internet also limit access for educators and psychologists.

Initially, major support for the development of basic and applied research in computerized testing applications came from the U.S. military and, later, the federal government's Office of Personnel Management (formerly the Civil Service Commission). In addition to military and governmental support, private organizations such as the Educational Testing Service and numerous test publishers actively developed and promoted computerized testing. In the 1970s, computer-assisted instruction (CAI) incorporated frequent assessment and feedback into programmed learning, primarily linear drill and practice programs. In the 1980s, multimedia and hypertext created networks of related text, graphics, audio files, or video clips in CAI that were integrated, interactive, flexible, and searchable. In the1990s, the Internet (also known as the Web) became a repository of thousands of interactive sites with multiple representations of information that included computerized assessment components in every field imaginable, including psychology and education.

Professional organizations such as the American Psychological Association (APA) and the National Association of School Psychologists (NASP) incorporated guidelines on computer utilization into professional training standards (APA's *Standards for Educational and Psychological Testing*, 1999; NASP's *Standards for Training and Field*

Placement Programs in School Psychology, 2000) and ethical guidelines (NASP's *Guidelines for Professional Ethics,* 2000).

At first, practitioners trained in the "old ways" of paper-and-pencil tests resisted using the new technology. Practitioners cited lack of appropriate equipment in the educational or clinical setting, lack of qualified university trainers, lack of high-quality software, lack of administrative support, and professional caution regarding research support for radical changes in professional functions (McCullough, 1985). Some resistance to change is still apparent. A 2001 study (Olson, 2001) of APA-accredited clinical and counseling programs found a median of only three computerized tests used in training programs with 25% of respondents reporting no computerized psychological tests in their training programs. However, special interest groups formed within professional organizations; for instance, the Computer and Technological Applications in School Psychology Committee (CTASP) of NASP was formed in 1982. CTASP produced newsletters, software reviews, inservice workshops, and information exchanges. CTASP also served to nudge its parent organization, NASP, into the computer age during the 1990s by producing daily newsletters during conventions, establishing e-mail as a communication tool, establishing a listserv for NASP members, and producing and maintaining a NASP Web site.

In the absence of leadership from the professional organizations or publishers, much of the early development and research in computerized assessment began at the "grassroots" level. Individual psychologists with access to personal computers developed numerous applications to meet their own professional needs (McCullough, 1985; Roid, 1986). These included test-scoring and interpretation programs; report-writing programs; statistical programs to assist in determining cutoff scores for learning disability discrepancy rules; creative applications of generic software, such as word processors and spreadsheets; and self-programmed simulations. Basic and applied research focused on computer-adapted or computer-assisted testing and direct assessment on the computer, usually following traditional paper-and-pencil models (Bug-

bee, 1996; Butcher, Perry, & Atlis, 2000; McCullough, 1985)

In the early 1980s, publishers began producing computerized assessment products such as test-scoring and interpretation programs; computer courseware that included computer-managed or computer-assisted testing; and computer-adapted testing programs in reading and mathematics. In the 1990s, most major standardized tests had accompanying computerized scoring programs available from the publishers. Computer-administered tests became available to measure cognitive, affective, social-emotional, perceptual, behavioral, and historical characteristics. During the 1990s, instructional software included "smart" computerized assessment that "learned" from an individual's responses and adjusted testing items accordingly, and utilized a variety of input and output modes (including verbal, visual, and tactile).

Computer assessment applications in psychology have primarily involved using the computer as a tool for routine clerical tasks such as test scoring and analysis, generating interpretive hypotheses for report writing, and data management and storage. Though computers provide the potential for radically altering assessment theories and practices, economic interests and a reluctance to change traditional practices impede the widespread adoption of innovative applications. Braden (1997) notes that theoretical complexity and computer technology are symbiotic, allowing measurement of constructs that can only be reliably measured with technology. For example, correct decision speed (CDS), a second-order factor in the Horn–Cattell cognitive theory, can only be measured reliably using computer paradigms (see Vernon, 1987, 1990). Braden suggests that technology may transform the use and interpretation of intelligence tests in five practical ways:

1. Developing theoretically complex tests with reduced clerical and computational demands.
2. Measuring elusive constructs such as CDS.
3. Including more integrated audio and video stimuli in tests.
4. Including statistical/actuarial procedures for ipsative profile analysis into scoring

software—allowing practitioners to understand the degree to which intraindividual variation affects criterion performance, and providing empirically grounded, computationally complex methods of interpretation.
5. Including aptitude–treatment interaction data as a minimum test validity standard in computerized scoring paradigms.

Some intelligence tests published in the late 1990s have included computer-administered forms (TechMicro, 1997). Tests that measure impulsiveness and reaction time associated with assessment of attention-deficit/hyperactivity disorder are also available (Campbell, D'Amato, Raggio, & Stephend, 1991; Rosen, 1995). However, the majority of field practitioners do not use these tests, preferring instead to continue with those with which they are more familiar, utilizing accompanying scoring programs to increase their efficiency at continuing traditional practices (an example of the QWERTY phenomenon[1]). The use of these computerized tests, especially in the schools, has been inhibited by a lack of appropriate and transportable equipment, lack of training and university trainers with knowledge of these tests, restricted access to the Internet in the school setting, and inconsistent results in research on their comparability with traditional procedures. Research on the implications of these technology developments for children and adolescents has tended to lag behind product development and distribution.

Utilization of technology for traditional assessment purposes usually emerges from the need for continuous or periodic assessment of a student's progress toward reaching academic or behavior goals. Computer-adapted testing, computer-based instruction that includes frequent assessment (e.g., CMI and CAI); computerized interviews; direct computer-assisted observation and recording of behavior; and computer simulations that record and track learning style or other cognitive and behavioral processes are means through which computerized assessment occurs. In addition, computerized scoring and interpretation of test results are a means of uniting empirical research on test score pattern analysis with verifiable behaviors or characteristics of the examinees.

Each of these technology-based procedures provides a tool for reaching evaluation goals. Each is defined and discussed below.

COMPUTERIZED ASSESSMENT APPLICATIONS

Computer-Adapted Testing

Computer-adapted testing starts with a database or large collection of facts, skills, and concepts from an array of subject areas placed into the memory banks or secondary storage devices of a computer. For any given area, the computer selects and tests a subset of skills, facts, or concepts, and the basal and ceiling levels are then determined for each area. The adapted or "tailored" part of the test program comes from the branching capabilities used to determine which questions should be asked of which persons. For example, questions about marriage would not be asked of a child. Sophisticated mathematical approaches (based on latent-trait theory or graphical modeling [GM] theory) are used to determine item presentation based on previous responses. For example, in a test of mathematical ability, a simple addition problem would not be presented to a person who had already correctly solved a complex algebraic equation. When testing is completed, the computer can then generate and sometimes monitor individualized educational plans or worksheets. In essence, computer-adapted testing is the ultimate criterion-referenced test (Wainer et al., 1990). By using examinees' response patterns to select items adaptively, computer-adapted testing can improve motivation, reduce testing time, and administer fewer items per examinee, all without sacrificing measurement accuracy (Almond & Mislevy, 1999).

"Latent-trait theory," which underlies computer-adapted testing, encompasses several mathematical models that express functional relationships between observable variables and the underlying hypothetical trait constructs that produce the observable variables. When latent trait theory is applied to tests of ability or achievement, it has become known as "item characteristic curve theory" or "item response theory" (IRT)—terms that are used interchangeably in the research literature. The item characteristic curve is the curve that portrays the probability of a correct response to a test item as a function of trait levels that produce those probabilities. IRT emphasizes both the role of the test item and the response of the examinees (Wainer et al., 1990; Weiss, 1983). IRT has been applied to the scoring of paper-and-pencil standardized tests to identify consistent patterns of responses and produce a more accurate estimate of ability than traditional number-correct scoring (Erdner, Guy, & Bush, 1998). By considering each item's characteristics, including its discrimination, location parameter, and "guessability," IRT scoring accounts for the fact that not all correct test answers are equally good indicators of a student's level of achievement (CTB/McGraw Hill, 1983). Some items may be correct because of guessing rather than knowledge of the content.

Latent trait theory consists of three elements:

1. A set of stimulus variables that is presented to individuals, such as test items on an ability test or achievement test, personality questionnaire items, or items on an attitude scale.
2. The responses of the individual when presented with these stimulus variables (the computer automatically records the response when a key is pressed).
3. Mathematical equations that describe the functional relationship between the observed response to the stimulus variables and the hypothesized underlying trait. These complex formulas allow inference of the performance of the individual on the hypothesized trait as a function of the characteristics of the stimulus variables (CTB/McGraw Hill, 1983; Weiss, 1983).

When the characteristics of the stimulus variables or test items are known, then latent-trait theory can estimate the unobservable trait levels for individuals based on their observed responses to the test items. Although adaptive testing is not dependent on IRT (Weiss, 1983), IRT is useful in the efficient implementation of adaptive testing. Graphic modeling (GM) theory has extended IRT to make inferences from complex multivariate dependencies (Almond & Mis-

levy, 1999). Complex assessment models are built by (1) defining unobservable variables to explain patterns of observable responses; (2) assembling tasks so that some sources of variation accumulate and others do not; and (3) using probability-based inference to manage accumulating information about an unobservable variable as assessment proceeds (Almond & Mislevy, 1999). The IRT model is primarily a task-centered model, while the GM model is a competency-centered model allowing more complex multivariate procedures that result in cross-modality competency comparisons.

Alfred Binet actually developed the first adaptive test, though his strategy was simplistic in comparison to computer-adapted tests based on IRT or GM theory. The Binet test (Form LM) used a variable entry point estimated by the examiner at the beginning of testing. Test items were scored as they were administered, and the correctness of the responses determined which items to administer next, branching up or down the levels of the test. The Binet test also had a variable termination criterion, meaning that different individuals were given tests of varying lengths, depending upon when they reached their "ceiling level."

Similar to Binet's application of adaptive testing, CAT has been developed to measure traits for individuals with a wide range of possible trait levels, but it has also been used for evaluating mastery. (For a more detailed discussion of latent-trait theory, see Lord & Novick, 1968; Wainer et al., 1990; Weiss, 1983. For a more detailed discussion of GM theory, see Almond & Mislevy, 1999.)

Instructional Delivery Systems

Instructional delivery systems include forms of computer-based instruction (e.g., CMI or CAI), information-processing tools, and concept mapping. (Concept mapping is discussed in more detail later.) CMI may be a part of CAI or an independent program. CMI uses and maintains records of frequent tests of mastery to select what to present next in the instructional program. A concept may be repeated, divided into smaller or easier tasks, or expanded upon, depending upon the individual's test performance. CMI does not rely solely on computer instruction, as

CAI does, but rather serves an overseer function. The computer may direct the student to read certain books, listen to certain tapes, see certain films, visit certain Web sites, or the like. When the assignments are completed, the student returns to the CMI program for testing and further assignments based on his or her test results. Since each student is managed individually, each can proceed at his or her own pace. The computer will summarize each student's progress and keep records for the teacher as well, including conducting an item analysis of its true–false and multiple-choice tests, and printing out reports on the group as a whole or on a selected individual. "Intelligent CAI" or "smart CAI" programs contain diagnostic tools that can identify patterns of error, select appropriate instructional content, adjust the level of difficulty, set the rate of progress through the lesson, and deliver the material in a format best suited to the student's learning style (Lieberman, 1985).

A computerized instructional delivery system consists of three major components: instructional objectives (input), delivery system (process), and learning outcomes (output). Each of these components has multiple complex dimensions (see Table 26.1), creating a challenge for evaluation of the system and for assessing learning outcomes (Jones & Paolucci, 1999). Typically, CAI systems have consisted of tutorial and drill-and-practice exercises with highly structured lessons that involve frequent testing to assess progress and determine which branch of the program to use next. Instruction usually follows a programmed instruction model, shaping the learning behavior by breaking instruction into small sequential steps, with frequent reviews and tests for mastery. Research has shown that the frequent feedback provided by these systems may increase student motivation, time on task, and achievement (Fletcher-Flinn, 1995; Niemiec, Sikorski, & Walberg, 1996).

TABLE 26.1. Complex Dimensions of Instructional Delivery Systems Affecting Assessment of Learning Outcomes

Instructional objectives	Delivery system	Learning outcomes
1. Learning domain	1. Locus of control	1. Cognitive skills
Cognitive	Instructor	Lower order
Affective	Lecturer	Knowledge
Psychomotor	Facilitator	Comprehension
2. Learner profile	Technology	Application
Cognitive style	Mediator	Higher order
Aptitude	Tutor	Analysis
Experience	Learner	Synthesis
Education level	Constructor	Evaluation
Achievement	Explorer	2. Affective
Motivation	2. Presence	Disposition
Attitude	a. Time	Perspective
Age	Synchronous	3. Psychomotor
Gender	Asynchronous	Capability
Ethnicity	b. Place	Performance mastery
3. Task	Colocated	
Concepts	Distance	
Rules	3. Media	
Principles	One medium	
	Multimedia	
	Hypermedia	
	Immersive	
	4. Connectivity	
	Information	
	Communication	
	Collaboration	

Note. From Jones & Paolucci (1999). Copyright 1999 by ISTE. Adapted by permission.

Modern CAI systems may employ multimedia, hypermedia, hypertext, and simulations in a multimodal and exploratory learning environment that is much more flexible, allowing more learner control and needing less teacher control than previous systems (Fletcher-Flinn, 1995).

The assessment of learning outcomes provides the major feedback mechanism within the instructional design process and is critical in evaluating the instructional system and its effectiveness. The information that is collected as evidence of learning achievement will depend upon the nature of the competency being measured. These measures may include cognitive tests (measures of intellectual skills), performance tests (measures of capability), and attitudinal tests (measures of disposition and perspective). The instrument and techniques used to assess these outcomes will depend upon the learning domain and objectives (e.g., text-based or oral formats for cognitive objectives, portfolios for performance objectives, or interviews for attitudinal objectives) (Jones & Paolucci, 1999; Seels & Glasgow, 1998). Table 26.1 summarizes some of the variables to consider when one is evaluating computerized instructional systems.

Studies that have evaluated CAI as a replacement for traditional classroom instruction have found mixed results. Though the effects of using hypermedia in instruction appear generally superior to those of non-hypermedia instruction as a whole, the effects may vary, depending on the type of instruction, content, age, or gender (Fletcher-Flinn, 1995; Liao, 1999; Lieberman, 1985). In studies that examined CAI as a supplement to, rather than a replacement for, traditional classroom instruction, significant positive effects on learning (as measured in standardized achievement test scores) were found, especially for students with lower achievement or slower learning rates and for males (Fletcher-Flinn, 1995; Liao, 1999; Lieberman, 1985). Meta analyses of this large body of research have summarized some evident trends, such as that found when studying 48 secondary school math and science CAI evaluations. Average test scores rose 0.32 of a standard deviation, which is equivalent to an increase from the 50th to the 63rd percentile (Kulik, Bangert, & Williams, 1983). Meta-analysis

mean effect sizes have increased in more recent studies. For example, the mean effect size for CAI across instructional levels (kindergarten through postsecondary) was 0.24 for the years 1987–1992, meaning that students receiving CAI scored 0.24 of a standard deviation higher than students not receiving CAI, or that the former students outperformed 60% of the later students. The 1990–1992 studies had an effect size of 0.33 (Fletcher-Flinn, 1995). The overall mean effect size for 1985–1995 studies with secondary students was 0.21, indicating that 58.2% of students receiving CAI did better than peers receiving only traditional instruction (Christmann, Badgett, & Lucking, 1997). The comparative effectiveness of CAI with secondary students is apparent in the following descending-order mean effect sizes: science, 0.64; reading, 0.26; music, 0.23; math, 0.18; vocational education, –0.08; and English, –0.42. Higher mean effect sizes possibly reflect the more sophisticated hypermedia CAI programs (science is one area where hypermedia excels), while the decreasing effect sizes across secondary content areas may reflect the different needs of secondary students (Christmann et al., 1997). First graders who used a CAI system for 20 minutes three times per week for an entire academic year showed significant reading gains over matched peers taught by traditional methods (Erdner et al., 1998). Children with learning disabilities, mild mental retardation, and serious emotional disturbances have also shown significant gains in reading, language, and math achievement when spending as little as 30 minutes per week using CAI lessons and tests (Chiang, 1978). Although mixed results have been reported, what appears to account for the effectiveness of CAI over traditional instruction is the better and more consistent quality of instruction provided by CAI. Frequent computerized assessment and feedback are integral parts of CAI.

Computerized Test Scoring and Analysis

Test scoring involves identifying responses as correct or incorrect, computing raw scores for each subtest of a battery, and then converting the raw scores to standard scores using norm tables prepared by the publisher/researcher. No other computerized assessment task has been embraced by psychologists so quickly as computerized scoring of tests. In 1995, 91% of all practicing psychologists engaged in at least some form of assessment (Watkins, Campbell, Nieberding, & Hallmark, 1995). In national surveys, computerized test scoring was clearly an early high-priority usage of computers by psychologists in the schools (Jacob & Brantley, 1987; McCullough & Wenck, 1984).

Computerized test scoring varies with the nature of the test being scored. Group tests have long been computer-scored, with literally millions of answer sheets processed each year, producing percentiles, stanines, normal curve equivalents, grade equivalents, normalized standard scores, IRT, or number-correct scores. Computerized scoring of individually administered psychological tests allows the derivation of complex scores such as factor scores; Bayesian-derived probability scores for low-base-rate behaviors such as suicide (Vanderplas & Vanderplas, 1979); item–option weighted scores (Roid, 1986); weighted scores from tailored, adapted, or multilevel tests calibrated with the three parameter model (Weiss, 1983); and sociometric ratings from entire classrooms contrasted with self-ratings and teacher ratings for individual students (Barclay, 1983). For psychological and vocational tests having complex and numerous scores, such as the MMPI, the Strong–Campbell Interest Inventory, the Tennessee Self Concept Scale, or the 16 Personality Factor Questionnaire (16PF), computer scoring provides a richness of interpretive data that could not otherwise be obtained without enormous effort (Roid, 1986).

A computer may score some test batteries easily because each response is clearly right or wrong, or is clearly part of one category or another. For example, arithmetic answers or answers on a rating scale have distinct and limited responses. These responses may be entered into the computer either directly by the examinee (on tests adapted to computer presentation, such as the MMPI and computer-adapted reading and math tests) or later an examiner, a clerk, or a computerized scanning device. The computer tabulates the score and converts it to the appropriate standard score. Other subtests require subjective scoring by the examiner, who must decide whether a response is acceptable, given certain parameters. For instance, a young child's language should not penalize him or her, and judgment is frequently necessary to determine correct responses. Gestures may have accompanied the response to make it more correct than incorrect, for example. Some computerized scoring programs are incorporating both qualitative and quantitative assessment results (Hammainen, 1994). The response may also receive a varying amount of credit, depending upon the nature of the response (concrete or abstract). Examples of these kinds of tests include achievement batteries and intelligence tests that involve verbal responses. For these tests, the examiner must compute the raw score for each subtest manually. The raw scores then are entered into the computer, which converts them into standard scores and may provide other statistical information as well, such as standard deviations, stanines, percentage of the population obtaining such scores, and so forth. Virtually all major standardized tests have computerized scoring programs available.

Most test-scoring programs depend on the examiner or clerk to type in raw data. Thus, individual subtests have to be scored in the traditional manner. The computer then displays the standardized scores accurately and in seconds. In some cases, the standard scores are accompanied by a written analysis of the scores; in other cases, a description of what the test measures is accompanied by a discussion of the subject's performance compared to the norm group and/or compared to him- or herself. Some programs can score multiple protocols at one time, while others can do only one at a time. Some programs allow data to be saved in a data bank for future reference and comparisons, and for incorporation into reports.

Some programs score more than one type of test—for instance, the Wechsler Intelligence Scale of Children—Third Edition (WISC-III), the Wide Range Achievement Test—3 (WRAT-3), and the Vineland Adaptive Behavior Scales—Revised. There may be a choice of tests to use in any combination, or it may be impossible to use the program without using all of the specific tests in the scoring program. Some scoring programs also require that all subtests be given in order to complete the scoring. Scoring programs that score multiple types of tests may also offer cross-test analysis and comparison, using a variety of statistical or clinical codes. For example, the McDermott Multidimensional Assessment of Children (M-MAC) program (McDermott & Watkins, 1985) followed an actuarial model that considered probability, sources of errors, empirical research, and accepted psychological theory in analyzing 22 different tests.

Computerized Test Interpretation

Computers can play a role in the more complex processes of test interpretation (Meehl, 1954). Debate was inspired by Meehl regarding the merits of actuarial/statistical (objective) decision making versus clinical judgment (subjective). Meehl contended that decisions based on objective data were more valid than subjective interpretations. Grove, Zald, Lebow, Smith, and Nelson (2000) conducted a meta-analysis of 136 studies and reported that there was a 10% accuracy advantage in using statistical prediction over clinical prediction.

Psychologists have long accepted computerized aggregate results for groups, such as national, district, or school norms or classroom summaries. However, applying computerized interpretation to individuals has raised concern about the bounds of acceptable clinical use. Ethical concerns have been raised (Jacob & Brantley, 1987; Zachary & Pope, 1984) and supported. Sixty-five percent of school psychologists surveyed in 1986, anticipated problems associated with computerized test scoring and interpretation (Jacob & Brantley, 1987). The validity of CBTI programs continues to be debated (Butcher et al., 2000; Eyde, Kowal, & Fishburne, 1991; Moreland, 1991).

Test-scoring and interpretation programs include publisher-authorized, privately produced, and public domain versions, and vary in quality and ease of use. The best test interpretation programs are designed on the basis of empirically validated decision rules and are intended for the use of trained professionals experienced with the test instrument and its supportive research. The worst of available programs include private and subjective narratives of individuals who developed the programs with limited reference to empirical studies.

Debate regarding computerized interpretation (Brantley, 1984; Butcher et al., 2000; Eyde et al., 1991; Jacob & Brantley, 1987; Matarazzo, 1983; McCullough & Wenck, 1984; Moreland, 1991; Roid, 1986) has included the following issues:

1. Advantages and disadvantages of computerized interpretation of tests, as compared to interpretation by a clinician working without a computer.
2. Legal and ethical concerns regarding responsibility for test interpretation and the effects of computerized interpretive reports in the hands of inexperienced or unqualified individuals, who may respond to the aura of objectivity and authority projected by a computerized report.
3. Insufficient validation of computerized reports, especially those that cannot be evaluated closely.
4. Identification and acceptance of "expert opinion" status with professional review of CBTI software at a level equal to that found with traditional research in professional journals.
5. Scoring-only versus descriptive versus clinician modeled versus clinical actuarial interpretations.
6. Reliance on computerized interpretation without regard to clinical judgment.

These concerns and others merit further discussion.

Advantages and Disadvantages of Computerized Interpretation

Advantages of computerized scoring and interpretation programs are as follows:

1. Scoring is much more consistent and accurate, and retrieval of norms from complex norms tables is greatly facilitated. Scoring errors may result from data entry error, or, more infrequently, from program defects (CTASP, 1987), but overall errors are greatly decreased with computerized scoring programs. Psychologists should check to be sure that data entry is accurate and that the resulting standard scores and profiles accurately describe the observed behavior.

2. Consistency as it relates to nonbiased assessment can be enhanced with the use of computerized interpretive programs. School psychologists have been shown to be influenced in their diagnostic decision making by positive or negative referral information about a child's intellectual, academic, and social abilities (Hersh, 1971); socioeconomic status (Matuszek & Oakland, 1979); and perhaps ethnicity or race (Frame, Clarizio, Porter, & Vinsonhaler, 1982; Matuszek & Oakland, 1979). McDermott (1980) found that diagnostic disagreement increased with higher levels of training and experience. Computerized interpretation programs offer conclusions that are neutral with respect to these biasing factors, and may even produce statistically adjusted data or cautions based on research with minorities. Again, the program merely offers suggestions for the psychologist to consider, but it may serve as a reminder to consider diagnostic conclusions that might not otherwise have been considered.

3. Scoring time is reduced significantly, saving the psychologist routine clerical work and freeing time for other, more rewarding professional pursuits. Some psychoeducational tests, like the Woodcock–Johnson—III Tests of Cognitive Abilities (Woodcock, McGrew, & Mather, 2001), are now only scored using a computer-scoring program. The computerized scoring program scores a protocol in less than a minute. A clerk can enter the raw scores and then provide a printout to the psychologist.

4. Interpreting multiscale tests is complex and involves numerous decision rules and reference to a constantly growing body of research. The computer can act as a memory aid and offer a variety of suggestions for possible interpretations of the material, perhaps helping the psychologist recall some possibilities that would not have been considered otherwise. The program may also offer some possible interpretations that make no sense at all, considering all the circumstances of the client. It becomes the psychologist's responsibility to maintain final authority over interpretation of the information collected.

5. Research showing moderator effects (i.e., the fact that certain age groups or ethnic groups have different ranges or patterns of scores) can be included in the computerized interpretation; again, this serves as a re-

minder for the psychologist to use caution when interpreting the data.

6. Numerous technical advances in profile analysis and statistical processing of scores are impractical to implement with a hand scoring method, since they require complex calculations by each clinician, with a high probability of calculation errors. The majority of clinicians do not have the time or motivation to do these calculations. Computerized scoring programs do the calculations and present the results for interpretation.

7. Flexibility in scheduling is an advantage of computerized assessment. Whether doing an intake assessment, high-stakes achievement testing, or career-vocational assessment, the test may be given frequently and taken at the convenience of the examinee. However, this does put the responsibility on the examinee to make the appointment well ahead of any deadlines that must be met. Computerized assessment does tend to be more expensive than conventional paper-and-pencil versions with the cost born by the examinee. This finding is in contrast to the fact that technology reduces the per-client costs for the test administrator. Insurance companies, especially managed care companies, may not pay for assessment and fee waivers may be needed for low-income examinees. Public agencies may balk at the costs involved, thus limiting the use of computerized tests.

8. Computerized assessment may provide immediate feedback, in some cases giving examinees the option to see their scores as soon as they finish. Other systems provide feedback to the professional who then translates it for the client using graphs or charts provided by the program. Ethical best practice demands that whatever and whenever feedback is provided, a qualified examiner is available to provide interpretive support.

Disadvantages of computerized scoring and interpretation programs include the following:

1. Equipment or trained personnel may be difficult if not impossible to obtain, or training time for psychologists and/or data entry clerks may strain already limited resources. The psychologist in the office who is known as the "computer buff" may find

him- or herself with additional uncompensated duties related to training, troubleshooting, and supervising the use of various programs. Priorities for equipment usage may need to be established.

2. Although the programs reflect current research and theory when purchased, they will require updating over time to remain current with the growing body of psychological research. Few programs make allowances for this fact. Without updating or attention to the need for updating, interpretations given today will still be the same 10 or 20 years from now, while theory has moved ahead.

3. Test-scoring and interpretation programs use advanced technology to introduce efficiency, greater accuracy, and greater consistency into current testing practices—testing practices that had their basis in an earlier period of technological and theoretical development. Computerized scoring and interpretation programs may serve to preserve practices that are outdated and no longer serve a rational function within a highly technical and computerized society. The cost of change and the widespread use of individual standardized tests may be used as arguments to resist change to a more efficient and practical mode of assessment. However, these are circular arguments and do not address the fact that there are technologically advanced alternatives to obtaining assessment information that may provide us with better diagnostic information, such as computer-adapted testing and computer simulations that record and track thinking processes. Using a computer to preserve practices that have only a historical basis to justify their existence requires careful examination and debate.

Unauthorized Use

Concern about unqualified users is related to issues of (1) controlling access to computerized programs, reports, or databases; (2) the ethical responsibilities of developers, distributors, and psychologist users; and (3) the concern that computer-generated reports have an air of objectivity and authority about them that might give them more weight than they should have in the hands of a client, a teacher, an administrator, or some other unqualified user. Most large publishing companies maintain strict procedures for individuals purchasing assessment products, including computerized scoring and interpretation programs. However, an institutional order is usually honored and may result in placement of materials in locations accessible to unqualified users.

Another concern is that a psychologist may give a client a computer report as the final psychological report without review or editing of its contents. National organizations such as APA (1999) and NASP (2000) have emphasized the responsibility of the *individual users* of computerized interpretive reports to be familiar with the research base of such reports, to refer to test manuals as needed, and to use appropriate caution in making decisions from these reports. A computerized interpretive report that is based on data only and is not reviewed for accuracy by the psychologist leaves the psychologist in jeopardy of an ethical violation. Alternatively, ignoring interpretations based on empirical findings rather than clinical judgment when the practitioner has no reason to believe that the findings are invalid for a client may also be an ethical violation, since these reports have been found to be more accurate than clinical judgment alone (Bersoff & Hofer, 1991). APA guidelines suggest that the validity and reliability of the computerized version of a test should be established and published by the developer, but computer-generated interpretations should be used only after professional review (APA, 1999; Bersoff & Hofer, 1991).

Bersoff and Hofer (1991) found court opinions related to copyright, client confidentiality, and use of computerized interpretations by nonpsychologists to be mixed and sometimes contradictory. They recommend that practitioners should maintain the prevailing "standard of care" to avoid charges of professional negligence. This "standard of care" is enunciated in professional associations' ethical guidelines relevant to computerized psychological testing. These guidelines include (1) user attention to evidence of program reliability and validity; (2) accurate data entry; (3) selection of a system appropriate to the client; (4) reasonable reliance and interpretation of the data; (5) assurance of client comfort with equipment and computerized procedures; and (6) knowledge of differential impact on clients, based on age, gender, ethnicity, and experience with computers.

The practitioner who uses computerized assessment must address the issues related to confidentiality of client electronic records and client privacy concerns also. If Web-based scoring services are used, data security is especially important. The Family Educational Rights and Privacy Act requires destruction of outdated assessment data. Assuming that this mandate includes electronic data may influence the selection of storage medium. Security procedures required for psychological records must be in place for electronic data to prevent access by unauthorized individuals. Alternatively, electronic data degeneration, accidental erasure, or other technological mishaps may endanger data integrity. Thus, secure backup procedures also need to be in place.

Documentation of Decision Rules

Validity studies should be performed and documented by the developers of computerized scoring and interpretive software. The APA's (1999) standards encourage developers to share adequate information with researchers in order for validation studies to proceed, but recognizes the proprietary rights of developers to withhold certain information that might endanger their copyright. Roid (1986) argues that documentation of the validity of decision rules is not incompatible with securing the rights to a program. Some central element of scoring or interpretive program logic could be withheld, but the validity of the program could be ascertained through studying the research base (including all references to published articles) and the numerical decision rules revealed in the documentation of the program, without one's having to know the entire operating specifications of a scoring and interpretive program (Butcher et al., 2000; Eyde et al., 1991; Moreland, 1991).

Campbell (1976) argued that research funding to expand and improve a computerized product—that is, to update the product in accord with the new research findings—is not usually supported by public or nonprofit foundation grants. Thus, if a commercial product is to be improved over time, revenues must be protected from erosion created by illegal copyright infringement or competing publishers. Experience has shown that an effective control is to withhold keys, norms, or portions of the interpretive decision rules.

Among the means by which to judge computerized scoring and interpretive programs are the quality and extent of the documentation. The documentation should clearly state the theoretical and research base of the program, and should provide examples of the logic and decision rules applied to the data. Limitations in the use of the program should also be clearly enunciated (Green, 1991; Moreland, 1991).

Insufficient Validation

Large and small publishers have produced interpretive programs including individual psychologists who produced them for their own personal use; the latter sometimes became public domain programs before publisher copyright lawsuits ended this practice. Each program usually has a particular theoretical orientation that is used to analyze data from a specific test or tests. For example, WISC-III analyses are available using the Sattler (1992, 2001). Kaufman (1980, 1994), or other clinical interpretation, or the McDermott (1982, 1990) statistical or actuarial method of interpretation. These analyses vary in the approach used to interpret the data, with each approach supported to some extent by research. One author may emphasize subtest-by-subtest interpretation, while another may emphasize groupings of subtests based on statistical correlations. Yet another may focus solely on Full Scale, Verbal, and Performance standard scores, ignoring individual subtest performance, or may emphasize standard errors of measurement and discrepancy formulas. Which of these analyses is valid? Computer simulations have proven useful in statistically analyzing the validity of interpretive models, such as Sattler's (2001). Macmann and Barnett (1997) used 5,000 cases in a computer simulation to critique the validity of the Sattler interpretive model and found significant deficiencies. They judged the model to be invalid and unable to accomplish its stated goals: "aptitude x treatment interactions involving the WISC III are unlikely to be found due to the unreliability of classifications for the identification of 'strengths' and 'weaknesses'" (p. 230).

In actual practice, practitioners may use a variety of interpretive approaches, depending upon the nature of the data and the training of the psychologist (Matuszek & Oakland, 1979). We have little research to tell us about the decision-making procedures followed by school psychologists in interpreting the complex array of data with which they work each day (Burns, 1998; de Mesquita, 1987).

There are few published validity studies of the diagnoses produced by these computerized scoring and interpretive programs. The M-MAC program, a sophisticated multitest scoring and interpretive program, had some validity studies supported by its publisher (Glutting, 1986; Hale & McDermott, 1984). However, the program was not updated when its tests were revised, and it is no longer published.

It should be noted that not every permutation of scores can be programmed into the computer. The programmer makes decisions about what are likely to be the most common patterns of scores and the most common interpretations of these patterns; a particular theory and body of research provide the guidance in making the choices. In addition, although there are some programs that attempt to include qualitative data with the quantitative, it is the psychologist's responsibility in using any program to be sure that his or her own professional judgment is always the key to appropriate interpretation of scores. The small number of validity and reliability studies makes it imperative for the psychologist to be alert to the kinds of diagnoses and interpretations being produced by the program. If the diagnoses start sounding alike, or do not discriminate fine differences in the data, there may be limits to using the program. The important point to remember is that these programs should only offer hypotheses to consider as potential interpretations of the data. Nothing in the program or printout should lead one to believe that the program is the final word on the performance of the individual.

Computer-Based Test Interpretation: Attaining "Expert" Status

A generic name for CBTI programs is "expert systems software." These programs have developed because of the research into artificial intelligence and complex computer languages that allow simulation of human thinking and decision-making processes. Expert systems software is used in the medical profession to diagnose illnesses and prescribe appropriate tests and treatment. It guides missiles, tracks satellites, and does environmental and weather studies and projections. In short, its growth in the psychology profession was to be expected. However, CBTI programs have not made optimal use of computer flexibility and power (Butcher et al., 2000). CBTI programs largely perform "look up and list out" functions. A broad range of interpretations are stored in the computer for various test indices, and the computer simply lists out the stored information for appropriate scale levels: Computers are not involved as much in decision making (Butcher et al., 2000). Although the interpretive statements contained in the reports have been shown to be comparable to practitioner-generated statements, analyses of computer-generated reports, such as one using the Exner interpretation system for the Rorschach, have indicated that the discriminant power of the CBTI for any single client was 5%, with 60% of the interpretive statements describing characteristics only of a "typical" outpatient. Thus research points to the importance of controlling the degree of generality in a report's descriptions to avoid the Barnum effect (Butcher et al., 2000). It should be noted that the practitioner-prepared reports might show similar outcomes.

One of the issues associated with expert systems/CBTI software is the issue of "Who is the expert?" A CBTI program is usually produced by a developer/programmer who represents a particular point of view or a particular publishing house or test. A tremendous amount of research-and-development time is required to produce an expert systems program that will interpret psychological data and its developers and producers expect some return on the investment of their time and money. Marketing strategies and advertisements attempt to generate as big a profit as possible. Frequently, advertisements for the program appear in mailboxes and journals long before research on the program has been published.

Psychological journals have been slow to recognize psychological computer programs as worthy of the same attention they give to traditional research. That is, validity or descriptive studies may be published, but seldom is the program itself sent out for review by peers, as is the case with traditional research. Although descriptions of various programs may appear in a "computer" review section of a journal, they are treated as book reviews—simply one person's opinion.

Disagreement exists in the measurement field on the means to determine validity in psychological applications such as CBTI and on the persons responsible for determining validity: publishers/developers or users (Cronbach, 1980; Mitchell, 1986). Moreover, the literature on evaluating the validity of CBTI programs has primarily focused on CBTI programs that interpret the MMPI and WISC III (Eyde et al., 1991; Faust & Ziskin, 1989; Guastello & Rieke, 1994; Moreland, 1985; Tsemberis, Miller, & Gartner, 1996). The APA's (1986) *Guidelines for Computer-Based Tests and Interpretations* volume focuses on CBTI personality assessment programs. CBTI programs now encompass much broader assessment areas than personality assessment, and the more complex programs interrelate and interpret more than one type of test (Sicoly, 1989). The M-MAC (McDermott & Watkins, 1985) was a good example of this latter type of CBTI program.

Moreland and Green (Moreland, 1985) established guidelines for evaluating the validity of CBTI programs. These guidelines have been challenged and expanded to incorporate issues raised by the more complex, multidimensional CBTI programs (Guastello & Rieke, 1994; McCullough, 1989; Moreland, 1985; Tsemberis et al., 1996). Many authors have sounded the alarm over the premature use of CBTI programs that have not been rigorously validated (Fowler & Butcher, 1986; Krug, 1989; Lanyon, 1984; Matarazzo, 1986; McCullough, 1985; Skinner & Pakula, 1986). Computer simulation methods were used to examine the reliability and validity of interpretations for Kaufman's "intelligent testing" approach to the WISC-III; analyses of decision reliability showed that Verbal–Performance IQ differences, factor index–score differences, and ipsative profile patterns on the WISC-III could not be interpreted with confidence (Macmann & Barnett, 1997). As reported earlier, the Sattler interpretive guidelines were also pronounced a "myth" (Macmann & Barnett, 1997).

Early computer newsletters attempted to fill the void by publishing edited and summarized software reviews that were done by several practitioners (CTASP, 1982–1989). Frequently feedback was given through these reviews that resulted in improvement of a program (CTASP, 1987). However, the payoff to the developer through status and recognition by peers, and perhaps credit toward tenure, was not the same as if the review were carried out by a recognized journal. Thus, by default, the developer and publisher can claim "expert" status in their advertising, with few to challenge them. There are specialized journals in educational, psychological, and computer technology that serve to publish information about new programs. For example, the Buros Institute publishes software reviews in the *Mental Measurement Yearbooks*. However, the majority of practitioners do not read these very technical journals regularly. There is a need for the "mainline" journals to recognize the contribution to psychology made by research and development in computerized assessment, and to accord computer program development the same status as that given to new test development or other research within the profession. Peer review of computer products would do much to encourage the development of superior products and to eliminate or warn practitioners about poor ones. The "expert" status would thus be earned through stringent peer review and not self-accorded.

Types of Scoring and Interpretive Programs

Roid and Gorsuch (1984) proposed a four-category typology that is useful in labeling and distinguishing among the various commercially available programs: (1) scoring-only, (2) descriptive, (3) clinician-modeled, and (4) clinical actuarial. Such descriptors aid in increasing user knowledge and expectations for the program, and each is discussed here.

Scoring-Only Programs

Quality and scoring features vary across programs. Some programs can score multiple protocols at one time, while others can score only one at a time. As noted earlier, time is saved with a multiscore program if more than one user scores tests with the program or if there is frequently more than one protocol to score at one time.

Some programs score more than one type of test, such as intelligence, achievement, and adaptive behavior scales, and then integrate the test results. The user may have multiple tests of each type from which to choose, or may be limited to the few that the program is designed to score. It is important to ascertain the minimum amount of information that must be entered to obtain results. For instance, some programs require that all subtest raw scores be entered in a particular domain in order to calculate the standard score and make the comparison. The program may not accept a "short-form" version of a test. At the same time, if a zero is entered for a nonadministered subtest, the resulting statistics may not be accurate. Appropriate statistics should accompany partial administrations. That is, if it is not possible to obtain a full-scale score with only a partial administration of the test, then a full-scale score should not be reported. The user should check the documentation to learn the limits and appropriate uses of the program (and the documentation should clearly state these limits). Research and statistical bases for cross-test analyses and comparisons should also be clearly explained and referenced.

Scoring and cross-test comparisons must follow psychometrically correct procedures. That is, grade equivalents should not be compared with standard scores, and grade or age equivalents should not be reported when it is inappropriate to do so (i.e., not substantiated by the test construction and standardization procedures). Printouts should be easy to read and should contain all relevant information. There should be a reminder printed that the text data must be interpreted by a professional trained to do so, and that the printout does *not* constitute a psychological report. It should also be possible to send the scoring report to either the screen, a storage devise, or the printer.

A desirable feature is the ability to transfer the data to permanent storage, preferably with the ability then to transfer it to a graphing, data management, or statistical program for further study (such as a pre–post examination, a compilation of group data, or a graphic representation for parent–teacher conferences).

The program itself should be technically sound. There should be error correction capability, ability to go both backward and forward through screen presentations, visually well-planned screen presentations, clear data entry procedures, and screen notification during data computations (not just a blank screen).

Descriptive Programs

When quantitative data are presented in descriptive programs, they are accompanied by descriptive words or sentences (such as "average," "significantly below average," or "indicates mastery of "), along with a printed profile or other graphic representation, and a list of score comparisons. Some programs with less sophisticated programming use a redundant format to report multiple-scale scores, using the same descriptors over and over. Research studies on the scaling properties of words, modifiers, adverbs, and verb phrases have empirically matched equivalent words and phrases (Hakel, 1968; Lichtenstein & Newman, 1967; Pohl, 1981). With a computer's capability of storing literally thousands of quantitative criteria and descriptive words to give the criteria meaning, sophisticated descriptive computer programs can be expected to produce a comprehensive report summarizing multiple indicators, incorporating a selection of descriptive words based on empirical studies of language, written in narrative paragraph composition, and describing statistical description of differences among subtest scores (Roid, 1986). An example from the Barclay Classroom Assessment System (Barclay, 1983) demonstrates the sophistication of such a program:

> The student is seen as having an outstanding thrust for achievement and is viewed as superior in persistence. She demonstrates impulsive, unpredictable and inconsistent behavior. She appears to be generally open and verbally expressive. In physical activities or working with her hands, she is seen as having an above average level of effort and perseverance. (Roid, 1986, p. 144)

The practitioner does need to be alert to sentences that overgeneralize and do not adequately discriminate the uniqueness of the profile. Overall accuracy may be good, but sentence-by-sentence analysis may indicate a number of irrelevant statements. As many as half of the statements in a CBTI report have been found to be irrelevant to case history information (Eyde et al., 1991). Furthermore, the length of the narratives and ratings of their overall accuracy have not shown a linear relationship. In a study of MMPI CBTI reports, the three systems with the highest accuracy ratings had relatively short or midrange narrative lengths (Eyde et al., 1991).

The profile or graph printed of the results can display in one picture an accurate representation of sophisticated statistical operations. The graphics can help to avoid overinterpretation of small differences between profile scales. Graphs can also display confidence intervals based on the standard error for each scale, percentile ranges, distributions of scores as they compare with the normal curve, and differences between each scale value and the mean of all the profile scale values as evidence of test scatter, while indicating which comparisons represent significant differences.

Clinician-Modeled Programs

Clinician-modeled CBTI programs may be programmed to reflect the interpretive process used by a renowned clinician, perhaps the person who designed the test that is being scored and interpreted. In essence, the computer attempts to simulate the thinking and decision-making logic of that particular person. A second type of clinician-modeled interpretive program is constructed from statistically analyzing groups of "expert" clinicians' opinions and building a computer model to simulate their thinking and decision making.

Clinician-modeled CBTI programs offer a consistent interpretive model—one whose theoretical and research base may be well known. For example, Dr. Lovick Miller, developer of the Louisville Behavior Checklist (Miller, 1981), participated in the development of an interpretive program by tape-recording his actual case interpretations. These were studied (Roid, 1986) to identify

decisions rules. A heuristic simulation was then designed on the computer. Through several cycles of development, results were entered into trial versions of the program and resubmitted to Dr. Miller for reinterpretation (without his awareness of which results were resubmissions). Examination of the fit between the objectively programmed rules and those actually used by Dr. Miller determined validation of the model. In addition, empirical research findings related to childhood rating scales such as the Louisville validated his interpretations. This same procedure has been shown to be highly accurate in personnel screening (Burroughs et al., 1999; Smith, 1968).

Clinical Actuarial Programs

Clinical actuarial programs developed for educational tests (McDermott, 1980, 1982, 1990) and psychological tests (Lachar, 1974) include extensive narrative descriptions and clinical hypotheses based on the clinical research findings for particular score patterns. Numerous multivariate statistical procedures that incorporate test and nontest information in the decision-making algorithms are part of these programs (Barclay, 1983; Eyde et al., 1991; McDermott & Watkins, 1985). The M-MAC (McDermott & Watkins, 1985), the Barclay Classroom Assessment System (Barclay, 1983), and several MMPI systems (Eyde et al., 1991) are examples of this technology.

Barclay (1983) incorporated 25 years of multivariate statistical studies of self-, peer, and teacher ratings of elementary students into a computerized interpretive program that provides a narrative, diagnostic, and prescriptive report on a given classroom. The computer analyzes and integrates a volume of information that would be clearly impractical to attempt by hand. For instance, sociometric choices by each class member are integrated with self-ratings, teacher ratings, and achievement scores. The resulting report can be up to 100 pages in length for a particular classroom. The narrative produced is one of high quality, as noted earlier.

Some of the most widely used clinical actuarial programs are those for the MMPI. Validity studies have found rates of accuracy of 79–90%, as rated by practitioners

(Eyde et al., 1991; Roid, 1986). However, in a study of computerized reports using adult norms to rate adolescent responses as opposed to using the adolescent norms, greater inaccuracy was found with the adult norms (20%) than the adolescent ones (10%) (Lachar, Klinge, & Grisell, 1976). Eyde and colleagues (1991) summarized their validity investigation of seven CBTI systems for the MMPI:

> Despite the large amount of empirical evidence available for the MMPI and its potential for actuarial prediction, the output of CBTI systems for the MMPI for individuals were found to vary significantly in their rated relevancy, accuracy and in their usefulness in case disposition, that is, diagnostic evaluation and disposition planning and accuracy. The quality of a CBTI system apparently depends on how the CBTI developer uses the MMPI's research literature and clinical lore. (p. 111)

The accuracy of the computerized descriptions can be assessed by a method of "replicated correlates (Lachar & Alexander, 1978; Lachar & Gdowski, 1979; Wirt, Lachar, Klinedinst, & Seat, 1977). Practitioners interview each client, then provide detailed ratings on a behavioral and symptom checklist. The clients complete the computer-scored inventory, such as the MMPI or the Personality Inventory for Children, and the scales are plotted onto a standard T-score profile. Each profile scale is divided into "elevations" or segments, such as $80T+$, $70T–79T$, $60T–69T$, $41T–59T$, and $40T$ and below (Roid, 1986). The frequency of each checklist description completed by the practitioner is then calculated for each elevation on the scale. The high-frequency checklist items then become correlates of a given scale. Findings are replicated on a new set of subjects, and only replicated checklist descriptors are used in the computerized report to describe a client's potential behavior or symptoms.

One means of increasing the validity and accuracy of computerized clinical actuarial reports is to tailor reports to a specific population, such as has been done with the 16PF in law enforcement (Dee-Burnet, Jones, & Krug, 1982) and marriage counseling (Krug, 1983) settings.

Computerized clinical actuarial programs produce detailed, objective, and authoritative-looking reports. Certainly they offer many of the advantages discussed above. The best of these programs come with extensive documentation, including detailed descriptions of the empirical bases for decision rules and narratives, and should have validity studies reported in the research literature. Most CBTI systems provide very little information on the development of the algorithm or the validity of the system. A user's guide is seldom provided (Eyde et al., 1991). It remains the practitioner's responsibility, however, to validate each computerized report for the individual client, and to make whatever changes or additions are necessary to insure accuracy. No CBTI program has been found to be 100% accurate. The practitioner must take into account all variables affecting the client, some of which may not be quantifiable for the computer (such as opportunities to succeed, environmental influences in the home or school, and individual responses to these factors).

Adapting Computerized Assessment to Meet Special Needs

Sometimes it is necessary to alter standardized test procedures in order to meet the needs of the client. In these cases, the individual's score cannot be assumed to be reliable or valid, and cannot be compared to the normative sample. The *Standards for Educational and Psychological Testing* volume (APA, 1999) requires demonstrated equivalency of modified test forms (e.g., computer-administered forms as opposed to paper–pencil forms).

Computerized assessment offers the possibility to develop alternate test forms that accommodate a variety of response formats, and also allow for automation of many administration and scoring procedures. Spoken stimulus items may be digitally recorded as well as spoken responses (Parshall, 2002). The timing of stimulus items can be systematized to provide an improved level of consistency in stimulus presentation. More efficient stimulus presentation can reduce testing time. Interactivity, as well as visual–auditory–kinesthetic stimulus and response sets, can increase attention to the task. Automated scoring and administration reduces coding and scoring errors, and results are available immediately. Computerized assessment can also reduce time spent on assessment by as much as 50% (Burroughs et al., 1999), thus reducing assessment costs as well.

Computer-administered tests may minimize any bias by the evaluator or social environment and reinforce the comparability of assessments across individuals (Haaf, Duncan, Skarakis-Doyle, Carew, & Kapitan, 1999). However, Ness and Lee (2001) found that people may read personality characteristics into a synthetic voice even when they know that it is made by a computer. When a computer voice mirrors their personalities (modulated by pitch, tone, and speed to reflect extrovert or introvert personalities), they like and may be more readily influenced by that voice. Client–computer interaction also may induce more spontaneous, less socially desirable responses than client–adult interviewer interaction (Haaf et al., 1999; Richman, Kiesler, Weisband, & Drasgow, 1999; Valla, Bergeron, & Smolla, 2000).

Automated adapted or alternative formats should be assessed for the cognitive, memory, and physical demands that may be added to the task. One example is automated scanning. Computers may present multiple stimuli by scanning through a number of selections. The scanning procedure is activated by a switch, sometimes attached to an eyelid or some body part over which the individual has some control; then a second switch (such as a second eye blink or finger tap) activates selection of the desired item (Bischof & Hedman, 1990). Compared with directly selecting an item response, automated scanning is a less efficient and a more time-consuming input method, due to the delay required for the scan to reach the preferred item (Bischof & Hedman, 1990; Haaf et al., 1999). Scanning involves a linear or sequential presentation of each item choice, increasing demands on cognitive and memory skills. The individual must locate the desired item, reject unwanted items, and attend to the cursor movement while timing the activation of the selection switch with the cursor movement to select the desired item. Responding to the scanner involves visual attention, reflective as opposed to impulsive responding, anticipation of the direction and pattern of the scan, and motivation to maintain attention. The energy re-

quired to attend and respond accurately, or to self-correct mistakes (if the software allows this), can quickly induce fatigue or escape/avoidance behavior as factors in the assessment.

Automated scoring is still in its infancy and results must be interpreted with caution. Whenever the technology is so sophisticated, the question becomes the extent to which the test becomes a measure of the neurocognitive demands of the technology (e.g. visual strength), as opposed to a measure of the task itself. Such factors as age, cognitive function, and attitudes toward or experience with computers, also may affect outcomes (Izquierdo-Porrera, Manchanda, Powell, Sorkin, & Bradham, 2002; Weber, Fritze, Schneider, Kuehner, & Maurer, 2002).

When computerized versions of standardized tests are developed, the performance demands associated with the computer use need to be investigated and reported in test manuals and published studies. Use of the modified computer version should not compromise validity. The computerized assessment must continue to measure what the original test was intended to measure, in order to establish the equivalency of the alternate format. In addition, scores obtained with the computerized assessment need to demonstrate developmental trends similar to those of the original, since developmental sensory–motor skills may affect the performance of younger children (Haaf et al., 1999). Haaf and colleagues (1999) reported on two computerized versions of the Peabody Picture Vocabulary Test—Revised (Dunn & Dunn, 1981). One version had children ages 4 years, 0 months to 8 years, 11 months use a trackball and selection button to select the correct picture from among four pictures that best represented an orally presented vocabulary word. A second version employed an automated scanning procedure in which each one of the four pictures was highlighted sequentially until the child pushed the selection button to select the correct choice. No significant differences were found for test condition or age when these two experimental conditions were compared with the results of the standardized administration to a matched randomly selected sample.

In addition, correlations between age and the computerized formats were quite similar to those obtained for the standard version, with no significant differences between these correlations (Haaf et al., 1999). For these normally developing subjects, motoric development related to computer use did not affect test performance. Anecdotal records indicated that the automated scanning version required the children to give greater attention to task for longer periods of time, resulting in verbalizations that indicated fatigue and lack of interest (Haaf et al., 1999). These children were also able to verbally indicate a desire to correct a response. Children without speech capability might require training in self correction techniques, with an unknown effect on test outcomes.

It is essential also to consider developmental progression of sensory-motor skills, including manual dexterity and hand–eye coordination, when one is considering employing computerized assessment with school-age children. The performance of children ages 5–10 years using various input devices, such as a mouse, joystick, and touch screen, has been studied (Scaife & Bond, 1991). Skills involved in the use of some computer input devices develop with increasing age. For example, older children demonstrate better control of a mouse and joystick than do younger children. By 8 years of age, mastery of the sensory–motor skills necessary for the use of a mouse or a joystick appears to be achieved, with no consistent improvement found to occur for these devices after this period. Children under 5 years of age also have difficulty with tasks that require their attention to temporal and spatial displacement, such as manipulating a mouse to effect a change on a screen; however, at the age of approximately 5 years, increased coordination skills result in improved performance (Scaife & Bond, 1991). Erdner and colleagues (1998) found that CAI increased the motivation and interest of 6-year-old children in learning to read.

Perhaps developers should stop trying to fit an old medium (paper and pencil) into a new medium that has significantly more powerful means to measure skills. That is, the QWERTY phenomenon seems to be at work here. Entirely new tasks are needed that don't tax the examinee but can still measure the construct adequately, perhaps even more efficiently and accurately. Rethinking needs to occur at the construct level, since technology allows measurement of content that is impossible to measure with paper and pencil.

Information Processing

In this information age, data are continually collected and stored. The total amount of data collected is doubling every 6 months through the use of highly automated computers with huge storage devices. Computers and other data-processing aids transform raw data into information. This information may then be used for decision making (e.g., a temperature control system for an office building may take measurements from hundreds of locations and control a vast array of heating and cooling machinery) (Moursund, 1999). Data collected from a state-mandated basic skills assessment may be used to make decisions about school district funding, individual school accountability status, individual teacher evaluation, or individual student placement or graduation. Data may be collected from multiple Internet sites around the world, analyzed and summarized by a student, and then placed in an electronic portfolio to become part of a performance assessment.

Computers can outperform people in many information-processing areas, but computers do *not* understand the human condition and what it means to be human. In other words, computers lack wisdom (Moursund, 1999). Weizenbaum (1976) agrees: "Since we do not now have any ways of making computers wise, we ought not now to give computers tasks that demand wisdom" (p. 25). Computer and information sciences have progressed from data processing to information processing, but they have not yet achieved knowledge processing. Through study and thinking activities, students transform information into personal knowledge. Students gain wisdom by integrating and then maturely analyzing their accumulated knowledge. Data, information, knowledge and wisdom form a continuous scale, with wisdom and data at the endpoints of this scale but not necessarily closely related.

Therefore, educators need to be careful about assessing and equating a student's utilization of good search strategies with acquired knowledge. Acquiring information has become easier with using search engines on the Internet. Assessment of a student's knowledge base must include an evaluation of how they have integrated that acquired information into their knowledge base. Students need to be assessed in environments in which they routinely use computers' information-processing capabilities to solve complex problems and accomplish difficult, challenging tasks. Assessment systems are needed that encourage students to move beyond just acquiring knowledge and into gaining wisdom (Moursund, 1999). Concept mapping or cognitive mapping is an innovative computerized assessment tool that helps to meet this need.

Concept Mapping

One electronic means for students to organize and communicate what they know in a visually rich environment is "concept mapping"—a process for representing concepts and their relationship in graphic form (Anderson-Inman & Ditson, 1999). Analogous to storyboards, flowcharts, or other diagramming techniques, concept maps are hierarchical representations of concepts and propositions that reflect both the content and the structure of a person's knowledge in a given domain. Concept maps provide a means to externalize or make visible the understanding of a concept and its relationship to other concepts. The software program Inspiration (Inspiration Software, 1988–1997) supports the production of electronic outlines as well as electronic diagrams, maps, and flowcharts. Anderson-Inman and colleagues have developed the *Concept-Mapping Companion, Second Edition* (Ditson, Kessler, & Anderson-Inman, 2001) to utilize electronic concept mapping as an assessment tool.

A unique form of curriculum-based assessment, concept maps visually portray the changes in an individual's understanding of a conceptual field over time. Conceptual formation tracking has three steps: (1) construct an initial map; (2) provide learning opportunities; and (3) refine the map using new concepts.

First, an initial map is constructed around a set of terms provided by the teacher or as a response to a more open-ended prompt, such as "Make a concept map showing what you know about x." The second and third steps are part of an iterative process during which the teacher provides instruction and students then revise their concept maps. By comparing this map with previous ones, the teacher or evaluator can track conceptual growth over time and assess the extent to which instruction is having the desired effect on student learning (Anderson-Inman & Ditson, 1999). Typically, the concept maps become much more complex with increasing knowledge making analysis very difficult and time-consuming. The *Concept-Mapping Companion* (Ditson, Kessler, and Anderson-Inman, 2001) electronically summarizes information about a given map (e.g., the number of symbols, links, and cross-links) and provides a list of the propositions and examples included in the map. A Likert scale allows the teacher or evaluator to record the accuracy of each proposition or example. Tests of interrater reliability show a high level of agreement (Kessler, Anderson-Inman, Ditson, & Morris, 1996).

Concept-mapping assessment provides an alternative approach to assessing students who have not responded well to the heavily text-centered world of school. Students who are good at concept mapping often excel on tests of spatial skills (Zeitz & Anderson-Inman, 1993) and might be described as learning best by visual means. The images used in concept mapping minimize the need for text and help students personalize their maps in ways that promote long-term retention of information (Anderson-Inman & Ditson, 1999; Anderson-Inman, Knox-Quinn, & Horney, 1996).

Computer-Administered Interviews

Garb (2000) pointed out that "using computers to make judgments and decisions in personality assessment can lead to dramatically improved reliability, a decrease in the occurrence of biases, and an overall increase in validity and reliability" (p. 36). Computerized interviews or questionnaires assist in identifying attitudes, beliefs, problem behavior areas, or etiological factors. They are found most often in university counseling centers, child guidance centers, and outpatient mental health centers. Computerized interviews usually involve an interactive program in which questions or stimuli are presented by a computer to an individual seated in front of the computer. The individual responds to the stimuli on a keyboard (sometimes specially altered with a yes–no or multiple-choice format), and subsequent stimuli are presented as a function of each individual's responses (Clavelle & Butcher, 1977; Farrell, 1999a, 1999b; Heppner, Kivlighan, & Good, 1994; McCullough, 1985).

The computerized interviewing system involves an interactive decision tree with paths selected according to the responses of the individual. For example, an initial presentation on the screen might be a listing of several different problem areas. If the individual selects "anxiety in the presence of other people" as one problem area, the next stimulus might be a list of social situations in which the subject might experience anxiety. If the subject indicates feeling anxious "around strangers," then the next presentation might inquire whether anxiety occurs with males and/or females or with large or small groups. This process continues for each problem area. Following the completion of the intake interview, the computer furnishes the clinician with a summary of problem areas, hypothesized causative factors, potential treatment strategies, hypothesized diagnostic categories, and other information of interest (Farrell, 1999a; Haynes & Wilson, 1979). Sophisticated systems accessible via the Internet or on computer servers allow online assessments, summary reports, treatment planning, and client tracking and verified follow-up reports (Farrell, 1999a, 1999b; Psychological Corporation, 1998).

In light of the explosive growth of telecommunications technology being used to solicit information, social-desirability-based distortion of responses to computerized administration of noncognitive instruments such as psychological inventories, attitude scales, or behavioral interviews was examined in a meta-analytic study (Richman et al., 1999). A near-zero overall mean effect size was obtained for computer versus paper-and-pencil questionnaires. When individuals are alone and can respond freely (i.e., backtrack to previous answers), there is less social-desirability-based distortion, as

respondents may be more comfortable and less wary of giving socially undesirable answers. Previously reported mixed or conflicting findings about the effect of the computer on socially desirable responding (Erdman, Klein, & Greist, 1985) appear to be explained in more recent studies that have employed more flexible interview systems, by moderating factors such as whether respondents are tested alone or in the presence of others, whether their responses are anonymous or personally identifiable, and whether they can backtrack (Richman et al., 1999). It should be noted that these studies were conducted primarily with adults, although some included adolescents.

Clients report that they feel less embarrassed or uncomfortable with a computerized interview than with a face-to-face therapist interviewer. Studies have shown that clients tend to be more honest (more willing to divulge socially undesirable behavior) when reporting sensitive behaviors (e.g., drug abuse, sexual activity) to a computer than when they are face to face with a human therapist. The type of assessment may affect the accuracy of the computerized interview. For instance, Richman and colleagues (1999) reported that "respondents displayed relatively less social desirability distortion on the computer when the measure was a behavioral measure, symptom checklist or an attitude scale (predicted effect size = −0.51) and more social desirability distortion in the computer interview when the measure was a personality scale (predicted effect size = −0.73)" (p. 767). However, client comfort with computerized interviews over face-to-face interviews may be challenged as more sophisticated computerized interviewing systems incorporate more "human" characteristics, such as voice-based interviews and increased interactivity (Naas, Moon, & Carney, 1999; Nass & Lee, 2001). Response bias may be introduced into computerized interviews by the choice of male or female voices, the personality ascribed to the voice, or by other social cues inherent in the programming.

A usual limitation of computerized interviews is the necessary requirement of being able to read text. A unique pictorial interview for 6- to 11-year-old children, the Interactive Dominic Questionnaire (Valla et al., 2000) is based on the *Diagnostic and Statistical Manual of Mental Disorders,* fourth edition (DSM-IV); it is an interactive cartoon on CD-ROM illustrating 90 situations, with a running time of 15 minutes. A voiceover describing a symptom asks a child how he or she would react. Children respond by clicking on "yes" or "no" boxes, thus disclosing their own reactions when they are faced with these situations. Each child's choices are recorded and automatically analyzed by the computer (Valla et al., 2000). This computerized interview screens for the most frequent DSM-IV mental health problems in young children such as ADHD, oppositional defiant disorder, conduct disorder, major depressive disorder, schizoaffective disorder, generalized anxiety disorder, and specific phobia. The interview blends pictures, sound and child-computer interaction in situations that represent children from different backgrounds, ethnicity, and genders.

Several benefits of computerized interviews have been identified (Farrell, 1999b; Haynes & Wilson, 1979; Powell, Wilson, & Hasty, 2002). They provide the following:

1. Substantial savings in professional time when intake interviews are an integral part of the assessment protocol.
2. Standardized information on a broad range of topics (e.g., physical complaints, mood, suicidal thoughts and behavior, hostility/anger, assertiveness, thought problems, sexual thoughts and behavior, substance use, work/career concerns, social support, independent recall of events, and other problem areas such as social relationships, sleep, life tasks).
3. Useful data to plan and monitor treatment design and implementation, and to evaluate treatment outcomes and effectiveness.
4. Reduced error variance associated with clinical interviews, since the method of presentation is constant across individuals, and variance attributed to interviewer fatigue, nonverbal cues, reactions to individuals' responses, or interviewer bias is reduced.
5. Detailed summary findings through computer analysis.
6. Useful, nonbiased, accurate, data for forensic purposes with young children

that does not interfere with independent recall of events.

As with any assessment procedure, the validity and reliability of the system and the data collected need to be examined. This can be accomplished through internal reliability checks during assessment, as well as by comparing derived data with data from other measurement instruments. Published reviews of validity studies on some programs are available (Farrell, 1999a, 1999b; Heppner et al., 1994; McCullough, 1985; Powell et al., 2002).

Limitations of computerized interview programs include these:

1. In crisis situations, the system may have to be abbreviated or bypassed; the determination of a crisis situation must be made by an intake interviewer.
2. System use is usually limited to individuals with "normal" cognitive functioning, or must be modified, since individuals with lower levels of cognitive functioning (e.g. young children, individuals with mental retardation, or long-term residents of psychiatric facilities) will experience difficulty reading written questions and/or responding according to directions.
3. Programs need to be flexible enough to handle the myriad of problems presented by clients without being overwhelming to either clients or clinicians.
4. Developer/programmer conceptual bias must be determined through studying the types of elicited responses that are constrained by the stimuli presented. System bias may be subtle—difficult to detect and difficult to overcome.

ISSUES IN COMPUTERIZED ASSESSMENT

As computerized assessment procedures become more prevalent, current and potential issues regarding microcomputer administration of psychological tests need to be addressed (Duthie, 1984; Garb, 2000; McCullough, 1985). These issues include validity, reliability, and equity; the response set of individuals to computers and resulting contamination of test results; cognitive-processing differences between paper-and-pencil and computerized assessment; screen format and equipment variability; control of testing materials and procedures; and the practicality of computerized assessment.

Validity, Reliability, and Equity

Validity and reliability of assessment results are critical issues for computerized assessment. Much research has focused on comparing paper-and-pencil versions of tests with their computerized counterparts (Bugbee, 1996; Herl, Chung, & Schacter, 1999; Mazzeo & Harvey, 1988; Tseng, Tiplady, Macleod, & Wright, 1998). In contrast to the traditional conceptualization of validity (e.g., content, criterion, construct), validity may be viewed as a unitary concept involving several types of evidence, including consequential validity and differential prediction (Mazzeo & Harvey, 1988; Messick, 1989). Consequential validity suggests that the consequences of test use as well as the implications of test interpretation must be considered. Differential prediction suggests the possibility that different prediction equations may be obtained for different groups (Sutton, 1997).

The Standards for Educational and Psychological Testing volume (APA, 1999) (specifically Standards 3.5 and 3.10) require test developers to address possible inequities in relation to cultural backgrounds and prior experiences, and to "ensure that intended inferences from test scores are equally valid for members of different groups of test takers" (p. 44). When developers are comparing the equivalence of scores on computerized versions of tests versus paper–pencil versions, the APA *Guidelines for Computer Tests and Interpretations* (1986) volume suggests:

> Scores from conventional and computer administrations may be considered equivalent when (a) rank orders of scores tested in alternative modes closely approximate each other, and (b) means, dispersions, and shapes of the score distributions are approximately the same or have been made approximately the same by rescaling the scores from the computer mode. (pp. 13–14)

Critics are concerned that inequities in paper–pencil assessment will be perpetuated in computerized assessment (Sutton, 1997). The APA (1986) approach focuses on group rather than individual differences, ignoring the fact that small group differences may have large individual implications, and it assumes that the status quo is an acceptable baseline. Sutton (1997) argues that computerized assessment research should "search for ways in which the computer testing technology could be used to improve testing by reducing inequities rather than replicating existing inequities. For example, the fewer number of items needed on adaptive tests means that the average time allowed per item can be lengthened." (p. 8). This could be useful to certain subgroups such as African Americans, Mexican Americans, and Puerto Ricans who have been shown to take more time to complete tests (Llabre & Froman, 1987).

Value judgments confound these two views of validity: equivalence versus minimizing group inequalities. With high-stakes testing such as state-mandated graduation examinations or college entrance examinations, the issues of whether a student's score is influenced by the mode of testing, or whether to minimize traditional inequities related to the artifacts in conventional testing, become important. Empirical evidence suggests that several characteristics of test takers, tests, and testing conditions affect outcomes of computerized assessment (Sutton, 1997). These characteristics are listed in Table 26.2.

TABLE 26.2. Characteristics That Affect Computerized Assessment Outcomes

Test takers	Tests	Testing conditions
Prior experience with computers	Time allotted to take the test	Setting of the computers
Attitudes toward computerized testing	Format and style of questions	Scheduling
Expectancies		Cost
Test-taking strategies		Immediate feedback

Test takers who are poor, members of ethnic minorities or females tend to have less experience with computers. A tutorial may be provided in high-stakes testing but may not make computer use automatic nor improve performance (Maki & Maki, 2002). Research is inconsistent on the effects of lack of experience (Sutton, 1997), perhaps due to the kind of tutorial, the range of experience present, or the design and complexity of the software. The more experience individuals have with computers, the more positive their attitudes toward computers at all levels of education (Sutton, 1991; Wu & Morgan, 1989). However, concomitant negative attitudes toward high-stakes testing may confound this finding.

Test takers' expectancies related to testing may be challenged by computer-adaptive testing where item difficulty is controlled. Low-achieving students may not be as discouraged because they do not encounter more difficult items, whereas high-achieving students with low assessments of their own ability might choose to answer questions wrong in order to get easier questions. For some high-achieving students used to performing well on standardized tests, computer-adapted testing may seem harder, as they won't encounter "easy" items. However, some research with a school district-wide computerized assessment system has found that these fears may be unfounded, as both teachers and students responded positively to adaptive testing (Kingsbury & Houser, 1999).

Traditional test-taking strategies have emphasized skipping or omitting items deemed difficult and returning to them later, then rechecking items as time permits. This strategy is not possible with computer-adapted testing because items may not be skipped and it is not possible to check items again once they are finished. New adaptive testing strategies are being promoted by testing companies, especially through Web sites, but access to this training is not universal.

Studies on the effects of varying test time limits are inconsistent, perhaps due to lack of control for ability levels of different groups and for small differences in the time allowed (Llabre & Froman, 1987). However, unlimited time to complete assessment resulted in no significant differences between European American and Hispanic

American groups. Unlimited time may be conceptually very different from "more" time for a test taker (Llabre, 1991).

Computerized assessment allows for a variety of formats, including highlighting or moving information, checking boxes in a table, marking a scale, completing a graph, choosing more than one answer, pointing and clicking on a map or anatomy diagram, creating a portfolio, or writing an essay. Gender and ethnic group differences have been found in various formats (Ben-Shakhar & Sinai, 1991; Boyken, 1982; Fletcher-Flinn, 1995; Liao, 1999; Slakter, Koehler, Hampton, & Grennell, 1971). For example, high task variability resulted in significantly higher scores for low-income African American students, but had no effect on low- and middle-income European American students (Allen & Boyken, 1991).

The settings in which computerized assessment occurs may influence anxiety or attitudes and may interact with gender, self-expectancies, and computer experience to affect computerized assessment performance (Sutton, 1997). High-stakes testing may occur in a public setting such as a computer lab, or in a semi-private setting such as in a workstation in a computer lab. For example, working in the presence of others did not affect men or women with high experience but women with low experience expressed more anxiety and performed less well while males with low experience showed the opposite effect (Robinson-Staveley & Cooper, 1990).

Computerized assessment may have negative, unintended, unpredictable consequences or unforeseen social consequences (Madaus, 1994). Empirical research is needed on the role and effects of differential experience, time limits, expectancies, adaptive test strategies, the public nature of computers in testing sites, and immediate feedback, on the validity and reliability of test results (Sutton, 1997)—especially in regards to high-stakes testing, where the decisions that are based on the test data could be life-changing.

Equivalency of Paper–Pencil versus Computerized Assessment

As computerized assessment procedures became more prevalent starting in the 1980s, professional organizations such as the American Psychological Association, American Educational Research Association, and the National Council of Measurement in Education created guidelines for developers and users of computer-based tests (APA, 1985, 1986, 1999). The APA guidelines indicate that validation studies must be performed by computer test developers to verify the equivalency to paper-and-pencil forms, particularly if norms from the paper-and-pencil version are to be used for the computerized assessments. Bugbee (1996) concluded that computer-based and paper-and-pencil assessments can be equivalent, but the test developer must take responsibility for conducting studies to show their equivalency.

Since the publication of the 1986 APA guidelines, several major studies have investigated the relationship between computerized assessments and paper-and-pencil assessments (Bugbee, 1996; Bunderson, Inouye, & Olsen, 1989; Mazzeo & Harvey, 1988; Wise & Plake, 1989). Mazzeo and Harvey (1988) concluded that computerized assessments are different from paper-and-pencil assessments in the following ways: (1) Omitted questions are not the same between the computerized and paper-and-pencil versions of a test; (2) test scores from computer-based personality inventories may yield lower test scores than paper-and-pencil measures; (3) speeded tests do not yield similar results between computerized and paper-and-pencil tests; (4) the enhanced visual interface along with audio–visual integration in computer-based assessments may make scores not equivalent with paper-and-pencil versions; and (5) tests with reading passages may be more difficult on computers.

The differences in omitted questions between computer-based and paper-and-pencil assessments were evaluated by Wise and Plake (1989), These authors suggested that computer-based assessments should (1) let test takers skip questions and answer them later, which is possible in most paper-and-pencil tests; (2) let users review previously answered questions to check for accuracy; and (3) allow users to change answers. In widely used high-stakes computer-adapted tests such as the GRE, however, it is not possible to carry out any of these three suggestions.

Several studies have examined the role anxiety plays in computer-based assessments as compared to paper-and-pencil assessments (Bernt, Bugbee, & Arceo, 1990; Ward, Hopper, & Hannafin, 1989; Wise & Plake, 1989). Bugbee (1996) pointed out that anxiety related to the use of computers tends to be a random variable across people, so any effects that anxiety could have on computer-based assessments would be just one portion of the error variance.

Response Set to Computers and Contamination of Test Results

There appears to be a mystique associated with computers—a projection of awe and power. Such characters as HAL in *2001—A Space Odyssey*, R2D2 in *Star Wars*, and TWIKKI in *Flash Gordon* are examples of emerging cultural computer archetypes for both children and adults (Duthie, 1984). In addition, some individuals may have had bad experiences with computers, such as being billed incorrectly, displaced from a job, or being told quite often and forcefully not to touch computer equipment available in a classroom or lab without permission and supervision. Some individuals may view the computer as an impersonal, powerful, inhuman beast, to the point where they fear it. In 1982, Mello estimated that 30% of office workers dreaded using computers. He classified the 5% of this group who showed severe, clinically significant phobic behaviors as "cyberphobes." However, over 20 years later, children and adolescents now experience computer technology as an integral and normal part of their lives; they readily use VCRs, video games, calculators, and personal computers, and technology is inextricably linked to their acquisition of knowledge. More recent studies have not found computer anxiety or use of Web-based assessment to be a significant factor in test results (Davis, 1999; Maki & Maki, 2002).

There are also powerful and subtle cultural and gender biases that may influence performance on computerized tests (Sutton, 1991, 1997). Anderson and colleagues (1984) found cultural and regional differences reflected in the greater prevalence and integration of computers into the curricula in wealthier, larger, urban school districts in the central, northern, and western parts of the United States. The children in these districts had more experience with computers, as would children with computers at home. One study found that past computer experience accounted for a significant amount of variance on an arithmetic reasoning test administered both as a paper-and-pencil test and as a computerized test (Lee, 1986). Experience with computers continues to be a factor to consider in using computerized assessment (Sutton, 1997).

Gender bias is documented by the fact that boys outnumber girls nearly 2:1 in enrollment in computer education classes and camps (Anderson et al., 1984). Male self-selection and female default in using computers have led to the computer center's becoming "male turf"—as socially inappropriate to girls as the boys' locker room (Lockheed & Frakt, 1984). Equity is a major issue in computer education (Anderson et al., 1984; Lipkin, 1984; Lockheed & Frakt, 1984; Miura & Hess, 1984; Schubert & Bakke, 1984) and should be considered as an influence on performance on computerized tests (Sutton, 1997).

Research on computer-assisted instruction has provided information on children's attitudes toward computers—an important variable in computerized assessment. Generally, children have shown quite positive attitudes toward computers and computer activities, usually expressing no fear and much enthusiasm about the technology (Lockheed & Frakt, 1984). However, attitudes may be less positive among girls and younger children, especially on the dimensions of ease of use and quality of the computer ("smart–stupid," "special–ordinary") (Williams, Coulombe, & Lievrouw, 1983). Gender differences tend to be strongest among adolescents in computer activity preferences. Girls prefer word processing, data bases, and graphics, while boys express more interest in further training in computer programming (Lockheed & Frakt, 1984). Most studies also have found increases in favorable attitudes toward computers after use (Lieberman, 1985; Romanczyk, 1986); this provides a strong argument for allowing adjustment and instruction time on the computer before using it as an assessment device (Sutton, 1997). Locating microcomputers in computer labs

and learning to program apparently contribute to increases in enthusiasm and positive attitudes toward computers (Lieberman, 1985). Use of the Internet and hypermedia programs has also been shown to increase positive attitudes toward computers (Sutton, 1997).

Cognitive Processing Differences

Three differences between paper-and-pencil administrations and computer administrations suggest that they may be separate cognitive tasks: (1) response time, (2) fatigue, and (3) presentation mode. It takes longer to take a paper-and-pencil test and requires some thought and writing skill to record the answer on the answer sheet. However, this task requirement may also allow some time for reflection upon the answer chosen. The computer requires only the pressing of a key—a response that can occur so quickly, it appears as a reflex response. Taking a test on a computer becomes a less complex task than a paper-and-pencil test. The response given so quickly may not represent the client's "best" response, merely the first one. Given this fact, it is possible that answers may be less thought out and more reflexive in nature. It is possible that different parts of the brain are involved in responding to the processing questions presented on a computer monitor.

Since tests administered on a computer can take less time (e.g., 30 minutes for a computerized MMPI as compared with more than an hour for the paper-and-pencil version), mental fatigue or lack thereof may affect test results to an unknown degree. Some of the variance in paper-and-pencil versus computerized results may be due to the computerized version's taking less time and effort to complete (leading to less mental fatigue) or due to the outcome's reflecting more impulsive "first-response" answers (because of the increased ease of responding). Some degree of the variance may also be due to different cognitive organization of the information presented under computerized conditions.

Many of the arguments against computerized assessment were made in the 1980s, when computer technology was in its infancy and the majority of people were not exposed to computers. As noted earlier, children have since grown up with Nintendos, Play Stations, and personal computers. Computers have been integrated into the majority of schools across the country. Children are taught in school how to "surf the Internet" to find information. Computers have become inextricably linked with knowledge acquisition. Perhaps, as noted earlier, if it is knowledge that is being assessed, it should be assessed more frequently in the mode in which it is acquired.

The visual and verbal content of computerized assessment may include more emphasis on hemispheric functions. The outcomes of the computerized assessment thus may be influenced by how the learning style of the individual accommodates the presentation mode. Computerized assessment can take advantage of the graphics capabilities of the computer. Verbal information can be presented in a variety of formats, such as imitating text on a book page, or (more likely) presenting it in a visually more pleasing manner with graphics, color, or different screen placements. The text may scroll out of sight. The individual may or may not have control over timing—that is, determining how long the text remains on the screen. These are variables that may also affect the cognitive processing of information and affect assessment outcomes.

Screen Format and Equipment Differences

Standardized formats are the rule with paper-and-pencil tests, but computerized tests often lack a standard presentation format. Some computers have 40, 64, or 80 characters printed on the video screen in a variety of type sizes, fonts, and presentation modes. Some are more readable than others. Some feature color displays with varying color backgrounds and type. Some are black and white, some green and black, some amber. Contrast varies with color and monitor settings. Research has shown color to be a powerful manipulator of attention, memory, and understanding (Durrett & Trezona, 1982); thus screen format or color may influence performance.

The presentation effect of the hardware (equipment) may be intimidating (large and businesslike), or nonstandard (a keyboard with large numbers only, with "stop" and "go" buttons in red and green), or confus-

ing (a keyboard with 92 keys, including multiple-function keys). The monitor may have a 17-inch screen or a 12-inch one. The monitor may reflect a glare from open windows, may be poorly lighted, or may be impossible to see at certain angles. There is a lack of standardization across and within computer systems, leading to a lack of standardization in presentation of the tests across individuals, and thus to serious reliability and validity problems.

Control of Testing Materials

A marketing strategy employed by many publishers involves a metered disk or chip that allows the administration of a certain number of tests or analyses (the number paid for). This is a form of copyright protection intended to insure that the test copyright holder gets a royalty, as if a consumable answer sheet were paid for and used up. The cost per computer-administered test is usually considerably more than that for its paper-and-pencil alternative—from $2 to $20 per administration, and more if an analysis is provided. These high costs may provide the motivation for unscrupulous individuals to break the copyright protection and have unlimited use of the software. Once this protection is broken, the program can be disseminated to unauthorized or untrained individuals, placing it totally out of the control of the psychology profession.

Evans (1979) addresses this issue in *The Micro Millennium*: "The vulnerability of the professions is tied up with their special strength—the fact that they act as exclusive repositories and disseminators of specialist knowledge" (p. 111). He expects the erosion of power of the established professions to be a striking feature of the "computer revolution." Professionals guard their secrets closely, Evans asserts,

> insisting on careful scrutiny and rigorous training of individuals who wish to enter their ranks. But this state of privilege can only persist as long as the special data and the rules for its administration remain inaccessible to the general public. Once the barriers which stand between the average person and this knowledge dissolve, the significance of the profession dwindles and power and status of its members shrink. Characteristically, the services that the profession originally offered

then become available at a very low cost. . . . In the final analysis, the raw material of a modern profession is nothing more than information, and the professional expertise lies simply in knowing the rules for handling or processing it." (p. 112)

An excellent example to illustrate this issue of professional control is the computerized intake interview, now commonly used in hospitals, psychiatric clinics, and doctors' offices. To the layperson, the questions a psychologist asks come from accumulated knowledge and insight, and give the impression that the psychologist is proceeding toward a goal with an understanding of the client's needs. On the basis of the interview, the psychologist may decide to gather more information through tests (computerized or otherwise), or may offer a preliminary hypothesis or diagnosis—a decision that will then lead to recommendations for interventions or remediation strategies. Although this may appear impressive to the layperson (especially if the hypothesis and recommendations "make sense"), in most cases the interview questions have become more or less formalized, the hypotheses generated fall into a relatively limited field of choices, and the recommendations follow automatically from the choice of hypotheses. As noted earlier, research has shown that people are more willing to confide in a computer than in a professional. There are perhaps thousands of "tests" and "psychological consultants" on the Web, varying markedly in quality. Protection of the public from unscrupulous or unqualified individuals giving inaccurate or questionable opinions or information is a major concern.

The point is that computer use may change the locus of control of some of the functions psychologists have been trained to perform. A computer may be able to carry out the routine and time-consuming clerical and record-keeping tasks. In doing so, it may free psychologists to have more meaningful contact with clients—to focus on decision making and interactions that require a human touch. Depending upon the nature of an individual psychologist's practice, this change in control of information processing may or may not be threatening, and may have as yet unknown effects upon the client–psychologist relationship. It will remove the psychologist one step from the data-gathering process. It is unclear what effect this would have on psychologists' work performance and the kind of decisions, interactions, and relationships formed with clients. Some psychologists have sounded warnings and encouraged fellow professionals to consciously consider the positive and negative ramifications of this change (Garb, 2000; Maddox, 1986; McCullough, 1990).

Practicality of Computer-Administered Tests

In a high-volume clinic, a centralized assessment center in a school district, a computer lab with a readily accessible multiple-terminal online server, an Internet or intranet network, or a dedicated psychological assessment computer system, computer-administered psychological tests may be practical. That is, they may be practical with adequate equipment and technical support if the number and type of computerized tests available are adequate to meet the evaluation needs of the setting. Kingsbury and Houser (1999) note that an increasing number of school districts have developed computer-adapted tests for the following purposes:

- Entry testing for new students transferring into or within the district.
- Diagnostic testing to identify areas of academic difficulty.
- Certification testing to verify that criteria to receive a diploma are met.
- Candidacy testing to determine a student's eligibility for services, such as entry into programs for talented and gifted students.
- Growth assessment to track academic progress in reading, mathematics, or science on a regular basis.
- Pretesting and posttesting before and after treatment or instruction.

Computer-based testing such as Kingsbury and Houser (1999) describe has the advantages of convenience in scheduling, increased testing opportunities, automated data collection, and prompt score reporting. In a setting with limited numbers of multipurpose computers (i.e., the computers are used for word processing, data management/record keeping, test scoring/analysis, statistics, and financial management), the use of this equipment for test administration may have to be prioritized in competition with other users. In addition, test data retrieval and storage are greatly facilitated with Internet or intranet accessibility, as opposed to the hazards and inefficiencies of disk-based retrieval and storage (Kingsbury & Houser, 1999), though security and data retention issues are raised.

Furthermore, for psychologists who traditionally go into a child's environment—the school building—to administer assessment batteries, computer equipment may vary from building to building. Availability and location may vary from no computers to a computer in every classroom to a computer lab that is never empty. Even with a laptop computer or PDA, finding a private location with ideal testing conditions (the principal's office does not qualify) often enters the realm of the impossible. Just finding a private place to administer the traditional battery sometimes enters that same realm. Portable computers offer a possible solution. Maintaining a constant power supply, either through careful attention to battery power or through finding a space with electrical outlets conveniently nearby, will be important in this case. Computerized assessment software choices may be dictated by the kind of equipment available, not necessarily by what was needed or desired.

Obviously, the use of computerized testing software in the same manner in which we have traditionally used paper-and-pencil tests presents some major problems. Perhaps it is time to consider different ways of meeting evaluation objectives. Instead of trying to figure out how to hook the jet up to the oxcart to reach evaluation goals, perhaps it is time to reevaluate whether we need the oxcart at all to get where we are going (to paraphrase Papert, 1980). Perhaps the question to ask regarding the practicality of computerized tests is this: Which or what kinds of computerized tests are practical and meet needs not now adequately served by paper-and-pencil tests? Do computerized tests add dimensions to assessment information that cannot be obtained from paper-and-pencil tests? Can this unique information be obtained in schools and clinic settings through already existing databases or through Internet or intranet communication networks?

Perhaps a practicality issue that really needs to be addressed before tremendous amounts of money and time are spent in developing computerized assessment programs that imitate paper-and-pencil tests is whether practices are being preserved that have no rational basis beyond their historical roots in an earlier period of technological and theoretical development. What is the need for IQ or standardized achievement tests if records of a child's progress are being updated regularly by a computer as part of a CAI or CAT program? What does the evaluation process add to this base of information, whether it is administered via computer or via paper and pencil?

To answer these questions, it is necessary to explore in more detail some of the options and research regarding computerized testing. There are some tasks that a computer appears better able to assess than a paper-and-pencil task. These include the skills required to use computer equipment, such as those sonar technicians must use as they make decisions based on radar- and computer-provided information (Cory, 1977). Cory (1977) found that short-term memory, sequential reasoning, interpreting visual displays, and working under distractions were measured with significantly more predictive validity on a computerized test than on a paper-and-pencil test. These were computerized tests developed specifically to measure the skills required in this specialized profession.

Computerized tests may also assess reading skills from a different perspective (Erdner et al., 1998; Freebody & Cooksey, 1985; Lally, 1981; McCullough, 1995). In a preliminary study of three children, Freebody and Cooksey (1985) studied simple timed responses to sets of words and word-like nonsense items, then accurately estimated vocabulary knowledge through word frequency and response time. Other studies have shown that individuals with larger amounts of domain-specific knowledge are able to access and organize that information faster in appropriate situations (Anderson, 1982; Feltovich, 1981; Neves & Anderson, 1981). The ability of the computer to track, time, and record responses opens up a means of assessment that focuses on the cognitive processes, not the outcome product. For example, in a simulation of a typical school psychology decision-making situation (a referral of a third-grade male who doesn't complete his assignments), experienced practitioners responded more quickly and with fewer, more relevant pieces of information than did inexperienced students (de Mesquita, 1987). Analysis of the thinking process is possible immediately with the computer record. Training in hypothesis generation and selection of relevant assessment questions and information can follow, and can be evaluated again and again with other simulations.

The implications of this research are that computerized assessment may be practical in evaluating factors related to the learning *process,* instead of focusing on outcome data as traditional paper-and-pencil tests must. Focusing on outcome data alone may not provide the insight necessary to detect inefficient thinking patterns or illogical choice of options. Individuals may arrive at the same outcome by following quite different cognitive and decision-making processes. The computer can record and represent the process underlying the created product, as is seen in the concept-mapping representations (Anderson-Inman & Ditson, 1999; 2001). It can make explicit the series of steps and missteps that has led to the creation of a particular object or result. The user leaves an audit trail of historical information that can be used to communicate, analyze, imitate, train, and clarify how an outcome occurred. It communicates *how* a result was achieved. Computerized assessment is the only vehicle that allows direct study of cognitive decision processes. The practicality of this information is only beginning to be recognized by researchers (Brown, 1985).

CHANGING INFORMATION MANAGEMENT PARADIGMS

Naturalistic Inquiry and Chaos Theory

Conducting a good assessment or evaluation requires doing four components well:

1. Asking good questions.
2. Observing and listening carefully.
3. Interpreting information to those who need it.

4. Propelling others to action by sharing information in simple, understandable terms.

Computerized assessment offers possibilities to improve each of these components, even to move to different paradigms of assessment. Via personal digital assistants, notebook computers, and/or networked or Web-based databases, data acquisition, processing, and output may provide immediate day-to-day or hour-to-hour trend analysis of a variety of activities (e.g., curriculum-based assessment, consultation activity, behavioral monitoring, or learning outcomes).

The QWERTY phenomenon (i.e., doing things the way they have always been done, only faster and more efficiently) is far too prevalent in computerized assessment practice. Assessment has a long history, with the scientific mode of inquiry as its foundation—that is, formulating hypotheses to answer questions, testing the hypotheses by collecting data in experimental or quasi-experimental conditions that break the problem into small parts, and analyzing the results (Guba & Lincoln, 1989). One paradigm, "naturalistic inquiry," focuses on the exploration, discovery, and understanding of natural processes and phenomena, while "chaos theory" emphasizes the prediction of idiographic, nonlinear, dynamic behavior (Heiby, 1995; Lincoln & Guba, 1985). In naturalistic inquiry, the investigator becomes part of the process and looks for patterns and relationships within all the interconnected parts of the problem. With chaos theory, measures of an individual are collected over a period of time (time series assessment); then vectors (often the simultaneous impact of several forces) are combined with a bifurcation point (a time in which there is some crucial change in behavior). Using mathematical models and emphasizing the interconnectedness of events, chaos theory may help to make sense of unstable and difficult-to-predict human behavior (Groth-Marnat, 2000).

Technology facilitates naturalistic or chaos-theory-based inquiry by being able to examine a large number of variables in complex ways. Large amounts of data may be collected and stored, while sophisticated tools analyze the complex relationships encountered. These technology tools may be called "decision support systems," "executive information systems," "online analytic processing," "structured query languages," "concept or knowledge mapping," "data mining," or "data warehousing" (Hanson, 1997). Concept mapping was discussed earlier; we describe some of the others below.

Decision Support Systems

Using decision support systems, decision makers "point and click" their way through complex data, answering one set of questions and immediately raising altogether new sets of questions in an interactive process of exploration, discovery, and understanding of information. Assessment specialists using these systems must be comfortable with the information systems and teach others how to use these technology-based tools to formulate better questions, because the nature of the information acquired is changed.

Touch-tone telephones may be used to collect both digital and voice data; to ask questions that require pressing a key to answer; or to record answers to open-ended questions via voice mail, then branch to other questions based on the response given. The technology analyzes all this data and provides immediate or next-day feedback. Timeliness and low cost aside, this technology may assist an individual with special needs for whom conventional tests are inappropriate or threatening, but who can and does handle touch-tone responding over a telephone.

Video links, as well as Internet- or Web-based databases, provide interactive connections. Numerous Web-based tests are available now, with the developer collecting data from each individual who takes the test. Sample representativeness becomes an issue, but may be controlled by collecting demographic information from each user or by controlling access to the site (Davis, 1999). Sample bias may be present, because those who are uncomfortable using the Web may choose not to take the test, or may take it but experience anxiety that negatively affects their scores. Interactive video, set up unobtrusively with a tiny digital camera, provides one-to-one, one-to-many, or many-to-many links, depending upon the purpose of the observation. The visual or audio data

thus collected can be analyzed qualitatively or quantitatively, anthropologically or ethnographically.

Longitudinal tracking provides information about the impact of educational programs and services on student learning and development, as individuals are monitored over time—before, during, and after their participation in a program or service. It is important to decide whom to track, what kinds of information to collect, what "points of contact" are available for data collection, and how the information will be acquired (Hanson, 1997). Several forms of automated data entry are possible, depending upon the nature of the tasks being observed; these include "swipe light pens," visual or auditory recognition systems, PDAs, or optical scan sheets.

A Continuum of Complexity in Computerized Assessment

Groth-Marnat (2000) imagines a continuum of complexity in computerized clinical assessment that begins with the simplest aspect, clerical efficiency (test scoring), and extends to novel assessment stimuli and interpretations.

1. *Clerical efficiency.* Data entry, scoring, and data storage.
2. *Interpretation.* Via either expert-derived or actuarial strategies, a much larger base for generating hypotheses can be developed.
3. *Innovative presentation of traditional test items.* Adaptive selection of test items based on item-response theory could increase the efficiency of assessment; based on a client's previous responses, irrelevant items could be skipped, or other areas could be explored in more depth.
4. *Networked norms.* Internet storage and reference to norms might be developed, such that norms could be tailored to each individual client, and each new client assessment could be stored in an ever-increasing database.
5. *Presentation of novel stimuli.* There are limitless ways in which test "items" might be presented. These might include virtual reality simulations, which are far more complex, rich, and lifelike than tra-

ditional paper–pencil tests (and have high face and ecological validity); tests may be interactive; actual interpersonal or task-related simulations may be presented; tests may be voice-activated; complex interpersonal responses might be noted and analyzed.

6. *Time series measures.* Instead of having one or two assessment sessions, examiners could attach computerized recording devices to a client to measure ongoing sequences of behaviors over a period of days or weeks; such information might be transferred to central data storage and integrated with additional assessment information (test results, demographics, medical records, etc.).

7. *Psychophysiological monitors.* Psychophysiological responses could be integrated with other forms of responses.

8. *Artificial intelligence.* Computers could "learn" from a wide number of sources (decision rules, research data, norms) and "experiences" (modal, as well as novel, clients; feedback on errors and successes), to become increasingly "intelligent."

9. *Each of these features might be integrated and interactive.* "The test site typically would be different from the site for processing the data" (Groth-Marnat, 2000, pp. 359–360).

Data Visualization

Data may be visualized as animated pictures rather than tables of numbers. Scientific methodology and traditional statistics focus primarily on confirmatory analyses providing numerical printouts that reduce and organize the data. Data visualization explores and displays data to create a visual analogy to the physical world that will enhance user insight and learning. The use of color, animation, and video software, as well as the use of one-, two-, and three-dimensional graphic data presentation techniques, enhances the ability to examine and make sense of very complex data. An example of data visualization techniques is seen each day in weather reports, which use a rich array of data visualization methodologies. A challenge is to keep a balance between presenting too much data and overwhelming the viewer (too much noise) and reducing the data to a single statistic that misrepresents reality (too much smoothing). This is analogous to providing information about cognitive strengths and weaknesses by reporting scores on 22 tests as opposed to an IQ score.

Hypertext and hypermedia may show data as simple as a one-dimensional histogram or as complicated as an animated, three-dimensional graphic image rotated over time to represent a fourth dimension of the information (Yu & Behrens, 1994). Animated, three-dimensional video graphics conveying complex information about the impact of numerous student services on the growth and development of students over time may be produced. By pointing and clicking through complex questions, assessors could evaluate which students benefited from which kinds of educational programs. Individual education programs (IEPs) would change dramatically.

Real-Time Data Interaction

Imagine sitting in a multidisciplinary team meeting and using a laptop computer and digital projector to interact with the data in real time. Rather than passively listening to a report of a student's assessment results, participants would actively participate in making sense of the student's data. Online analytic processing comes with the ability to "submit commands to the statistical software, analyze the data, generate data tables, charts, or graphs, and have them displayed to the 'consumer' audience on command" (Hanson, 1997, p. 7). An important component of interactive data analysis is getting the participants involved in generating assessment and evaluation questions (Lincoln & Guba, 1985). Once participants generate questions, the evaluator submits the commands to analyze the data into the laptop computer, and the results appear on the projection screen for all to see.

Traditionally, the assessment specialist tries to anticipate what questions will be asked. Inevitably, someone asks "Did you look at . . . ?" The interactive data analysis tools help the data consumer to formulate relevant kinds of questions. Tufte (1990) summarizes it best: "The world is complex, dynamic, multidimensional: the paper is static, flat. How are we to represent the rich visual world of experience and measurement on mere flatland?"(p. 9).

Another data support system, data warehousing, provides assessment results summarized in aggregate or disaggregate formats with tables, charts, and graphs. This format is useful for annual reports or analyzing trends in data. This format is also found in many computerized scoring programs for standardized tests. It may be applied to qualitative data, such as voice mail responses or video clips. A program evaluation report or student evaluation could include video clips of the student participating in a program or audio recordings of the student's evaluations of the program experience.

A structured query language (SQL) is a data support system that allows decision makers to formulate questions, query the information database, and analyze the results. As the questions become more refined, the process becomes iterative, and the questions can narrow the data to a very specific focus. A decision maker has control over the data summary format, creating whatever presentation format is needed.

Yet another data support system, data mining, is a systematic approach to analyzing and presenting data that includes these steps: sampling data; exploring and analyzing data; modifying or transforming data; modeling or simulating a decision; and presenting information.

The data-mining process uses naturalistic methodologies to analyze real-time data. For example, in a program evaluation, data from students who did and did not participate in a particular service is converted into a database, and factor analysis, correspondence analysis, or clustering techniques are used to identify subgroups of students who benefited from participating in the program. Then differences between the two groups are explored. In the modification phase, the database is queried to identify new variables or new groupings of students who benefited from the educational program; for example, it can be determined whether males, low-income students, or bilingual students benefited more than other groups. Additional variables might be added to better understand these differences. In the next phase, the analysis done in earlier stages may be validated or tested against a holdout sample

from the first step, or a cross-validation with a new cohort of participants may be analyzed (Hanson, 1997). Again, qualitative and quantitative data may be used.

Automated Data-Recording Systems

During the last half of the 1990s, there was an increased availability of pen-based PDAs (e.g., Newtons, Palm Pilots, etc.). PDAs have several advantages over desktop computers, such as greater portability and a more natural interface. PDAs are not tied to a traditional keyboard, mouse, and monitor configuration as a personal computer is. Rather, PDAs are small enough to fit into a pocket or a purse for the ultimate in portability. PDAs also allow the user to enter text via a stylus tapped onto a pictured keyboard, an attached portable keyboard, or by writing characters that approximate the letters of the alphabet. All data can be easily uploaded or downloaded to a desktop computer. Current top-of-the-line models have color screens; interchangeable, programmable modules; and wireless telephone and Internet access.

PDAs were not originally intended to replace desktop computers or portable laptop computers. Instead, they provided the user with a portable platform and set of tools for performing everyday common tasks (e.g., a calendar, a Rolodex, a to-do list, etc.). Increasingly sophisticated PDAs do replace laptop computers, cameras, and telephones, as they are used for wireless and often verbal-generated telecommunications such as access to the Internet and email, telephone transmission, data gathering and disseminating, digital image recording and displaying, and word processing, database and spreadsheet use. Third-party vendors have developed a variety of applications that can be loaded on PDAs, such as behavioral observation or rating forms and questionnaires.

In clinical trials of early PDAs, test users reported preferences for the PDAs over paper and pencil for tasks such as diary entries and questionnaires, and the age of the test users did not seem to affect satisfaction levels (Drummond, Ghosh, Ferguson, Brackenridge, & Tiplady, 1995; Tiplady, 1994). Tseng and colleagues (1998) investigated the effects of mood on the performance of a battery of cognitive tests via paper and pencil, the Newton PDA, or computer presentations. They found that "computer anxiety" may affect the results of cognitive function, but that the effects appear to be minimized with PDAs as compared to desktop computers.

Automated relational databases are used increasingly to maintain special education records. Software programs are commercially available that have all special education forms stored in a digital format. Special education personnel, including school psychologists, are increasingly using these databases to manage the ever-increasing amount of paperwork for multidisciplinary team meetings, as well as to track student progress and mandated timelines for reassessment. Imagine having the assessment information needed at one's fingertips in a PDA downloaded from a desktop computer or via the Internet.

Automated data-recording systems may have two basic modes of operation: parallel and serial input. Each emphasizes different aspects of the observation process and results in a different classification of data. In parallel systems, more than one event can be recorded at a time. For instance, an event key is depressed at the onset of an event and released upon termination. These data are stored in real time to facilitate the retrieval of duration data, and multiple events can be recorded easily, especially if videotaping is available. For example, the videotape may be viewed several times in order to obtain multiple pieces of information. In serial systems, only one character can be recorded at a time. Such a system is particularly useful in the natural environment when the observer wishes to record the sequential occurrence of a large number of events. Automated data systems may be judged on several criteria, including the ability to provide complete information; type and size of memory or storage capabilities; ease of obtaining data analysis; portability; ability to synchronize separate data records; the means used to transmit data; adaptability to various environments; and speed of transmission (Fitzpatrick, 1977).

There are also statistical packages designed to analyze the behavioral data collected and transmitted to computers through automated data collection systems.

The software provides (1) a sorting function that combines and selects events and portions of records; (2) a counting and summing function that tabulates frequencies of selected events, durations, or rates, and constructs histograms; and (3) an organizational description function that computes temporal relationships and histograms (computer data printouts) between pairs of selected events and detects nonrandom occurrences of selected events (Fitzpatrick, 1983). It is possible to construct a simple program for a microcomputer that will record elapsed time and frequency data (Romanczyk, 1986), so that data can be entered directly into the computer without having to be transferred from another device. For example, the data can be entered easily on a portable or stationary computer located conveniently in the classroom, with a teacher or aide pressing certain keys to indicate beginning or ending behaviors.

Recording errors are possible with automated systems, and automated systems are limited in the manner in which data can be classified. It may be difficult to code subject groupings, subject characteristics, several concomitant behaviors, or the behavior of more than one subject. More research is needed into sources of error in and the potentialities of these systems.

FUTURE TRENDS IN COMPUTERIZED ASSESSMENT

Test Administration

Three trends will continue to evolve. First, test developers will increasingly make use of the Internet and portable computing devices to distribute and support computerized scoring programs. It is more cost-effective for a user and publishers to download a computer software program directly onto a hard drive than to receive the program on some type of storage media. Second, online versions of computer-adapted psychoeducational and psychological tests will be made available to qualified users via the Internet. Issues of test security and continued profitability for the test publishers will be resolved. The proliferation of tests that have migrated to the Internet will continue to grow. Third, the type of behavior or construct measured and the manner in which traditional constructs are measured or defined will change as technology allows measurement of process as well as outcomes. Qualitative and quantitative data will be collected. The results of a brain scan may find their way into a lesson plan designed to meet unique learning needs (Dehaene, Spelke, Stanescu, Pinel, & Tsivkin, 1999; Pugh, Shaywitz, & Shaywitz, 2000; Richards et al., 1999).

There are several advantages to tests' being available online. First, all testing materials will be accessible wherever there is a computer or other device that has Internet access (and, increasingly, this is wireless access). Second, the cost of providing the test product to the end user should be reduced as easels, test booklets, and carrying cases become relics of the past. (Although these savings have not been passed onto the consumer thus far, publishers argue that high development costs must be covered.) Third, with permission of the end user, test data without identifying information can be gathered from a continual stream of users. Data can be used to generate norms from very specific segments of the population that may not always be included in standardization samples.

There are also several roadblocks to online testing. Test publishers need to become convinced that selling access to a traditional psychological test via the Internet can be as profitable as selling paper and pencil versions. From the users' perspective, concerns about confidentiality will need to be resolved. For example, when a psychological test is administered via the Internet, some procedures will need to be in place to insure that an individual's test results will not be stored on an insecure server or sent over insecure information transport means that are accessible by other parties. Safeguards need to be in place as well to confirm the identity of the test taker.

A major, predicted change in test administration is the integration of quantitative and qualitative test results using computerized assessment. In the late 1990s, paper-and-pencil tests such as the Cognitive Assessment System (Naglieri & Das, 1997), the Developmental Neuropsychological Assessment (Korman, Kirk, & Kemp, 1998), and the Wechsler Intelligence Scale for Children—Third Edition as a Process Instrument (Kaplan, Fein, Kramer, Delis, & Morris, 1999), included qualitative as well as quantitative test scores. There is an increased interest not only in quantifying a examinee's performance compared to a normative group, but also in evaluating what strategies the examinee has used to obtain those scores. Computerized assessment can keep track of many variables beyond a raw score (response latency, error patterns, etc.).

Direct assessment of cognitive functioning via complex brain studies of many kinds hold promise for understanding how humans learn and remember; what the brain normally does as people read, calculate, and estimate; and what goes wrong when people have difficulty with these tasks (Pugh et al., 2000). This computerized assessment (which collects brain functioning data during the performance of specific tasks) may provide important information about the role of memory, attention, emotion, and motivation in learning as well as contributing to the development of identification and intervention strategies related to learning disabilities, attention-deficit disorders, dyslexia, and other learning impairments.

Report Writing

At the turn of the 21st century, speech recognition software was starting to become a viable product. The processing speeds of personal computers and PDAs, the increased size of memory, and software improvements have made speech recognition software easier to use and more accurate. School psychologists may use speech recognition software to help them write psychological reports and to dictate IEP meeting minutes. The science fiction concept of HAL in *2001: A Space Odyssey* (i.e., a computer that could interact with humans via speech) is now a reality. In the future, voice recognition software will allow us to interact fully with computers.

Information Access

Our ability to multitask and access information via wireless telecommunication technology has increased dramatically since the dawn of the 21st century. The next revolution beyond the personal computer is that of wireless technologies. In 2003, it is common to have integrated, wireless Internet access, cellular phone communication, digital video recording (both still and moving), and basic productivity software applications on a PDA. A device that fits into a shirt pocket has more power and productivity power than the computers in the mid–20th century that occupied whole buildings. Access to information grows exponentially daily. The challenge is not access to information but how to efficiently identify, sort, and critically analyze sources and data.

Several innovations have been mentioned previously in this chapter, including using the computer to assess skills in ways not possible with paper-and-pencil tests. To elaborate further, computer technology is changing rapidly, becoming more powerful and sophisticated, and incorporating other technologies that expand its capabilities still further. This includes DVD or video disk–computer interactive programs. Research with this combination of technologies has produced programs that administer a picture preference test (Morf, Alexander, & Fuerth, 1981) or assess and teach communication skills to individuals who are deaf (Thorkildsen, 1982). An innovative instructional method that has assessment implications involves presenting a typical social interaction scene, then interacting with the computer to stop the video action to have the student decide what happens next. Depending upon the selection, the video disk presents the consequences of that choice nearly instantaneously. Social skills training modules utilizing this technology have been developed (Thorkildsen, Lubke, Myette, & Parry, 1985–1986). Instead of asking children questions about social–emotional development, it would be possible to assess their skills directly with this type of simulation.

Computer simulations offer school psychologists an opportunity to assess skill levels more directly in a variety of areas. The computer keeps track of a child's responses, leaving a psychologist free to observe, question, and interact with the child without having to write everything down, which interferes with free-flowing interaction.

Despite standardization problems with equipment, computerized test administration will continue to expand to include a wide variety of tests. Innovative test makers are likely to make use of such technological devices as touch screens, light pens, voice synthesizers and recorders, toggle levers, biofeedback physiological recorders, DNA analyzers, and voice pattern recognizers. For instance, a voice-operated version of the MMPI allows the client to respond "True" or "False" vocally to items presented on the screen (Richards, Fine, Wilson, & Rogers, 1983).

Computer-adapted testing will continue to expand. To illustrate one application of IRT theory and CAT, Carroll (1987) described the report of the National Assessment of Educational Progress on national assessments in reading. Standard deviation points from –2 to +2 on the 0–500 scale were described in relation to reading levels—for instance, Rudimentary (150), Basic (200), Intermediate (250), Adept (300), and Advanced (350). Another example is the use of IRT to do pattern analysis on national standardized group tests, such as the Comprehensive Test of Basic Skills, and to report the results in ways that have direct implications for instructional planning (Erdner et al., 1998).

Test Scoring

Computers will assume an increasing role in test scoring as more complex scoring systems for educational and psychological tests are implemented. These include (1) continuous norming (Zachary & Gorsuch, 1985); (2) answer-until-correct scoring for achievement or ability tests (Wilcox, 1981); (3) problem-solving error analysis scoring for achievement tests (Birenbaum & Tatsuoka, 1982); (4) item–option weighting (Downey, 1979); (5) graphical modeling and item response theory modeling for computer-adapted testing (Tufte, 1990); and (6) chaos-based theory mathematical models for predicting unstable behavior (Heiby, 1995). This has been an area in which psychologists have readily accepted computer technology, because it has allowed greater consistency and accuracy of scoring, and has improved efficiency while eliminating a routinized chore. Test scoring has become so complex that some widely used tests cannot be hand-scored anymore, for example, the Woodcock–Johnson Psycho-Educational

Assessment Battery—Third Edition (Woodcock et al., 2001).

Test Interpretation

Technology advances will allow more sophisticated CBTI programs. Future interpretations of computer-manipulated data may include (1) matching test profiles with criterion group profiles and using multivariate statistics to determine how they fit (Roid, 1986); (2) establishing predictive links between two or more tests (Zachary, Crumpton, & Spiegel, 1985); (3) linking test score patterns with verifiable behaviors or characteristics of examinees (Roid, 1986); (4) linking data on aptitude–treatment interactions or traits with behavior intervention data to predict what instruction will be beneficial to what children under what conditions (McCullough, Hopkins, & Bowser, 1982); (5) linking developmental factors with universal crises (such as rejection by a best friend or intervention effectiveness data to increase accuracy of recommended educational changes (McCullough et al., 1982); and (6) producing intervention effectiveness data to increase accuracy of recommended educational changes (McCullough et al., 1982). For example, a psychologist could input data showing impulsive responding. The computer would draw upon its data base to describe possible intervention strategies, with the additional information that plan A (a cognitive-behavioral strategy) has an 80% chance of success, that plan B (a token economy) has a 40% chance, and that plan C (a computer simulation) has not been tried before. Psychoeducational recommendations would be supported with research-based information.

SUMMARY AND CONCLUSIONS

Computerized assessment offers psychologists a sophisticated tool, but it is a tool with limits. A computer does only what it is programmed to do. Since we humans are not perfect yet, neither are our tools. The limits on the system are human limits, mistakes, misinterpretation, misuse, and children who do not fit the system. Psychologists must always regard computerized tests and interpretations with caution, in order to avoid falling victim to their objective and authoritative air. "High-tech/high-touch" has been shown to be important in instructional computer research (Metzger, Ouellette, & Thormann, 1984), where children highly motivated to use the computers still demanded the teacher's attention and touch. There is too much information to be gained from personal human interaction for us ever to turn assessment over completely to computers. Yet, used as a creative tool, the computer may be able to give us insights into behavior and allow us to observe learning processes directly, rather than just outcomes. As the benefits of incorporating this tool into our repertoire of professional behaviors accumulate, we can choose to adapt computers to help us do what we do now more efficiently, or we can choose to use the technology creatively and change and improve what we do now. We can hitch the jet to the oxcart, or we can choose to soar.

NOTE

1. The QWERTY phenomenon refers to the fact that the typewriter keyboard was designed when typewriters had metal rods that had to strike the paper. Typists who typed too fast got the rods jammed together. So the keyboard was designed to slow down typists by putting the most frequently used letters farther apart. Other arrangements of keys have been shown to facilitate faster typing, but the QWERTY keyboard lives on in electronic keyboards.

REFERENCES

Allen, B. A., & Boyken, A. W. (1991). The influence of contextual factors on Afro-American and Euro-American children's performance: Effects of movement opportunity and music. *International Journal of Psychology, 26*(3), 373–387.

Almond, R. G., & Mislevy, R. J. (1999). Graphical models and computerized adaptive testing. *Applied Psychological Measurement, 23*(3), 223–237.

American Psychological Association (APA), American Educational Research Association (AERA), & National Council on Measurement in Education (NCME). (1999). *Standards for educational and psychological testing.* Washington DC: American Psychological Association.

American Psychological Association (APA), Committee on Professional Standards and Committee on Psychological Tests and Assessment. (1986). *Guidelines for computer-based tests and interpretations.* Washington, DC: Author.

Anderson, J. R. (1982). Acquisition of cognitive skill. *Psychological Review, 89,* 369–406.

Anderson, R. E., Welch, W. W., & Harris, L. J. (1984). Inequities in opportunities for computer literacy. *The Computing Teacher, 11*(8), 10–12.

Anderson-Inman, L., & Ditson, L. (1999). Computer-based concept mapping: A tool for negotiating meaning. *Learning and Leading with Technology, 26*(8), 6–13.

Anderson-Inman, L., Knox-Quinn, C., & Horney, M. A. (1996). Computer-based strategies for students with learning disabilities: Individual differences associated with adoption level. *Journal of Learning Disabilities, 29*(5), 461–484.

Barclay, J. R. (1983). A meta-analysis of temperament-treatment interactions with alternative learning and counseling treatments. *Development Review, 2*(4), 410–443.

Ben-Shakhar, G., & Sinai, Y. (1991). Gender differences in multiple-choice tests: The role of differential guessing tendencies. *Journal of Educational Measurement, 28*(1), 23–35.

Bennett, R. E. (1999). Using new technology to improve assessment. *Educational Measurement, 18*(3), 5–12.

Bernt, F. M., Bugbee, A. C., & Arceo, R. D. (1990). Factors influencing student resistance to computer administered testing. *Journal of Research on Computing in Educaton, 22*(3), 265–275.

Bersoff, D. N., & Hofer, P. J. (1991). Legal issues in computerized psychological testing. In T. B. Gutkin & S. L. Wise (Eds.), *The computer and the decision-making process* (pp. 225–243). Hillsdale, NJ: Erlbaum.

Birenbaum, M., & Tatsuoka, K. (1982). The effect of a scoring system based on the algorithm underlyng the students' response patterns on the dimensionality of achievement test data of the problem solving type. *Journal of Educational Measurement, 20,* 17–26.

Bischof, J., & Hedman, G. (1990). Computer access. In G. Hedman (Ed.), *Rehabilitation technology* (pp. 99–121). Binghamton, NY: Haworth Press.

Boyken, A. W. (1982). Task variability and the performance of black and white school children: Vervistic explorations. *Journal of Black Studies, 12,* 469–485.

Braden, J. P. (1997). The practical impact of intellectual assessment issues. *School Psychology Review, 26*(2), 242–248.

Brantley, J. (1984). *Review of computerized Wechsler analysis programs.* Paper presented at the annual convention of the National Association of School Psychologists, Philadelphia.

Brown, J. S. (1985). Process versus product: A perspective on tools for communal and informal electronic learning. In M. Chen & W. Paisley (Eds.), *Children and microcomputers: Research on the newest medium* (pp. 248–266). Beverly Hills, CA: Sage.

Bugbee, A. C. (1996). The equivalence of paper-and-pencil and computer-based testing. *Journal of Research on Computing in Education, 28,* 282–299.

Bunderson, C. V., Inouye, D. K., & Olsen, J. B. (1989). The four generations of computerized educational measurement. In R. L. Linn (Ed.), *Educational measurement* (3rd ed., pp. 367–407). New York: American Council on Education/Macmillan.

Burns, D. J. (1998). *A computer simulation investigation of preschool psychoeducational decision-making by school psychologists.* Unpublished doctoral dissertation, Northern Arizona University.

Burroughs, W. A., Murray, J., Wesley, S. S., Medina, D. R., Penn, S. L., Gordon, S. R., & Catello, M. (1999). Easing the implementation of behavioral testing through computerization. In F. Drasgow & J. B. Olson-Buchanan (Eds.), *Innovations in computerized assessment* (pp. 221–248). Mahwah, NJ: Erlbaum.

Butcher, J. N., Perry, J. N., & Atlis, M. M. (2000). Validity and utility of computer-based test interpretation. *Psychological Assessment, 12*(1), 6–18.

Campbell, D. P. (1976). Author's reaction to Johnson's review. *Measurement and Evaluation in Guidance, 9,* 45–56.

Campbell, J. W., D'Amao, R. C., Raggio, D. J., & Stephend, K. D. (1991). Construct validity of the computerized continuous performance test with measures of intelligence, achievement and behavior. *Journal of School Psychology, 29*(2), 143–150.

Carroll, J. B. (1987). The national assessments in reading: Are we misreading the findings? *Phi Delta Kappan, 68,* 424–430.

Center for Electronic Studying. (1998). *Concept-mapping companion.* Eugene, OR: International Society for Technology in Education.

Chiang, A. (1978). *Demonstration of the use of computer-assisted instruction with handicapped children.* Arlington, VA: RMC Research Corporation.

Christmann, E., Badgett, J., & Lucking, R. (1997). Microcomputer-based computer-assisted instruction within differing subject areas: A statistical deduction. *Educational Computing Research, 16*(3), 281–296.

Clavelle, P. R., & Butcher, J. N. (1977). An adaptive typological approach to psychiatric screening. *Journal of Consulting and Clinical Psychology, 45,* 851–859.

Computer and Technological Applications in School Psychology Committee (CTASP). (1982–1989). *CTASP Newsletter.* Washington, DC: National Association of School Psychologists.

Cory, C. H. (1977). Relative utility computerized versus paper–pencil tests for predicting job performance. *Applied Psychological Measurement, 1,* 551–564.

Cowden, D. J. (1946). An application of sequential analysis to testing students. *Journal of the American Statistical Association, 41,* 547–556.

Cronbach, L. J. (1980). *Validity on parole: How can we go straight?* In W. B. Schrader (Ed.), *Measuring achievement: Progress over a decade. Proceedings of the 1979 ETS Invitational Conference* (pp. 99–108). San Francisco: Jossey-Bass.

CTB/McGraw Hill. (1983). *Comprehensive Test of Basic Skills: Test coordinator's handbook.* Monterey, CA: Author.

Davis, R. N. (1999). Web-based administration of a personality questionnaire: Comparison with traditional methods. *Behavior Research Methods, Instruments, and Computers, 31*(4), 572–577.

Dee-Burnet, R., Jones, E. F., & Krug, S. (1982). *Law enforcement assessment and development report manual.* Champaign, IL: Institute for Personality and Ability Testing.

de Mesquita, P. (1987). *The information processing and diagnostic decision making of school psychologists while solving a computer-simulated diagnostic referral problem.* Paper presented at the annual convention of the National Association of School Psychologists, New Orleans, LA.

Ditson, L. A., Kessler, R., & Anderson-Inman, L. (2001). *Concept-Mapping Companion, Second Edition.* Eugene, OR: International Society for Technology in Education.

Downey, R. G. (1979). Item-option weighting of achievement tests: Comparative study of methods. *Applied Psychological Measurement, 3,* 453–461.

Drummond, H. E., Ghosh, S., Ferguson, A., Brackenridge, D., & Tiplady, B. (1995). Electronic quality of life questionnaires: A comparison of pen-based electronic questionnaires with conventional paper in a gastrointestinal study. *Quality of Life Research, 4,* 2–7.

Dunn, L. M., & Dunn, L. M. (1981). *Peabody Picture Vocabulary Test—Revised manual.* Circle Pines, MN: American Guidance Service.

Durrett, J., & Trezona, J. (1982). How to use color displays effectively: The elements of color vision and their implications for programmers. *Pipeline, 7*(2), 13–16.

Duthie, B. (1984). A critical examination of computer-administered psychological tests. In M. D. Schwartz (Ed.), *Using computers in clinical practice: Psychotherapy and mental health applications* (pp. 135–140). New York: Haworth Press.

Erdman, H. P., Klein, M. H., & Greist, J. H. (1985). Direct patient computer interviewing. *Journal of Consulting and Clinical Psychology, 53,* 760–773.

Erdner, R. A., Guy, R. F., & Bush, A. (1998). The impact of a year of computer assisted instruction on the development of first grade learning skills. *Educational Computing Research, 18*(4), 369–386.

Evans, C. (1979). *The micro millennium.* New York: Viking Press.

Eyde, L. D., Kowal, D. M., & Fishburne, F. J., Jr. (1991). The validity of computer-based test interpretations of the MMPI. In T. B. Gutkin & S. L. Wise (Eds.), *The computer and the decision-making process* (pp. 75–133). Hillsdale, NJ: Erlbaum.

Farrell, A. (1999a). Development and evaluation of problem frequency scales from Version 3 of the Computerized Assessment System for Psychotherapy Evaluation and Research. *Journal of Clinical Psychology, 55*(4), 447–464.

Farrell, A. D. (1999b). Evaluation of the Computerized Assessment System for Psychotherapy Evaluation and Research (CASPER) as a measure of treatment effectiveness in an outpatient training clinic. *Psychological Assessment, 11*(3), 345–358.

Faust, D., & Ziskin, J. (1989). Computer-assisted psychological evaluation as legal evidence: Some day my prints will come. *Computers in Human Behavior, 5*(1), 23–36.

Feltovich, P. J. (1981). *Knowledge based components of expertise in medical diagnosis* (Technical Report No. PDS–2). Pittsburgh, PA: University of Pittsburgh, Learning Research and Development Center.

Fitzpatrick, L. M. (1983). BEHAVE—an automated data analysis system for observed events. *Behavior Research Methods and Instrumentation, 15,* 452–455.

Fletcher-Flinn, C. M. (1995). The efficacy of computer assisted instruction (CAI): A meta-analysis. *Educational Computing Research, 12*(3), 219–242.

Fowler, R. D., & Butcher, J. N. (1986). Critique of Matarazzo's views on computerized testing: All sigma and no meaning. *American Psychologist, 41,* 94–96.

Frame, R., Clarizio, H. F., Porter, A. C., & Vinsonhaler, J. R. (1982). Interclinician agreement and bias in school psychologists' diagnostic and treatment recommendations for a learning disabled child. *Psychology in the Schools, 19,* 319–327.

Freebody, P., & Cooksey, R. W. (1985). Computer assessment of reading vocabulary; A preliminary study of the relationship between knowledge, word frequency and response time. *Reading Psychology, 6,* 157–168.

Garb, H. N. (2000). Computers will become increasingly important for psychological assessment: Not that there's anything wrong with that! *Psychological Assessment, 12*(1), 31–39.

Glutting, J. J. (1986). The McDermott Multidimensional Assessment of Children: Applications to the classification of childhood exceptionality. *Journal of Learning Disabilities, 19*(6), 321–384.

Green, B. F., Jr. (1970). Comments on tailored testing. In W. H. Holtzman (Ed.), *Computer-assisted instruction, testing, and guidance* (pp. 245–273). New York: Harper & Row.

Green, B. F. (1991). Guidelines for computer testing. In T. B. Gutkin & S. L. Wise (Eds.), *The computer and the decision-making process* (pp. 245–273). Hillsdale, NJ: Erlbaum.

Groth-Marnat, G. (2000). Visions of clinical assessment: Then, now, and a brief history of the future. *Journal of Clinical Psychology, 56*(3), 349–365.

Grove, W. M., Zald, D. H., Lebow, B., Smith, E., & Nelson, C. (2000). Clinical versus mechanical prediction: A meta-analysis. *Psychological Assessment, 12,* 19–30.

Guastello, S. J., & Rieke, M. L. (1994). Computer-based test interpretations as expert systems: Validity and viewpoints from artificial intelligence theory. *Computers in Human Behavior, 10*(4), 435–455.

Guba, E. G., & Lincoln, Y. (1989). *Fourth generation evaluation.* Thousand Oaks, CA: Sage.

Haaf, R., Duncan, B., Skarakis-Doyle, E., Carew, M., & Kapitan, P. (1999). Computer-based language assessment software: The effects of presentation and response format. *Language, Speech, and Hearing Services in Schools, 30*(1), 68–74.

Hakel, M. D. (1968). How often is often? *American Psychologist, 23,* 533–534.

Hale, R. L., & McDermott, P. A. (1984). Pattern

analysis of an actuarial stategy for computerized diagnosis of childhood exceptionality. *Journal of Learning Disabilities, 17,* 30–37.

Hammainen, L. (1994). Computerized support for neuropsychological test interpretation in clinical situations. *The Clinical Neuropsychologist, 8,* 167–185.

Hanson, G. R. (1997, Summer). Using technology in assessment and evaluation. *New Directions in Student Services, 78,* 31–44.

Haynes, S. N., & Wilson, C. C. (1979). *Behavioral assessment: Recent advances in methods, concepts, and applications.* San Francisco: Jossey-Bass.

Heiby, E. M. (1995). Chaos theory, nonlinear dynamical models, and psychological assessment. *Psychological Assessment, 7,* 5–9.

Heppner, P., Kivlighan, D., & Good, G. (1994, July). Presenting problems of university counseling center clients: A snapshot and multivariate classification scheme. *Journal of Counseling Psychology, 41,* 315–324.

Herl, H. E., Jr., O'Neil, H. F., Chung, G. K. W. K., & Schacter, J. (1999). Reliability and validity of a computer-based knowledge mapping system to measure content understanding. *Computers in Human Behavior, 15,* 315–333.

Hersh, J. B. (1971). Effects of referral information on testers. *Journal of Counseling and Clinical Psychology, 37*(1), 116–122.

Inspiration Software. (1988–1997). *Inspiration* [Computer software]. Portland, OR: Author.

Izquierdo-Porrera, A. M., Manchanda, R., Powell, C. S., Sorkin, J. D., & Bradham, D. D. (2002). Factors influencing the use of computer technology in the collection of clinical data in a predominantly African-American population. *Journal of the American Geriatrics Society, 50*(8), 1411–1415.

Jacob, S., & Brantley, J. C. (1987). Ethical-legal problems with computer use and suggestions for best practices: A national survey. *School Psychology Review, 16,* 69–77.

Jones, T. H., & Paolucci, R. (1999). Research framework and dimensions for evaluating the effectiveness of educational technology systems on learning outcomes. *Journal of Research on Computing in Education, 32*(1), 17–27.

Kaplan, E., Fein, D., Kramer, J., Delis, D., & Morris, R. (1999). *WISC-III as a Process Instrument (WISC-III PI).* San Antonio, TX: Psychological Corporation.

Kaufman, A. S. (1994). *Intelligent testing with the WISC-III.* New York: Wiley.

Kessler, R., Anderson-Inman, L., Ditson, L. A., & Morris, J. D. (1996). *Evaluating concept maps in traditional and electronic environments.* New York: American Educational Research Association.

Kingsbury, G. G., & Houser, R. L. (1999). Developing computerized adaptive tests for school children. In F. Drasgow & J. B. Olson-Buchanan (Eds.), *Innovations in computerized assessment* (pp. 93–115). Mahwah, NJ: Erlbaum.

Korman, M., Kirk, U., & Kemp, S. (1997). *NEPSY.* San Antonio, TX: Psychological Corporation.

Krug, S. (1983). *Marriage Counseling Report manual.* Champaign, IL: Institute for Personality and Ability Testing.

Krug, S. (1989, August). *Solid state psychology: The impact of computerized assessment on the science and practice of psychology.* Paper presented at the annual convention of the American Psychological Association, New Orleans, LA.

Kulik, J. A., Bangert, R. L., & Williams, G. W. (1983). Effects of computer-based teaching on secondary school students. *Journal of Educational Psychology, 75,* 19–26.

Lachar, D. (1974). Accuracy and generalizability of an automated MMPI interpretation system. *Journal of Clinical and Consulting Psychology, 42,* 267–273.

Lachar, D., & Alexander, R. S. (1978). Veridicality of self report: Replicated correlates of the Wiggins MMPI content scales. *Journal of Consulting and Clinical Psychology, 46,* 1349–1356.

Lachar, D., & Gdowski, M. C. L. (1979). *Actuarial assessment of child and adolescent personality: An interpretive guide for the Personality Inventory for Children profile.* Los Angeles, CA: Western Psychological Services.

Lachar, D., Klinge, V., & Grisell, J. L. (1976). Relative accuracy of automated MMPI narratives generated from adult norm and adolescent norm profiles. *Journal of Consulting and Clinical Psychology, 44,* 20–24.

Lally, M. (1981). Computer-assisted teaching of sight-word recognition for mentally retarded school children. *American Journal of Mental Deficiency, 85,* 383–388.

Lanyon, R. I. (1984). Personality assessment. *Annual Review of Psychology, 35,* 667–701.

Lee, J. A. (1986). Effects of past computer experience on computerize aptitude test performance. *Educational and Psychological Measurement, 46,* 727–733.

Liao, Y.-K. C. (1999). Effects of hypermedia on students' achievement: A meta-analysis. *Journal of Educational Multimedia and Hypermedia, 8*(3), 255–277.

Lichtenstein, S., & Newman, J. R. (1967). Empirical scaling of common verbal phrases associated with numerical probabilities. *Psychonomic Science, 9,* 563–564.

Lieberman, D. (1985). Research on children and microcomputers: A review of utilization and effects studies. In M. Chen & W. Paisley (Eds.), *Children and microcomputers: Research on the newest medium* (pp. 59–86). Beverly Hills, CA: Sage.

Lincoln, Y., & Guba, E. G. (1985). *Naturalistic inquiry.* Thousand Oaks, CA: Sage.

Lipkin, J. (1984). Computer equity and computer educators (you). *The Computing Teacher, 11*(8), 19–21.

Llabre, M. M. (1991). Time as a factor in the cognitive test performance of Latino college students. In G. D. Keller, J. R. Deneer, & R. J. Magallan (Eds.), *Assessment and access: Hispanics in higher education* (pp. 95–104). Albany: State University of New York Press.

Llabre, M. M., & Froman, T. W. (1987). Allocation of time to test items: A study of ethnic differences. *Journal of Experimental Education, 55,* 137–140.

Lockheed, M. E., & Frakt, S. B. (1984). Sex equity: Increasing girls' use of computers. *The Computing Teacher, 11*(8), 16–18.

Lord, F. M., & Novick, M. R. (1968). *Statistical theories of mental test scores.* Reading, MA: Addison-Wesley.

Macmann, G. M., & Barnett, D. W. (1997). Myth of the master detective: Reliability of interpretations for Kaufman's "intelligent testing" approach to the WISC III. *School Psychology Quarterly, 12*(3), 197–234.

Madaus, G. (1994). A technological and historical consideration of equity issues associated with proposals to change the nation's testing policy. *Harvard Educational Review, 64*(1), 76–95.

Maddox, C. D. (1986). Microcomputers in education: Problems and cautions. *Techniques, 2*(1), 9–14.

Maki, W. S., & Maki, R. H. (2002). Multimedia comprehension skill predicts differential outcomes of Web-based and lecture courses. *Journal of Experimental Psychology—Applied, 8,* 1, 85–98.

Matarazzo, J. D. (1986). Response to Fowler and Butcher on Matarazzo. *American Psychologist, 41,* 96.

Matarazzo, J. M. (1983). Computerized psychological testing [Editorial comment]. *Science,* p. 221.

Matuszek, P. A., & Oakland, T. (1979). Facts influencing teachers and psychologists recommendations regarding special class placement. *Journal of School Psychology, 17,* 116–125.

Mazzeo, J., & Harvey, A. L. (1988). *The equivalence of scores from automated and conventional educational and psychological tests: A review of the literature* (CBR No. 87-8, ETS RR No. 88-21). Princeton, NJ: Educational Testing Service.

McCullough, C. S. (1985). Best practices in computer applications. In A. Thomas & J. Grimes (Eds.), *Best practices in school psychology* (pp. 301–310). Kent, OH: National Association of School Psychologists.

McCullough, C. S. (1989, March). *Evaluating the validity of computer-based test interpretation programs.* Paper presented at the annual convention of the National Association of School Psychologists, Boston.

McCullough, C. S. (1990). Computerized assessment. In C. Reynolds & R. Kamphaus (Eds.), *Handbook of psychological and educational assessment of children: Intelligence and achievement* (pp. 723–747). New York: Guilford Press.

McCullough, C. S. (1995). Using computer technology to monitor student progress and remediate reading problems. *School Psychology Review, 24*(3), 426–439.

McCullough, C. S., Hopkins, S., & Bowser, P. (1982). *Measuring potential: Uses and abuses of computers in school psychology.* Des Moines: Iowa Department of Public Instruction.

McCullough, C. S., & Wenck, S. (1984). Current microcomputer applications in school psychology. *School Psychology Review, 13,* 429–439.

McDermott, P. A. (1980). Congruence and typology of diagnoses in school psychology: An empirical study. *Psychology in the Schools, 17,* 12–24.

McDermott, P. A. (1982). Actuarial assessment systems for the grouping and classification of school children. In C. R. Reynolds & T. B. Gutkin (Eds.), *The handbook of school psychology* (pp. 243–272). New York: Wiley.

McDermott, P. A. (1990). Applied systems: Actuarial assessment. In T. B. Gutkin & C. R. Reynolds (Eds.), *The handbook of school psychology* (2nd ed., pp. 526–558). New York: Wiley.

McDermott, P. A., & Watkins, M. W. (1985). *The McDermott Multidimensional Assessment of Children.* Cleveland, OH: Psychological Corporation.

Meehl, P. E. (1954). *Clinical versus statistical prediction: A theoretical analysis and a review of the evidence.* Minneapolis: University of Minnesota Press.

Mello, J. P., Jr. (1982). Deep in your heart it creeps. *80 Micro, 33,* 373–374.

Messick, S. (1989). Validity. In R. L. Linn (Ed.), *Educational measurement* (3rd ed., pp. 13–103). New York: Macmillan.

Metzger, M., Ouellette, D., & Thormann, J. (1984). *Learning disabled students and computers: A teacher's guidebook.* Eugene, OR: International Council for Computers in Education.

Miller, L. C. (1981). *Louisville Behavior Checklist manual.* Los Angeles, CA: Western Psychological Services.

Mitchell J. V., Jr. (1986). Measurement in the larger context: Critical current issues. *Professional Psychology: Research and Practice, 17*(6), 544–550.

Miura, I. T., & Hess, R. D. (1984). Enrollment differences in computer camps and summer classes. *The Computing Teacher, 11*(8), 22–23.

Moreland, K. L. (1985). Validation of computer-based test interpretations: Problems and prospects. *Journal of Consulting and Clinical Psychology, 53*(6), 816–825.

Moreland, K. L. (1991). Assessment of validity in computer-based test interpretations. In T. B. Gutkin & S. L. Wise (Eds.), *The computer and the decision-making process* (pp. 43–74). Hillsdale, NJ: Erlbaum.

Morf, M., Alexander, P., & Fuerth, T. (1981). Fully automated psychiatric diagnosis: Some new possibilities. *Behavior Research Methods and Instruments, 13,* 413–416.

Moursund, D. (1999). Data, information, knowledge, wisdom. *Learning and Leading with Technology, 26*(8), 4–5.

Nass, C., & Lee, K. M. (2001). Does computer-synthesized speech manifest personality?: Experimental tests of recognition, similarity-attraction, and consistency-attraction. *Journal of Experimental Psychology, 7,* 171–181.

Naas, C., Moon, Y., & Carney, P. (1999). Are people polite to computers?: Responses to computer-based interviewing systems. *Journal of Applied Social Psychology, 29*(5), 1093–1110.

Naglieri, J. A., & Das, J. P. (1997). Intelligence revised: The planning, attention, simultaneous, successive (PASS) cognitive processing theory. In R. F. Dillon (Ed.), *Handbook on testing* (pp. 136–163). Westport, CT: Greenwood Press.

National Association of School Psychologists. (2000). *Guidelines for professional ethics.* Washington, DC: Author.

National Association of School Psychologists. (2000, July). *Standards for training and field placement programs in school psychology.* Washington, DC: Author.

Neves, D. M., & Anderson, J. R. (1981). Knowledge compilation: Mechanisms for automatization of cognitive skills. In J. R. Anderson (Ed.), *Cognitive skills and their acquisition* (pp. 57–84). Hillsdale, NJ: Lawrence Erlbaum.

Niemiec, R. P., Sikorski, C., & Walberg, H. J. (1996). Learner-control effects: A review of reviews and a meta-analysis. *Educational Computing Research, 15*(2), 157–174.

Olson, K. R. (2001). Computerized psychological test usage in APA-accredited training programs. *Journal of Clinical Psychology, 57*(6), 727–736.

Papert, S. (1980). *Mindstorms: Children, computers and powerful ideas.* New York: Basic Books.

Parshall, C. K., & Balizet, S. (2002). Audio computer-based tests (CBTs): An initial framework for the use of sound in computerized tests. *Educational Measurement: Issues and Practice. 20*(2), 5–15.

Pohl, N. F. (1981). Scale considerations in using vague quantifiers. *Journal of Experimental Education, 49,* 235–240.

Powell, M. B., Wilson, J. C., & Hasty, M. K. (2002). Evaluation of the usefulness of "Marvin": A computerized assessment tool for investigative interviewers of children. *Computers in Human Behavior, 18*(5), 577–592.

Psychological Corporation. (1998). *OPTAIO* [Computer software]. San Antonio, TX: Author.

Quality Education Data. (2002a). *Internet usage in teaching 2002–2003* (7th ed.). Denver, CO: Author.

Quality Education Data. (2002b). *Technology purchasing forecast 2002–2003* (8th ed.). Denver, CO: Author.

Richards, J. S., Fine, P. R., Wilson, T. L., & Rogers, J. T. (1983). A voice-operated method for administering the MMPI. *Journal of Personality Assessment, 47,* 167–170.

Richman, W. L., Kiesler, S., Weisband, S., & Drasgow, R. (1999). A meta-analytic study of social desirability distortion in computer-administered questionnaires, traditional questionnaires and interviews. *Journal of Applied Psychology, 53*(5), 754–775.

Robinson-Staveley, K., & Cooper, J. (1990). Mere presence, gender, and reactions to computers: Studying human–computer interaction in the social context. *Journal of Experimental Social Psychology, 26,* 168–183.

Roid, G. H. (1986). Computer technology in testing. In B. S. Plake, J. C. Witt, & J. B. Mitchell (Eds.), *The future of testing: Buros–Nebraska symposium on measurement and testing* (pp. 29–69). Hillsdale, NJ: Erlbaum.

Roid, G. H., & Gorsuch, R. L. (1984). Development and clinical use of test interpretive programs on microcomputers. In M. D. Schwartz (Ed.), *Using computers in clinical practice: Psychotherapy and mental health applications* (pp. 141–150). New York: Haworth Press.

Romanczyk, R. G. (1986). *Clinical utilization of mi-crocomputer technology.* New York: Pergamon Press.

Rosen, L. D. (1995). Three ADHD tests prove computerized technology vital tool for clinicians. *The National Psychologist, 4,* 20–21.

Sattler, J. M. (1992). *Assessment of children's intelligence* (3rd ed.). San Diego, CA: Author.

Sattler, J. M. (2001). *Assessment of children: Cognitive applications* (4th ed.). San Diego, CA: Author.

Scaife, M., & Bond, R. (1991). Developmental changes in children's use of computer input devices. *Early Child Development and Care, 69,* 19–38.

Schubert, J. G., & Bakke, T. (1984). Practical solutions to overcoming equity in computer use. *The Computing Teacher, 11*(8), 28–30.

Seels, B., & Glasgow, Z. (1998). *Making instructional design decisions.* Englewood Cliffs, NJ: Educational Technology Publications.

Sicoly, F. (1989). Computer-aided decisions in human services: Expert systems and multivariate models. *Computers in Human Behavior, 5*(1), 47–60.

Skinner, H. A., & Pakula, A. (1986). Challenge of computers in psychological assessment. *Professional Psychology, 17*(1), 44–50.

Slakter, M. J., Koehler, R. A., Hampton, S. H., & Grennell, R. I. (1971). Sex, grade level and risk taking on objective examinations. *Journal of Experimental Education, 39*(3), 65–68.

Smith, R. D. (1968). Heuristic simulation of psychological decision processes. *Journal of Applied Psychology, 52,* 325–330.

Sutton, R. E. (1991). Equity and computers in the schools: A decade of research. *American Educational Research Journal, 61,* 475–503.

Sutton, R. E. (1997). Equity and high stakes testing: Implications for computerized testing. *Equity and Excellence in Education, 30,* 5–15.

TechMicro. (1997). *The Computer-Optimized Multimedia Intelligence Test (C.O.M.I.T.).* [Online]. Available: http://www.computertests.com/index.htm [1999, December 28].

Thorkildsen, R. J. (1982). *Review of the use of computer technology in special education settings.* Unpublished manuscript, University of Oregon.

Thorkildsen, R. J., Lubke, M. M., Myette, B. M., & Parry, J. D. (1985–1986). Artificial intelligence: Applications in education. *Education Research Quarterly, 10*(1), 2–9.

Tiplady, B. (1994). The use of personal digital assistants in performance testing in psychopharmacology. *British Journal of Clinical Pharmacology, 37,* 523–527.

Tsemberis, S., Miller, A. C., & Gartner, D. (1996). Expert judgments of computer-based and clinician-written reports. *Computers in Human Behavior, 12*(1), 167–175.

Tseng, H.-M., Tiplady, B., Macleod, H. A., & Wright, P. (1998). Computer anxiety: A comparison of pen-based personal digital assistants, conventional computer and paper assessment of mood and performance. *British Journal of Psychology, 89*(4), 599–610.

Tufte, E. R. (1990). *Envisioning information.* Cheshire, CT: Graphics Press.

Valla, J.-P., Bergeron, L., & Smolla, N. (2000). The Dominic-R: A pictorial interview for 6 to 11 year old children. *Journal of the American Academy of Child and Adolescent Psychiatry, 39*(1), 85–93.

Vanderplas, J. M., & Vanderplas, J. H. (1979). Multiple versus single-index predictors of dangerousness, suicide, and other rare behaviors. *Psychological Review, 45,* 343–349.

Vernon, P. A. (1987). *Speed of information processing and intelligence.* Norwood, NJ: Ablex.

Vernon, P. A. (1990). An overview of chronometric measures of intelligence. *School Psychology Review, 19*(4), 399–410.

Wainer, H., Dorans, H. J., Flaugher, R., Green, G. F., Mislevy, R. J., Steinberg, L., & Thissen, D. (1990). *Computerized adaptive testing: A primer.* Hillsdale, NJ: Erlbaum.

Ward, T. J., Jr., Hopper, S. R., & Hannafin, K. M. (1989). The effect of computerized tests on the performance and attitudes of college students. *Journal of Educational Computing Research, 5*(3), 327–333.

Watkins, C. E., Campbell, V. L., Nieberding, R., & Hallmark, R. (1995). Contemporary practice of psychological assessment by clinical psychologists. *Professional Psychology: Research and Practice, 26,* 54–60.

Weber, B., Fritze, J., Schneider, B., Kuehner, T. & Maurer, K. (2002). Bias in computerized neuropsychological assessment of depressive disorders caused by computer attitude. *Acta Psychiatrica Scandinavica, 105*(2), 126–130.

Weiss, D. J. (1983). *New horizons in testing: Latent trait test theory and computerized adaptive testing.* New York: Academic Press.

Weizenbaum, J. (1976). *Computer power and human reason: From judgment to calculation.* San Francisco: Freeman.

Wilcox, R. R. (1981). Solving measurement problems with an answer-until-correct scoring procedure. *Applied Psychological Measurement, 5,* 399–414.

Williams, F., Coulombe, J., & Lievrouw, L. (1983). Children's attitudes toward small computers: A preliminary study. *Educational Communication and Technology Journal, 31*(1), 3–7.

Wirt, R. D., Lachar, D., Klinedinst, J. K., & Seat, P. D. (1977). *Multidimensional description of child personality: A manual for the Personality Inventory for Children.* Los Angeles, CA: Western Psychological Services.

Wise, S. L., & Plake, B. S. (1989). Research on the effects of administering tests via computers. *Educational Measurement: Issues and Practice, 8*(3), 5–10.

Woodcock, R. McGrew, K., & Mather, N. (2001). *Woodcock–Johnson III Tests of Cognitive Abilities.* Itasca, IL: Riverside.

Wu, Y.-K., & Morgan, M. (1989). Computer use, computer attitudes, and gender: Differential implications of micro and mainframe usage among college students. *Journal of Research on Computing in Education, 21,* 214–228.

Yu, C. H., & Behrens, J. T. (1994). *The visualization of multi-way interactions and high-order terms in multiple regression.* Paper presented at the annual meeting of the Psychometric Society, Urbana-Champaign, IL.

Zachary, R. A., Crumpton, E., & Spiegel, D. F. (1985). Estimating WAIS-R IQ from the Shipley Institute of Living Scale. *Journal of Clinical Psychology, 41,* 86–94.

Zachary, R. A., & Gorsuch, R. L. (1985). Continuous norming: Implications for the WAIS-R. *Journal of Clinical Psychology, 41,* 86–94.

Zachary, R. A., & Pope, K. S. (1984). Legal and ethical issues in the clinical use of computerized testing. In M. D. Schwartz (Ed.), *Using computers in clinical practice: Psychotherapy and mental health applications* (pp. 151–166). New York: Haworth Press.

Zeitz, L., & Anderson-Inman, L. (1993). *Computer-based concept mapping in a high school science class: The effects of student characteristics.* Atlanta, GA: American Educational Research Association.

27

Assessing the Psychological and Educational Needs of Children with Moderate and Severe Mental Retardation

CHRISTINE W. BURNS

An important distinction must be made between "assessment" and the narrower term "testing." Assessment is a process that enables one to analyze critically and evaluate the nature of children's characteristics. Assessment may involve tests, interviewing, observation of behavior in natural or structured settings, and recording of physiological functions. Tests represent a specific aspect of the assessment process. Anastasi (1968) defines a test as "an objective and standardized measure of a sample of behavior" (p. 21). This chapter focuses on the assessment of children with moderate and severe mental retardation.

GOALS AND LIMITATIONS OF ASSESSMENT

The psychological and educational assessment of children with moderate and severe retardation may be defined in terms of three goals: (1) diagnosis, (2) documentation of status or progress, and (3) planning or prescribing intervention. A diagnostic goal is appropriate when it is necessary to determine whether a child's performance reflects established criteria for the diagnosis of men-

tal retardation. Normative instruments are typically used to yield information to confirm or disconfirm the diagnosis. When there is a need to verify a child's current status or change in status from one occasion to another, the goal of assessment is that of documenting status or progress. The goal of planning or prescribing interventions involves assessment to obtain a profile of a child's unique strengths and deficits from which an intervention program can be developed. The American Association on Mental Retardation (AAMR) recommends two additional purposes for assessment: identifying supports and evaluating the effects of added supports (AAMR, 1992). The additional goals identified by AAMR highlight a shift toward a more ecological and values-driven assessment (Siegel-Causey & Allinder, 1998). This emphasis shifts away from the limitations of the individual to the impact environmental factors have on how independently the person is able to function in a variety of settings.

Underlying these goals is the basic assumption of psychological assessment: that the instruments used are valid for the purpose selected and will document accurately the skills, traits, attributes, or behaviors of

671

interest. A number of factors, however, limit this assumption for those with moderate and severe mental retardation. These limitations may affect the formulation of referral questions, the selection of instruments and/or techniques, and the degree of confidence with which inferences can be drawn about assessment results. Limitations are imposed by definitional issues, child characteristics, examiner characteristics, and measurement issues.

Definitional Issues

There is a lack of consensus on the definitions of basic terms. Labels such as "severe disability," "moderate impairment," "moderate retardation," or "multiple handicaps" have frequently been used to describe a child who is developmentally disabled in some way. The variability of labels applied to "special children" (Simeonsson, 1986) has contributed to the confusion and to the difficulties in generalization of assessment and treatment results.

The most widely endorsed definition for "mental retardation" has been set forth by the AAMR:

> Mental retardation refers to substantial limitations in present functioning. It is characterized by significantly subaverage intellectual functioning, existing concurrently with related limitations in two or more of the following applicable adaptive skill areas: communication, self-care, home living, social skills, community use, self-direction, health and safety, functional academics, leisure and work. Mental retardation manifests before age 18. (AAMR, 1992, p. 5)

Children with mental retardation present with substantial limitations in conceptual, practical, and social intelligence; however, other personal capabilities (such as health and temperament) may not be affected. Subaverage intelligence is defined as an IQ of approximately 70 to 75 or below, based upon the performance on an individually administered test of intelligence. The required limitations in adaptive skills are more closely related to the child's intellectual limitations than to other factors, such as cultural or linguistic diversity or sensory limitations. It is necessary to provide evidence of limitations in at least two adaptive

areas, therefore demonstrating a more generalized limitation and thus reducing the probability of any measurement error (AAMR, 1992). The AAMR definition subclassifies mental retardation according to its intensity and the nature of needed supports. The *Diagnostic and Statistical Manual of Mental Disorders,* fourth edition (DSM-IV) subclassifies mental retardation into four degrees of severity, as presented in Table 27.1.

Child Limitations

Mentally retarded children are very likely to have impaired functioning in more than one area. Limitations that affect the psychological assessment of these children can be grouped into two categories: internal and external limitations. Limitations of an internal nature are those that affect a child's level of responsiveness and reactivity. Levels of arousal, or state, may vary widely from extended periods of sleep and drowsiness to a state of agitation and excessive activity for those with severe disabilities. Such variability may be reflective of neurological insults (Touwen & Kalverboer, 1973). It may also be an expression of the effects of medications administered to manage seizures or other medical conditions. The variability of state may contribute to different performances from one observation to the next (Simeonsson, 1986).

Limitations of an external nature include aspects of a child's sensory and/or motor functioning. For example, impairments of vision, kinesthesis, or hearing may limit the child's performance and expression in the assessment process. Sensory impairments or processing disorders restrict or alter the ways in which messages from others are received and responses expressed (Efron,

TABLE 27.1. DSM-IV Classification System for Mental Retardation

Level of functioning, based on IQ	Classification
50–55 to approximately 70	Mild retardation
35–40 to 50–55	Moderate retardation
20–25 to 35–40	Severe retardation
Below 20 or 25	Profound retardation

1981). Children with moderate to severe mental retardation frequently lack the experience that other children gain from interacting with their environment, as well as the opportunities for incidental learning (Cote & Smith, 1983). Some of the differences in experiences are the direct results of severe impairments (e.g., decreased or distorted sensory input, lack of mobility, decreased social contact) (Stillman & Battle, 1986). Repetitive, rhythmic habit patterns such as rocking, head banging, and head rolling, which are found to varying degrees in these children, constitute another limitation of an external nature (Kravitz & Boehm, 1971). These behaviors severely limit a child's ability to attend to the stimuli presented by the examiner, and therefore interfere with accurate assessment of the child's abilities.

Examiner Limitations

Examiners frequently lack the special knowledge or skills to carry out the psychological assessment of those with moderate and severe mental retardation. Graduate training programs, in their clinical assessment classes and practicum experiences, emphasize assessment of those individuals with mild mental disabilities; little exposure is provided to the moderately and severely retarded populations. An examiner's personal orientation may also limit adequate assessment of these populations. Such personal bias may result in misidentification of the problems and in inappropriate domains being selected for assessment. Although complete objectivity may be difficult to achieve, awareness of one's personal orientation as a source of bias in assessment may help to reduce this aspect of examiner limitations.

Measurement Limitations

There are few practical instruments for assessing individuals with severe mental retardation. In addition, normative tables generally do not permit the estimation of functioning levels for this population. For example, the Wechsler Intelligence Scale for Children—Third Edition (WISC-III; Wechsler, 1991) does not permit calculation of a Full Scale IQ below 40. The Stanford–Binet Intelligence Scale: Fourth Edition (Thorn-

dike, Hagen, & Sattler, 1986) does permit calculations of IQs below 40; however, it is important to note that these values are extrapolated data. There were no children in the standardization sample functioning at this low level. Extrapolated test scores are not appropriate for individual diagnosis, because their reliability is unknown.

Current psychological assessment procedures can be grouped into three major strategies on the basis of the approach to assessment. The three approaches are psychometric, behavioral, and qualitative-developmental. With any particular strategy, the focus of the assessment may be categorized within one of four domains: cognitive, communicative, personal/social, and behavioral functioning.

PSYCHOMETRIC ASSESSMENT

Defining Psychometric Assessment

Psychometric assessment enables one to quantify a child's characteristics and compare these quantitative values against a norm or standard. The interpretation of variability in mental abilities through profile analysis can provide valuable information for educational and therapeutic programming.

Selected Measures

The number of psychometric measures available is vast. No attempt is made here to provide a comprehensive review of all such instruments; however, this section reviews a sampling of psychometric measures of intellectual functioning and adaptive behavior that are appropriate for different developmental ages. The Wechsler scales, the Stanford–Binet, and the Kaufman Assessment Battery for Children (K-ABC; Kaufman & Kaufman, 1983a, 1983b) are all well established and are specifically described elsewhere in this volume.

Intellectual Functioning
Infancy

The Bayley Scales of Infant Development— Second Edition (BSID-II) battery (Bayley, 1993) provides a standardized assessment of cognitive and motor development for young children 1 month through 42 months of age. The BSID-II was renormed on a stratified random sample of 1,700 children (850 boys and 850 girls) grouped at 1-month intervals on the variables of age, sex, region, race/ethnicity, and parental education. Data are provided in the manual on numerous clinical samples: children who were born prematurely, had frequent otitis media, had the HIV antibody, were prenatally exposed to drugs, were asphyxiated at birth, were developmentally delayed, had autism, or had Down's syndrome.

The Mental Scale yields a normalized standard score called the Mental Development Index, which evaluates a number of abilities: sensory-perceptual acuities, discriminations, and response; acquisition of object constancy; memory, learning, and problem solving; vocalization, beginning of verbal communication; basis of abstract thinking; habituation; mental mapping; complex language; and mathematical concept formation. The Motor Scale yields a Psychomotor Development Index and assesses the following skills: degree of body control, large-muscle coordination, finer manipulative skills of the hands and fingers, dynamic movement, dynamic praxis, postural imitation, and stereognosis. A Behavior Rating Scale is also available. This 30-item scale rates the child's relevant test-taking behaviors, and measures the following factors: attention/arousal, orientation/engagement, emotional regulation, and motor quality.

The BSID-II has moderate to high internal-consistency reliability coefficients for the Mental Scale (average = .88; range = .78 to .93), Motor Scale (average = .84; range = .75 to .87), and Behavior Rating Scale Total Score (average = .88; range = .82 to .92) across the 17 age groups represented in the standardization sample. Test–retest reliability coefficients are more variable. Behavior Rating Scale coefficients are consistently lower than stability coefficients for the Mental Scale and Motor Scale (median interval was 4 days). Strong correlations between the Mental Development Index, the Wechsler Preschool and Primary Scale of Intelligence—Revised (.73), and the McCarthy Scales of Children's Abilities (.79) provide evidence for criterion validity for children at the older age range (36–42

months) of the BSID-II. The manual presents data from exploratory factor analyses of the Behavior Rating Scale. The analysis provides support for a two-factor model for young infants (1–5 months) and a three-factor model for older infants and children (6–42 months).

The BSID-II and its predecessor (the original BSID) have been used widely with developmentally delayed infants and young children, as well as with older individuals whose severity of disability places them in the functional range of the scales. However, it is important to indicate the qualifications that apply to the use of infant scales with older children and adults.

Early Childhood

The Miller Assessment for Preschoolers (MAP; Miller, 1988) is a brief yet comprehensive preschool screening instrument that identifies children who exhibit mild to moderate developmental delays. Developmental domains assessed include neural foundations, coordination, verbal tasks, nonverbal tasks, and complex tasks. The MAP may be used in cases of more severe developmental deviations to provide a developmental overview and to delineate patterns of strengths and needs.

The MAP was designed for children 2 years, 9 months to 5 years, 8 months of age. The test is individually administered in about 30–40 minutes. The standardization was conducted on 1,200 preschoolers in nine U.S. census regions; the sample was stratified by age, race, sex, size of residence community, and socioeconomic factors. Percentiles for six age groups for overall performance and for five performance indices are provided.

Middle Childhood/Adolescence

The Wechsler scales and the Stanford–Binet are the instruments most frequently used with this age group.

Adaptive Behavior

Although many definitions of "adaptive behavior" have been proposed, the term can be defined simply as the performance of daily activities required for social and personal sufficiency. It is an age-related construct; adaptive behavior skills increase with age. Adaptive behavior is identified by the standards of others and within the social context where the child functions (Kamphaus & Frick, 1996). Witt and Martens (1984), in a review of the various definitions and interpretations of adaptive behavior, noted that most definitions (1) consider adaptive behavior to be age- and culture-specific and (2) include such areas as independent functioning, social responsibility, and cognitive development. Adaptive behavior can be conceptualized as a single-factor or a multifactor construct (Widaman, Stacy, & Borthwick-Duffy, 1993). The results of factor-analytic studies are divergent; therefore, firm conclusions about the structure of adaptive behavior cannot be drawn (Stinnnett, Fuqua, & Coombs, 1999).

Adaptive behavior instruments are generally used for two purposes (Cone & Hawkins, 1977; Taylor, 1985). The first purpose is to identify those individuals who vary significantly from normal" expectations in such areas as independent functioning and socialization. These tests or instruments, sometimes referred to as "descriptive" (Cone & Hawkins, 1977), are used to make classification/placement decisions as well as to identify general strengths and weaknesses. The majority of the descriptive instruments for assessing adaptive behavior are standardized on nondisabled individuals.

Another set of instruments yields much more specific information related to the identification of educational/instructional objectives. Cone and Hawkins (1977) refer to these instruments as "prescriptive"; they are often developed for and standardized on more severely disabled children. In comparison to descriptive tests, prescriptive tests usually include more specific and sequential items related to a smaller number of areas. Instruments do exist that include both descriptive and prescriptive items. For a comprehensive coverage of the issues involved in assessing adaptive behavior, the reader should consult a special edition of the *Journal of Special Education* (edited by Kamphaus, 1987).

In contrast to earlier definitions of mental retardation, there are now 10 individual adaptive behavior areas that can be considered when making a diagnosis of mental retardation; as mentioned earlier, an individual must show limitations in at least two of these areas. The Adaptive Behavior Assessment System (ABAS; Harrison & Oakland, 2000) is the first test to assess all 10 of the adaptive skills areas specified by the AAMR and the DSM-IV: Communication; Community Use; Functional Academics; Home Living; Health and Safety; Leisure; Self-Care; Self-Direction; Social; and Work. The instrument is appropriate for ages 5–89. Three forms are available—a parent form, a teacher form, and an adult form. The ABAS yields general adaptive composites as well as test age equivalents.

The Adaptive Behavior Scale—School: Second Edition (ABS-S:2; Lambert, Nihira, & Leland, 1993) is the most recent in a series of revisions of the original American Association on Mental Deficiency (AAMD) scale. The ABS-S:2 consists of two parts. Part One is organized developmentally and designed to evaluate a person's skills and habits in nine behavior domains: Independent Functioning; Physical Development; Economic Activity; Language Development; Numbers and Time; Prevocational Activity; Self-Direction; Responsibility; and Socialization. These domains are important to the understanding of the development of personal independence and personal responsibility in daily living. Part Two comprises seven domains that pertain to personality and behavior disorders: Social Behavior; Conformity; Trustworthiness; Stereotyped and Hyperactive Behavior; Self-Abusive Behavior; Social Engagement; and Disturbing Interpersonal Behavior. The rater responds to a 3 point Likert scale that typifies the frequency with which the individual performs certain behaviors (i.e., "never," "occasionally," and "frequently").

The ABS-S:2 was standardized on a sample of 2,074 individuals with mental retardation and 1254 without mental retardation. Raw scores can be converted into scaled scores ($M = 10$, $SD = 3$), percentile rank scores, and age equivalents for all nine Part One domains. Similarly, standard scores and percentile rank scores can also be derived for the seven Part Two domains. Three factor scores can be calculated from Part One items: Personal Self-Sufficiency, Community Self-Sufficiency, and Personal–Social Responsibility. Part Two items contribute to two factor scores: Social Adjustment and Personal Adjustment. Factor scores are converted into standard scores ($M = 100$, $SD = 15$) and percentile rank scores. Coefficient alphas were higher for the sample with mental retardation; alphas ranged from .82 (Prevocational/Vocational Activity domain) to .98 (Independent Functioning domain, Personal Self-Sufficiency factor, and Community Self-Sufficiency factor). Moderate correlations between Part One domains/factors, the Vineland Adaptive Behavior Scales (VABS; see below), and the Adaptive Behavior Inventory provide evidence for the ABS-S:2's criterion-related validity. The results suggest overlap among the scales in measuring the construct of adaptive behavior, but each scale is also measuring something distinct from the others.

The Comprehensive Test of Adaptive Behavior (CTAB; Adams, 2000a) evaluates how well students with physical and mental disabilities function independently in their environments. It was designed as both a descriptive and a prescriptive test of adaptive behavior. The CTAB includes 500 empirically sequenced items that measure adaptive behavior across six areas: (1) Self-Help Skills, (2) Home Living Skills, (3) Independent Living Skills, (4) Social Skills, (5) Sensory and Motor Skills, and (6) Language Concepts and Academic Skills. The CTAB uses a combination of an examiner test form and a parent/guardian survey to build a profile of an individual's adaptive behavior across. all the settings in which he or she lives, works, and learns. The CTAB is designed to be used with individuals ages 5–60. The entire CTAB standardization form was administered to over 6,000 individuals with mental retardation. The standardization sample included children, adolescents, and adults in schools, community-based programs, and institutions. Norms are reported as standard scores, percentile ranks, and age equivalents. The CTAB is inappropriate for typically developing individuals, because skills are not sequenced in "normal" developmental order.

Validity studies revealed that the CTAB total score correlated .55 and .38 with the WISC-R (Wechsler, 1974) and Form L-M of the Stanford–Binet Intelligence Scale (Terman & Merrill, 1973), respectively, and .68

with the Vineland Social Maturity Scale (Doll, 1965). Interrater reliability coefficients for all CTAB categories, subcategories, and total test ranged from .89 to .99, with a median value of .98. Test–retest reliability coefficients ranged from .81 to .99, with a median value of .95. Internal-consistency correlations (coefficient alpha), provided separately for males and females at seven age levels for each CTAB category, were all uniformly high; they ranged from .78 to .995, with a median correlation of .98. Standard errors of measurement (SEMs) for each CTAB category were reported separately for males and females with mental retardation—for each of seven different age levels (ranges = 5–6 to 19–22 years) of individuals enrolled in school, and for each of seven different age levels (ranges = 10–14 years to 60+ years) of individuals not enrolled in school. The SEMs were generally low, ranging from 1.7 to 5.2 for the school-enrolled sample and 1.9 to 4.8 for the non-school-enrolled sample.

The Comprehensive Test of Adaptive Behavior—Revised (CTAB-R; Adams, 2000a) is designed to assess individuals from birth to age 60. The standardization norms included children, adolescents, and adults in schools, community-based facilities, and residential facilities. Gender-specific items are included (497 male items and 524 female items). No other information is available regarding this revision at this time.

The Normative Adaptive Behavior Checklist (NABC; Adams, 2000b) is a brief descriptive test that quickly identifies individuals with adaptive behavior deficits. The NABC contains 120 items that measure adaptive behaviors across the same six skill areas as the CTAB. It was normed on 6,130 individuals from infancy through age 21; all items were also administered to an additional 6,000 individuals with mental and physical disabilities. The norms are reported as standard scores, percentile ranks, and age equivalents. Validity data reported in the test manual were limited to data collected on the CTAB. Interrater reliability estimates for individual domains and the total test score were high, ranging from .96 to .99. Test–retest reliability coefficients ranged from .79 to .99 (.79 for the Independent Living Skills domain and .99 for Self-Help Skills, Language Concepts and Academic

Skills, and the total score). Internal-consistency correlations (coefficient alpha) were uniformly high, with a median correlation of .985. SEMs were generally quite low (2.1 or less for the subcategories, 4.9 or less for the total domain scores).

The Normative Adaptive Behavior Checklist—Revised (NABC-R; Adams, 2000b) is an updated version of the NABC, using the AAMR (1992) definition of mental retardation. The NABC-R was normed on over 12,000 students with and without mental retardation from birth to age 21. Norms are reported as standard scores, percentile rank scores, and age equivalents. No other information is available at this time regarding the revision.

The Scales of Independent Behavior— Revised (SIB-R) battery (Bruinink, Woodcock, Weatherman, & Hill, 1996) constitutes an individually administered measure of functional independence and adaptive functioning in school, home, employment, and community settings. The SIB-R can be used from early infancy to mature adult levels (80 years of age and older). The instrument is organized into four adaptive behavior skill clusters (Motor, Social Interaction and Communication, Personal Living, and Community Living) and three maladaptive behavior indexes (Internalized, Asocial, and Externalized). A Full Scale score is obtained from the adaptive skill clusters, and a Maladaptive Behavior Index can be derived from the maladaptive behavior indexes. A 40-item short form is available for individuals at any developmental level, and an Early Development scale of adaptive behavior is available for children from early infancy through 6 years old or for older individuals with severe disabilities whose developmental levels are below 8 years of age. The normative data for the SIB-R were gathered from 2,182 individuals in 15 states and more than 60 communities. The norms are given as age equivalents, percentile ranks, and standard scores ($M = 100$, $SD = 15$).

Split-half, test–retest, and interrater reliabilities are reported in the manual. Split-half reliabilities ranged from .84 to .98 for the four adaptive skill clusters and Full Scale scores. Test–retest reliabilities over a 4-week interval ranged from .96 to .98 for the adaptive behavior clusters and from .80 to .83 for the maladaptive behavior indexes. Interrater

reliabilities were based upon independent ratings by teachers and teacher aides. SIB-R cluster and Broad Independence score correlations between raters ranged from .88 to .97. The reliability coefficients for the three maladaptive behavior indexes were .57 (Internalized), .87 (Asocial), and .78 (Externalized). Both construct and criterion-related validity data were reported. There were high correlations (mostly in the .90s) between the original SIB and the SIB-R, except in those areas that were truncated in a particular sample (e.g., motor and toileting skills for adolescents and adults). The authors thus concluded that the earlier validity studies on the original SIB would be generalizable in evaluating the validity of the SIB-R. Analyses indicated that the SIB-R adaptive behavior scores are strong developmental measures of adaptive behavior; most of the coefficients were in the 90s, with the exception of areas with highly restricted score ranges for adolescents and adults. Criterion-related validity was established by correlating the original SIB and the original ABS-S (r's = .66 to .8 1). Correlations between the SIB-R and the Woodcock–Johnson—Revised (WJ-R) Broad Cognitive Ability score ranged from .64 to .82 for all ages without disabilities. Criterion-related validity data were cited in the manual for individuals with disabilities, correlating the SIB and WJ-R cognitive ability scores, with a median correlation of .85. The SIB maladaptive behavior indexes and the Quay–Peterson Revised Behavior Problem Checklist scales showed correlations ranging from –.66 to .12.

The VABS (Sparrow, Balla, & Cicchetti, 1984), mentioned earlier, constitute a revision of the Vineland Social Maturity Scale (Doll, 1935, 1965); they assess the personal and social sufficiency of individuals from birth to adulthood. There are three versions of the VABS: the Interview Edition, Survey Form; the Interview Edition, Expanded Form; and the Classroom Edition. Each version measures adaptive behavior in four domains: Communication, Daily Living Skills, Socialization, and Motor Skills. In addition, the Survey Form and Expanded Form include a Maladaptive Behavior domain. Each form of the VABS requires a respondent familiar with the behavior of the individual to answer behavior-oriented questions posed by a trained interviewer or to complete a questionnaire. The Survey Form contains 297 items administered over a 20- to 60-minute period. The Expanded Form, which takes approximately 60–90 minutes to administer, contains 577 items, including the 297 items of the Survey Form. The Classroom Edition contains 244 items, designed for children from 3 years, 0 months to 12 years, 11 months of age. It provides an assessment of adaptive behavior in the classroom. The form is to be completed by the classroom teacher in approximately 20 minutes.

The Survey Form and Expanded Form of the VABS provide norm-referenced information based on the performance of a representative national standardization sample of about 4,800 disabled and nondisabled individuals. Separate norms are provided for children and adults with mental retardation, emotional disturbances, and physical disabilities. The Classroom Edition was also standardized on a representative sample of about 3,000 students, ages 3 years, 0 months to 12 years, 11 months. The norms are represented as standard scores ($M = 100$ and $SD = 15$) for the four domain scores and for the Adaptive Behavior Composite. National percentile ranks, stanines, and age equivalents are also reported.

Split-half, test–retest, and interrater reliabilities are reported in the manual. Median split-half reliabilities for the Survey Form were as follows: Communication domain, $r_{xx} = .89$; Daily Living Skills domain, $r_{xx} = .90$; Socialization domain, $r_{xx} = .86$; Motor Skills domain, $r_{xx} = .83$; Adaptive Behavior Composite, $r_{xx} = .94$; and Maladaptive Behavior domain, $r_{xx} = .86$. Test–retest reliabilities after a 2- to 4-week interval were in the .80s and .90s for the Survey Form. Interrater reliability coefficients for the Survey Form and Expanded Form ranged from .62 to .75. SEMs ranged from 3.4 to 8.2 over the four domains on the Survey Form and from 2.2 to 4.9 for the Adaptive Behavior Composite. On the Expanded Form, standard errors of measurement ranged from 2.4 to 6.2 over the four domains and from 1.5 to 3.6 for the Adaptive Behavior Composite.

Concurrent validity was established by correlating the VABS with a variety of tests. A correlation of .55 was reported with the original Vineland. Correlations between the Vineland Adaptive Behavior Composite and the K-ABC Mental Processing Composite and Achievement scale were .32 and .37, respectively. Correlations with the WISC or WISC-R were .52 for children with emotional disturbances, .70 for children with visual impairments, and .47 for children with hearing impairments.

BEHAVIORAL/ECOLOGICAL ASSESSMENT

Elements of Behavioral Assessment

Behavioral assessment provides valuable assessment methods for evaluating the educational and psychological needs of those with moderate and severe mental retardation. Behavioral assessment is an approach to gathering data about an individual that emphasizes environmental and/or organismic control over behavior, reliance on direct observation of behavior, the use of multiple assessment methods, and consideration of the temporal and contextual basis within which the target behavior is embedded (Mash, 1979). The methods of behavioral assessment include observation in the natural environment (using event recording, interval recording, duration recording, etc.); the use of permanent products (e.g., accident reports, videotapes of client behavior for future behavior analysis); behavioral checklists of client behavioral excesses and deficits; and the use of enactment analogues (e.g., role playing) (Powers, 1985; Powers & Handleman, 1984).

Behavioral assessment is idiographic in application. Controlling variables, response covariations, and treatment strategies are understood to be specific to the individual (Powers, 1985). This is in contrast to the previously discussed nomothetic assessment (psychometric assessment), which leads to generalizations about an individual's performance in comparison to that of a normative group.

Behavioral assessment has multiple functions, including (1) allowing predictions of future behavior under particular circumstances; (2) facilitating evaluation of specific behavioral excesses, deficits, or skills; (3) transforming vague problems into specific questions; (4) providing information on the individual's resources for change; and (5) serving as a pretreatment measure for the rate of responding (Kanfer & Nay, 1982).

With the use of Kanfer and Saslow's (1969) "stimulus–organism–response–contingencies of reinforcement–consequence" (S-O-R-K-C) analysis, the assessment of children with moderate and severe mental retardation takes on a multidimensional, multisituational focus. Powers (1985) has noted that this model is an improvement over the antecedent–behavior–consequence (A-B-C-) paradigm for these populations, because of the importance of the contingencies and schedules of reinforcement (K) and the organism (O). Attention to organismic variables emphasizes that an individual's physiological conditions and prior learning histories are to be considered in the assessment and treatment planning (Powers & Handleman, 1984).

Behavioral assessment should take on an ecological/systems perspective. First, when assessing the target behavior (the molecular level of assessment), attention should be given to stimulus (S) and consequence (C) variables. Relevant stimulus conditions include time, place, and setting. The next level of analysis is a molar analysis (i.e., an analysis of the molar contexts within which the behavior is embedded is conducted; Powers, 1985). Within these different environments, there may be resources that facilitate or hinder the production or nonproduction of the behavior.

Children with moderate and severe mental retardation exhibit disturbances in developmental rate or sequence of language, motor, cognitive, perceptual, and adaptive functioning; therefore, when one is conducting a behavioral assessment with such a child, attention to both typical and atypical developmental sequences is critical.

Objectives of Behavioral Assessment

The four objectives of behavioral assessment noted by Nelson and Hayes (1981) can provide a framework for the behavioral assessment of moderately and severely retarded children. The four steps are (1) identification of target behaviors; (2) determination of controlling variables, both environmental and organismic; (3) development of the intervention plan; and (4) evaluation of the effects of intervention. Both molecular and molar levels of behavior analysis are integrated into the assessment.

Identification of the Target Behavior

When one is identifying a target behavior, several criteria should be met in the definition of the behavior. The definition should be objective, clear, and complete (Hawkins & Dobes, 1977).

Determination of Controlling Variables

The second step is accomplished by applying the S-O-R-K-C analysis (Kanfer & Saslow, 1969). Three major classes of controlling variables exist: current environmental variables (stimuli and consequences), organismic variables, and contingencies of reinforcement (Nelson & Hayes, 1979). In addition, when one is assessing children with moderate and severe mental retardation, schedules of reinforcement and responses are important.

Stimuli

Stimulus (S) antecedents are those environmental conditions that precede the target behavior and that are presumed to exert some control over emission of the target behavior. These variables can be identified by initially informally recording all events and interactions immediately preceding the target behavior.

Organismic Variables

Organismic (0) variables include biological states, such as hunger, fatigue, health, and sensory acuity (Nelson & Hayes, 1979); genetic, biochemical, or neurological variables (Mash & Terdal, 1997); and prior learning histories (Powers & Handleman, 1984). These variables should be included in the assessment, so that the resultant intervention reflects the specific behavioral excesses or deficits under the control of biological or genetic factors (Powers, 1985).

Responses

The assessment of the child's responses (R) to antecedent or consequent stimuli includes specification of at least five dimensions: frequency, duration, topography, pervasiveness, and magnitude (Powers, 1985).

Contingencies of Reinforcement

Schedules of reinforcement (Ferster & Skinner, 1957) and the contingencies of reinforcement (K) (Kanfer & Saslow, 1969) influence the rate, correctness, durability, topography, or potency of a child's response. Several contingencies of reinforcement are relevant for these populations, including variation of reinforcement (Egel, 1981), stimulus-specific reinforcement (Litt & Schreibman, 1981), variation of intertrial interval (Koegel, Dunlap, & Dyer, 1980), and stimulus variation during the task (Dunlap & Koegel, 1980).

Consequences

Consequences (C) are defined functionally: Reinforcing consequences increase the likelihood that behavior will increase or maintain over time; aversive consequences increase the likelihood that behavior will decrease over time.

A variety of methods can be used to collect data for the S-O-R-K-C analysis, including direct observation, behavioral checklists, archival data, and third-party interviews (Kazdin, 2001; Ollendick & Hersen, 1984; Powers & Handleman, 1984).

Development of an Intervention Plan

The purpose of the third step is to collect information on the various situational contexts within which the target behavior occurs. Several objectives have been identified for this ecological analysis (Kanfer & Saslow, 1969; Powers & Handleman, 1984). These include (1) clarifying the problem situation by determining who supports and who objects to the behavior; (2) assessing reinforcers and punishers that are salient for the child, and determining which individuals have been effective in reinforcing or punishing behavior in the past; (3) assessing the child's developmental status for biological and physical changes that might limit functioning, and the child's social status for affiliations and community resources that might contribute to the acquisition and

maintenance of more adaptive behavior; (4) assessing the extent of self-control, conditions necessary for self-control, and situations (persons, places, events) that cause a breakdown in self-control; (5) assessing social relationships for significant others who elicit appropriate (and inappropriate) behavior, and determining which reinforcers are operative in social situations; and (6) assessing sociocultural and environmental correlates to the target behavior, including prevailing cultural norms and physical environments that elicit appropriate or inappropriate behavior. Failure to account for the ecological resources and constraints may increase the likelihood that interventions will not generalize across persons or settings or maintain over time (Powers, 1985).

Evaluation of the Effects of Intervention

The evaluation occurs both during and after the intervention. The evaluation should include two elements: selection of practical dependent measures, and the choice of an appropriate design (Nelson & Hayes, 1979).

QUALITATIVE-DEVELOPMENTAL ASSESSMENT

Defining Qualitative Assessment

Qualitative assessment differs from psychometric assessment in its non-normative focus; the focus is on analyzing the nature and state of development, not on comparing a child's performance with that of a standardization group. Qualitative and behavioral assessment differ in their focus in that behavioral assessment focuses on functional rather than structural or developmental aspects (Simeonsson, 1986).

Three objectives define those assessment implications unique to the qualitative approach: (1) analysis of cognitive structures, (2) documentation of developmental competence, and (3) identification of stage of functioning.

In qualitative assessment, one analyzes the cognitive structures or processes the child demonstrates to solve problems that are encountered, whether through sensory–motor means or through mental operations. For example, the focus of assessment is not on the child's level of arithmetic achievement, but rather on the operations the child uses to solve problems. In qualitative-developmental assessment, the focus is on the documentation of competence—on describing the characteristics demonstrated by a child, regardless of his or her impairment or disability. Designation of the stages of development is another common feature of theories of qualitative development. Identification of children in terms of stages of functioning is useful descriptively in order to plan developmentally sequenced treatments (Simeonsson, 1986). The usefulness of this approach may be seen with a group of children classified as "severely mentally retarded" who have a homogeneous label, but may in fact be heterogeneous in regard to level of qualitative function.

Selected Measures and Procedures

The number of measures based on qualitative-developmental theories that have been developed into formal instruments is quite limited; however, a plethora of informal measures and procedures have been described in the literature (Simeonsson, 1986).

Cognition

The goal of qualitative assessment of cognition is to identify the nature and level of the child's learning. The domains assessed differ from stage to stage, as they reflect the changing developmental structures of cognition in the child.

The most widely used measure of sensory–motor development is the infant Psychological Development Scale (Uzgiris & Hunt, 1975). The scale covers development in the areas of Object Permanence, Object Means, Limitation, Causality, Objects in Space, and Schemes. Functional levels are defined for each of the areas in terms of one of the six substages of the sensory–motor period. Another instrument that has been applied with this population is the Albert Einstein Scales of Sensori Motor Intelligence (Corman & Escalona, 1969). Three subscales are included: Prehension, Object Permanence, and Spatial Relationships.

Assessment of preoperational development focuses on the emergence of representational competence and its expression, in common as well as unique domains of thought (Simeonsson, 1986). Preoperational reasoning is characterized by intuitive and egocentric thinking, expressed in artificialism, animism, and syncretism. Measures in this area are drawn from the clinical and empirical literature. Piaget's original writings on the child's conception of time (1927/1971), reality (1937/1971), the world (1926/1975), and movement (1946/1971) provide illustrations of clinical interviews and procedures.

Assessment of cognition at the concrete operational level has centered around the "conservation task" developed by Piaget. The conservation task assesses the child's ability to demonstrate the reversibility of thought, inherent in mental operations. In the basic conservation assessment paradigm, equivalence of mass, number, or length, for example, is established for two sets of obejcts by a child. A perceptual transformation is then made of the objects. The child's task is to determine whether the essential quality (mass, number, length) is conserved in spite of the perceptual transformation.

Inhelder (1968) addresses the diagnosis of reasoning in children with mental retardation. Persons who only reach the stage of concrete operations are defined as mildly mentally retarded. Those who only reach the preoperational stage at maturity are defined as moderately or severely retarded; those who do not develop beyond the sensory–motor stage at maturity are defined as profoundly retarded. Persons with mental retardation fail to achieve formal operations at maturity; therefore, no description of the assessment of formal operations is provided within this chapter.

Personal–Social Functioning

The assessment of personal and social characteristics from a qualitative-developmental perspective focuses primarily on the way in which the child constructs social reality (Simeonsson, 1986). At the sensory–motor level, emerging self–other differentiation can be assessed through observation of the child's use of toys (Lowe, 1975). Assessment of personal and social skills at the preoperational and later stages has been conducted with perspective-taking tasks—for example, Urberg and Docherty's (1976) five role-taking tasks, or Secord and Peevers's (1973) person perception interview.

Behavior

The Carolina Record of Individual Behavior (CRIB; Simeonsson, Huntington, Short, & Ware, 1982) was designed to encompass the sensory–motor level of functioning, and therefore is suitable for young children or for those functioning at a very low developmental level. It consists of three sections (A, B, and C); A addresses developmental characteristics, and B and C document behavioral characteristics. The CRIB was derived in part from items on the Infant Behavior Record of the original BSID (Bayley, 1969). The CRIB is an observational measure and can be completed either on the basis of observing the administration of a developmental measure such as the BSID-II (Bayley, 1993), or on the basis of a period of systematic interaction with the child.

A qualitative measure of behavior that includes the sensory–motor stage as well as the preoperational stage is that of peer play development. The child–peer interaction is scored along physical dimensions such as proximity and use of objects, and along social dimensions such as reciprocity and communication (Parten, 1932).

For those individuals functioning at or above the preoperational stage, problem solving is an applicable assessment domain. Shure and Spivack (1972) have developed a measure of problem-solving skills that consists of a series of problem situations described or illustrated to a child, who is then asked to list the steps he or she would take to solve the problem.

Measures such as the Imaginary Audience Scale (IAS; Elkind & Bowen, 1979) may be valuable in the assessment of disabled adolescents and young adults, whose impairments and limited social experiences may contribute to unrealistic perceptions of themselves and their peers. The IAS presents common social situations requiring the respondent to indicate a preferred way of resolving a personal dilemma (e.g., unaffected, accepting, self-conscious). A feature of potential significance for those with mental retardation is that half of the items measure

"abiding self" (permanent traits) and half measure "transient self" (situational factors) (Simeonsson, 1986). Analyses across these dimensions may be useful in identifying the extent to which self-appraisal of adolescents with mental retardation is a function of factors seen as permanent and unchangeable (e.g., impairment) and those seen as situational and changeable (e.g., social experience).

SUMMARY

The present chapter has described psychometric, behavioral/ecological, and qualitative-developmental approaches to the assessment of the moderately and severely mentally retarded. All approaches can be used to assess this population within a variety of domains, including cognition and social–emotional functioning.

The task of assessing children with moderate and severe mental retardation is a challenging one. The assessment process should be guided by flexibility—that is, matching strategies and domains to achieve specific assessment objectives for a particular child. Flexible methodology is necessary to assess the complex individual differences of these populations.

REFERENCES

American Association on Mental Retardation (AAMR). (1992). *Mental retardation: Definition classification, and systems of support* (9th ed.). Washington, DC: Author.

American Psychiatric Association. (1994). *Diagnostic and statistical manual of mental disorders* (4th ed.). Washington, DC: Author.

Adams, G. L. (2000a). *Comprehensive Test of Adaptive Behavior—Revised.* Seattle, WA: Educational Achievement Systems.

Adams, G. L. (2000b). *Normative Adaptive Behavior Checklist—Revised.* Seattle, WA: Educational Achievement Systems.

Anastasi, A. (1968). *Psychological testing* (3rd ed.). New York: Macmillan.

Bayley, N. (1969). *Bayley Scales of Infant Development.* New York: Psychological Corporation.

Bayley, N. (1993). *Bayley Scales of Infant Development—Second Edition.* San Antonio, TX: Psychological Corporation.

Bruinink, R. H., Woodcock, R. W., Weatherman, R.F., & Hill, B. K. (1996). *The Scales of Independent Behavior—Revised.* Chicago: Riverside.

Cone, J., & Hawkins, R. (1977). *Behavioral assessment: New directions in clinical psychology.* New York: Brunner/Mazel.

Corman, H. H., & Escalona, S. K. (1969). Stages of sensorimotor development: A replication study. *Merrill–Palmer Quarterly, 15,* 35 1–361.

Cote, K. S., & Smith, A. (1983). Assessment of the multiply handicapped. In R. T. Jose (Ed.), *Understanding low vision* (pp. 379–401). New York: American Foundation for the Blind.

Doll, E. A. (1935). A genetic scale of social maturity. *American Journal of Orthopsychiatry, 5,* 180–188.

Doll, E. A. (1965). *Vineland Social Maturity Scale.* Circle Pines, MN: American Guidance Service.

Dunlap, G., & Koegel, R. L. (1980). Motivating autistic children through stimulus variation. *Journal of Applied Behavior Analysis, 13,* 619–627.

Efron, M. (1981). Vision assessment and implications. In S. R. Walsh & R. Holzberg (Eds.), *Understanding and educating the deaf–blind/severely and profoundly handicapped* (pp. 73–84). Springfield, IL: Charles C Thomas.

Egel, A. L. (1981). Reinforcer variation: Implications for motivating developmentally disabled children. *Journal of Applied Behavior Analysis, 14,* 345–350.

Elkind, D., & Bowen, R. (1979). Imaginary audience behavior in children and adolescents. *Developmental Psychology, 15,* 36–44.

Ferster, C. B. & Skinner, B. F. (1957). *Schedules of reinforcement.* New York: Appleton-Century-Crofts.

Harrison, P., & Oakland, T. (2000). *Adaptive Behavior Assessment System (ABAS).* San Antonio, TX: Psychological Corporation.

Hawkins, R. P., & Dobes, R. W. (1977). Behavioral definitions in applied behavior analysis: Explicit or implicit. In B. C. Etzel, J. M. Le Blanc, & D. M. Baer (Eds.), *New developments in behavioral research: Theorv. methods, and applications* (pp. 167–188). New York: Wiley.

Inhelder, B. (1968). *The diagnosis of reasoning in the mentally retarded.* New York: Day.

Kamphaus, R. W. (Ed.). (1987). Adaptive behavior [Special issue]. *Journal of Special Education, 21*(1).

Kamphaus, R. W., & Frick, P. J. (1996). *Clinical assessment of child and adoldescent personality and behavior.* Needham Heights, MA: Allyn & Bacon.

Kanfer, F. H., & Nay, W. R. (1982). Behavioral assessment. In G. T. Wilson & C. M. Franks (Eds.), *Contemporarv behavior therapy: Conceptual and empirical foundations* (pp. 367–402). New York: Guilford Press.

Kanfer, F. H., & Saslow, G. (1969). Behavioral diagnosis. In C. M. Franks (Ed.), *Behavior therapy: Appraisal and status* (pp. 417–444). New York: McGraw-Hill.

Kaufman, A. S., & Kaufman, N. L. (1983a). *Kaufman Assessment Battery for Children: Administration and scoring manual.* Circle Pines, MN: American Guidance Service.

Kaufman, A. S., & Kaufman, N. L. (1983b). *Kaufman Assessment Battery for Children: Interpretive manual.* Circle Pines, MN: American Guidance Service. th

Kazdin, A. E. (2001). *Behavior modification in applied setting* (6th ed.). Belmont, CA: Wadsworth/Thomson.

Koegel, R. L., Dunlap, G., & Dyer, K. (1980). Intertrial interval duration and learning in autistic children. *Journal of Applied Behavior Analysis, 13,* 91–96.

Kravitz, H., & Boehm, J. J. (1971). Rhythmic habit patterns in infancy: Their sequence, age of onset and frequency. *Child Development, 42,* 399–413.

Lambert, N., Nihira, K., & Leland, H. (1993). *AAMR Adaptive Behavior Scale—School* (2nd ed.). Austin, TX: Pro-Ed.

Litt, M. D., & Schreibman, L. (1981). Stimulus-specific reinforcement in the acquisition of receptive labels by autistic children. *Analysis and Intervention in Developmental Disabilities, 1,* 171–186.

Lowe, M. (1975). Trends in the development of representative play. *Journal of Child Psychology and Psychiatry, 16,* 35–47.

Mash, E. J. (1979). What is behavioral assessment? *Behavioral Assessment, 1,* 23–29.

Mash, E. J., & Terdal, L. G. (Eds.). (1997). *Behavioral assessment of childhood disorders* (3rd ed.). New York: Guilford Press.

Miller, L. J. (1988). *Miller Assessment for Preschoolers.* San Antonio, TX: Psychological Corporation.

Nelson, R. O., & Hayes, S. C. (1979). Some current dimensions of behavioral assessment. *Behavioral Assessment, 1,* 1–16.

Nelson, R. O., & Hayes, S. C. (1981). Nature of behavioral assessment. In M. Hersen & A. Bellack (Eds.), *Behavioral assessment: A practical handbook* (2nd ed., pp. 3–37). New York: Pergamon Press.

Ollendick, T. H., & Hersen, M. (1984). An overview of child behavioral assessment. In T. H. Ollendick & M. Hersen (Eds.), *Child behavioral assessment: Principles and procedures* (pp. 3–19). New York: Pergamon Press.

Powers, M. D. (1985). Behavioral assessment and the planning and evaluation of intervention for developmentally disabled children. *School Psychology Review, 14,* 155–161.

Powers, M. D., & Handleman, J. 5. (1984). *Behavioral assessment of severe developmental disabilities.* Rockville, MD: Aspen.

Parten, M. B. (1932). Social participation among preschool children. *Journal of Abnormal and Social Psychology, 27,* 243–269.

Piaget. J. (1971). *The child's conception of movement and speed.* New York: Ballantine Books. (Original work published 1946)

Piaget, J. (1971). *The child's conception of time.* New York: Ballantine Books. (Original work published 1927)

Piaget. J. (1971). *The construction of reality in the child.* New York: Ballantine Books. (Original work published 1937)

Piaget. J. (1975). *The child's conception of the world.* Totowa, NJ: Littlefield, Adams. (Original work published 1926)

Secord, B. H., & Peevers, P. F. (1973). Developmental changes in attributions of descriptive concepts to persons. *Journal of Personality and Social Psychology, 27,* 120–128.

Shure, M., & Spivack, G. (1972). Means–ends thinking, adjustment, and social class among elementary school-aged children. *Journal of Consulting and Clinical Psychology, 38,* 348–353.

Siegel Causey, E. & Allinder, R. M. (1998). Using alternative assessment for students with severe disabilities: Alignment with best practices. *Education and Training in Mental Retardation and Development Disabilities, 33,* 168–178.

Simeonsson, R. J. (1986). *Psychological and developmental assessment of special children.* Boston: Allyn & Bacon.

Simeonsson, R. J., Huntington, G. S., Short, R. J., & Ware, W. (1982). The Carolina Record of Individual Behavior: Characteristics of handicapped infants and children. *Topics in Early Childhood Special Education, 2,* 43–55.

Sparrow, S., Balla, D., & Cicchetti, D. (1984). *Vineland Adaptive Behavior Scales.* Circle Pines, MN: American Guidance Service.

Stillman, R., & Battle, C. (1986). Developmental assessment of communicative abilities in the deaf–blind. In D. Ellis (Ed.), *Sensory impairments in mentally handicapped people* (pp. 319–335). San Diego, CA: College-Hill Press.

Stinnett, T. A., Fuqua, D. R., & Coombs, W. T. (1999). Construct validity of the AAMR Adaptive Behavior Scale—School: 2. *School Psychology Review, 28,* 31–43.

Taylor, R. L. (1985). Measuring adaptive behavior: Issues and instruments. *Focus on Exceptional Children, 18*(2), 1–8.

Terman, L. M., & Merrill, M. A. (1973). *Stanford–Binet Intelligence Scale: 1972 norms edition.* Boston: Houghton Mifflin.

Thorndike, R. L., Hagen, E. P. & Sattler, J. M. (1986). *Stanford–Binet Intelligence Scale: Fourth Edition.* Chicago: Riverside.

Touwen, B. C. L., & Kalverboer, A. F. (1973). Neurological and behavioral assessment of children with minimal brain dysfunction. *Seminars in Psychiatry, 5,* 79–94.

Urberg, K. A., & Docherty, E. M. (1976). Development of role-taking skills in young children. *Developmental Psychology, 12,* 198–204.

Uzgiris, I. C., & Hunt, J. (1975). *Ordinal Scales of Intellectual Development.* Urbana: University of Illinois Press.

Wechsler, D. (1974). *Wechsler Intelligence Scale for Children—Revised.* New York: Psychological Corporation.

Wechsler, D. (1991). *Wechsler Intelligence Scale for Children—Third Edition.* San Antonio, TX: Psychological Corporation.

Widaman, K. F., Stacy, A. W., & Borthwick-Duffy, S. A. (1993). Construct validity of dimensions of adaptive behavior: A multitrait–multimethod evaluation. *American Journal on Mental Retardation, 98,* 219–234.

Witt, J., & Martens, B. (1984). Adaptive behavior: Tests and assessment issues. *School Psychology Review, 13,* 478–484.

28

Assessment of Children for Intervention Planning Following Traumatic Brain Injury

BARBARA A. ROTHLISBERG
RIK C. D'AMATO
BLANCA N. PALENCIA

Brain trauma is the leading cause of death and disability in industrialized nations. In the United States alone, from 1 to 3 million individuals per year suffer some type of brain injury. About 10% of those injured experience long-term impairment in functioning, with a higher percentage encountering some shorter-term difficulty in communication, thinking, and/or an aspect of daily living (Kraemer & Blacher, 1997; Ylvisaker & Feeney, 1998). Of those individuals recovering from traumatic brain injury (TBI), a significant proportion are children and adolescents who, having survived accidents or abusive situations, must then deal with potential changes in their academic and social skills. Before 1990—when TBI was recognized as a category of exceptional educational need in PL 101-476, the Individuals with Disabilities Education Act (IDEA) of 1990—children who had an acquired brain injury and showed persistent educational difficulties were served under other educational disability classifications. These classifications included learning disabilities, emotional disturbances, mental disabilities, other health impairments, or physical disabilities; students received related services under those categories. Unfortunately, often

this assistance was unable to address the scope and sequence of the students' expected course of recovery (Waaland & Kreutzer, 1988). Since recognition of TBI as an educational disability, the numbers of students so designated has increased steadily. For example, between academic years 1993–1994 and 1994–1995, the U.S. Department of Education noted a 33% increase in the number of students classified as having TBI (from 5,395 to 7,188 students ages 6–21; U.S. Department of Education, 1996). Although listed as only 0.1% of the total number of students identified, the fact that this group of students is growing indicates that more attention must be paid to the assessment and treatment of learners with TBI within a school setting. The diversity of cognitive strengths and weaknesses associated with brain damage, and the unique patterns of recovery possible within this group, make students with TBI particularly challenging to current educational practice (Blake & Fewster, 2001; Lehr, 1990). TBI can cause an enduring disability that needs ongoing educational evaluation and modification of the methods of instruction to help students adapt to the expectations of the school setting. Unfortunately, there is no one common need or impairment shared by individuals with TBI; it may be more a category of etiology than a category of disability (Ylvisaker, 1993).

DEFINITIONS ASSOCIATED WITH TBI

"TBI" is usually defined as brain damage occurring after birth because of accidents, assaults, and/or abuse, whereas damage caused by infections, tumors, metabolic disorders, toxins, and/or anoxic injuries is referred to as "nontraumatic brain injury" (Savage & Wolcott, 1994). Some professionals prefer to use the term "acquired brain injury" instead of "TBI," because they think that the term "acquired" clarifies the difference between children born with congenital or degenerative brain conditions and those who are affected later (Kolb & Whishaw, 1990; Lezak, 1995; Savage & Wolcott, 1994). Whatever one's preference for a specific definition, federal law currently excludes congenital and degenerative brain injury and birth trauma from the educationally related TBI designation. Students with nontraumatic brain injury may qualify for special education services under the educational diagnostic category of "other health impairments."

Classifications of Head Injury

Head injury is often classed as either "open" or "closed." (Although individuals who have suffered a head injury do not always have a brain injury, for purposes of this discussion the terms "brain injury" and "head injury" are used synonymously.) Open head injury involves the penetration of the dural lining that covers and protects the brain by either a missile (bullet) or a depressed skull fracture, resulting in localized damage (Blosser & DePompei, 1994). Closed head injury (CHI) is nonpenetrating and usually follows a blunt blow to the skull. Often two subtypes of CHI are identified: "nonacceleration" and "acceleration" injuries. Nonacceleration injuries are less common and require a moving object to strike a stationary skull (e.g., a baseball striking a spectator at a game). Because the head is not itself in motion, the damage is typically less severe in nonacceleration head

injuries than in acceleration injuries. Acceleration (and deceleration) injuries arise when the moving skull is suddenly shifted (as in "shaken baby syndrome" or in vehicular accidents) (Blosser & DePompei, 1994; Ylvisaker & Feeney, 1998). Such sudden shifts can cause the brain to compress against the inside of the skull at the site of impact and at the opposite side of the skull as the brain bounces back from the initial impact point.

When acceleration (and deceleration) injuries occur, damage and its effects can be more difficult to predict. Rotational as well as linear forces on the shifting brain inside the skull can increase the likelihood of injury. For example, the frontal lobes are extremely vulnerable in CHI. The sharp inner ridges of the skull can cause shearing injuries to cerebral tissue. The twisting and tearing of tissue can damage nerve axons, disrupting neural connections. Axonal damage may not be observed on typical brain scans. Such diffuse damage often results in coma (Blosser & DePompei, 1994). Given the interconnectedness of neural systems in the brain, the impairments following this type of traumatic injury can include decreased ability to process information, difficulty focusing attention, slowed speech and motoric responses, and difficulty in integrating and organizing information (Blosser & DePompei, 1994; Kurlychek, Boyd, & Walker, 1997; Stratton & Gregory, 1994; Ylvisaker & Feeney, 1998). This type of cellular damage can also explain the diversity of impairments observed in individuals with TBI; no two individuals will experience the same type and degree of diffuse neural damage (Blosser & DePompei, 1994; Kurlychek et al., 1997; Ylvisaker & Feeney, 1998).

Aside from the injury site, other factors can affect later development and function in children who experience TBI. These secondary events complicate the initial trauma. These include hemorrhage or disruption in cerebral blood flow, brain swelling, hypoxia, and seizure activity, as well as other injuries elsewhere to the body. The extent to which these secondary events occur or are controlled affect expected recovery (Bigler, 1990; Blosser & DePompei, 1994; Rosenthal & Ricker, 2000; Ylvisaker & Feeney, 1998). Two commonly used methods of gauging the severity of brain injury are the presence of coma (its depth and duration) and posttraumatic amnesia (PTA—the elapsed time between the injury and an individual's recovery of continuous memory; Hynd & Willis, 1988; Lezak, 1995). Injured individuals who do not experience coma, or who are comatose only briefly, usually display less residual damage than individuals who experience lengthy comas or PTA. Other meaningful prognostic indicators include age at injury, premorbid intelligence, psychiatric history, and any abnormal neuroradiological and/or neurological findings (Bigler, 1990; Johnson, 1992; Lezak, 1995; Rosenthal & Ricker, 2000). An awareness of prognostic indications is important for school personnel, because they will help to define how the injury may be expected to influence the child's future academic and interpersonal behavior. Type and severity of injury, the child's premorbid adjustment and age at injury, the length of recovery, and the child's current medical status are all factors in the educational consequences a cerebral trauma may cause for a child (Bigler, 1990; Cronin, 2001; Medical Economics Data, 1993).

Some investigators have suggested that the risk of TBI is not random but may be related to the premorbid characteristics of the children so affected. That is, many children who later experience TBI were characterized before the injury as exhibiting some learning difficulties, impulsivity, or hyperactivity. An individual child's preference for higher-risk behaviors may increase the probability that trauma can occur; however, even under these circumstances, there is no behavioral or personality profile that assures no risk of such an injury (Blosser & DePompei, 1994; Kraemer & Blacher, 1997; Ylvisaker & Feeney, 1998).

Consequences of Brain Injury

The cognitive and behavioral consequences of brain injury during the developmental period are complicated by the expected maturation of the central nervous system and the types of traumas to which children are exposed. In infancy (when head injury due to shaking and falls is most common), the growth and changes in brain structure are rapid, and the most functional and concrete cognitive abilities are established. Later in life, when cognition begins to shift to more complex and abstract activities, vehicular accidents are the most common causes of brain damage. The nature and the timing of the cerebral insult may disrupt the normal progression of cerebral development in unpredictable ways (Haley, Cioffi, Lewin, & Baryza, 1990). This means that "the injured brain is no longer normal and one cannot assume that any changes taking place will be just like those seen in normally developing brains" (Johnson, 1992, p. 404). Severity and location of the brain lesion(s) (affecting cortical and/or subcortical areas) will influence a child's prognosis, particularly if the frontal lobes are compromised in some way (Lezak, 1995; Prigatano, 1987). Most severe changes in cerebral integrity will alter all areas of the student's life (e.g., home, school, community, interpersonal) (Begali, 1994; Cronin, 2001; Utah TBI Task Force, 1994).

Unfortunately, much of what is understood about brain–behavior relations is based on adult models (Fletcher & Taylor, 1984); however, injury during nervous system development can have greater ramifications for a child's prognosis than it can for an adult's (Lehr, 1990). There is less predictability between severity of damage and long-term recovery when children are injured than when adults are injured. Some children with generalized and apparently severe damage show few residual behavioral difficulties, whereas others with seemingly limited damage experience profound academic and adaptive problems (Fletcher & Taylor, 1984; Stratton & Gregory, 1994). In addition, early injury can disrupt the acquisition of more complex cognitive behaviors—almost as if the bridge between foundational abilities and more sophisticated learning capacities has been severed. Early damage may not even yield observable difficulties until the function associated with the damaged area is supposed to mature (Cronin, 2001; Lehr, 1990; Russell, 1993; Waaland & Kreutzer, 1988; Ylvisaker & Feeney, 1998).

After severe injury, students with TBI will show unique patterns of disturbance in thinking and behavior. Again, depending on the site and extent of injury, executive functioning, memory, attention, reasoning, language, motor skills, and control of emotional behavior may be impaired. Ylvisaker and Feeney (1998) have particularly emphasized the range of executive functions that may be compromised due to diffuse axonal damage. They define "executive functions" as "those responsible for regulating all aspects of deliberate, nonautomatic, nonroutine behavior" (p. 53). Such impairments will present challenges to an affected student's learning in ways neither the student nor the school can fully anticipate (Ylvisaker et al., 2001).

Executive Function Impairments

Because the axons in and between frontal and limbic areas of the brain are often affected in CHI, and because the executive functions on which the individual depends for mature strategic behavior develop in frontal areas, the importance of evaluation and treatment planning related to executive skills is paramount (Ylvisaker & Feeney, 1998). Goal setting, planning and organizing, problem solving, and the ability to evaluate one's own performance have all been identified as potential deficit areas in cases of severe TBI (Blosser & DePompei, 1994; Ylvisaker & Feeney, 1998). Related to these mechanisms of purposeful action can be impairments in initiation and inhibition. Initiation deficits involve the learner's inability to act in a social or cognitive situation even when he or she possesses the necessary knowledge of rules and procedures that would lead to a successful response, whereas inhibition deficits can result in socially inappropriate behavior, impulsiveness, and disorganized responses in both behavior and communication (Stratton & Gregory, 1994; Ylvisaker & Feeney, 1998). The effects of the loss of the ability to initiate or inhibit action cannot be understated. First, if a child was injured in early childhood, difficulty in these behavioral responses and in other aspects of executive function may not be anticipated; the frontal areas of the brain mature later than other areas, supporting the findings of delayed impairment in TBI. Second, difficulties in initiation and inhibition may be misdiagnosed as due to other causes (ranging from laziness to conduct disorder), leading to inappropriate and unsuccessful interventions (Ylvisaker & Feeney, 1998).

Memory Impairments

The functional capacity of memory is commonly affected by TBI (Kraemer & Blacher, 1997). For example, memory for facts and basic knowledge (declarative memory), and even the consciousness that an event or instructional situation has occurred (explicit memory), are particularly vulnerable to injury. The result of damage may be most telling in the difference between remote memory (for information learned/events occurring before the injury) and recent memory (for information presented/events occurring since injury). Students with TBI may not be able to remember multistep directions or consolidate new learning. Also, they may need help to retrieve information in long-term storage (Blosser & DePompei, 1994; Kraemer & Blacher, 1997). Many children with TBI can do well on measures of previous learning; however, they may be limited in their comprehension of current and future learning opportunities (Cronin, 2001; Kraemer & Blacher, 1997; Ylvisaker & Feeney, 1998).

Attentional Difficulties

Attentional skills can be characterized in several ways; however, TBI often causes youngsters to have problems in sustaining their awareness of learning situations, and also in dividing their attention between tasks (e.g., listening and taking notes) (Kraemer & Blacher, 1997). Besides issues of focus, the students may have difficulty with distractibility and with filtering out nonessential stimulation from the learning situation (Blosser & DePompei, 1994). When considered together with impulsivity and other frontal lobe problems, students who experience deficits in attention and arousal will have a difficult time completing academic tasks successfully.

Reasoning Deficits

Strongly related to executive functioning, reasoning difficulties can make students with TBI particularly vulnerable to academic failure. Students are likely to be confused when they return to school, because the learning process is "different" from their earlier experiences. Students with TBI may show gaps in their understanding of concepts; they may seem able to handle complex material, when in fact basic skills have been disrupted (Ylvisaker, Szekeres, & Hartwick, 1994). Some cognitive abilities will be preserved, whereas others may be severely disrupted, adding a variability to the students' aptitude for integrating and solving problems that probably was not present premorbidly (Kraemer & Blacher, 1997).

Language Impairments

Children with TBI may experience a host of language and communication problems, from difficulty in name retrieval and fluency of speech to difficulty in pragmatic communication skills. Stratton and Gregory (1994) have emphasized that effective communication is a "brain-wide" process and is not restricted to left-hemisphere integrity. Instead, nonverbal (i.e., ability to read facial expressions), emotional, and verbal skills all influence communicative success. According to Stratton and Gregory, some researchers suggest that individuals with TBI exhibit deficits more associated with language "use" than with "form." That is, students with TBI may appear to understand phonology and grammar adequately, but show persistent difficulty in organizing their own speech or comprehending correctly the connected discourse of others (Blosser & DePompei, 1994; Stratton & Gregory, 1994; Ylvisaker & Feeney, 1998).

Motor Impairments

Movement difficulties often accompany brain damage. Spasticity (muscle tightness), tremor, and problems with coordinated sequences of movement of both fine and gross motor muscle groups can affect students' fluidity of movement in things like walking, writing, and forming speech sounds (Cronin, 2001; Kraemer & Blacher, 1997).

Emotional/Behavioral Difficulties

As noted, the complexity of connections between cortical and subcortical brain areas can allow serious brain trauma to manifest its effect across multiple systems. When areas of the brain involved with emotion, reasoning, memory, and planning are influenced by an injury, impulsivity, aggressiveness, disinhibition, and emotional lability can result. Thus typical methods of discipline can be ineffective, because a student with TBI does not associate his or her behavior with dictated consequences, or even recall or connect past behavioral sequences with the current situation (Blake & Fewster, 2001; Kraemer & Blacher, 1997). In addition, the child's loss of his or her sense of subjective self (the preinjury self) can be confusing and pronounced. Poor awareness of social situations, problems with language comprehension, inappropriate actions or comments, and other changes in response can lead to modified reactions by friends and teachers. The behavioral and emotional consequences of TBI are probably the most obvious and troubling for the child and for significant others (e.g., parents, siblings, peers, teachers) (Cronin, 2001; Kraemer & Blacher, 1997; Kreutzer, Serio, & Bergquist, 1994; Stratton & Gregory, 1994; Ylvisaker & Feeney, 1998).

TBI presents a challenge to all stakeholders in the educational process. The student with TBI may present with multidimensional learning needs, because the brain operates as a functional system where neural connections tie together structures engaged in everything from autonomic activities to planful integration of new information with stored knowledge. The consequences of injury depend on such variables as age, personality, recovery time, and support systems, as well as on actual damage to the brain. Recovery is uncharted, because all individuals have unique patterns of injury. Given all these factors, treatment of students with TBI offers different challenges to family and educational institutions than does treatment of "nonacquired" disabilities. The pace of recovery for students with TBI is expected to slow dramatically after 18–36 months postinjury; however, new learning needs may appear years later as expected maturation of cerebral structures is impeded by residual damage. Consequently, educational plans for these students may need frequent revision to insure successful academic growth. Similarly, repeated assessments of learning capabilities may be needed to monitor changes in skills and the effectiveness of instructional techniques (Cohen, 1986; Cronin, 2001; Lehr, 1990).

NEUROPSYCHOLOGICAL ASSESSMENT OF CHILDREN WITH TBI

When a neurologically based condition (such as TBI) exists, the emphasis for evaluation shifts from specific diagnosis to considerations for long-term treatment, both educationally and for functional life skills. Sophisticated imaging techniques such as computerized tomography (CT) imaging, magnetic resonance imaging (MRI), and functional magnetic resonance imaging (FMRI) all have helped in understanding the association of structural damage in brain injury with later behavioral differences. However, though imaging technology has improved the understanding of brain–behavior relations, the particular pattern of strengths and weaknesses that an individual will exhibit will not be evident from those procedures alone. Instead, more traditional neuropsychological and psychoeducational test score patterns and the learner's reaction to the assessment setting may better establish the actual extent of damage and degree of disability the student will experience. Neuropsychologically oriented testing can elaborate on the individual's capacity in many functional areas (e.g., problem solving, memory) and help with educational programming (Kurlychek et al., 1997).

A Psychometric or Quantitative Approach to Assessment Data

Traditionally, neuropsychologists identified themselves as belonging to certain schools or taking certain approaches to clinical data (Mapou, 1995). A psychometric, product-oriented, or quantitative approach to neuropsychology uses standard performance data to assess individuals within and across all the functional domains to be measured, by comparing the findings to those for a normative group (Lezak, 1995). This actuarial interpretation is designed to detect whether an individual's performance is discrepant from that of others who are performing within the normal range. Patterns of performance are usually considered in four ways (Jarvis & Barth, 1994; Reitan & Wolfson, 1985; Selz, 1981): (1) level of performance (relative to normative standards); (2) pattern of performance (uniqueness of strengths and weaknesses); (3) lateral differ-

ences (comparisons of motor, sensory, and hemispheric differences for each side); and (4) pathognomonic signs (indications of abnormal responses or brain damage). Proponents of this school typically recommend a standard or fixed battery of tests in order to analyze an individual's strengths and weaknesses. Battery assessment—as with the various forms of the Halstead–Reitan Neuropsychological Battery (HRNB) (e.g., Halstead–Reitan Neuropsychological Test Battery, Halstead–Reitan Neuropsychological Battery for Older Children, Reitan–Indiana Test Battery; Reitan & Wolfson, 1985; Teeter & Semrud-Clikeman, 1997) or the Luria–Nebraska Neuropsychological Battery (LNNB; Golden, 1981, 1989)—involves the same set of subtests or instruments for each person tested (Hynd & Semrud-Clikeman, 1990; Hynd & Willis, 1988). This standard battery format insures that all significant behavioral domains are covered in the assessment and that results can be interpreted within set guidelines, because a battery offers a normative data base to which test profiles can be compared (Reitan & Wolfson, 1995). The HRNB family of measures is arguably the most commonly used with adults and children. It includes tests that were chosen according to their ability to predict brain dysfunction (Teeter & Semrud-Clikeman, 1997).

A Qualitative Approach to Assessment Data

A purely qualitative approach to neuropsychological assessment sees the scope and purpose of assessment in a different light. Practitioners recognize the range of diversity in individual performance on neuropsychological and common psychological tests and techniques, and use that individuality to guide assessment. A classic proponent of the qualitative approach, Luria (1980), viewed assessment from a case study perspective. A set of unique and individualized procedures, questions, or tasks geared to the specifics of the case shaped Luria's evaluation process (for an outline of Luria's method, see Hynd & Semrud-Clikeman, 1990). Luria was interested in how brain damage could disrupt or alter the functional system of organization he had proposed, and he used his process-oriented techniques to direct his hypotheses about his patients (Luria, 1973, 1980).

Luria emphasized that a functional systems approach best explains brain activity. Complex cognitive processes are actually based on systems of connections organized throughout various levels of the nervous system. Within such a "functional complex," the learner's response to a given stimulus may be channeled along many axonal routes, depending on the established neural pathways of the individual. Thus function no longer could be assigned to a particular structure or group of cells in the brain, but was viewed as the result of an adaptable system of elements that could be interchangeable, depending on the situation (Luria, 1973, 1980). Luria proposed a functional pluripotentialism of brain structures. This suggests that no cell aggregate or structure in the brain is solely responsible for a specific function, but that structures systematically interconnect with other systems and play a role in multiple types of tasks. Thatcher and John (1977) conceived of this nervous system arrangement as a mosaic engaged in analyzing input and planning action, and as a system of interconnections whose purpose is to establish balance between the individual and his or her environment.

Luria described the functional systems of the brain in terms of three basic units. The first unit is primarily concerned with energy level or wakefulness. It consists of the upper and lower portions of the brain stem, particularly the reticular formation. This unit is intended to adjust cortical tone so that stimuli are adequately filtered or perceived. Injury to this unit may cause attentional problems, disorganization, or sleep disruptions (Teeter & Semrud-Clikeman, 1997). The second unit involves the analysis, storage, and coding of information; it includes the temporal, parietal, and occipital regions of the cortex. Within the second unit, functions are developmentally govern and are divided into three zones. Primary zones record sensory information, whereas secondary zones organize and code the inputs. The tertiary zones then integrate and synthesize information from various sources (e.g., vision, hearing, touch). There is hemispheric specialization in the secondary and tertiary zones, so that analysis of language is predominantly a left-hemispheric responsibility, whereas analysis of music may be ascribed more to the right hemisphere. Injury to this unit can involve problems with integration of knowledge and/or memory difficulties. The third unit, the frontal region, is also subdivided into three zones. The primary zone deals with simple motor output; the secondary with sequencing of movements; and the tertiary with planning, organization, and implementation of conscious action. Luria attributed the highest-level functions to the third unit of the brain. It is the last to mature, but has extensive connections to other brain areas (Jørgensen & Christensen, 1995; Teeter & Semrud-Clikeman, 1997). Damage to the frontal regions can disrupt problem solving and/or abilities to initiate or inhibit behavioral sequences.

Luria's hypotheses on brain organization and his study of associated functions have suggested that assessment must be specialized to understand the variations in the behavior of individuals who have experienced brain injury. Unfortunately, with a purely qualitative view of assessment, the psychometric rigor available to quantitative methods is lost. Efforts to standardize the Lurian method of analysis (e.g., the LNNB) have not been entirely successful (Teeter & Semrud-Clikeman, 1997).

A Flexible Approach to Neuropsychological Assessment

Frankly, a flexible approach to assessment that combines elements of purely quantitative and qualitative aspects of case material when TBI is involved is likely to offer the best overall picture of a child's status and potential learning ability (Mapou, 1995). Because children show distinctive patterns of learning and behavioral characteristics, it is improbable that any given test (or even battery of tests), in isolation, can capture the range of skills exhibited by an individual. For example, it has been noted that TBI often affects the frontal areas of the brain that are involved with executive functions (e.g., planning, organizing, and initiating action). Executive functions are difficult to isolate and focus on with standardized test procedures; supplemental "real-world" exercises may be the only way to truly understand the extent to which such brain functions have been affected by trauma (Kurlychek et al., 1997).

Similarly, because severe brain trauma can influence all aspects of an individual's life, it is important to understand the contexts in which the person must function to make predictions about behavior or plan rehabilitation or treatment options (McCaffrey & Puente, 1992; Rosenthal & Ricker, 2001; Teeter & Semrud-Clikeman, 1997). Teeter and Semrud-Clikeman (1997) have articulated the need for a broad-band view of the assessment of children with their transactional model of neuropsychological assessment. The transactional model frames the description of a brain trauma and its behavioral consequences within the context of the learner's previous adjustment, expected developmental changes, and the quality of interpersonal supports available (e.g., family, community, school) (Blosser & DePompei, 1991, 1994). The approach recognizes that the individual is in constant interaction with the external world, so any intervention—be it medical, pharmacological, academic, or behavioral—must be seen in an ecological context (Teeter & Semrud-Clikeman, 1997).

Data on the functioning of different cognitive and behavioral systems provide vital information to school psychologists and other professionals who must plan rehabilitation programs for children with TBI in schools and assist families in adapting to these children. Conclusions drawn by clinicians from assessment information will guide the interventions recommended. D'Amato, Rothlisberg, and Leu Work (1999) have pointed out that the value of any evaluation is grounded in its ability to offer effective interventions that help a child to function better in both academic and social situations. The knowledge gained from neuropsychologically related instruments enriches and broadens the standard evaluations given in educational settings, so that not only is a baseline of intellectual and academic achievement available, but a clearer understanding of perceptual, memory, and processing potentials is possible. The performance results from neuropsychological measures can suggest strategies to help maximize the learner's cognitive and behavioral strengths and ac-

complish important educational objectives (Hartlage & Reynolds, 1981).

Behavioral Systems to Be Assessed

Different authors have recommended different subsets of systems for neuropsychological analysis. According to Luria (1980), an evaluation has to be comprehensive and must measure the full range of abilities subserved by the brain. The systems provided in Table 28.1 are useful when developing interventions in academic settings. Evaluation of these cognitive and behavioral systems is assisted with the use of neuropsychological and psychological tests. A partial listing of measures that can be used to examine children's ability to function in academic and social settings is available in Table 28.2. Assessment should consist of a range of techniques: review of records, direct observation of the learner in classroom and social settings, interviews with the student and involved adults, and both objective and subjective measures. Multiple sources of information (e.g., student, parent, teacher) and multiple settings (incorporating home, school, and community sites) should be considered (Sachs, 1991; Utah TBI Task Force, 1994).

Dynamic Assessment of Learner Capacities

Although the student's scores on standardized instruments can give useful information about the differences between the student's premorbid and postinjury abilities in terms of the knowledge retained, test scores often do not predict actual classroom performance by students with TBI (Harrington, 1990; Waaland & Kreutzer, 1988; Ylvisaker et al., 2001). Standardized testing is controlled by the examiner, who presents consistent, well-defined tasks to the examinee. The regimentation of the standardized procedures offers clearly articulated expectations for the learner—something that is not typically the case in a normal classroom environment. In an uncontrolled classroom situation, students with TBI can quickly overload on information and learning expectations. They are often uncertain about how to organize their time or the information being presented to them. Gaps in knowledge caused by injury can also exacerbate the students' uncertain-

TABLE 28.1. Systems to Be Formally and Informally Assessed in Neuropsychological Evaluations for TBI

System	Components
Sensory-perceptual abilities	Visual, auditory, tactile/kinesthetic, integrated (two or more components concurrently)
Motor functions	Fine motor, gross motor, strength, coordination, lateral preference
Intellectual/cognitive abilities	*Verbal functions:* Language, reasoning, memory, learning, numerical ability, integrative functioning
	Nonverbal functions: Perceptual organization, reasoning, memory, learning, integrative functioning, spatial manipulation and construction
Processing	Visual, motoric, auditory, spatial, linguistic/verbal, simultaneous, sequential
Communication and language	Receptive and expressive vocabulary, speech and language level, written language
Academic achievement	Preacademic skills, reading decoding and comprehension, mathematical calculations and reasoning
Personality/behavior/family	*Adaptive behavior:* Daily living, development, play/recreation
	Social environment: Parental and sibling relationships, community relationships
Environmental fit	Learner coping style, frustration tolerance, learning environment, peer and community reactions, learner competencies, teacher and staff knowledge, teacher and staff reactions

Note. Based on D'Amato & Rothlisberg (1997) and D'Amato, Rothlisberg, and Rhodes (1997).

ty. Therefore, to detect the degree of actual learning difficulties that a student with TBI is experiencing, modifications of testing procedures and testing the limits of performance are recommended (Clark & Hostetter, 1995; Cohen, 1986; Harrington, 1990; Ylvisaker et al., 1994). Some modifications include the following:

- Changing instructions to include more prompts or clues to the problem solution.
- Changing response mode (visual or verbal; recall or recognition).
- Varying environmental noise or distractors.
- Varying difficulty level of task to determine frustration tolerance.
- Varying abstractness of questions or tasks.
- Assessing response to frequent versus infrequent feedback.

Looking specifically at how well the student can adapt his or her learning skills to the fluid situations commonly present in class-

rooms will give added information to teachers who may not know what to expect about the student's new tolerance for instruction. Information on rate of learning, potential differences in instructional and response mode, tolerance for ambiguity, and response to structured versus unstructured situations may suggest ways in which teaching methods can be adjusted to accommodate the student's needs (Harrington, 1990; Ylvisaker et al., 1994).

An assessment procedure has utility only insofar as it leads to successful interventions. Unfortunately, even with a comprehensive evaluation of behavioral, cognitive, social, emotional, and contextual domains using multiple methods, the translation of data into workable interventions is tenuous at best (Rothlisberg, 1992). Current thinking in the diverse fields of the social sciences acknowledges that an understanding of human learning is multifaceted and contextual. Indeed, theories of learning have moved from a functional orientation through behavioral, information-processing, and cognitive to

TABLE 28.2. Instruments and Procedures Commonly Used to Evaluate Neuropsychological Functions in Students with TBI

System	Instrument/Procedure
Sensory-perceptual abilities	Child and classroom observations; developmental history; mental status examination; Motor-Free Visual Perception Test; Reitan–Kløve Sensory-Perception Examination (from the Halstead–Reitan Neuropsychological Battery, or HRNB); Reitan–Kløve Tactile Form Recognition Test (HRNB); Tactile–Visual (from the Luria–Nebraska Neuropsychological Battery, or LNNB); vision and hearing screenings
Motor functions	Bender–Gestalt Test of Visual–Motor Integration; Detroit Tests of Learning Ability—Third Edition (Motoric Composite); Developmental Test of Visual–Motor Integration; Finger Oscillation Test (HRNB); Grip Strength (HRNB); Kaufman Assessment Battery for Children (K-ABC, Nonverbal scale); McCarthy Scales of Children's Abilities (Motor scale); Motor Skills (LNNB); Purdue Pegboard, Tactile Performance Test (HRNB); Wechsler Intelligence Scale for Children—Third Edition (WISC-III, selected Performance subtests)
Intellectual/cognitive abilities	Battelle Developmental Inventory; Bayley Scales of Infant Development—Second Edition; Category Test (HRNB); Das–Naglieri Cognitive Assessment System; Differential Ability Scales; K-ABC; Kaufman Adolescent and Adult Intelligence Test; WISC-III; Wechsler Adult Intelligence Scale—Third Edition
Attention/concentration/memory	Benton Visual Retention Test—Revised; Children's Auditory Verbal Learning Test—Children's Version; Children's Auditory Learning Test; Detroit Tests of Learning Ability—Third Edition; FULD Object Memory Test; Rey Auditory Verbal Learning Test; Rhythm Test (HRNB); Test of Memory and Learning; Wechsler Memory Scale—Third Edition; Wide Range Assessment of Memory and Learning; Wisconsin Card Sorting Test
Communication and language skills	Aphasia Screening Test (HRNB); Bracken Basic Concepts Scale—Revised; Controlled Oral Word Association (Word Fluency); Peabody Picture Vocabulary Test—Third Edition; Receptive/Expressive Language (LNNB); Revised Token Test; Test of Adolescent Language; Test of Language Development; Test of Written Language
Processing	*Auditory/verbal processing:* Detroit Tests of Learning Ability—Third Edition; Peabody Picture Vocabulary Test—Third Edition; Seashore Rhythm Test (HRNB); Reitan–Kløve Sensory-Perception Examination (HRNB); Speech Sound Perception Test (HRNB) *Visual/spatial processing:* Aphasia Screening Test (HRNB); Detroit Tests of Learning Ability—Third Edition; Matrix Analogies Test; Motor-Free Visual Perception Test; Test of Nonverbal Intelligence—Second Edition; visual acuity screening
Academic achievement	Differential Ability Scales; Kaufman Test of Educational Achievement; Key Math Diagnostic Arithmetic Test—Revised; Peabody Individual Achievement Test—Revised; Reading, Writing, Arithmetic (LNNB); Wechsler Individual Achievement Test; Woodcock Reading Mastery Test—Revised; Woodcock–Johnson Psycho-Educational Battery—III: Achievement
Personality/behavior/family and environmental fit	Behavior Assessment System for Children; Behavior Evaluation Scales; Burks Behavior Rating Scales; Child Behavior Checklist; classroom observations; clinical interview with child or adolescent; Family Environment Scale; home visit and interview; interview with teacher; Minnesota Multiphasic Personality Inventory—2; Personality Inventory for Children; Revised Children's Manifest Anxiety Scale; sentence completion tests; Thematic Apperception Tests; Vineland Adaptive Behavior Scales

Note. Based on D'Amato, Rothlisberg, and Rhodes (1997).

variations of constructivist and sociocultural approaches (Cobb & Yackel, 1990; Mayer, 1996). The idea that learning is purposeful and derives meaning from the individual learner's interactions and previous experiences complicates treatment efforts. A "one size fits all" approach to instructional modification is particularly questionable for students with TBI, because a common pattern of strengths and weaknesses or recovery does not exist (Prigatano, 1990; Ylvisaker & Feeney, 1998; Ylvisaker et al., 2001).

INTERVENTION PLANNING FOR CHILDREN FOLLOWING TBI

Traditionally, the primary focus of clinical neuropsychology has been the identification of patterns of behavioral deficits associated with brain impairment, whereas rehabilitation has focused on the management of deficits to maximize the level of functioning in everyday life activities (e.g., dressing, walking, eating). Particularly in dealing with children with TBI, intervention plans must address not only adaptive skills, but those cognitive and social capacities that let children learn and function in the school and broader community. Unlike injured adults, who are working to recapture disrupted abilities to the greatest extent possible, children with TBI are challenged to develop increasingly sophisticated patterns of behavior despite the presence of central nervous system damage. In these cases, the knowledge available from neuropsychology's understanding of brain–behavior relations must be merged with what is known about rehabilitation and educational practice. All the dimensions or contexts of a child's life come into play when one is testing hypotheses about the best intervention plan to meet the learner's needs (Cronin, 2001; Ylvisaker & Feeney, 1998).

Much of what is known about neuropsychological rehabilitation has involved adult patients. Only recently, with the medical and educational communities' increasing awareness about the incidence of children with TBI, researchers and school practitioners have recognized the potential for rehabilitative services within a school environment. Unfortunately, few studies have addressed the outcome of rehabilitation efforts for children with head trauma (Ewing-Cobbs, Miner, Fletcher, & Levin, 1989; Klonoff, Clark, & Klonoff, 1993). Although one must acknowledge the important differences between the consequences of TBI in children and in adults, the experience gained from the rehabilitation of adult patients has formed the basis from which guidelines for pediatric rehabilitation can be generated. Therefore, understanding rehabilitation in children begins with rehabilitation programs geared toward adults.

Foundations of Rehabilitation

The neuropsychological rehabilitation of adults began in earnest during World War I (Boake, 1991; Teuber, 1966). Goldstein initiated the formal study of cognitive disturbances resulting from cerebral lesions, based on his clinical assessment and rehabilitation of German soldiers suffering from head wounds (Boake, 1991). Luria's work during World War II with Soviet soldiers who had penetrating head wounds furthered the understanding of the cognitive and behavioral consequences of brain trauma, and led him to develop his influential theory of the organization of higher cortical functions (Luria, 1973, 1980).

Luria theorized that the destruction of links between functional units of the brain would disrupt higher mental processes. The degree and type of disruption would depend on the location of the lesion site. The overlapping and interconnected aspects of Luria's functional approach to brain organization helped to explain the diversity of responses to brain trauma witnessed in adults, but it also suggested that partial restoration of lost or damaged abilities could occur if a different "route" or subsystem could be established to transmit information within the brain. Luria's ideas offered a model on which many current techniques in cognitive rehabilitation are based (Ben-Yishay & Diller, 1983; Ben-Yishay & Prigatano, 1990; Christensen & Uzzell, 1987).

Holistic Cognitive Rehabilitation

A holistic approach to rehabilitation advocates that the perspectives of neuropsychology, clinical psychology, psychology, and psychiatry be integrated to help understand the behavioral disturbances resulting from TBI (Prigatano et al., 1986). Both cognitive and personality disturbances are recognized as having a profound influence on a person's ability to return to work and reestablish interpersonal relationships after a severe brain injury has occurred. Therefore, a holistic view of rehabilitation argues that social skill training and psychotherapy should accompany efforts at cognitive treatment (Prigatano, 1990). A pilot program of holistic neuropsychological rehabilitation for soldiers with brain injury was established in Israel in 1974. This treatment program was under the direction of Ben-Yishay (Boake, 1991; Ben-Yishay & Prigatano, 1990), who brought its concept to the United States in 1977, when Ben-Yishay and Diller established the New York University (NYU) Head Trauma Rehabilitation Program. The NYU program has since served as a model for the development of other rehabilitation centers across the country.

Holistic programs such as the NYU Rehabilitation Program focus on areas of functioning that have been found to predict the best outcomes in self-care and daily life functional competence, vocational attainment, and interpersonal skills/social adjustment (Ben-Yishay & Prigatano, 1990). The variables that have best predicted later functioning in this model are the person's ability to control his or her emotional reactions and to interact with others in socially appropriate ways (Ben-Yishay & Prigatano, 1990; Prigatano, 2000).

In the NYU Rehabilitation Program, treatment takes place in a therapeutic community that consists of patients, their families, and the rehabilitation team over the course of a 20-week period. Each period of treatment includes a phase of initial evaluation and intensive treatment, and a phase designed to extend treatment results beyond the confines of the program. Extended treatment emphasizes vocational preparation, so that the chance for productive employment is increased. After successful completion of occupational trials, actual employment and postdischarge follow-up are implemented (Ben-Yishay & Prigatano, 1990).

Prigatano and colleagues (1986) replicated Ben-Yishay's holistic model at the Neuropsychological Rehabilitation Program in Oklahoma. Their approach emphasizes the social milieu as an important factor in patient outcomes. In a social milieu program, individuals with TBI and their families are placed in a therapeutic setting with professional staff members who provide educational and emotional support designed to enhance the patients' cognitive, interpersonal, and social outcomes (Prigatano, 1997). All staffers work together to help individuals with TBI and their families reach their respective goals. Goals may include preparation for improvement in appropriate social interactions, memory strategies, academic skills, family cohesiveness, and occupational proficiency.

Although important, cognitive rehabilitation is only one aspect of holistic rehabilitation (Prigatano, 1997). A holistic approach also includes psychotherapy; establishment of the therapeutic milieu, and formation of a working alliance with patients and their families; education; and protected work trials. Thus the approach attempts to respond to the total cognitive and psychosocial needs of the individual with TBI, and sees that individual within the contexts in which he or she must function.

Ben-Yishay and the NYU group proposed that intervention actually progresses along six clinical/cognitive stages of growth for the individual who has been injured. Stage 1 is engagement, where the goal is to improve the person's alertness, attention, and concentration. Stage 2 focuses on having the individual develop an awareness of the consequences of the brain injury and begin to adjust to the resulting changes. Stage 3 involves the mastering of necessary cognitive tasks, whereas stage 4 offers control of available compensatory strategies. Stage 5 addresses acceptance of the limits of one's ability to compensate and involves reorientation of future expectations. Stage 6 suggests the establishment of an identity that involves the successful resolution of the previous stages (Ben-Yishay & Diller, 1983). Holistic rehabilitation attempts to help the individual resolve the issues surrounding his or her injury and function as adequately as possible in day-to-day settings.

Holistic Rehabilitation in Schools

Fletcher-Janzen and Kade (1997) have proposed adapting the holistic approach to rehabilitation for use with children who have experienced TBI. A holistic view of rehabilitation to pediatric brain injury could be employed in schools, because it not only offers a response to the cognitive and physical changes experienced by students with TBI, but acknowledges the changes in personality, emotionality, and adaptive behavior. Considering neurodevelopmental issues and psychotherapeutic interventions in a school setting would broaden the treatment currently given and would highlight the dynamic interactions that can occur among physical, cognitive, and psychosocial deficits in an educational situation (Fletcher-Janzen & Kade, 1997; Ylvisaker et al., 1994).

If one were to apply a holistic method of treatment to children, a natural context for rehabilitative services would be the school. Children with TBI face many difficulties when reentering schools (Blake & Fewster, 2001; Clark, 1997). However, if the social milieu approach advocated by Prigatano were implemented in an educational setting, the community of service providers (psychologist, counselors, teachers, administrators, and support staff) could help children with TBI and their families to cope better with the cognitive and behavioral consequences of the injury (Farmer, Clippard, Luehr-Wiemann, Wright, & Owings, 1997). Just as Prigatano and colleagues (1986) have argued that psychotherapeutic interventions are needed to deal holistically with adults who have experienced TBI, the psychosocial adjustment of children with TBI will be enhanced if the emotional and cognitive rehabilitation go hand in hand in the school setting. The focus (particularly for younger children) would be the acquisition and retention of academic and social skills, rather than the vocational orientation for adults. Efforts would be made to use compensatory methods in the mastery of both academic and social tasks, to support the child as he or she deals with the long-term changes caused by injury, and to offer opportunities for learning success and reasonable control over decision making.

Ylvisaker and Feeney (1998) offer a version of holistic functional rehabilitation that demonstrates the advantages of a school-based intervention program in meeting the needs of the total learner with TBI. Their functional approach to rehabilitation emphasizes real-world goals in academic, interpersonal, and personal realms; views assessment and intervention as a collaborative enterprise; builds on the individual's existing strengths; pursues growth goals in natural contexts, using naturally occurring interpersonal supports (family, friends, teachers); and strives to make the individual as self-directed and responsible as possible. Interventions feature positive apprenticeship relationships for learning and the creation of a learning environment that supports opportunities for effective problem solving in a range of situations.

The rehabilitative schemes presented offer a general philosophy of intervention that can guide the process that families and schools can undertake when working with students who have experienced TBI. However, other dimensions of intervention can enrich teachers' and other staff members' understanding of the educational process for these students. Teachers may presume that teaching students with TBI is very different from teaching other students, or they may expect that a few well-practiced techniques will "correct" the learning problems that are exhibited. They may not be prepared for the process of discovering workable instructional methodology or the idea that the methods used for teaching may need periodic review to match a student's recovery of function (Madigan, Hall, & Glang, 1997; Todis, Glang, & Fabry, 1997). The best-informed intervention choice is likely to be made after various possible hypotheses about the student's responses to learning tasks or social situations are tested (Ylvisaker & Feeney, 1998). Thus openness to intervention options and awareness of the multidimensionality of treatment programs are useful in programming (Ylvisaker et al., 2001).

The SOS Intervention Model

D'Amato and Rothlisberg (1997) have introduced an approach that can be likened to broad levels of intervention: the "structure, organization, and strategies" (SOS) approach to intervention. The SOS model attempts to allow for the typical responses of students with TBI to the school environment, and to frame the suggestions for addressing student needs at different layers of external versus internal influence. The levels of structure, organization, and strategies are distinguished by the degree of external control or accommodation needed to bring order into the life experiences of students whose injuries have impaired their natural capacity to direct aspects of their learning. "Structure" primarily refers to the degree of physical reorganization dictated for maximal learning, whereas "organization" refers to broad instructional methods used to establish order and relevance to the student's learning setting. "Strategies" are attempts to instruct the student in the benefits of various planning and self-monitoring schemes.

Within each intervention level, suggestions for remediation, adaptation, or alternative method of instruction can be considered and used in interaction with the functional domain under consideration (e.g., memory, attention, academic skill). The student's unique characteristics have to be considered in fashioning an actual educational response.

Structure

TBI can lead to a sense of disorientation, frustration, and low tolerance for environmental change, particularly during the initial months of recovery. As the child struggles to make sense out of his or her altered perception of the world and altered level of competence, greater environmental stability may need to be created to help the student function. Reducing distractions, providing clear expectations for acceptable behavior, and establishing a stable daily routine will allow for a sense of security (Utah TBI Task Force, 1994; Ylvisaker & Feeney, 1998). A secure and consistent environment allows the student to focus attentional resources on the demands of learning, not survival, in the school environment. Reinforced structure can include elements such as the following:

• *A home–school partnership.* Misconceptions about the consequences of cerebral injury in childhood are typical for parents and school personnel alike (Clark, 1997; Todis et al., 1997). Effective school reentry requires that all parties have basic knowl-

edge about the possible effects of the injury. Supportive communication with parents helps the family as the child begins his or her recovery (Cohen, 1986;Waaland & Kreutzer, 1988). A family–school partnership will also help teachers and classmates understand the consequences of an injury (Blake & Fewster, 2001).

• *Work-release programming.* Parents and school staff will need to plan for transition into the working world for adolescents with TBI. Students with learning difficulties may find meaningful employment difficult to secure (Rojewski, 1992; Scuccimarra & Speece, 1990). The day-to-day work routine will need to be discussed and practiced (Ylvisaker & Feeney, 1998). Vocational educators and adult service providers in the community will probably be enlisted to improve the relevance of the student's individual educational plan for long-term vocational adjustment and to act as models and mentors (Reiff & deFur, 1992; Rojewski, 1992; Sachs & Redd, 1993).

• *Teacher stability.* Because continuity of programming is essential, a teaching staff trained to work with students recovering from TBI is important. Students can benefit from working with the same teacher or group of teachers for more than 1 year at a time. Extended time together that fosters trust in the learning environment may be more important than learning the traditional educational content (Savage, 1987).

• *Consistent behavioral routines.* Students with TBI often have difficulty following directions and making use of independent time. Consistency and scheduling reliability can help strengthen self-control (Adams et al., 1991; Harrington, 1990; Telzrow, 1990). Routine is extremely important, as are clear expectations for behavior. Traditional behavioral techniques may not be effective with students who have experienced TBI, because such techniques require children to remember cause–effect relations and often to focus on the behavioral consequences of an action (Cohen, 1986). Ylvisaker and Feeney (1998) have recommended that attention to the antecedents of behaviors can be more important than consequences to behavioral success. Scripts for situations can eliminate uncertainty and return control to a student. Brief, clear rules and expectations for performance will help eliminate confusion and increase the student's sense of competence.

• *Controlled environmental stimulation.* Some students with TBI learn better independently in quiet classrooms, whereas others like the interaction with other active learners. Study carrels, headphones, ear plugs, and special learning areas can provide the level of stimulation needed for optimal learning to take place. Classmates and/or school staff can monitor and help students who are poorly oriented to the physical aspects of the school. For example, students with TBI may not react well to frequent class changes or to unstructured study hall time, both of which are typical in high schools. Assistance with the setting reduces confusion and reinforces appropriate activity. This structural component also is important with vocational planning. Recognition that appropriate workplace accommodations may mean minimization of background activity can help individuals and their potential employers become more aware of the components of the job setting and its match with worker characteristics (Sachs & Redd, 1993).

• *Physical endurance and stamina.* TBI may mean that a student tires easily, so the length of the school day may need modification, or a rest time may need to be provided (Begali, 1994). Revised class selection and assignments also may be needed, to allow for a simpler class schedule or alternate course requirements (Rosen & Gerring, 1986). For older working students, issues of productivity levels and work schedules may need to be addressed (Rojewski, 1992).

• *Emotional support.* Students recovering from TBI may have great difficulty adjusting to their new persona and to the reactions of others. They may feel abandoned by friends and misunderstood by teachers and parents (Blake & Fewster, 2001; Deaton, 1990; Rojewski, 1992; Russell, 1993). They may not even recognize themselves. Therefore, counseling and support groups are often needed and should be integrated into the total treatment plan (Prigatano et al., 1986). "Chill-out time" may be appropriate for some students who need to remove themselves from a situation in which control has been lost, in order to regain emotional balance (Ylvisaker & Feeney, 1998).

Organization

Organization, a close ally of structure, can be defined as providing students who have experienced TBI with the necessary environmental cues and aids to foster acquisition of new learning and help them to retrieve previous knowledge (Telzrow, 1990). The consequences of a student's TBI may include a decreased ability to organize and plan activities, and the student will therefore require organizational modifications for his or her work (Adams et al., 1991; Utah TBI Task Force, 1994).

• *Instructional tactics.* Disruptions of a child's ability to plan activities, complete tasks, and gather information are common after TBI. Teachers must adjust to the fact that a student returning to school with a brain injury may need to reacquaint him- or herself with the procedure of *how* to learn, not *what* to learn (Cohen, 1986). The student's procedural knowledge needs to be evaluated. Does the student know the actions necessary to complete a task? Students with TBI need to learn not only planning skills, but those needed for coping if the plan fails, and for revising a plan if required (Savage & Wolcott, 1994). Planning for and coping with change should be important components in the curriculum.

A set routine and organizational cues will aid students in detecting important elements of lessons. Advance organizers, objective sheets (including key words and concepts), clearly specified guidelines for instruction, and multimodal cues can counteract some students' attentional difficulties and consolidate their learning (Ewing-Cobbs, Fletcher, & Levin, 1986; Rosen & Gerring, 1986; Telzrow, 1990). Practice with and repetition of activities, as well as feedback on performance, can also strengthen students' confidence (Prigatano, 1990). Moreover, students with TBI appreciate the element of choice in activities. Often they feel that they have lost control of themselves and their every activity. Choice may reduce challenging behaviors and improve participation in academic and social tasks (Ylvisaker & Feeney, 1998).

• *Organized assignments.* Teachers also can help students with TBI by allowing modifications to the students' workload.

Expectations for normal performance in the classroom or on the job may need to be adjusted. For example, poor note-taking skills may be compensated for by allowing a student to tape lectures or duplicate another student's notes. Progress can be monitored through an assignment notebook or weekly study plan.

Teachers' expectations for assignments and examinations will need to be reviewed. Extended deadlines or smaller task units may help students manage work. A student may also need alternate means of assessment, because recall is typically weaker than recognition of information with this group (Rosen & Gerring, 1986). Discussion with the student about options for assignments and exams may improve the student's response to work requirements.

• *Life skills curriculum.* Educational relevance is especially critical in planning for students with TBI who have deficits in functional skills. Activities pertinent to everyday living should be incorporated in the curriculum (Savage & Wolcott, 1994; Whitten, D'Amato, & Chittooran, 1992). Again, planning and carrying out routines of behavior will increase a learner's comfort level with tasks and can improve the sense of personal competence.

• *Career education.* Transitional programs that stress career education and job training may be particularly critical for students who suddenly find themselves at a different functional level after TBI. Students may need the opportunity to practice vocational skills in a structured setting with many opportunities for observational learning, practice, and feedback (Sachs & Redd, 1993). Modeled experiences, job shadowing, on-the-job training, and/or internships can ease an individual into the vocational setting (Rojewski, 1992).

Strategies

In tandem with organization and structure, teachers should offer their students instruction in the development of learning strategies (D'Amato & Rothlisberg, 1997). Swanson (with Hoskyn & Lee, 1999) showed that differences in effect size between students with and without learning disabilities were smaller for instructional interventions when strategy instruction was involved than

when other forms of treatment were employed. Unfortunately, effective strategies for students without learning difficulties were not the same as those for students with learning disabilities, nor were they generalized across different learning conditions. Brain injury may disrupt the learning process itself, and memory deficits can exacerbate difficulties in instruction. Although educational programming often focuses on content (e.g., reading, writing, and mathematics), the cognitive correlates of learning (e.g., attention, impulse control) are disrupted with TBI (Blosser & DePompei, 1991; Telzrow, 1990; Waaland & Kreutzer, 1988). Strategy instruction helps students select problem-solving methods and tactics to make learning more efficient.

• *Instructional method adaptations.* Most often, student profiles reflect academic deficiencies and not useful strategies for dealing with information. Learning styles can relate to kinesthetic, visual, or auditory modalities, as well as to hemispheric processing styles such as simultaneous or sequential approaches (Hartlage & Telzrow, 1983; Telzrow, 1985). Structuring tasks or instructing students in alternative approaches to solving problems or completing work will benefit all learners in the classroom (see Harrington, 1990; Telzrow, 1990). Often, just asking a student how he or she plans to accomplish an assignment reveals important information about problem-solving options; however, students do not always understand or implement the best way(s) for them to learn.

• *Compensation.* Intractable skill deficits that do not respond to even extensive instruction are often a clue that a deficit area is involved. It is important to work with students by using the competencies that have been maintained despite injury. Compensatory approaches are methods that advocate working around blocks in a child's learning process (Gaddes & Edgell, 1994).

• *Remediation.* Direct instruction in certain academic areas can be helpful, although students with TBI often do not benefit from a content-based method. Practice in the content area across a variety of situations can bolster academic confidence for students (Gaddes & Edgell, 1994; Prigatano, 1990).

• *Peer modeling.* Allowing a child with TBI to learn from peers, rehearse appropriate behavior, and receive feedback on the success of behavior is invaluable not only to that child, but to others as well. Classmates who have a difficult time understanding the differences in the student after injury can display little tolerance for the student's new responses (Lehr, 1990). Therefore, peer modeling may help both the student with TBI and his or her classmates to adapt to the long-term behavioral differences the student can exhibit.

• *Social skill programming.* Some students with TBI may need very concrete lessons in appropriate social behavior. Behavior after injury may appear immature and inappropriate. Parents, teachers, and peers can help by providing practice and feedback on the quality of the students' reactions to environmental events. Given that the school day allows for extensive observation of student socialization, school personnel can tailor social skills training groups to discuss and practice the needed social and interpersonal competencies (Deaton, 1990). However, it should be remembered that some children with TBI suffer not from social skill deficits, but from impairments in initiation caused by frontal lobe injury. In such a case, initiation of social interaction or of questioning in cognitive situations must come from someone other than the learner with TBI. Peer training and natural classroom situations allow the student the opportunity to ease into social and academic interactions (Ylvisaker & Feeney, 1998).

Domains of Intervention

To this point, intervention with students who have TBI has been discussed in terms of a general philosophy of rehabilitation and the level of attack that may be involved in adjusting the routine of school experience or the instructional context to the learner's requirements. At least one other dimension to intervention should be considered—that of the domain in which modifications could occur. Just as assessment samples broadly from brain-related systems (see Table 28.1), so too can treatment focus on different aspects of activity, from sensory–motor competence to the ability to deal with new learning demands.

Sensory-Perceptual Abilities

Forming the basis of what a child understands, and associated with Luria's second unit of the brain, sensory-perceptual abilities can influence the success with which students take in and process sensory information. Although visual and hearing acuity may be displayed, the child may not be able to make sense of or integrate inputs. There may be a disconnection between what is seen or heard and the meaning of this information for the learner. Traditionally, this has led to multisensory approaches to learning. Specific tactics to improve understanding often involve using two or more sensory options to support instruction. Consequently, written instructions or demonstrations will be presented to supplement oral presentation of material, or hands-on, tactile/kinesthetic experiences will be used to make information more "real" to the student.

Motor Functions

Housed in the frontal area of the brain (Luria's third unit), the motor system controls both fine and gross motor movements. Fine motor skills that can be affected with injury include motor movements governing speech production, fluid writing, shoe tying, or any activity that requires finger or vocal agility. Gross motor patterns of behavior are involved with fluid walking, skipping, or picking up and holding objects. Particularly when a child must integrate visual or auditory perceptions with motor outputs (e.g., while taking notes from a lecture or copying information from text), motor difficulties will become more troublesome. The fluidity and intentionality of movements may be compromised and restrict the student's response speed and options. Besides appropriate physical therapy, modifications to the curriculum could include compensating for motor problems by allowing oral responses or pointing rather than written work; tape-recorded presentations or test answers; cooperative learning settings, where the child contributes information but is not responsible for recording it; and adaptive technology, which will prevent less precise movements from hindering the child's ability to express ideas and needs.

Intellectual and/or Cognitive Abilities

As mentioned previously, retraining or using compensatory practices to further rehabilitation is only an emerging strategy in reintegrating children with TBI into the school environment (Wedding, Horton, & Webster, 1986). This is a broad-based "brain-wide" domain that can include elements of memory, language, and a host of problem-solving and reasoning skills. Deficits in cognitive abilities often present themselves in an individual's difficulty in adapting to and learning from complex learning situations (Blosser & DePompei, 1994; Ylvisaker & Feeney, 1998). Such a student is unwilling or unable to initiate a response to a task or follow it through to completion. Here, strategy training and metacognitive routines are suggested. These might include modeling of and training in problem-solving processes, and also scripting routines and situations so that the student is aware of actions' potential consequences.

Memory, Learning, and Processing

Often subsumed by the cognitive domain, the memory, learning, and processing areas of the brain deal with foundational capacities that can interrupt the acquisition of new information or the recall of old. For example, attentional difficulties, impulsivity, or poor social judgment may detract from the intent of instructive efforts in school. Working with the student to point out or highlight key information, integrate it in context, and organize the way similar tasks may be accomplished may move him or her along in the learning process.

Memory is impossible to assess in the abstract. There is always some context, content, or perception to which it is connected. Likewise, memory is multifaceted; different theories divide memory skills in different ways, and so interventions with memory as a focus may take several forms. Strategy selection may focus on verbal or nonverbal aspects of memory, or on the length of retention (short, intermediate, or long) (Gaddes & Edgell, 1994; Lezak, 1995), but is governed by accessing those parts of the cerebral system that are most intact to "rewire" functioning (i.e., Luria's functional systems approach). Therefore, mnemonic

devices, spatial/visual prompts, or alternative response methods (recognition vs. recall) could be implemented to reduce confusion (Gouvier, Webster, & Blanton, 1986). Ylvisaker and Feeney (1998) advocate scripting, planning books, and discussion of daily schedules as means of offering control to students with TBI, who often forget commitments.

Communication and Language

Communication is a key skill not only cognitively and socially, but in terms of rehabilitative strategies (Blosser & DePompei, 1994). Adaptations may involve speech and language therapy, modification of instructions and response demands, and communicative devices (e.g., pictorial labels and picture boards). Language impairments at the pragmatic level also can offer extreme challenges to students who must navigate social and vocational situations. Consequently, language prompts and modeling activities by educational staff and peers may lessen the confusion students with TBI experience when they do not understand the nuances of speech (Blosser & DePompei, 1994; Stratton & Gregory, 1994; Ylvisaker & Feeney, 1998).

Academic Achievement

Knowledge gained from a flexible assessment of academic areas can be integrated here into classroom practice. Todis and colleagues (1997) have noted that although there is no exact method or curriculum for teaching students with TBI, existing information does suggest practices that are not conducive to learning. Inappropriate instruction includes things like textbook- or workbook-driven lessons (instead of lessons based on student understanding); fragmented or disconnected learning activities, with no clearly stated learning objectives; fragmented schedules driven by special events, resource room schedules, or just general organizational confusion on the part of the teacher; and ineffective behavior management procedures or methods of motivation in the classroom. Modifications to the classroom should be context-based and should foster consistency of expectation and maximum self-regulation. Guides are available that address the needs of students with TBI (e.g., Clark & Hostetter, 1995; Savage & Wolcott, 1994), but general suggestions on classroom requirements include things like modifying the pace and repetition of instructions; modeling and offering assistance on the development of student organizational skills and strategies; and modifying assignments or feedback given to increase awareness of the student's learning success.

Personality, Behavior, and the Family

Severe brain damage affects all aspects of a learner's life. The person must adjust to a new persona and face the expectations of others who remember the person "as he or she was." Instead of improving with time, the changed reality may actually get worse as latent learning difficulties (i.e., lack of mature planning abilities) emerge (Szekeres & Meserve, 1994). Thus, as holistic rehabilitation models suggest (Prigatano, 1990), the psychotherapeutic needs of the student must be integrated with cognitive needs in the individualized treatment plan. A large part of the support felt by students will come from their families; consequently, intervention efforts within the school must also fit family needs. Helping the family come to grips with the changes TBI has caused through supportive counseling; suggesting consistency of treatment approaches between home and school; helping parents and siblings in the development of management skills; and linking families to national organizations all will help lessen the helplessness felt by family members (Sachs, 1991).

Environmental Fit

As mentioned in connection with the SOS model, structural adaptations may be appropriate to help the student adjust to TBI. Rehabilitation experts have noted that the degree of comfort and routine in the individual's life will affect the progress of recovery and educational/vocational success (Prigatano, 1990; Szekeres & Meserve, 1994; Ylvisaker & Feeney, 1998). Safety, consistency of routine, the physical environment (e.g., closeness to the teacher), structure of the day and its length, and willingness of the teacher and classmates to provide the cues

and models necessary to strengthen positive cognitive, social, and self-regulatory behaviors will all be key in the student's ability to reintegrate him- or herself into school life and make the best of intervention efforts.

CONCLUSIONS

The educational implications of TBI may actually improve the understanding of brain–behavior relations in the educational, psychological, and medical professions. No other educational disability demands more of rehabilitative professionals and the resources available for teaching and learning. TBI's variable severity, uneven course, and ramifications for the contexts in which a student must function test accepted notions of educational evaluation and intervention. Many children who are severely injured will never be the same as they were before injury. Moreover, no two children with TBI will manifest the same deficits or follow the same course of recovery. The question then becomes whether educational settings can respond to this acquired disability and adapt learning environments to address these unique students' needs. To succeed in this arena will mean that education truly ascribes to the idea of developing individual education programs and child-driven learning.

REFERENCES

Adams, L., Carl, C. A., Covino, M. E., Filbin, J., Knapp, J., Rich, J. P., Warfield, M. A., & Yenowine, W. (1991). *Guidelines paper: Traumatic brain injuries.* Denver: Colorado Department of Education, Special Education Services Unit.

Begali, V. (1994). The role of the school psychologist. In R. C. Savage & G. F. Wolcott (Eds.), *Educational dimensions of acquired brain injury* (pp. 453–474). Austin, TX: Pro-Ed.

Ben-Yishay, Y., & Diller, L. (1983). Cognitive remediation. In M. Rosenthal, E. R. Griffith, M. R. Bond, & J. D. Miller (Eds.), *Rehabilitation of the adult and child with traumatic brain injury* (pp. 225–240). Philadelphia: Davis.

Ben-Yishay, Y., & Prigatano, G. P. (1990). Cognitive remediation. In M. Rosenthal, E. R. Griffith, M. R. Bond, & J. D. Miller (Eds.), *Rehabilitation of the adult and child with traumatic brain injury* (2nd ed., pp. 393–409). Philadelphia: Davis.

Bigler, E. D. (1990). Neuropathology of traumatic brain injury. In E. D. Bigler (Ed.), *Traumatic brain* injury: *Mechanisms of damage, assessment, intervention, and outcome* (pp. 13–49). Austin, TX: Pro-Ed.

Blake, C., & Fewster, D. (2001). Providing a creative and effective learning environment for students with traumatic brain injury at the middle and high school levels. *International Journal of Adolescence and Youth, 10*(1–2), 117–133.

Blosser, J. I., & DePompei, R. (1991). Preparing education professionals for meeting the needs of students with traumatic brain injury. *Journal of Head Trauma Rehabilitation, 6*(1), 73–82.

Blosser, J. L., & DePompei, R. (1994). *Pediatric traumatic brain injury: Proactive intervention.* San Diego, CA: Singular.

Boake, C. (1991). History of cognitive rehabilitation following head injury. In J. S. Kreutzer & P. H. Wehman (Eds.), *Cognitive rehabilitation for persons with traumatic brain injury: A functional approach* (pp. 112–147). Baltimore: Brookes.

Christensen, A.-L., & Uzzell, B. (Eds.). (1987). *Neuropsychological rehabilitation.* Boston: Kluwer.

Clark, E. (1997). Children and adolescents with traumatic brain injury: Reintegration challenges in educational settings. In E. D. Bigler, E. Clark, & J. Farmer (Eds.), *Childhood traumatic brain injury: Diagnosis, assessment, and intervention* (pp. 191–211). Austin, TX: Pro-Ed.

Clark, E., & Hostetter, C. (1995). *Traumatic brain injury: Training manual for school personnel.* Longmont, CO: Sopris West.

Cobb, P., & Yackel, E. (1990). Constructivist, emergent, and sociocultural perspectives in the context of developmental research. *Educational Psychologist, 31,* 175–190.

Cohen, S. B. (1986). Educational reintegration and programming for children with head injuries. *Journal of Head Trauma Rehabilitation, 1*(4), 22–29.

Cronin, A. F. (2001). Traumatic brain injury in children: Issues in community function. *American Journal of Occupational Therapy, 55*(4), 377–384.

D'Amato, R. C., & Rothlisberg, B. A. (1997). How education should respond to students with traumatic brain injuries. In E. D. Bigler, E. Clark, & J. E. Farmer (Eds.), *Childhood traumatic brain injury: Diagnosis, assessment, and intervention* (pp. 213–237). Austin, TX: Pro-Ed.

D'Amato, R. C., Rothlisberg, B. A., & Leu Work, P. (1999). Neuropsychological assessment for intervention. In C. R. Reynolds & T. B. Gutkin (Eds.), *Handbook of school psychology* (3rd ed., pp. 452–475). New York: Wiley.

D'Amato, R. C., Rothlisberg, B. A., & Rhodes, R. L. (1997). Utilizing a neuropsychological paradigm for understanding common educational and psychological tests. In C. R. Reynolds & E. Fletcher-Janzen (Eds.), *Handbook of clinical child neuropsychology* (2nd ed., pp. 270–294). New York: Plenum Press.

Deaton, A. V. (1990). Behavioral changes strategies for children and adolescents with traumatic brain injury. In E. D. Bigler (Ed.), *Traumatic brain injury* (pp. 231–249). Austin, TX: Pro-Ed.

Ewing-Cobbs, L., Fletcher, J. M., & Levin, H. S. (1986). Neurobehavioral sequelae following head injury in children: Educational implications. *Journal of Head Trauma Rehabilitation, 1*(4), 57–65.

Ewing-Cobbs, L., Miner, M. E., Fletcher, J. M., & Levin, H. S. (1989). Intellectual, motor, and language sequelae following closed head injury in infants and preschoolers. *Journal of Pediatric Psychology, 14,* 531–547.

Farmer, J. E., Clippard, D. S., Luehr-Wiemann, Y., Wright, E., & Owings, S. (1997). Assessing children with traumatic brain injury during rehabilitation: Promoting school and community reentry. In E. D. Bigler, E. Clark, & J. Farmer (Eds.), *Childhood traumatic brain injury: Diagnosis, assessment, and intervention* (pp. 33–61). Austin, TX: Pro-Ed.

Fletcher, J. M., & Taylor, H. G. (1984). Neuropsychological approaches to children: Towards a developmental neuropsychology. *Journal of Clinical Neuropsychology, 6,* 39–56.

Fletcher-Janzen, E., & Kade, H. D. (1997). Pediatric brain injury rehabilitation in a neurodevelopmental milieu. In C. R. Reynolds & E. Fletcher-Janzen (Eds.), *Handbook of clinical child neuropsychology* (2nd ed., pp. 452–481). New York: Plenum Press.

Gaddes, W. H., & Edgell, D. (1994). *Learning disabilities and brain function* (3rd ed.). New York: Springer-Verlag.

Golden, C. J. (1981). The Luria–Nebraska Children's Battery: Theory and formulation. In G. W. Hynd & J. E. Obrzut (Eds.), *Neuropsychological assessment and the school-age child: Issues and procedures* (pp. 277–302) New York: Grune & Stratton.

Golden, C. J. (1989). The Nebraska Neuropsychological Battery. In C. R. Reynolds & E. Fletcher-Janzen (Eds.), *Handbook of clinical child neuropsychology* (pp. 193–204). New York: Plenum Press.

Gouvier, D., Webster, J. S., & Blanton, P. D. (1986). Cognitive retraining with brain-damaged patients. In D. Wedding, A. M. Horton, & J. S. Webster (Eds.), *The neuropsychology handbook: Behavioral and clinical perspectives* (pp. 278–324). New York: Springer.

Haley, S. M., Cioffi, M. I., Lewis, J. E., & Baryza, M. J. (1990). Motor dysfunction in children and adolescents after traumatic brain injury. *Journal of Head Trauma Rehabilitation, 5*(4), 77–90.

Harrington, D. E. (1990). Educational strategies. In M. Rosenthal, E. R. Griffith, M. R. Bond, & J. D. Miller (Eds.), *Rehabilitation of the adult and child with traumatic brain injury* (2nd ed., pp. 476–492). Philadelphia: Davis.

Hartlage, L. C., & Reynolds, C. R. (1981). Neuropsychological assessment and individualized instruction. In G. W. Hynd & J. E. Obrzut (Eds.), *Neuropsychological assessment and the school-aged child* (pp. 355–378). New York: Grune & Stratton.

Hartlage, L. C., & Telzrow, C. F. (1983). The neuropsychological bases of educational intervention. *Journal of Learning Disabilities, 16,* 521–528.

Hynd, G. W., & Semrud-Clikeman, M. (1990). Neuropsychological assessment. In A. S. Kaufman (Ed.), *Assessing adolescent and adult intelligence* (pp. 638–695). Boston: Allyn & Bacon.

Hynd, G. W., & Willis, W. G. (1988). *Pediatric neuropsychology.* New York: Grune & Stratton.

Individuals with Disabilities Education Act (IDEA) of 1990, PL 101-476, 20 U.S.C. § 1400 (1990).

Jarvis, P. E., & Barth, J. B. (1994). *The Halstead–Reitan Neuropsychological Battery: A guide to interpretation and clinical applications.* Odessa, FL: Psychological Assessment Resources.

Johnson, D. A. (1992). Head injured children and education: A need for greater delineation and understanding. *British Journal of Educational Psychology, 62,* 404–409.

Jørgensen, K., & Christensen, A.-L. (1995). The approach of A. R. Luria to neuropsychological assessment. In R. L. Mapou & J. Spector (Eds.), *Clinical neuropsychological assessment: A cognitive approach* (pp. 217–236). New York: Plenum Press.

Klonoff, H., Clark, C., & Klonoff, P. S. (1993). Long-term outcome of head injuries: A 23 year follow up study of children with head injuries. *Journal of Neurology, Neurosurgery and Psychiatry, 56,* 410–415.

Kolb, B., & Whishaw, I. Q. (1990). *Fundamentals of human neuropsychology* (3rd ed.). New York: Freeman.

Kraemer, B. R., & Blacher, J. (1997). An overview of educationally relevant effects, assessment, and school reentry. In A. Glang, G. H. S. Singer, & B. Todis (Eds.), *Students with acquired brain injury: The school's response* (pp. 3–31). Baltimore: Brookes.

Kreutzer, J. S., Serio, C. D., & Bergquist, S. (1994). Family needs after brain injury: A quantitative analysis. *Journal of Head Trauma Rehabilitation, 9,* 104–115.

Kurlychek, R. T., Boyd, T. M., Walker, N. M. (1997). The role of neuropsychology in educating students with ABI. In A. Glang, G. H. S. Singer, & B. Todis (Eds.), *Students with acquired brain injury: The school's response* (pp. 109–122). Baltimore: Brookes.

Lehr, E. (1990). *Psychological management of traumatic brain injuries in children and adolescents.* Rockville, MD: Aspen.

Lezak, M. D. (1995). *Neuropsychological assessment* (3rd ed.). New York: Oxford University Press.

Luria, A. R. (1973). *The working brain.* New York: Penguin Books.

Luria, A. R. (1980). *Higher cortical functions in man* (2nd ed.). New York: Basic Books.

Madigan, K. A., Hall, T. E., & Glang, A. (1997). Effective assessment and instructional practices for students with ABI. In A. Glang, G. H. S. Singer, & B. Todis (Eds.), *Students with acquired brain injury: The school's response* (pp. 123–183). Baltimore: Brookes.

Mapou, R. L. (1995). Introduction. In R. L. Mapou & J. Spector (Eds.), *Clinical neuropsychological assessment: A cognitive approach* (pp. 1–16). New York: Plenum Press.

Mayer, R. E. (1996). Learners as information processors: Legacies and limitations of educational psychology's second metaphor. *Educational Psychologist, 31,* 151–162.

McCaffrey, R. J., & Puente, A. E. (1992). Overview, limitations, and directions. In R. J. McCaffrey & A. E. Puente (Eds.), *Handbook of neuropsychological assessment: A biopsychosocial perspective* (pp. 511–520). New York: Plenum Press.

Medical Economics Data. (1993). *The PDR family guide to prescription drugs.* Montvale, NJ: Author.

Prigatano, G. P. (1990). Recovery and cognitive retraining after cognitive brain injury. In R. D. Bigler (Ed.), *Traumatic brain injury: Mechanisms of damage, assessment, intervention, and outcome* (pp. 273–296). New York: Longman.

Prigatano, G. P. (1997). Learning from our successes and failures: Reflections and comments on "Cognitive rehabilitation: How it is and how it might be." *Journal of the International Neuropsychological Society, 3,* 497–499.

Prigatano, G. P. (2000). A brief overview of four principles of neuropsychological rehabilitation. In A. Christensen & B. P. Uzzell (Eds.), *International handbook of neuropsychological rehabilitation: Critical issues in neuropsychology* (pp. 115–125). Dordrecht, Netherlands: Kluwer Academic.

Prigatano, G. P., Fordyce, D. J., Zeiner, H. K., Roueche, J. R., Pepping, M., & Wood, B. C. (1986). *Neuropsychological rehabilitation after brain injury.* Baltimore: Johns Hopkins University Press.

Reiff, H. B., & deFur, S. (1992). Transition for youths with learning disabilities: A focus on developing independence. *Learning Disability Quarterly, 15,* 237–249.

Reitan, R. M., & Wolfson, D. (1985). *The Halstead–Reitan Neuropsychological Test Battery: Theory and clinical interpretation.* Tucson, AZ: Neuropsychology Press.

Rojewski, J. W. (1992). Key components of model transition services for students with learning disabilities. *Learning Disability Quarterly, 15,* 135–150.

Rosen, C. D., & Gerring, J. P. (1986). *Head trauma: Educational reintegration.* San Diego, CA: College-Hill Press.

Rosenthal, M., & Ricker, J. (2000). Traumatic brain injury. In R. G. Robert & T. R. Elliott (Eds.), *Handbook of rehabilitation psychology* (pp. 49–74). Washington, DC: American Psychological Association.

Rothlisberg, B. A. (1992). Integrating psychological approaches to intervention. In R. C. D'Amato & B. A. Rothlisberg (Eds.), *Psychological perspectives on intervention: A case study approach to prescriptions for change* (pp. 190–198). New York: Longman.

Russell, N. K. (1993). Educational considerations in traumatic brain injury: The role of the speech–language pathologist. *Language, Speech, and Hearing Services in Schools, 24,* 67–75.

Sachs, P. R. (1991). *Treating families of brain-injury survivors.* New York: Springer.

Sachs, P. R., & Redd, C. A. (1993). The Americans with Disabilities Act and individuals with neurological impairments. *Rehabilitation Psychology, 38,* 87–101.

Savage, R. C. (1987). Educational issues for the head-injured adolescent and young adult. *Journal of Head Trauma Rehabilitation, 2*(1), 1–10.

Savage, R. C., & Wolcott, G. F. (Eds.). (1994). *Educational dimensions of acquired brain injury.* Austin, TX: Pro-Ed.

Scuccimarra, D. J., & Speece, D. L. (1990). Employment outcomes and social integration of students with mild handicaps: The quality of life two years after high school. *Journal of Learning Disabilities, 23,* 213–219.

Selz, M. (1981). The Halstead–Reitan Neuropsychological Batteries for Children. In G. W. Hynd & J. E. Obrzut (Eds.), *Neuropsychological assessment and the school-age child: Issues and procedures* (pp. 195–235). New York: Grune & Stratton.

Stratton, M. C., & Gregory, R. J. (1994). After traumatic brain injury: A discussion of consequences. *Brain Injury, 8,* 631–645.

Swanson, H. L., with Hoskyn, M., & Lee, C. (1999). *Interventions for students with learning disabilities: A meta-analysis of treatment outcomes.* New York: Guilford Press.

Szekeres, S. F., & Meserve, N. F. (1994). Collaborative intervention in schools after traumatic brain injury. *Topics in Language Disorders, 15,* 21–36.

Teeter, P. A., & Semrud-Clikeman, M. (1997). *Child neuropsychology: Assessment and interventions for neurodevelopmental disorders.* Needham Heights, MA: Allyn & Bacon.

Telzrow, C. F. (1985). The science and speculation of rehabilitation in development neuropsychological disorders. In L. C. Hartlage & C. F. Telzrow (Eds.), *The neuropsychology of individual differences: A developmental perspective* (pp. 271–307). New York: Plenum Press.

Telzrow, C. F. (1990). Management of academic and educational problems in traumatic brain injury. In E. D. Bigler (Ed.), *Traumatic brain injury* (pp. 251–272). Austin, TX: Pro-Ed.

Teuber, H.-L. (1966). Kurt Goldstein's role in the development of neuropsychology. *Neuropsychologia, 4,* 299–310.

Thatcher, R. W., & John, E. R. (1977). *Functional neuroscience* (Vol. 1). Hillsdale, NJ: Erlbaum.

Todis, B., Glang, A., & Fabry, M. A. (1997). Family–school–child: A qualitative study of the school experiences of students with ABI. In A. Glang, G. H. S. Singer, & B. Todis (Eds.), *Students with acquired brain injury: The school's response* (pp. 33–72). Baltimore: Brookes.

U.S. Department of Education. (1996). *To assure the free appropriate public education of all children with disabilities: Eighteenth Annual Report to Congress on the Implementation of the Individuals with Disabilities Education Act.* Washington, DC: U.S. Government Printing Office.

Utah TBI Task Force. (1994). *Utah traumatic brain injuries training for school personnel: Trainers manual.* Salt Lake City: Utah State Office of Education.

Waaland, P. K., & Kreutzer, J. S. (1988). Family response to childhood traumatic brain injury. *Journal of Head Trauma Rehabilitation, 3*(4), 51–63.

Wedding, D., Horton, A. M., & Webster, J. S. (Eds.). (1986). *Handbook of clinical and behavioral neuropsychology.* New York: Springer.

Whitten, J. C., D'Amato, R. C., & Chittooran, M. M. (1992). A neuropsychological approach to intervention. In R. C. D'Amato & B. A. Rothlisberg (Eds.), *Psychological perspectives on intervention: A case study approach to prescriptions for change* (pp. 112–136). New York: Longman.

Ylvisaker, M. (1993). *Assessment and treatment of traumatic brain injury with school age children and adults.* Buffalo, NY: EDUCOM.

Ylvisaker, M., & Feeney, T. J. (1998). *Collaborative brain injury intervention.* San Diego, CA: Singular.

Ylvisaker, M., Szekeres, S. F., & Hartwick, P. (1994). A framework for cognitive intervention. In R. C. Savage & G. F. Wolcott (Eds.), *Educational dimensions of acquired brain injury* (pp. 35–67). Austin, TX: Pro-Ed.

Ylvisaker, M., Todis, B., Glang, A., Urbanczyk, B., Franklin, C., DePompei, R., Feeney, T., Maxwell, N. M., Pearson, S., & Tyler, J. S. (2001). Educating students with TBI: Themes and recommendations. *Journal of Head Trauma Rehabilitation, 16*(1), 76–93.

Index